DIAGNOSTIC
NEURORADIOLOGY

Pathology contributions from

H. Okazaki and B. Scheithauer, *Slide Atlas of Neuropathology*,
Gower Medical Publishing (by permission of Mayo Foundation
and Gower-Mosby)

H. Okazaki, Fundamentals of Neuropathology, ed 2, Igaku-Shoin Medical publishers

Royal College of Surgeons of England, *Slide Atlas of Pathology*
(by permission of the Royal College and Gower Medical Publishing)

Armed Forces Institute of Pathology, Washington, D.C.
Archives, Departments of Radiologic Pathology and Neuropathology
Yakovlev Collection
Rubinstein Collection

E. Tessa Hedley-Whyte, M.D.
Professor of Pathology, Harvard Medical School
Neuropathologist, Massachusetts General Hospital
(material from the Charles S. Kubik Laboratory for Neuropathology)

Emmanuel Ross, M.D. (deceased)
Professor of Pathology, Loyola University School of Medicine

Jeannette J. Townsend, M.D.
Professor of Pathology and Neurology
University of Utah School of Medicine

Bruce Horten, M.D.
Attending Pathologist, Lenox Hill Hospital, New York

Carol K. Petito, M.D.
Professor of Pathology, University of Miami School of Medicine

Ellsworth C. Alvord, Jr., M.D.
Professor of Pathology, University of Washington School of Medicine

Scott R. VandenBerg, M.D.
Associate Professor of Pathology, University of Virginia
School of Medicine

The Rubinstein Collection, University of Virginia
School of Medicine

Peter C. Burger, M.D.
Professor of Pathology
The Johns Hopkins University School of Medicine

Lawrence E. Becker, M.D.
Professor of Pathology and Pediatrics, University of Toronto

Jacqueline Flament-Durand
Professor of Pathology, Universite Libre de Bruxelles

Anatomy contributions from

Wolfgang Rauschning, M.D., Ph.D.
Professor of Orthopaedics, Uppsala University

Victor M. Haughton, M.D.
Professor of Radiology, Medical College of Wisconsin

Robert A. Chase, M.D.
Emile Holman Professor of Surgery and Anatomy
The David Bassett Collection, Stanford University

DIAGNOSTIC NEURORADIOLOGY

Anne G. Osborn, M.D., F.A.C.R.
Professor of Radiology
University of Utah School of Medicine
Salt Lake City, Utah
and
Nycomed Visiting Professor in Diagnostic Imaging
Armed Forces Institute of Pathology
Washington, D.C.

Illustrated by
Julian Maack, M.F.A., C.M.I.
Director, Department of Medical Illustration
University of Utah School of Medicine

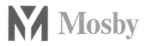

Mosby

St. Louis Baltimore Boston Chicago London Madrid Philadelphia Sydney Toronto

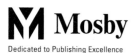

Publisher: George Stamathis
Editor: Anne S. Patterson
Developmental Editor: Carolyn Malik
Project Manager: Carol Weis
Senior Production Editor: Florence Achenbach
Designer: Betty Schulz

Printed in the United States of America
Composition by The Clarinda Company
Printing/binding by Von Hoffmann Press

Mosby–Year Book, Inc.
11830 Westline Industrial Drive
St. Louis, Missouri 63146

Library of Congress Cataloging in Publication Data

Osborn, Anne G., 1943-
    Diagnostic neuroradiology / Anne G. Osborn ; Illustrated by Julian
Maack.
        p.   cm.
    Includes bibliographical references and index.
    ISBN 0-8016-7486-7
    1. Nervous system--Imaging.   2. Nervous system--Pathophysiology.
I. Title.
    [DNLM: 1. Central Nervous System Diseases--diagnosis.
2. Diagnostic Imaging.   WL 141 081d 1994]
RC349.D520798   1994
616.8'04754--dc20
DNLM/DLC
for Library of Congress   93-37717
                                                            CIP

95 96 97 / 9 8 7 6 5 4

To my husband, sweetheart, best friend, and eternal companion Ron
With love and thanks for your unwavering support and enthusiasm.
You make the trip worthwhile.

Foreword

There is no doubt about it—Anne Osborn loves to teach. Her many accomplishments attest to that fact: four textbooks of neuroradiology, countless lectures delivered throughout the world from Washington to the Peoples' Republic of China, and the acclaim of radiology residents and medical students who have attended her lectures and conferences at the University of Utah and at the Armed Forces Institute of Pathology where she was Distinguished Scientist, 1989-1990, and has since served as Sterling Visiting Professor.

Dr. Osborn has not forgotten what it was like to be a resident, and her approach to this book was guided by her extensive experience in teaching residents. She knows what they must know to be competent radiologists and which topics strike fear in their hearts. Her day-to-day interaction with clinicians and her many lectures at postgraduate courses have also attuned her to what practicing radiologists and other clinicians seek in a major textbook of neuroradiology. She can sift out what is important and teach it with memorable analogies drawn from her vast personal knowledge of mythology, sports, history, popular culture, art, and cooking. Her lectures are filled with beautiful concise word slides and radiographs carefully matched with color pathologic specimens. Who can forget how she uses her swirling shoulder length hair to illustrate that "caput medusa" of a venous angioma or her slide of a piece of cauliflower dipped in ranch dressing to make one remember the gross pathologic appearance of an epidermoid tumor?

All the elements that have seasoned her lectures over the past years have been distilled into *Diagnostic Neuroradiology*. She addresses the subjects that are most difficult for radiologists in training such as the changes over time in the appearance of blood on the magnetic resonance scan. As with all the sections in this book, she approaches the problem from the point of view of the clinician, radiologist, medical physicist, and pathologist, and discusses it in detail with well-chosen radiographs, photographs, and her trademark "boxes" that provide easy-to-remember important summaries along the way. Color is used liberally, creating a gallery for the pathologic sections that she has laboriously collected from colleagues all over the world. Her prose is crisp and witty but deadly serious in its content.

Not just a textbook of neuroradiology, this is a vast fund of information on embryology, anatomy, pathology, and surgery of the central nervous system. Dr. Osborn knows the importance of these disciplines to the understanding of their radiologic correlates, and she has taken great pains to integrate them by the use of superb diagrams and drawings created to her specifications by her long-time colleague and medical illustrator, Mr. Julian Maack.

To say that the text is well documented would be a gross understatement. References are plentiful and timely—many appeared in periodicals only three months before publication of the book.

Radiology residents, practicing radiologists, other clinicians, and neuroscientists will find much of value in Osborn's *Diagnostic Neuroradiology*. It is considerably more than an atlas of interesting cases. It is a comprehensive systematic study of the nervous system, visually pleasing, with a rhyme and reason that make it both informative and easy to read. One would expect no less from one of the radiology's premier teachers.

Michael S. Huckman, M.D.
Professor of Radiology
Director of Neuroradiology
Department of Diagnostic Radiology
Rush Medical College
Chicago, Illinois

Preface

iagnostic Neuroradiology was created first and foremost as a teaching text. My goal was to write a reasonably comprehensive—but not exhaustive—book that would present the anatomy, pathology, and multimodality imaging manifestations of CNS diseases in a format that is readable and easily understood by residents, practicing radiologists, and clinical neuroscientists. Common entities and important but less frequently encountered lesions are delineated. Where appropriate, line diagrams and anatomic drawings have been created to illustrate these lesions. Extensive references are included at the end of each chapter for more in-depth study and have been updated within 3 months of publication.

Because I am convinced that neuropathology forms the best foundation for understanding the imaging manifestations of CNS diseases, each entity is introduced by a brief discussion of its gross and microscopic pathology. As a resource, I have used and referred extensively to three excellent neuropathology textbooks. For a succinct introduction and overview, I recommend H. Okazaki's *Fundamentals of Neuropathology,* second edition (Igaku-Shoin, 1989) and P.C. Burger et al, *Surgical Pathology of the Nervous System and its Coverings,* third edition (Churchill Livingstone, 1991). The consummate reference text on brain tumors is, of course, Russel and Rubinstein's *Pathology of Tumours of the Nervous System,* fifth edition (Williams & Wilkins, 1989).

Some gross pathologic specimens are illustrated and are courtesy of neuropathologic colleagues. Because *Diagnostic Neuroradiology* is primarily a neuroimaging text, the pathology illustrations are perforce relatively limited. I have made a modest attempt at demonstrating some of the more important radiologic-pathologic correlations. If this brief introduction whets your appetite for more, look for the forthcoming Mosby book by Dr. Okazaki and colleagues (scheduled publication date in 1995).

The extracranial head and neck is certainly an important aspect of neuroradiology. However, because of space limitations and the availability of several excellent textbooks in this area, I have chosen to limit *Diagnostic Neuroradiology* to skull and brain, spine and cord. Technical aspects of neuroradiology (e.g., diagnostic and interventional angiographic procedures, MR physics and pulse sequences, and so forth) are not discussed; other excellent texts that cover these areas are readily available. Finally, you will note that MR scans are simply referred to as T1-, PD-, or T2-weighted sequences. Purists will wince but—believing that simplifying has its advantages—I have chosen to keep the captions as short as possible, focusing instead on the imaging features and diseases themselves.

I hope that you will find reading *Diagnostic Neuroradiology* enjoyable and educational.

Anne G. Osborn
Salt Lake City, Utah

Acknowledgments

Each of us is a reflection not only of our own knowledge and experience, but the influence, work, and thought processes of others. I acknowledge with gratitude and affection the heritage of those who trained me in neuroradiology: William Marshall, Leslie Zatz, Dixon Moody, and Joseph Poole (deceased). Their excitement about, and enthusiasm for, CNS imaging prompted my decision in 1974 to join the rapidly growing subspecialty of neuroradiology. Although I was never formally one of his fellows, Derek Harwood-Nash has been a wonderful role model and has had a profound influence on my academic career.

A unique mid-career influence resulted from my sabbatical year as Distinguished Scientist at the Armed Forces Institute of Pathology, 1989-1990. The A.F.I.P. is a special place. Its faculty is comprised of military and civilian physicians who are renowned for their diagnostic acumen and teaching skills. Observing my colleagues in the Department of Radiologic Pathology has added immeasurably to my teaching skills and effectiveness. To Alan Davidson, Jim Buck, Jim Smirniotopoulos, Dick Moser, Mark Kransdorf, and Melissa Rosado de Christenson: thank you. Thanks also to the radiologists and residents from around the world whose contributions to the archives of this wonderful institution have created an unparalleled resource. Some cases in this text are from these extensive archives.

From neuropathology colleagues at the A.F.I.P., as well as in many distinguished institutions, I learned just how important knowing the gross pathology of CNS lesions is for understanding neuroimaging findings. Selected cases used in this text are kindly furnished by these colleagues and are gratefully acknowledged. We have attempted to trace their "genealogy" and hopefully have them appropriately credited. Other cases are from the exquisite *Slide Atlas of Neuropathology* and *Slide Atlas of Pathology*, by Drs. Okazaki, Scheithauer, and the Royal College of Surgeons of England respectively. Dr. Peter Burger et al. have permitted the use of some cases from their excellent text, *Surgical Pathology of the Nervous System and its Coverings*. Archives and collections that have also been invaluable resources are the Archives of the A.F.I.P., the Rubinstein Collections, Yakovlev Collection, Archives of the C.S. Kubik Laboratory for Neuropathology at the Massachusetts General Hospital, and the neuropathology teaching archives at the University of Utah.

My neuroradiology colleagues at the University of Utah, H. Ric Harnsberger, John Jacobs, and Wayne Davis not only assembled cases for our teaching file, but helped with ideas and manuscript suggestions, and provided clinical coverage for me during the heavy writing periods. Richard S. Boyer, Virgil Condon, and colleagues at the Primary Childrens' Medical Center in Salt Lake City contributed numerous pediatric cases; their input and acumen is gratefully acknowledged.

Over the years, other Utah colleagues and groups have also contributed numerous cases to our neuroradiology teaching file, which formed the basis for much of this book. Thanks are extended to Pat Luers, Steve Hunt et al. at Cottonwood Hospital Medical Center; Duane Blatter et al. at LDS Hospital; Wendell Gibby, Doug Wing, and Bruce McIff at Utah Valley Medical Center; Mark Fruin and colleagues at Holy Cross Hospital; Jim Jones, St. Benedict's Hospital; Juan Fuentes, McKay-Dee Hospital; Ben Fulton; and Jack Zahniser.

Some cases I used in the text have appeared in contributions I and my associates have made to various course syllabi, collections, and trade reviews. Acknowledged with thanks are the American College of Radiology and the Neuroradiology Learning File, the Radiological Society of North America (special and categorical courses), *MRI Decisions*, the Nycomed Foundation, and the NICER Series on Diagnostic Imaging.

Thanks are extended to Mary and Jack Wheatley. Their generous support of the University of Utah Department of Radiology for my educational outreach activities made it possible for me to devote the intense time and effort required to complete this undertaking. Finally, thanks to Drs. Loevner and Carlton Roos for assistance in proofreading the text for the second printing.

A.G.O.

Contents

PART ONE

Brain development and congenital malformations

with:
Richard S. Boyer

Normal Brain Development and General Classification of Congenital Malformations

Formation of the human central nervous system (CNS) is a continuous, immensely complicated process with repeated cycles of development, modeling and remodeling, and modification and modulation that begin in early fetal life.[1] Knowledge of basic CNS development is essential for understanding congenital malformations of the brain and spine encountered in modern clinical radiology practice.

An in-depth discussion of neuroembryology is beyond the scope of this text. For a more detailed, concise delineation, Keith L. Moore's basic embryology textbook, *The Developing Human*,[2] is suggested. Dr. Moore has generously permitted use of the drawings reprinted in this chapter.

NORMAL BRAIN DEVELOPMENT

The basic events of CNS cytogenesis and morphogenesis are summarized in the box, p. 5.

Neurulation

At its very early stages the human embryo is basically a simple bilaminar disk. At about 2 weeks of embryonic life the neural plate appears on the dorsal aspect of the disk as an area of focal ectodermal proliferation (Fig. 1-1, *A*). At approximately 18 days of gestation the neural plate invaginates, forming the neural groove (Fig. 1-1, *B*). The lateral portions of this groove then thicken and proliferate, forming paired elevations called the neural folds (Fig. 1-1, *C* and *D*). The edges of these folds bend medially toward each other, eventually making contact and closing over the top of the neural groove to form the neural tube (Fig. 1-1, *C* to *F*).

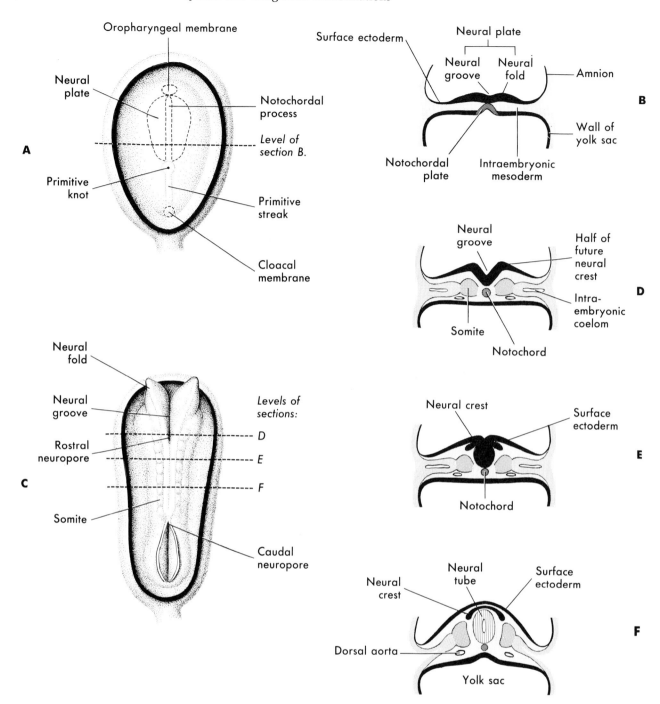

Fig. 1-1. Diagrams illustrating formation of the neural crest and folding of the neural plate into the neural tube. **A,** Dorsal view of an embryo of about 18 days, exposed by removing the amnion. **B,** Transverse section of this embryo showing the neural plate and early development of the neural groove. The developing notochord is also shown. **C,** Dorsal view of an embryo of about 22 days. The neural folds have fused opposite the somites but are widely spread out at both ends of the embryo. The rostral and caudal neuropores are indicated. Closure of the neural tube occurs initially in the region corresponding to the future junction of the brain and spinal cord. **D** to **F,** Transverse sections of this embryo at the levels shown in **C** illustrating formation of the neural tube and its detachment from the surface ectoderm. Note that some neuroectodermal cells are not included in the neural tube but remain between it and the surface ectoderm as the neural crest. These cells first appear as paired columns on the dorsolateral aspect of the neural tube, but they soon become broken up into a series of segmental masses. (From K.L. Moore, *The Developing Human,* W.B. Saunders, 1988.)

The proximal two thirds of the neural tube thickens to form the future brain; the caudal one third represents the future spinal cord. The neural tube lumen will become the brain ventricular system (see subsequent discussion) and the central canal of the spinal cord.[2]

Neural Tube Closure

Closure of the neural tube begins in the hindbrain region and proceeds in a "zipperlike" fashion toward both ends of the embryo[3] (Fig. 1-1, C). Ciliated epithelial cells lining the neural tube begin to secrete a watery liquid that distends the brain cavity, while the flaring cephalic end of the CNS constricts to form the primary brain vesicles.[1] Failure of neural tube apposition in concert with fluid pressure that is inadequate to enlarge and form the ventricles properly is thought to result in the Chiari II malformation (*see* Chapter 2).

Formation of Brain Vesicles and Flexures

After the rostral neuropore closes, three hollow fluid-filled expansions are formed: the forebrain (prosencephalon), midbrain (mesencephalon), and hindbrain (rhombencephalon) (Fig. 1-2). The hindbrain continues caudally into a tubelike cylinder with a narrow central lumen, the future spinal cord.[4] Subsequent constriction and bending of the cephalic end of the neural tube forms the telencephalon (future cerebral hemispheres), diencephalon (thalamus, hypothalamus), mesencephalon (tectum, midbrain), metencephalon (pons, cerebellum), and myelencephalon (medulla) (Fig. 1-2). Three major flexures, the midbrain, pontine, and cervical flexures, divide the developing brain into cerebrum, cerebellum, and spinal cord (Fig. 1-3).[4a]

Disturbance in the process of differentiating the cerebral vesicles results in the spectrum of holoprosencephalies, whereas anomalies in cerebellar hemispheric growth and development result in various forms of cerebellar dysgenesis and, probably, the Dandy-Walker spectrum as well. It is worth noting that the cerebellar vermis is formed from midline fusion of the hemispheric primordia, beginning superiorly and continuing inferiorly. Therefore when the vermis is hypoplastic (as in Dandy-Walker malformations), only its superior lobules are present.

Neuroembryology in a Nutshell

Neural plate forms
Neural plate invaginates, producing neural folds
Neural folds appose in midline to form neural tube
Tube closes like zipper, beginning in hindbrain area
Tube constricts and bends, forming:

prosencephalon	telencephalon (future hemispheres)
	diencephalon (thalamus, hypothalamus)
mesencephalon	mesencephalon (tectum, midbrain)
	metencephalon (pons, cerebellum)
rhombencephalon	myelencephalon (medulla)

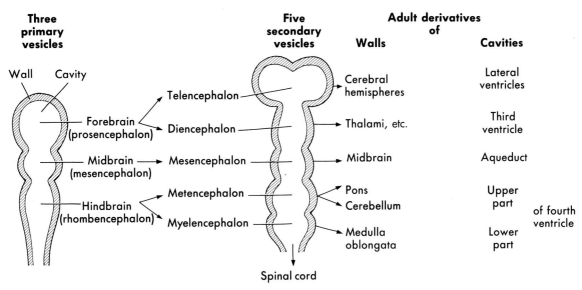

Fig. 1-2. Diagrammatic sketches of the brain vesicles indicating the adult derivatives of their walls and cavities. The rostral (anterior) part of the third ventricle forms from the cavity of the telencephalon; most of the third ventricle is derived from the cavity of the diencephalon. (From K.L. Moore, *The Developing Human*, W.B. Saunders, 1988.)

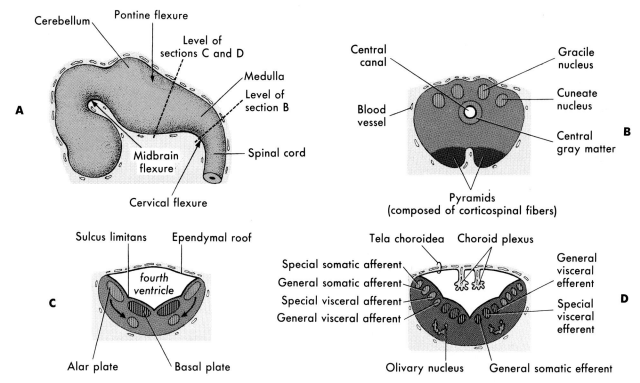

Fig. 1-3. **A,** Sketch of the developing brain at the end of the fifth week showing the three primary divisions of the brain and the brain flexures. **B,** Transverse section through the caudal part of the myelencephalon (developing closed part of the medulla). **C** and **D,** Similar sections through the rostral part of the myelencephalon (developing "open" part of the medulla) showing the position and successive stages of differentiation of the alar and basal plates. The arrows in **C** show the pathway taken by neuroblasts from the alar plates to form the olivary nuclei. (From K.L. Moore, *The Developing Human,* W.B. Saunders, 1988.)

Disjunction of Cutaneous and Neural Ectoderm

Immediately after neural tube closure, the superficial ectoderm of each side separates from the underlying neural ectoderm and then closes over it (Fig. 1-1, *F*). This separation of ectodermal from neural tissue is extremely important and is known as disjunction. The two portions of superficial ectoderm then fuse to establish the integrity of the superficial ectoderm (future skin).[5] The future meninges, neural arches, and paraspinal muscles are formed from mesenchyme that migrates dorsally between the neural tube and the skin.

Premature separation or nondisjunction both result in severe anomalies. If the disjunction of the neural and cutaneous ectoderm occurs too early, adjacent mesenchyme can enter the neural groove. These mesenchymal cells give rise to spinal cord lipomas and participate in forming lipomyelomeningoceles. More focal failure of disjunction results in a persisting epithelial-lined communication between the ectoderm and neural tube derivatives, i.e., a dermal sinus. A larger area of nondisjunction results in an open neural tube that is continuous dorsally with cutaneous ectoderm, i.e., myelocele or myelomeningocele.[5]

Forebrain Formation

Formation and maturation of the brain neocortex is a complex but orderly process that involves neuronal proliferation, differentiation, and migration. The cerebral hemispheres first appear as bilateral outpouchings, or diverticulae, of the telencephalon at approximately 35 days of gestation (Fig. 1-4). As these cerebral vesicles expand, cellular layers develop within their walls to form the germinal matrix from which the neurons and glial cells will arise. Swellings around the third ventricle form the diencephalon, i.e., the thalamus and hypothalamus (Fig. 1-5).

Neuronal formation. Formation of the embryonic cortex begins with production of neuronal and glial precursors in the germinal zones that line the lateral and third ventricles.[6] The germinal matrix forms at about 7 weeks' gestational age and involutes at about

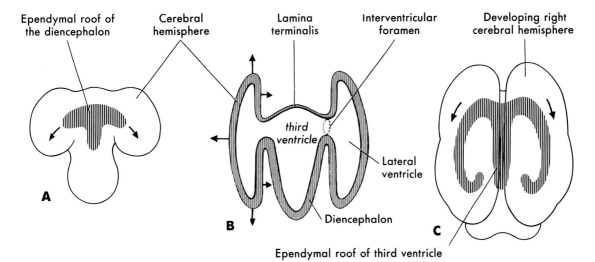

Fig. 1-4. A, Sketch of the dorsal surface of the forebrain indicating how the ependymal roof of the diencephalon is carried out to the dorsomedial surface of the cerebral hemispheres. **B,** Diagrammatic section of the forebrain showing how the developing cerebral hemispheres grow from the lateral walls of the forebrain and expand in all directions until they cover the diencephalon. The arrows indicate some directions in which the hemispheres expand. The rostral wall of the forebrain, the lamina terminalis, is very thin. **C,** Sketch of the forebrain, as viewed anteriorly, showing how the ependymal roof is finally carried into the temporal lobes as a result of the C-shaped growth pattern of the cerebral hemispheres. (From K.L. Moore, *The Developing Human,* W.B. Saunders, 1988.)

28 to 30 weeks, although it persists in the form of focal cell clusters up to weeks 36 through 39.[7] Cells form in the germinal matrix, differentiate, and then migrate peripherally along specialized radial glial fibers that span the entire thickness of the hemisphere from the ventricular surface to the pia.[6]

Neuronal migration. With the exception of the outer layer, neurons migrate from the germinal matrix to cortex in an "inside-out" sequence: those that will form the deepest cortical layer (layer 6) migrate first, followed by layers 5, 4, 3, and, finally, layer 2. This migration and layering process occurs from weeks 6 to 7 through 24 to 26, when the full six-layered cortex is achieved.[7] A brain insult during neuronal migration can result in abnormalities ranging from lissencephaly (smooth brain) to schizencephaly (split brain), polymicrogyria, and laminar or focal heterotopias.

Cerebral commissures. As the cerebral cortex is developing, commissural fibers connect corresponding areas of the cerebral hemispheres with each other. These commissures develop between approximately 8 and 17 weeks gestation, contemporaneous with many other major cerebral structures.[8] The most important of the commissural fibers cross in the lamina terminalis, the rostral end of the forebrain[2] (Fig.

1-6). The largest of the interhemispheric communications is the corpus callosum, connecting neocortical areas. The corpus callosum forms from front to back except for the rostrum, which forms last. An insult to the developing brain can result in complete or partial callosal agenesis. When partial, the splenium and rostrum are always affected.[9]

Midbrain Formation

The midbrain (mesencephalon) undergoes less change than any other part of the developing brain, excepting the caudal hindbrain.[2] The neural canal narrows and becomes the cerebral aqueduct (Fig. 1-7, *D*). Neuroblasts from the alar plate of the midbrain form the tectum and colliculi; those from the basal plate form the tegmentum (Fig. 1-7, *B*).[2]

Hindbrain Formation

The hindbrain (rhombencephalon) is composed of a rostral segment (metencephalon) and a caudal segment (myelencephalon). The metencephalon gives rise to the pons and cerebellum, and the myelencephalon becomes the medulla.[2] Development of the pons and cerebellum is illustrated in Figure 1-7.

Spine and Spinal Cord Formation

The spinal cord and spinal canal are formed by a complex process called canalization and retrogressive

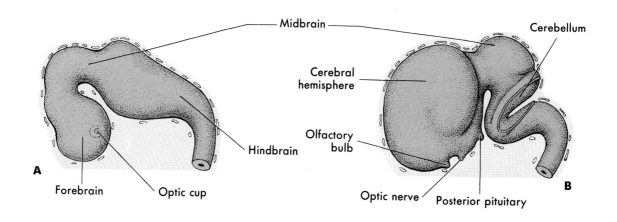

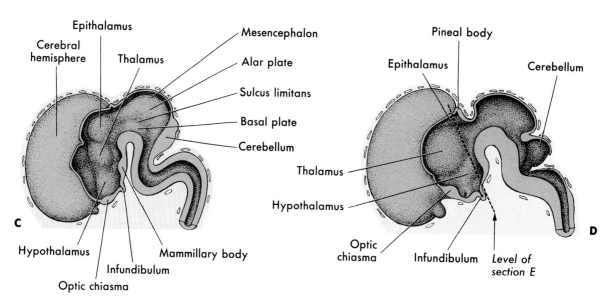

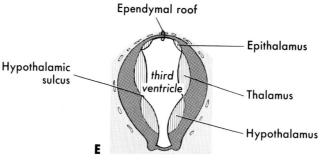

Fig. 1-5. A, External view of the brain at the end of the fifth week. **B,** Similar view at 7 weeks. **C,** Median section of this brain showing the medial surface of the forebrain and midbrain. **D,** Similar section at 8 weeks. **E,** Transverse section through the diencephalon showing the epithalamus dorsally, the thalamus laterally, and the hypothalamus ventrally. (From K.L. Moore, *The Developing Human,* W.B. Saunders, 1988.)

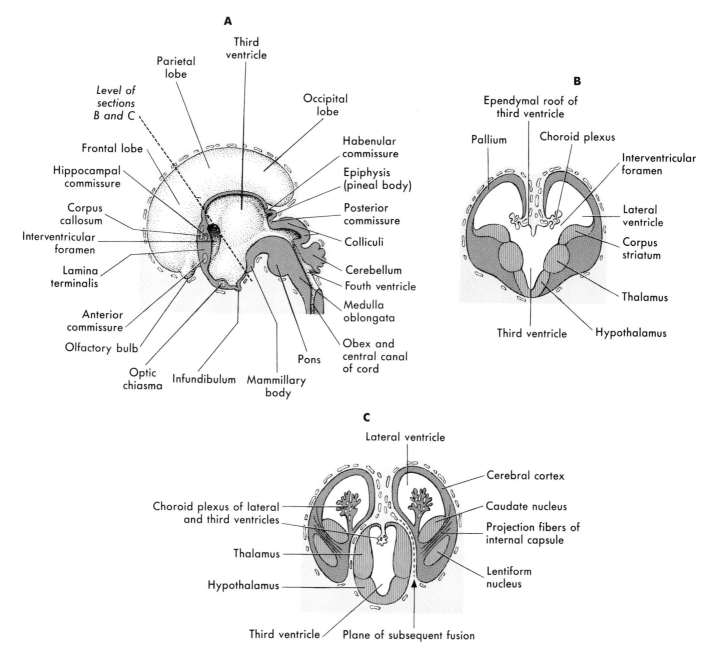

Fig. 1-6. A, Drawing of the medial surface of the forebrain of a 10-week embryo show-ing the diencephalic derivatives, the main commissures, and the expanding cerebral hemispheres. **B,** Transverse section through the forebrain at the level of the interven-tricular foramen showing the corpus striatum and the choroid plexuses of the lateral ventricles. **C,** Similar section at about 11 weeks showing division of the corpus striatum into caudate and lentiform nuclei by the internal capsule. The developing relationship of the cerebral hemispheres to the diencephalon is also illustrated. (From K.L. Moore, *The Developing Human*, W.B. Saunders, 1988.)

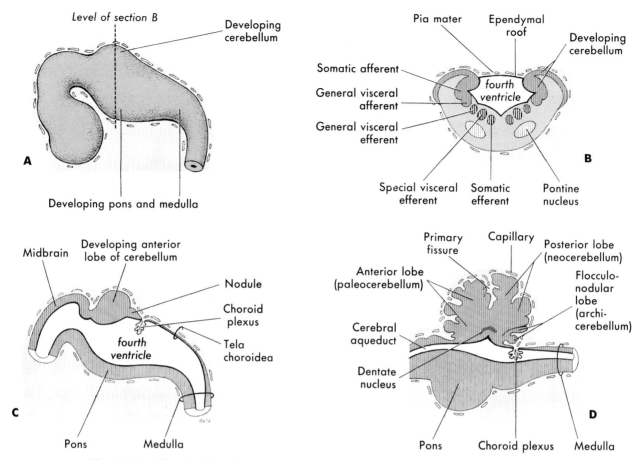

Fig. 1-7. A, Sketch of the developing brain at the end of the fifth week. **B,** Transverse section through the metencephalon (developing pons and cerebellum) showing the derivatives of the alar and basal plates. **C** and **D,** Sagittal sections of the hindbrain at 6 and 17 weeks, respectively, showing successive stages in the development of the pons and cerebellum. (From K.L. Moore, *The Developing Human,* W.B. Saunders, 1988.)

differentiation (the latter applies only to the distal cord). A caudal cell mass forms and then cavitates. If the caudal cell mass fails to form properly, sacral agenesis and caudal regression syndromes result. If it forms but differentiates abnormally, teratomas and spinal canal lipomas occur. Abnormal retrogressive differentiation results in the spectrum of tethered cord, ranging from simple low-lying conus to thick filum and fatty filum with lipoma.

GENERAL CLASSIFICATION OF CENTRAL NERVOUS SYSTEM MALFORMATIONS

Congenital malformations of the brain, spine, and spinal cord are numerous; over 2000 different congenital cerebral malformations have been described. One third of all major embryologic anomalies involve the CNS; over 75% of fetal deaths have cerebral malformations.[10] Various chromosomal and DNA repair disorders that result in CNS anomalies have been identified; the neurogenetics and imaging findings in the more common syndromes have been delineated

by Kumar et al.[11] These are summarized in Table 1-1.

Several different systems have been developed to categorize and classify CNS congenital malformations but most are based on the system devised by DeMyer and modified by Volpe,[12] arranging disorders according to the estimated time of onset of morphologic derangements. Useful modifications have been made by van der Knaap and Valk,[13] as well as Boyer.[14] All these systems divide malformations according to the major developmental stages of the human brain: dorsal and ventral induction, neuronal proliferation, migration, organization, and myelination. Thus specific congenital CNS anomalies that can often be recognized on neuroimaging studies are related to the timing of specific neuroembryologic events. Therefore we will discuss the major identifiable CNS congenital anomalies in this manner. The major events in normal CNS development with anomalies resulting from disruptions at various embryonic stages are listed in Table 1-2. A simplified classification is presented in the box.

Table 1-1. Chromosomal, DNA repair disorders

Type	CNS manifestations	Associated anomalies	Comments
Autosomal aberrations *Trisomies*			
21 (Down syndrome)	Mental retardation, generalized brain atrophy; Alzheimer's; underdeveloped temporal, inferior frontal gyri	Brachycephaly; hypotelorism; hypoplastic maxillae, nose; skull base deformities; cervical spinal stenosis, atlantoaxial dislocation	Most common chromosomal disorder
18 (Edwards syndrome)	Gyral dysplasias (microgyria), hyperplasias; cerebellar hypoplasia; sometimes callosal agenesis, Chiari II; choroid plexus cysts	Dolichocephaly; lowset ears; microphthalmia; micrognathia; hypertelorism	Second most common trisomy, <10% survive beyond 1 year
13 (Patau syndrome)	Alobar holoprosencephalies; arrhinencephaly, cerebellar dysplasias, hypoplasias	Microcephaly; major ocular abnormalities (colobomas, microphthalmia)	Survival <9 months; may develop retinoblastoma
9	Subependymal, choroid plexus cysts; Dandy-Walker; progressive hydroencephalus	Micrognathia; bulbous nose; skeletal, cardiac anomalies	
Partial autosomal monosomies			
Short arm deletion chromosome 4	Midline defects, cerebellar anomalies, gyration disorders	Cardiac defects; severe facial anomalies	Death often from congestive heart failure
Short arm deletion chromosome 5 (Cri-du-chat syndrome)	Severe mental deficiency	Microcephaly; hypertelorism, congenital heart disease	Characteristic catlike cry
Long arm deletion chromosome 15 (Prader-Willi syndrome)	Mental retardation (mid-moderate)	Truncal obesity; short stature; hypogonadism	
Short arm deletion chromosome 17 (Miller-Dieker syndrome)	Lissencephaly; absent/hypoplastic corpus callosum; profound mental retardation	Microcephaly; dysmorphic facies; cardiac defects	Severe growth deficiency
Sex chromosome aberrations *Sex chromosome increases*			
X: 47, XXY syndrome (Klinefelter)	Mental retardation (variable; increases with increasing number of X chromosomes)	Testicular atrophy, small penis; lack of secondary sex characteristics; gynecomastia	Most common cause of male hypogonadism
Y: 47, XYY syndrome			
Sex chromosome decreases			
X: 45, X syndrome (Turner)	No major CNS anomalies, dysfunction	Short stature, webbed neck; aortic coarctation; infertility; mild hearing impairment, occasional ptosis	Significant mental impairment should prompt search for other disorders

Data from Kumar AJ et al: Chromosomal disorders: background and neuroradiology, *AJNR* 13:577-593, 1992. *Continued.*

Table 1-1—cont'd. Chromosomal, DNA repair disorders

Type	CNS manifestations	Associated anomalies	Comments
Fragile X Syndrome	Cognitive, behavioral disabilities; vermian cerebellar hypoplasias	Hyperactivity; speech disorders	Second most commonly recognized genetic cause of mental retardation in males (Down is first); most female patients have normal intelligence
DNA repair defects			
Cockayne's Syndrome	Calcifications in lentiform, dentate nuclei common; cerebral, cerebellar, brainstem atrophy common; cerebral white matter lesions	Microcephaly; abnormal facies; kyphoscoliosis in some	Inherited as autosomal recessive traits; can't repair DNA damage
Ataxia Telangiectasia	Cerebellar atrophy; lentiform calcifications; pachygyria; white matter lesions	Multisystem telangiectasias; immunodeficiencies	High risk of lymphoreticular neoplasms
Xeroderma Pigmentosa	Cerebral, cerebellar atrophy mental retardation	Ataxia, choreoathetosis, spasticity	
Fanconi's Anemia	Not reported	Progressive pancytopenia	Predisposition to malignancy
Bloom's Syndrome	Not reported	Abnormal facies; immunodeficiencies	Growth deficiency; predisposition to malignancy

Table 1-2. Congenital malformations of the brain and spine

Developmental stage	Gestational age	Normal events	Disorders
Dorsal induction *Primary neurulation*	3-4 weeks	Notochord, chordal mesoderm induce neural plate Neural plate closes dorsally, forming neural tube Tube closes, beginning at medulla, proceeds rostrally and caudally	Neural tube defects: Craniorachischisis Anencephaly Myeloschisis Cephalocele Myelomeningocele Chiari malformations Hydromyelia
Secondary neurulation	4-5 weeks	Notochord, mesodermal interactions form dura, pia, vertebrae, skull	Occult dysraphic disorders: Myelocystocele Diastematomyelia Meningocele/lipomeningocele Lipoma Dermal sinus with/without cyst Tethered cord/tight filum terminale

Modified from Boyer R: MR in brain formation and malformation. *Sem US, CT, MR* 9:183-185, 1988.

Table 1-2—cont'd. Congenital malformations of the brain and spine

Developmental stage	Gestational age	Normal events	Disorders
Secondary neurulation—cont'd			Anterior dysraphic lesions (e.g., neurenteric cyst) Caudal regression syndrome
Ventral induction	5-10 weeks	Prechordal mesoderm induces face, forebrain Cleavage of prosencephalon (forebrain); formation of optic vesicles, olfactory bulbs/tracts Telencephalon (endbrain) gives rise to cerebral hemispheres, ventricles, putamen, caudate Diencephalon (between-brain) gives rise to thalami, hypothalamus, globus pallidus Rhombencephalon gives rise to cerebellar hemispheres, vermis Myelencephalon (cordbrain) gives rise to medulla and pons	Holoprosencephalies: Alobar Semilobar Lobar Septooptic dysplasia Arrhinencephaly Facial anomalies Cerebellar hypoplasias/dysplasias (?Chiari IV) Joubert syndrome Rhombencephalosynapsis Tectocerebellar dysplasia Dandy-Walker malformation
Neuronal proliferation, differentiation, histogenesis	2-4 months	Germinal matrix forms at 7 weeks; cellular proliferation forms neuroblasts, fibroblasts, astrocytes endothelial cells Chorod plexus is formed and CSF production begins	Microencephaly Megalencephaly Neurocutaneous syndromes NF-1, NF-2 Tuberous sclerosis Sturge-Weber VonHippel-Lindau Neurocutaneous melanosis Ataxia-telangiectasia Others Aqueductal stenosis Arachnoid cysts Congenital vascular malformations Congenital neoplasms
Cellular migration	2-5 months	Neuroblasts migrate from germinal matrix along radial glial fibers Cortical layers form from deep to superficial Gyri, sulci form Commissural plates form corpus callosum, hippocampal commissure	Schizencephaly Open lip Closed lip Lissencephaly Pachy/polymicrogyria Heterotopias Callosal agenesis Without lipoma With lipoma Lhermitte-Duclos disease

Continued.

Table 1-2—cont'd. Congenital malformations of the brain and spine

Developmental stage	Gestational age	Normal events	Disorders
Neural organization	6 months-postnatal	Neuronal alignment, orientation, layering; dendrites proliferate; synapes form	
Myelination, maturation	6 months-adulthood	Oligodendrocytes produce myelin Peak myelin formation from 30 weeks gestation to 8 months postnatal Corpus callosum develops further; attains adult configuration at birth	Metabolic disorders Dysmyelinating disorders
Acquired degenerative, toxic, inflammatory lesions	Any stage	Secondarily acquired injury to otherwise normally formed structures	Hydranencephaly Hemiatrophy Multicystic encephalomalacia Periventricular leukomalacia

---

Simplified Classification of Brain Malformations

Disorders of organogenesis

Neural tube closure
Diverticulation/cleavage
Sulcation/cellular migration
Abnormalities of size
Destructive lesions

Disorders of histogenesis

Neurocutaneous syndromes

Disorders of cytogenesis

Congenital neoplasms

REFERENCES

1. Angevine JB Jr: General principles of neurogenesis, *BNI Quarterly* 5:19-28, 1989A.
2. Moore KL: *The Developing Human,* ed 4, pp 364-401, Philadelphia, WB Saunders Co, 1988.
3. Barkovich AJ: Congenital malformations of the brain. In *Pediatric Neuroimaging,* pp. 77-147, New York, Raven Press, 1990.
4. Angevine JB Jr: Morphogenesis of the central nervous system, *BNI Quarterly* 5:17-27, 1989A.
4a. Hansen PE, Ballesteros MC, Soila K et al: MR imaging of the developing human brain, *RadioGraphics* 13:21-36, 1993.
5. Naidich TP, Raybaud C: Embryogenesis of the spine and spinal cord, *Riv di Neuroradiol* 5(suppl 2):101-112, 1992.
6. Barkovich AJ: Formation, maturation and disorders of the brain neocortex, *AJNR* 13:423-446, 1992.
7. Gerard NJ, Raubaud CA: In vivo MRI with fetal brain cellular migration, *J Comp Asst Tomogr* 16:265-267, 1992.
8. Barkovich AJ, Norman D: Anomalies of the corpus callosum: correlation with further anomalies of the brain, *AJNR* 9:493-501, 1988.
9. Barkovich AJ: Apparent atypical callosal dysgenesis: analysis of MR findings in six cases and their relationship to holoprosencephaly, *AJNR* 11:333-339, 1990.
10. Poe LB, Coleman LL, Mahmud F: Congenital central nervous system anomalies, *RadioGraphics* 9:801-826, 1989.
11. Kumar AJ, Naidich TP, Stetten G et al: Chromosomal disorders: background and neuroradiology, *AJNR* 13:577-593, 1992.
12. Volpe JJ: Normal and abnormal human brain development, *Clinics in Perinatology* 4:3-30, 1977.
13. Van der Knaap, Valk J: Classification of congenital abnormalities of the CNS, *AJNR* 9:315-326, 1988.
14. Boyer RS: MR in brain formation and malformation, *Sem US, CT, MR* 9:183-185, 1988.

Disorders of Neural Tube Closure

Chiari Malformations
   Chiari I
   Chiari II
   Chiari III
   Chiari IV
Cephaloceles
   Occipital and Parietal
   Sincipital and Sphenopharyngeal
   Nasal Cephaloceles, Dermoids, and Gliomas
   Atretic Cephaloceles
Corpus Callosum Anomalies
   Corpus Callosum Agenesis
   Corpus Callosum Lipoma

he formation of the brain and spinal cord is referred to as dorsal induction (*see* Table 1-1). The two general stages of dorsal induction are primary and secondary neurulation. Primary neurulation involves the formation of the brain and upper spine; secondary neurulation refers to formation of the distal spine.[1]

Disorders of primary neurulation are mostly neural tube closure defects and early central nervous system (CNS) anomalies, typically occurring at around 3 or 4 gestational weeks. These include Chiari malformations, cephaloceles, and myelomeningoceles. During secondary neurulation, interactions between the notochord and mesoderm form the skull, dura, pia, and vertebrae. These occur at 4 to 5 gestational weeks. Abnormalities of secondary neurulation result in spinal dysraphic disorders that range from simple, isolated anomalies such as spina bifida occulta to more complex malformations such as meningocele and lipomeningocele, neurenteric cysts, dermal sinus, and the caudal regression syndromes. Only the skull and brain anomalies will be discussed here; congenital anomalies of the spine and spinal cord are delineated in Chapter 19.

CHIARI MALFORMATIONS

German pathologist Hans Chiari described congenital hindbrain anomalies in which cerebellar tissue descends into the cervical canal. In 1891 he described an anomaly, now designated as Chiari type I, consisting of elongated peglike cerebellar tonsils displaced into the upper cervical canal. In 1896 he described a second type of hindbrain anomaly, known as Chiari type II, in which the vermis, pons, medulla, and an elongated fourth ventricle were displaced inferiorly into the cervical canal.[2] He also reported a single case of cervical spina bifida combined with multiple cerebellar and brainstem anomalies that has since been called a Chiari type III malformation.[3] Some authors have added a fourth type of hindbrain abnormality to the group of Chiari malformations, but the so-called Chiari IV malformation is actually a form of severe cerebellar hypoplasia and occurs during a later stage of development[4] (*see* Chapter 4).

Chiari I Malformation

Pathology. Chiari I malformation (sometimes termed *congenital tonsillar ectopia*) is a relatively simple anomaly that is unassociated with other congenital brain malformations. In contrast to the Chiari II malformation (see subsequent discussion), in this disorder the vermis, fourth ventricle, and medulla are normal or only minimally deformed. Elongated, pointed, "peglike" cerebellar tonsils are displaced inferiorly through the foramen magnum into the upper cervical spinal canal (Fig. 2-1).

Tonsillar position and clinical presentation. Statistically significant differences in tonsillar position with age normally occur. In general, the cerebellar tonsils ascend with increasing age. In the first decade of life, 6 mm should be used as the criterion for tonsillar ectopia. This decreases to 5 mm in the second

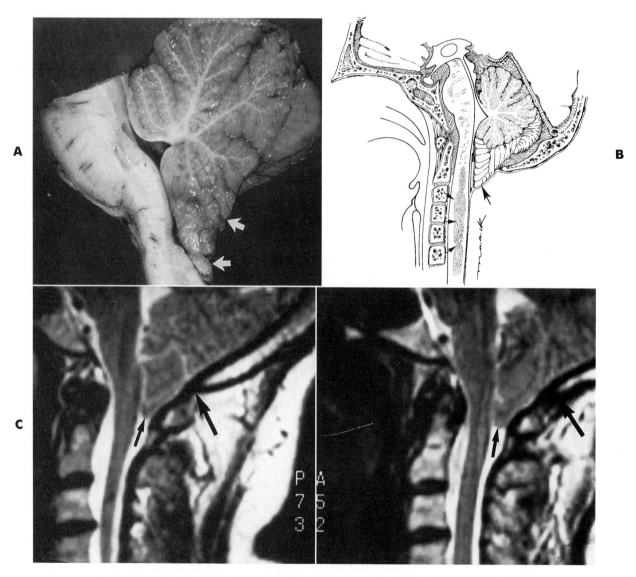

Fig. 2-1. A, Gross pathologic specimen of Chiari I malformation, lateral view. Note the peglike low-lying tonsils *(arrows)*. Only minimal deformities of the fourth ventricle and vermis are present. **B,** Anatomic diagram of the Chiari I malformation. Pointed, low-lying tonsils are seen *(large black arrow)*. Syringohydromyelia is indicated by the small black arrows. **C,** Sagittal T2-weighted MR scans in a patient with an incidental finding of Chiari I malformation. The foramen magnum is indicated by the large black arrows. The cerebellar tonsils *(small black arrows)* lie 10 mm below the foramen magnum. **(A,** Courtesy E. C. Alvord, Jr.)

and the third decades, to 4 mm between the fourth to the eighth decades, and to 3 mm by the ninth decade.[5]

Symptomatic patients with Chiari I malformation often present with long-tract signs and other symptoms that mimic demyelinating disease. As a group, patients with brainstem or cerebellar signs have the largest mean inferior tonsillar displacement. In a recent series, herniations greater than 12 mm were invariably symptomatic. However, nearly 30% of patients with tonsillar displacements ranging from 5 to 10 mm below the foramen magnum were asymptomatic.[6]

Associated abnormalities. Chiari I malformation is usually not associated with other brain anomalies. However, spinal cord, skull base, and spine lesions are common in this disorder.

Spinal cord. Accumulation of cerebrospinal fluid (CSF) within the spinal cord is a frequent finding in patients with Chiari I (Figs. 2-1, *B,* and 2-2). Simple distention of the ependymal-lined central canal is classically termed *hydromyelia.* Dissection of CSF through the ependyma to form paracentral cavitations within the cord is termed *syringomyelia.* The distinction between these two conditions is not possible on imaging studies and is sometimes difficult to establish even after detailed histologic examination.[7] Therefore the term *syrinx,* or *syringohydromyelia,* is used subsequently to describe any pathologic CSF-containing cord cavity, whether or not it is continuous with the central canal.

A *syrinx* is present in 20% to 40% of all patients with Chiari I. If only symptomatic patients are considered, the occurrence of associated syringohydromyelia is even higher, ranging from 60% to 90%.[6,8] The cervical spinal cord is the common site, although occasionally patients with Chiari I have a lesion that involves the entire cord. An isolated thoracic cord syrinx is uncommon.

The etiology of the *hydrosyringomyelia* associated with Chiari malformations is unknown but is likely

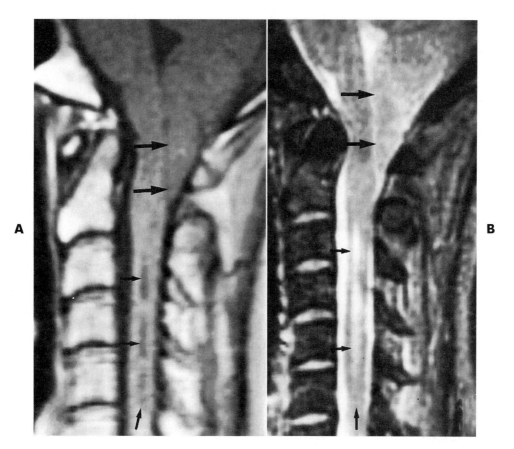

Fig. 2-2. Sagittal T1-weighted **(A)** and T2-weighted **(B)** MR scans in a patient with Chiari I malformation. The peglike, low-lying tonsils are indicated by the large black arrows. A collapsed syrinx of the cervical spinal cord is present *(small black arrows).* This 40-year-old female had a 3-year history of long tract signs. Cranial MR scan had been requested to evaluate for demyelinating disease. No evidence for multiple sclerosis was seen on T2WI of the brain.

secondary to pathologic cerebrospinal fluid dynamics. Postulated causes include posterior compression at the foramen magnum and anterior indentation of the medulla and cord secondary to basilar invagination.[9] Some studies show that syrinx is more frequent in patients with moderate degrees of cerebellar tissue herniation.[8,10] Others report little correlation between increasing tonsillar descent and more extensive or distended syrinxes.[11]

Skull base and spine. Osseous anomalies are seen in about one quarter of all patients with Chiari I malformation and include atlantooccipital assimilation, platybasia, basilar invagination, and fused cervical vertebrae (Klippel-Feil)[6] (*see* box, *below*).

Imaging. Tonsillar configuration and position, as well as the presence of associated hydrosyringomyelia, are easily detected on sagittal T1- and T2-weighted MR scans (Figs. 2-1, *C,* and 2-2). CT is less satisfactory for assessing tonsillar position and configuration unless intrathecal contrast is used.

Chiari II Malformation

Etiology. Chiari II malformation is a complex anomaly with skull, dura, brain, spine, and cord manifestations. Although its exact etiology is unknown, recent evidence suggests that the fetal neural folds fail to neurulate completely, leaving a dorsal opening. Consequently, the developing spinal cord walls do not appose properly and abnormal drainage of CSF through the dehiscent neural tube into the amniotic cavity results. The primitive ventricular system then decompresses and collapses. Because the primitive ventricular system is inadequately distended, this alters the inductive effect of pressure and volume on the surrounding mesenchyme, adversely affecting endochondral bone formation. An abnormally small posterior fossa is the result.[12]

Subsequent development of the cerebellum and brain stem within the abnormally small posterior fossa leads to upward herniation, resulting in an enlarged tentorial incisura and dysplastic tentorium, and to downward herniation of the cerebellar vermis and brain stem through an enlarged foramen magnum into the upper cervical canal.[12,13] Other related cerebral and skull anomalies observed in the Chiari II malformation (such as a large massa intermedia, corpus callosum dysgenesis, and the so-called lückenschädel, or lacunar skull) have also been accounted for by this unified theory.

Pathology and imaging manifestations. The spectrum of abnormalities in Chiari II malformation is very broad, with many different findings reported (*see* box, p. 19). The Chiari II malformation has abnormalities of the following:

1. Skull and dura
2. Hindbrain, cerebellum, and midbrain
3. Cerebrospinal fluid spaces
4. Cerebral hemispheres
5. Spine and spinal cord

It is helpful to consider these abnormalities separately.

Skull and dura. The pathologic changes of Chiari II malformation are shown schematically in Figure 2-3. Normal membranous bone formation of the calvarial vault requires distention of the underlying brain and ventricular system that is lacking in the Chiari II malformation. Radial growth of the developing calvarium is profoundly altered.[12] The result is the so-called *lacunar skull* (lückenschädel).

The gross pathology and plain film radiographic appearance of lacunar skull are striking (Figs. 2-4 and 2-5). Focal calvarial thinning and a "scooped-out" appearance are typical. These skull changes are most striking at birth and tend to diminish with age. Because the defects are not caused by hydrocephalus, their resolution is unrelated to surgical intervention and ventricular shunting. Lacunar skull should be distinguished from prominent convolutional markings that can occur normally or with hydrocephalus after sutural closure. In the latter instance, other changes of increased intracranial pressure such as sellar erosion should be present.

CT and MR scans of infants with a Chiari II malformation also demonstrate scalloping and thinning of the inner calvarial table. Although the most obvious manifestations of lacunar skull resolve by about 6 months of age, subtle calvarial thinning and scal-

---

Chiari I Malformation

Peglike, pointed tonsils displaced into upper cervical canal

At least 6 mm in first decade of life
10-30 years: 5 mm
30-80 years: 4 mm

Associated anomalies

Brain
  Usually none
Ventricles
  Mild/moderate hydrocephalus (20%-25%)
Spinal cord
  Syringomyelia in 30%-60% of all patients; 60%-90% in symptomatic patients
Skeletal anomalies in 25%
  Basilar invagination (25%-50%)
  Klippel-Feil (5%-10%)
  Atlantooccipital assimilation (1%-5%)

Chiari II Malformation

Skull and dura

Calvarial defects (lacunar skull, or lückenschädel)
Small posterior fossa with low-lying transverse sinuses
Fenestrated falx
Heart-shaped incisura with hypoplastic tentorium
Gaping foramen magnum
Concave clivus, petrous ridges

Brain

Inferiorly displaced vermis
Medullary spur and kink
Beaked tectum
Interdigitated gyri
Cerebellum "creeps" around brainstem and "towers" through wide tentorial incisura
Associated anomalies: callosal dysgenesis, heterotopias, polymicrogyria, stenogyria

Ventricles

Whole system: hydrocephalus in 90%
Fourth: elongated, tubelike, inferiorly displaced
Third: large massa intermedia; may be high riding if corpus callosum absent
Lateral: colpocephaly; scalloped, pointed walls

Spine and cord

Myelomeningocele in nearly 100%
Syringohydromyelia 50%-90%
Diastematomyelia
Segmentation anomalies in <10%; incomplete C1 arch

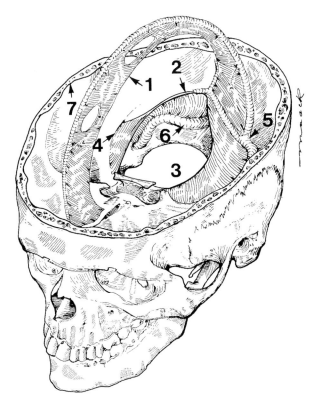

Fig. 2-3. Anatomic drawing depicting the skull and dural abnormalities seen in the Chiari II malformation. *1*, Hypoplastic, fenestrated falx cerebri. *2*, Wide, "heart-shaped" tentorial incisura. *3*, Gaping foramen magnum. *4*, Concave petrous ridges. *5*, Low-lying torcular Herophili. *6*, Low-lying transverse sinuses, small posterior fossa. *7*, Lückenschädel (lacunar) skull.

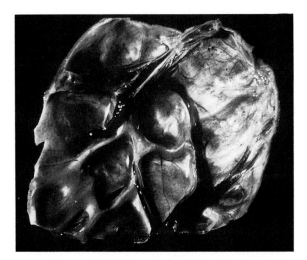

Fig. 2-4. Gross specimen of the calvarium from a patient with Chiari II malformation shows striking changes of lückenschädel (lacunar) skull. (From archives of Armed Forces Institute of Pathology, Washington, D.C.)

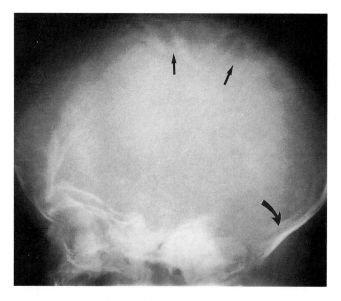

Fig. 2-5. Lateral plain film radiograph of a newborn with Chiari II shows the typical "scooped-out" changes of lacunar skull *(small arrows)*. Note small posterior fossa with low-lying transverse sinuses *(curved arrow)*.

loping may persist into adulthood (Fig. 2-6, *B*). Other skull abnormalities seen in Chiari II include an abnormally small and shallow posterior fossa with low-lying transverse sinuses and torcular herophili. The foramen magnum is unusually large (gaping) (Fig. 2-6, *A*), and the posterior aspects of the petrous temporal bones are often concave (Fig. 2-6, *C*). The clivus also develops abnormally and is often short, with a concave configuration similar to the petrous ridges.

The dural folds that form the falx cerebri and tentorium cerebelli are frequently dysplastic in the Chiari II malformation. The tentorium arises laterally from the low-lying transverse sinuses and is often defi-

cient, producing a widened or "heart-shaped" incisura (Figs. 2-3 and 2-7). The falx may be thinned, hypoplastic, or fenestrated. The interhemispheric fissure often has an irregular, serrated appearance because apposing gyri cross the midline and even interdigitate (Figs. 2-8 and 2-9).

Hindbrain, cerebellum, and midbrain. The gross parenchymal pathology of Chiari II is shown in Figure 2-10, *A;* an anatomic diagram summarizing the features of this malformation is illustrated in Figure 2-10, *B.* Hindbrain and cerebellar abnormalities in Chiari II are a constant (Fig. 2-11, *A*). The medulla and cerebellum are displaced downward into the upper cervical canal for a variable distance. The inferi-

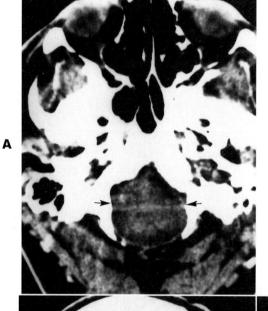

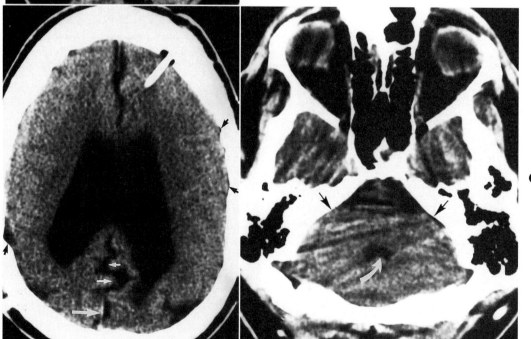

Fig. 2-6. Axial CT scans in a 27-year-old patient with Chiari II malformation. **A,** Gaping foramen magnum is indicated by the arrows. **B,** Section through the lateral ventricles shows the hypoplastic, fenestrated falx cerebri *(large white arrow)* with interdigitating gyri *(small white arrows)* that cross the midline, giving a "serrated" appearance to the interhemispheric fissure. Note that the inner table of the skull shows some persisting subtle areas of scalloped calvarial thinning *(black arrows)*. **C,** Black arrows indicate the concave petrous ridges; the curved arrow indicates the tube-shaped fourth ventricle seen within the abnormally small posterior fossa.

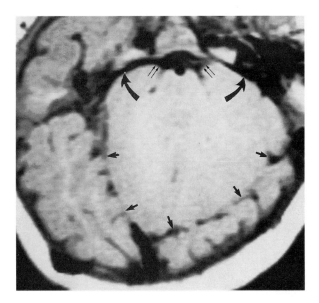

Fig. 2-7. Axial T1-weighted MR scan in a patient with Chiari II malformation shows a gaping, somewhat "heart-shaped" tentorial incisura (*single, small arrows*) that appears completely plugged with the upwardly herniating cerebellum. The cerebellar hemispheres extend anteromedially (*double arrows*) and almost completely engulf the brainstem. The petrous ridges are concave (*curved arrows*).

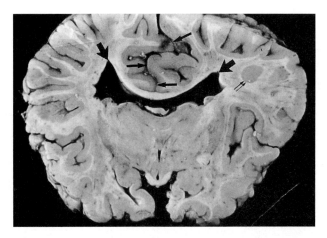

Fig. 2-8. Coronal anatomic section of the cerebral hemispheres and lateral ventricles in Chiari II. Note hypoplastic falx with interdigitating gyri (*small arrows*) and "scalloped," or pointed, ventricular margins (*large arrows*). Also note heterotopic gray matter (*double arrows*) and thinned corpus callosum.

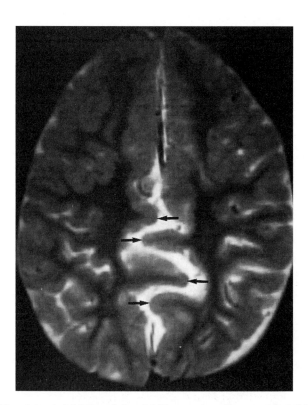

Fig. 2-9. Axial T2-weighted MR scan in a 7-year-old child with Chiari II malformation shows a hypoplastic, fenestrated falx cerebri with striking interdigitating gyri (*arrows*).

orly displaced cerebellar tissue is typically the vermian nodulus, uvula, and pyramis.[13a] The medulla is inferiorly kinked in 70% of all cases and may lie as low as the upper thoracic canal. Formation of a medullary "spur" and "kink" with the cervical spinal cord are characteristic. Occasionally, ectopic choroid plexus from the fourth ventricle is present. Sagittal postcontrast T1WIs show an enhancing nodule at the tip of the caudally displaced cerebellar vermis that should not be mistaken for a pathologic mass.[13b]

The displaced vermis and medulla form a "cascade" of displaced tissue that protrudes through the gaping foramen magnum to lie behind the spinal cord (Figs. 2-10 and 2-11). The cerebellar hemispheres and vermis also herniate upward (towering cerebellum) (Fig. 2-12) through the widened incisura that, in turn, appears completely plugged with the displaced cerebellar tissue (Fig. 2-7). In addition to the cephalad-caudad displacement of posterior fossa contents, the cerebellar hemispheres often extend anteromedially around the brainstem (Fig. 2-7). In particularly severe cases the pons and medulla are nearly engulfed by the cerebellum.

Midbrain anomalies are various. The tectal plate is often pointed or "beaked" (Fig. 2-11). The tectal deformity is caused by pressure from the superiorly herniated cerebellum.

Cerebrospinal fluid spaces. Abnormalities of the ventricles are seen in over 90% of all patients with Chiari II malformation. The fourth ventricle is displaced caudally and is typically small, elongated, and somewhat tubular, lacking a normal-appearing dorsum or fastigium (Fig. 2-10, *B*). The third ventricle is frequently large with a very prominent massa inter-

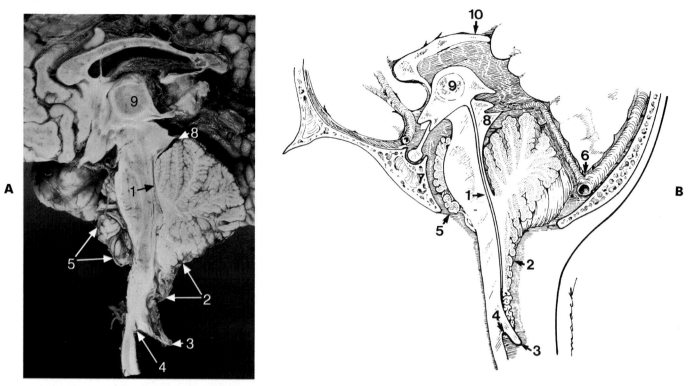

Fig. 2-10. Gross pathologic specimen **(A)** and anatomic diagram **(B)** demonstrate findings of Chiari II malformation. *1,* Elongated, tubelike fourth ventricle. *2,* "Cascade" of inferiorly displaced vermis and choroid plexus *(arrows). 3,* Medullary "spur." *4,* Medullary "kink." *5,* Cerebellar hemispheres "creep" anteriorly around brainstem. *6,* Low-lying torcular herophili, transverse sinuses. *7,* Concave clivus. *8,* "Beaked" tectum. *9,* Large massa intermedia. *10,* Partial callosal agenesis. (**A,** Modified from Naidich TP et al: The Chiari II malformation: Part IV. The hindbrain deformity, *Neuroradiol* 25:179-197, 1983.)

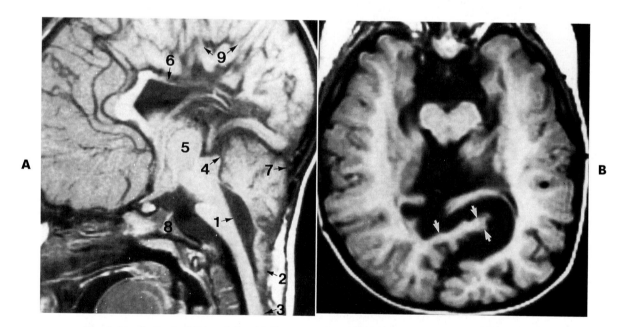

Fig. 2-11. A, Sagittal T1-weighted MR scan in Chiari II malformation. *1,* Elongated, tubelike fourth ventricle. *2,* "Cascade" of inferiorly displaced vermis behind medulla. *3,* Medullary spur. *4,* "Beaked" tectum. *5,* Large massa intermedia. *6,* Partial agenesis of corpus callosum. *7,* Low-lying torcular herophili. *8,* Concave clivus. *9,* Narrow, constricted gyri (stenogyria). **B,** Axial T1-weighted MR scan shows gross gyral interdigitation and stenogyria *(arrows)*.

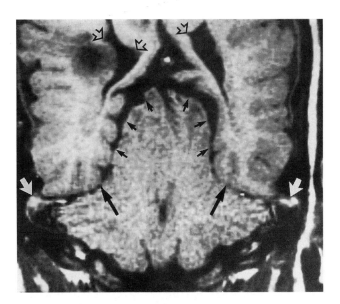

Fig. 2-12. Coronal T1-weighted MR scan in a patient with Chiari II malformation shows low-lying transverse sinuses *(white arrows)* and a very small posterior fossa. A hypoplastic tentorium cerebelli with gaping incisura *(large black arrows)* is present with "towering cerebellum" *(small black arrows)*. The lateral ventricles have a serrated or scalloped appearance *(open arrows)*.

media (Fig. 2-11). The lateral ventricles vary in size from normal to markedly enlarged. The atria and occipital horns are often disproportionately enlarged (a condition termed *colpocephaly*) (Fig. 2-13, *A*). The margins of the lateral ventricles have a serrated or scalloped appearance that often persists after shunting (Fig. 2-12), and the frontal horns are frequently pointed anteroinferiorly (Fig. 2-13, *B*). Aqueductal stenosis may also occur with Chiari II malformations.

The subarachnoid spaces in patients with Chiari II are also usually altered. The cisterna magna is small or inapparent (Figs. 2-6, *A*, and 2-11, *A*), and the interhemispheric fissure frequently appears irregular or serrated secondary to fenestration or hypoplasia of the falx cerebri with secondary gyral interdigitation (Figs. 2-8 and 2-9).

Cerebral hemispheres. A spectrum of parenchymal abnormalities, commonly sulcation and gyration disorders such as polymicrogyria and gray matter heterotopias, contracted narrow gyri (stenogyria), and corpus callosum dysgenesis, are all seen in Chiari II malformations (Fig. 2-11).

Spine and spinal cord. Various spine and cord anomalies are associated with the Chiari II malforma-

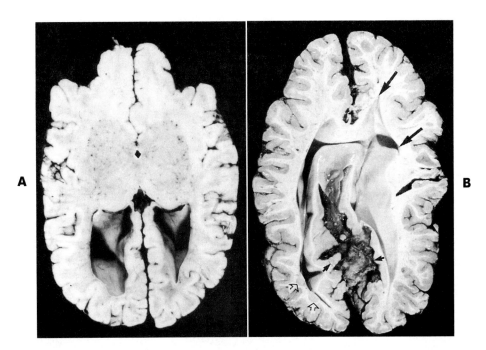

Fig. 2-13. Two gross pathology specimens showing abnormalities of the lateral ventricles in Chiari II malformation. **A,** The atria and lateral ventricles are disproportionately enlarged (colpocephaly). Agenesis of the corpus callosum is also present. **B,** Enlarged lateral ventricles have a scalloped, pointed appearance *(large arrows)*. The posterior interhemispheric fissure is abnormal, with constricted narrow gyri (stenogyria) *(small arrows)*. Callosal agenesis is also present, with gray matter heterotopias *(outlined arrows)*. (**A,** Courtesy Rubinstein Collection, University of Virginia Department of Pathology. **B,** Courtesy E. Tessa Hedley-Whyte.)

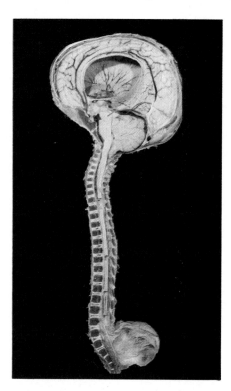

Fig. 2-14. Whole gross neuraxis specimen of Chiari II malformation. Note tethered cord and myelomeningocele. (Courtesy Royal College of Surgeons of England and Gower Medical Publishing.)

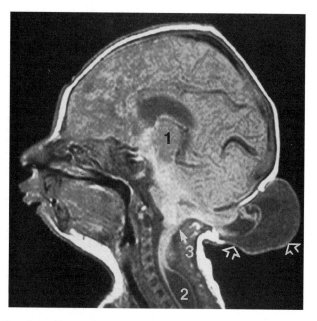

Fig. 2-15. Sagittal T1-weighted MR scan in a patient with Chiari III malformation. Note features of Chiari II that include *(1)* a large massa intermedia, *(2)* cervical syrinx, and *(3)* cerebellar tissue herniated inferiorly through the foramen magnum into the upper cervical canal. A low occipital encephalocele *(open arrows)* contains herniated, dysplastic-appearing cerebellar tissue. (Courtesy M. Castillo. Reprinted with permission from *AJNR 13:* 107-113, 1992.)

tion. Myelomeningocele is present in virtually all cases[14] (Fig. 2-14). Syringohydromyelia and diastematomyelia also often accompany Chiari II malformations (*see* Chapter 19). Lipomyelomeningocele, however, is not typically associated with the Chiari II malformation.

Chiari III Malformation

Pathology. The definition of Chiari III malformation has been expanded recently to include patients with hindbrain herniation into a low occipital or high cervical encephalocele in combination with features of the Chiari II malformation.[15] Encephaloceles in Chiari III contain various amounts of brain. Cerebellum and occipital lobes are common cephalocele contents; occasionally the medulla and pons are also herniated. The herniated tissue is strikingly abnormal and often nonfunctioning because of necrosis, gliosis, fibrosis, and the presence of heterotopias.

Imaging. MR readily establishes the presence, and the contents, of cephaloceles (Fig. 2-15).[16] It is particularly important to recognize position of the brain stem, medulla, and potential anomalies of venous drainage associated with the encephalocele. Herniation of the fourth and lateral ventricles is also often present.

Chiari IV Malformation

Chiari IV malformation is discussed under cerebellar hypoplasias and dysplasias (*see* Chapter 4).

CEPHALOCELES

Pathology. A skull defect in association with herniated intracranial contents is termed a *cephalocele*.[17] If the herniation contains solely leptomeninges and CSF it is termed a *meningocele*.[18] Cephaloceles in which the protruding structures consist of leptomeninges, CSF, and brain are termed *meningoencephaloceles*. Cephaloceles can be congenital or acquired (e.g., posttraumatic, surgical); only congenital cephaloceles are considered here (*see* box).

Incidence. Cephaloceles occur approximately 1 to 3 times in 10,000 live births. The different types of cephaloceles show significant geographic variations, as well as substantial differences in race and gender.[18] Occipital cephaloceles predominate in individuals of white European or North American origin, whereas sincipital (frontoethmoidal) lesions are more common in Southeast Asians and aboriginal Australians.[19] In North America, about 70% to 90% of all cephaloceles are occipital, with 5% to 10% each found in the parietal and frontal areas. Basal encephaloceles are the rarest form of encephalocele.

Cephaloceles

Occipital

Up to 80%-90% of all cephaloceles in white North Americans, Europeans
Female predominance
Association with neural tube defects (myelomeningocele, 7%; diastematomyelia, 3%)
Cyst contents variable

Parietal

10%-15% of cephaloceles in white North Americans, Europeans
Male predominance
Frequently associated with midline brain anomalies (corpus callosum agenesis, Dandy-Walker malformation, lobar holoprosencephaly)

Transsphenoidal

Uncommon
Associated with sellar, endocrine abnormalities; agenesis corpus callosum

Sincipital (frontoethmoidal)

Most common in Southeast Asians
Male predominance
Not generally associated with neural tube defects

Nasal

Crista galli absent/eroded
Foramen cecum enlarged
Various cyst contents

Summarized from Naidich TP, Altman NR, Braffman BH et al: Cephaloceles and related malformations, *AJNR* 13:655-690, 1992.

Associated abnormalities. Although various neural anomalies are associated with cephaloceles (see subsequent discussion), most cephaloceles do not occur as part of known syndromes.[18] A prominent exception is Meckel syndrome, in which cystic dysplastic kidneys and cardiac anomalies are associated with orofacial clefting and occipital cephaloceles.[20] Skull defects in fetal or neonatal cephaloceles are nearly always found in the midline. Off-midline lesions usually indicate an association with amniotic band syndrome.[21]

Occipital and Parietal Cephaloceles

Occipital cephaloceles originate between the foramen magnum and the lambda. They are often large and have highly variable contents.[18] Brain within these cephaloceles is usually dysplastic and gliotic cerebellum. In severe cases the midbrain and part of the ventricular system may also be contained within the cephalocele. Occipital cephaloceles can be associated with neural tube defects such as the Chiari II and III malformations[16] (Figs. 2-15 and 2-16). Dandy-Walker malformation, cerebellar dysplasias, diastematomyelia, and Klippel-Feil syndrome are also associated with occipital cephaloceles.[17]

Parietal cephaloceles arise from a skull defect between the lambda and bregma. They are commonly associated with midline brain anomalies such as absent corpus callosum (Fig. 2-17), Dandy-Walker malformation (Fig. 2-17; *see* Fig. 4-6), lobar holoprosencephaly, and Chiari II malformation.[18]

Sincipital and Sphenopharyngeal Cephaloceles

Sincipital (frontoethmoidal) cephaloceles lie between the nasal and ethmoid bones. They typically show no association with neural tube defects.[18] Transsphenoidal (sphenopharyngeal) meningoencephaloceles occur in association with numerous distortions of the sellar and parasellar structures, as well as endocrine abnormalities. They are also frequently associated with callosal agenesis (Fig. 2-18).

Nasal Cephaloceles, Dermoids, and Gliomas

Nasal cephaloceles, as well as nasal dermoids and nasal "gliomas," occur when a dural diverticulum that traverses the prenasal space and normally connects the superficial ectoderm of the developing nose with the developing brain fails to regress. Resulting anomalies range from dermal sinus, dermoid and epidermoid to nasal cephaloceles, and so-called nasal gliomas (which are usually sequestrations of dysplastic or heterotopic glial tissue). Nasoethmoidal encephaloceles are identified as complex masses of mixed soft tissue and CSF that are contiguous with intracranial structures, typically through a widened calvarial opening.[22]

The crista galli is very important in the differential diagnosis of congenital nasal masses. If it is present but split, the mass is typically a dermoid (Fig. 2-19). If it is absent or eroded and the foramen cecum is enlarged, the lesion is a cephalocele (Fig. 2-20).

Atretic Cephaloceles

Sometimes termed *meningocele manque*, atretic meningoceles are regarded as *formes fruste* of meningoencephaloceles.[18] They consist of a skin-covered subcutaneous lesion that consists of meningeal and ectopic foci of glial or other CNS tissues such as anomalous blood vessels.[23] Their importance lies in the high incidence of associated anomalies such as cerebrooculomuscular (Walker-Warburg) syndrome. The major differential diagnosis of atretic cephalocele is sinus pericranii or dermoid cyst. Sinus pericranii is filled with venous blood and varies in size. Dermoid cysts typically do not enhance following contrast administration, whereas sinus pericranii enhances strongly.

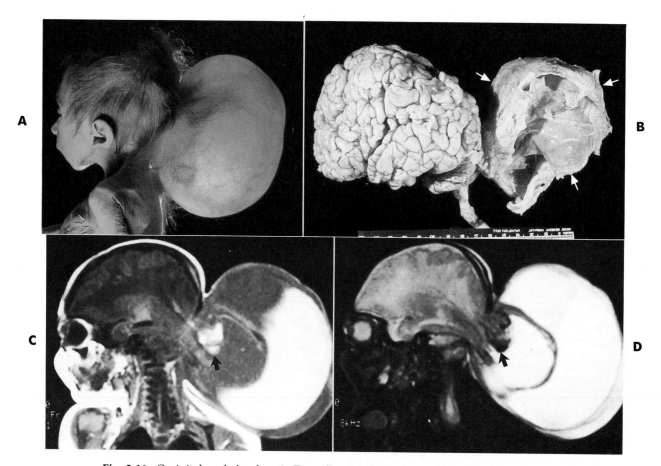

Fig. 2-16. Occipital cephaloceles. **A,** Transillumination and, **B,** gross specimen of an autopsy case. Note disorganized, dysplastic brain within the cephalocele *(arrows).* Sagittal **(C)** T1- and **(D)** T2-weighted MR scans in a newborn with a large occipital cephalocele show dysplastic brain *(arrows).* (**A** and **B,** Courtesy E. Tessa Hedley-Whyte. **C** and **D,** Courtesy W. Gibby.)

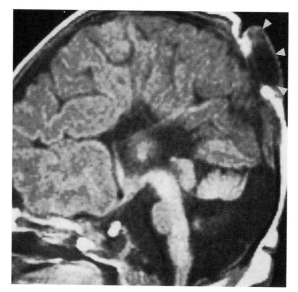

Fig. 2-17. Sagittal T1-weighted MR scan in a patient with a small parietal cephalocele *(arrowheads).* Note coexisting Dandy-Walker malformation and corpus callosum agenesis.

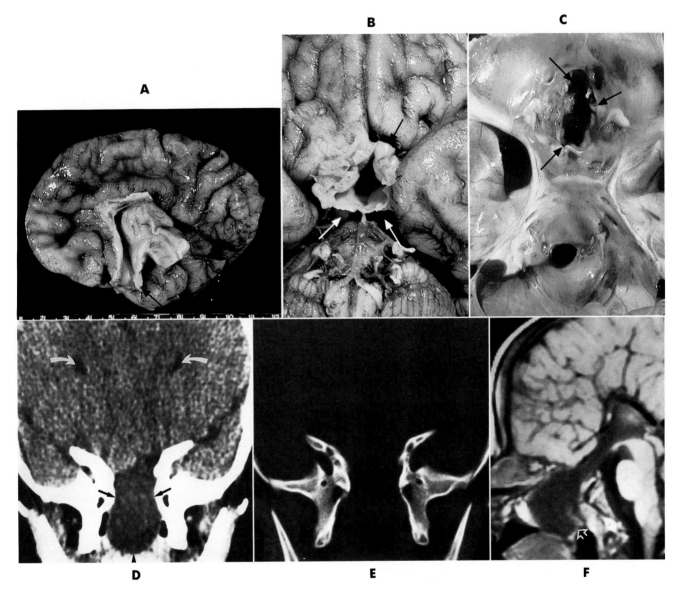

Fig. 2-18. Basal cephaloceles. **A** to **C,** Autopsy specimen of Walker-Warburg syndrome with sphenoid cephalocele and pachygyria. The third ventricle and hypothalamus (**A** and **B,** *arrows*) are herniated through a defect in the basisphenoid (**C,** *arrows*). **D** to **F,** Imaging studies in a patient with a nasopharyngeal (sphenoid-type) cephalocele. Coronal CT scan without contrast enhancement shows a large CSF-containing mass (**D,** *black arrows*) that extends inferiorly through a wide defect in the basisphenoid bone. Note agenesis of the corpus callosum, indicated by the widely spaced lateral ventricles *(curved white arrows).* **E,** Bone detail shows the widely dehiscent sphenoid bone. **F,** Sagittal T1-weighted MR scan shows the cephalocele. Although the cephalocele consists mostly of CSF, a small amount of herniated brain tissue is present *(open arrow).* Note agenesis of the corpus callosum with radiating, spoke-wheel arrangement of the gyri around the high-riding third ventricle. (**A** to **C,** Courtesy E. Tessa Hedley-Whyte.)

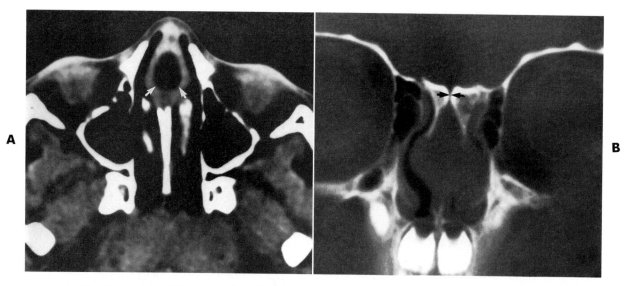

Fig. 2-19. Axial CT scan with soft tissue **(A)** and coronal osseous **(B)** windows shows nasal dermoid *(white arrows)* with splitting of the crista galli *(black arrows)*.

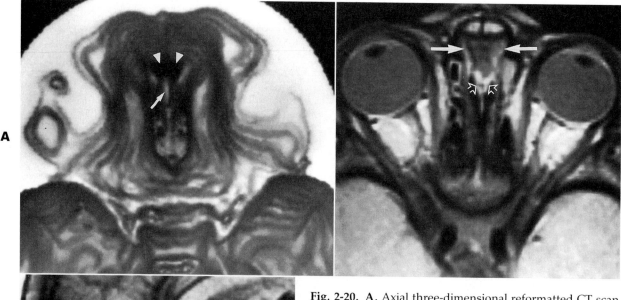

Fig. 2-20. A, Axial three-dimensional reformatted CT scan in a patient with a nasal cephalocele shows foreshortened crista galli *(arrow)* and an enlarged foramen cecum *(arrowheads)*. **B,** Axial balanced MR scan shows soft tissue mass *(white arrows)* anterior to the deformed crista galli *(open arrows)*. **C,** Sagittal T1-weighted MR scan shows skull base defect *(arrows)* anterior to the high signal of the marrow-filled foreshortened crista galli.

CORPUS CALLOSUM ANOMALIES

The corpus callosum forms from anterior to posterior except for the rostrum, which is formed last (*see* Chapter 1). Callosal agenesis can be complete or partial; when partial, the splenium and rostrum are always missing.[24] Hypogenesis can be associated with absence of other commissural tracts such as the anterior and hippocampal commissures.[25] A complete but atrophic or hypoplastic corpus callosum results from an insult to the cerebral cortex or white matter after the corpus callosum is completely formed, i.e., by 18 to 20 gestational weeks.[24]

Corpus Callosum Agenesis

Pathology. In complete callosal agenesis the entire corpus callosum, as well as the cingulate gyrus and sulcus, are absent. Sulci and gyri on the medial hemispheric surface thus appear to have a radial, or spokelike, configuration around a high-riding, elevated third ventricle (Fig. 2-21, *A*).[25a] Because white matter axons do not cross the corpus callosum they course longitudinally instead of transversely. Bundles of these white matter tracts called Probst bundles, indent and invaginate into the superomedial aspects of the lateral ventricles (Fig. 2-21, *B*).

With partial callosal agenesis the rostrum and splenium are absent or hypoplastic and the genu and body are present to various degrees (see subsequent discussion).

Imaging (*see* box). In complete callosal agenesis the lateral ventricles appear widely separated and nonconverging. On axial CT and MR scans they appear to lie parallel to each other and often have small, pointed frontal horns with disproportionately en-

---

Corpus Callosum Agenesis

Pathology, imaging

High-riding third ventricle open superiorly to interhemispheric fissure, with or without dorsal cyst
Radial, spokelike orientation of gyri
Parallel, nonconverging lateral ventricles
Longitudinal white matter tracts (Probst bundles) indent superomedial lateral ventricles
Colpocephaly (dilated occipital horns) common

Associated abnormalities in 50%*

Chiari II
Migration disorders (heterotopias, lissencephaly, schizencephaly)
Cephaloceles
Dandy-Walker malformation
Holoprosencephalies
Azygous anterior cerebral artery
Lipoma

*From Barkovich AJ, Norman D: Anomalies of the corpus callosum: correlation with further anomalies of the brain, *AJNR* 9:493-501, 1988.

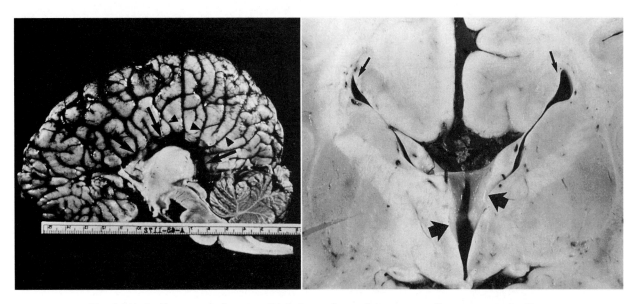

B

Fig. 2-21. A, Gross pathology, sagittal view, of complete corpus callosum agenesis. Note absence of the cingulate gyrus with high-riding third ventricle (*large arrows*) and the radial or "spoke-like" orientation of the gyri (*arrowheads*). **B,** Coronal gross pathology specimen with callosal agenesis shows high-riding third ventricle (*large arrows*) that is contiguous dorsally with the interhemispheric fissure. The longitudinal-oriented white matter tracts, the Probst bundles (*small arrows*), indent the medial margins of the lateral ventricles. (**A,** From archives of Armed Forces Institute of Pathology. **B,** Courtesy J. Townsend.)

larged occipital horns (colpocephaly) (Figs. 2-13, *A*, 2-22, and 2-23).

On coronal CT and MR scans the medial borders of the parallel lateral ventricles appear concave and are indented by the longitudinally oriented fiber tracts (*Probst bundles*) (Fig. 2-24, *B* and *C*). On axial studies the Probst bundles are seen as prominent bands of white matter medial to the nonconverging lateral ventricles (Fig. 2-25, *A* and *B*). The third ventricle is elevated and lies between the widely separated lateral ventricles. The third ventricle itself is

continuous superiorly with the interhemispheric fissure (Fig. 2-25, *C*). A dorsal interhemispheric cyst may be present (Figs. 2-23, 2-25, and 2-26). Extraaxial cysts associated with callosal agenesis should be differentiated from intraaxial midline cysts such as porencephalic cyst, dorsal cysts with holoprosencephaly, and simple upward extension of the third ventricle in corpus callosum agenesis.[26]

On sagittal MR studies, complete callosal agenesis is seen as absence of an identifiable cingulate gyrus and sulcus with gyri that radiate outward from the

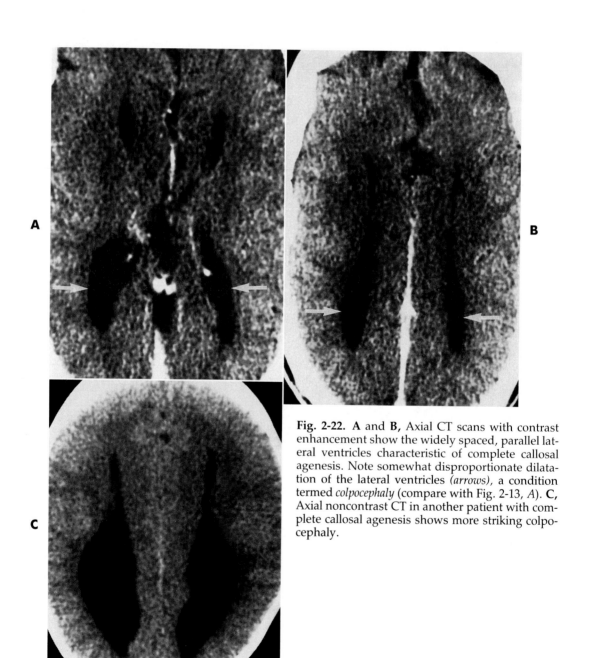

Fig. 2-22. A and **B,** Axial CT scans with contrast enhancement show the widely spaced, parallel lateral ventricles characteristic of complete callosal agenesis. Note somewhat disproportionate dilatation of the lateral ventricles *(arrows)*, a condition termed *colpocephaly* (compare with Fig. 2-13, *A*). **C,** Axial noncontrast CT in another patient with complete callosal agenesis shows more striking colpocephaly.

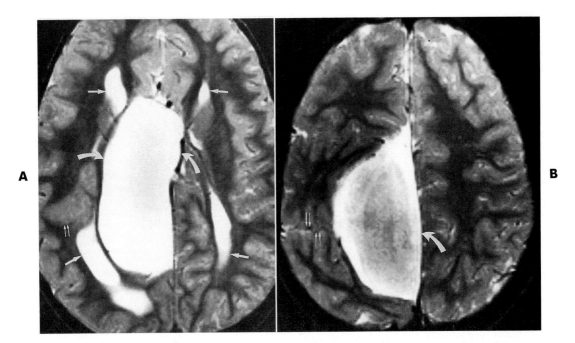

Fig. 2-23. **A** and **B,** Axial T2-weighted MR scans in a patient with complete callosal agenesis show widely spaced lateral ventricles *(straight arrows).* A moderately large dorsal interhemispheric cyst is present *(curved arrows).* Note an accompanying anomaly, unilateral schizencephaly with heterotopic gray matter *(double arrows).*

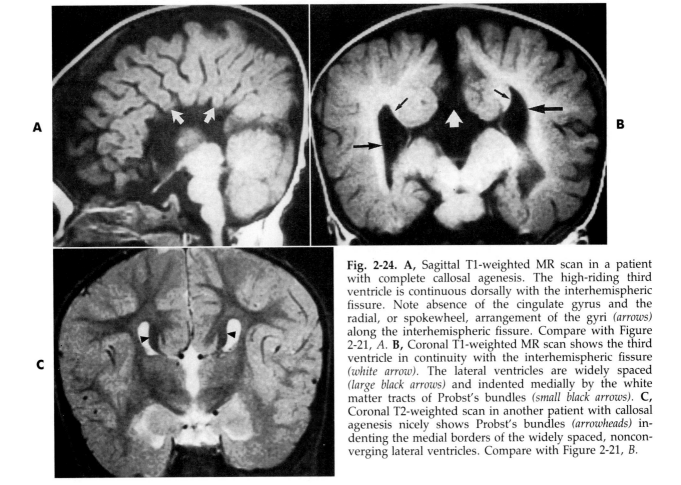

Fig. 2-24. A, Sagittal T1-weighted MR scan in a patient with complete callosal agenesis. The high-riding third ventricle is continuous dorsally with the interhemispheric fissure. Note absence of the cingulate gyrus and the radial, or spokewheel, arrangement of the gyri *(arrows)* along the interhemispheric fissure. Compare with Figure 2-21, *A.* **B,** Coronal T1-weighted MR scan shows the third ventricle in continuity with the interhemispheric fissure *(white arrow).* The lateral ventricles are widely spaced *(large black arrows)* and indented medially by the white matter tracts of Probst's bundles *(small black arrows).* **C,** Coronal T2-weighted scan in another patient with callosal agenesis nicely shows Probst's bundles *(arrowheads)* indenting the medial borders of the widely spaced, nonconverging lateral ventricles. Compare with Figure 2-21, *B.*

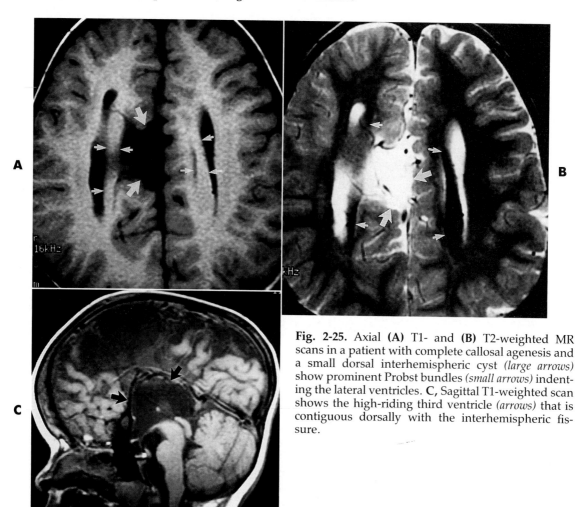

Fig. 2-25. Axial **(A)** T1- and **(B)** T2-weighted MR scans in a patient with complete callosal agenesis and a small dorsal interhemispheric cyst *(large arrows)* show prominent Probst bundles *(small arrows)* indenting the lateral ventricles. **C,** Sagittal T1-weighted scan shows the high-riding third ventricle *(arrows)* that is contiguous dorsally with the interhemispheric fissure.

high-riding third ventricle (Fig. 2-24, *A*). If the corpus callosum is only partially dysgenetic, the genu and body are present and the splenium and rostrum are absent (Fig. 2-27).

Associated abnormalities. In nearly half of all cases, callosal dysgenesis is associated with other cerebral anomalies.[24] These include azygous anterior cerebral artery, Chiari II (Fig. 2-11, *A*) and Dandy-Walker malformations (*see* Figs. 2-17 and 4-4), arachnoid cysts, heterotopias, cephaloceles (Fig. 2-31), schizencephaly (Fig. 2-23), colobomas, miscellaneous midline facial and other skeletal anomalies, and Aicardi syndrome (females with agenesis of the corpus callosum, ocular abnormalities, and infantile spasms).[27-29]

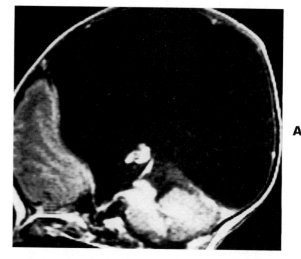

Fig. 2-26. Agenesis of the corpus callosum with a very large dorsal interhemispheric cyst. **A,** Sagittal T1-weighted MR scan shows the third ventricle is contiguous superiorly with the large CSF-containing dorsal cyst. **B** and **C,** Axial T1-weighted scans show enlarged but well-formed lateral and third ventricles. The thalami are separated, and a complete interhemispheric fissure is present, distinguishing this condition from alobar and semilobar holoprosencephaly.

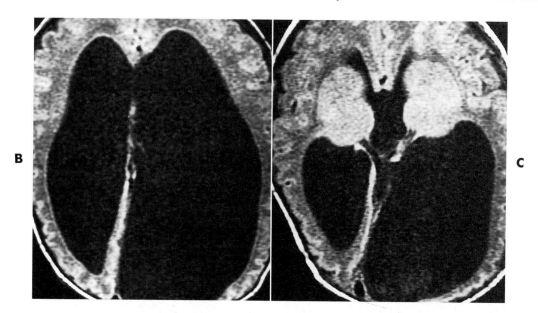

Fig. 2-26, cont'd. For legend see previous page.

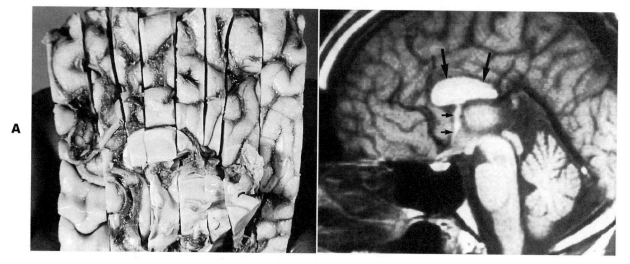

Fig. 2-27. **A,** Gross pathologic specimen and **B,** sagittal T1-weighted MR scan show the findings of partial callosal agenesis. The body and genu are present *(large arrows),* whereas the splenium and rostrum are missing. *Small arrows* indicate the lamina terminalis. (**A,** Courtesy E. C. Alvord, Jr. **B,** Courtesy W. Gibby.)

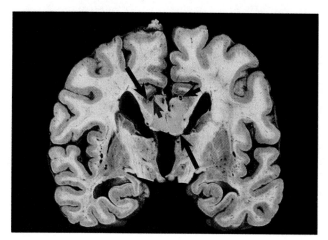

Fig. 2-28. Gross pathology of callosal agenesis with a large bulky tubulonodular lipoma *(large arrows).* Note anterior cerebral artery branches within the mass *(small arrows).* (From Okazaki H: Fundamentals of Neuropathology, ed 2, Igaku-Shoin Medical Publishers, New York, 1989.)

CORPUS CALLOSUM LIPOMA

Pathology. Intracranial lipomas are thought to represent persistence of the meninx primativa, a mesenchymal neural crest derivative, and are a type of brain malformation rather than a true neoplasm.[15] Thirty percent of all intracranial lipomas occur in the callosal area. Half of these occur with various degrees of callosal dysgenesis.

Two types of callosal lipomas have been described: an anterior bulky tubulonodular variety that is frequently associated with forebrain and rostral callosal anomalies (Fig. 2-28) and a more posterior ribbonlike curvilinear lipoma that is generally seen with a normal or nearly normal corpus callosum (Fig. 2-29).[30,31]

Imaging. Plain film radiographs classically show a low density midline mass associated with curvilinear calcifications (Fig. 2-30). CT scans demonstrate the characteristic findings of callosal agenesis associated with a fatty density mass that is variably calcified. Signal intensity on MR scans is typically that of fat, i.e., high signal on T1-weighted scans with low signal on T2-weighted studies. Prominent vessels often course directly through the more bulky anterior callosal lipomas (Fig. 2-31). Curvilinear lipomas are common incidental findings, seen as a C-shaped linear lesion abutting a normal or nearly normal corpus callosum (Fig. 2-32).

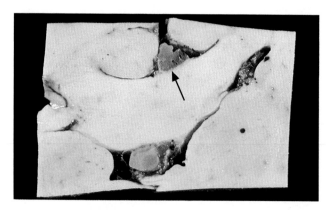

Fig. 2-29. Coronal gross pathology of a small, ribbonlike curvilinear lipoma *(arrow)*. Note intact corpus callosum. (From archives of Armed Forces Institute of Pathology.)

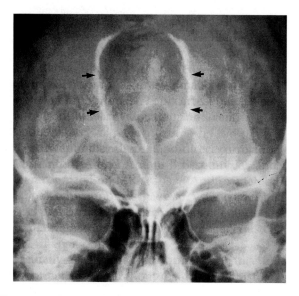

Fig. 2-30. Plain skull film, PA view, with the bilateral curvilinear calcifications *(arrows)* classically associated with corpus callosum agenesis with lipoma. Note that the center of the lesion appears somewhat low density because of the fat-containing lipoma.

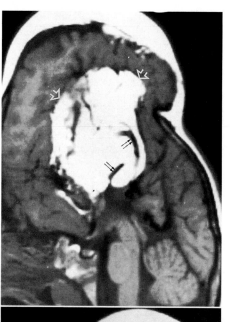

A

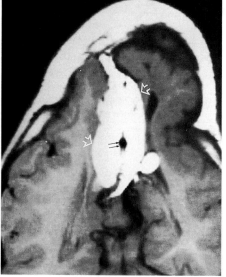

B

Fig. 2-31. For legend see p. 35.

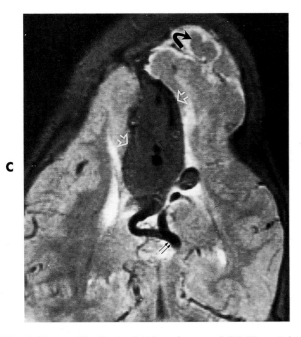

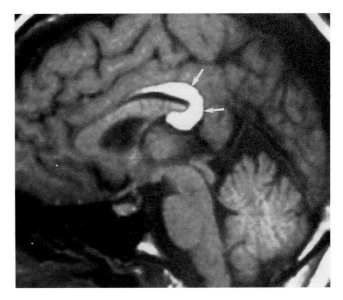

Fig. 2-31, cont'd. Sagittal **(A)** and coronal **(B)** T1-weighted MR scans in a patient with callosal agenesis and a large vertex encephalocele. A bulky, tubulonodular-type lipoma *(white arrows)* is present that is traversed by an azygous anterior cerebral artery *(double black arrows)*. **C,** Coronal T2-weighted scan shows that the encephalocele contains dysplastic brain *(curved black arrow)*.

Fig. 2-32. Sagittal T1-weighted MR scan with incidental finding of a posterior, ribbonlike curvilinear lipoma *(arrows)* that lies just above the body and splenium of a nearly normal corpus callosum. This type of lipoma is typically seen with a normal corpus callosum (contrast with Fig. 2-29 in which the bulky, anterior tubulonodular lipoma is seen with complete callosal agenesis).

REFERENCES

1. Castillo M, Dominguez R: Imaging of common congenital anomalies of the brain and spine, *Clin Imaging* 16:73-88, 1992.
2. Pitman HW: The Chiari crisis, *BNI Quarterly* 6:10-16, 1990.
3. Castillo M, Quencer RM, Dominguez R: Chiari III malformation: imaging features, *AJNR* 13:107-113, 1992.
4. Byrd SE, Osborn RE, Radkowski MA et al: Disorders of midline structures: holoprosencephaly, absence of corpus callosum and Chiari malformations, *Sem US, CT, MR* 9:201-215, 1988.
5. Mikulis DJ, Diaz O, Egglin TK, Sanchez R: Variance of the cerebellar tonsils with age: preliminary report, *Radiology* 183:725-728, 1992.
6. Elster AD, Chen MYM: Chiari I malformations: clinical and radiologic reappraisal, *Radiology* 183:347-353, 1992.
7. Milhorat TH, Johnson WD, Miller JI et al: Surgical treatment of syringomyelia based on magnetic resonance imaging criteria, *Neurosurgery* 31:231-245, 1992.
8. Pillay PK, Awad IA, Little JR, Hahn JF: Symptomatic Chiari malformation in adults: a new classification based on magnetic resonance imaging with clinical and prognostic significance, *Neurosurg* 28:639-645, 1991.
9. Muhonen MG, Menzes AH, Sawin PD, Weinstein SL: Scoliosis in pediatric Chiari malformations without myelodysplasia, *J Neurosurg* 77:69-77, 1992.
10. Stovner W, Rinck P: Syringomyelia in Chiari malformations: relation to extent of cerebellar tissue herniation, *Neurosurgery* 31:913-917, 1992.
11. Clifton AG, Stevens JM, Kendall BE: Idiopathic and Chiari-associated syringomyelia in adults: observation on cerebrospinal fluid pathway at the foramen magnum using static MRI, *Neuradiol* 33(suppl):167-169, 1991.

12. McLone DG, Naidich TP: Developmental morphology of the subarachnoid space, brain vasculature, and contiguous structures, and the cause of the Chiari II malformation, *AJNR* 13:463-482, 1992.
13. McLone DG, Knepper PA: The cause of Chiari II malformation: a unified theory, *Pediat Neurosci* 15:1-12, 1989.
13a. Naidich TP: Chiari II malformation. In Weinberg PE, editor: Neuroradiology Test and Syllabus, part 1, set 28, pp 213-215, American College of Radiology Professional Self-evalution and Continuing Education Program, Reston, 1990.
13b. Stark JE, Clasier CM: MR demonstration of ectopic fourth ventricular choroid plexus in Chiari II malformation, *AJNR* 14:618-621, 1993.
14. Vandertop WP, Asai A, Hoffman HJ et al: Surgical decompression for symptomatic Chiari II malformation in neonates with myelomeningocele, *J Neurosurg* 77:541-544, 1992.
15. Barkovich AJ: Congenital malformations of the brain. In *Pediatric Neuroimaging,* pp 77-147, New York, Raven Press, 1990.
16. Castillo M, Quencer RM, Dominguez R: Chiari III malformation: imaging features, *AJNR* 13:107-113, 1992.
17. Emery JL, Kalhan SC: The pathology of exencephalus, *Dev Med Child Neurol* 12:91-64, 1970.
18. Naidich TP, Altman NR, Braffman BH et al: Cephaloceles and related malformations, *AJNR* 13:655-590, 1992.
19. Simpson DA, David DJ, White J: Cephaloceles: treatment, outcome and antenatal diagnosis, *Neurosurg* 15:14-21, 1984.
20. Goldstein RB, LaPidus AS, Filly RA: Fetal cephaloceles: diagnosis with US, *Radiology* 180:803-808, 1991.
21. Mahony BS, Filly RA, Callen PW et al: The amniotic band syndrome: antenatal diagnosis and potential pitfalls, *Am J Obstet Gynec* 152:63-68, 1985.

22. Barkovich AJ, Vandermarck P, Edwards MSB, Cagen PH: Congenital nasal masses: CT and imaging features in 16 cases, *AJNR* 12:105-116, 1991.

23. Martinez-Lage JF, Sola J, Casas C et al: Atretic cephalocele: the tip of the iceberg, *J Neurosurg* 77:230-235, 1992.

24. Barkovich AJ, Norman D: Anomalies of the corpus callosum: correlation with further anomalies of the brain, *ASNR* 9:493-501, 1988.

25. Barkovich AJ: Apparent atypical callosal dysgenesis: analysis of MR findings in six cases and their relationship to holoprosencephaly, *AJNR* 11:333-339, 1990.

25a. Georgy BA, Hesselink JR, Jernigan TL: MR imaging of the corpus callosum, *AJR* 160:949-955, 1993.

26. Mori K: Giant interhemispheric cysts associated with agenesis of the corpus callosum, *J Neurosurg* 76:224-230, 1992.

27. Curnes JT, Laster DW, Koubek TD et al: MRI of corpus callosal syndromes, *AJNR* 7:617-622, 1986.

28. Baierl P, Markl A, Thelen M, Laub MC: MR imaging in Aicardi syndrome, *AJNR* 9:805-806, 1988.

29. Hall-Craggs MA, Harbord MG, Finn JP et al: Aicardi syndrome: MR assessment of brain structure and myelination, *AJNR* 11:532-536, 1990.

30. Truwit CL, Barkovich AJ: Pathogenesis of intracranial lipoma: an MR study in 42 patients, *AJNR* 11:665-675, 1990.

31. Tart RP, Quisling RG: Curvilinear and tubulonodular varieties of lipoma of the corpus callosum: an MR and CT study, *J Comp Asst Tomogr* 15:809-810, 1991.

Disorders of Diverticulation and Cleavage, Sulcation and Cellular Migration

DISORDERS OF DIVERTICULATION AND CLEAVAGE: HOLOPROSENCEPHALIES AND RELATED DISORDERS

During the fourth gestational week, the neural tube forms three primary brain vesicles: the forebrain (prosencephalon), midbrain (mesencephalon), and hindbrain (rhombencephalon). During the fifth week the forebrain further divides into two secondary vesicles: the telencephalon and the diencephalon (*see* Fig. 1-2). Anlage of the telencephalon and diencephalon separate by day 32; partial division of the telencephalon into two cerebral hemispheres occurs by the end of the fifth fetal week.

Complete or partial failure in division of the developing cerebrum (prosencephalon) into hemispheres and lobes results in the holoprosencephalies.[1] In holoprosencephaly, there is failure of lateral cleavage into distinct cerebral hemispheres and failure of transverse cleavage into diencephalon and telencephalon.[2]

Prosencephalic abnormalities are directly related to the mesenchymal tissue of the prechordal mesoderm. This tissue is responsible for cleavage of the telencephalon and development of the midline facial structures.[3] The majority of patients with moderate or severe forms of holoprosencephaly also have facial anomalies. As stated by DeMyer and paraphrased by Harwood-Nash, "The face predicts the brain."[4]

Holoprosencephaly is classically divided into three types by degree of brain cleavage (Table 3-1):
1. Alobar holoprosencephaly (most severe)
2. Semilobar holoprosencephaly (moderately severe)
3. Lobar holoprosencephaly (mildest form)

In fact, these disorders form a continuum with no sharp division between the different types.

Table 3-1. Holoprosencephalies

Finding	Alobar	Semilobar	Lobar
Craniofacial anomalies	Severe	Variable	Absent or mild
Ventricles	Monoventricle	Rudimentary occipital horns	Squared-off frontal horns
Septum pellucidum	Absent	Absent	Absent
Falx cerebri	Absent	Partial	Well formed
Interhemispheric fissure	Absent	Partial	Present; some anteroinferior fusion
Thalami, basal ganglia	Fused	Partially separated	Separated

Alobar Holoprosencephaly

A "holoprosencephalic" appearance of the ventricular system is normal in early fetal development. At about 4 weeks of gestation, the primitive ventricles appear as a single relatively undifferentiated cavity (*see* Fig. 1-4). In the most severe form of holoprosencephaly, alobar holoprosencephaly, there is persistence of this primitive central monoventricle.

Pathology and imaging manifestations. Alobar holoprosencephaly is characterized by nearly complete lack of ventricular and hemispheric cleavage. The brain is basically an undifferentiated holosphere with a central monoventricle and fused thalami (Fig. 3-1). Imaging studies show a completely unsegmented rim of brain that surrounds a largely undifferentiated central CSF-filled cavity (Fig. 3-2). There is no interhemispheric fissure, falx cerebri, or corpus callosum (Figs. 3-2, *A*, and 3-3, *A* to *C*). A large posterior midline cyst is often present (Fig. 3-3, *D* and *E*).[5] This should be distinguished from callosal agenesis with dorsal third ventricular interhemispheric cyst (*see* Fig. 2-26, *A*). Here, the interhemispheric fissure is complete, the falx is present, and the frontal horns have a bicornuate appearance[6] (Fig. 3-3, *F*).

Associated abnormalities. Severe craniofacial anomalies are seen in most cases of alobar holoprosencephaly. These include cyclops with rudimentary displaced nose (ethmocephaly) and monkeylike head with defective nose and severe hypotelorism (cebocephaly).[3] Reported extracranial abnormalities include polydactyly, renal dysplasia, omphalocele, and hydrops.[5] Most neonates with holoprosencephaly who die soon after birth have associated major congenital malformations. Several chromosomal abnormalities have been reported with cyclopia or holoprosencephaly, most commonly trisomy 13.[3]

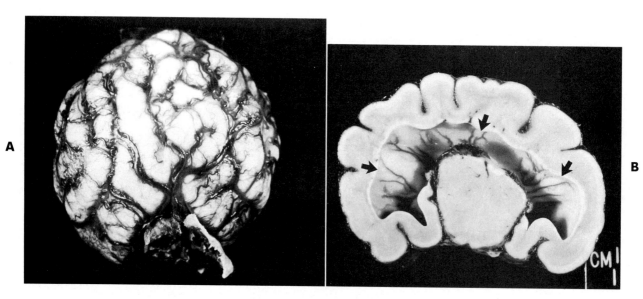

Fig. 3-1. Gross pathology of alobar holoprosencephaly. **A,** Intact brain shows a completely unsegmented holosphere. **B,** Coronal cut section shows a central monoventricle (*arrows*) The thalami are fused, the falx is absent, and there is no interhemispheric fissure. (From archives of the Armed Forces Institute of Pathology.)

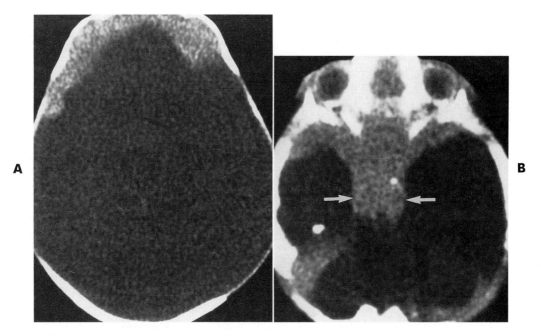

Fig. 3-2. **A** and **B,** Axial noncontrast CT scans of alobar holoprosencephaly. The basal ganglia are fused (**B,** *arrows*), and a large CSF-filled monoventricle fills most of the intracranial cavity. The interhemispheric fissure and falx cerebri are absent.

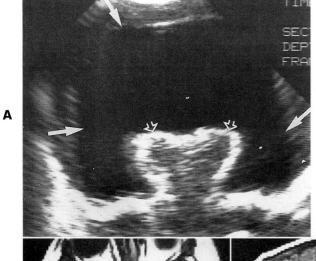

Fig. 3-3. **A** to **E,** Imaging studies in alobar holoprosencephaly. Coronal ultrasound **(A)** and T1-weighted MR **(B)** scans show a central horseshoe-shaped monoventricle *(large arrows)* with fused thalami centrally *(open arrows).* There is no falx or interhemispheric fissure. The corpus callosum is absent. **C** and **D,** Axial T1-weighted MR scans show the fused thalami *(open arrows)* and large central CSF-filled ventricular cavity that is almost completely undifferentiated. A dorsal interhemispheric cyst is present *(black arrows),* also demonstrated on the sagittal T1-weighted scan **(E,** *arrows).* (**A** to **D,** From archives of the Armed Forces Institute of Pathology.)

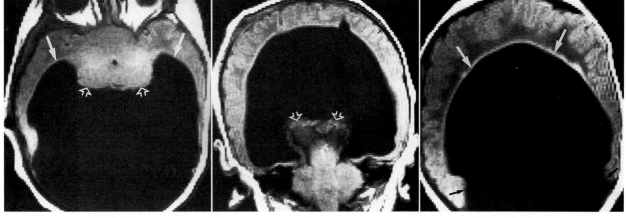

B   C   D   *Continued.*

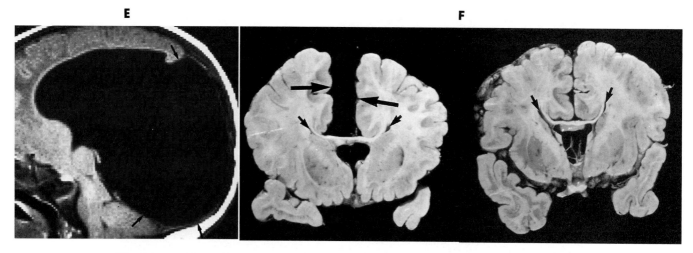

Fig. 3-3, cont'd. F, Coronal gross specimen of callosal agenesis with an interhemispheric cyst *(large arrows)* shown for comparison. Note the bicornuate appearance of the lateral ventricles *(small arrows)*. The thalami are completely separated and the interhemispheric fissure is well developed (**E,** From archives of Armed Forces Institute of Pathology. **F,** Courtesy E. Tessa Hedley-Whyte.)

Semilobar Holoprosencephaly

Pathology and imaging. Semilobar holoprosencephaly is intermediate in severity. There is partial but interrupted attempt at brain diverticulation. A somewhat H-shaped monoventricle with partially developed occipital and temporal horns is common. A rudimentary falx cerebri and incompletely formed interhemispheric fissure are often seen, with partial or complete fusion of the basal ganglia (Fig. 3-4).

Associated abnormalities. In general, facial anomalies are either absent or are milder than those associated with alobar holoprosencephaly. Facial lesions commonly seen with various degrees of semilobar holoprosencephaly include hypotelorism, as well as median and lateral cleft lip.[3]

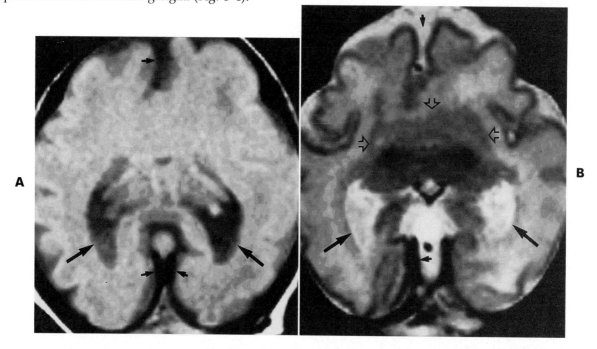

Fig. 3-4. Axial **(A)** T1- and **(B)** T2-weighted MR scans in an infant with severe semilobar holoprosencephaly. Primitive occipital horns are present *(large black arrows)* and a partial, rudimentary interhemispheric fissure is identified *(small black arrows)*. The basal ganglia are fused (**B,** *open arrows*).

Lobar Holoprosencephaly

Pathology and imaging. In this form of holoprosencephaly there is nearly complete brain cleavage. The ventricles appear well lobulated. Absence of the septum pellucidum gives a squared-off or boxlike configuration to the frontal horns (Fig. 3-5). Separation of the basal ganglia is seen. A nearly completely formed interhemispheric fissure and falx cerebri are present, although their most anteroinferior aspects may be absent and the frontal lobes fused inferiorly across the midline (Figs. 3-5 and 3-6). An azygous anterior cerebral artery may be present (Fig. 3-7).

Rarely, the inferior frontal lobes are separated and the posterior frontal or parietal regions are continuous across the midline, so-called middle interhemispheric fusion. This variant of holoprosencephaly is associated with other abnormalities such as neuronal migration anomalies, callosal dysgenesis, and hypoplastic anterior falx cerebri.[6a]

Associated abnormalities. The optic vesicles and olfactory bulbs may be hypoplastic. Mild hypotelorism can be seen, but severe facial anomalies are rare.

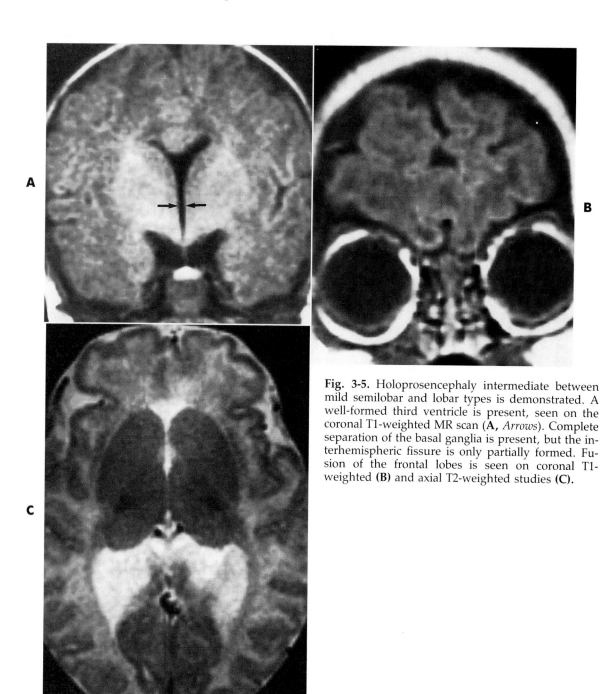

Fig. 3-5. Holoprosencephaly intermediate between mild semilobar and lobar types is demonstrated. A well-formed third ventricle is present, seen on the coronal T1-weighted MR scan (**A,** *Arrows*). Complete separation of the basal ganglia is present, but the interhemispheric fissure is only partially formed. Fusion of the frontal lobes is seen on coronal T1-weighted (**B**) and axial T2-weighted studies (**C**).

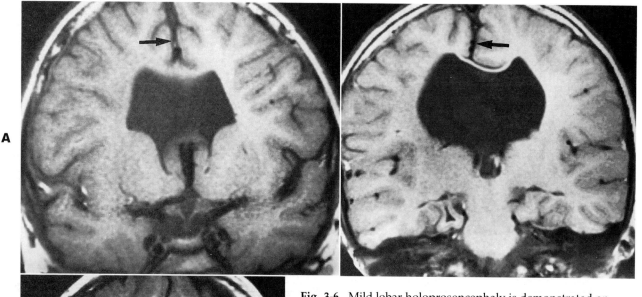

Fig. 3-6. Mild lobar holoprosencephaly is demonstrated on coronal (**A** and **B**) and axial (**C**) T1-weighted scans. Note the relatively well-formed falx cerebri and interhemispheric fissure *(large black arrows)*. The basal ganglia are separated by the third ventricle *(open arrow)*. A small area of persistent fusion in the anteroinferior frontal lobe region is seen *(small black arrows)*.

Septooptic Dysplasia

Pathology and imaging. Septooptic dysplasia (de Morsier syndrome) can be considered a very mild form of lobar holoprosencephaly. Absence or dysgenesis of the septum pellucidum in conjunction with optic nerve hypoplasia are the basic components (Fig. 3-8, *A*). Imaging studies in these patients typically show squared-off frontal horns without a septum pellucidum dividing the lateral ventricles (Fig. 3-8, *B*).

Associated abnormalities. Two anatomic subsets of septooptic dysplasia have been identified. One is associated with schizencephaly. In this group the ventricles are normal, a remnant of the septum pellucidum is present, and the white matter of the optic radiations appears normal. The clinical symptoms in this group are seizures and visual symptoms. The second group does not have associated schizenceph-

aly, exhibits diffuse white matter hypoplasia with ventriculomegaly, has complete absence of the septum, and typically presents clinically with symptoms of hypothalamic-pituitary dysfunction.[7]

Dysplasia or absence of the septum pellucidum is also associated with other brain anomalies, including aqueductal stenosis, Chiari II malformation, cephaloceles, callosal agenesis, porencephaly, and hydranencephaly.[8]

Arhinencephaly

Pathology and imaging. In arhinencephaly the olfactory bulbs and tracts are absent (Fig. 3-9, *A*). Coronal MR scans show olfactory sulci but no olfactory bulbs or tracts (Fig. 3-9, *B*).

Associated abnormalities. Arhinencephaly is actually a spectrum of disorders. Although isolated olfactory aplasia can occur, it is usually part of a complex cerebral and somatic malformation syndrome. Most, although not all, cases of holoprosencephaly are associated with absent olfactory bulbs and tracts. Olfactory aplasia also occurs in some genetic conditions such as Kallmann's syndrome (anosmia, hypogonadism, and mental retardation).[9]

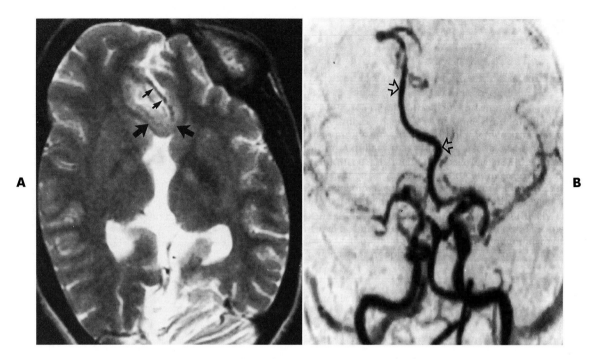

Fig. 3-7. Lobar holoprosencephaly with azygous anterior cerebral artery (ACA). **A,** Axial T2-weighted scan shows minimal fusion of the frontal lobe cortex *(large arrows)*. The azygous ACA is indicated by the small arrows. **B,** MR angiogram shows the azygous ACA *(open arrows)*. (Courtesy Joel Curé.)

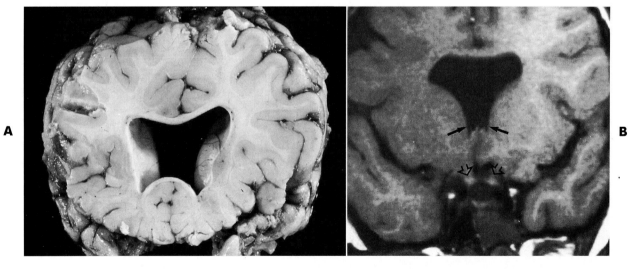

Fig. 3-8. Gross coronal gross pathology specimen **(A)** and coronal T1-weighted MR scan **(B)** show characteristic findings of septooptic dysplasia. The absent septum pellucidum with a squared-off appearance to the frontal horns is indicated by the small black arrows. The optic nerves *(open arrows)* are mildly hypoplastic. (**A,** Courtesy J. Townsend.)

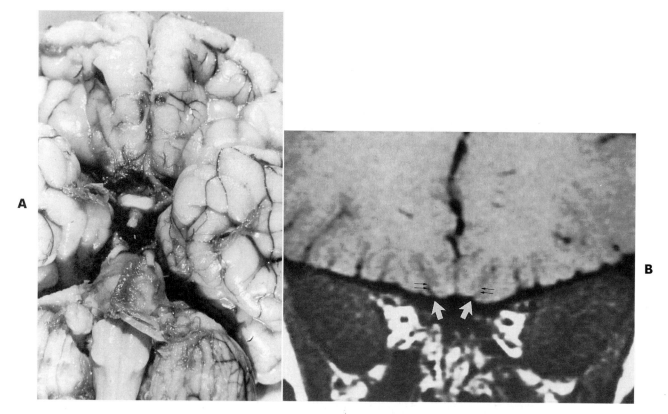

Fig. 3-9. **A,** Gross pathologic specimen of arhinencephaly. The olfactory bulbs are absent. **B,** Coronal T1-weighted MR scan in a patient with arhinencephaly shows absence of the olfactory bulbs in their usual position below the olfactory sulci *(arrows)*. (**A,** Courtesy Rubinstein Collection, Armed Forces Institute of Pathology.)

SULCATION AND CELLULAR MIGRATION

Beginning with the seventh gestational week, neuronal and glial precursors are generated in the germinal matrix that lines the lateral and third ventricles. These young neurons then migrate along the radial glial fibers that extend from the ventricle to brain surface. There is a direct correspondence between the site of cell proliferation within the germinal zone and location within the cerebral cortex.[2] Disruption in the normal process of neuronal generation and cellular migration results in a spectrum of brain malformations.[10] These are divided into several types, depending on the timing and severity of the arrest of neuronal migration.[2]

Lissencephaly

Etiology and pathology. The developing brain of a 16 or 17 week fetus normally has a smooth, "agyric" appearance with shallow sylvian fissures and almost no surface sulcation (Fig. 3-10, *A* to *C*). Lissencephaly, or "smooth brain," refers to brains with absent or poor sulcation (Fig. 3-10, *D*). Lissencephaly can be complete (synonymous with agyria) or incomplete, where a few shallow sulci are present. In the latter case, it is synonymous with agyria-pachygyria,

or nonlissencephalic cortical dysplasia (see subsequent discussion).

Intrauterine infections can also result in a smooth, lissencephalic-appearing brain (see Chapter 16).

Imaging findings. Imaging studies in children with so-called type I lissencephaly show colpocephaly and a thickened cortex with broad, flat gyri, smooth gray-white matter interface, and straight oblique or shallow sylvian fissures, giving a figure eight appearance[11] (Fig. 3-11). If intrauterine infection has resulted in lissencephaly, parenchymal calcifications can be present as well (Fig. 3-12). A second type of lissencephaly, type II, has been described as an agyric, severely disorganized unlayered cortex[10] with poor corticomedullary demarcation.[12] MR studies in patients with type II lissencephaly show thickened cortex that has a polymicrogyric appearance associated with hypomyelination of the underlying white matter. A third type of lissencephaly, the cerebrocerebellar type, occurs without a figure eight configuration and has microcephaly, moderately thick cortices, enlarged ventricles, and hypoplastic cerebellum and brain stem.[11]

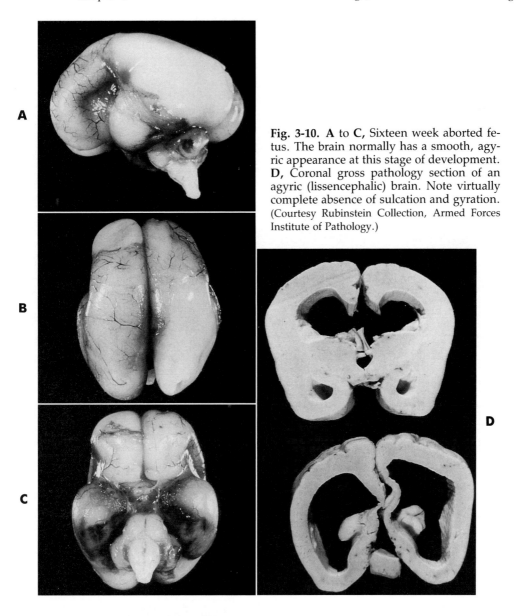

Fig. 3-10. A to C, Sixteen week aborted fetus. The brain normally has a smooth, agyric appearance at this stage of development. **D,** Coronal gross pathology section of an agyric (lissencephalic) brain. Note virtually complete absence of sulcation and gyration. (Courtesy Rubinstein Collection, Armed Forces Institute of Pathology.)

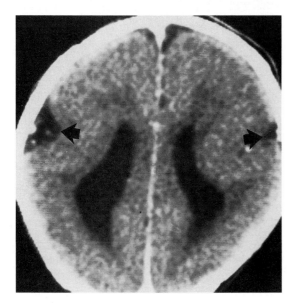

Fig. 3-11. Contrast-enhanced axial CT scan of lissencephaly. The sylvian fissures are shallow *(arrows)*, giving the brain a figure eight appearance. The virtual absence of surface sulcation is characteristic for lissencephaly.

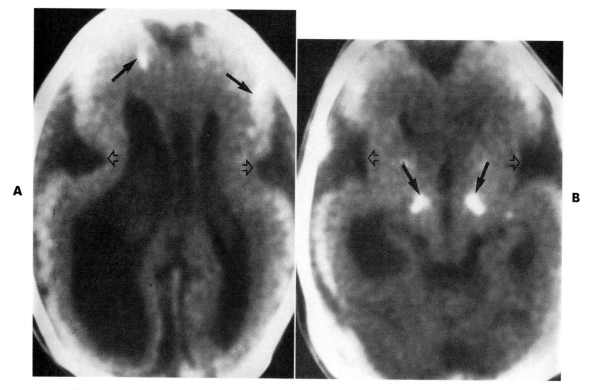

Fig. 3-12. Axial noncontrast CT scans through the midventricular **(A)** and basal ganglionic **(B)** levels in a newborn with intrauterine TORCH. Note the small, agyric brain with shallow sylvian fissures **(A,** *open arrows)* and figure eight appearance. Dystrophic calcification in the basal ganglia and subcortical white matter *(black arrows)* is also present.

Associated abnormalities. Miller-Dieker syndrome is associated with type I lissencephaly. Type II lissencephaly is associated with Walker-Warburg syndrome. These patients have ocular malformations, cephaloceles, and profound congenital hypotonia[13] (Fig. 3-13; *see* Fig. 2-18, *A* to *C*). Fukuyama's congenital muscular dystrophy (cerebro-oculo-muscular syndrome) is probably part of this spectrum as well.[10,11] Fukuyama's congenital muscular dystrophy may also have migrational malformations (pachygyria/polymicrogyria) and delayed myelination.[14]

Nonlissencephalic Cortical Dysplasias

The agyria-pachygyria complex has recently been reclassified into a more general category, nonlissencephalic cortical dysplasia, because the terms *pachygyria* and *polymicrogyria* actually are histologic descriptions and can be difficult to distinguish on MR examination.[15] The cortical dysplasias can be either diffuse or focal, unilateral or bilateral.

Pathology and imaging. Gross pathologic and imaging appearance in the nonlissencephalic cortical dysplasias varies from a diffusely thickened, abnormal cortex that has an irregular, "bumpy" gyral pattern (polymicrogyria) and relative paucity of underlying white matter (Figs. 3-14 and 3-15) to more focal areas of thickened, flattened cortex (pachygyria) (Figs. 3-16 and 3-17). Approximately one quarter of patients with nonlissencephalic cortical dysplasias

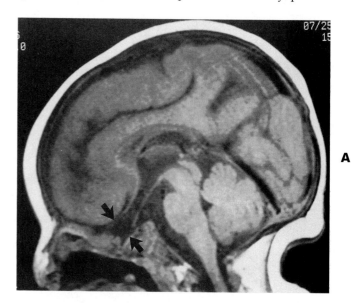

Fig. 3-13 A. For legend, see next page.

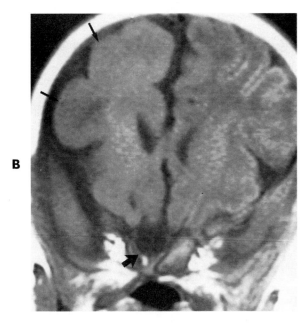

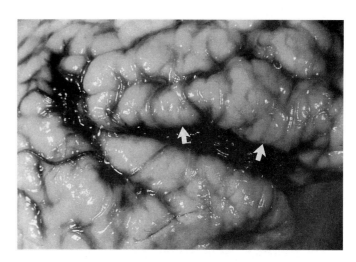

Fig. 3-13, cont'd. Sagittal **(A)** and coronal **(B)** T1-weighted MR scans in a patient with Walker-Warburg syndrome, sphenoethmoidal cephalocele *(large arrows)*, and lissencephaly. The right hemisphere has a disorganized appearance, with thickened, nearly agyric cortex *(small arrows)* and poor gray-white matter demarcation. (Courtesy Joel Curé.)

Fig. 3-14. Gross pathology specimen, lateral view, demonstrating foci of multiple small, "bumpy" gyri along the sylvian fissure characteristic of polymicrogyria *(arrows)*.

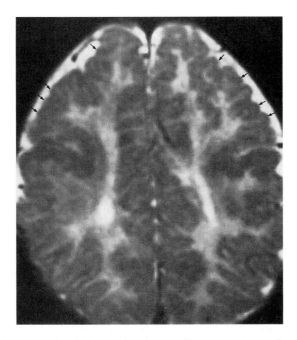

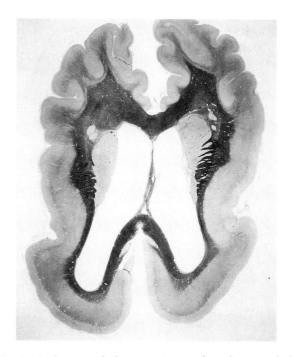

Fig. 3-15. Axial T2-weighted scan demonstrating polymicrogyria *(arrows)* with a relative paucity of underlying white matter.

Fig. 3-16. Gross pathology specimen of nonlissencephalic cortical dysplasia. Some comparatively more normal sulcation and gyration is present in the frontal lobes, but both sylvian fissures are shallow and the parietooccipital cortex is almost completely agyric. (Courtesy Yakovlev Collection, Armed Forces Institute of Pathology.)

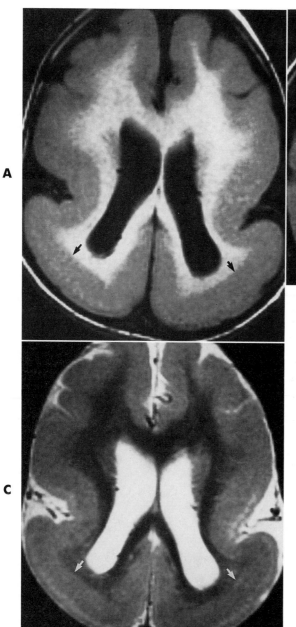

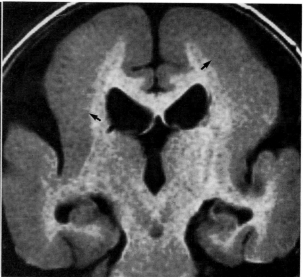

Fig. 3-17. Axial **(A)** and coronal **(B)** T1-weighted MR scans of nonlissencephalic cortical dysplasia. Note the shallow sylvian fissures and thickened, nearly agyric-appearing cortex *(arrows)*. **(C)** T2-weighted axial scan shows the paucity of normal white matter and the thickened cortex with smooth gray-white interface.

Laminar heterotopias. If diffuse arrest of neuronal migration occurs, a layer of neurons is interposed between the ventricle and cortex. Alternating layers of gray and white matter are seen in this "band," or "laminar," form of heterotopia (Fig. 3-18).[16] The abnormally located gray matter is isointense with cortical gray matter on all imaging sequences (Fig. 3-19).

Nodular heterotopias. These abnormalities of cellular migration can also be either diffuse or focal. A striking form of nodular heterotopia occurs when multiple small foci of gray matter are seen in the subependymal region (Figs. 3-20 and 3-21). The differential diagnosis is subependymal nodules (SENs) seen with tuberous sclerosis (TS). In TS the nodules are irregularly shaped and often calcified on CT studies. On MR studies, SENs are not precisely isointense with cortical gray matter and occasionally show enhancement after contrast administration. In contrast, heterotopias parallel cortex in signal on all MR imaging sequences and do not enhance.[17]

have abnormalities of the underlying white matter, usually seen as foci of increased T2 signal, that suggest the presence of gliosis.[15]

Heterotopias

Gray matter heterotopias are collections of otherwise normal neurons in abnormal locations secondary to arrest of neuronal migration along the radial glial fibers.[10] Heterotopias can be bandlike (laminar) or nodular, focal, or diffuse.

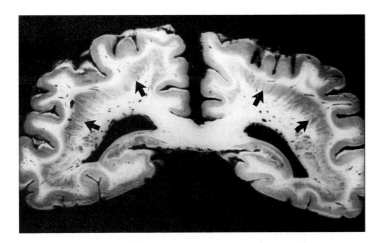

Fig. 3-18. Gross pathology specimen, coronal section, demonstrating laminar (band) heterotopic gray matter *(large black arrows)*. The layers of gray matter alternate with the white matter, giving a laminated or "target" appearance to the brain. (From archives of the Armed Forces Institute of Pathology.)

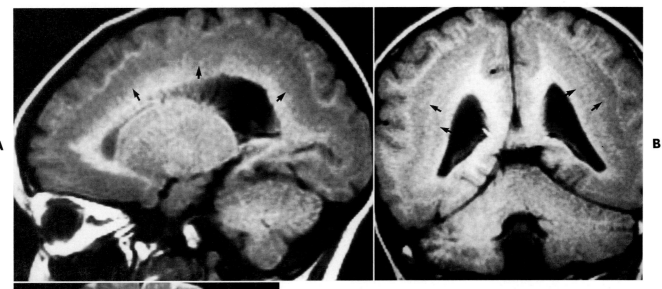

Fig. 3-19. Sagittal **(A)** and coronal **(B)** T1-weighted and axial T2-weighted **(C)** MR scans in a patient with band heterotopia. Bands of gray matter alternate with the white matter. The layered, laminated appearance of multiple bands of heterotopic gray matter *(arrows)* is particularly striking in this case.

Peters

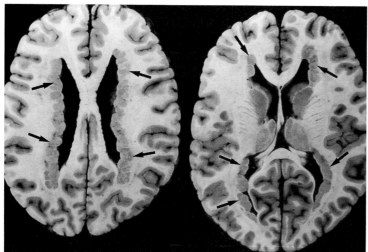

Fig. 3-20. Axial gross pathology specimen of diffuse subependymal nodular heterotopia. The lateral ventricles appear studded with multiple foci of heterotopic gray matter *(arrows)*. (Courtesy Okazaki H, Scheithauer B: *Slide Atlas* of *Neuropathology*, Gower Medical Publishing Company).

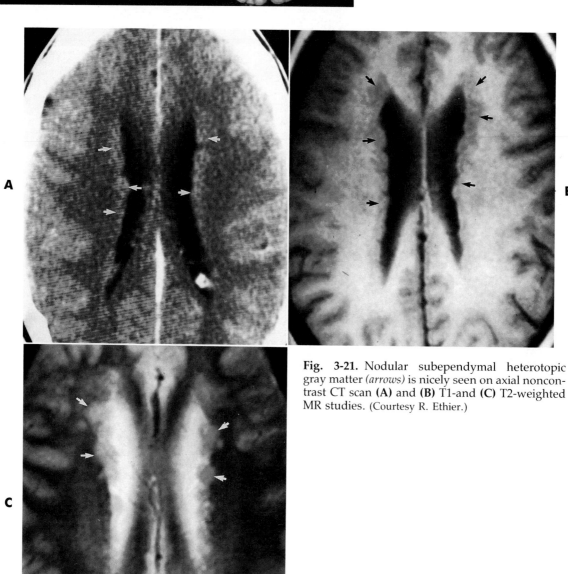

Fig. 3-21. Nodular subependymal heterotopic gray matter *(arrows)* is nicely seen on axial noncontrast CT scan **(A)** and **(B)** T1-and **(C)** T2-weighted MR studies. (Courtesy R. Ethier.)

Pathology and imaging. Heterotopias that are more focal have a variable appearance. They can deform the cerebral hemispheres and indent adjacent ventricles (Fig. 3-22). Again, the signal on MR imaging is isointense with gray matter on all sequences.

No enhancement is seen following contrast administration. When masses of heterotopic gray matter are located more peripherally near the cortex, they may be associated with prominent anomalous cortical draining veins (Figs. 3-23 and 3-24).

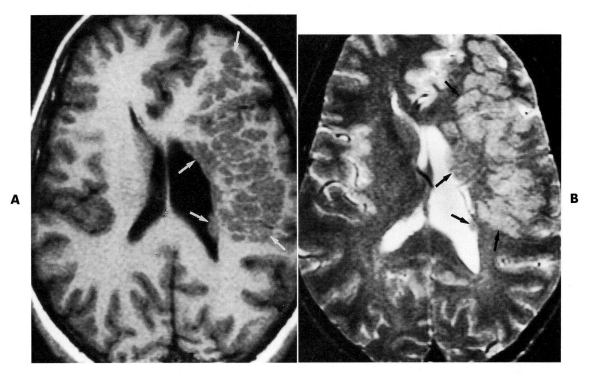

Fig. 3-22. Axial **(A)** T1- and **(B)** T2-weighted MR scan of focal heterotopic gray matter. Masses of gray matter (*arrows*) indent the lateral ventricle.

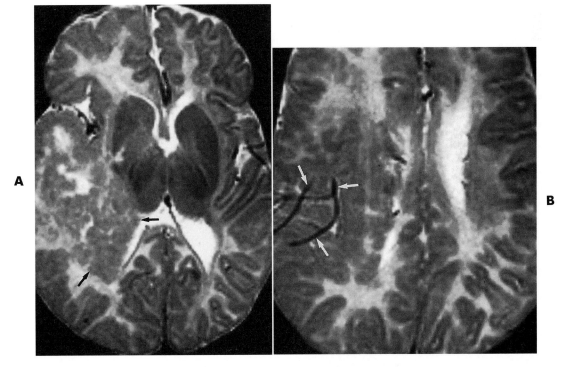

Fig. 3-23. Axial T2-weighted MR scans of heterotopic gray matter **(A)** *(black arrows)* with prominent anomalous cortical draining veins **(B)** *(white arrows)*.

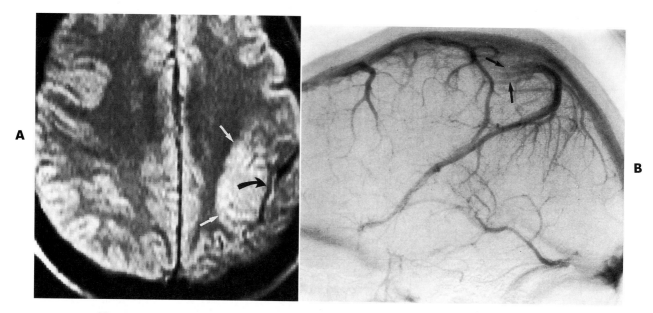

Fig. 3-24. A, Long TR/short TE axial MR scan shows a mass of heterotopic gray matter *(white arrows)* with prominent cortical draining veins *(black arrow)*. **B,** Internal carotid angiogram, lateral view, venous phase, shows the anomalous cortical draining veins *(arrows)*.

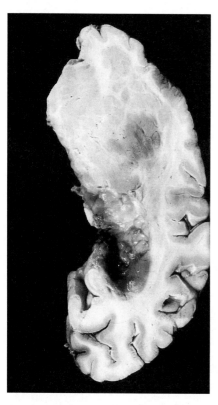

Fig. 3-25. Axial gross pathology specimen of dysplastic cerebral hemisphere. No identifiable frontal horn of the lateral ventricle can be seen, and the frontal lobe is composed of dysplastic, disorganized heterotopic gray matter. No sylvian fissure is present. (From archives of Armed Forces Institute of Pathology.)

Occasionally part or all of a cerebral hemisphere can be completely dysplastic, with absence of normal sulcation and sylvian fissure (Fig. 3-25). In extreme cases, no lateral ventricle can be identified and the hemisphere consists entirely of dysplastic, disorganized masses of gray matter with hypoplastic white matter (Fig. 3-26).[17a] These cases can resemble an intracranial mass, especially if the ipsilateral ventricle is absent or severely deformed. Biopsy of tissue from these dysplastic hemispheres may lead to the erroneous diagnosis of gangliocytoma (*see* Chapter 14).

Schizencephaly

Pathology. Schizencephaly (split brain) is a gray matter-lined cerebrospinal fluid-filled cleft that extends from the ependymal surface of the brain through the white matter to the pia (Fig. 3-27). Two types are recognized: type I, or *closed-lip schizencephaly*, in which the cleft walls are in apposition, and type II, or *open lip schizencephaly*, in which the walls are separated. In either instance the cleft is lined by heterotopic gray matter. The clefts can be unilateral or bilateral, symmetric or asymmetric.[18]

Imaging. CT scans of closed-lip schizencephaly may show only a slight outpouching, or "nipple," at the ependymal surface of the cleft (Fig. 3-28). The full thickness cleft, or pial-ependymal seam, may be dif-

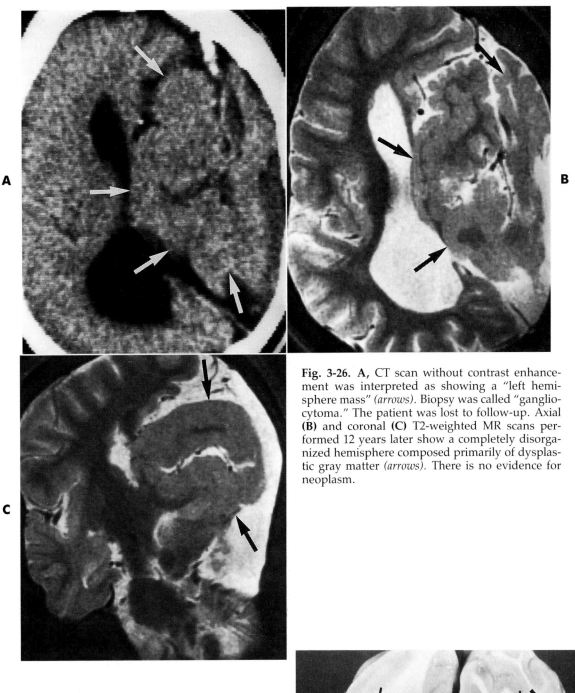

Fig. 3-26. **A,** CT scan without contrast enhancement was interpreted as showing a "left hemisphere mass" *(arrows)*. Biopsy was called "gangliocytoma." The patient was lost to follow-up. Axial **(B)** and coronal **(C)** T2-weighted MR scans performed 12 years later show a completely disorganized hemisphere composed primarily of dysplastic gray matter *(arrows)*. There is no evidence for neoplasm.

Fig. 3-27. Coronal gross brain specimen demonstrates bilaterally symmetrical schizencephalic clefts *(large arrows)*. Note abnormal heterotopic gray matter *(small arrows)* that lines the full-thickness clefts. (Courtesy E. Ross.)

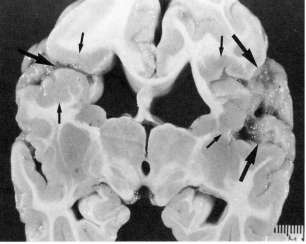

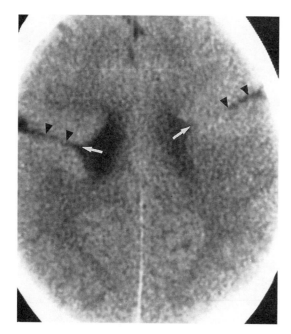

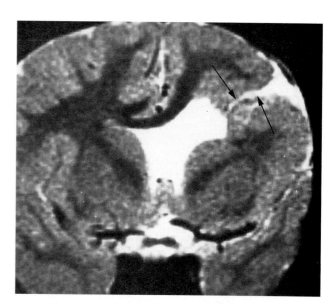

Fig. 3-28. Axial CT scan without contrast enhancement shows bilateral closed-lip schizencephaly. Note the out-pouchings, or "nipples," of CSF *(arrows)* and the gray matter-lined pial-ependymal seams *(arrowheads)*.

Fig. 3-29. Coronal T2-weighted MR scan of unilateral closed-lip schizencephaly. The pial-ependymal seam *(arrows)* is easily identified.

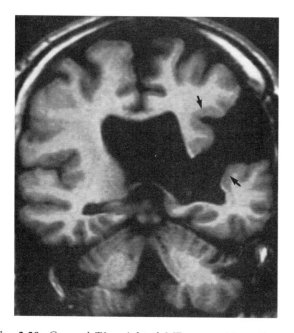

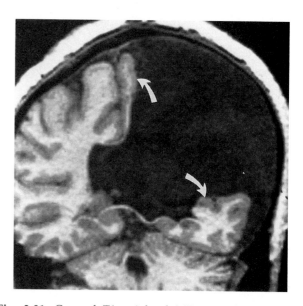

Fig. 3-30. Coronal T1-weighted MR scan with unilateral, open-lip schizencephaly. The full-thickness cleft extends from the ventricle to the surface of the brain and is lined with gray matter *(arrows)*.

Fig. 3-31. Coronal T1-weighted MR scan shows a very large unilateral open-lip schizencephaly. Gray matter *(arrows)* lines the cleft. (Courtesy P. Van Tassel and Joel Curé.)

ficult to detect on CT scans but is easily discernible on MR studies (Fig. 3-29). Open-lip schizencephaly has a larger, more apparent gray matter-lined CSF cleft (Fig. 3-30). Occasionally the schizencephalic clefts are very large (Figs. 3-31 and 3-32).

The imaging differential diagnosis of schizencephaly is porencephalic cyst. Because porencephalic cysts result from insults to otherwise normally developed brain, the CSF space is lined by gliotic white matter, not dysplastic heterotopic cortex (Fig. 3-33).

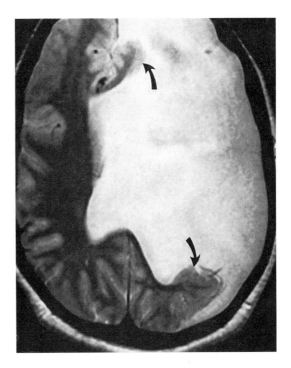

Fig. 3-31, cont'd.   Axial T2-weighted MR scan shows a very large unilateral open-lip schizencephaly. Gray matter (*arrows*) lines the cleft.   (Courtesy P. Van Tassel and Joel Curé.)

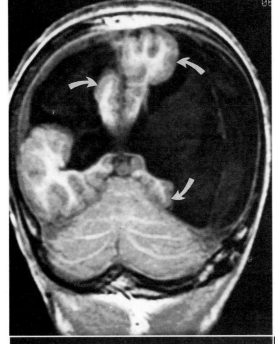

Fig. 3-32. Coronal T1- (**A**) and coronal and axial T2-weighted (**B** and **C**) MR scans show large bilateral open-lip schizencephalic clefts that are lined by abnormal gray matter *(arrows)*. (Courtesy P. Van Tassel and J. Curé.)

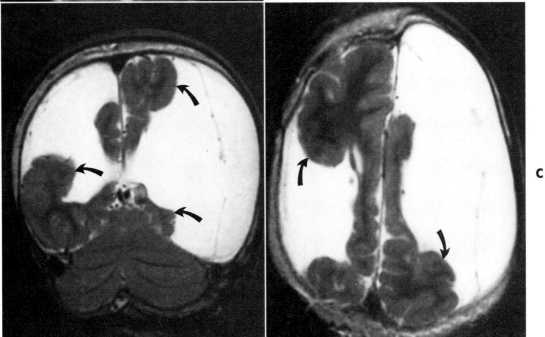

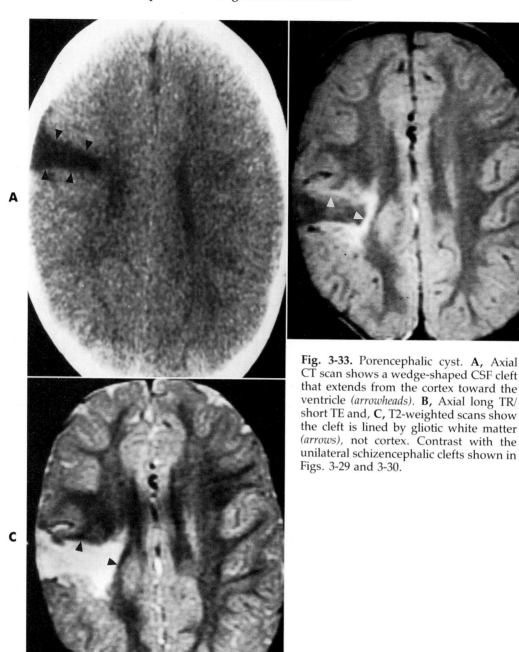

Fig. 3-33. Porencephalic cyst. **A,** Axial CT scan shows a wedge-shaped CSF cleft that extends from the cortex toward the ventricle *(arrowheads).* **B,** Axial long TR/ short TE and, **C,** T2-weighted scans show the cleft is lined by gliotic white matter *(arrows),* not cortex. Contrast with the unilateral schizencephalic clefts shown in Figs. 3-29 and 3-30.

Unilateral Megalencephaly

Pathology. *Unilateral megalencephaly* is a term that describes hamartomatous overgrowth of part or all of one cerebral hemisphere associated with localized neuronal migrational anomalies of various severity.[19] The hemisphere is enlarged compared to the opposite normal side. Heterotopic gray matter is common and sulcation is frequently abnormal. The ipsilateral ventricle is often enlarged (Fig. 3-34) and the white matter may be either hyperplastic (Fig. 3-35) or hypoplastic (Fig. 3-36).[2] Ultrasonography typically shows the enlarged ventricle and midline shift. Homogeneous parenchymal echogenicity with decreased sulcation of the affected hemisphere can also be seen.[19]

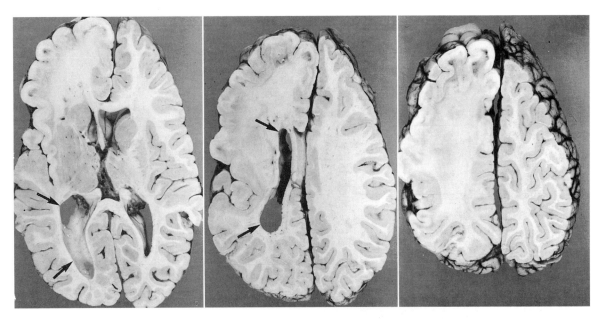

Fig. 3-34. Gross pathology of unilateral megalencephaly. The left hemisphere is enlarged, with hyperplastic white matter. The ipsilateral lateral ventricle is enlarged *(arrows).* (Courtesy B. Horten.)

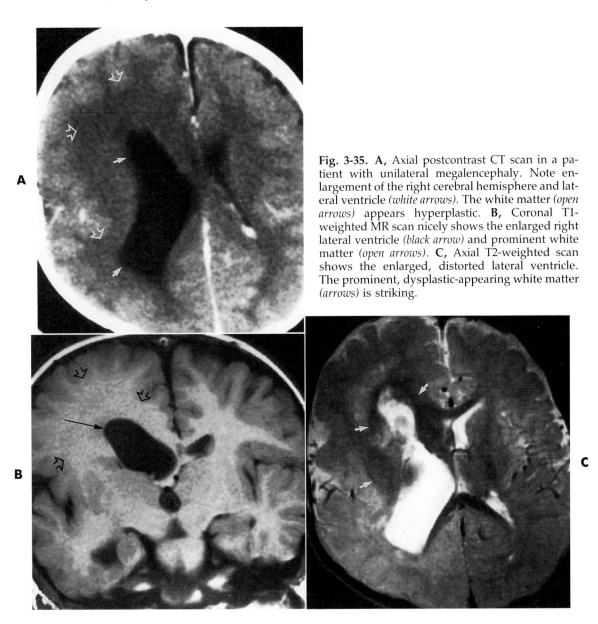

Fig. 3-35. A, Axial postcontrast CT scan in a patient with unilateral megalencephaly. Note enlargement of the right cerebral hemisphere and lateral ventricle *(white arrows).* The white matter *(open arrows)* appears hyperplastic. **B,** Coronal T1-weighted MR scan nicely shows the enlarged right lateral ventricle *(black arrow)* and prominent white matter *(open arrows).* **C,** Axial T2-weighted scan shows the enlarged, distorted lateral ventricle. The prominent, dysplastic-appearing white matter *(arrows)* is striking.

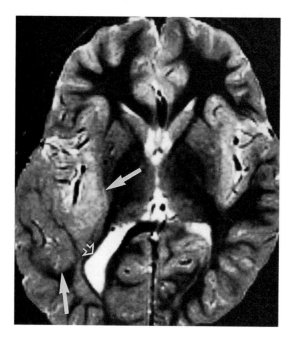

Fig. 3-36. Axial T2-weighted MR scan in a patient with long-standing seizures and right-sided unilateral megalencephaly. Note enlargement of the ipsilateral occipital horn *(open arrow)*. In this particular case, the white matter in the parietooccipital region is hypoplastic and the gray matter around the sylvian fissure and insula is thickened with abnormal sulcation *(white arrows)*.

REFERENCES

1. Byrd SE, Osborn RE, Radkowski MA et al: Disorders of midline structures: holoprosencephaly, absence of corpus callosum, and Chiari malformations, *Sem US, CT, MR* 9:201-215, 1988.

2. Barkovich AJ: Congenital malformations of the brain. In *Pediatric Neuroimaging*, pp 77-147, New York, Raven Press, 1990.

3. McGahan JP, Nyberg DA, Mack LA: Sonography of facial features of alobar and semilobar holoprosencephaly, *AJR* 154:143-148, 1990.

4. DeMyer W: Classification of cerebral malformations, *Birth Defects* 7:78-93, 1971.

5. Nyberg DA, Mack LA, Bronster A et al: Holoprosencephaly: prenatal sonographic diagnosis, *AJNR* 8:871-878, 1987.

6. Young JN, Oakes WJ, Hatten HP Jr: Dorsal third ventricular cyst: an entity distinct from holoprosencephaly, *J Neurosurg* 77:556-561, 1992.

6a. Barkovich AJ, Quint DJ: Middle interhemispheric fusion: an unusual variant of holoprosencephaly, *AJNR* 14:431-440, 1993.

7. Barkovich AJ, Fram EK, Norman D: Septo-optic dysplasia: MR imaging, *Radiology* 171:189-192, 1989.

8. Barkovich AJ, Norman D: Absence of the septum pellucidum: a useful sign in the diagnosis of congenital brain malformations, *AJNR* 9:1107-1114, 1988.

9. Louis DN, Arriagada PV, Hyman BT, Hedley-Whyte T: Olfactory dysgenesis in hypoplasia: a variant in the arhinenencephaly spectrum? *Neuroradiology* 42:179-182, 1992.

10. Barkovich AJ, Gressens P, Evrard P: Formation, maturation, and disorders of brain neocortex, *AJNR* 13:423-446, 1992.

11. Dietrich RB, Demos D, Kocit et al: Lissencephaly: MR and CT appearances with different subtypes, *Radiol* 185(suppl):123, 1992.

12. Kimura S, Kobayashi T, Sasaki Y et al: Congenital polyneuropathy in Walker-Warburg syndrome, *Neuropediatrics* 23:14-17, 1992.

13. Rhodes RE, Hatten HP Jr, Ellington KS: Walker-Warburg syndrome, *AJNR* 13:123-126, 1992.

14. Aihara M, Tanabe Y, Kato K: Serial MRI in Fukuyama type congenital muscular dystrophy, *Neuroradiology* 34:396-398, 1992.

15. Barkovich AJ, Kjos BO: Nonlissencephalic cortical dysplasias: correlation of imaging findings with clinical deficits, *AJNR* 13:95-103, 1992.

16. Barkovich AJ, Jackson DE Jr, Boyer RS: Band heterotopias: a newly recognized neuronal migration anomaly, *Radiol* 171:455-458, 1989.

17. Barkovich AJ, Chuang SH, Norman D: MR of neuronal migration anomalies, *AJNR* 8:1009-1017, 1987.

17a. Castillo M, Kwock L, Scatliff J et al: Proton MR spectroscopic characteristics of a presumed giant subcortical heterotopia, *AJNR* 14:426-429, 1993.

18. Barkovich AJ, Kjos BO: Schizencephaly: correlation of clinical findings with MR characteristics, *AJNR* 13:85-94, 1992.

19. Babyn P, Chuang S, Daneman A, Withers C: Sonographic recognition of unilateral megalencephaly, *J Ultrasound Med* 11:563-566, 1992.

Posterior Fossa Malformations and Cysts

Dandy-Walker Complex
    Dandy-Walker Malformation
    Dandy-Walker Variant
Miscellaneous Posterior Fossa Cysts
    Mega Cisterna Magna
    Posterior Fossa Arachnoid Cyst
Miscellaneous Cerebellar Hypoplasias/Dysplasias
    Chiari IV Malformation
    Joubert's Syndrome
    Rhombencephalosynapsis
    Tectocerebellar Dysraphia
    Lhermitte-Duclos Disease

DANDY-WALKER COMPLEX

In the past, posterior fossa cystic malformations have been divided into Dandy-Walker malformation, Dandy-Walker variant, mega cisterna magna, and posterior fossa arachnoid cysts. Based on the results of multiplanar MR imaging, the Dandy-Walker malformation and variant are now thought to represent a continuum of developmental anomalies on a spectrum that has been designated the "Dandy-Walker complex."[1]

The Dandy-Walker (D-W) complex is characterized by cystic dilatation of the fourth ventricle and an enlarged posterior fossa with upward displacement of the lateral sinuses, tentorium, and torcular Herophili

associated with varying degrees of vermian aplasia or hypoplasia.[2] Because the vermis is present in cases of mega cisterna magna and posterior fossa arachnoid cyst, these are considered separately from the Dandy-Walker malformation.

Dandy-Walker Malformation

Etiology. The exact origin of the D-W malformation is unknown. Theories include failure of development of the anterior medullary velum (embryonic roof of the fourth ventricle), atresia of the fourth ventricular outlet foramina, and delayed opening of the foramen of Magendie. Insults of varying severity to both the developing cerebellar hemispheres and fourth ventricle are currently thought to be the genesis of this anomaly.[1]

Pathology and imaging. Pathologic and radiologic findings in D-W are summarized in the box, p. 60. Gross pathology of D-W is shown in Figure 4-1. An anatomic diagram that depicts the major abnormalities characterizing D-W is shown in Figure 4-2. Dandy-Walker malformations have abnormalities of the following:
    1. Skull and dura
    2. Ventricles and posterior fossa CSF spaces
    3. Cerebellum, vermis, and brainstem
It is helpful to consider separately these different manifestations.

Dandy-Walker Malformation

Skull and dura

Large posterior fossa
High tentorial insertion (lambdoid-torcular inversion)
High transverse sinuses

Ventricles and CSF spaces

Fourth ventricle floor present; ventricle open dorsally to large posterior fossa cyst
Hydrocephalus in 80%

Cerebellum, vermis, brainstem

Vermian, cerebellar hemispheric hypoplasia
Vermian remnant anterosuperiorly everted above cyst
Cerebellar hemispheres winged anterolaterally in front of cyst
Brainstem may be hypoplastic, compressed
Heterotopias, cerebellar dysplasias common

Associated CNS anomalies

Corpus callosum agenesis in 20%-25%
Heterotopias, gyral anomalies, schizencephaly
Cephaloceles

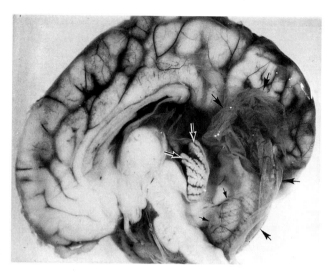

Fig. 4-1. Gross pathologic specimen, lateral view, of Dandy-Walker malformation. The fourth ventricle is open dorsally to a large posterior fossa cyst *(large black arrows)*. The tiny remnant of the vermis *(black and white arrows)* is everted anterosuperiorly over the large cyst. The hypoplastic cerebellar hemispheres are indicated by the small black arrows. (Courtesy E. C. Alvord, Jr.)

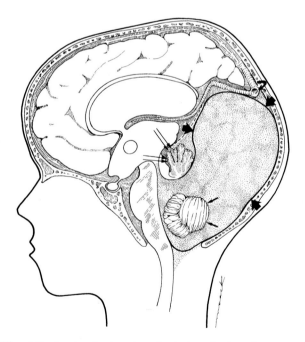

Fig. 4-2. Anatomic drawing depicting the key features of Dandy-Walker malformation. A large posterior fossa cyst *(large black arrows)* is present, elevating the confluence of the sinuses (torcular Herophili) *(curved arrow)*. The hypoplastic vermis *(double arrows)* is everted over the posterior fossa cyst. The cerebellar hemispheres *(small black arrows)* are hypoplastic.

Skull and dura. In contrast to Chiari II, in which the posterior fossa is abnormally small, in D-W the posterior fossa is strikingly enlarged, with abnormally high position of the straight sinus, torcular Herophili, and tentorium (Fig. 4-3, *A* and *B*). This produces the classic findings of lambdoid-torcular inversion on plain films (Fig. 4-3, *C*) and elevation of the torcular herophili, tentorial apex, and transverse sinuses on angiographic (Fig. 4-3, *D*) and MR studies (Figs. 4-3, *E*, and 4-4).

Ventricles and posterior fossa CSF spaces. The floor of the fourth ventricle is present, the cystically dilated fluid-filled ventricle balloons posteriorly behind (Fig. 4-4, *A*) and between widely separated, variably hypoplastic cerebellar hemispheres (Fig. 4-4, *B*). In severe cases the cyst occupies most of the enlarged posterior fossa. Generalized obstructive hydrocephalus is present in about 80% of patients with D-W. If callosal agenesis coexists with D-W, dilatation of the occipital horns (colpocephaly) can sometimes be identified (Fig. 4-4, *C* and *D*).

Cerebellum, vermis, and brainstem. Varying degrees of cerebellar and vermian hypoplasia are present in D-W. The spectrum ranges from complete vermian absence in one quarter of cases to mild hypoplasia. The vermian remnant typically appears rotated and elevated above the posterior fossa cyst (Figs. 4-1, 4-2, and 4-4, *A*). The cerebellar hemispheres also demonstrate varying degrees of hypoplasia. Only minimal hypoplasia may be present (Fig. 4-5). In more severe cases, the cerebellar hemispheres

A   **B**

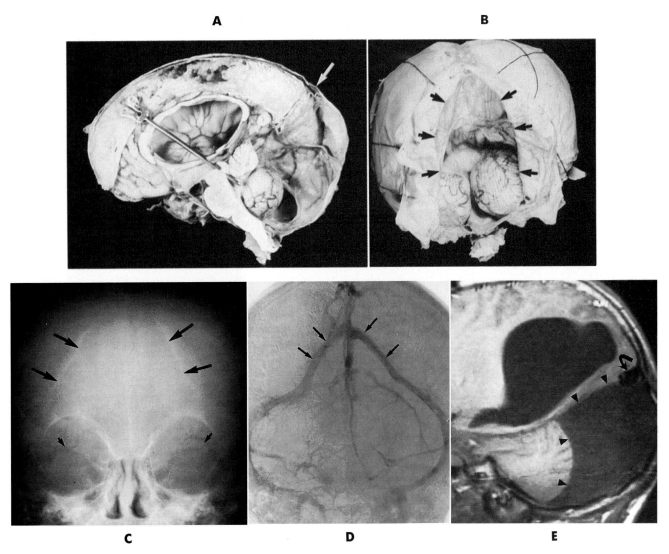

C   **D**   **E**

Fig. 4-3. Gross pathology specimen, lateral (**A**) and dorsal (**B**) views, with dura and dural sinuses intact. Note high position of the torcular and transverse sinuses *(arrows)* elevated over the large posterior fossa cyst. **C,** Plain film skull radiograph, PA view, shows elevation of the torcular Herophili and transverse sinuses *(large black arrows)* above the lambdoid sutures *(small black arrows)* in this patient with Dandy-Walker (D-W) malformation. **D,** AP view of subtracted posterior fossa angiogram, venous phase, in a patient with D-W malformation. The sinus confluence and lateral sinuses *(arrows)* are elevated above the lambda. **E,** Off-midline sagittal T1-weighted MR scan in another patient with D-W malformation shows the large posterior fossa cyst *(arrowheads)* elevating the torcular and transverse sinuses *(curved arrow)*. (**A** and **B,** Courtesy E. Ross. **D,** Reprinted from Osborn AG, *Introduction to Cerebral Angiography,* Harper and Row, 1980.)

appear "winged outward" and displaced anterolaterally against the petrous portion of the temporal bone[2] (Fig. 4-4, *B*). The brainstem may be hypoplastic (Fig. 4-6) or compressed. Cerebellar disorganization and heterotopias are sometimes associated.

Associated abnormalities. Other CNS abnormalities are present in 70% of cases with D-W.[3] These include corpus callosum agenesis (Figs. 2-17 and 4-5, *B*) or dysgenesis with or without dorsal interhemispheric cyst; migrational abnormalities with gray matter heterotopias (Fig. 4-4, *B*), clefts, polymicrogy-

ria and agyria, and occipital cephaloceles[4] (Fig. 2-17). In patients with subtorcular occipital cephaloceles there is often communication between the posterior fossa cyst and the cephalocele (Fig. 4-6).

Non-CNS anomalies associated with the Dandy-Walker malformation include polydactyly and cardiac anomalies, among others.[5]

Dandy-Walker Variant

Pathology and imaging. The so-called Dandy-Walker variant is mild vermian hypoplasia with a variably sized cystic space caused by open commu-

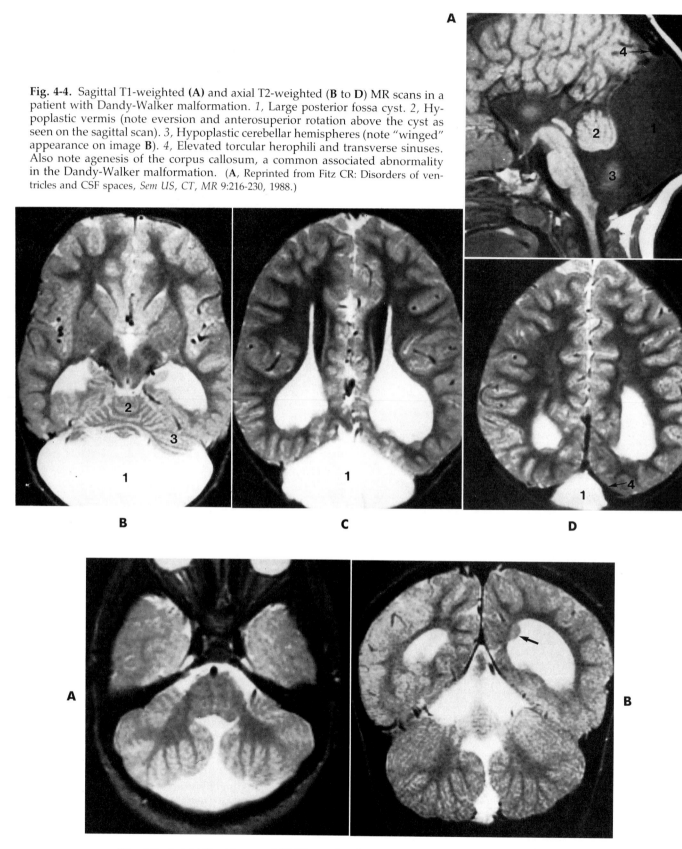

Fig. 4-4. Sagittal T1-weighted **(A)** and axial T2-weighted **(B** to **D)** MR scans in a patient with Dandy-Walker malformation. *1,* Large posterior fossa cyst. *2,* Hypoplastic vermis (note eversion and anterosuperior rotation above the cyst as seen on the sagittal scan). *3,* Hypoplastic cerebellar hemispheres (note "winged" appearance on image **B**). *4,* Elevated torcular herophili and transverse sinuses. Also note agenesis of the corpus callosum, a common associated abnormality in the Dandy-Walker malformation. **(A,** Reprinted from Fitz CR: Disorders of ventricles and CSF spaces, *Sem US, CT, MR* 9:216-230, 1988.)

Fig. 4-5. Axial **(A)** and coronal **(B)** T2-weighted MR scans in a patient with Dandy-Walker malformation. Only mild cerebellar hemispheric hypoplasia is present with a relatively small posterior fossa cyst. Agenesis of the corpus callosum with colpocephaly is present. Note periventricular heterotopic gray matter *(arrow).*

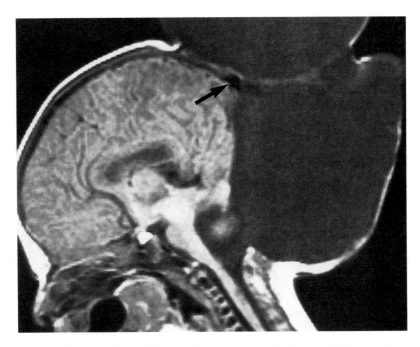

Fig. 4-6. Sagittal T1-weighted MR scan in a patient with Dandy-Walker malformation. The posterior fossa cyst communicates directly with a large occipital cephalocele. Note high position of the torcular herophili *(arrow)*.

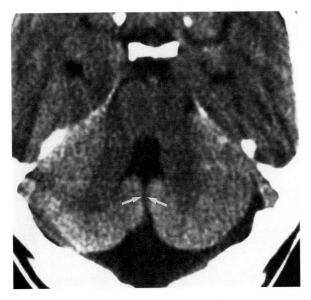

Fig. 4-7. Axial CT scan without contrast enhancement of a so-called Dandy-Walker "variant." The inferior vermis is hypoplastic and the fourth ventricle communicates dorsally with an enlarged cisterna magna through a slitlike opening that creates the characteristic "key-hole" deformity *(arrows)* seen in this condition.

nication of the posteroinferior fourth ventricle and cisterna magna through an enlarged vallecula (Fig. 4-7). The fourth ventricle is often slightly to moderately enlarged but the posterior fossa is typically normal size.[3] The inferior vermian lobules are variably hypoplastic; the brain stem is usually normal. Al-

though hydrocephalus may be present, the third and lateral ventricles are usually normal.

MISCELLANEOUS POSTERIOR FOSSA CYSTS
Mega Cisterna Magna

Pathology and imaging. In mega cisterna magna the vermis is intact and the cerebellar hemispheres are normally formed. The fourth ventricle typically appears normal (Figs. 4-8 and 4-9). A large cisterna magna is present and may extend above the vermis to the straight sinus (Fig. 4-10). Occasionally the posterior fossa can appear quite enlarged, with prominent scalloping of the occipital squamae (Figs. 4-9 and 4-10).[2] In such cases the distinction between mega cisterna magna and posterior fossa arachnoid cyst may be difficult unless intrathecal contrast is used. An enlarged but otherwise normal cisterna magna is readily opacified following contrast instillation into the lumbar subarachnoid space.

Posterior Fossa Arachnoid Cyst

Pathology and imaging. Posterior fossa arachnoid cysts (PFAC) are CSF-filled masses enclosed within split layers of the arachnoid. Here the fourth ventricle and vermis are normally formed but displaced by the cyst (Fig. 4-11). Imaging studies show a nonenhancing mass that closely parallels CSF in attenuation and signal intensity (Fig. 4-12). The differential diagnosis of posterior fossa arachnoid cyst includes the Dandy-Walker complex, mega cisterna magna, and

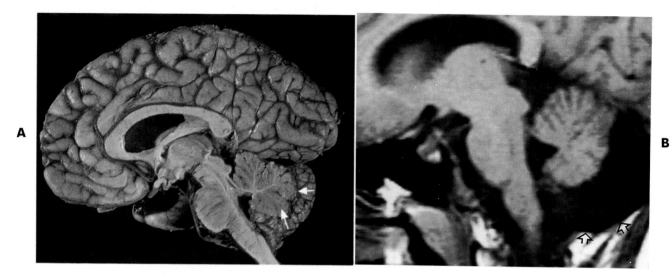

Fig. 4-8. A, Gross pathology specimen of mega cisterna magna. Note the intact vermis *(arrows)*. The approximate location of the inner table of the occiput is indicated by the dotted lines. **B,** Sagittal T1-weighted MR scan of mega cisterna magna *(arrows)*. The vermis is intact and the fourth ventricle appears normal. (**A,** Courtesy E. Tessa Hedley-Whyte.)

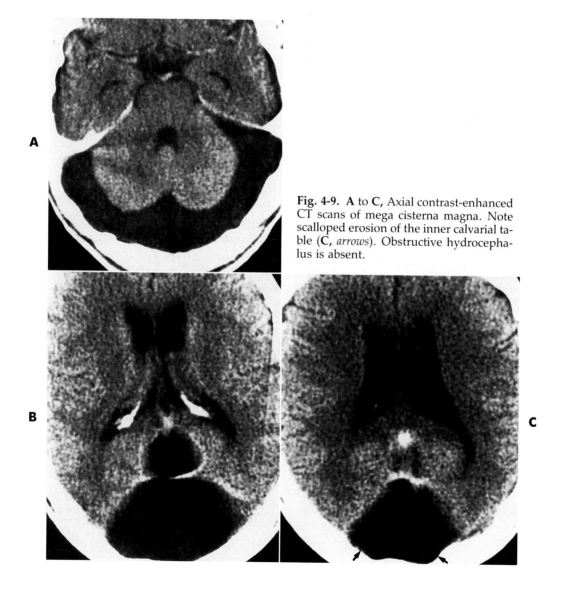

Fig. 4-9. A to **C,** Axial contrast-enhanced CT scans of mega cisterna magna. Note scalloped erosion of the inner calvarial table (**C,** *arrows*). Obstructive hydrocephalus is absent.

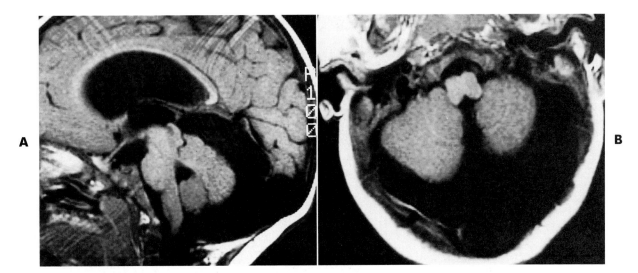

Fig. 4-10. Sagittal **(A)** and axial **(B)** T1-weighted MR scans of mega cisterna magna. The vermis is intact. The enlarged CSF space extends superiorly above the vermis to the straight sinus. Mild enlargement of the lateral ventricles is seen. This case would be difficult to distinguish from some cases of posterior fossa arachnoid cyst.

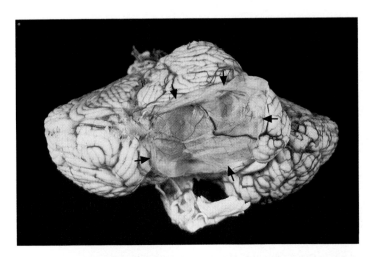

Fig. 4-11. Gross pathology specimen of posterior fossa arachnoid cyst *(arrows)*. Note that the vermis and cerebellum are present but deformed. (Courtesy Rubinstein Collection, University of Virginia Department of Pathology.)

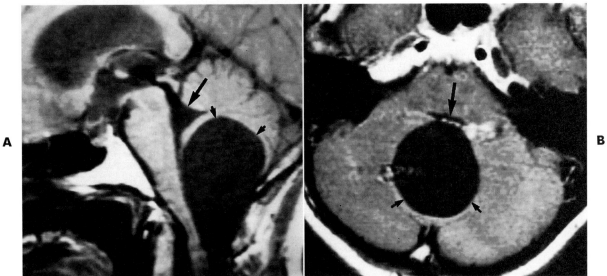

Fig. 4-12. Sagittal **(A)** and axial **(B)** T1-weighted MR scans show a classic posterior fossa arachnoid cyst *(small black arrows)*. Note normally formed but displaced fourth ventricle *(large black arrows)* and vermis.

Table 4-1. Differential diagnosis of posterior cysts and cystlike masses

Finding	Dandy-Walker malformation	Dandy-Walker variant	Mega cisterna magna	Posterior fossa arachnoid cyst
Location	Occupies most of posterior fossa	Midline posterior	Midline, posterior; typically minimal/absent extension in front of cerebellopontine angle	Posterior midline; cerebellopontine angle
Fourth ventricle	Floor present; open dorsally to large cyst	"Keyhole" appearance	Normal	Normal but displaced
Vermis	Absent/hypoplastic; everted over cyst	Inferior lobules hypoplastic, otherwise normal	Normal	Normal but distorted
Obstructive hydrocephalus	Common	Absent	Absent	Variable
Enhancement after contrast	Absent	Absent	Absent	Absent
Calcification	Absent	Absent	Absent	Absent
Cyst density/signal	CSF	CSF	CSF	~CSF
Margins	Smooth	Smooth	Smooth	Smooth
Skull	Large posterior fossa; lambdoid-torcular inversion	Normal	Inner table may be scalloped	Usually normal

other benign nonneoplastic masses such as inflammatory and enterogenous cysts. Cystic neoplasms (hemangioblastoma, pilocytic astrocytoma) and cystlike tumors such as dermoid and epidermoid also should be considered in the differential diagnosis of PFACs. Comparative imaging findings in these disorders are summarized in Table 4-1.

MISCELLANEOUS CEREBELLAR HYPOPLASIAS/DYSPLASIAS
Chiari IV Malformation

Pathology and imaging. Severe cerebellar hypoplasia has sometimes been termed *Chiari IV malformation*. Findings in this very rare entity include absent or severely hypoplastic cerebellum, small brainstem, and large posterior fossa cerebrospinal fluid spaces (Fig. 4-13).

Associated abnormalities. In contrast to Dandy-Walker malformation, obstructive hydrocephalus and other CNS anomalies are usually absent.

Joubert's Syndrome

Pathology and imaging. Joubert's syndrome is an autosomal recessive disorder characterized by a dysgenetic vermis that appears split or segmented and disorganized[6,7] (Fig. 4-14). The inferior and superior cerebellar peduncles are often small, and the fourth ventricular roof consequently appears superiorly convex on sagittal MR scans. Hydrocephalus is not a feature of this syndrome.

Associated abnormalities. CNS anomalies reported with Joubert's syndrome include callosal dysgenesis, congenital retinal dystrophy, and oculomotor abnormalities. Marked global developmental delay is typical. Non-CNS disorders include neonatal breathing abnormalities, polydactyly, and cystic kidney disease.[7]

Rhombencephalosynapsis

Pathology and imaging. Rhombencephalosynapsis is a rare posterior fossa malformation that consists

Enterogenous cyst	Inflammatory cyst	Dermoid	Epidermoid tumor	Cystic neoplasm
Anterior to brainstem	Any location	Midline, fourth ventricle	Cerebellopontine angle; fourth ventricle	Vermis, cerebellum
Normal	Normally formed; may be distorted	Normal but distorted/displaced	Normal but distorted/displaced	Normal but displaced
Normal	Normal	Normal but distorted	Normal but distorted	Normal but distorted
Absent	Variable	Variable	Variable	Common
Absent	Common	Uncommon	Unusual	Common
Absent	Common	Common	Unusual	Common
Equal or slightly higher than CSF	Often slightly hyperdense/intense compared to CSF	Iso/hypodense on NECT; often like fat on MR	Equal or slightly higher than CSF	Often hyperdense/hyperintense compared to CSF
Smooth	Smooth	Smooth/lobulated	Irregular, frondlike	Smooth/lobulated
Normal	Normal	May have sinus tract	Normal	Normal

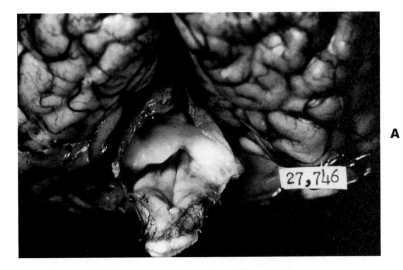

Fig. 4-13. A, Gross pathology specimen of Chiari IV malformation/severe cerebellar hypoplasia. (**A,** Courtesy J. Townsend.)   *Continued.*

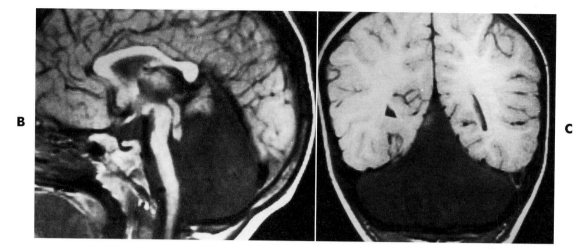

Fig 4-13, cont'd. Sagittal **(B)** and coronal **(C)** T1-weighted MR scans in another case show virtually complete cerebellar aplasia, small brainstem, and a CSF-filled posterior fossa that is normal in size. There is no evidence for hydrocephalus.

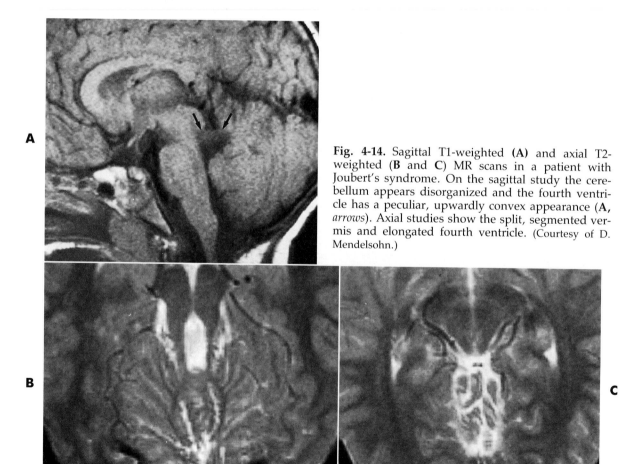

Fig. 4-14. Sagittal T1-weighted **(A)** and axial T2-weighted **(B** and **C)** MR scans in a patient with Joubert's syndrome. On the sagittal study the cerebellum appears disorganized and the fourth ventricle has a peculiar, upwardly convex appearance **(A,** *arrows*). Axial studies show the split, segmented vermis and elongated fourth ventricle. (Courtesy of D. Mendelsohn.)

of vermian agenesis or hypogenesis combined with midline fusion of the cerebellar hemispheres and peduncles, and apposition or fusion of the dentate nuclei and variable fusion of the colliculi.[7a] (Fig. 4-15).

Associated abnormalities. Supratentorial anomalies that occur with rhombencephalosynapsis vary widely. The cerebral hemispheres may be normal or nearly normal. Ventriculomegaly is common. Absent septum pellucidum, anterior commissure hypoplasia, fused thalami, dysgenetic or deformed corpus callosum, schizencephaly, and cephalocele have been reported.[7a-9]

Tectocerebellar Dysraphia

Pathology and imaging. This rare anomaly consists of vermian hypoplasia or aplasia, occipital, cephalocele, and dorsal traction of the brainstem. The hypoplastic cerebellar hemispheres are rotated, lying ventrolateral to the brainstem.[10]

Lhermitte-Duclos Disease

Pathology. Lhermitte-Duclos disease, also termed *dysplastic gangliocytoma of the cerebellum*, is an uncommon cerebellar dysplasia that is characterized by a unique pattern of cellular disorganization, hypertrophied granular-cell neurons, and axonal hypermyelination in the molecular layer of the cerebellum.[11] There is gross thickening of the cerebellar folia without or with mass effect (Fig. 4-16). Dysplastic gangliocytoma can be focal or diffuse.

Imaging findings. On CT scans, Lhermitte-Duclos disease can mimic posterior fossa neoplasm. The typ-

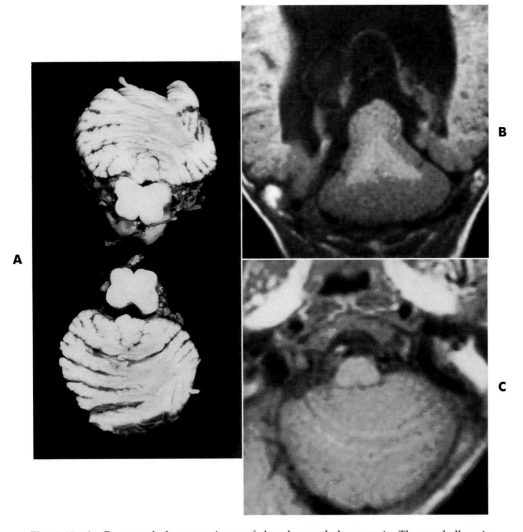

Fig. 4-15. A, Gross pathology specimen of rhombencephalosynapsis. The cerebellum is fused across the midline. Coronal **(B)** and axial **(C)** T1-weighted MR scans in a patient with rhombencephalosynapsis. Note midline fusion of cerebellar hemispheres and lack of normal vermis. (**A,** Courtesy Rubinstein Collection, University of Virginia Department of Pathology. **B** and **C,** Courtesy D. Brown.)

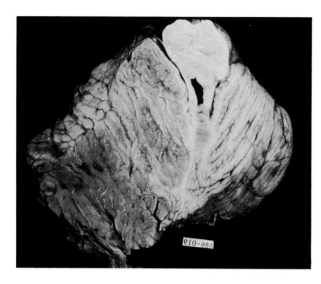

Fig. 4-16. Gross pathology specimen of Lhermitte-Duclos disease. The cerebellar folia appear thickened and enlarged. Moderate mass effect is present. (From archives of the Armed Forces Institute of Pathology.)

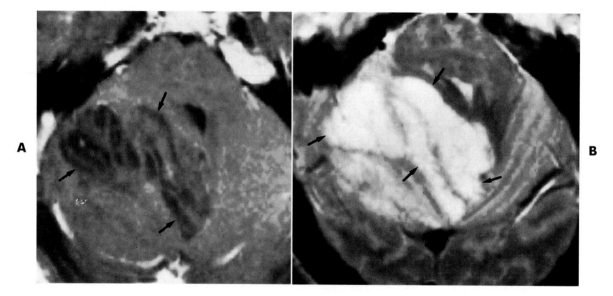

Fig. 4-17. A, Axial postcontrast T1-weighted MR scan in a patient with Lhermitte-Duclos disease. A laminated-appearing hypointense nonenhancing mass *(arrows)* is present that compresses and displaces the fourth ventricle. **B,** T2-weighted study shows the thickened hyperintense enlarged folia *(arrows)* that are characteristic of this disorder. (Courtesy J.R. Gussler.)

ical appearance is that of a poorly delineated hypo- or isodense posterior fossa lesion that does not enhance following contrast administration. Mass effect and displacement of the fourth ventricle may occur. Calcification and hydrocephalus may also be present.[12]

MR studies demonstrate a low signal, nonenhancing mass on T1-weighted studies (Fig. 4-17, *A*). A very characteristic laminated, or folial, pattern of increased signal is seen on T2-weighted scans and should suggest the diagnosis (Fig. 4-17, *B*).[11]

Associated abnormalities. Lhermitte-Duclos disease may exist in isolation. It has also been associated with an uncommon neurocutaneous syndrome, Cowden disease (multiple hamartoma syndrome).[13,14] Other reported associations include megalencephaly, polydactyly, local gigantism, heterotopias, and cutaneous hemangiomata.[15]

REFERENCES

1. Barkovich AJ, Kjos BO, Norman D, Edwards MS: Revised classification of posterior fossa cysts and cystlike malformations based on the results of multiplanar MR imaging, *AJNR* 10:977-988, 1989.
2. Altman NR, Naidich TP, Braffman BH: Posterior fossa malformations, *AJNR* 13:691-724, 1992.
3. Kollias SS, Prenger EC, Becket WW Jr et al: Posterior fossa cystic malformations: possible pitfalls in radiographic diagnosis, *Radiol* 185(suppl):403, 1992.
4. Bindal AK, Storrs BB, McLone DG: Occipital meningioceles in patients with the Dandy-Walker syndrome, *Neurosurg* 28:844-847, 1992.
5. Raimondi AJ, Sato K, Shimoji T: *The Dandy-Walker syndrome,* pp. 1-75, Basel: Karger Press, 1984.
6. Freide RL, Boltshauser E: Uncommon syndromes of cerebellar vermis aplasia, I. Joubert syndrome, *Dev Med Child Neurol* 20:758-763, 1978.
7. Kendall B, Kingsley D, Lambert SR et al: Joubert syndrome: a clinico-radiological study, *Neuroradiol* 31:502-506, 1990.
7a. Simmons G, Damiano TR, Truwit CL: MRI and clinical findings in rhombencephalosynapsis, *J Comp Asst Tomogr* 17:211-214, 1993.
8. Truwit CL, Barkovich AJ, Shanahan R, Maroldo TV: MR imaging of rhombencephalosynapsis, *AJNR* 12:957-965, 1991.
9. Savolaine ER, Fadell RJ, Patel YP: Isolated rhombencephalosynapsis diagnosed by magnetic resonance imaging, *Clin Imaging* 15:125-129, 1991.
10. Freide RL: Uncommon syndromes of cerebellar vermis aplasia, II: Tectocerebellar dysraphia with occipital encephalocele, *Dev Med Child Neurol* 20:758-763, 1978.
11. Shanley DJ, Vassallo CJ: Atypical presentation of Lhermitte-Duclos disease: preoperative diagnosis with MRI, *Neuroradiol* 34:102-103, 1992.
12. Ashley DG, Zee C-S, Chandrasoma PT, Segall HD: Lhermitte-Duclos disease: CT and MR findings, *J Comp Asst Tomogr* 14:984-987, 1990.
13. Padberg GW, Schot JDL, Vielvoye GJ et al: Lhermitte-Duclos disease and Cowden disease: a single phakomatosis, *Ann Neurol* 29:517-523, 1991.
14. Williams DW, Elster AD, Ginsberg LE, Stanton C: Recurrent Lhermitte-Duclos disease: report of two cases and association with Cowden's disease, *AJNR* 13:287-290, 1992.
15. Vieco PT, del Carpio-O'Donovan R, Melanson D et al: Dysplastic gangliocytoma (Lhermitte-Duclos disease): CT and MR imaging, *Pediatr Radiol* 22:366-369, 1992.

Disorders of Histogenesis: Neurocutaneous Syndromes

Neurocutaneous syndromes are also known as phakomatoses (the Greek roots of the word *phakomatosis* have been described—with varying degrees of accuracy—as meaning birthmark, lentil bean, freckle, or spot).[1] This heterogeneous group of disorders generally has central nervous system and, for the most part, cutaneous manifestations. Many of the neurocutaneous syndromes also have prominent visceral and connective tissue abnormalities. Several different phakomatoses have been described; the major, and some of the more interesting but less-common, neurocutaneous syndromes are listed above. Only the principal disorders will be discussed in depth; some of the uncommon neurocutaneous syndromes are described briefly.

NEUROFIBROMATOSIS

Neurofibromatosis is not a single entity but is actually a group of heterogeneous diseases.[2] Although several variants of neurofibromatosis have been proposed, to date the National Institutes of Health (NIH) Consensus Development Conference has defined only two distinct types: Neurofibromatosis type 1 (NF-1, von Recklinghausen disease, sometimes termed peripheral neurofibromatosis) and neurofibromatosis type 2 (NF-2, bilateral acoustic schwannomas or "central" neurofibromatosis).[3] Because NF-1 often has central lesions and NF-2 can occasionally have peripheral manifestations the terms central and peripheral neurofibromatosis have been discarded.

Neurofibromatosis Type 1 (von Recklinghausen Disease)

Incidence and inheritance. NF-1 is the most common of all the phakomatoses and accounts for more than 90% of all neurofibromatosis cases. NF-1 is one of the most common single gene congenital syndromes, with a reported incidence of one in 2000 to

3000 live births. The responsible gene is on the long arm of chromosome 17. A high mutation rate occurs at this locus because approximately 50% of patients with NF-1 are new mutations in whom a family history of the disease is absent. Inheritance is autosomal dominant with high penetrance but very variable expressivity.[1]

Diagnostic criteria. Diagnosis of NF-1 is established when two or more of the following findings are present[3]:

Six or more 5 mm or larger cafe-au-lait spots
One plexiform neurofibroma *or* two or more neurofibromas of any type
Two or more pigmented iris hamartomas (so-called Lisch nodules)
Axillary or inguinal region freckling
Optic nerve glioma
First-degree relative with NF-1
Presence of a characteristic bone lesion (e.g., dysplasia of the greater sphenoid wing, pseudarthrosis)

To date, the Consensus Panel criteria have not been revised to include the characteristic MR findings reported in NF-1 (see subsequent discussion).

Pathology and imaging. Lesions in NF-1 may include the following:

Neoplasms
    Optic nerve glioma
    Nonoptic gliomas
    Plexiform neurofibroma
    Neurofibrosarcoma
Nonneoplastic "hamartomatous" lesions
    White matter lesions
    Basal ganglia lesions
Skull and meningeal dysplasias, other osseous lesions
Spine, cord, and nerve root lesions
Miscellaneous lesions (including non-CNS)
    Eye and orbit abnormalities
    Vascular abnormalities
    Visceral, endocrine tumors

CNS manifestations occur in 15% to 20% of all patients with NF-1 (*see* box).

Many somatic manifestations of NF-1 are age related; external stigmata may be subtle or absent in very young children. Cutaneous lesions and tumors at all sites generally increase in size and number with increasing age.[2]

Neoplasms. The increased risk of developing a CNS neoplasm in a patient with von Recklinghausen neurofibromatosis has been estimated to be four times that of the general population.[4] The neoplasms reported in NF-1 are typically lesions of neurons and astrocytes.[1,5]

Neurofibromatosis Type 1

Synonyms
NF-1, Von Recklinghausen disease (obsolete: "peripheral" neurofibromatosis)

Incidence
1:2000-3000 (>90% of all NF cases)

Inheritance
Autosomal dominant
High penetrance, variable expressivity
Chromosome 17

Clinical
Prominent cutaneous manifestations

CNS lesions in 15%-20%
Brain: lesions of neurons, astrocytes
    Optic nerve glioma
    Nonoptic gliomas (usually low-grade astrocytomas)
    Nonneoplastic "hamartomatous" lesions
        Basal ganglia
        White matter
Spinal cord/roots/peripheral nerves
    Nonneoplastic "harmartomatous" cord lesions
    Cord astrocytoma
    Neurofibromas of spinal/peripheral nerves
        Scattered
        Plexiform
Osseous/dural lesions
    Hypoplastic sphenoid wing
    Sutural defects
    Kyphoscoliosis
    Dural ectasia
    Meningioceles
Ocular/orbital manifestations
    Optic nerve glioma
    Lisch nodules in iris
    Buphthalmos (cow eye, or macrophthalmia)
    Retinal phakomas
    Plexiform neurofibroma (CNV_1 most common)
Vascular lesions
    Progressive cerebral arterial occlusions
    Aneurysms
    Vascular ectasia
    Arteriovenous fistulae, malformations

Non-CNS lesions
Visceral, endocrine tumors
Musculoskeletal lesions (outside skull, spine)
    "Ribbon ribs"
    Tibial bowing
    Pseudoarthroses
    Focal overgrowth of digit, ray, or limb

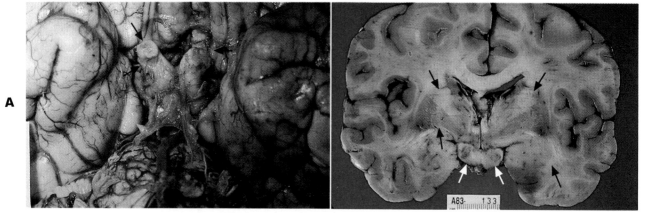

Fig. 5-1. A, Gross pathologic specimen of the brain, seen from below, of a patient with neurofibromatosis type I (NF-1). Bilateral optic nerve gliomas *(arrows)* are present. **B,** Coronal cut section shows that the glioma involves the optic chiasm *(large arrows)*. Also seen are multiple basal ganglionic and white matter hamartomatous lesions *(small arrows)*, characteristic of NF-1. (Courtesy C. Petito.)

The common CNS tumor in NF-1 is *optic nerve glioma*, occurring in 5% to 15% of cases, although only about one quarter of all patients with optic nerve gliomas have NF-1.[6] Optic nerve gliomas can involve one or both optic nerves and commonly extend into the chiasm (Figs. 5-1 and 5-2). Posterior involvement of the optic tracts, lateral geniculate body, and optic radiations occurs but is less common (Fig. 5-3).[7] Most optic nerve gliomas are histologically benign, low-grade astrocytomas (usually the pilocytic type) that behave clinically more like hamartomas than malignant neoplasms,[1,8] although up to 20% of all chiasmal gliomas in children may behave aggressively with fatal results.[9]

Imaging of optic nerve gliomas and their posterior extension is best delineated by magnetic resonance imaging. Most of these neoplasms are hypo- to isointense on T1-weighted scans and show increased signal on T2WI. Contrast enhancement is variable; en-

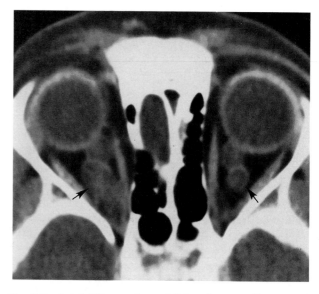

Fig. 5-2. Axial CT scan in a child with neurofibromatosis type 1 shows bilateral optic nerve gliomas *(arrows)*.

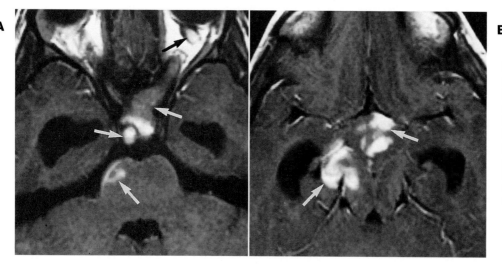

Fig. 5-3. Postchiasmatic spread of optic nerve glioma in a patient with neurofibromatosis type 1. Axial (**A** and **B**) and sagittal **(C)** postcontrast T1-weighted MR scans show that the left optic nerve glioma extends posteriorly into the chiasm, hypothalamus, medial temporal lobe, and pons *(arrows)*.

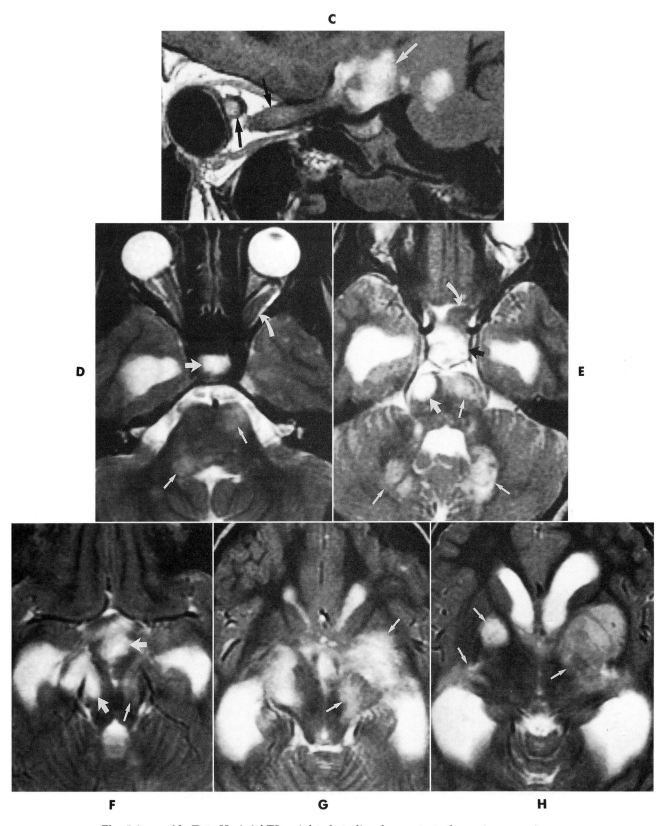

Fig. 5-3, cont'd. D to H, Axial T2-weighted studies demonstrate the optic nerve glioma *(curved arrows)*, which appears slightly hypointense to gray matter, the very hyperintense chiasmatic and retrochiasmatic involvement *(large arrows)*, and numerous hamartomatous foci of slightly less intense signal in the white matter and basal ganglia *(small arrows)*.

hancement is typically absent or minimal in most cases with opticochiasmatic involvement but can occasionally be striking, particularly when extension along the posterior optic pathway is present (Fig 5-3).

Nonoptic gliomas have an increased frequency of occurrence in NF-1. Most are low-grade, relatively benign astrocytomas of the brain stem, tectum, and periaqueductal regions, although more anaplastic astrocytomas do occur (Fig. 5-4). Nonastrocytic gliomas associated with NF-1 are very uncommon; a few cases of intracranial ependymoma have been reported but are uncommon.[10]

Plexiform neurofibromas are a hallmark of NF-1 and are diagnostic of von Recklinghausen neurofibromatosis. They are found in about one third of all patients with NF-1.[11] Plexiform neurofibromas are multiple, tortuous, wormlike masses that arise along the axis of a major nerve. They are unencapsulated and tend to infiltrate and separate the normal nerve fascicles, producing a fusiform appearance.[12]

Plexiform neurofibromas in the head and neck commonly occur along the first (orbital) division of the trigeminal nerve. They often are associated with sphenoid wing dysplasia and middle cranial fossa arachnoid cyst or prominent subarachnoid spaces. Plexiform neurofibromas frequently extend posteriorly to involve the cavernous sinus but typically do not extend posteriorly beyond Meckel's cave.

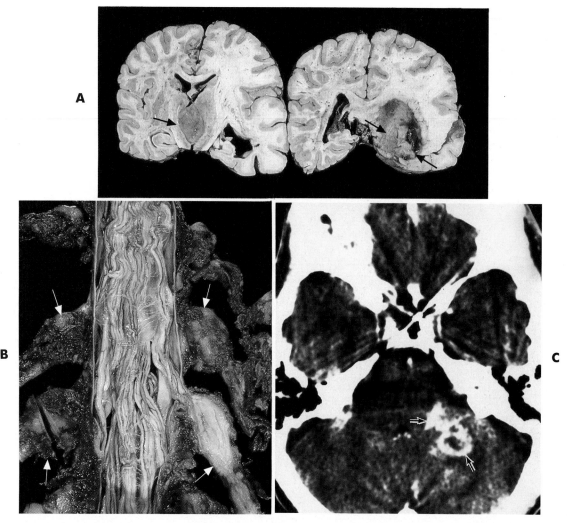

Fig. 5-4. A and **B,** Gross pathologic specimens in a patient with neurofibromatosis type I (NF-1) and glioblastoma multiforme. **A,** Coronally sectioned brain shows the hemorrhagic, necrotic tumor in the deep basal ganglia *(arrows).* **B,** Spinal cord shows multiple nerve root tumors *(arrows).* **C,** Contrast-enhanced axial CT scan in another patient with NF-1. Artifact from surgical clip is seen in the sellar region; chiasmatic biopsy several years before the current study disclosed pilocytic astrocytoma. A poorly delineated, contrast-enhancing posterior fossa mass *(open arrows)* is seen. Anaplastic astrocytoma was found at craniotomy. (**A** and **B,** Courtesy E. Tessa Hedley-Whyte.)

CT scans show a poorly delineated mass in the high deep masticator space that often involves the orbit and cavernous sinus. On MR scans, plexiform neurofibromas are typically isointense with muscle on T1-weighted sequences and enhance strongly following contrast administration (Fig. 5-5).[13]

Sarcomatous degeneration of peripheral soft-tissue neurofibromas is estimated to occur in 5% to 15% of all patients with NF-1. Malignant peripheral nerve sheath tumors in the head and neck arise from the supraorbital or maxillary branches of CN V and may diffusely invade the skull base. A neurofibrosarcoma of the spinal nerve roots can invade the spine (see subsequent discussion).

Nonneoplastic "hamartomatous" lesions. Benign brain parenchymal abnormalities are observed in nearly 80% of all patients with NF-1[14] (Figs. 5-1 and 5-6 to 5-9). Multiple lesions in the basal ganglia, optic radiations, brainstem, and cerebral peduncles are common.[2,5] Pathologically these lesions are foci of *hyperplastic* or *dysplastic glial proliferation* and considered malformative rather than neoplastic.[5a]

Ninety per cent of the white matter lesions in NF-1 show no mass effect or enhancement after contrast administration. Although the white matter lesions may increase in size or number in early childhood, they typically diminish with age; some are occasionally observed into adulthood, however (Fig. 5-7).[14]

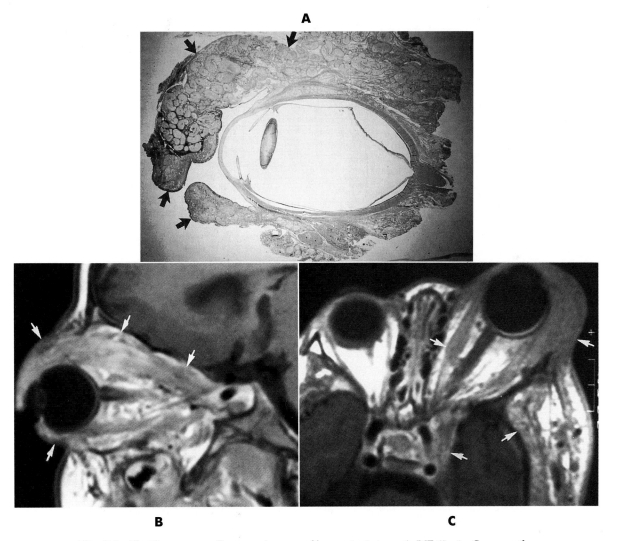

Fig. 5-5. Plexiform neurofibromas in neurofibromatosis type 1 (NF-1). **A,** Gross pathologic specimen of the eye and periorbital soft tissues in a patient with NF-1. Buphthalmos (cow eye) is present with a large plexiform neurofibroma of the eyelid *(arrows)*. Sagittal **(B)** and axial **(C)** T1-weighted MR scans with contrast enhancement show the poorly delineated plexiform neurofibroma infiltrating the soft tissues of the eyelid, high deep masticator space, retrobulbar soft tissues, and cavernous sinus *(arrows)*. **(A** to **C,** Courtesy B. Haas and A. Hidayat.)   *Continued.*

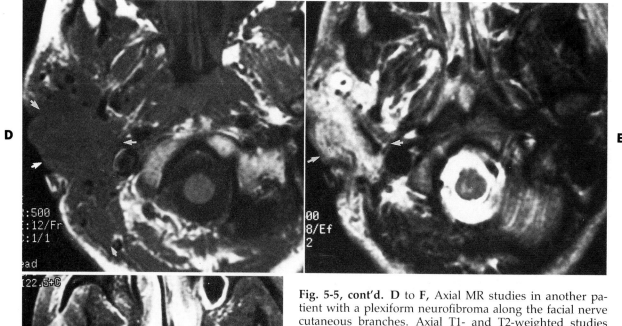

Fig. 5-5, cont'd. D to **F,** Axial MR studies in another patient with a plexiform neurofibroma along the facial nerve cutaneous branches. Axial T1- and T2-weighted studies show the diffusely infiltrating nature of the lesion (**D** and **E,** *arrows*). Postcontrast fat suppression scan (**F,** *arrows*) shows the lesion enhances strongly. (**D** to **E,** Courtesy K. Reynard.)

Uncommonly, moderate mass effect can be observed (Fig. 5-9) and contrast enhancement can occur (Fig. 5-8, *F* and *G*).

The significance of the high signal intensity lesions that enhance following contrast administration remains undetermined.[5a] Caution against aggressive operative and adjuvant therapy for brain stem lesions in these patients has been recommended because the few cases that have come to biopsy or autopsy have largely demonstrated benign pathology.[10,15]

In a recent longitudinal series, none of the white matter lesions seen in NF-1 evolved into a neoplasm.[14] Interval MR imaging follow-up of atypical lesions (large size, mass effect, contrast enhancement, proximity to an optic pathway glioma) is recommended.[2]

Basal ganglia lesions, primarily involving the globus pallidus, have also been observed in patients with documented NF-1. On CT scans they are seen as relatively well-defined unilateral or bilateral lesions that do not enhance following contrast administration.[16] On MR studies, high intensity basal ganglia foci are seen on T1-weighted sequences (Figs. 5-8, *B,* and 5-9, *A*). They are somewhat hyperintense on T2WI (*see* Fig. 5-3, *A*). The lesions typically do not exhibit mass effect, edema, or contrast enhancement and do not show progression.[17] Uncommonly, some increase in signal after contrast administration can be observed (Fig. 5-7). The basal ganglia lesions may represent a different histology from the white matter lesions because their morphology and signal characteristics are often slightly different from the brain stem and cerebellar abnormalities previously discussed (Fig. 5-3).[5]

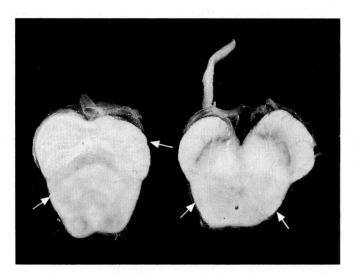

Fig. 5-6. Gross pathology of brainstem and pons in neurofibromatosis type 1. The pons and midbrain have numerous foci of gliosis, delayed myelination, and hamartomatous change *(arrows)*. (From archives of the Armed Forces Institute of Pathology.)

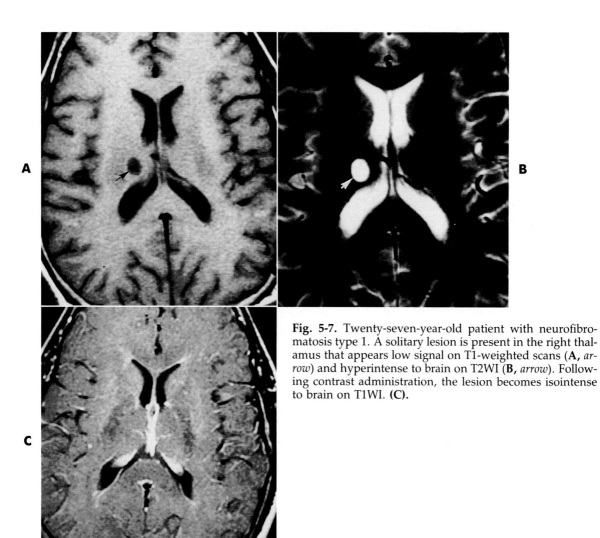

Fig. 5-7. Twenty-seven-year-old patient with neurofibromatosis type 1. A solitary lesion is present in the right thalamus that appears low signal on T1-weighted scans (**A**, *arrow*) and hyperintense to brain on T2WI (**B**, *arrow*). Following contrast administration, the lesion becomes isointense to brain on T1WI. (**C**).

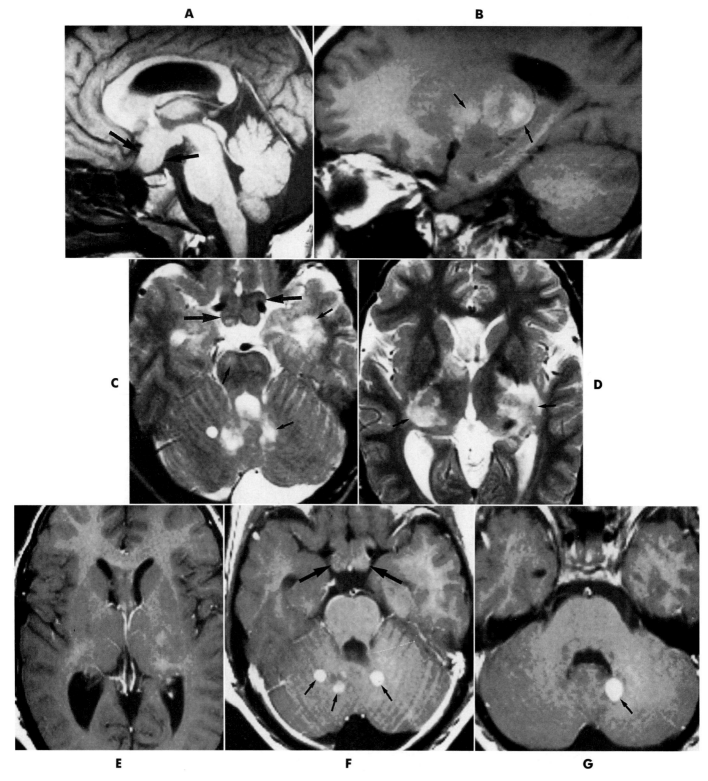

Fig. 5-8. MR scans in a child with neurofibromatosis type 1. **A** and **B,** Sagittal T1-weighted scans without contrast enhancement show opticochiasmatic glioma (**A,** *black arrows*) and high-signal foci in the basal ganglia and thalami (**B,** *black arrows*). **C,** and **D,** Axial T2-weighted scans show the chiasmatic glioma is low signal (**C,** *large black arrows*). Also seen are multiple foci of increased signal in the medulla, pons, cerebellum, thalami, and septum pellucidum (**C** and **D,** *small black arrows*). **E** to **G,** Postcontrast T1-weighted scans show that the supratentorial lesions and optic chiasm mass (**F,** *large black arrows*) do not enhance, whereas some—but not all—of the posterior fossa lesions show increased signal (**F** and **G,** *small black arrows*).

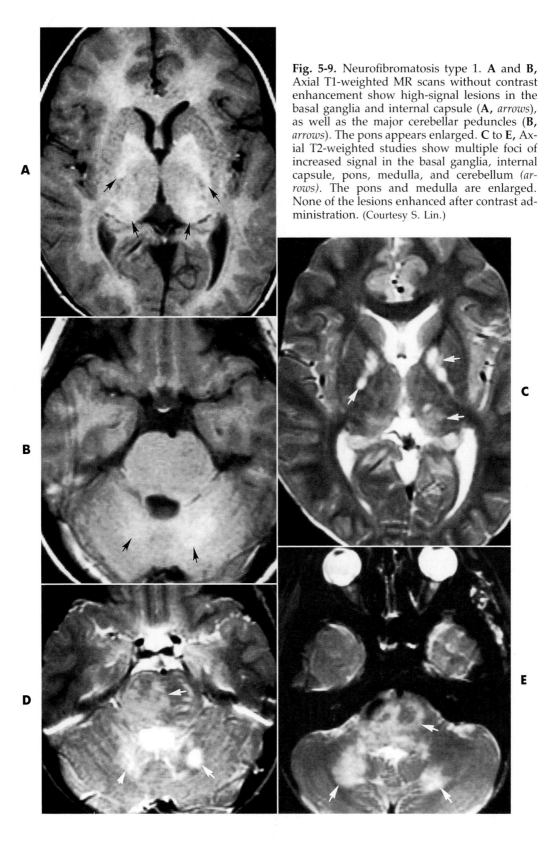

Fig. 5-9. Neurofibromatosis type 1. **A** and **B,** Axial T1-weighted MR scans without contrast enhancement show high-signal lesions in the basal ganglia and internal capsule (**A,** *arrows*), as well as the major cerebellar peduncles (**B,** *arrows*). The pons appears enlarged. **C** to **E,** Axial T2-weighted studies show multiple foci of increased signal in the basal ganglia, internal capsule, pons, medulla, and cerebellum (*arrows*). The pons and medulla are enlarged. None of the lesions enhanced after contrast administration. (Courtesy S. Lin.)

Skull, meningeal, and osseous lesions. Skull and dural lesions are common in patients with NF-1.[17a] These include macrocrania, *hypoplasia of the greater sphenoid ala* with temporal lobe herniation into the orbit (Figs. 5-10, *A*, 5-11, and 5-12), *calvarial defects* (Fig. 5-10, *B*) (the lambdoid suture is a characteristic location), and *dural ectasia.* Enlargement of the internal auditory canals can sometimes be seen in patients with NF-1; this is secondary to dysplastic dural enlargement, not acoustic schwannoma (which is a feature of NF-2). Other reported distinctive osseous lesions in NF-1 include focal overgrowth of a digit, ray, or an entire limb, tibial bowing, "ribbon ribs," and pseudoarthrosis.[1]

Spine, spinal cord, and nerve root. Radiologic abnormalities of the spine in patients with NF-1 are common, occurring in 60% of patients.[18] Osseous, dura, nerve root, and cord lesions occur.

The common spinal abnormality is enlargement of one or more neural foramina, seen in nearly 60% of NF-1 patients. Most often this is secondary to the presence of a *neurofibroma* along the exiting nerve root (see subsequent discussion); less commonly it is caused by dural ectasia or arachnoid cyst. Scalloping of the posterior vertebral bodies is seen in 10% (Fig. 5-13). This finding is nearly always secondary to *dural dysplasia,* not neurofibroma.[18]

Spinal deformities, typically *kyphoscoliosis* (Fig. 5-13, *A*), also occur, as do *meningoceles.* Multilevel outpouchings of dura and CSF can be seen. Occasionally, meningoceles can become quite large, particularly in the thoracic region.[19,20] The osseous and dural lesions seen in NF-1 most likely represent independent derivatives of a common mesenchymal dysplasia.[21]

Asymptomatic intradural extramedullary masses, typically neurofibromas, are present in nearly 20% of NF-1 patients.[18] So-called dumbbell tumors are found on the exiting spinal nerves of 13% to 20% of patients with NF-1. Histologically these are also neurofibro-

A

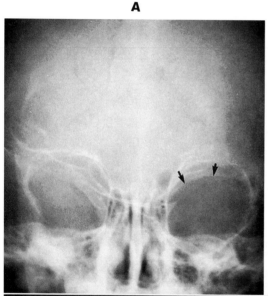

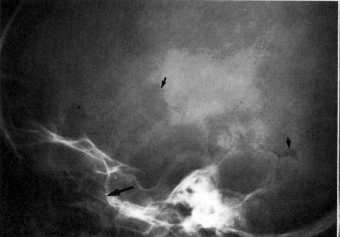

B

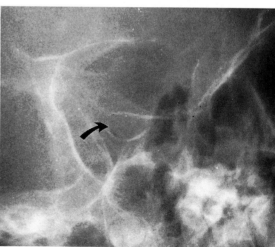

C

Fig. 5-10. PA **(A)** and lateral **(B)** plain skull films in a patient with neurofibromatosis type 1 show the characteristic findings produced by sphenoid wing hypoplasia. On frontal views the orbit appears "empty" **(A,** *arrows);* on lateral views, only a single curvilinear line is seen representing the normal greater sphenoid wing **(B,** *large arrow).* The other sphenoid wing is absent. In addition to sphenoid hypoplasia, other characteristic skull changes include sutural defects **(B,** *small arrows).* Oblique view **(C)** shows enlarged optic canal *(arrow).* The patient had an optic nerve glioma.

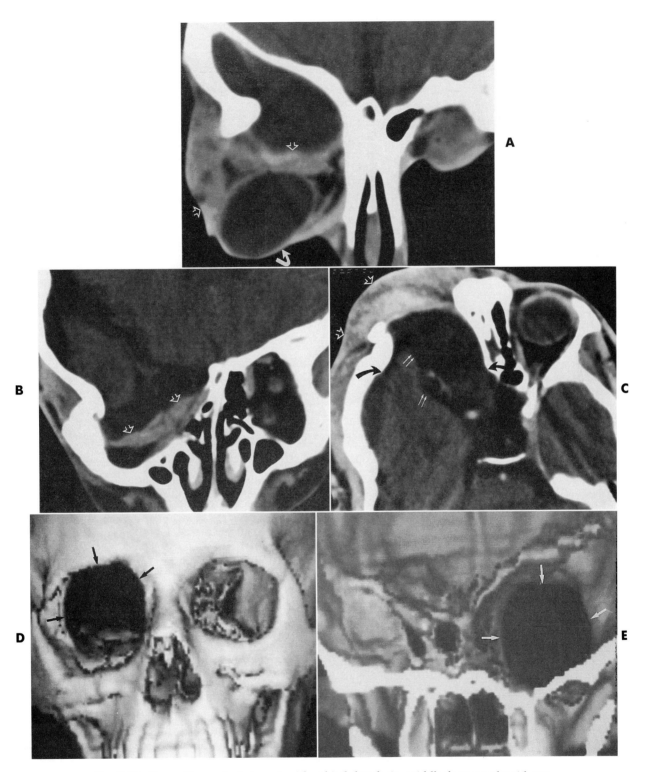

Fig. 5-11. Neurofibromatosis type 1 with orbital dysplasia, middle fossa arachnoid cyst, plexiform neurofibroma, and buphthalmos. **A** and **B,** Coronal CT scans show the enlarged globe *(curved arrow)* and plexiform neurofibroma *(open arrows)*. **C,** Axial CT scan shows the absent sphenoid wing with arachnoid cyst *(double arrows)* and temporal lobe protruding through the dehiscent sphenoid bone *(curved arrows)* into the orbit. The plexiform neurofibroma is indicated by open arrows. Reformatted 3-D shows the enlarged, "empty" orbit *(arrows)* as seen anteriorly **(D),** as well as from the posterior, endocranial aspect **(E).** (Courtesy I. Tarwal and M. Shroff.)

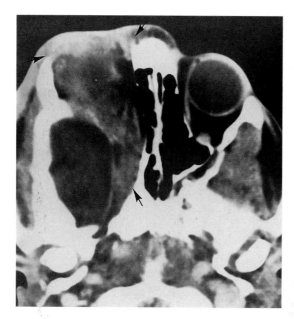

Fig. 5-12. Axial postcontrast CT scan in a patient with neurofibromatosis type 1 shows striking sphenoid wing hypoplasia, and plexiform neurofibroma *(arrows)*.

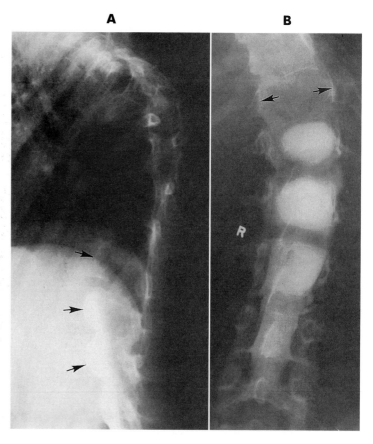

Fig. 5-13. Lateral **(A)** and AP **(B)** postmyelogram plain films in a patient with neurofibromatosis type 1. Note marked thoracic kyphoscoliosis and extreme posterior vertebral scalloping secondary to dural dysplasia (**A**, *arrows*). Widened interpediculate distance secondary to the pronounced dural dysplasia is also present (**B**, *arrows*).

mas.[22] Radiologically the nerve root tumors in NF-1 tend to be relatively small and scattered (Fig. 5-14). Multiple arachnoid cysts may also develop and protrude along the course of these roots, mimicking tumors.[1]

Spinal cord lesions are seen on MR studies in 14% of NF-1 patients.[18] Intramedullary tumors are typically low grade *astrocytoma*. *"Hamartomatous" lesions* similar to those identified in the basal ganglia and cerebral white matter may occasionally be identified on high-resolution T2-weighted studies (Fig. 5-15).

Miscellaneous lesions. Ocular lesions identified in NF-1 include Lisch nodules of the iris, foci of astrocytic proliferation in the retina, and buphthalmos (macrophthalmia, or cow-eye) (Figs. 5-5 and 5-11).

Vascular abnormalities are also associated with von Recklinghausen neurofibromatosis. Whereas renal and gastrointestinal system lesions are common, involvement of the craniocerebral vessels is relatively rare. More than 85% of the reported cerebrovascular lesions are of a purely occlusive or stenotic nature,[23] including *progressive cerebral arterial occlusive disease* with "moyamoya" pattern of collateral circulation [24] (Fig. 5-16, *A* and *B*). Histologic examination of the affected vessels usually discloses advanced intimal, and occasionally medial, dysplasia with marked luminal narrowing.[25]

Aneurysms are the second most frequently reported vascular abnormality in NF-1 (Fig. 5-16, *C* and *D*).[26-28] *Nonaneurysmal vascular ectasias* (Fig. 5-16, *C* and *D*)

and arteriovenous fistulae or malformations (Fig. 5-16, *E*) can also occur in association with NF-1.[29]

Non-CNS lesions. Visceral and *endocrine tumors* have been reported in about 4% of patients with NF-1.[11]

Neurofibromatosis Type 2

Inheritance and incidence. Neurofibromatosis type 2, also known as NF-2 or "bilateral acoustic schwannomas," is a distinct form of the disease that must be separated clinically and radiographically from NF-1.[6] It too is transmitted with autosomal dominant inheritance but has been identified with defects of chromosome 22. NF-2 is much less common than NF-1, occurring approximately once in 50,000 live births.

Diagnostic criteria. The NIH Consensus Committee has also defined clinical criteria for NF-2. Bilateral masses of the eighth cranial nerves are diagnostic. A patient is also considered to have NF-2 if there is a

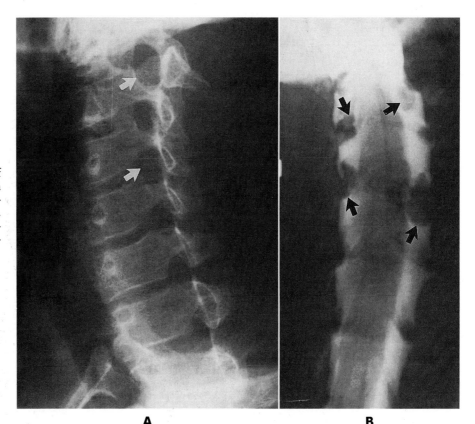

A

B

Fig. 5-14. A, Oblique plain film of the cervical spine in a patient with neurofibromatosis type 1 shows enlarged neural foramina *(arrows).* **B,** Myelogram shows small extramedullary intradural filling defects secondary to neurofibromas *(arrows).*

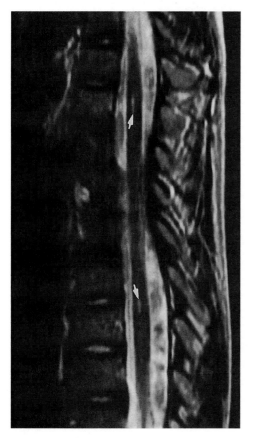

Fig. 5-15. Sagittal T2-weighted fast spin-echo MR scan in a patient with neurofibromatosis type 1 and thoracic kyphoscoliosis shows multiple intramedullary foci of increased signal *(arrows).* Note that the cord is not enlarged; the lesions did not enhance after contrast administration and probably represent benign white matter lesions similar to those often observed in the brain.

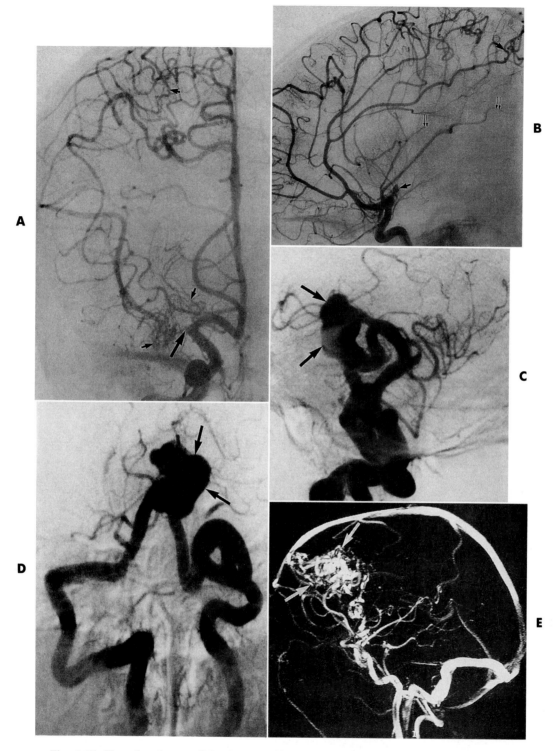

Fig. 5-16. Vascular abnormalities in neurofibromatosis type 1 (NF-1). **A** and **B,** Seven-year-old child with NF-1 and acute left-sided hemiplegia at age 2. Right carotid angiogram, AP **(A)** and lateral **(B)** views, shows occlusion of the right proximal middle cerebral artery **(A,** *large arrow*) with basilar and cortical collateral blood flow *(small arrows)* to the M1 segment and some of the distal MCA branches. Stenoses, slow antegrade flow, and frank occlusions in more distal vessels are also present *(double arrows).* **C** and **D,** A 54-year-old oriental male with NF-1. Lateral **(C)** and AP **(D)** vertebral angiogram shows marked vascular ectasia, tortuosity, and a giant basilar artery aneurysm *(arrows).* **E,** Phase-contrast MR angiogram in a 27-year-old female with NF-1 shows an arteriovenous malformation *(arrows).* (**A** and **B,** Courtesy D. Harwood-Nash. **C** and **D,** Courtesy M.H. Teng.)

first-degree relative with NF-2 plus either a single eighth nerve mass or any two of the following: schwannoma, neurofibroma, meningioma, glioma, or juvenile posterior subcapsular lens opacity.[1,3] NF-1 and NF-2 are compared in the boxes, *right* and p. 73.

Cutaneous manifestations are much less common in NF-2 compared to NF-1. Therefore NF-2 patients are often older at the time of initial diagnosis. Cafe-au-lait spots are absent or few; cutaneous neurofibromas and Lisch nodules are not features of NF-2.

Pathology and imaging. CNS lesions eventually develop in virtually all patients with NF-2 and include the following:
1. Neoplasms
   Cranial nerves
   Meninges
2. Nonneoplastic intracranial calcifications
3. Spinal cord and nerve root tumors

Neoplasms. Type 2 neurofibromatosis seems to be associated with tumors of Schwann cells and meninges (Figs. 5-17, *A*, and 5-18).[5] *Intracranial schwannomas* most frequently involve the vestibulocochlear nerves (Figs. 5-17, *A*, and 5-18, *A* and *E*); from 2% to 10% of all patients with acoustic nerve tumors have NF-2.[30] Bilateral acoustic schwannomas are the hallmark of NF-2 and diagnostic of this condition (Figs. 5-18, *A*; 5-20, *B*; and 5-21, *F*). Unilateral acoustic tumors typically arise from the vestibular nerve and displace the facial and cochlear nerves around the tumor capsule. In NF-2 patients these nerves often en-

---

Neurofibromatosis Type 2

Synonyms:

NF-2, bilateral acoustic schwannomas (obsolete: "central" neurofibromatosis)

Incidence

1:50,000

Inheritance

Autosomal dominant
Chromosome 22

Clinical

Cutaneous manifestations rare

CNS lesions in ~100%

Brain: lesions of schwann cells, meninges
    CN VIII schwannomas most common (bilateral acoustic schwannomas diagnostic for NF-2); multiple schwannomas of other cranial nerves highly suggestive of NF-2)
    Meningiomas; often multiple
    Nonneoplastic intracranial calcifications (especially choroid plexus)
Spinal cord/roots
    Cord ependymomas
    Multilevel, bulky schwannomas of exiting roots
    Meningiomas
Spine
    Secondary changes (expansion, erosion secondary to cord/root tumors)

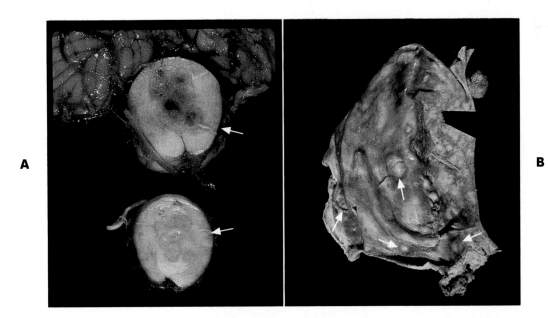

A   **B**

Fig. 5-17. Gross pathology specimens from a patient with neurofibromatosis type 2 (NF-2). **A,** Bilateral acoustic schwannomas were present; one is cut across and shown here *(arrows).* **B,** The dura over the convexity and parasagittal area contains multiple meningiomas *(arrows).* (Courtesy E. Tessa Hedley-Whyte.)   *Continued.*

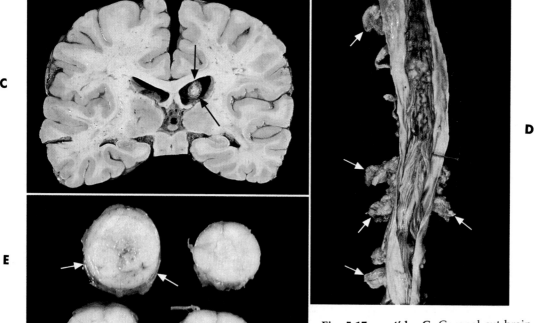

Fig. 5-17, cont'd.   C, Coronal cut brain specimen shows abnormally enlarged, calcified choroid plexus (arrow). D, The spinal cord is enlarged. Multiple, rounded, nerve root schwannomas are present (arrows). E, Cut section through the spinal cord demonstrates ependymoma (arrows). (Courtesy E. Tessa Hedley-Whyte.)

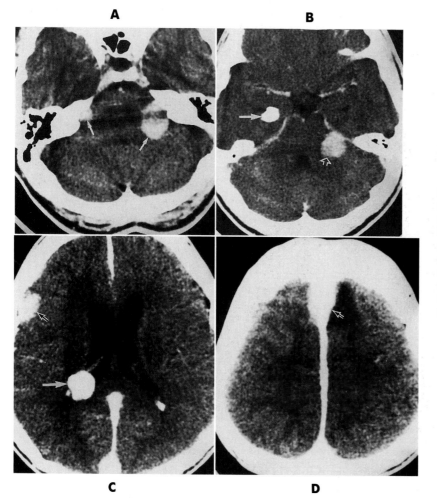

Fig. 5-18. Postcontrast axial CT scans in a patient with neurofibromatosis type 2 (NF-2). Typical lesions of NF-2 include bilateral eighth nerve schwannomas (A, arrows); schwannomas of other cranial nerves (trigeminal schwannoma in B, open arrow); nonneoplastic choroid plexus calcifications (B and C, white arrows), and multiple meningiomas (C and D, black and white arrows).

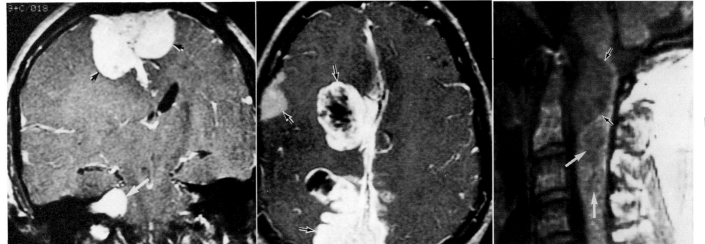

E | F, G

Figure 5-18, cont'd. Five years later, postcontrast MR scans show progression of the lesions. The left-sided vestibulocochlear schwannoma has been resected; the lesion in the right cerebellopontine angle is larger (**E,** *white arrow*). The meningiomas have grown larger (**E** and **F,** *black and white arrows*). Cervical spine MR scan without contrast enhancement shows another meningioma at the craniocervical junction (**G,** *black and white arrows*) and an intramedullary lesion (**G,** *white arrows*) that at surgery was found to be an ependymoma.

ter the tumor directly or are engulfed by the mass. The bilateral acoustic tumors in NF-2 also sometimes invade the cochlea and temporal bone. Stereotactic radiosurgery may be a viable, even preferred, treatment option in some of these patients.[31]

The trigeminal nerve is the next most frequently involved nerve in NF-2 (Fig. 5-18, *B*). Although isolated schwannomas can occur spontaneously along other cranial nerves (with the exception of the olfactory and optic nerves, which are really brain tracts), presence of an oculomotor, trochlear, or abducens nerve tumor should prompt investigation for NF-2 (Figs. 5-19 and 5-22, *C*). Involvement of more than one cranial nerve by schwannoma should also raise the suspicion for NF-2 (Figs. 5-18 and 5-19).

On imaging studies, schwannomas tend to appear

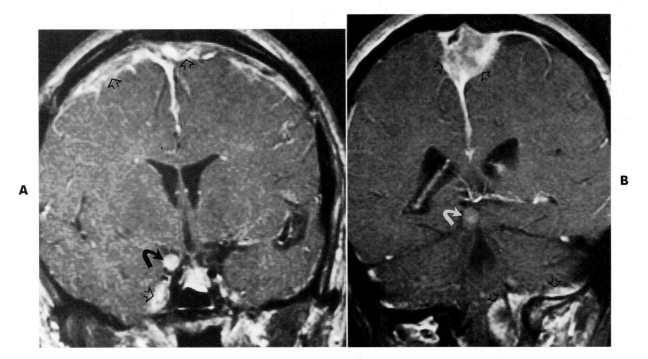

A | B

Fig. 5-19. Coronal postcontrast T1-weighted MR scans in a patient with neurofibromatosis type 2 show multiple meningiomas *(open arrows),* as well as schwannomas of the oculomotor (**A,** *curved arrow*) and trochlear (**B,** *curved arrow*) nerves.

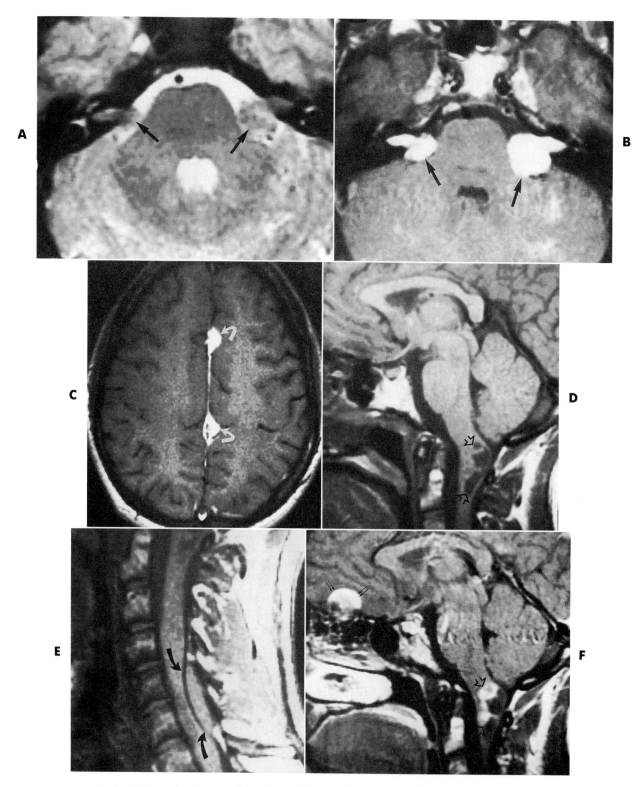

Fig. 5-20. Twenty-six-year-old patient with neurofibromatosis type 2 (NF-2). Precontrast axial T2-weighted (**A**) and postcontrast T1-weighted scans (**B** and **C**) show bilateral eighth nerve schwannomas (**A** and **B**, *arrows*) and multiple meningiomas (**C**, *arrows*). Also present on precontrast sagittal T1-weighted scans of the brain and cervical spine are an intraaxial lesion at the cervicomedullary junction (**D**, *arrows*) and an extraaxial lesion at the midcervical level (**E**, *arrows*). Postcontrast scan (**F**) showed strong but inhomogeneous enhancement of the intramedullary mass *(open arrows)* and an unsuspected planum sphenoidale mass *(double arrows)*. The cervicomedullary junction mass is a spinal cord ependymoma; the planum sphenoidale and extraaxial cervical masses are meningiomas.

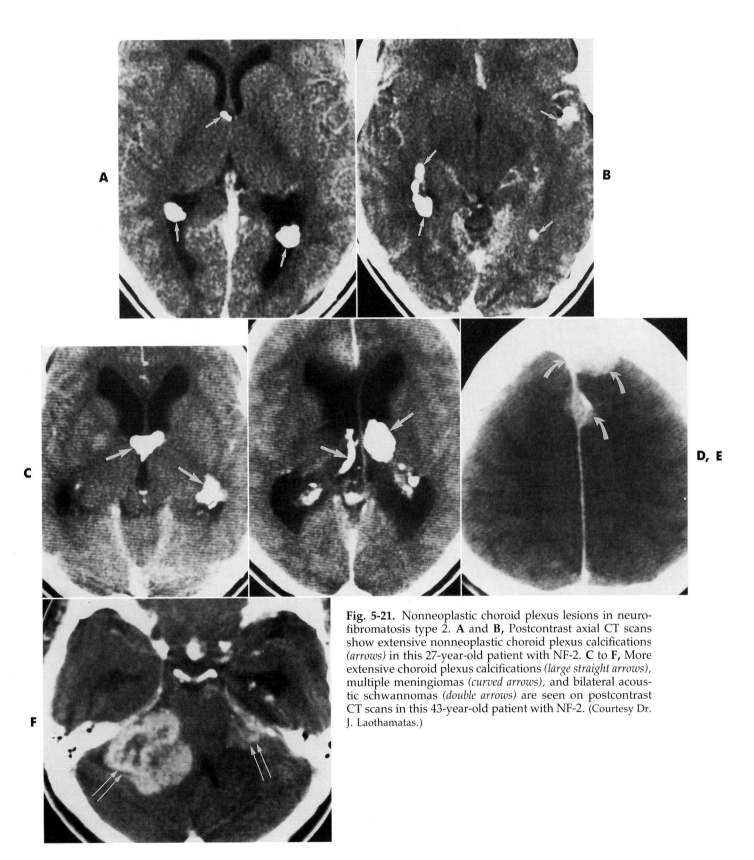

Fig. 5-21. Nonneoplastic choroid plexus lesions in neurofibromatosis type 2. **A** and **B,** Postcontrast axial CT scans show extensive nonneoplastic choroid plexus calcifications *(arrows)* in this 27-year-old patient with NF-2. **C** to **F,** More extensive choroid plexus calcifications *(large straight arrows),* multiple meningiomas *(curved arrows),* and bilateral acoustic schwannomas *(double arrows)* are seen on postcontrast CT scans in this 43-year-old patient with NF-2. (Courtesy Dr. J. Laothamatas.)

rounded and focal. Because they often undergo cystic degeneration and hemorrhage, their attenuation characteristics on CT and signal on MR are frequently somewhat heterogeneous. Schwannomas tend to be iso- or hypodense compared to brain on NECT and show strong but occasionally inhomogeneous enhancement following contrast administration (Fig. 5-18, *A*). On MR studies they appear as well-delineated masses that are iso- to hypointense compared to brain on T1-weighted scans and iso- to hyperintense on balanced and T2WI. Strong but heterogeneous enhancement is typical (Fig. 5-20).[13] Two thirds of asymptomatic children with NF-2 skin/spine lesions or one parent with the disease have an eighth cranial nerve schwannoma on contrast-enhanced MR scans.[31a]

Intracranial meningiomas are also common in NF-2. They are often multiple (Figs. 5-17 to 5-22). Intracranial tumors other than schwannomas and meningiomas are not a feature of NF-2.

Nonneoplastic intracranial lesions. *Unusual calcifications* in the choroid plexus (Figs. 5-17, *C*, and 5-21), cerebellar cortex, and, occasionally, on the surface of the cerebral cortex are a feature of NF-2.[32]

Spinal cord and nerve root. Spine lesions in NF-2 are very common. Multiple intradural, extramedullary soft tissue masses are identified in most patients and are typically *meningiomas* (Fig. 5-20, *E*) or *schwannomas* (Fig. 5-22, *A*).[18] Multilevel masses along the exiting spinal nerve roots can be features of both NF-1 and NF-2 (Figs. 5-17, *D*, and 5-23). In NF-2 cases these are usually schwannomas;[22,33a,33] tissue from these tumors, as well as sporadic spinal schwanno-

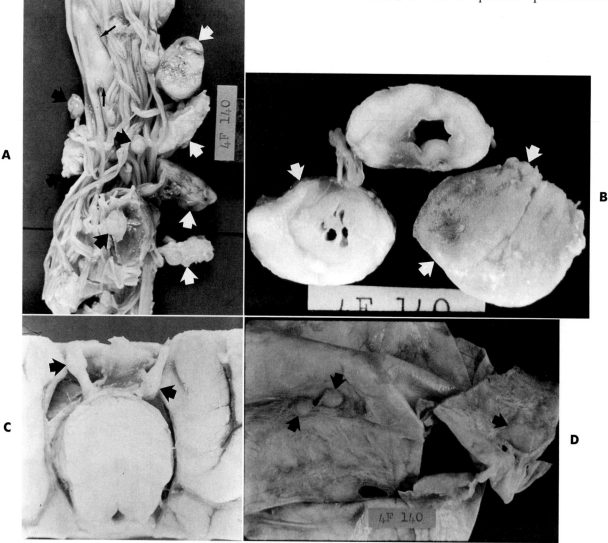

Fig. 5-22. Gross pathology of spine and cord lesions in a patient with neurofibromatosis type 2. **A,** Multiple spinal schwannomas *(large black arrows)* and meningioma *(small black arrows)* are seen. **B,** A spinal cord ependymoma is present. This patient also had bilateral oculomotor nerve schwannomas (**C,** *arrows*) and multiple intracranial meningiomas (**D,** *arrows*). (Courtesy Rubinstein Collection, University of Virginia Department of Pathology.)

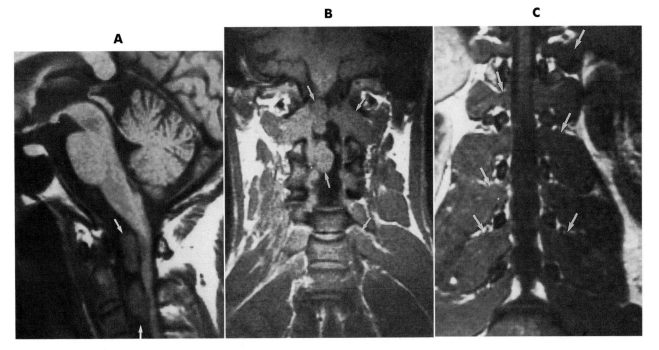

Fig. 5-23. Sagittal **(A)** and coronal **(B)** cervical, as well as coronal lumbar **(C),** T1-weighted MR scans in a patient with neurofibromatosis type 2 show multilevel, bilateral bulky fusiform lesions *(arrows)* along the exiting spinal nerve roots.

mas, shows chromosome 22 deletions, suggesting that a locus on this gene may be responsible for schwann cell tumorigenesis regardless of location in the CNS.[34]

Imaging studies of peripheral nerve root schwannomas show a well-delineated encapsulated mass that is intermediate signal intensity on T1-weighted studies and hyperintense on T2WI. Intense enhancement following contrast administration is typical. Sonographic evaluation discloses well-defined hypoechoic lesions that show distal sound enhancement.[35]

Intramedullary tumors are common in NF-2. These are typically *ependymomas* (Figs. 5-18, *G;* 5-19, *D* to *F;* and 5-22, *B*).[18] Osseous abnormalities are common in NF-2 patients and—in contrast to NF-1—secondary to tumors of the spinal cord or nerve roots, not dural dysplasia.

Segmental neurofibromatosis

Although chromosomal linkage studies document only two genetically distinct types of neurofibromatosis, clinical evidence supports the existence of several additional subtypes of the disease.[2] Segmental neurofibromatosis (NF-5) is a rare form of neurofibromatosis in which the cutaneous and neural changes are confined to one region of the body. Pain and pruritus (due to the large numbers of mast cells in the neurofibromas) are the presenting symptoms in most of these patients.[6,36] Regional involvement of the lumbosacral plexus and scalp have been reported in

NF-5.[36,37] The genetics and the relationship of segmental neurofibromatosis to von Recklinghausen disease are undetermined.

TUBEROUS SCLEROSIS

Incidence and inheritance. Tuberous sclerosis (Bourneville disease) is an autosomal dominant disorder with variable expressivity and high penetrance that demonstrates widespread potential for hamartomatous growths in multiple organ systems. Tuberous sclerosis (TS) has an approximate incidence of 1:10,000 to 50,000, although a *forme fruste* of the disease is probably much more common.[2]

Considerable genetic heterogeneity in TS has been reported. A gene locus on the 9q32-34 region has been found for approximately one third of families.[38] Other TS cases may result from spontaneous mutation of a chromosome 11 locus,[2] whereas a still-unidentified locus elsewhere in the genome may account for the majority of familial TS cases.[38]

Diagnostic criteria. The classic clinical triad of a papular facial nevus (the so-called adenoma sebaceum that is neither an adenoma nor contains sebaceous glands), seizures, and mental retardation is found in less than half the patients.[39] Hence the radiologic hallmarks of this disorder are very important and are now universally accepted as sufficient for diagnosis.[40] The clinical and pathologic features of TS are summarized in the box, p. 94.

Pathology and imaging. The pathogenesis of the CNS lesions in TS is unknown but is thought to be associated with disordered migration of dysgenetic neurons along abnormal radial glial fibers.[41,42] Four major categories of intracranial lesions in TS are recognized as follows[41]:

1. Cortical tubers
2. White matter abnormalities
3. Subependymal nodules
4. Subependymal giant cell astrocytoma

Microscopic examination shows that all four types of lesions have giant cell clusters with various degrees of neuronal and astrocytic differentiation.[42]

Cortical tubers. Cortical hamartomas, or "tubers," are the most characteristic lesions of TS at pathologic examination (Fig. 5-24). They are detected on the MR studies of 95% of patients with TS. Nearly 80% are identified solely by their abnormal signal; 20% also expand and distort the affected gyri.[42] MR appearance of cortical tubers varies with age. In neonates and young children, cortical tubers are hyperintense to premyelinated white matter on T1WI and hypointense on T2-weighted scans (Fig. 5-25). In older children and adults the lesions are iso- to hypointense on T1WI and hyperintense to both gray and white matter on balanced and T2-weighted scans. Enhancement following contrast administration occurs in less

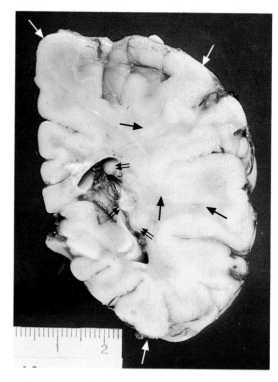

Fig. 5-24. Gross pathology of brain lesions in tuberous sclerosis. Cortical tubers (*white arrows*), white matter lesions (*small single arrows*), and subependymal nodules (*double arrows*) are all shown. (Courtesy C. Petito.)

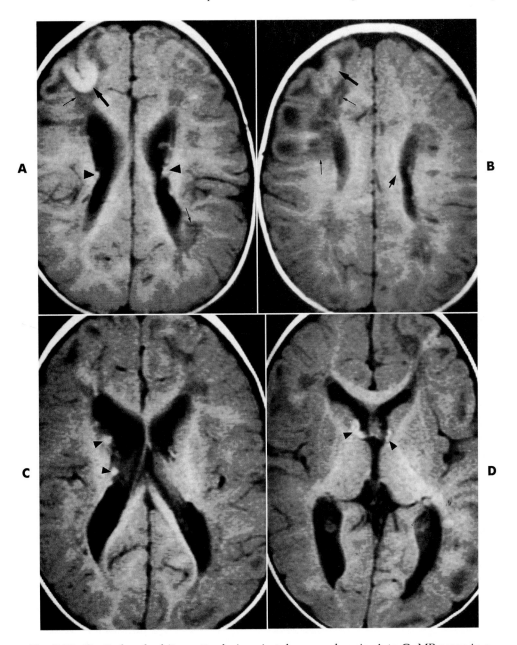

Fig. 5-25. Cortical and white matter lesions in tuberous sclerosis. **A** to **G,** MR scans in a 3-month-old child with tuberous sclerosis. Cortical tubers appear mildly to moderately hyperintense compared to premyelinated white matter on the T1-weighted studies (**A** to **D,** *large arrows*) but quite hypointense on T2WI (**E** to **G,** *black arrows*). Multiple white matter lesions are seen that are primarily hypointense (**A** to **D,** *small arrows*) to adjacent brain on T1-weighted scans. Most of the lesions appear strikingly hyperintense on T2WI (**E** to **G,** *small arrows*). Multiple subependymal nodules are also seen; these are primarily hyperintense on T1WI (**A** to **D,** *arrowheads*) and hypointense on T2WI (**E** to **G,** *arrowheads*). *Continued.*

than 5% of patients and does not indicate neoplasia because cortical tubers do not undergo malignant degeneration.[42]

Cortical tubers also show age-related changes on CT scans. In infants they appear as peripheral lucencies within broadened cortical gyri and tend to become isodense in older children and adults. Calcifi-

cation of these lesions also increases with age (Fig. 5-25, *H* and *I*); calcification is rare in infants. By age 10, 50% of patients have calcified cortical tubers.[43]

White matter lesions. Four distinct patterns of white matter lesions on MR imaging have been reported: straight or curvilinear bands that extend from the ventricle through the cerebrum toward the cor-

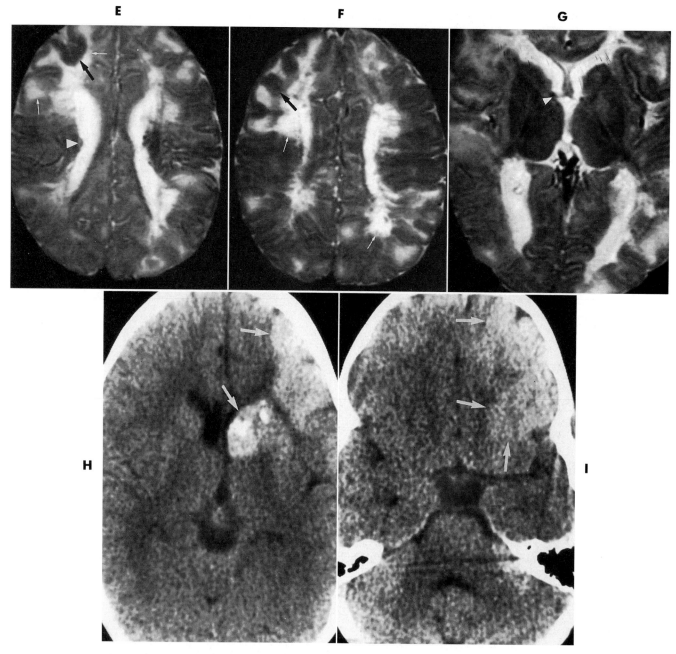

Fig. 5-25, cont'd. H and **I,** Axial CT scans without contrast enhancement in a 6-year-old child with tuberous sclerosis (TS) show a calcified, wedge-shaped hamartoma *(arrows)* that extends the full thickness from the subependymal area to cortex.

tex (Fig. 5-25, *A* to *G);* wedge-shaped lesions (Fig. 5-25, *H* and *I);* nonspecific "tumefactive" or conglomerate foci; and cerebellar radial bands. Like the cortical tubers, in older children and adults these lesions are all typically iso- to hypointense to white matter on T1WI and hyperintense to both gray and white matter on T2-weighted scans (Fig. 5-25, *A* to *G).* In infants the white matter lesions are hyperintense on short TR scans and hypointense to unmyelinated

white matter on T2-weighted studies. Approximately 12% of white matter lesions show enhancement after contrast administration.[42] These lesions are histologically benign and are believed to represent *disorganized, dysplastic white matter* or *dysmyelinated foci* with lines of migration disorder.[44]

Subependymal   nodules   (SENs). *Subependymal hamartomas* are found in 95% of patients with TS. Nearly two thirds are located near the caudate nu-

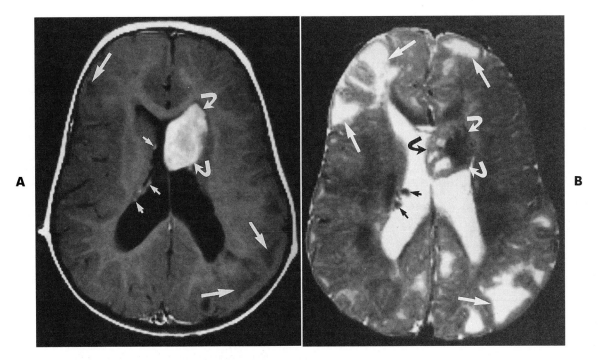

Fig. 5-26. Four-year-old child with tuberous sclerosis and subependymal giant cell astrocytoma. Postcontrast axial **(A)** T1- and **(B)** T2-weighted MR scans show benign white matter lesions *(large arrows)*, small subependymal nodules along the striothalamic groove *(small arrows)*, and a subependymal giant cell astrocytoma *(curved arrows)*.

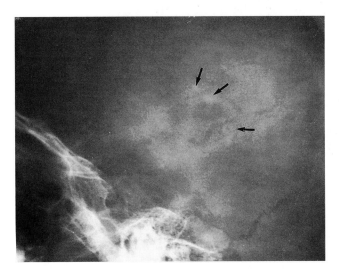

Fig. 5-27. Lateral plain film radiograph in a 10-year-old child shows periventricular calcifications *(arrows)*.

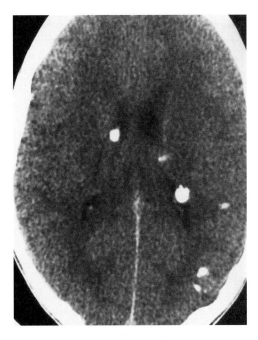

Fig. 5-28. Axial noncontrast CT scan in a patient with tuberous sclerosis shows both subependymal and parenchymal calcifications.

cleus along the striothalamic groove of the lateral ventricles just behind the foramen of Monro (Figs. 5-25 and 5-26); less common sites within the lateral ventricles include the atria and temporal horns. Third and fourth ventricular SENs are very infrequent. On MR studies, SENs appear as irregular nodules jutting into the CSF-filled ventricles. Signal is variable but is usually hypointense to white matter on T2WI because of calcification. In neonates these lesions are typically not calcified but may appear hyperintense to adjacent

unmyelinated white matter on T1WI (Fig. 5-25). Detectable calcification of SENs on plain film radiographs is unusual before the age of 2 years (Fig. 5-27). CT scans delineate periventricular and parenchymal calcifications in TS particularly well (Fig. 5-28).

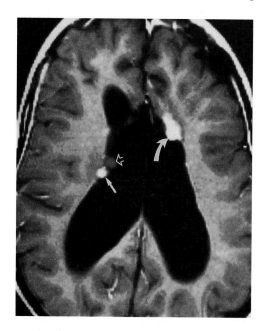

Fig. 5-29. Axial postcontrast T1-weighted MR scan in a patient with tuberous sclerosis who had a subependymal giant cell astrocytoma partially removed. Some residual tumor *(curved arrow)* is present. Two subependymal nodules are clearly identified; one enhances following contrast *(straight arrow)* but the other does not *(open arrow)*.

Between 30% and 80% of all SENs enhance after contrast administration[42,42a] (Fig. 5-29). Enhancement of a SEN does not denote neoplastic transformation[45]; periodic follow-up scans of enhancing lesions near the foramen of Monro are indicated because subependymal giant cell astrocytomas occur in this area.[46]

Subependymal giant cell astrocytomas (SGCAs). The incidence of SGCAs in TS is about 15%; most if not all patients with a subependymal giant cell astrocytoma have TS. All SGCAs appear to be located at or near the foramen of Monro. SGCAs are frequently calcified, appear heterogeneous on CT and MR scans, and show intense but somewhat inhomogeneous enhancement following contrast administration (Fig. 5-26).[42] SGCAs enlarge with time but are histologically benign. Associated obstructive hydrocephalus is common and is the most common cause of symptoms in patients with SGCA.

Miscellaneous CNS lesions. *Retinal hamartomas* are present in over half of all TS patients but typically do not impair vision unless they involve the macula or cause vitreous hemorrhage.[47] Mild nonobstructive ventricular enlargement is seen in 25% of patients with TS.[42] Vascular abnormalities have also been reported in association with tuberous sclerosis. Progressive degenerative changes in large elastic arteries, particularly the thoracic and abdominal aorta, may lead to *aneurysm* formation.[48] Vascular dysplasia with progressive *occlusion* of the craniocervical

vessels has also been reported in association with a "moyamoya" pattern of collateral circulation.[49]

Non-CNS lesions. Multisystem involvement with TS is common. Extracranial lesions are found in the cutaneous tissues (facial angiofibromas, peri- or subungual fibromas, hypomelanotic macules, shagreen patches), kidneys (renal cysts, angiomyolipomas in 40% to 80% of cases), heart (rhabdomyomas, found in 30%), lungs (cystic lymphangiomyomas, chronic fibrosis, 1%), liver (leiomyomas, adenomas), spleen and pancreas (adenomas), musculoskeletal system (present in 50% of patients; lesions are primarily multiple bone islands in the diploic space, pelvis, and spine; cysts and undulating periosteal new bone of the metatarsals, metacarpals, and phalanges are also sometimes seen), and vascular system (rarely involved; when present, aneurysms and nonatheromatous stenoses are characteristic).[50]

STURGE-WEBER SYNDROME

Etiology and pathology. Sturge-Weber syndrome (encephalotrigeminal angiomatosis) is a sporadically occurring phakomatosis characterized by a "port-wine" vascular nevus flammeus in the trigeminal nerve distribution (the first division is most frequently affected), leptomeningeal venous angiomatosis, seizures, dementia, hemiplegia, hemianopsia, buphthalmos, and glaucoma *(see box, p. 100).*[51] The precise etiology of Sturge-Weber syndrome (SWS) is unknown, but it is probably due to faulty development of cortical venous drainage.

Pathologic findings are those of a plexus of multiple small thin-walled telangiectatic capillaries or venules that lies along the brain in the subarachnoid space between the pia and arachnoid membranes (Fig. 5-30, *A*).[1] A paucity of normal cortical draining veins results in venous stasis and vascular congestion with hypoxia of the affected cortex. Slowly progressive atrophy of the brain underlying the angioma occurs, with dystrophic calcification in the middle layers of the cortical gray matter (Fig. 5-30, *B*). The angioma itself is not calcified.

Imaging. Intracranial calcification is the common radiologic manifestation of SWS. Detectable calcification before 2 years of age is uncommon. Skull films demonstrate the so-called tram-track pattern of calcification, caused by *calcification in apposing gyri* on either side of an intervening dilated sulcus (Fig. 5-31). On CT, curvilinear calcifications in a gyral pattern are observed (Fig. 5-32). These are most prominent in the occipital and posterior parietal lobes ipsilateral to the facial angioma. Progressive *cortical atrophy* is commonly seen with secondary manifestations such as ipsilateral calvarial thickening and enlargement of the paranasal sinuses and mastoid.

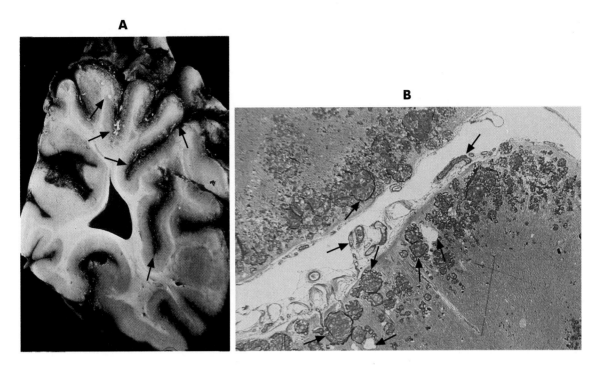

Fig. 5-30. A, Gross pathology specimen of Sturge-Weber syndrome. A plexus of thin-walled vessels occupies the subarachnoid space between the gyri *(large arrows)*. Dystrophic calcification is present in the underlying shrunken cortex *(small arrows)*. **B,** Microscopic section shows the leptomeningeal angioma *(large arrows)*, encephalomalacic changes in the underlying cortex *(curved arrows)*, and dystrophic calcifications *(small arrows)*. (Courtesy Rubinstein Collection, Armed Forces Institute of Pathology.)

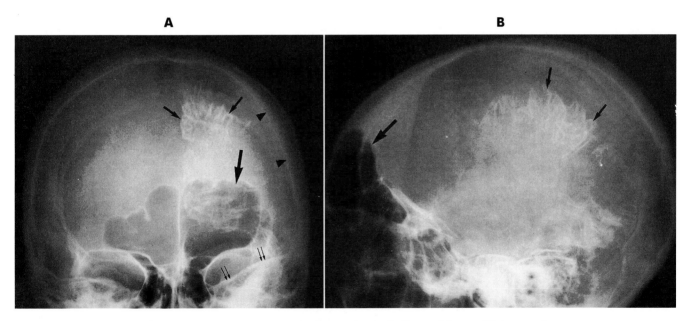

Fig. 5-31. PA plain skull radiograph shows classic findings of Sturge-Weber syndrome. "Tram-track" calcifications *(small arrows)* are present with secondary signs of cerebral hemiatrophy, including thick calvarium *(arrowheads)*, enlarged frontal sinus *(large arrows)*, and elevated petrous temporal bone *(double arrows)*.

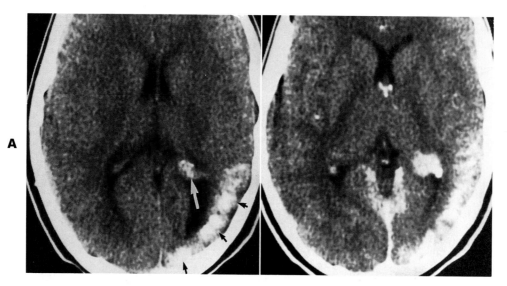

Fig. 5-32. Precontrast **(A)** and postcontrast **(B)** axial CT scans in a patient with SWS demonstrate the classical findings of parietooccipital cortical calcifications *(black arrows)* and enlarged choroid plexus *(white arrow)*. Note ipsilateral cerebral atrophy. Contrast enhancement in this case is minimal.

Sturge-Weber Syndrome

Synonym

Encephalotrigeminal angiomatosis

Inheritance

None (sporadic occurrence)

Clinical

Vascular nevus flammeus (port wine stain) in CN V distribution (V_1 most frequent)

Etiology

Normal cortical venous drainage fails to develop

Pathology

Leptomeningeal angiomatous vascular plexus with secondary dystrophic cortical changes

Imaging manifestations

Calcification
    Located in cortex underlying angioma
    Unusual before 2 years of age
    Often gyriform, curvilinear
    Most common in parietal, occipital lobes
Atrophy
    Atrophic cortex with dystrophic Ca^{++}
    Adjacent subarachnoid spaces enlarged
    Secondary skull changes
        Thickened diploic space
        Ipsilateral frontal sinus enlarged
        Enlarged mastoid with elevated petrous ridge
Enhancement may occur in ipsilateral choroid plexus, angioma, chronically ischemic cortex, or all three areas
Enlarged medullary, supependymal veins
Ocular lesions
    Buphthalmos
    Scleral/choroidal angiomata

Enhancement following contrast administration can be observed on both CT and MR. The *pial angioma* often enhances (Fig. 5-33),[52,52a] but gyral enhancement (Fig. 5-34), possibly due to cortical ischemia, and striking ipsilateral *choroid plexus enhancement* from collateral venous drainage may be observed as well (Figs. 5-34 to 5-36). Very *prominent medullary* and *subependymal veins* may be identified in some cases of SWS (Figs. 5-33 and 5-36).[52a] MR angiography in combination with MR imaging can give detailed information regarding the vascular anomalies in SWS.[52b]

Associated abnormalities. About one third of the patients with SWS have ocular abnormalities. Congenital glaucoma with buphthalmos is seen in 10% to 30%; scleral and choroidal angiomata have also been reported.[1] SWS can also be associated with the angio-osteo-hypertrophy of Klippel-Trenaunay syndrome (see subsequent discussion).

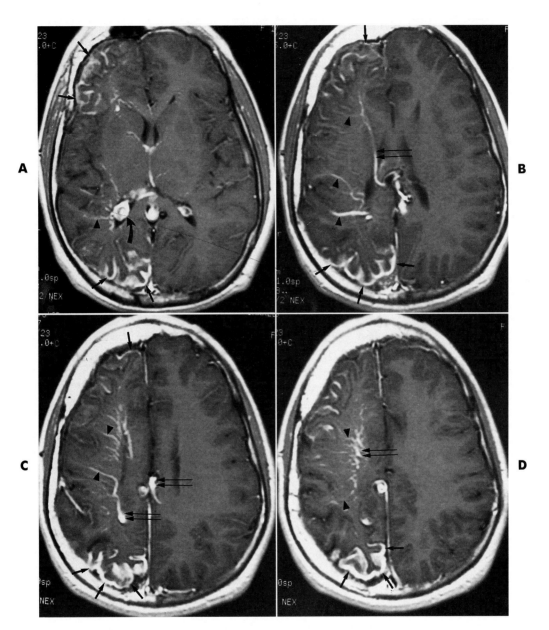

Fig. 5-33. Sturge-Weber syndrome (SWS). **A** to **D,** Axial postcontrast MR scans show mild atrophy of the right hemisphere. The pial leptomeningeal angioma enhances strongly *(small arrows)*. Multiple prominent medullary veins in the deep white matter are seen *(arrowheads)* that drain into numerous enlarged subependymal veins *(double arrows)*. The ipsilateral choroid plexus is also enlarged (**A,** *curved black arrow*).

Continued.

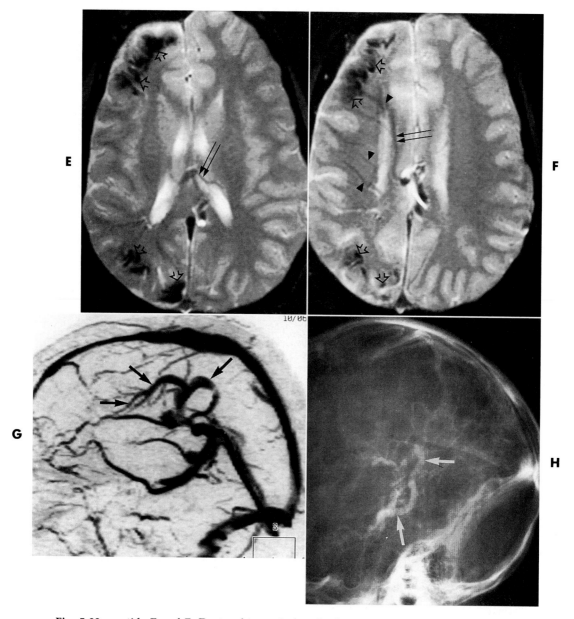

Fig. 5-33, cont'd. E and **F,** Dystrophic cortical and subcortical calcification is well demonstrated on the T2-weighted studies *(open arrows)*. The enlarged medullary veins are indicated by the arrowheads, and the prominent subependymal veins are indicated by the double arrows. **G,** MR "venogram" shows paucity of normal cortical draining veins and strikingly enlarged subependymal veins *(arrows)*. **H,** Carotid angiogram, lateral view, venous phase, in another patient with SWS shows prominent subependymal veins *(arrows)*. (**A** to **F,** Courtesy Joel Curé.)

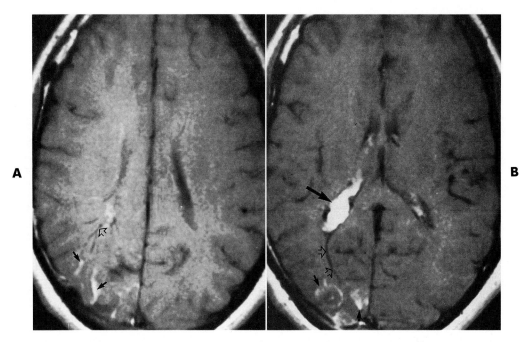

Fig. 5-34. Postcontrast axial T1-weighted MR scans in a patient with Sturge-Weber syndrome (SWS) show foci of gyral enhancement (*small arrows*), an enlarged, strongly enhancing choroid plexus *(large arrow)*, and prominent vascular channels in the medullary white matter that represent collateral pathways for cortical venous drainage *(open arrows)*. (Courtesy D. Brown and R. Benedikt.)

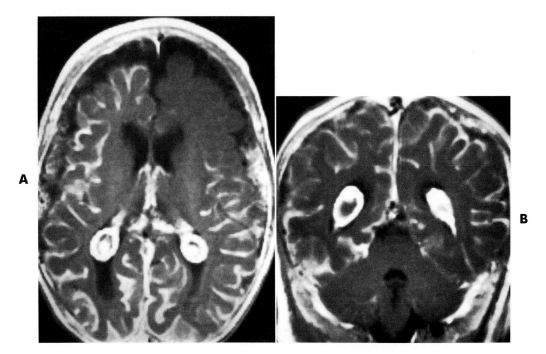

Fig. 5-35. Axial **(A)** and coronal **(B)** postcontrast T1-weighted MR scans in a patient with bilateral Sturge-Weber syndrome (SWS). The enhancement of the angiomas and choroid plexus bilaterally is striking. (From Benedikt RA, Brown DC, Walker R et al: Sturge-Weber syndrome: cranial MR imaging with Gd-DTPA, *AJNR* 14:409-415, 1993.)

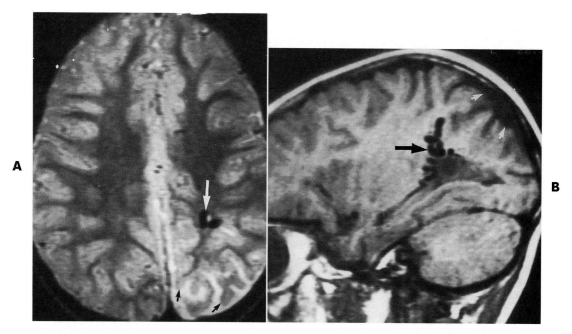

Fig. 5-36. Axial T2-weighted **(A)** and sagittal T1-weighted **(B)** MR scans show strikingly enlarged medullary veins *(large arrows)* in a patient with Sturge-Weber syndrome. Cortical atrophy is indicated by the small arrows. (Courtesy W. Gibby.)

VON HIPPEL-LINDAU SYNDROME

Inheritance. Von Hippel-Lindau syndrome (VHL) is an autosomal dominant disorder with incomplete penetrance that has variable manifestations. It is linked to a defect on the short arm of chromosome 3.[53]

Diagnostic criteria. The clinical diagnosis of VHL is based on the presence of multiple hemangioblastomas of the CNS, one hemangioblastoma plus a visceral manifestation, or one central or visceral manifestation in a patient with an affected first-order family member.[54]

Age, presentation. Age at presentation is variable but is very uncommon before puberty. If a retinal angioma is present, patients typically become symptomatic in their 20s; patients with hemangioblastomas of the brain and spinal cord commonly become symptomatic in their mid- to late 30s; and renal cell carcinoma develops by the early to midforties.

Pathology and imaging. VHL is a multisystem disease that is characterized by cysts, angiomas, and neoplasms of the CNS and abdominal viscera[55,56] *(see box)*. Several different lesions have been described in VHL. Common lesions and their approximate incidences[56-59] are as follows:
  Retinal angiomas (40% to 50%)
  Hemangioblastomas (40% to 80%)
  Cerebellum (75% of hemangioblastomas in VHL)
  Spinal cord (25% of hemangioblastomas in VHL)
  Visceral cysts and neoplasms (50% to 70%)

Von Hippel-Lindau Syndrome
Inheritance
Autosomal dominant
Incomplete penetrance, variable expressivity
Chromosome 3
Clinical
Age at presentation varies with differing manifestations but uncommon before midteens
Multisystem manifestations
CNS
Cerebellar, spinal cord, retinal hemangioblastomas common; supratentorial rare
Non-CNS
Visceral cysts
Neoplasms
Renal cell carcinoma (25% to 40%)
Pheochromocytoma (10%)

Ocular lesions. Retinal angiomas are found in 50% to 60% of patients with VHL, are multiple in approximately one third, and bilateral in up to half of all cases.[41] The retinal lesions are elevated, yellowish-red masses with a single dilated tortuous feeding artery and an enlarged draining vein.[60] Diagnosis is readily apparent at fundoscopic examination; in the absence of hemorrhage and subretinal exudate, imaging findings may be subtle or absent.

Cerebellar hemangioblastoma. Cerebellar heman-

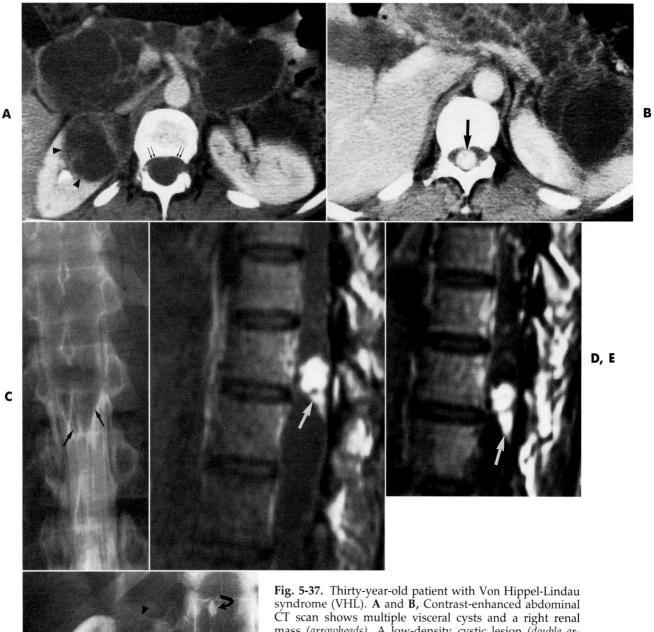

Fig. 5-37. Thirty-year-old patient with Von Hippel-Lindau syndrome (VHL). **A** and **B,** Contrast-enhanced abdominal CT scan shows multiple visceral cysts and a right renal mass *(arrowheads).* A low-density cystic lesion *(double arrows)* with enhancing nodule *(large arrow)* is seen within the spinal canal. **C,** AP myelogram shows an intramedullary mass *(arrows)* that expands the conus medullaris. **D,** and **E,** Postcontrast sagittal T1-weighted MR scans show cystic spinal cord hemangioblastoma. The enhancing nodule is indicated by arrows. **F,** Angiogram shows the largely avascular renal mass *(arrowheads).* The vascular nodule of the spinal hemangioblastoma is indicated by the curved arrow. (Courtesy J.F. Lally.)

gioblastomas represent between 7% and 12% of all posterior fossa tumors. Cerebellar hemangioblastomas are found in up to two thirds of patients with VHL,[6,41] whereas about one fourth of patients with hemangioblastomas have VHL.[2] Most hemangioblastomas are detected between 20 and 50 years of age and are quite rare in children.

More than 90% of all hemangioblastomas occur in the posterior fossa.[61] The most common location is the cerebellum (65%); brainstem and spinal cord are less common sites (20% and 15%, respectively).[2] A subpial location is typical.[56] Multiple lesions are present in 10% of all patients with hemangioblastoma and are considered diagnostic of VHL.[6] Multiple lesions are seen in 42% of patients with VHL-associated hemangioblastoma.[58]

On CT scans, about 80% of cerebellar hemangioblastomas appear cystic, with an isodense, noncalcified mural nodule that shows strong enhancement after contrast administration. The cyst wall is composed of compressed, gliotic tissue that typically does not show contrast enhancement. Solid tumors occur in 20% of all cases (Fig. 5-37). The uncommon supratentorial hemangioblastomas are more often solid than cystic.[61]

On MR scans, hemangioblastomas usually show prolonged T1 and T2, although their signal can be complex if hemorrhage has occurred.[56] The common appearance is that of a cerebellar hemispheric or vermian cyst that has a somewhat higher signal than CSF. An isointense mural nodule that shows strong, uniform enhancement after contrast administration is typical. "Flow voids" in the afferent and efferent vessels supplying the tumor can often be detected (*see* Fig. 14-42).[56]

On cerebral angiography the typical hemangioblastoma has an intensely vascular nodule with a dense, prolonged vascular stain. Early draining veins may occasionally be seen. A large avascular mass effect representing the associated cyst is common.

Spinal cord hemangioblastoma. Intramedullary hemangioblastomas are seen in about 10% to 30% of patients with VHL. The common appearance is that of a syrinxlike cyst with an isointense nodule that enhances strongly after contrast material is administered (Fig. 5-37).

Non-CNS lesions. Visceral cysts and neoplasms are common in VHL (Fig. 5-37). Renal cell carcinoma is the most frequent tumor (found in up to 50% of patients), followed by pheochromocytoma (seen in 10% to 15% of cases).[59]

OTHER NEUROCUTANEOUS SYNDROMES
Wyburn-Mason Syndrome

Wyburn-Mason syndrome is an entity that is also referred to as unilateral retinocephalic vascular mal-

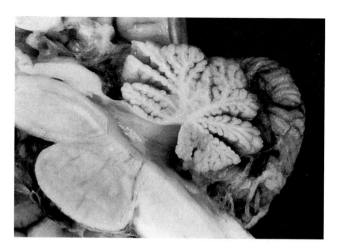

Fig. 5-38. Gross pathology specimen from a patient with ataxia-telangiectasia. Note the marked cerebellar atrophy. (Courtesy L. Becker.)

formations. Cutaneous vascular nevi, retinal and optic nerve vascular malformations, and ipsilateral cerebral arteriovenous malformations involving the visual pathways and midbrain are characteristic (*see* Fig. 10-4).[62,63] The lesions are typically unilateral, although bilateral manifestations have been reported.[64]

Ataxia-Telangiectasia

Also known as Louis-Bar syndrome, ataxia-telangiectasia (A-T) is an heredofamilial syndrome of uncertain origin that consists of oculocutaneous telangiectasias and cerebellar ataxia.[65] Ataxia typically begins in childhood, although the facial and conjunctival telangiectasias may not appear until later.[6] Pathologic CNS hallmarks of A-T are marked, progressive cerebellar atrophy predominately affecting the anterior vermis (Fig. 5-38). There is an increased incidence of malignant neoplasms and susceptibility to infections reported with this syndrome.[65]

Rendu-Osler-Weber Disease

Rendu-Osler-Weber disease (ROW) is also known as hereditary hemorrhagic telangiectasia (HHT). This autosomal dominant neurocutaneous syndrome is characterized by multiple mucocutaneous and visceral vascular abnormalities. The vascular lesions include (1) telangiectasias (primarily found in the skin and mucosa) (Fig. 5-39); (2) arteriovenous malformations and fistulae, found mainly in the liver (30% of all patients), lungs (15% to 20%) (Fig. 5-40, *A* and *B*), brain (28%) (Fig. 5-40 *C* to *F*), and spine (8%); and (3) aneurysms that can involve any size vessel.[66-68] Nearly half the cases with neurologic complications are due to pulmonary arteriovenous fistulae (AVFs). These cause paradoxical thrombi, gas, or septi emboli or produce thrombosis secondary to polycythemia.[69-71] The remaining neurologic symptoms in ROW are due to intracranial vascular malfor-

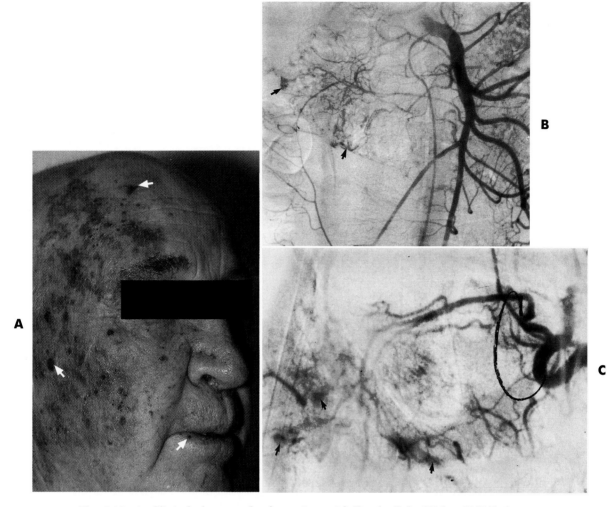

Fig. 5-39. A, Clinical photograph of a patient with Rendu-Osler-Weber (ROW) disease and multiple mucocutaneous telangiectasias *(arrows).* **B,** AP superior mesenteric and **C,** lateral external carotid angiograms in another patient with ROW show multiple mucosal telangiectasias *(arrows).* (**B** and **C,** Courtesy T.H. Newton.)

mations, hepatic encephalopathy, or cerebral abscess.[72]

Although multiple arteriovenous malformations are rare, about one third of these patients have either ROW or Wyburn-Mason syndrome.[63,73]

Epistaxis occurs in 85% of all patients with ROW.[74] The mucocutaneous lesions of ROW are typically capillary telangiectasias.

Klippel-Trenaunay-Weber Syndrome

Klippel-Trenaunay syndrome (KTS) is an angio-osteo-hypertrophy, i.e., it consists of overgrowth of bone and blood vessels.[1,75] KTS is characterized by a large angiomatous nevus, hypertrophy of soft tissue or overgrowth of bone (or both), venous varicosities, and anomalies of the fingers and toes.[76] Several KTS patients have been described who also exhibit prominent CNS findings that are identical to Sturge-Weber syndrome. The combined disease is then referred to as Klippel-Trenaunay-Weber syndrome and exhibits the findings of cutaneous angiomata, soft-tissue or bony hypertrophy, and leptomeningeal vascular malformation.[6]

Meningioangiomatosis

Meningioangiomatosis (MA) is a rare neurocutaneous angiodysplasia that is part of a spectrum of hamartomatous, meningeal-based lesions that involve the meninges, blood vessels, and adjacent brain.[6] Pathologic features include proliferation of meningeal tissue and blood vessels. Cortical meningovascular fibroblastic proliferation is present with infiltration of the underlying brain along the Virchow-Robin spaces (Fig. 5-41, *A*). On CT, a peripheral calcified lesion with variable mass effect and some degree of enhancement after contrast administration is typical. MR scans show an iso- to slightly hypodense cortical mass that has heterogeneous signal on T2WI. En-

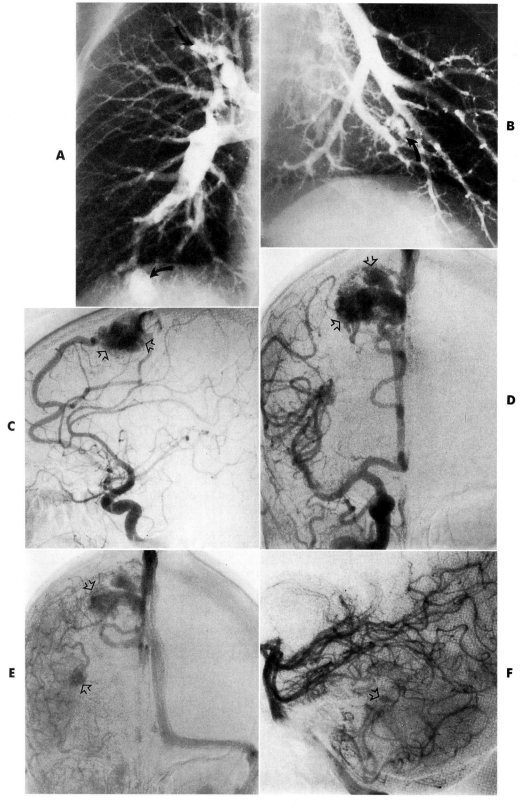

Fig. 5-40. Rendu-Osler-Weber disease. Right **(A)** and left **(B)** pulmonary angiograms show multiple arteriovenous fistulae *(arrows)*. Lateral **(C)** and AP **(D** and **E)** carotid and lateral vertebral **(F)** angiograms show multiple intracranial arteriovenous malformations *(arrows)*.

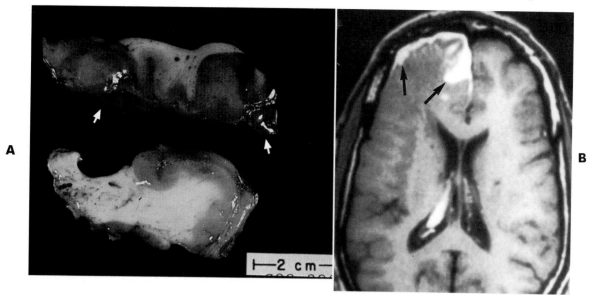

Fig. 5-41. A, Gross surgical specimen of meningioangiomatosis. Note proliferation of thickened, hyperplastic vascular meninges *(arrows)* overlying the cortex. **B,** Axial post-contrast MR scan in the same patient shows striking leptomeningeal enhancement in the area of meningioangiomatosis *(arrows)*. (From archives of the Armed Forces Institute of Pathology.)

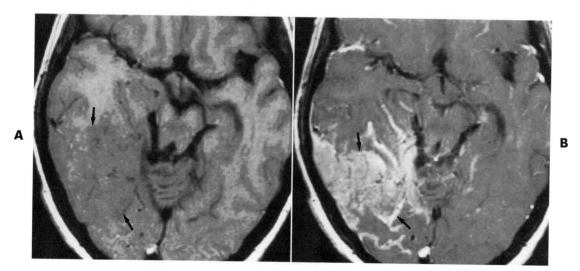

Fig. 5-42. Pre- **(A)** and post-contrast **(B)** axial T1-weighted MR scans in a patient with neurocutaneous melanosis. The lesions are isointense with gray matter **(A,** *arrows)* and show striking increase in signal after contrast administration **(B,** *arrows)*. (Courtesy D. Baleriaux.)

hancement following contrast may be striking (Fig. 5-41, *B*). In most cases, cerebral angiography is either normal or shows an avascular mass.[77,78] MA may be a *forme fruste* of neurofibromatosis.

Neurocutaneous Melanosis

Neurocutaneous melanosis (NCM) is a rare neuroectodermal dysplasia that is characterized by multiple congenital pigmented or giant hairy cutaneous nevi in conjunction with leptomeningeal proliferation of melanin-producing cells.[79] Approximately 40% of

patients develop primary malignant melanoma of the CNS.[6] Reported imaging findings on T1-weighted MR scans include an iso- or hyperintense meningeal-based mass that enhances strongly after contrast administration (Fig. 5-42).[79,80]

Epidermal Nevus Syndrome

Epidermal nevi are congenital skin lesions consisting of slightly raised ovoid or linear plaques.[81] Several different epidermal nevus syndromes have been described.[6] The most common is the **linear sebaceous**

nevus syndrome (of Jadassohn). Hemimegalencephaly, gyral malformations (pachy/polymicrogyria, heterotopias), mental retardation, seizures, unilateral megalencephaly, and facial hemihypertrophy have been reported.[81,82,82a] In some patients with **epidermal nevus syndrome** (ENS), ocular abnormalities such as ptosis, colobomas, Coats disease, and pseudopapilledema occur.[83] In others, CNS vascular abnormalities such as infarcts, vascular dysplasias with segmental stenoses, and alternating areas of dilatation, arteriovenous malformations, and aneurysms can be seen.[84] **Blue rubber bleb nevus** syndrome typically has bluish discolored skin and mucocutaneous lesions. Multiple intracranial venous angiomas and sinus pericranii are features of this syndrome (*see* Chapter 7).

Basal Cell Nevus (Gorlin) Syndrome

Basal cell nevus (Gorlin-Goltz) syndrome is inherited as a highly penetrant autodomal dominant trait with variable expressivity. It consists of multiple basal cell carcinomas of the skin, odontogenic keratocysts of the jaw, and various skeletal anomalies such as bifid ribs.[85] Intracranial abnormalities include lamellar dural calcification (Fig. 5-43), callosal agenesis, and CNS neoplasms. Medulloblastoma, meningioma, astrocytoma, and craniopharyngioma have been reported with Gorlin syndrome.[86]

Miscellaneous Melanocytic Phakomatoses

Hypomelanosis of Ito (HI) is a rare neurocutaneous syndrome that is characterized by bizarre hypopigmented skin lesions. CNS lesions occur in approx-

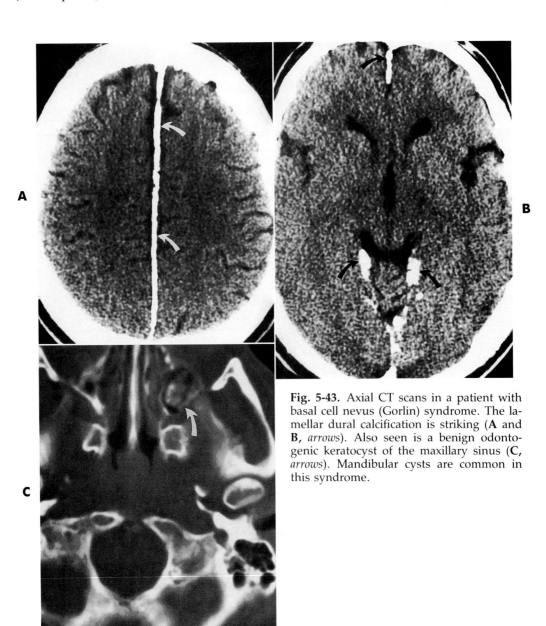

Fig. 5-43. Axial CT scans in a patient with basal cell nevus (Gorlin) syndrome. The lamellar dural calcification is striking (**A** and **B,** *arrows*). Also seen is a benign odontogenic keratocyst of the maxillary sinus (**C,** *arrows*). Mandibular cysts are common in this syndrome.

imately 50% of patients with HI and include hemimegalencephaly, white matter abnormalities similar to those seen with leukodystrophies, disordered cortical lamination with gray matter heterotopias, and diffuse atrophy.[87] **Nevus of Ota syndrome** is also known as oculodermal melanosis. Characteristic blue-gray lesions in the trigeminal nerve dermatomes are seen in association with abnormal meningeal pigmentation that is confined to the dura and calvarial periosteum, sparing the pia. Other reported abnormalities include choroid and ciliary body melanomas and primary CNS malignant melanomas.[6] **Incontinentia pigmenti** is an uncommon neurocutaneous disorder that appears in infancy. Erythematous vesicular skin lesions that later become verrucous and pigmented are seen. CNS manifestations include microcephaly, hydrocephalus, optic nerve atrophy, skull deformities, and optic nerve atrophy.[6] **Cellular blue nevus** is a variant of blue nevus that arises in the dermis and may extend locally to involve the intracranial structures.[88]

Cowden disease

Also known as multiple hamartoma syndrome, Cowden disease is a rare hereditary condition that is characterized by multiple hamartomas and neoplasms of ectodermal, mesodermal, and endodermal origin. Skin and mucous membrane lesions are common. Thyroid, breast, colon, and adnexal cysts and tumors, as well as neuromas, neurofibromas, and meningiomas, have been described. There is a recently reported association of Cowden disease with Lhermitte-Duclos disease.[89,90]

REFERENCES

1. Smirniotopoulos JG, Murphy FM: The phakomatoses, *AJNR* 13:725-746, 1992.
2. Elster AD: Radiologic screening in the neurocutaneous syndromes: strategies and controversies, *AJNR* 13:1078-1082, 1992.
3. National Institute of Health Consensus Development Conference: Neurofibromatosis Conference Statement, *Arch Neurol* 45:579-588, 1988.
4. Sorenson SA, Mulvihill JJ, Nielsen A: Long term follow-up of Von Recklinghausen neurofibromatosis: survival and malignant neoplasms, *New Engl J Med* 314:1010-1015, 1986.
5. Aoki S, Barkovich AJ, Nishimura K et al: Neurofibromatosis types 1 and 2: cranial MR findings, *Radiology* 172:527-534, 1989.
5a. Zimmerman RA, Yachnis AT, Rorke CB et al: Pathology of findings of cerebral high signal intensity in two patients with type 1 neurofibromatosis, *Radiol* 185(suppl):123, 1992.
6. Pont MS, Elster AD: Lesions of skin and brain. Modern imaging of the neurocutaneous syndromes, *AJR* 158:1193-1203, 1992.
7. Menor F, Marti-Bonmati L, Mulas F et al: Imaging considerations of central nervous system manifestations in pediatric patients with neurofibromatosis type 1, *Pedit Radiol* 21:389-394, 1991.
8. Brown EW, Riccardi VM, Mawad M et al: MR imaging of optic pathways in patients with neurofibromatosis, *AJNR* 8:1031-1036, 1987.
9. Imes RK, Hoyt WY: Childhood chiasmal gliomas: update of the facts of patients in the 1969 San Francisco Study, *Br J Ophthalmol* 70:179-182, 1986.
10. Raffel C, McComb JG, Bodner S, Gilles FE: Benign brain-stem lesions in pediatric patients with neurofibromatosis: case reports, *Neurosurg* 25:959-964, 1989.
11. Huson SM, Harper PS, Compston DA: Von Recklinghausen neurofibromatosis: a clinical and population study in southeast Wales, *Brain* 111:1355-1381, 1988.
12. Suh J-S, Abenoza P, Galloway HR et al: Peripheral (extracranial) nerve tumors: correlation of MR imaging and histologic findings, *Radiology* 183:341-346, 1992.
13. Beges C, Revel MP, Gaston A et al: Trigeminal neuromas: assessment of MRI and CT, *Neuroradiol* 34:179-183, 1992.
14. Sevick RJ, Barkovich AJ, Edwards MSB et al: Evolution of white matter lesions in neurofibromatosis type 1: MR findings, *AJR* 159:171-175, 1992.
15. Rubinstein LJ: The malformative central nervous system lesions in the central and peripheral forms of neurofibromatosis: a neuropathological study of 22 cases, *Ann NY Acad Sci* 486:14-29, 1986.
16. Menor F, Marti-Bonmati L: CT detection of basal ganglia lesions in neurofibromatosis type 1: correlation with MRI, *Neuroradiol* 34:305-307, 1992.
17. Mirowitz SA, Sarton K, Gado M: High-intensity basal ganglia lesions on T1-weighted MR images in neurofibromatosis, *AJNR* 10:1159-1163, 1989.
17a. DiMario FJ Jr, Bowers P, Jagjivan B et al: Analysis of skull anthropometric measurements in patients with neurofibromatosis type 1, *Invest Radiol* 28:116-120, 1993.
18. Egelhoff JC, Bates DJ, Ross JS et al: Spinal MR findings in neurofibromatosis types 1 and 2, *AJNR* 13:1071-1077, 1990.
19. Bensaid AH, Dietermann JL, Kastler B et al: Neurofibromatosis with dural ectasia and bilateral symmetrical pedicular clefts: report of two cases, *Neuroradiol* 34:107-109, 1992.
20. Nakasu Y, Minouchi K, Hatsuda N et al: Thoracic meningiocele vs neurofibromatosis: CT and MR findings, *J Comp Asst Tomogr* 15:1062-1064, 1991.
21. So CB, Li DKB: Anterlateral cervical mengiocele in association with neurofibromatosis: MR and CT studies, *J Comp Asst Tomogr* 13:692-695, 1992.
22. Halliday AL, Sobel RA, Martuza RL: Benign spinal nerve sheath tumors: their occurrence sporadically and in neurofibromatosis types 1 and 2, *J Neurosurg* 74:248-253, 1991.
23. Sobata E, Ohkuma H, Suzuki S: Cerebrovascular disorders associated with von Recklinghausen's neurofibromatosis: a case report, *Neurosurg* 22:544-549, 1988.
24. Battistella PA, Monciotti C, Carra S et al: Neurofibromatosi di von Recklinghausen e vasculopatia arteriosa cerebrale, *Riv di Neuroradiol* 5(Suppl 1):147-150, 1992.
25. Woody RC, Perrot LJ, Beck SA: Neurofibromatosis cerebral vasculopathy in an infant: clinical, neuroradiographic, and neuropathologic studies, *Pediatr Path* 12:613-619, 1992.
26. Negoro M, Nakaya T, Terashima K, Sugita K: Extracranial vertebral artery aneurysm with neurofibromatosis, *Neuroradiol* 31:533-536, 1990.
27. Gomori JM, Weinberger G, Shachar E, Freilich G: Multiple intracranial aneurysms and neurofibromatosis: a case report, *Australas Radiol* 35:271-273, 1991.
28. Muhonen MG, Godersky JC, VanGilder JC: Cerebral aneurysms associated with neurofibromatosis, *Surg Neurol* 36:470-475, 1992.
29. Schievink WI, Piepgras DG: Cervical vertebral artery aneurysms and arteriovenous fistulae in neurofibromatosis type 1: case reports, *Neurosurg* 29:760-765, 1991.
30. Baldwin D, King TT, Chevretton E, Morrison AW: Bilateral cerebellopontine angle tumors in neurofibromatosis type 2, *J Neuosurg* 74:910-915, 1991.

31. Linskey ME, Lunsford LD, Flickinger JC: Tumor control after stereotactic radiosurgery in neurofibromatosis patients with bilateral acoustic tumors, *Neurosurg* 31:829-838, 1992.

31a. Mautner V-F, Tatagiba M, Guthoffer R et al: Neurofibromatosis 2 in the pediatric age group, *Neurosurg* 33:92-96, 1993.

32. Mayfrank L, Moyadjer M, Wullich B: Intracranial calcified deposits are part of the diagnostic spectrum of neurofibromatosis type 2, *Neuroradiol* 33(Suppl):601-603, 1991.

32. Li MH, Holtas S: MR imaging of spinal neurofibromatosis, *Acta Radiol* 32, fasc 4:279-285, 1991.

33. Fontaine B, Hansen MP, VonSattel JP et al: Loss of chromosome 22 alleles in human sporadic spinal schwannomas, *Ann Neurol* 29:183-186, 1991.

34. Sintzoff SA Jr, Bank WO, Gevenois PA et al: Simultaneous neurofibroma and schwannoma of the sciatic nerve, *AJNR* 13:1249-1252, 1992.

35. Freidman DP: Segmental neurofibromatosis (NF-5): a rare form of neurofibromatosis, *AJNR* 12:971-972, 1991.

36. Trattner A, David M, Hodak E: Segmental neurofibromatosis, *J Ann Acad Dermatol* 23:1-38, 1990.

37. Haines JL, Short MP, Kwiatkowski DJ et al: Localization of one gene for tuberous sclerosis within 9q32-9q34, and further evidence for heterogeneity, *Am J Human Genetics* 49:764-772, 1991.

38. Seidenwurm DJ, Barkovich AJ: Understanding tuberous sclerosis, *Radiology* 183:23-24, 1992.

39. Gomez MR: Criteria for diagnosis in tuberous sclerosis, Gomez MR (ed), *Tuberous Sclerosis,* ed 2, pp 9-19, New York: Raven, 1988.

40. Braffman BH, Bilaniuk CT, Zimmerman RA: MR of central nervous system neoplasia of the phakomatoses, *Sem Roentgenol* 25:198-217, 1990.

41. Braffman BH, Bilaniuk CT, Zimmerman RA: MR of central nervous system neoplasia of the phakomatoses, *Sem Roentgenol* 25:198-217, 1990.

42. Braffman BH, Bilaniuk LT, Naidich TP et al: MR imaging of tuberous sclerosis: pathogenesis of this phakomatosis. Use of gadopentetate dimeglumine, and literature review, *Radiology* 183:227-238, 1992.

42a. Menor F, Marti-Bonnati L, Mulas F et al: Neuroimaging in tuberous sclerosis: a clinicoradiological evaluation in pediatric patients, *Pediatr Radiol* 22:485-489, 1992.

43. Kingsley D, Kendall B, Fitz C: Tuberous sclerosis: a clinicoradiological evaluation of 110 cases with particular reference to atypical presentation, *Neuroradiol* 28:171-190, 1986.

44. Iwasaki S, Nakagawa H, Kichikawa K et al: MR and CT of tuberous sclerosis: linear abnormalities in the cerebral white matter, *AJNR* 11:1029-1034, 1990.

45. Wippold FJ II, Baber WW, Gado M et al: Pre- and post-contrast MR studies in tuberous sclerosis, *J Comp Assist Tomogr* 16:69-72, 1992.

46. Abbruzzese A, Bianchi MC, Puglioli M et al: Astrocitomi gigantocellulari nella sclerosi tuberosa, *Riv de Neuroradiol* 5(suppl 1):111-116, 1992.

47. Dotan SA, Trobe SD, Gebarski SS: Visual loss in tuberous sclerosis, *Neuroradiology* 41:1915-1917, 1991.

48. Ng S-H, Ng K-K, Pai S-C, Tsai C-C: Tuberous sclerosis with aortic aneurysm and rib changes: CT demonstration, *J Comp Asst Tomogr* 12:666-668, 1988.

49. Imaizumi M, Nukada T, Yoneda S et al: Tuberous sclerosis with moya-moya disease: case report, *Med J Osaka Univ* 28:345-353, 1978.

50. Bell DG, King BF, Hattery RR et al: Imaging characteristics of tuberous sclerosis, *AJR* 156:1081-1086, 1991.

51. Elster AD, Chen MYM: MR imaging of Sturge-Weber syndrome, *AJNR* 11:685-689, 1990.

52. Yeakley JW, Woodside M, Fernstermacher MJ: Bilateral neonatal Sturge-Weber-Dimitri disease: CT and MR findings, *AJNR* 13:1179-1182, 1992.

52a. Benedikt RA, Brown DC, Ghaed VN et al: Sturge-Weber syndrome: cranial MR imaging with Gd-DTPA, *AJNR* 14:409-415, 1993.

52b. Vogl TJ, Stemmler J, Bergman C et al: MR and MR angiography of Sturge-Weber syndrome, *AJNR* 14:417-425,1993.

53. Hosoe S. Brauch H, Latif F et al: Localization of the von Hippel-Lindau disease to a small region of chromosome 3, *Genomics* 8:634-640, 1990.

54. Filling-Katz MR, Choyke PL, Patronas NJ et al: Radiologic screening for von Hippel-Lindau Disease: the role of Gd-DTPA enhanced MR imaging of the CNS, *J Comp Asst Tomogr* 13:743-755, 1989.

55. Sato Y, Waziri M, Smith W et al: Hippel-Lindau Disease: MR imaging, *Radiology* 166:241-246, 1988.

56. Ho VB, Smirniotopoulos JG, Murphy FM, Rushing EJ: Radiologic-pathologic correlation: hemangioblastoma, *AJNR* 13:1343-1352, 1992.

57. Huson SM, Harper PS, Hourihan MD et al: cerebellar hemangioblastoma and von Hippel-Lindau disease, *Brain* 109:1297-1310, 1986.

58. Neuman HPH, Eggert HR, Scheremet R et al: Central nervous system lesions in von Hippel-Lindau syndrome, *J Neurol, Neurosurg, Psychiatr* 55:898-901, 1992.

59. Levine E, Collins DL, Horton WA, Schimke RN: CT screening of the abdomen in von Hippel-Lindau disease, *AJR* 139:505-510, 1982.

60. Burk RR: Von Hippel-Lindau disease (angiomatosis of the retina and cerebellum), *J Am Opt Assn* 62:382-387, 1991.

61. Ginzburg BM, Montanera WJ, Tyndel FJ et al: Diagnosis of von Heppel-Lindau disease in a patient with blindness resulting from bilateral optic nerve hemanglioblastoma, *AJR* 159:403-405, 1992.

62. Kikuchi K, Kowada M. Sakamoto T et al: Wyburn-Mason syndrome: report of a rare case with computed tomographic and angiographic evaluations, *CT: J Comp Tomogr* 12:111-115, 1988.

63. Willinsky RA, Lasjaunias P, Terbrugge K, Burrows P: Multiple cerebral arteriovenous malformations (AVMs), *Neuroradiol* 32:207-210, 1990.

64. Patel V, Gupta SC: Wyburn-Mason syndrome, *Neuroradiol* 31:544-546, 1990.

65. Muras I, Bernini ML, Bernini FP: Neurodiagnostica dell'atassia-telangiectasia de Louis-bar, *Riv di Neuroradiol* 5(suppl 1):93-95, 1992.

66. Sobel D, Norman D: CNS manifestations of hereditary hemorrhagic telangiectasia, *AJNR* 5:569-573, 1984.

67. Ralls PW, Johnson MB, Radin R et al: Hereditary hemorrhagic telangiectasia: findings in the liver with color Doppler sonography, *AJR* 159:59-61, 1992.

68. Aesch B, Lioret E, deToffel B, Jan M: Multiple cerebral angiomas and Rendu-Osler-Weber disease: case report, *Neurosurg* 29:599-602, 1991.

69. Desai SP, Rees C, Jinkins JR: Paradoxical cerebral emboli associated with pulmonary arteriovenous shunts: report of three cases, *AJNR* 12:355-359, 1991.

70. Caroli M, Arienta C, Rampini PM, Balbi S: Recurrence of brain abscess associated with asymptomatic arteriovenous malformation of the lung, *Neurochirurgia* 35:167-170, 1992.

71. Roman G, Fisher M, Perl DP, Poser CM: Neurological manifestations of hereditary hemorrhagic telangiectasia (Rendu-Osler-Weber disease): report of two cases and review of the literature, *Ann Neurol* 4:130-144, 1978.

72. John PR: Early childhood presentation of neurovascular disease in hereditary hemorrhagic telangiectasia, *Pediatr Radiol* 22:140-141, 1992.

73. Iizuka Y, Lasjaunias P, Garcia-Monaco R et al: Multiple cerebral arteriovenous malformations in children (15 patients), *Neuroradiol* 33:538, 1991.

74. Lasjaunias P, Berenstein A: *Surgical Neuroangiography.* Vol 2, pp 379-383, New York: Springer-Verlag, 1987.

75. Taira T, Tamura Y, Kawamura H: Intracranial aneurysm in a child with Klippel-Trenaunay-Weber syndrome: case report, *Surg Neurol* 36:303-306, 1991.

76. McGrory BJ, Amadio PC, Dobyns JH et al: Anomalies of the fingers and toes associated with Klippel-Trenaunay syndrome, *J Bone Joint Surg* 73:1537-1546, 1991.

77. Tien RD, Osumi A, Oakes JW et al: Meningioangiomatosis: CT and MR findings, *J Comp Asst Tomogr* 16:361-365, 1992.

78. Aizpuru RN, Quencer RM, Norenberg M et al: Meningio-angiomatsosis: clinical, radiologic and histopathologic correlation, *Radiol* 179:819-821, 1991.

79. Rhodes RE, Friedman HS, Halter HP Jr et al: Contrast-enhanced MR imaging of neurocutaneous melanosis, *AJNR* 12:380-382, 1991.

80. Sebag G, Dubois J, Pfister P et al: Neurocutaneous melanosis and temporal lobe tumor in a child: MR study, *AJNR* 12:699-700, 1991.

81. Pavone L, Curatolo P, Rizzo R et al: Epidermal nevus syndrome, *Neurology* 41:266-271, 1991.

82. Sarwar M, Schafer ME: Brain malformation in linear nervus sebaceous syndrome: an MR study, *J Comp Asst Tomogr* 12:338-340, 1988.

82a. Cavenagh EC, Hart BL, Rose D: Association of linear sebaceous nevus syndrome and unilateral megalencephaly, *AJNR* 14:405-408, 1993.

83. Campbell SH, Patterson A: Pseudopapilledema in the linear naevus syndrome, *Br J Ophthal* 76:372-374, 1991.

84. Dobyns WB, Garg BP: Vascular abnormalities in epidermal nervus syndrome, *Neuroradiology* 41:276-278, 1991.

85. Lovin JD, Talarico CL, Wegert SL et al: Gorlin's syndrome with associated odontogenic cysts, *Pediatr Radiol* 21:584-587, 1991.

86. Schultz SM, Twickler DM, Wheeler DE, Hagen TD: Ameloblastoma associated with basal cell nervus (Gorlin) syndrome: CT findings, *J Comp Asst Tomogr* 11:901-904, 1987.

87. Williams DW III, Elster AD: Cranial MR imaging in hypomelanosis of Ito, *J Comp Asst Tomogr* 14:981-983, 1990.

88. Nakano S, Kinoshita K: MR of cellular blue nevus, AJNR 9:807, 1988.

89. Padberg GW, Schot JDL, Vielvoye GJ et al: Lhermitte-Duclos disease and Cowden disease: a single phakomatosis, *Ann Neurol* 29:517-523, 1991.

90. Williams DW III, Elster AD, Ginsberg LE, Stanton C: Recurrent Lhermitte-Duclos disease: report of two cases and association with Cowden's disease, *AJNR* 13:287-290, 1992.

PART TWO

CEREBRAL VASCULATURE: NORMAL ANATOMY AND PATHOLOGY

with
Wayne L. Davis
John Jacobs

Normal Vascular Anatomy

U nderstanding normal brain vascular anatomy is fundamental to neuroimaging. Thorough familiarity with the craniocerebral vessels and their vascular territories provides the requisite anatomic background for understanding the imaging manifestations of brain hemorrhage, trauma, and vascular diseases. Although an exhaustive description of all vessels and possible variants is beyond the scope of this text, the major vessels and commonly encountered variants, as well as rare but important anomalies, are described here.

ARTERIAL ANATOMY
Aortic Arch and Great Vessels

Aortic arch. Familiarity with normal aortic arch anatomy and branching patterns, as well as commonly encountered anatomic variants, is necessary for safe, successful transfemoral catheterization of the cerebral vessels.[1]

Three major branches arise from the outer curve of the human aortic arch. These vessels are the innominate, left common carotid, and left subclavian arteries (Fig. 6-1).[2]

Innominate artery. The innominate artery (IA), also known as the brachiocephalic trunk, is typically the first vessel that arises from the aortic arch (Fig. 6-1). Shortly after its origin the IA bifurcates into the right subclavian and right common carotid arteries (Fig. 6-2).

Right subclavian artery. Major branches of the right subclavian artery (SCA) are the right vertebral and internal mammary arteries and the thyrocervical and costocervical trunks (Figs. 6-1, *B*, and 6-2). An aberrant right SCA is a common arch anomaly and occurs in 0.5% to 1.0% of all cases. In this instance it is the last instead of the first brachiocephalic vessel arising from the aortic arch.[1]

Right vertebral artery. The right vertebral artery (VA) originates as the first RSCA branch. The right VA is the dominant vertebral artery in about 25% of cases. Several anomalous origins of the right VA have been described, but all are uncommon.[3]

Right common carotid artery. The right common carotid artery (CCA) arises from the proximal IA at various distances from the aortic arch. Occasionally the RCCA arises directly from the aortic arch (usually when the right SCA is aberrant) (Fig. 6-3). At the midcervical level, typically around the C3 to C5 level, the right CCA bifurcates into the external and internal carotid arteries.

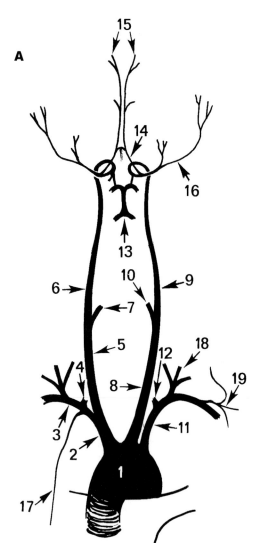

A

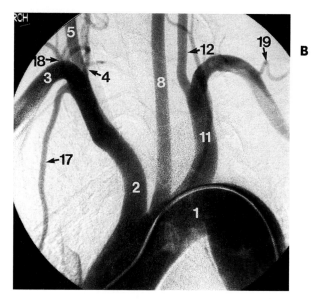

B

Fig. 6-1. A, Anatomic drawing of the aortic arch and great vessels with their major branches. **A,** *1,* Aortic arch. *2,* Innominate artery (brachiocephalic trunk). *3,* Right subclavian artery (SCA). *4,* Right vertebral artery (VA). *5,* Right common carotid artery (CCA). *6,* Right internal carotid artery (ICA). *7,* Right external carotid artery. (ECA). *8,* Left CCA. *9,* Left ICA. *10,* Left ECA. *11,* Left SCA. *12,* Left VA. *13,* VAs unite to form basilar artery (BA). *14,* Circle of Willis. *15,* Anterior cerebral artery (ACAs). *16,* Middle cerebral artery (MCA). *17,* Internal mammary artery. *18,* Thyrocervical trunk. *19,* Costocervical trunk. **B,** Digital subtraction (1024 × 1024) aortic arch angiogram, left anterior oblique view, shows normal great vessel origins and branching patterns. (**A,** From Osborn AG: *Handbook of Neuroradiology,* Mosby-Year Book, 1991.)

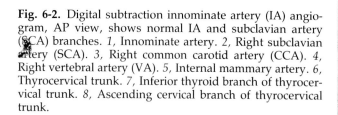

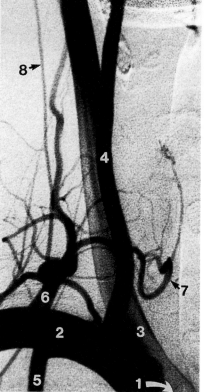

Fig. 6-2. Digital subtraction innominate artery (IA) angiogram, AP view, shows normal IA and subclavian artery (SCA) branches. *1,* Innominate artery. *2,* Right subclavian artery (SCA). *3,* Right common carotid artery (CCA). *4,* Right vertebral artery (VA). *5,* Internal mammary artery. *6,* Thyrocervical trunk. *7,* Inferior thyroid branch of thyrocervical trunk. *8,* Ascending cervical branch of thyrocervical trunk.

Left common carotid artery. The left common carotid artery (CCA) is normally the second major vessel originating from the aortic arch. Frequent variants include a common origin with the IA. The left CCA can also arise directly from the IA. The left CCA may occasionally be hypoplastic or absent. In the latter case, the external and internal carotid arteries arise directly from the aortic arch. Very rarely, a nonbifurcating carotid artery gives origin to all branches that usually arise from the ECA.[4,5]

Left subclavian artery. The left SCA is usually the last branch that arises from the aortic arch (Fig. 6-1). The major left SCA branches are the left vertebral artery, the thyrocervical trunk, and the costocervical trunk (Fig. 6-3).

Left vertebral artery. The left VA is the first SCA branch; it is the dominant vertebral artery in 50% to 60% of cases. In an additional 25% the right and left VAs are approximately equal in size.[1] Anomalous origin of the left VA directly from the aortic arch is seen in about 5% of cases. When the left VA has an arch origin it is often the nondominant vertebral artery.

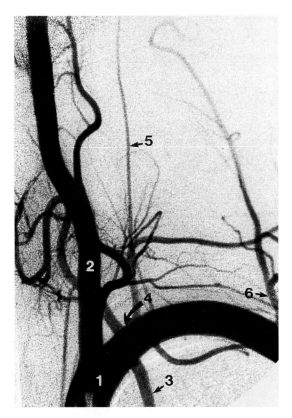

Fig. 6-3. Digital subtraction left subclavian angiogram, AP view, shows the left SCA and its branches. *1,* Left subclavian artery (SCA). *2,* Left vertebral artery (VA). *3,* Internal mammary artery. *4,* Thyrocervical trunk. *5,* Ascending cervical branch of thyrocervical trunk. *6,* Costocervical trunk.

Carotid Arteries

External carotid artery. The external carotid artery (ECA) is the smaller of the two terminal common carotid artery branches. The ECA typically supplies most extracranial structures of the head and neck (Fig. 6-4, *A*).[6] The ECA branches, territories supplied, and functional hemodynamic balance between adjacent arterial trunks are quite variable.[7] Proximal branches that arise from the ECA are shown in Fig. 6-4, *B;* the distal and terminal ECA branches are illustrated in Fig. 6-5, *A* and *B*.

Superior thyroid artery. The superior thyroid artery supplies the larynx and most of the upper thyroid gland (Fig. 6-4). The inferior thyroid and isthmus are supplied by branches of the thyrocervical trunk (Fig. 6-2) or a small branch from the aortic arch, the *arteria thyroidea ima.* Separate branches for the superior larynx and thyroid gland may also arise directly from the ECA.[6]

Ascending pharyngeal artery. The ascending pharyngeal artery has various origins but typically arises from the CCA bifurcation or the proximal ECA (Fig. 6-4). It supplies the nasopharynx, oropharynx, and the middle ear, and has hypoglossal and jugular branches that supply cranial nerves IX, X, and XI. It has some meningeal supply and also muscular branches that anastomose with vertebral artery branches.[6]

Lingual artery. The lingual artery (Fig. 6-4) supplies the tongue, floor of the mouth, submandibular gland, and part of the mandible. It may arise from a common lingual-facial trunk.

Facial artery. The facial artery exists in hemodynamic balance with other ECA arterial pedicles such as the maxillary artery.[7] It usually supplies the face, palate, lip, and cheek. The angular branch of the facial artery anastomoses with orbital branches of the ophthalmic artery and thus provides a potential source of collateral blood flow to the internal carotid system.

Occipital artery. The occipital artery supplies the posterior scalp, upper cervical musculature, and posterior fossa meninges (Fig. 6-4). Like the ascending pharyngeal artery, it has numerous potential anastomoses with the vertebral artery.

Posterior auricular artery. This small vessel supplies the pinna, external auditory canal, and scalp.

Superficial temporal artery. The superficial temporal artery (STA) is one of two distal terminal ECA branches (Figs. 6-4, *A,* and 6-5). It supplies part of the scalp and ear. On cerebral angiograms the STA should be distinguished from the middle meningeal artery. The STA has a characteristic hairpin turn where it crosses the zygomatic arch (Fig. 6-5, *B*). A major STA branch, the **transverse facial artery,** often supplies part of the deep face and cheek. The trans-

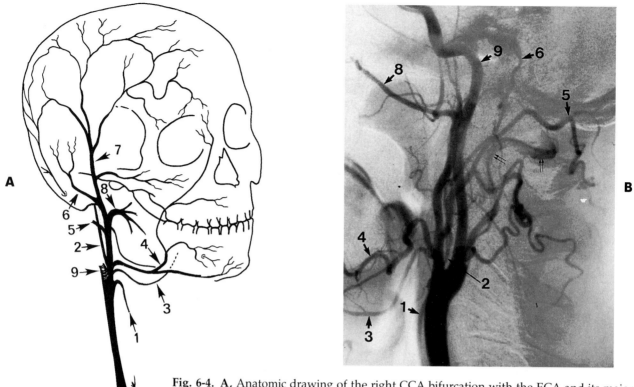

Fig. 6-4. **A,** Anatomic drawing of the right CCA bifurcation with the ECA and its major branches. Oblique view. *1,* Superior thyroidal artery. *2,* Ascending pharyngeal artery. *3,* Lingual artery. *4,* Facial artery. *5,* Occipital artery. *6,* Posterior auricular artery. *7,* Superficial temporal artery. *8,* Maxillary artery. *9,* Internal carotid artery. **B,** Left common carotid angiogram, lateral view, shows the major ECA branches. Note transient opacification of the ipsilateral vertebral artery *(double arrows)* via anastomoses with ECA muscular branches. (**A,** From Osborn AG: *Handbook of Neuroradiology,* Mosby-Year Book, 1991.)

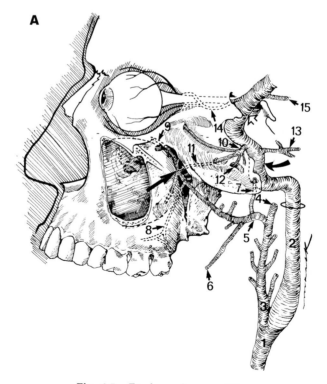

Fig. 6-5. For legend see p. 121.

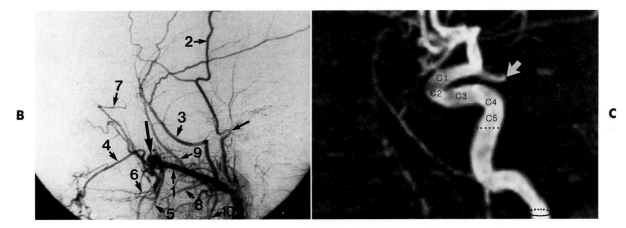

Fig. 6-5, cont'd. A, Anatomic diagram of the CCA bifurcation, ICA segments, and ECA branches. The large arrow points to the distal maxillary artery bifurcation into its deep branches within the pterygopalatine fossa. The sphenopalatine artery origin is hidden, medial to the maxillary artery. The circle around the internal carotid artery denotes its entrance into the petrous carotid canal. The curved arrow marks the beginning of the cavernous ICA. Near the anterior clinoid process the ICA pierces the dura *(open arrow)*. *1,* Common carotid artery. *2,* Internal carotid artery. *3,* External carotid artery. *4,* Superficial temporal artery (cut off). *5,* Maxillary artery. *6,* Inferior alveolar artery. *7,* Middle meningeal artery. *8,* Descending palatine artery. *9,* Infraorbital artery. *10,* Inferolateral trunk (note anastomosis with the maxillary artery, an ECA branch, via the artery of the foramen rotundum). *11,* Artery of the foramen rotundum. *12,* Artery of the foramen ovale. *13,* Meningohypophyseal trunk. *14,* Ophthalmic artery. *15,* Posterior communicating artery. **B,** Digital subtraction ECA angiogram, lateral view, shows the distal ECA branches. Within the pterygopalatine fossa *(large arrow)* the maxillary artery divides into its terminal branches to the maxillary sinus and orbit. *1,* Maxillary artery. *2,* Superficial temporal artery (small arrow denotes hairpin turn over the zygomatic arch). *3,* Middle meningeal artery. *4,* Infraorbital artery. *5,* Descending palatine artery. *6,* Sphenopalatine artery. *7,* Anterior deep temporal artery. *8,* Transverse facial artery. *9,* Middle deep temporal artery. *10,* Inferior alveolar artery. **C,** Lateral reprojected image from multiple overlapping thin slab MR angiogram shows the distal ICA and its segments. The approximate exocranial opening of the carotid canal is indicated by the dotted black line (compare with **A**). The cavernous ICA segments are named and numbered. Note a prominent posterior communicating artery *(arrow)*.

verse facial artery may also arise directly from the ECA.[6]

Internal maxillary artery. Deep branches of the internal maxillary artery (IMA) are shown in Fig. 6-5. In hemodynamic balance with the facial artery, the IMA supplies deep facial structures such as the muscles of mastication, palate and maxilla, sinuses, nose, and orbit. Through its middle and accessory meningeal branches, the IMA also supplies part of the cranial meninges. The IMA has numerous important anastomoses with the internal carotid artery (via the inferolateral trunk in the cavernous sinus) and ophthalmic artery (via ethmoidal branches) (see subsequent discussion).

Internal carotid artery. The internal carotid artery (ICA) is divided into several somewhat arbitrary segments (Fig. 6-6, *A*). The first two segments are extracranial: the carotid bulb and the cervical ICA segment. The third ICA segment is intraosseous. This part of the ICA lies within the petrous temporal bone.

The distal two segments are the cavernous and intracranial (supraclinoid) ICA segments.

Carotid bulb. The carotid bulb includes the distal 2 to 4 cm of the CCA, the bulbous dilatation at the ICA origin, and a 2- to 4-cm segment beyond the bifurcation (Figs. 6-5 and 6-6). Common carotid angiograms show the proximal ICA enlargement that forms the carotid bulb (Fig. 6-6, *A*). Flow at the CCA bifurcation is complex, and flow distal to the bulb is normally laminar (Fig. 6-6, *B*).[8] Flow reversal within the posterior bulb is normal; it is depicted on color flow doppler ultrasound (Fig. 6-6, *C*).

Cervical segment. The ascending, or cervical, ICA typically has neither narrowings nor dilatations, almost never branches, and does not taper.[8] From its origin at the CCA bifurcation, the ICA initially lies posterolateral to the ECA. As the cervical ICA ascends, it crosses behind and then medial to the ECA. In about 10% of cases the ICA originates from the CCA bifurcation medial to the ECA.[1]

Cervical ICA anomalies. Anomalous ECA branch-

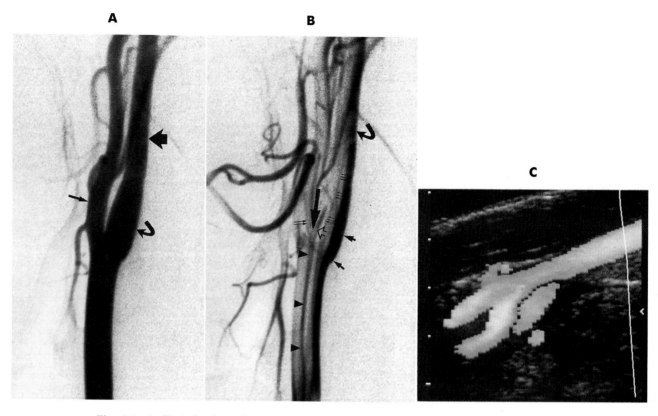

Fig. 6-6. A, Digital subtraction common carotid angiogram, early arterial phase, lateral view. The ICA *(large arrow)* arises posterior to the ECA. The carotid bulb *(curved arrow)* is normal. **B,** Late arterial phase shows the intravascular flow patterns described by Kerber et al.[8] The central slipstream *(arrowheads)* strikes the carina of the CCA bifurcation *(large arrow),* then sends most of its flow *(open arrow)* into the anterior part of the proximal ICA. The remainder *(double arrows)* of the stream passes into the ECA. Relatively stagnant flow in the carotid bulb *(small arrows)* pushes the posterior slipstream *(triple arrows)* anteriorly. Normal laminar flow is reestablished distally in the second ICA segment *(curved arrow).* **C,** Color flow doppler ultrasound scan shows a normal CCA bifurcation. Flow reversal in the posterior carotid bulb, shown in blue, is normal. **(C,** Courtesy D. Priest.)

es sometimes arise from the cervical ICA; persistent embryonic vessels may anastomose with the vertebrobasilar system (see subsequent discussion).

Petrous segment. The intraosseous segment begins where the ICA enters the carotid canal in the petrous temporal bone. Within the temporal bone the ICA first makes an anteromedial right angle bend, then bends again as it courses cephalad to enter the cavernous sinus (Fig. 6-5, *A* and *C*).

The intrapetrous ICA has tympanic branches that supply the middle ear. An inconstant branch, the **vidian artery** (artery of the pterygoid canal), courses through the foramen lacerum and vidian canal to anastomose with branches of the ECA. A small but important branch, the **caroticotympanic artery,** supplies the middle and inner ear.

The intrapetrous ICA can be aberrant, with a posterolateral instead of anteromedial course through the temporal bone. In this case the **aberrant ICA** traverses the hypotympanum, where it appears as a pulsatile retrotympanic mass. An aberrant ICA has a sharply angled, more posterolateral course that can be readily identified on CT scans (Fig. 6-7, *A*), as well as conventional cerebral angiograms (Fig. 6-8) and MR angiography (Fig. 6-7, *B*). Recognition of this normal anatomic variant and differentiation of an aberrant ICA from a glomus tympanicum paraganglioma is essential. Unwitting biopsy of this normal vascu-

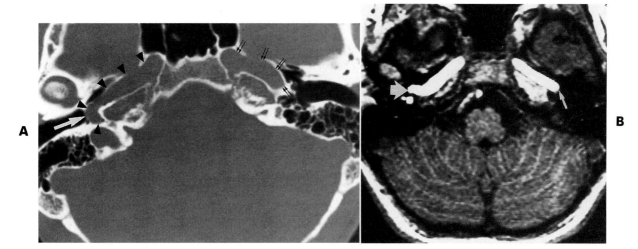

Fig. 6-7. A, Axial CT scan in a patient with pulsatile tinnitus. The right ICA has an aberrant course and traverses the hypotympanum where it is seen as a soft tissue mass *(white arrows)* adjacent to the inferior aspect of the cochlear promontory. Compare aberrant course of the right ICA *(arrowheads)* with the normal left ICA *(double arrows)* on the axial view. **B,** A patient who has pulsatile tinnitus had a vascular-appearing mass behind the right tympanic membrane. Screening MR angiography was performed. Axial source image (SPGR 60) shows an aberrant right ICA *(large arrow).*

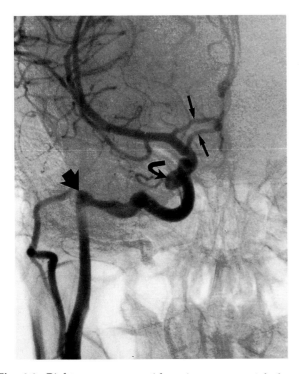

Fig. 6-8. Right common carotid angiogram, arterial phase, AP view in a patient with pulsatile tinnitus. Numerous vascular abnormalities are present. The ICA is aberrant, with an abnormally superolateral course *(large arrow).* There is duplication of the horizontal anterior cerebral artery *(small arrows).* The inferior A1 duplicated segment has an infraoptic origin. A small cavernous ICA aneurysm is present *(curved arrow).* There is an increased incidence of saccular aneurysms with many such vascular anomalies.

lar variant has disastrous clinical consequences that range from life-threatening hemorrhage to cerebral infarction.[9]

Another rare but important intratympanic vascular anomaly, a **persistent stapedial artery** (PSA), is caused by an intrapetrous embryonic vascular channel, the stapedio-hyoid artery. A PSA originates from the petrous ICA and, in the majority of reported cases, is enclosed within a bony canal on the cochlear promontory.[10] In these cases the PSA terminates as the middle meningeal artery. CT shows absence of the ipsilateral foramen spinosum.[11] A PSA may course across or through the footplate of the stapes, complicating prosthetic surgery.[10]

Cavernous segment. The cavernous segment (Fig. 6-5, *C*) begins where the ICA exits from the carotid canal at the petrous apex and terminates at its entrance into the intracranial subarachnoid space adjacent to the anterior clinoid process. The precise point at which the ICA pierces the dura is difficult to determine on routine angiograms alone, although MR imaging may be helpful.[12]

The cavernous ICA is further subdivided and numbered as follows (Fig. 6-5, *A* and *C*):

The ascending cavernous (C5) portion extends from the endocranial opening of the carotid canal to the beginning of the first (posterior) ICA genu.

The C4 portion is the genu itself, or the portion between the ascending and horizontal (C3) ICA segments.

The horizontal, or C3 portion, lies between the posterior and anterior 90 degree bends (second genu).

The anterior genu, or C2 portion, extends between the horizontal segment and remainder of the intracavernous ICA, termed the C1 segment.

The cavernous ICA has several small but important branches. The **meningohypophyseal artery** (posterior trunk) arises near the junction of the C4 and C5 segments (Fig. 6-5, A). Although it is seen in virtually 100% of anatomic dissections, this artery is normally seen only if high quality digital or film subtraction angiograms are used (*see* Fig. 6-21, C). The posterior trunk has branches that supply the posterior pituitary gland (*inferior hypophyseal branch*), tentorium (*marginal tentorial branch* or *artery of Bernasconi and Cassinari*), cavernous sinus and clival dura, and sometimes cranial nerves III to VI.[13] The meningohypophyseal artery enlarges to supply dural vascular malformations (Fig. 6-9) or neoplasms that involve the tentorium, cavernous sinus, or clivus.

The **inferolateral trunk** (lateral mainstem artery) arises inferolaterally from the C4 segment of the cavernous ICA and supplies cranial nerves III, IV, VI, and the gasserian ganglion (CN V), as well as the cavernous sinus dura. The inferolateral trunk (ILT) anastomoses with branches of the internal maxillary artery, providing collateral circulation between the ECA and ICA systems[14] (Fig. 6-9). The ILT is usually seen on the lateral view of subtracted cerebral angiograms (see Fig. 6-21, C). The ILT may become enlarged with vascular neoplasms or malformations or as a source of collateral blood supply to the ECA (Fig. 6-9).

Small *capsular branches* arise from the distal C3 or C2 ICA segment to supply part of the anterior pituitary gland. These tiny vessels are usually not identified on normal cerebral angiograms.

Intradural segment. The ICA pierces the dura adjacent to the anterior clinoid process (Fig. 6-5, A). Before it terminates in the anterior and middle cerebral arteries the ICA gives off superior hypophyseal, ophthalmic, posterior communicating, and anterior choroidal arteries.

The **superior hypophyseal trunk** arises from the posteromedial aspect of the supraclinoid ICA. It courses across the ventral surface of the optic chiasm to terminate in the pituitary stalk and gland. It also sends small branches to the chiasm and hypothalamus.[15] Numerous anastomoses with hypophyseal branches from the contralateral ICA form a vascular network termed the *superior hypophyseal plexus.* Unless pathologically enlarged, the capsular and hypophyseal vessels are usually not visualized on routine cerebral angiograms.[16]

The **ophthalmic artery** (OA) arises from the anterosuperior ICA medial to the anterior clinoid process (Fig. 6-5, A). In the majority of cases the OA origin is intradural. The OA passes anteriorly through the optic canal, initially lying below the optic nerve. It then crosses superomedially over the nerve to supply the globe (via the central retinal and ciliary arteries). The OA also has dural branches (anterior falcine and recurrent meningeal arteries) and orbital branches. Its orbital branches have a reciprocal blood supply and numerous anastomoses with the ECA.

Anomalies of the OA include an intracavernous origin; the OA gives rise to the middle meningeal artery in 0.5% of cases.[1]

The **posterior communicating artery** (PCoA) arises from the posterior aspect of the intradural ICA just below the anterior choroidal artery (Fig. 6-5, A and C). The PCoA courses posterolaterally above the oculomotor nerve (CN III) to join the posterior cerebral artery. Small branches of the PCoA, the anterior thalamoperforating arteries, supply parts of the optic chiasm, thalamus and hypothalamus, and pituitary stalk.

The common PCoA anomaly is hypoplasia, seen in nearly one third of anatomic dissections.[17] Next common is persistence of its embryonic configuration

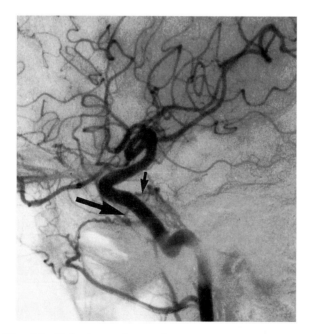

Fig. 6-9. Right internal carotid angiogram, arterial phase, lateral view, in a patient with a dural AVM at the skull base. The inferolateral trunk *(large arrow)* and meningohypophyseal trunk *(small arrow)* are enlarged.

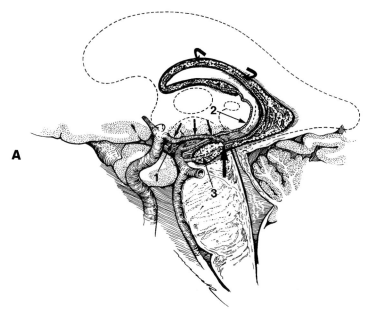

A

Fig. 6-10. A, Anatomic diagram of the anterior choroidal artery (AChA). *1,* AChA. *2,* Medial posterior choroidal artery (MPChA). *3,* Lateral posterior choroidal artery (LPChA). Small arrows indicate cisternal AChA. Large arrow indicates the "plexal point," where the AChA enters the choroidal fissure of the temporal horn. **B** and **C,** Digital subtraction internal carotid angiograms from separate cases demonstrate the AChA. **B,** Lateral angiogram. **C,** AP study. Cisternal AChA segment *(open arrow).* Plexal point *(large arrow).* Intraventricular AChA as it courses posterosuperiorly around the thalamus *(small arrows).*

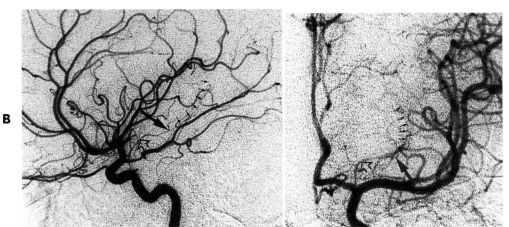

B

C

(the so-called fetal origin of the posterior cerebral artery), seen in 20% to 25% of all cases (*see* Fig. 6-21, C). Junctional dilatations (infundibuli) are seen at the PCoA origin in 6%[18] (*see* Fig. 9-16, *D*). Other PCoA anomalies such as duplication are rare.

The **anterior choroidal artery** (AChA) arises from the ICA a few millimeters above the PCoA. Occasionally their origins are reversed.[19]

The AChA has cisternal and intraventricular segments (Figs. 6-10 and 6-11). The AChA initially courses within the suprasellar cistern under the optic tract and posteromedially around the temporal lobe uncus.[20]

Just before reaching the lateral geniculate body the AChA angles sharply laterally and enters the choroidal fissure of the temporal horn.[21] This abrupt kink is represented by the angiographic "plexal point" (Fig. 6-10). The intraventricular AChA segment supplies the choroid plexus of the lateral ventricle. The actual wall of the lateral ventricle is usually not supplied by the AChA.[22]

The AChA exists in reciprocal vascular supply with the lateral (LPChA) and medial (MPChA) posterior choroidal arteries (Fig. 6-11). In the common pattern the AChA supplies choroid plexus in the temporal horn and part of the atrium. AChA branches usually supply the optic tract and cerebral peduncle, as well as the uncal and parahippocampal gyri of the temporal lobe.[23,24] Perforating AChA branches may also supply part of the thalamus and posterior limb of the internal capsule (see Fig. 6-16). Although multiple anastomoses exist among the various AChA segments,[24] as well as with LPChA and MPChA branches, these are quite variable.[25]

True AChA anomalies are uncommon. Aplasia is very rare. AChA hypoplasia and hyperplasia are seen in 3% and 2.3% of cases, respectively. In the hyperplastic variant the AChA vascular territory includes part of the usual posterior cerebral artery distribution.[25]

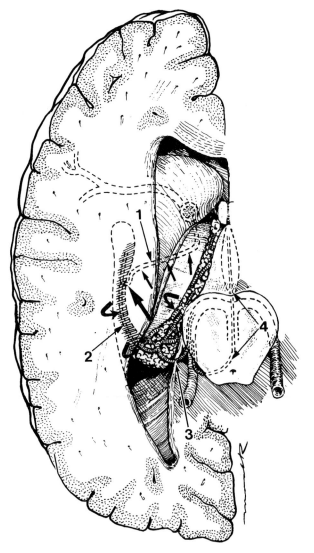

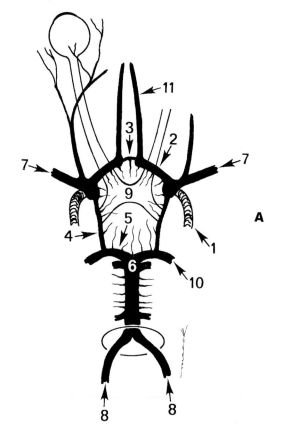

Fig. 6-12. For legend see p. 127.

Fig. 6-11. Anatomic diagram of the anterior and posterior choroidal arteries depicts their reciprocal relationship. *1,* Anterior choroidal artery (AChA). Cisternal AChA segment *(small black arrows).* The "plexal point" where AChA enters the choroidal fissure of the lateral ventricle *(large black arrow). 2,* Intraventricular AChA is in reciprocal hemodynamic balance with branches of the lateral posterior choroidal artery (LPChA) *(curved black arrows). 3,* LPChA is shown as it originates from the posterior cerebral artery (PCA). *4,* Medial posterior choroidal artery (MPChA) originates from PCA and courses superomedially to the third ventricle choroid plexus.

Circle of Willis

Components. The circle of Willis is an interconnecting arterial polygon that surrounds the ventral surface of the diencephalon adjacent to the optic nerves and tracts.[1] The normal circle of Willis is shown diagramatically, anatomically, and angio-

graphically in Figure 6-12. The following vessels comprise the circle of Willis:

1. The two ICAs
2. The horizontal (A1) segments of both anterior cerebral arteries
3. The anterior communicating artery
4. The two posterior communicating arteries
5. The horizontal (P1) segments of both posterior cerebral arteries
6. The basilar artery

The ICAs, ACAs, ACoA, and their branches are sometimes termed the *anterior circulation;* the basilar bifurcation, PCAs, and PCoAs are collectively termed the *posterior circulation.*[17]

In normal patients the entire circle of Willis is only occasionally visualized on a single injection during cerebral angiography (Fig. 6-12, *C*). Contrast-enhanced spiral CT with maximum intensity projection can be used to obtain "angiographic" images of the circle and its major branches[26; 26a,b] (Fig. 6-13). Other noninvasive techniques for visualizing these vessels include magnetic resonance angiography (MRA) and transcranial doppler ultrasound.

Time-of-flight MRA sequences with multiple overlapping thin slab techniques[27,28] nicely depict the cir-

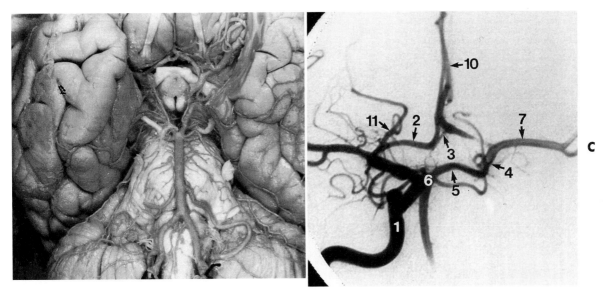

Fig. 6-12, cont'd. Anatomic diagram **(A)** and gross anatomic specimen **(B)** depict the circle of Willis. Note penetrating arteries that arise from the circle of Willis to supply numerous structures at the base of the brain. *1,* Internal carotid artery (ICA). *2,* Horizontal (A1) anterior cerebral artery segment. *3,* Anterior communicating artery (ACoA). *4,* Posterior communicating artery (PCoA). *5,* P1 segment of posterior cerebral artery (PCA). *6,* Basilar artery (BA) bifurcation. *7,* Middle cerebral artery (MCA; not part of the circle of Willis). *8,* Vertebral arteries (VAs; also not part of the circle of Willis). *9,* Optic chiasm. *10,* P2 (postcommunicating) PCA segment. *11,* A2 (postcommunicating) ACA segment. **C,** Digital subtraction right internal carotid angiogram, arterial phase, AP view. Transient contrast reflux fills the entire circle of Willis. **(A,** Modified from Osborn AG: *Handbook of Neuroradiology,* Mosby-Year Book, 1991. **B,** From Bassett DL: *A Stereoscopic Atlas of Human Anatomy,* section 1: the central nervous system. Courtesy Bassett Collection, R. Chase (curator), Stanford University.)

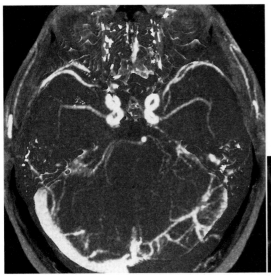

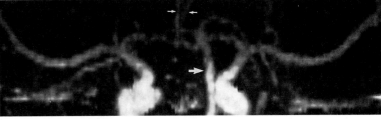

Fig. 6-13. CT "angiographic" image of the normal circle of Willis. **A,** Axial maximum intensity projection shows the major vessels of the circle. The off-midline BA bifurcation into the PCAs and segments of the ICAs and M1 MCA are seen. The ACAs are slightly obscured in this projection by bone artifact. Also note prominent filling of the right transverse sinus and multiple veins overlying the tentorium. **B,** Frontal projection of the circle of Willis after selecting a region of interest that removed the major posterior dural sinuses. The ICAs are seen bifurcating into the anterior and middle cerebral arteries. The off-midline BA is also clearly seen bifurcating into the PCAs *(large arrow).* In this projection the ACAs are clearly seen with both the A1 and A2 segments *(small arrows).* (Courtesy M.P. Marks.)

A

B

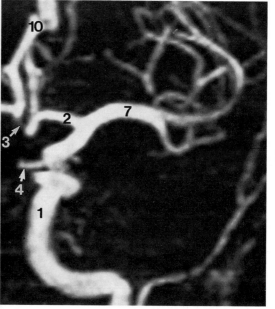

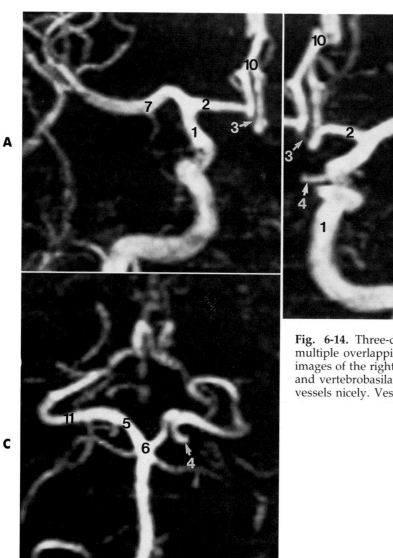

Fig. 6-14. Three-dimensional time-of-flight MRA using multiple overlapping thin slab technique. Reprojected AP images of the right **(A)** and left **(B)** internal carotid arteries and vertebrobasilar artery **(C)** show the major intracranial vessels nicely. Vessels are labeled as in Fig. 6-12.

cle of Willis (Fig. 6-14). Phase contrast MRA adds useful information about the hemodynamics of normal and abnormal blood flow in the circle[27,29] (Figs. 6-15). Transcranial doppler sonography (TCD) can also be used to assess flow velocities and detect perfusion disturbances in the proximal intracerebral vessels.[30]

Branches. Several small vessels arise from the circle of Willis to supply the optic chiasm and tracts, infundibulum, hypothalamus, and other important structures at the base of the brain (Fig. 6-12, *A*). These important vessels are the medial lenticulostriate arteries (from the A1 ACA segment), thalamoperforating and thalamogeniculate arteries (from the PCoA, basilar tip, and proximal PCAs), and perforating

branches (from the ACoA).[31] Vascular territories of these small perforating vessels and the major intracranial arteries are depicted in Fig. 6-16.

Normal variants. A complete circle of Willis in which no component is absent or hypoplastic is seen in only 20% to 25% of cases; anomalies of the posterior circle are seen in nearly 50% of all anatomic specimens.[17] Common normal variants include hypoplasia of one or both posterior communicating arteries (34%), a hypoplastic or absent A1 anterior cerebral artery segment, and "fetal" origin of the posterior cerebral artery from the ICA with hypoplastic or absent P1 segment (17%) (*see* Fig. 6-21, *C*). Infundibular dilatations at the PCoA origin from the ICA are present in 10% of cases.[30]

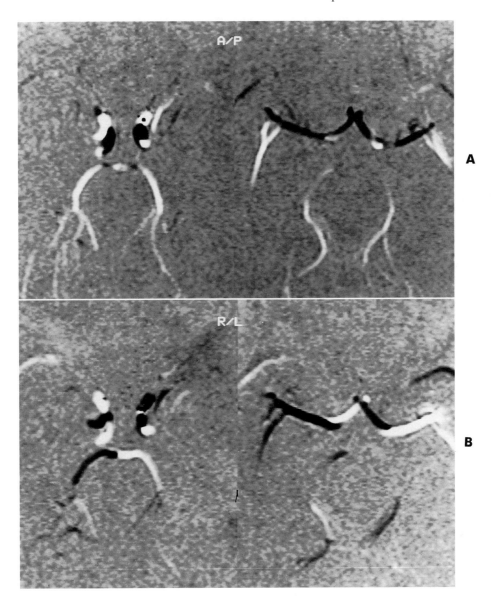

Fig. 6-15. Velocity (flow directional) images of the normal circle of Willis. **A,** In this case, two slices are obtained with anterior/posterior, phase/velocity encoding. They demonstrate a normal flow pattern within the circle of Willis. Flow anterior to posterior is encoded with white signal, and flow posterior to anterior is encoded with black signal. **B,** Right/left phase velocity encoding also demonstrates normal flow pattern around the circle of Willis. These scans were obtained with a velocity encoding value (VENC) of 80 cm/sec.

Anomalies. Congenital absence of one or both ICAs is rare.[32] Intrasellar intercarotid communicating arteries are common if one ICA is absent. Although this is an uncommon anomaly, it is important to identify its presence when considering cerebrovascular or transphenoidal surgery.[33] There is also a high incidence of intracranial aneurysm associated with ICA agenesis.

Carotid-vertebrobasilar anastomoses. These anomalies represent persistent embryonic circulatory patterns. Channels between the embryonic aorta (which eventually forms the caudal carotid artery) and the paired longitudinal neural arteries (which eventually form the basilar and vertebral arteries) may fail to regress, resulting in a congenital carotid-basilar or vertebral anastomosis[34] (Fig. 6-17).

The most common carotid-basilar anastomosis is the persistent **primitive trigeminal artery** (PTA). This anomaly is present in 0.1% to 0.6% of cerebral angiograms. Bilateral PTAs are extremely rare.[35]

In utero the embryonic trigeminal artery supplies the basilar artery before the posterior communicating and vertebral arteries develop. As these vessels emerge, the PTA normally disappears.[36]

BRAIN VASCULAR TERRITORIES

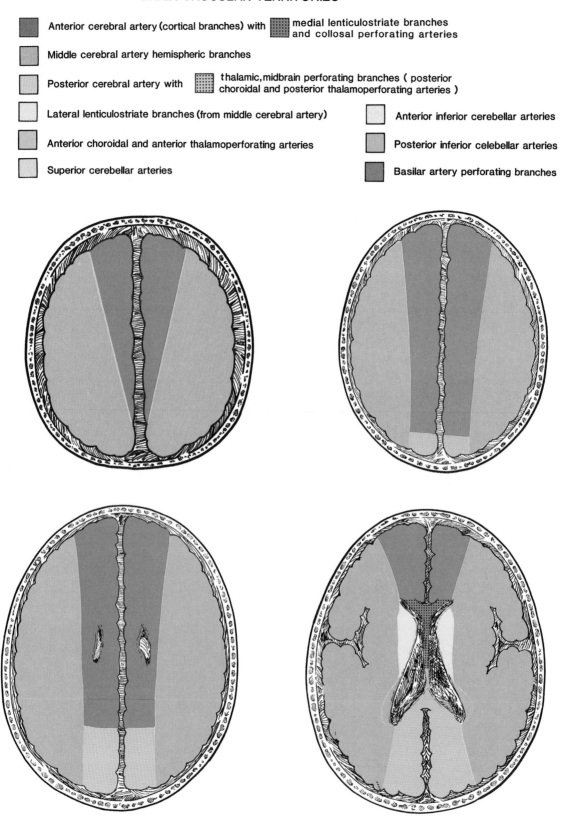

Anterior cerebral artery (cortical branches) with | medial lenticulostriate branches and collosal perforating arteries

Middle cerebral artery hemispheric branches

Posterior cerebral artery with | thalamic, midbrain perforating branches (posterior choroidal and posterior thalamoperforating arteries)

Lateral lenticulostriate branches (from middle cerebral artery)

Anterior inferior cerebellar arteries

Anterior choroidal and anterior thalamoperforating arteries

Posterior inferior celebellar arteries

Superior cerebellar arteries

Basilar artery perforating branches

Fig. 6-16. Approximate vascular territories of the cerebral arteries and their branches, as well as posterior fossa vessels. There is considerable variability in these territories, particularly in the basal ganglia, midbrain, and posterior fossa. For example, vascular supply to the medulla is depicted here as arising from basilar artery perforating branches and the posterior inferior cerebellar artery, but penetrating branches from the vertebral artery and anterior inferior cerebellar artery may supply the medulla. (Adapted and modified from M. Savoiardo: *The vascular territories of the carotid and vertebrobasilar systems*. Diagrams based on CT studies of infarcts, *Ital J Neurol Sci* 7:405-409, 1986.)

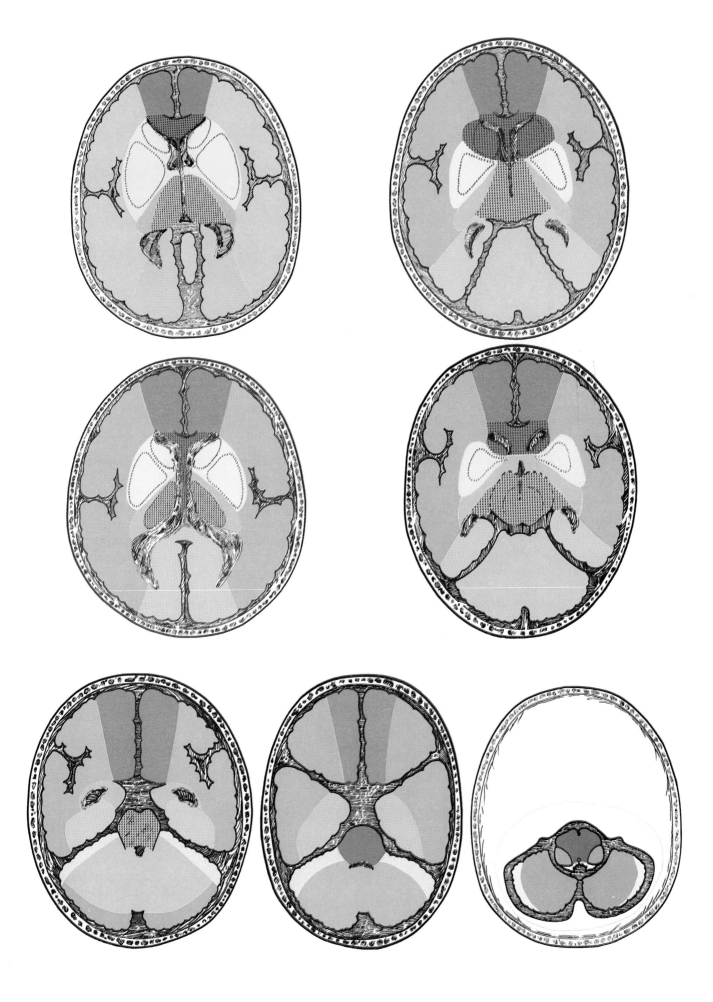

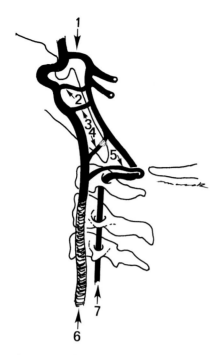

Fig. 6-17. Anatomic diagram illustrating different embryonic carotid-basilar anastomoses. Lateral view. *1,* Posterior communicating artery. *2,* Persistent trigeminal artery. *3,* Acoustic (otic) artery. *4,* Hypoglossal artery. *5,* Proatlantal intersegmental artery. *6,* Internal carotid artery. *7,* Vertebral artery. (From Osborn AG: *Handbook of Neuroradiology,* Mosby-Year Book, 1991.)

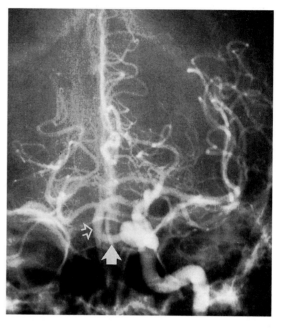

Fig. 6-18. Left internal carotid angiogram, arterial phase, AP view. A persistent trigeminal artery (PTA) is indicated by the white arrow. The PTA courses posteromedially from the ICA and anastomoses with the distal basilar artery *(open arrow).*

A PTA arises where the ICA exits the carotid canal and enters the cavernous sinus. It then runs posterolaterally along the trigeminal nerve (41%) or crosses over or through the dorsum sellae (59%) before joining the basilar artery[37,37a] A PTA is usually associated with small posterior communicating and vertebral arteries and a hypoplastic basilar artery caudal to the anastomosis.[1] PTAs have an increased incidence of intracranial aneurysms and vascular malformations.[38]

PTAs are readily identified on routine cerebral angiograms (Fig. 6-18) and have characteristic findings on contrast-enhanced CT scans, standard spin-echo MR imaging (Fig. 6-19), or MR angiography.[36-38]

The second most common persistent carotid-vertebral anastomosis is the persistent **primitive hypoglossal artery** (PHA). This anomalous vessel courses through the hypoglossal canal, parallels CN XII through part of its course, and connects the cervical ICA with the basilar artery (Fig. 6-20). A PHA is demonstrated in 0.027% to 0.26% of cerebral angiograms and often associated with an intracranial aneurysm. When present, a PHA is functionally a single artery that supplies the brainstem and cerebellum.[39]

Less common persistent carotid-vertebrobasilar anastomoses are the **persistent otic artery** (POA) and the **proatlantal intersegmental artery** (PIA). POAs are very rare and are seen as a short arterial segment originating from the petrous ICA. The POA projects medially ,through the internal auditory meatus and joins the caudal basilar artery. Because the vertebral arteries may be hypoplastic or absent a POA may be the major or sole arterial supply to the basilar artery.[34] A PIA is a suboccipital anastomosis between the ECA or cervical ICA and a vertebral artery. A PIA typically courses between the arch of C1 and the occiput.

Cerebral Arteries

The distal internal carotid artery usually terminates by bifurcating into the anterior and middle cerebral arteries. The posterior cerebral arteries typically arise from the basilar artery, less commonly from the ICA.

Anterior cerebral artery (ACA). The ACA is the smaller of the two terminal ICA branches.[40] The ACA has several major segments, each of which has important branches (Figs. 6-21 and 6-22).

Horizontal (A1) segment. The A1 segment extends medially from the ACA origin to its junction with the ACoA (Fig. 6-22). Deep perforating branches, the **medial lenticulostriate arteries,** arise from the A1 segment and pass cephalad through the anterior perforated substance. These small vessels usually sup-

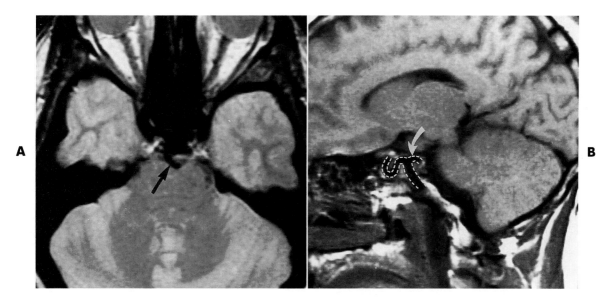

Fig. 6-19. Two cases of persistent trigeminal artery demonstrated on routine spin-echo MR. **A,** Long TR/short TE (proton density-weighted) axial MR scan shows a small PTA *(arrow).* **B,** Sagittal T1-weighted MR scan of a trigeminal artery *(arrow).* The ICA/PTA complex is outlined by dotted white lines. In sagittal plane this complex resembles the Greek letter tau (τ). (**B,** Courtesy A. Fortner. Reprinted with permission from *J Comp Asst Tomogr* 12:847-850, 1988.)

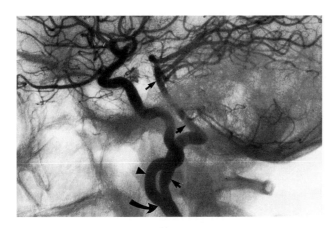

Fig. 6-20. Common carotid angiogram, arterial phase, lateral view, shows a primitive hypoglossal artery (PHA) *(arrows)* that arises from the cervical ICA *(arrowhead)* and supplies the posterior fossa vasculature. Note point at which the PHA originates from the ICA *(open arrow).* (From archives of the Armed Forces Institute of Pathology.)

ply the head of the caudate nucleus and anterior limb of the internal capsule.[41]

A2 segment. This segment includes the ACA from its junction with the ACoA to its bifurcation into the pericallosal and callosomarginal arteries (Fig. 6-22). The A2 segment courses cephalad in the cistern of the lamina terminalis and curves around the corpus callosum genu. The **recurrent artery of Heubner** is a lenticulostriate branch that typically arises from the proximal A2 segment (50% of cases). Sometimes the

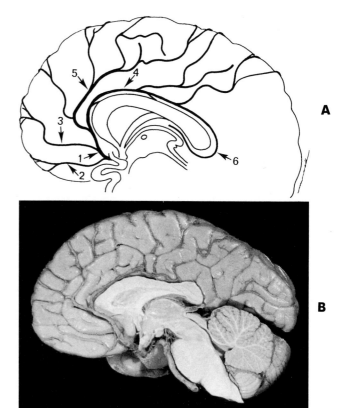

Fig. 6-21. A, Lateral anatomic diagram of the anterior cerebral artery (ACA) and its major branches. **B,** Gross anatomic specimen of the right cerebral hemisphere shows the ACA. *1,* A2 (postcommunicating) ACA segment. *2,* Orbitofrontal artery. *3,* Frontopolar artery. *4,* Pericallosal artery. *5,* Callosomarginal artery. *6,* Splenial artery.

Continued.

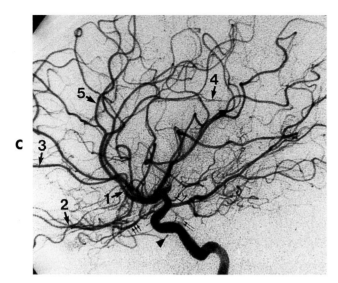

Fig. 6-21, cont'd. C, Digital subtraction internal carotid angiogram, midarterial phase, lateral view. ACA branches are numbered as in **A**. Fetal origin of the PCA is indicated by the open arrow. Cavernous and supraclinoid ICA branches shown include the meningohypophyseal trunk *(double arrows)*, the inferolateral trunk *(arrowhead)*, and the ophthalmic artery *(triple arrows)*. *1,* A2 (postcommunicating) ACA segment. *2,* Oarbitofrontal artery. *3,* Frontopolar artery. *4,* Pericallosal artery. *5,* Callosomarginal artery. *6,* Splenial artery. (**A,** From Osborn AG: *Handbook of Neuroradiology,* Mosby-Year Book, 1991. **B,** From Bassett DL: *A Stereoscopic Atlas of Human Anatomy,* section 1: the central nervous system. Courtesy Bassett Collection, R. Chase (curator), Stanford University.)

recurrent artery arises from A1 (44%) or, less commonly, the ACoA.[42] Two cortical vessels, the **orbitofrontal** and **frontopolar arteries** also arise from A2. As the A2 segment courses superiorly within the interhemispheric fissure, it bifurcates near the callosal genu into the two main terminal ACA branches, the **pericallosal** and **callosomarginal arteries.**

Cortical (A3) branches and vascular territory. Classically, cortical ACA branches are considered to supply the anterior two thirds of the medial hemispheric surfaces plus a small superior area that extends over the convexities (Fig. 6-16). Recent studies indicate that the major cerebral artery territories have considerable normal variability.[43,44] Vascular distribution of the hemispheric ACA branches with usual, minimum, and maximum territories of supply is depicted in Fig. 6-23.

Anterior communicating artery (ACoA). The ACoA is technically part of the circle of Willis, not a true ACA branch. However, most investigators treat the ACA and ACoA as a single complex.[42]

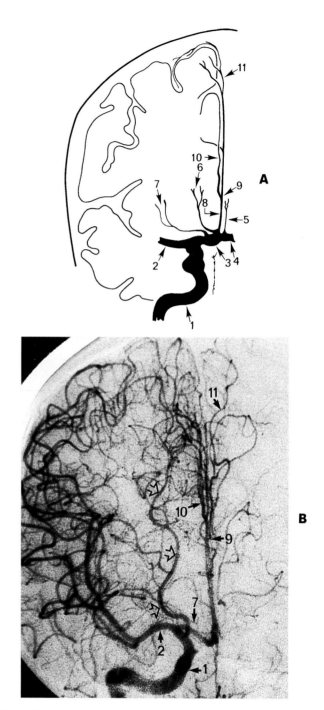

Fig. 6-22. Anteroposterior anatomic drawing **(A)** and arterial phase internal carotid angiogram **(B)** show the ACA and its branches. *1,* Internal carotid artery. *2,* Middle cerebral artery. *3,* Horizontal (A1) ACA segment. *4,* Anterior communicating artery (ACoA). *5,* Small ACoA branch to basal ganglia, corpus callosum genu. *6,* Medial lenticulostriate arteries. *7,* Recurrent artery of Heubner. *8,* A2 segment of ACA. *9,* ACA bifurcation. *10,* Pericallosal artery. *11,* Callosomarginal artery. Fetal origin of the posterior cerebral artery from the internal carotid artery *(open arrows).* (**A,** From Osborn AG: *Handbook of Neuroradiology,* Mosby-Year Book, 1991.)

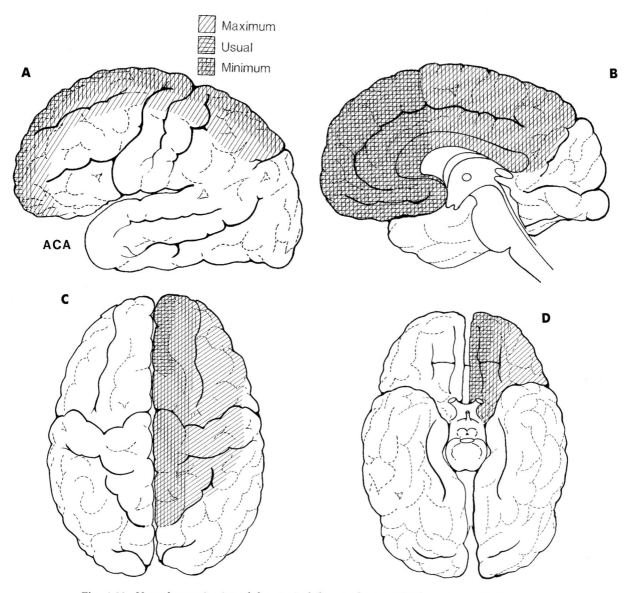

Fig. 6-23. Vascular territories of the cortical (hemispheric) ACA branches with the maximum, usual, and minimum distributions as delineated by van der Zwan.[44] **A,** Lateral view; **B,** medial view; **C,** superior view; and **D,** base view.

Perforating branches. Small perforating ACoA branches are almost invariably present. These tiny but nevertheless important vessels may supply parts of the lamina terminalis and hypothalamus, anterior commissure, fornix, septum pellucidum, paraolfactory gyrus, the subcallosal region, and the anterior part of the cingulate gyrus (Fig. 6-16). Occasionally these branches may even supply part of the medial hemisphere beyond the callosal genu.[45] Although rarely seen on routine cerebral angiograms, they sometimes can be visualized on superselective stud-

ies and are often encountered during microsurgical approaches to ACoA aneurysms.[42]

Variants and anomalies. Anatomic variations in the ACA-ACoA complex are present in approximately one third of anatomic dissections. Common variations are **hypoplastic** or **absent A1 segment,** seen in 5% to 18% and **duplicated ACoA,** seen in 10% of all cases.[42]

An **azygous ACA** is a solitary unpaired vessel that arises as a single trunk from the confluence of the horizontal (A1) segments of the right and left

ACAs.[46] A true azygous ACA is rare and is often associated with other intracranial anomalies such as lobar holoprosencephaly (see Fig. 3-7) and saccular aneurysm.[47] More commonly, a **bihemispheric ACA** sends a variable number of branches to the contralateral hemisphere. Here, separate right and left ACA vessels are present, but one is dominant and sends branches to both hemispheres, whereas the other is hypoplastic and may terminate in an orbitofrontal or frontopolar branch.

Other ACA variants such as infraoptic origin and A1 fenestration or duplication are uncommon (see Fig. 6-8). Infraoptic ACA origin and duplicated ACA are associated with an increased incidence of saccular aneurysms.[47,48] Fenestrated arteries have the same incidence of intracranial aneurysms as other circle of Willis bifurcation points.[48a]

Middle cerebral artery. The middle cerebral artery (MCA) is the larger of the two terminal ICA branches.

Like the ACA, the MCA is divided into several major segments (Fig. 6-24).

Horizontal (M1) segment. The horizontal MCA segment extends laterally from its origin at the ICA bifurcation to its bifurcation or trifurcation at the sylvian fissure (Fig. 6-25). Deep perforating branches, the **lateral lenticulostriate arteries,** arise from M1 and course superiorly to supply the lentiform nucleus, as well as part of the internal capsule and caudate nucleus (Figs. 6-25 to 6-27).[44]

Insular (M2) segment. At its genu the MCA divides into its insular (M2) branches. These loop over the insula and then pass laterally to exit from the sylvian fissure (Fig. 6-24, *B* and *C*).

Opercular (M3) segments. These are the MCA branches as they emerge from the sylvian fissure and ramify over the hemispheric surface (Figs. 6-25 and 6-27). Classically, much of the cerebral cortex and white matter is supplied by MCA branches (Fig. 6-16).[49,50] Recent studies indicate wide variability in

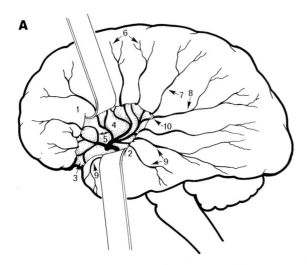

A

Fig. 6-24. **A,** Lateral anatomic diagram of the brain showing the middle cerebral artery (MCA) and its hemispheric branches. **B** and **C,** Anatomic dissections of the MCA branches within the sylvian fissure, seen from lateral **(B)** and superior **(C)** perspectives. *1,* Operculum of frontal lobe. *2,* Operculum of temporal lobe. *3,* Sylvian fissure (pulled or dissected apart). *4,* Insula. *5,* Insular (M2) MCA branches. *6,* Precentral and postcentral sulcal MCA branches. *7,* Posterior parietal artery. *8,* Angular artery. *9,* Temporal branches. *10,* Sylvian point. (**A,** From Osborn AG: *Handbook of Neuroradiology,* Mosby-Year Book, 1991. **B** and **C,** From Bassett DL: *A Stereoscopic Atlas of Human Anatomy,* section 1: the central nervous system. Courtesy Bassett Collection, R. Chase (curator), Stanford University.)

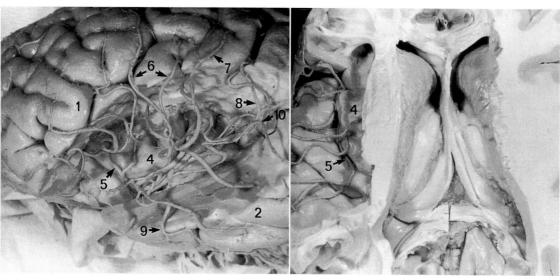

B   **C**

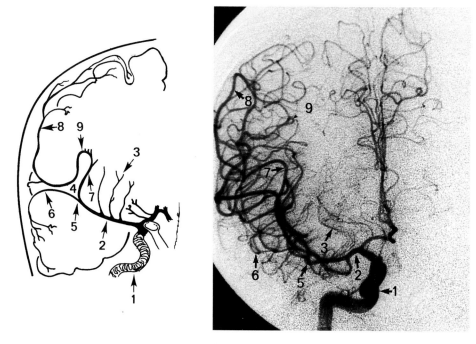

Fig. 6-25. Anteroposterior anatomic drawing **(A)** and internal carotid angiogram **(B)** show the MCA and its branches. *1*, Internal carotid artery. *2*, Horizontal (M1) MCA segment. *3*, Lateral lenticulostriate arteries. *4*, Sylvian fissure. *5*, MCA bifurcation. *6*, Anterior temporal artery. *7*, M2 (sylvian) segments of MCA hemispheric branches. *8*, M3 (opercular) MCA branches. *9*, Sylvian point. (**A**, From Osborn AG: *Handbook of Neuroradiology*, Mosby-Year Book, 1991.)

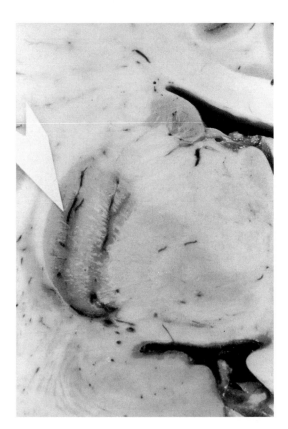

Fig. 6-26. Gross anatomy of the lateral lenticulostriate arteries *(arrow)* as they course within the putamen. (Courtesy E. Ross.)

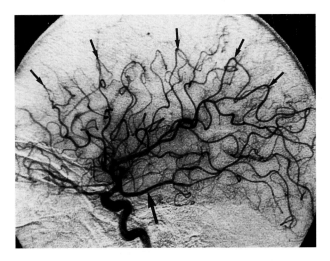

Fig. 6-27. A, Digital subtraction left internal carotid angiogram, midarterial phase, lateral view. The A1 ACA segment is hypoplastic and the posterior cerebral artery *(large arrow)* has a fetal origin from the ICA. Because the ACA does not fill from the left ICA, an unobstructed view of the MCA hemispheric (opercular) branches and their vascular distribution *(small arrows)* is seen.

Continued.

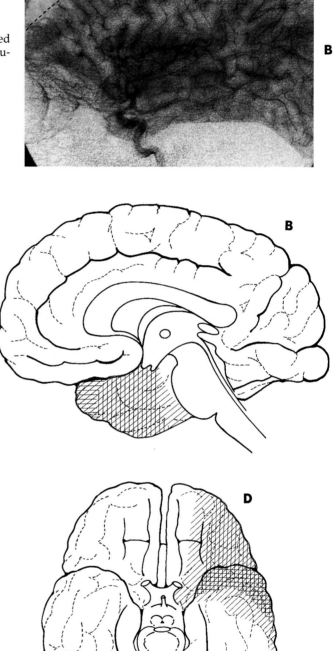

Fig. 6-27, cont'd.   B, Capillary phase shows the watershed between the anterior and middle cerebral artery distributions *(dotted line).*

B

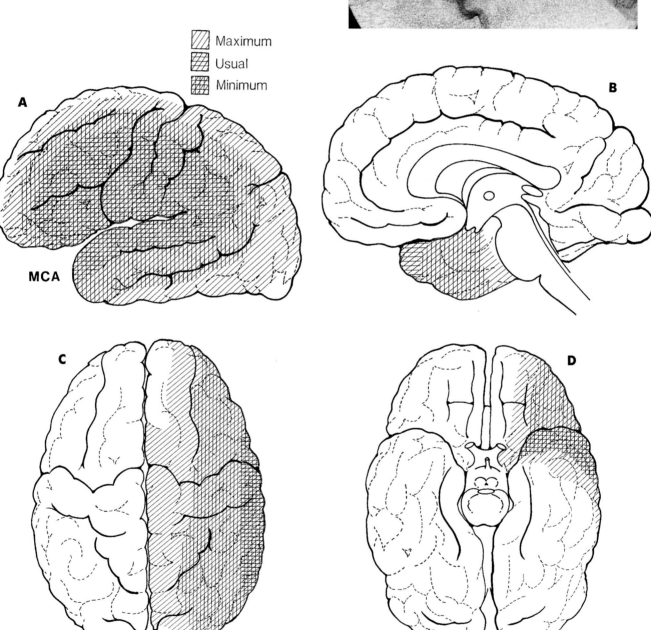

Fig. 6-28. Vascular territory of the MCA hemispheric branches with the maximum, usual, and minimum distributions as delineated by van der Zwan.[44] **A,** Lateral view; **B,** medial view; **C,** superior view; and **D,** base view.

all cerebral vascular distributions, including that of the MCA.[44] The usual, minimum, and maximum vascular territories supplied by MCA hemispheric branches are shown in Fig. 6-28.

Variants and anomalies. MCA anomalies are less frequently seen than variations in other major intracranial arteries. Fenestration, duplication, single-trunk, and accessory arteries are all uncommon, seen in less than 5% of cases.[51]

Posterior cerebral artery. In most cases the posterior cerebral arteries (PCAs) originate from the basilar artery bifurcation (Figs. 6-12 and 6-29). The major PCA segments and their branches are as follows.[51a]

Precommunicating (P1 or peduncular) segment. This short segment of the PCA extends laterally from its origin at the basilar bifurcation to its junction with the PCoA. **Posterior thalamoperforating arteries** arise from the basilar bifurcation and P1 segments, then pass cephalad and dorsally to supply the diencephalon (thalamus) and midbrain[52] (Figs. 6-30, *B,* and 6-31, *B*). The **medial posterior choroidal artery** (MPChA) originates either from P1 or the proximal P2 segment and runs anteromedially along the roof of the third ventricle. It supplies the tectal (collicular) plate, part of the midbrain and posterior thalamus, pineal gland, and tela choroidea of the third ventricle (Figs. 6-30 and 6-31, *D*).

Ambient (P2) segment. This perimesencephalic

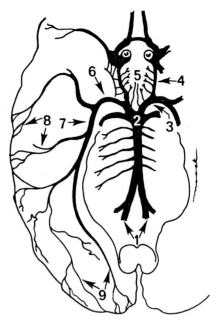

Fig. 6-29. Anatomic drawing of the base of brain showing the basilar artery, posterior cerebral arteries (PCAs), and circle of Willis. *1,* Vertebral arteries. *2,* Basilar artery. *3,* P1 segment of PCA. *4,* Posterior communicating artery. *5,* Small branches (thalamoperforating arteries) arise from the circle of Willis and basilar tip to supply base of brain. *6,* P2 PCA segment. *7,* P3 PCA segment. *8,* Temporal branches of PCA. *9,* Occipital branches with calcarine artery *(medial arrow).* (From Osborn AG: *Handbook of Neuroradiology,* Mosby–Year Book, 1991.)

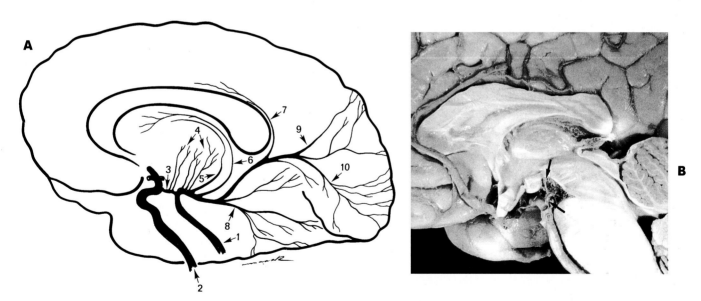

Fig. 6-30. A, Anatomic drawing of the medial cerebral hemisphere surface showing the PCA and its branches. *1,* Basilar artery. *2,* ICA. *3,* PCoA. *4,* Thalamoperforating arteries. *5,* Medial posterior choroidal artery. *6,* Lateral posterior choroidal artery. *7,* Splenial artery. *8,* Posterior temporal artery. *9,* Posterior parietal artery. *10,* Occipital artery. **B,** Midline anatomic dissection shows thalamoperforating branches *(arrows)* arising from the basilar artery bifurcation and proximal PCAs to supply the midbrain. (**A,** From Osborn AG: *Handbook of Neuroradiology,* Mosby–Year Book, 1991. **B,** From Bassett DL: *A Stereoscopic Atlas of Human Anatomy,* section 1: the central nervous system. Courtesy Bassett Collection, R. Chase (curator), Stanford University.)

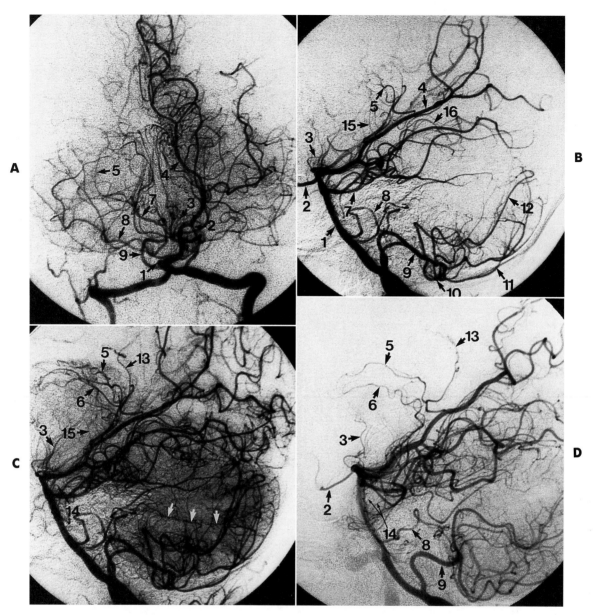

Fig. 6-31. AP **(A)** and lateral early **(B)** and late arterial phase **(C)** digital subtraction vertebral angiograms show the posterior cerebral artery and posterior fossa vasculature. The right posterior cerebral artery is not visualized because it has a "fetal" origin from the ipsilateral internal carotid artery (*see* Fig. 6-49). The great horizontal fissure of the cerebellum is shown (**C,** *white arrows*). **D,** Lateral vertebral angiogram in another patient shows the choroidal and posterior splenial arteries particularly well. *1,* Basilar artery (BA). *2,* Posterior communicating artery (PCoA). *3,* Posterior thalamoperforating arteries. *4,* Posterior cerebral artery (PCA). *5,* Lateral posterior choroidal artery (LPChA). *6,* Medial posterior choroidal artery (MPChA). *7,* Superior cerebellar arteries (SCA). *8,* Anterior inferior cerebellar artery (AICA). *9,* Posterior inferior cerebellar artery (PICA). *10,* Tonsillar branches of PICA. *11,* Hemispheric branches of PICA. *12,* Inferior vermian branches of PICA. *13,* Splenial branch of PCA. *14,* Pontine perforating BA branches. *15,* Thalamogeniculate branches of PCA. *16,* Superior vermian branches of SCA.

segment extends from the PCA-PCoA junction posteriorly around the midbrain, coursing above the trochlear nerve and tentorial incisura. Its major branch is the **lateral posterior choroidal artery** (LPChA). The LPChA can originate either from P2 or proximal cortical branches. The LPChA courses over the pulvinar of the thalamus and supplies the posterior thalamus and lateral ventricular choroid plexus (Figs. 6-30 and 6-31, *D*). The MPChAs, LPChAs, and AChAs anastomose with each other and have reciprocal vascular territories (*see* Fig. 6-11).[23,53]

Thalamogeniculate arteries (TGAs) arise from the

crural (ambient, or P2) PCA segment and supply the medial geniculate body, pulvinar, brachium of the superior colliculus, crus cerebri, and, occasionally, the lateral geniculate body (Fig. 6-31, *B* and *C*).[54]

Quadrigeminal (P3) segment. This segment of the PCA runs behind the midbrain within the quadrigeminal plate cistern (Fig. 6-29). **Inferior temporal arteries** supply the undersurface of the temporal lobe in reciprocal relationship with temporal branches of the MCA. The **parietooccipital artery** supplies the posterior one third of the interhemispheric surface in reciprocal relationship with the ACA branches. Part of the posterolateral cortex can also be supplied by this PCA branch. The **calcarine artery** supplies the occipital pole and visual cortex. **Posterior pericallosal**

(splenial) arteries supply the splenium of the corpus callosum and anastomose with their counterparts from the ACA (Figs. 6-30 and 6-31, *D*).[50]

Vascular distribution. Vascular distribution of the PCA is quite variable because its branches share reciprocal relationships with the MCA (particularly in the temporal lobe), ACA, and AChA.[44] In the most common situation, the medial and superior boundary between the PCA and the ACA is located in the parietooccipital sulcus. From the lateral view, the PCA area of supply typically extends on a line through the inferior temporal gyrus.[44] The usual, minimum, and maximum vascular territories of the PCA and its branches are depicted on Figs. 6-16 and 6-32.

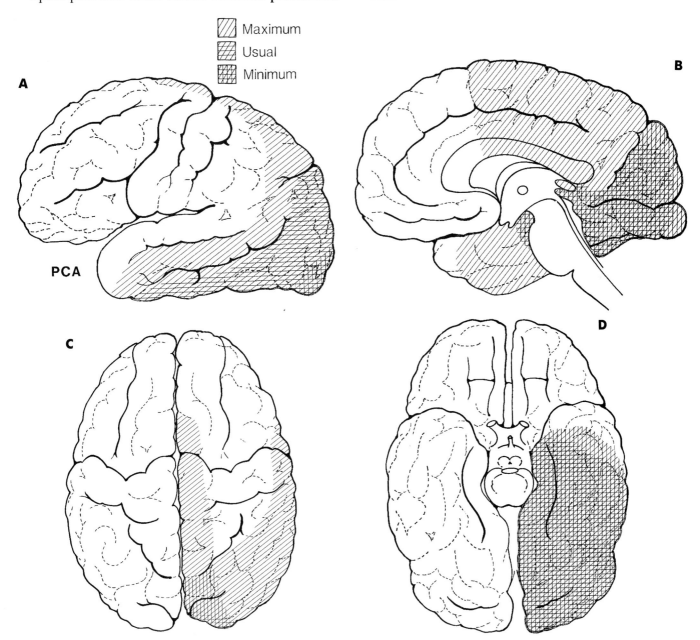

Fig. 6-32. Vascular distribution of the PCA cortical branches with maximum, usual, and minimum territories as delineated by van der Zwan.[44]

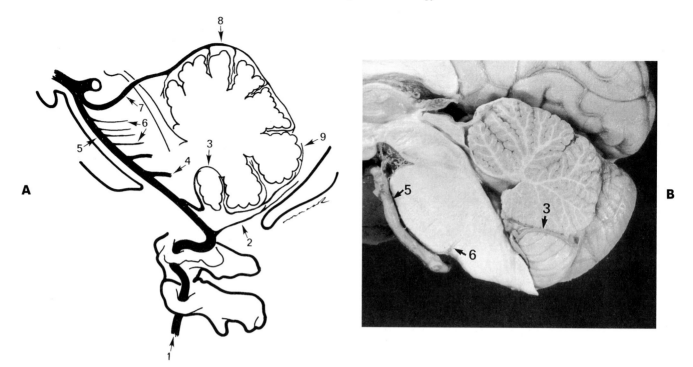

Fig. 6-33. A, Lateral anatomic drawing of the infratentorial arteries. **B,** Anatomic dissection of the posterior fossa vasculature, midline lateral view, shows the superior vermian artery and the posterior inferior cerebellar artery with its inferior vermian branches. *1,* Vertebral artery. *2,* Posterior meningeal artery. *3,* Posterior inferior cerebellar artery. *4,* Anterior inferior cerebellar artery (cut off). *5,* Basilar artery. *6,* Pontine perforating branches. *7,* Superior cerebellar artery. *8,* Superior vermian artery. *9,* Inferior vermian artery. (**A,** From Osborn AG: *Handbook of Neuroradiology,* Mosby-Year Book, 1991. **B,** From Bassett DL: *A Stereoscopic Atlas of Human Anatomy,* section 1: the central nervous system. Courtesy Bassett Collection, R. Chase (curator), Stanford University.)

Variants and anomalies. **Fetal origin of the PCA** from the ICA instead of the basilar artery is the most common anomaly, seen in 15% to 20% of cases (*see* Fig. 6-21, *C*). **Carotid-basilar anastomoses** may also result in the carotid system, supplying the PCA via a trigeminal artery or other persistent embryonic anastomotic vessel (see previous discussion).

Posterior Fossa Arteries

Vertebral arteries. The vertebral arteries (VAs) usually originate from their respective subclavian arteries; the left VA is usually the dominant vessel (50% to 60% of cases).[55] The VAs course cephalad to enter the transverse foramina, typically at C6. They ascend directly to C2 where they turn laterally, then superiorly, through the C1 vertebral foramina (Fig. 6-33, *A*). After looping posteriorly along the atlas, each VA passes superomedially through the foramen magnum. Within the posterior fossa, usually anterior to the medulla, the VAs unite to form the basilar artery (Fig. 6-34; *see* Fig. 6-12, *A* and *B*).[56]

Extracranial VA branches. Numerous small segmental spinal, meningeal, and muscular branches arise from the VA. Abundant anastomoses between VA and ECA muscular, thyrocervical, and, sometimes, costocervical branches are present (*see* box). The **posterior meningeal artery** (PMA) usually arises from the VA as it courses along the posterior arch of the atlas. Occasionally the PMA may originate from the ECA (usually the occipital artery or ascending pharyngeal artery) or even the posterior inferior cerebellar artery.[57] The PMA supplies the falx cerebelli and can become greatly enlarged with dural vascular malformations or neoplasms (Fig. 10-24, *C*).

Intracranial VA branches. The **anterior spinal artery** joins with its homologue from the opposite VA and courses caudally for a variable distance in the anteromedial sulcus of the cervical cord.

The **posterior inferior cerebellar artery** (PICA) typically arises as a single trunk from the distal VA (Figs. 6-35 and 6-36).[58] The PICA has the following five segments (Fig. 6-35, *B,* and 6-36, *C*)[50]:

1. An anterior medullary segment in front of the medulla
2. A lateral medullary segment that courses alongside the medulla caudally to the level of CNs IX-XI

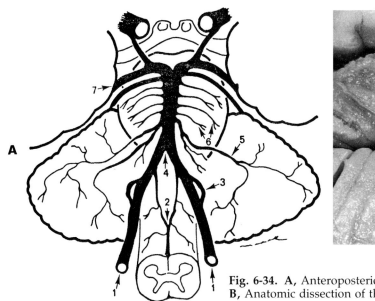

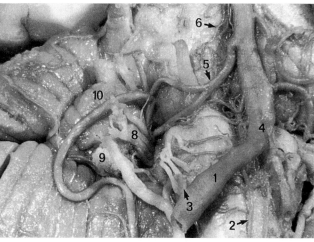

Fig. 6-34. A, Anteroposterior anatomic drawing of the vertebrobasilar circulation. **B,** Anatomic dissection of the posterior fossa vasculature, anterior view. *1,* Vertebral arteries. *2,* Anterior spinal arteries. *3,* posterior inferior cerebellar artery (PICA). *4,* Vertebral arteries unite to form basilar artery (BA). *5,* Anterior inferior cerebellar artery (AICA). *6,* Pontine perforating BA branches. *7,* Posterior cerebral arteries. *8,* Cranial nerves VII and VIII. *9,* Choroid plexus emerging from foramen of Luschka. *10,* Flocculus. (**A,** From Osborn AG: *Handbook of Neuroradiology,* Mosby-Year Book, 1991. **B,** From Bassett DL: *A Stereoscopic Atlas of Human Antomy,* section 1: the central nervous system. Courtesy Bassett Collection, R. Chase (curator), Standord University.)

3. A tonsillomedullary segment that courses around the inferior half of the cerebellar tonsil
4. A telovelotonsillar segment in the cleft between the tela choroidea and inferior medullary velum rostrally and the superior pole of the tonsil caudally
5. Cortical or hemispheric branches

PICA branches supply the choroid plexus of the fourth ventricle (Fig. 6-35, *B*), posterolateral medulla, cerebellar tonsil, inferior vermis, and posteroinferior surface of the cerebellar hemisphere (Fig. 6-35, *C*).[59,59a]

Variants and anomalies. Persistent embryonic carotid-vertebral anastomoses were discussed previously. In 5% of cases the left VA has an aortic arch origin. A hypoplastic VA is common, seen in up to 40% of normal angiograms[60] (Fig. 6-36). In 1% of cases the VA terminates in the PICA. VA duplication or fenestration occasionally occurs. There may be an increased incidence of associated aneurysms and vascular malformations in some cases[61] (Fig. 9-4).

Numerous anomalous origins of the PICA have been reported.[62,63] One of the most common is an extracranial PICA origin from the VA. In these cases the PICA arises below the foramen magnum. Anomalous PICAs are also associated with an increased incidence of intracranial aneurysms.[64]

Basilar artery. The right and left VAs unite to form the basilar artery (BA) (Fig. 6-34, *B*). The BA then courses cephalad in front of the pons and ter-

---

Extracranial to Intracranial Vascular Anastomoses

Maxillary artery to internal carotid artery (ICA) via:

  Middle meningeal artery to ethmoidal branches of ophthalmic artery
  Artery of the foramen rotundum to inferolateral trunk of ICA
  Accessory meningeal artery to inferolateral trunk
  Vidian artery to intratemporal ICA
  Anterior and middeep temporal arteries to ophthalmic artery via lacrimal, palpebral, or muscular branches

Occipital artery to vertebral artery (via muscular and radicular branches of the first and second cervical segments)

Ascending pharyngeal artery to vertebral artery (via musculospinal branches) at C3 level

Ascending pharyngeal artery to internal carotid artery (via petrous and cavernous branches)

Facial artery to internal carotid artery (via angular branch of facial to orbital branches of ophthalmic artery)

Posterior auricular artery to internal carotid artery (via stylomastoid artery)

Extracranial-intracranial surgical bypass (typically superficial temporal or occipital artery to middle cerebral)

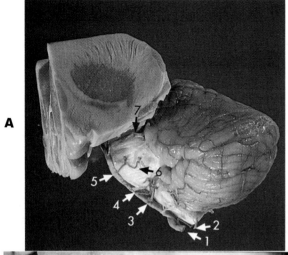

A

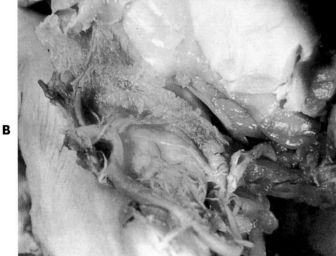

B

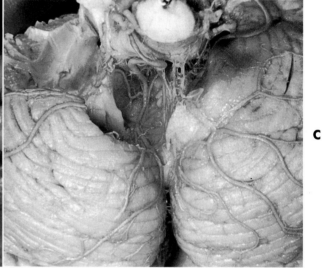

C

Fig. 6-35. Anatomic dissections demonstrate the posterior fossa vasculature. Same key as Fig. 6-33. **A,** Lateral view of the major posterior fossa vessels. **B** and **C,** Posterior inferior cerebellar artery (PICA) and its branches. **B,** Close-up view of the dissected PICA. The basilar artery has been removed. The five PICA segments plus branches to the choroid plexus of the fourth ventricle, medulla, and vermis tonsil are demonstrated. Compare with Fig. 6-36, *C.* **C,** Inferior view of the cerebellar hemispheres with the tonsil removed shows PICA and its hemispheric branches. (From Bassett DL: *A Stereoscopic Atlas of Human Anatomy,* section 1: the central nervous system. Courtesy Bassett Collection, R. Chase (curator), Stanford University.)

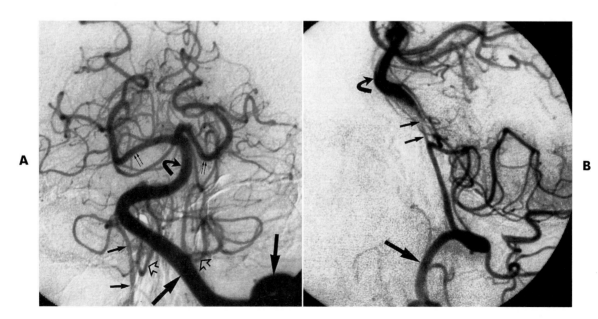

A

B

Fig. 6-36. For legend see p. 145.

Fig. 6-36, cont'd. A, Digital subtraction left vertebral angiogram, arterial phase, AP view. The left VA *(large arrows)* is dominant. The basilar artery *(curved arrow)* and its terminal branches, the two PCAs, are shown by the double arrows. Both PICAs are opacified *(open arrows)*. Contrast has refluxed into the hypoplastic distal right VA segment *(small arrows)*. **B,** Right vertebral angiogram, midarterial phase, lateral view, shows a small right VA *(large arrow)* and a hypoplastic distal VA segment *(small arrows)* between the PICA origin and the basilar artery *(curved arrow)*. **C,** Late arterial phase demonstrates small right VA *(large arrow)* and the five PICA segments: *1,* anterior medullary segment; *2,* lateral medullary segment; *3,* tonsillomedullary (inferior) segment; *4,* telovelotonsillar segment; *5,* cortical and hemispheric branches. The hypoplastic distal VA segment is indicated by the small unnumbered arrow.

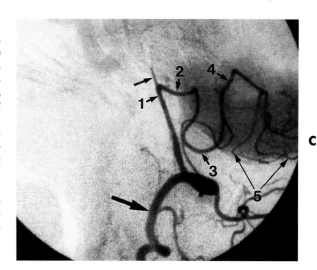

minates in the interpeduncular cistern by dividing into the posterior cerebral arteries (Figs. 6-12, *B;* 6-34, *B;* and 6-36, *A*).

The BA averages about 3 cm in length and 1.5 to 4 mm in width[17]; diameters greater than 4.5 mm should be considered abnormal.[65] The normal BA lies in the pontine cistern within a space delimited by the lateral margins of the clivus and dorsum sellae; extension beyond these confines indicates the presence of dolichoectasia.[65]

Branches. The first major branch of the BA is the **anterior inferior cerebellar artery** (AICA) (Figs. 6-31, 6-34, and 6-35, *A*). In 60% to 75% of cases the AICA arises from the BA as a single vessel.[66,67] The AICA courses posterolaterally within the cerebellopontine angle cistern toward the internal auditory canal (IAC). A few millimeters from its origin, the AICA is usually crossed by the abducens nerve (CN VI).[55] Near the IAC meatus, the AICA is typically anteroinferior to the facial and vestibulocochlear nerves (CNs VII and VIII).[67] The AICA supplies these nerves, as well as the inferolateral pons, middle cerebellar peduncle, flocculus, and anterolateral (petrosal) surface of the cerebellar hemisphere[59] (Fig. 6-16).

The **superior cerebellar arteries** (SCAs) arise near the BA apex and curve posterolaterally around the pons and mesencephalon below the tentorial incisura and CNs III and IV (Figs. 6-31 and 6-33). The SCAs supply the entire superior surface of the vermis and cerebellar hemispheres (Fig. 6-35, *A*), as well as much of the deep cerebellar white matter and dentate nuclei (Fig. 6-16).[59,68]

Short and long segment circumflex **perforating branches** arise along the entire length of the BA, although the majority are found in its cephalic portion (Figs. 6-31; 6-33, *A;* and 6-34, *A*).[55, 68a] These supply the ventral pons and rostral brainstem.[52] The BA terminates by dividing into the paired **posterior cerebral**

arteries (PCAs). The vascular territories supplied by the basilar pontine perforating branches, AICA, PICA, and the SCAs are depicted in Fig. 6-16.

Variations and anomalies. Persistent embryonic carotid-vertebrobasilar anastomoses have already been described. SCAs can arise from the PCA or even directly from the ICA. If the PCA has a fetal origin, the distal BA may be hypoplastic. Occasionally a fenestrated BA can be identified and is associated with an increased incidence of saccular aneurysms. Other anomalies are very uncommon.

VENOUS ANATOMY

The cerebral venous system is composed of dural sinuses and superficial cortical and deep (medullary white matter and subependymal) veins (Fig. 6-37). The venous vasculature is much more variable than its arterial counterpart.

Dural Sinuses

Superior sagittal sinus. The superior sagittal sinus (SSS) is a midline structure situated in-between the inner table of the skull superiorly and the leaves of the falx cerebri laterally. It is lined by endothelium that is continuous with that of the superficial cortical veins, most of which are between 0.1 and 1 mm in diameter (Fig. 6-37, *B*).[69] There are no valves in the SSS.

The SSS typically originates near the crista galli anteriorly and extends posteriorly to its confluence with the straight and lateral sinuses (Figs. 6-37, *A* and 6-38, *B*). The rostral aspect of the SSS may be hypoplastic or atretic (Fig. 6-39). In such cases, substitute intradural venous channels course posteriorly in the parasagittal region, receiving prominent tributaries from the cerebral cortex. This anomaly is seen in 6% to 7% of cases and should not be mistaken for pathologic occlusion.[70]

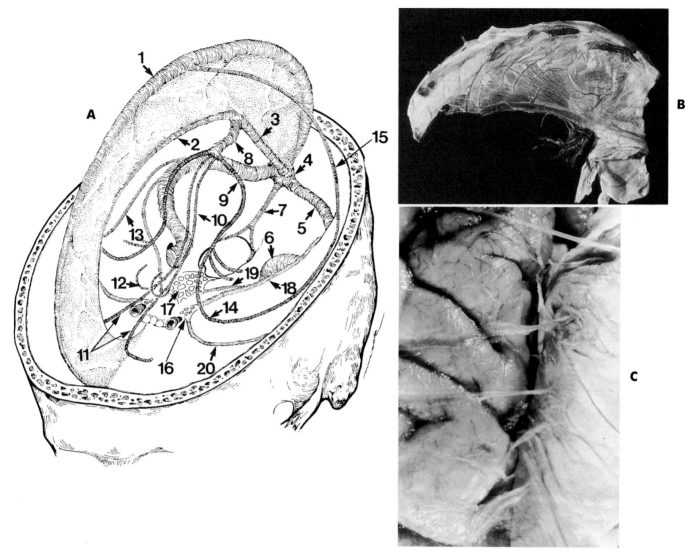

Fig. 6-37. A, Anatomic diagram of the cerebral venous system. *1.* Superior sagittal sinus (SSS). *2.* Inferior sagittal sinus (ISS). *3.* Straight sinus (SS). *4.* Torcular herophili (sinus confluence). *5.* Transverse sinus (TS). *6.* Sigmoid sinus. *7.* Occipital sinus (OS). *8.* Vein of Galen. *9.* Basal vein of Rosenthal (BVR). *10.* Internal cerebral veins (ICVs). *11.* Septal veins. *12.* Thalamostriate veins (TSVs). *13.* Vein of Labbe. *14.* Superficial middle cerebral vein (SMCV). *15.* Vein of Trolard. *16.* Cavernous sinus. *17.* Clival venous plexus. *18.* Superior petrosal sinus (SPS). *19.* Inferior petrosal sinus (IPS). *20.* Sphenoparietal sinus. **B,** Autopsy specimen with falx cerebri and tentorium cerebelli shows the major dural sinuses. **C,** Close-up view of the cortical veins as they cross the subdural space to enter the SSS. (**B,** Courtesy E. Tessa Hedley-Whyte. **C,** Courtesy E. Ross.)

Inferior sagittal sinus. The inferior sagittal sinus (ISS) is an inconstantly identified channel that runs in the inferior free margin of the falx cerebri. The ISS joins with the vein of Galen to form the straight sinus (Figs. 6-37; 6-38, *A;* and 6-40).

Straight sinus. The straight sinus (SS) is enclosed by the confluence of dura from the falx cerebri and tentorium cerebelli (Fig. 6-37 and 6-40, *A*). In most cases a line drawn along the SS is tangential to the upper aspect of the splenium of the corpus callo-

sum.[71] The SS courses backward and downward toward its confluence with the SSS, where they form the torcular Herophili (confluens sinuum) (Fig. 6-40, *B* and *C*).

The SS may be hypoplastic or absent. In such cases an accessory falcine sinus is usually present.

Transverse and occipital sinuses. The venous confluence (torcular Herophili) divides into the transverse (lateral) and occipital sinuses (Fig. 6-37, *A*). The transverse sinuses course laterally around the tento-

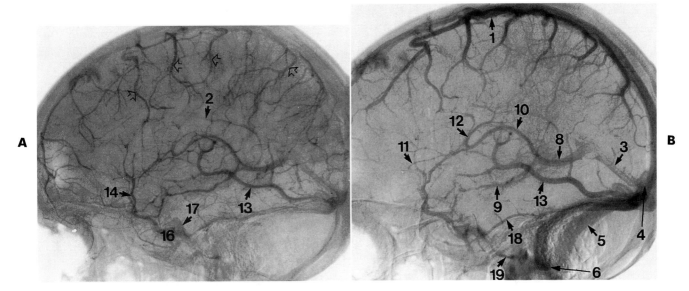

Fig. 6-38. Left internal carotid angiogram, early **(A)** and late **(B)** venous phases, lateral view. The early phase shows the superficial cortical veins well; the later venous phase shows the subependymal veins and dural sinuses. Some of the unnamed superficial cortical veins are indicated by the *open arrows*. Same key as Fig. 6-37.

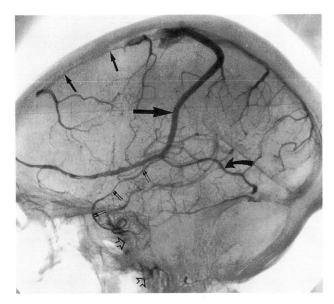

Fig. 6-39. Right internal carotid angiogram, venous phase, lateral view, showing hypoplasia of the rostral superior sagittal sinus *(small arrows)*. A very large anastomotic vein of Trolard is present *(large arrow)*. This is a normal anatomic variant and should not be mistaken for dural sinus thrombosis. Prominent drainage into the pterygoid and deep facial venous plexuses is indicated by the open arrows. A small vein of Labbé is shown *(curved arrow)*. The superficial middle cerebral veins are indicated by double arrows.

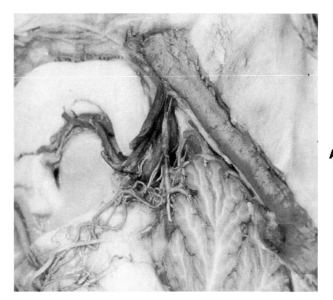

Fig. 6-40. A, Anatomic dissection showing the internal cerebral vein, vein of Galen, and inferior and superior sagittal sinuses as seen from behind. (**A**, From Bassett DL: *A Stereoscopic Atlas of Human Anatomy*, section 1: the central nervous system. Courtesy Bassett Collection, R. Chase (curator), Stanford University.) *Continued.*

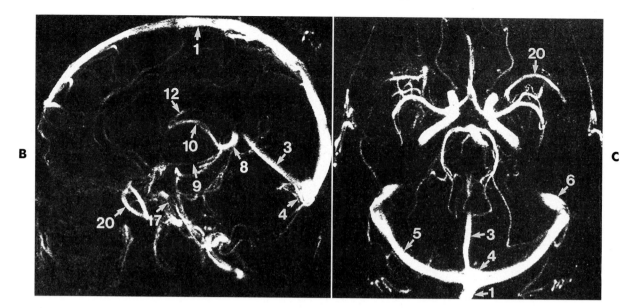

Fig. 6-40, cont'd. Phase contrast MRA study with lateral (**B**) and submentovertex (**C**) views shows the deep cerebral veins and major dural sinuses. Same key as Fig. 6-37.

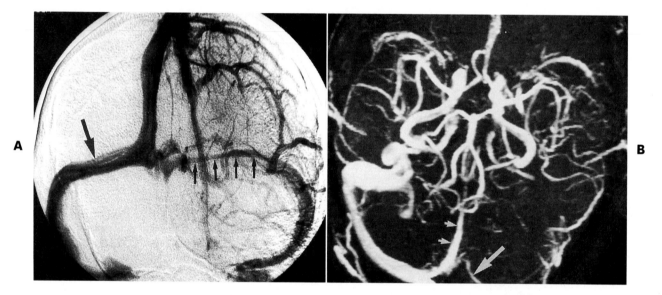

Fig. 6-41. Variations in transverse sinus (TS) anatomy are illustrated by these two cases. **A,** Digital subtraction left internal carotid angiogram, venous phase, AP view. The right TS is dominant *(large arrow)* and the left TS is hypoplastic *(small arrows)*. **B,** Multiple overlapping thin slab MR angiogram shows a hypoplastic left TS *(large arrow)* and a very prominent occipital sinus *(small arrows)*.

rial attachment to the calvarium. In half the cases the transverse sinuses (TS) are well formed bilaterally and the occipital sinus (OS) is rudimentary or absent.

Asymmetry of the TSs is common (50% to 80% of cases); the right TS is usually the dominant drainage pattern (Fig. 6-41, *A*). Agenesis of part or all of a TS occurs in 1% to 5% of cases and should not be mistaken for dural sinus occlusion. In such instances the OS may appear very prominent[72] (Fig. 6-41, *B*). The

OS courses anteroinferiorly from the torcular to the foramen magnum.

Tentorial sinuses. Numerous tentorial sinuses drain into the dural sinuses near the torcular herophili and may appear quite prominent on contrast-enhanced CT or MR studies (Fig. 6-42). These venous channels may provide significant drainage for the adjacent cerebellar hemispheres and cerebellum.[73] They

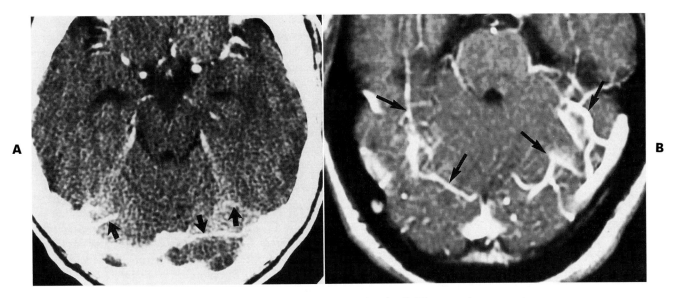

Fig. 6-42. Axial postcontrast CT **(A)** and T1-weighted MR **(B)** scans show prominent tentorial sinuses *(arrows)*, a normal finding.

can also become enlarged significantly if the SS or SSS is occluded (*see* Chapter 11).

Sigmoid sinuses. Near the posterolateral wall of the petrous temporal bone the TSs turn inferiorly to form the sigmoid sinuses. The sigmoid sinuses continue inferiorly into the jugular bulb at the skull base, where they are joined by the inferior petrosal sinus and tributaries from the clival venous plexus.

Cavernous sinuses. The cavernous sinuses are complex multiseptated laterosellar extradural venous spaces. A true venous "cavernous" sinus, i.e., one in

which a large blood-filled channel extends from the lateral wall of the cavernous sinus to the sella and completely surrounds the intracavernous cranial nerves and internal carotid artery, is uncommon.[74] The cavernous sinus is usually a highly variable collection of venous channels. The ICA and cranial nerves III, IV, V1 and V2, and VI either course within the sinus itself or are contained in its lateral dural wall (Fig. 6-43).

The cavernous sinuses receive the superior and inferior ophthalmic veins and communicate with each other via intercavernous sinuses. They also communicate posteriorly with the periclival venous plexus,

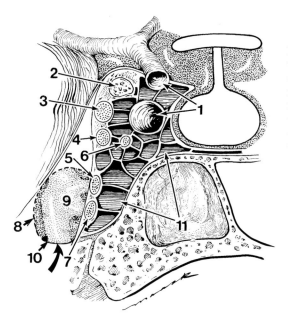

Fig. 6-43. Anatomic diagram of the cavernous sinus, AP view. Note the multiseptated venous channels. Meckel's cave, a diverticulum of dura and cerebrospinal fluid that invaginates into the cavernous sinus around the trigeminal nerve, is shown by dotted lines. Note that Meckel's cave is therefore a continuation of the posterior fossa subarachnoid space that is covered by the dura and venous channels of the cavernous sinus. *1,* Internal carotid artery (cut across). *2,* Anterior clinoid process. *3,* CN III (oculomotor). *4,* CN IV (trochlear). *5,* CN V1 (ophthalmic division, trigeminal nerve). *6,* CN VI (abducens nerve). *7,* CN V2 (maxillary division, trigeminal nerve). *8,* Meckel's cave. *9,* Gasserian (semilunar or trigeminal) ganglion. *10,* CN V3 (mandibular division, trigeminal nerve). Note that CN V3 exits Meckel's cave inferiorly through the foramen ovale *(curved black arrow)* and technically does not traverse the cavernous sinus. *11,* Septated venous channels that comprise the cavernous sinus.

superolaterally with the sigmoid sinus via the superior petrosal sinus, inferiorly with the jugular bulb via the inferior petrosal sinuses and deep facial veins via the pterygoid venous plexus, and laterally with venous sinuses along the sphenoid wing (Figs. 6-37 and 6-38).

Cerebral Veins

The cerebral veins are typically divided into two basic groups: superficial (cortical) veins and deep veins. These will be considered briefly and followed by a discussion of posterior fossa venous anatomy.

Superifical cortical veins. These are usually quite small and highly variable. Near the vertex these veins cross the potential subdural space to enter the SSS (Figs. 6-37 and 6-38, *A*). At this point they are subject to rupture and spontaneous or traumatic hemorrhage.

Most of the superficial cortical veins are unnamed, although the following three are often identified:
1. **Superficial middle cerebral vein** (which runs along the sylvian fissure)
2. **Vein of Trolard** (a large anastomotic cerebral vein that courses cephalad from the sylvian fissure to the SSS)
3. **Vein of Labbe** (this vessel courses posterolaterally from the sylvian fissure to the transverse sinus)

Deep cerebral veins. The deep cerebral veins include medullary veins, subependymal veins, the basal veins, and the vein of Galen.

Medullary veins. The subcortical and deep white matter are drained by medullary veins that originate 1 to 2 cm below the cortex and course centrally toward the subependymal veins surrounding the cerebral ventricles. These medullary veins may become enlarged in vascular malformations, vascular neoplasms, and as a collateral venous drainage channel. The perivascular spaces that surround the medullary veins may also become quite prominent.

Subependymal veins. The subependymal veins surround the lateral ventricles and receive venous blood from the medullary veins of the centrum semiovale. Several subependymal veins are named. Among them are the **thalamostriate vein** (which courses over the caudate nucleus) and the **septal vein** (which courses posteriorly from the frontal horn along the septum pellucidum). These two veins join, typically near the foramen of Monro, to form the **internal cerebral vein** (ICV). The ICVs are paired paramedian structures that run posteriorly in the velum interpositum just above the roof of the third ventricle.

The deep cerebral veins are easily identified on late venous phase cerebral angiograms (Fig. 6-38, *B*), as well as contrast-enhanced CT or MR scans (Fig. 6-44) and MR angiograms (Fig. 6-40).[75,76]

Basal veins. The ICVs receive prominent tributaries from the medial temporal lobes, the **basal veins of Rosenthal** (BVRs). The BVRs course posterosuperiorly in the ambient cisterns and, with the ICVs, form the vein of Galen (Fig. 6-44, *A*).

Vein of Galen. The vein of Galen (great cerebral

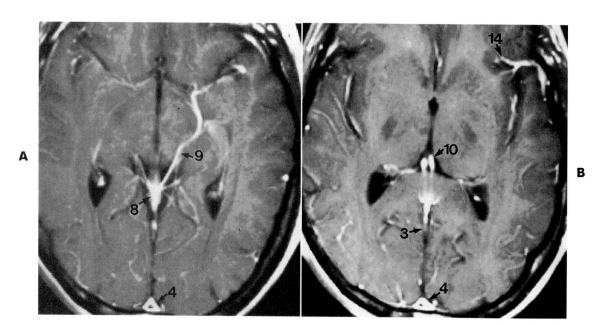

Fig. 6-44. A to **C,** Axial postcontrast T1-weighted MR scans show normal deep subependymal veins. Same key as Fig. 6-57.

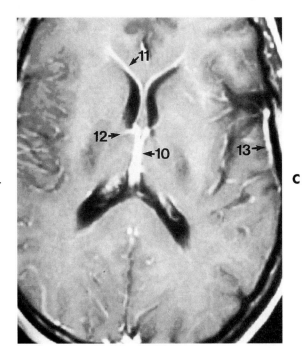

Fig. 6-44, cont'd. For legend see p. 150.

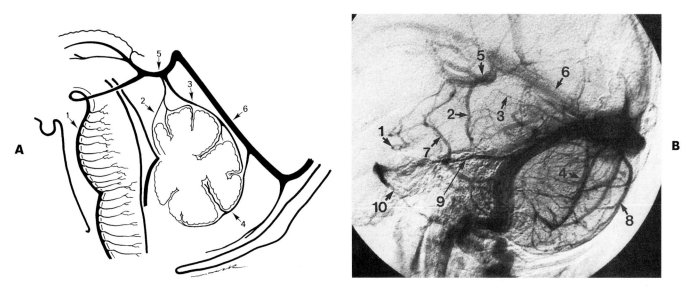

Fig. 6-45. A, Lateral anatomic drawing of the major posterior fossa veins. **B,** Digital subtraction left vertebral angiogram, venous phase, lateral view, depicts the posterior fossa veins. *1,* Anterior pontomesencephalic veins. *2,* Precentral cerebellar vein. *3,* Superior vermian vein. *4,* Inferior vermian vein. *5,* Vein of Galen. *6,* Straight sinus. *7,* Lateral mesencephalic vein (not shown). *8,* Cerebellar hemispheric veins (not shown). *9,* Superior petrosal sinus (not shown). *10,* Clival venous plexus (not shown). (**A,** From Osborn AG: *Handbook of Neuroradiology,* Mosby-Year Book, 1991).

vein) is a prominent venous channel that curves posteriorly under the splenium of the corpus callosum. The vein of Galen and the inferior sagittal sinus unite to form the straight sinus. The ICVs and dural sinuses are particularly well visualized on phase contrast MRA (Fig. 6-40, *B*).

Posterior fossa veins (Fig. 6-45). The **anterior pontomesencephalic vein** is actually a plexus of numerous small veins that lie along the surface of the pons and mesencephalon. The **precentral cerebellar vein** lies in front of the cerebellar vermis just above and behind the roof of the fourth ventricle. **Superior** and **inferior vermian veins** drain the cerebellar vermis; **hemispheric veins** drain the hemispheres. Vermian and hemispheric veins are tributaries of the tentorial sinuses, as well as the straight and transverse sinuses.

REFERENCES

1. Osborn AG: *Introduction to Cerebral Angiography*, pp 33-48. Harper and Row, Hagerstown, 1980.
2. Zamir M, Sinclair P: Origin of the brachiocephalic trunk, left carotid and left subclavian arteries from the arch of the human aorta, *Invest Radiol* 26:128-133, 1991.
3. Wasserman BA, Mikulis DJ, Manzione JV: Origin of the right vertebral artery from the left side of the aortic arch proximal to the origin of the left subclavian artery, *AJNR* 13:355-358, 1992.
4. Morimoto T, Nitta K, Kazekawa K, Hashizume K: The anomaly of a non-bifurcating cervical carotid artery, *J Neurosurg* 72:130-132, 1990.
5. Lambiase RE, Haas RA, Carney WI Jr, Ragg J: Anomalous branching of the left common carotid artery with associated atheroscleratic changes: a case report, *AJNR* 12:187-189, 1991.
6. Lasjaunias PL, Choi IS: The external carotid artery: functional anatomy. *Riv de Neuroradiol* 4(Suppl 1):39-45, 1991.
7. Russell EJ: Functional angiography of the head and neck, *AJNR* 7:927-936, 1986.
8. Kerber CW, Heilman CB: Flow dynamics: the internal carotid artery: I. Preliminary observations using a transparent elastic model, *AJNR* 13:173-180, 1992.
9. Sesana WE, Oliveira CA: Internal carotid artery simulating a middle ear mass, *Ann Otol Rhinol Laryngol* 102:71-73, 1993.
10. Pahor AL, Hussain SSM: Persistent stapedial artery, *J Laryngol Otr* 106:254-257, 1992.
11. Guinto FC Jr, Garrabrant EC, Radcliffe WB: Radiology of the presistent stapedial artery, *Radiol* 105:365-369, 1972.
12. Brant-Zawadzki M: Routine MR imaging of the internal carotid artery siphon: angiographic correlation with cervical carotid lesions, *ANJR* 11:467-471, 1990.
13. Tran-Dinh H: Cavernous branches of the internal carotid artery: anatomy and nomenclature, *Neurosurg* 20:205-210, 1987.
14. Capo H, Kupersmith MJ, Berenstein A et al: The clinical importance of the inferolateral trunk of the internal carotid artery, *Neurosurg* 28:773-778, 1991.
15. Gibo H, Kobayashi SH, Kyoshima K, Hokama M: Microsurgical anatomy of the arteries of the pituitary stalk and gland as reviewed from above, *Acta Neurochirurgica* (Wien) 90:60-66, 1988.
16. Decaminada N, Hacker H: Masse sellari e parasellari non di origine ipofisaria, *Riv di Neuroradiol* 4:313-321, 1991.
17. Saeki N, Rhoton AL Jr: Microsurgical anatomy of the upper basilar artery and the posterior circle of Willis, *J Neurosurg* 46:563-578, 1977.
18. Bisaria K: Anomalies of the posterior communicating artery and their potential clinical significance, *J Neurosurg* 60:572-576, 1984.
19. Moyer DJ, Flamm ES: Anomalous arrangement of the origins of the anterior choroidal and posterior communicating arteries, *J Neurosurg* 76:1017-1018, 1992.
20. Marinkovic SV, Milisavljevic MM, Vuckovic VD: Microvascular anatomy of the uncus and the parahippocampal gyrus, *Neurosurg* 29:809-814, 1991.
21. Hodes JE, Aymard A, Casasco A et al: Embolization of arteriovenous malformations of the temporal lobe via the anterior choroidal artery, *ANJR* 12:779-780, 1991.
22. Mohr JP, Steinke W, Timsit SG et al: The anterior choroidal artery does not supply the corona radiata and lateral ventricular wall, *Stroke* 22:1502-1507, 1991.
23. Fujii K, Lenkey C, Rhoton AL Jr: Microsurgical anatomy of the choroidal arteries: Lateral and third ventricles, *J Neurosurg* 52:165-188, 1980.
24. Dowd CF, Halbach VV, Barnwell SL et al: Particulate embolization of the anterior choroidal artery in the treatment of cerebral arteriovenous malformations, *AJNR* 12:1055-1061, 1991.

25. Takahashi S, Suga T, Kawata Y, Sakamoto K: Anterior choroidal artery: angiographic analysis of variations and anomalies, *AJNR* 11:719-729, 1990.
26. Napel S, Marks MP, Rubin GD et al: CT angiography with spiral CT and maximum intensity projection, *Radiol* 185:607-610, 1992.
26a. Marks MP, Napel S, Jordan JE, Enzmann DR: Diagnosis of carotid artery disease: preliminary experience with maximum-intensity-projection spiral CT, *AJR* 160:1267-1271, 1993.
26b. Dillon EH, van Leeuwen MS, Fernandez MA, Mali WPTM: Spiral CT angiography, *AJR* 160:1273-1278, 1993.
27. Huston J III, Ehman RL: Comparison of time-of-flight and phase-contrast MR neuroangiographic techniques, *Radio-Graphics* 13:9-19, 1993.
28. Davis WL, Warnock SH, Harnsberger HR et al: Intracranial MRA: Single volume vs. multiple thin slab 3D time-of-flight acquisition, *J Comp Asst Tomogr* 17:15-21, 1993.
29. Ross MR, Pelc NJ, Enzmann DR: Qualitative phase contrast MRA in the normal and abnormal circle of Willis, *AJNR* 14:19-25, 1993.
30. Haring HP, Rotzer HK, Reindl et al: Time course of cerebral blood flow velocity in central nervous system infections: a transcranial Doppler sonography study, *Arch Neurol* 50:98-101, 1993.
31. Pedroza A, Dujovny M, Artero JC et al: Microanatomy of the posterior communicating artery, *Neurosurg* 20:228-235, 1987.
32. Quint D, Silbergleit R: Congenital absence of the left internal carotid artery, *Radiol* 182:477-481, 1992.
33. Udzura M, Kobayashi H, Taguchi Y, Sekino H: Intrasellar intercarotid communicating artery associated with agenesis of the right internal carotid artery: case report, *Neurosurg* 23:770-773, 1988.
34. Reynolds AF Jr, Stovring J, Turner PT: Persistent otic artery, *Surg Neurol* 13:115-117, 1980.
35. Okada Y, Shima T, Nishida M et al: Bilateral persistent trigeminal arteries presenting with brain-stem infarction, *Neuroradiol* 34:283-286, 1992.
36. Silbergleit R, Mehta BA, Barnes RD II et al: Persistent trigeminal artery detected with standard MRI, *J Comp Asst Tomogr* 17:22-25, 1993.
37. Schuierer G, Laub G, Huk WJ: MR angiography of the persistent trigeminal artery: report on two cases, *AJNR* 11:1131-1132, 1990.
37a. Ohshiro S, Inoue T, Hamada Y, Matsuno H: Branches of the persistent primitive trigeminal artery: an autopsy case, *Neurosurg* 32:144-148, 1993.
38. Fortner AA, Smoker WRK: Persistent primitive trigeminal artery aneurysm evaluated by MR imaging and angiography, *J Comp Asst Tomogr* 12:847-850, 1988.
39. Kanai H, Nagai H, Wakabayashi S, Hashimoto N: A large aneurysm of the persistent primitive hypoglossal artery, *Neurosurg* 30:794-797, 1992.
40. Muller HR, Brunholz CHR, Radu EW, Buser M: Sex and side differences of cerebral arterial caliber, *Neuroradiol* 33:212-216, 1991.
41. Ghika JA, Bogousslavsky J, Regli F: Deep perforators from the carotid system, *Arch Neurol* 47:1097-1100, 1990.
42. Nathal E, Yasui N, Sampei T, Suzuki A: Intraoperative anatomical studies in patients with aneurysms of the anterior communicating artery complex, *J Neurosurg* 76:629-634, 1992.
43. Damasio H: A computed tomographic guide to the identification of cerebral vascular territories, *Arch Neurol* 40:138-142, 1983.
44. van der Zwan A, Hillen B, Tulleken CAF et al: Variability of the major cerebral arteries, *J Neurosurg* 77:927-940, 1992.
45. Vincentelli F, Lehman G, Caruso G et al: Extracerebral course of the perforating branches of the anterior communicating ar-

tery: microsurgical anatomical study, *Surg Neurol* 35:98-104, 1991.

46. Schick RM, Rumbaugh CL: Saccular aneurysm of the azygos anterior cerebral artery, *AJNR* 10:S73, 1989.

47. Cennamon J, Zito J, Chalif DJ et al: Aneurysm of the azygos pericallosal artery: diagnosis by MR imaging and MR angiography, *AJNR* 13:280-282, 1992.

48. Suzuki M, Onuma T, Sakurai Y et al: Aneurysms arising from the proximal (A1) segment of the anterior cerebral artery, *J Neurosurg* 76:455-458, 1992.

48a. Sanders WP, Sorek PA, Mehta BA: Fenestration of intracranial arteries with special attention to associated aneurysms and other anomalies, *AJNR* 14:675-680, 1993.

49. Berman SA, Hayman LA, Hinck VC: Correlation of CT cerebral vascular territories with function: 3. middle cerebral artery, *AJNR* 5:161-166, 1984.

50. Berman SA, Hayman LA, Hinck VC: Cerebrovascular territories. In LA Hayman: *Clinical Brain Imaging: Normal Structure and Functional Anatomy*, pp 402-416, Mosby-Year Book, St. Louis, 1992.

51. Vinansky F, Dujovny M, Ausman JI et al: Anomalies and variations of the middle cerebral artery: a microanatomical study, *Neurosurg* 22:1023-1027, 1988.

51a. Gerber CJ, Neil-Dwyer G, Evans BT: An alternative surgical approach to aneurysms of the posterior cerebral artery, *Neurosurg* 32:928-931, 1993.

52. Barkhoff F, Valk S: "Top of the basilar" syndrome: a comparison of clinical and MR findings, *Neuroradiol* 30:293-298, 1988.

53. Timurkaynak E, Rhoton AL Jr, Barry M: Microsurgical anatomy and operative approaches to the lateral ventricles, *Neurosurg* 19:689-723, 1986.

54. Milisavljevic MM, Marinkovic SV, Gibo H, Puskas LF: The thalamogeniculate perforators of the posterior cerebral artery: the microsurgical anatomy, *Neurosurg* 28:923-930, 1991.

55. Schronz C, Dujovny M, Ausman JI et al: Surgical anatomy of the arteries of the posterior fossa, *J Neurosurg* 65:540-544, 1986.

56. Osborn AG: Posterior fossa vasculature: In *Handbook of Neuroradiology*, pp 61-67. Year Book Medical Publishers, 1990.

57. Tanohata K, Maehara T, Noda M et al: Anamalous origin of the posterior meningial artery from the lateral medullary segment of the posterior inferior cerebellar artery, *Neuroradiol* 29:89-92, 1987.

58. Lister JR, Rhoton AL Jr, Matososhima T, Peace DA: Microsurgical anatomy of the posterior inferior cerebellar artery, *Neurosurg* 10:170-199, 1982.

59. Savoiardo M, Bracchi M, Passerini A, Visciana A: The vascular territories of the cerebellum and brainstem: CT and MR study, *AJNR* 8:199-209, 1987.

59a. Friedman DP: Abnormalities of the posterior inferior cerebellar artery: MR imaging findings, *AJR* 160:1259-1263, 1993.

60. Arnold V, Lehrmann R, Kursawe HK, Luckel W: Hypoplasia of vertebralasilar arteries, *Neuroradiol* 33(suppl):426-247, 1991.

61. Tran-Dinh HD, Soo YS, Jayasinghe LS: Duplication of the vertebrovasilar system, *Australian Radiol* 35:220-224, 1991.

62. Takasato Y, Hayashi H, Kobayashi T, Hashimoto Y: Duplicated origin of right vertebral artery with rudimentary and accessory left vertebral arteries, *Neuroradiol* 34:287-289, 1992.

63. Ahuja A, Graves VB, Crosby DL, Strothu CM: Anomalous origin of the posterior inferior cerebellar artery from the internal carotid artery, *AJNR* 13:1625-1626, 1992.

64. Manabe H, Oda N, Ishii M, Ishii A: The posterior inferior cerebellar artery originating from the internal carotid artery, associated with multiple aneurysms, *Neuroradiol* 33:513-515, 1991.

65. Smoker WRK, Price MJ, Keyes WD et al: High-resolution computed tomography of the basilar artery: I. normal size and position, *AJNR* 7:55-60, 1986.

66. Naidich TP, Kricheff II, George AE, Lin JP: The normal anterior inferior cerebellar artery, *Radiol* 119:355-373, 1976.

67. Martin RG, Grant JL, Peace D et al: Microsurgical relationships of the anterior inferior cerebellar artery and the facial-vestibulocochlear nerve complex, *Neurosurg* 6:483-507, 1980.

68. Cormier PJ, Long ER, Russell EJ: MR imaging of posterior fossa infarctions: vascular territories and clinical correlates, *RadioGraphics* 12:1079-1096, 1992.

68a. Marinkovic SV, Gibo H: The surgical anatomy of the perforating branches of the basilar artery, *Neurosurg* 33:80-87, 1993.

69. Anders BT, Dujovny M, Mirchandani HG, Ausman JI: Microsurgical anatomy of the venous drainage into the superior sagittal sinus, *Neurosurg* 24:514-520, 1989.

70. Kaplan HA, Brosder J: Atresia of the rostral superior sagittal sinus: substitute parasaggital venous channels, *J Neurosurg* 38:602-607, 1973.

71. Hasegawa M, Yamasita J, Yamashima T: Anatomical variation of the straight sinus on magnetic resonance imaging: the infratentorial suprasellar approach to pineal region tumors, *Surg Neurol* 36:354-359, 1991.

72. Dora F, Zileli T: Common variations of the lateral and occipital sinuses at the confluens sinuum, *Neuroradiol* 20:23-27, 1980.

73. Matsushima T, Suzuki SO, Fukui M et al: Microsurgical anatomy of the tentorial sinuses, *J Neurosurg* 71:923-928, 1989.

74. Bonneville JF, Catten F, Racle A et al: Dynamic CT of the laterosellar extradural venous spaces, *AJNR* 10:535-542, 1989.

75. Mattle HP, Wentz KU, Edelman RR et al: Cerebral venography with MR, *Radiol* 178:453-458, 1991.

76. Chakeres DW, Schmalbrock P, Brogan M et al: Normal venous anatomy of the brain: demonstration with gadopentetate dimeglumine in enhanced 3-D MR angiography, *AJNR* 11:1107-1118, 1991.

Intracranial Hemorrhage

Intracranial hemorrhage (ICH) is a common cause of acute neurologic deterioration and a frequent indication for emergent neuroimaging. Because ICH also complicates the presentation and appearance of many CNS lesions, it is important to understand the pathophysiology and imaging of intracerebral blood clots before discussing the lesions themselves.

In this chapter we first review thrombosis, clot formation, and the evolution of ICH. Factors that influence the CT and MR appearance of acute, subacute, and chronic hemorrhage are then delineated. Finally we briefly discuss the major nontraumatic causes of intracranial hemorrhage and their imaging spectra.

Traumatic brain injury and the secondary effects of head injury are discussed in the following chapter (Chapter 8).

PATHOPHYSIOLOGY OF INTRACRANIAL HEMORRHAGE
Origin of Bleeding

Intracerebral hemorrhage (ICH) is commonly arterial in origin, arising not only from the primary arterial site but also from smaller vessels around the expanding hematoma margin.[1] Cortical veins and dural sinuses are less common sources of ICH.

Thrombosis, Clot Formation, and Hemorrhage Evolution

Thrombosis and clot formation are complex dynamic processes in which gross structure and macroscopic composition of thrombi change with time. Physiologic processes such as clot retraction, cellular infiltration, and fibrinolysis[2] plus red blood cell morphology, hemoglobin denaturation, and the development of blood degradation products interact to affect the MR appearance of ICH (Fig. 7-1, *A*).

Immediate effects of hemorrhage. An intracerebral hematoma is initially liquid, composed of 95% to 98% oxygen-saturated hemoglobin.[3] Within seconds after loss of vessel integrity, platelet thrombi form and erythrocyte aggregation in the extravasated

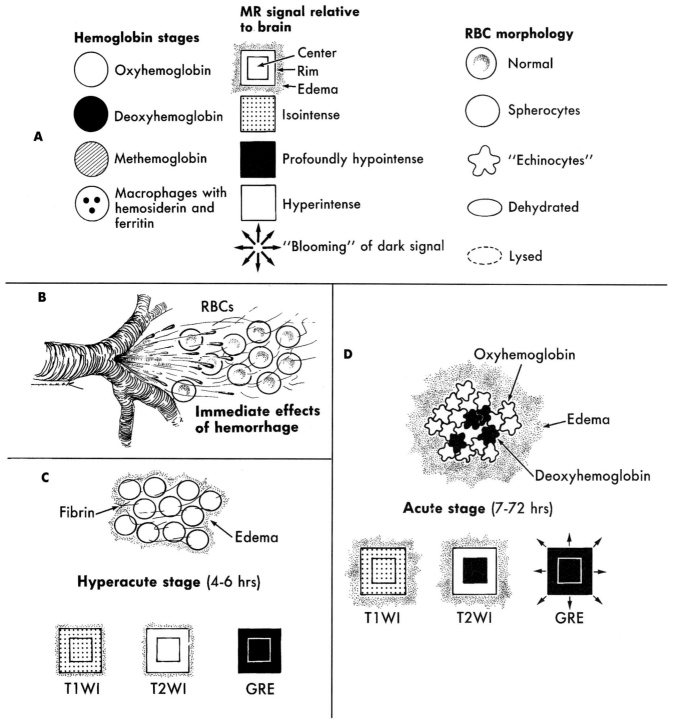

Fig. 7-1. Anatomic diagrams depict the time course of intracranial hemorrhage (ICH) and the MR appearance of blood clots at different stages of evolution. This simplified representation combines the concepts delineated by several investigators. **A,** Key to red blood cell (RBC) morphologic changes and blood degradation products with MR signal relative to brain in Figs. 7-1, **B** to **H. B,** Immediate effects of hemorrhage. If coagulation is normal, a hemostatic plug is formed almost immediately after loss of blood vessel wall integrity. **C,** Hyperacute stage. The clot is an inhomogeneous matrix of fibrin and activated platelets with trapped RBCs and leukocytes interspersed with watery serum. At about 4 to 6 hours, RBCs begin to lose their biconvex shape and become spherical. **D,** Acute stage. Clot retraction and hemoconcentration with RBC packing occurs. The RBCs continue to change shape, shrinking and forming "echinocytes." Intracellular oxyhemoglobin undergoes oxidation to deoxyhemoglobin. Edema surrounds the clot.

Continued.

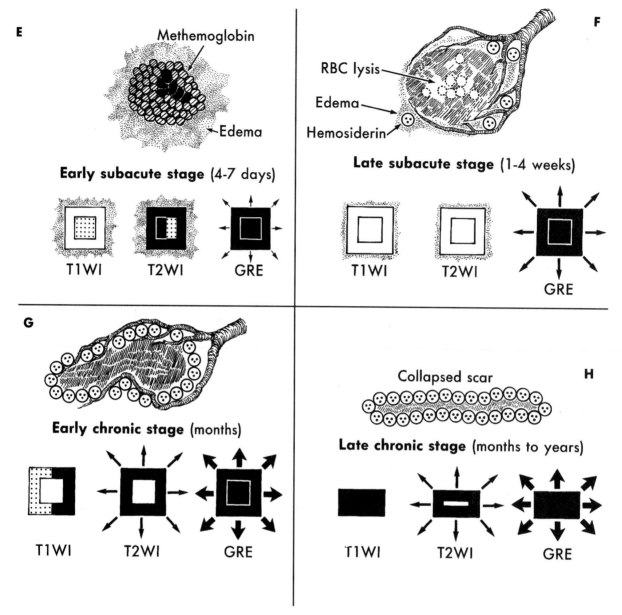

Fig. 7-1, cont'd.   E, Early subacute stage. The RBC echinocytes lose their spicules and become tiny spherocytes. Hemoglobin oxidative denaturation continues. The center of the clot is profoundly hypoxic. Surrounding edema remains intense. **F,** Late subacute stage. At around 1 week following the initial hemorrhage, RBC lysis occurs. Some misshapen RBC "ghosts" are present in the pool of extracellular liquid that contains free dilute methemoglobin. Edema diminishes and neovascular proliferation with reactive inflammatory changes around the clot begins. These sprouting capillaries initially have a deficient blood-brain barrier. *See* Fig. 7-2. **G,** Early chronic stage. The hematoma cavity gradually shrinks and inflammatory changes diminish as the blood vessels surrounding the clot mature. Edema disappears. The clot wall contains ferritin- and hemosiderin-laden macrophages. *See* Fig. 7-3. **H,** Late chronic stage. This stage can last for months to years, especially in adults. The hematoma now consists of a slitlike fibrotic scar that contains iron storage products in macrophages. A small central pool that contains extracellular methemoglobin may be present. *See* Fig. 7-19.

blood begins. An unretracted fibrin mass is formed first as plasma clotting factors convert soluble proteins into a gel matrix. This creates a complex inhomogeneous mass that contains erythrocytes, white blood cells, and small platelet clumps interspersed with protein-rich serum (Fig. 7-1, *B*).

Hyperacute hemorrhage. Over the next 4 to 6 hours, peripheral edema begins to develop and hemoconcentration ensues as the protein clot retracts, packing the red blood cells (RBCs) to a hematocrit of approximately 70% to 90%.[4] During the hyperacute stage the hematoma still contains intact biconcave RBCs with oxygenated hemoglobin.

Glucose depletion in the hematoma center occurs over the next several hours. As their energy source is diminished, the extravasated RBCs gradually lose their biconcave shape and become spherical (Fig. 7-1, *C*).[5] Significant changes in protein concentration also occur during this stage as molecular cross-linking proceeds and free water within the clot diminishes.

Acute hemorrhage. By 12 to 48 hours after clot formation begins, the RBCs become significantly dehydrated. As they shrink and lose their spherical shapes,[6] trapped RBCs acquire irregular spiculated projections and form "echinocytes."[5]

Hemoglobin desaturation also occurs. By 24 to 72 hours, most intracerebral hematomas contain shrunken but intact erythrocytes with high concentrations of deoxygenated intracellular hemoglobin (Fig. 7-1, *D*).[7] Edema surrounding the clot is pronounced at this stage.

Subacute hemorrhage. The *early* subacute phase of ICH begins within a few days after the initial hemorrhage. Oxidative denaturation of hemoglobin progresses and deoxyhemoglobin is gradually converted to methemoglobin (MetHb) (Fig. 7-1, *E*). Because the blood clot interior is profoundly hypoxic, these changes first occur around the periphery and then progress centrally.

The *late* subacute phase begins at around 1 week. Hemoglobin oxidation and cell lysis begin at the clot periphery. The shrunken, crenated RBCs gradually lyse and release MetHb into the extracellular space (Figs. 7-1, *F*, and 7-2). Edema slowly subsides and mass effect gradually diminishes.

Changes also appear in the brain surrounding the clot as perivascular inflammatory reaction ensues and macrophages collect in the clot wall (Figs. 7-1, *F*, and 7-3). These secondary reactive changes account for the ring enhancement often observed on contrast-enhanced CT and MR studies of resolving hematomas[8] (*see* Fig. 7-12).

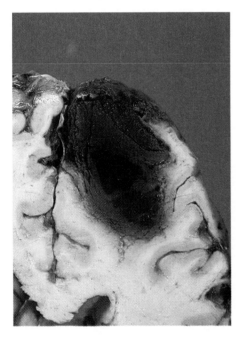

Fig. 7-2. Autopsy specimen shows posttraumatic left frontal lobe hematoma. At about 1 week following the traumatic event, the subacute hematoma contains a central liquified clot surrounded by reactive inflammatory changes. (Courtesy J. Townsend.)

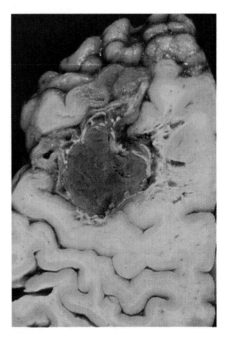

Fig. 7-3. Gross pathologic specimen of organizing hematoma, early chronic stage. The vascularized clot wall is well formed and the hematoma cavity has begun to shrink. Edema is diminishing. (Courtesy E. Ross.)

Early chronic hemorrhage. White matter edema surrounding the hematoma disappears as inflammation regresses. Vascular proliferation encroaches on the hematoma cavity, gradually reducing its size (Fig. 7-1, *G*). Peripheral reactive astrocytosis becomes pronounced.[8] At this stage the resolving clot contains a relatively uniform pool of dilute extracellular MetHb surrounded by a vascularized wall that contains activated macrophages. The macrophages in the hematoma wall contain at least two iron-storage substances: ferritin and hemosiderin.[9]

Late chronic hemorrhage. Chronic hematomas are cystic or collapsed slitlike cavities surrounded by a dense collagenous capsule (Fig. 7-1, *H*). With progressive neovascular proliferation in the wall, the acellular hematoma is gradually replaced by a vascularized fibrotic matrix containing ferritin- and hemosiderin-laden macrophages. In infants, these iron-positive macrophages may eventually disappear almost completely, whereas in adults, a small hemosiderin- or ferritin-laden scar may persist for years.[10]

IMAGING OF INTRACRANIAL HEMORRHAGE
Computed Tomography

The appearance of uncomplicated intracranial hemorrhage on computed tomography (CT) is comparatively straightforward.

Acute hemorrhage
Physiology. On CT studies only one factor, electron density, determines image contrast. There is a linear relationship between CT attenuation and hematocrit, hemoglobin concentration, and protein content. Because the hematocrit of an acute retracted clot is around 90% and the globin (protein) component of hemoglobin has a high mass density,[11] fresh intracerebral blood clots typically appear hyperdense on CT when compared to normal brain (Fig. 7-4).

The contributions to clot density from calcium and protoporphyrin are negligible; iron accounts for less than 0.5% of hemoglobin by weight and contributes comparatively little to the hyperdensity of acute intracerebral hematomas (ICHs) on nonenhanced CT scans.[12]

Typical CT appearance. CT demonstration of an acute clot is a function of its density, volume, location, and relationship to surrounding structures, as well as technical factors such as slice thickness, window width, and scan angle.[12] Small petechial hemorrhages or thin, linear clots adjacent to the calvarium or skull base may be difficult to detect. Window widths between 150 to 250H are helpful in separating small peripheral hematomas from the dense overlying skull (Fig. 7-5).

The CT density of a clot is independent of its location unless the blood is mixed with other fluids (e.g., cerebrospinal fluid). Thus acute epidural and subdural hematomas, subarachnoid hemorrhage, and parenchymal clots are all usually hyperdense to brain.[12] If patients have normal coagulation function but blood is accumulating very rapidly, unretracted semiliquid clot may be present. This results in hypodense areas within the generally hyperdense acute hematoma, the so-called swirl sign (Fig. 7-6).[12] If contrast is administered during brisk ongoing hemor-

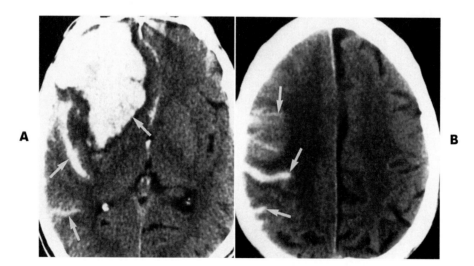

Fig. 7-4. Acute intracranial hemorrhage. **A** and **B,** Axial CT scans in another patient with intracranial hemorrhage caused by a ruptured right middle cerebral artery aneurysm (not shown). Here acute hemorrhage appears as hyperdense collections within the right frontal lobe, sylvian fissure, and subarachnoid spaces *(arrows)*.

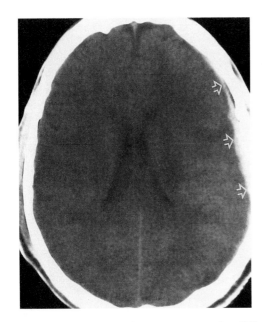

Fig. 7-5. Thin, linear acute hematomas can be difficult to detect if they are adjacent to other high density structures like the calvarial vault. Wide window width shows this SDH *(arrows).*

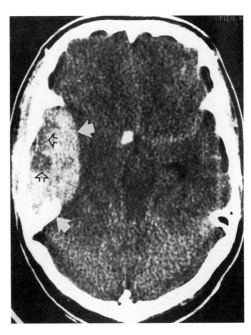

Fig. 7-6. Axial CT scan without contrast enhancement shows a large epidural hematoma (EDH) *(white arrows).* The central low density area *(open arrows)* represents unretracted hyperacute hemorrhage.

rhage, contrast extravasation can occasionally be detected on CT scans.[12]

Atypical CT appearance. Systemic disease processes can complicate the CT appearance of acute ICHs. Occasionally acute ICHs appear isodense with adjacent brain. Acute hematomas will be isodense if the hematocrit (and therefore protein concentration) is sufficiently low. This occurs with extreme anemia, i.e., when the hemoglobin concentration drops to 8 to 10 g/dl.[13,14]

Coagulation disorders can also alter clot formation (see subsequent discussion). Hemostasis may be altered so radically that normal clotting and lytic reactions are delayed or absent.[5] Hemorrhagic diatheses can be caused by a lack of coagulation factors (e.g., hemophilia) and defects in fibrin deposition, abnormal platelet function, poor vascular integrity, or excessive fibrinolytic activity resulting in an unstable clot.[15]

With abnormal clotting function, failure of clot retraction may result in a relatively isodense acute ICH (Fig. 7-7). Fluid-fluid levels within clots can also occur. They are present in up to 50% of patients when hemorrhage results from a coagulopathy (Fig. 7-8).[15a] Iatrogenic ICH complicating thrombolytic therapy for acute myocardial infarction often has an unusual appearance with relatively low density clot and fluid-fluid levels[16,17] (see subsequent discussion).

Subacute hemorrhage

Physiology. The attenuation of uncomplicated intracerebral hematomas decreases with time, diminishing at an average of 1.5H per day.[12] Resolving intraparenchymal clots first liquefy and then resorb, with the process starting at the periphery and progressing centrally. Proliferating capillaries around the clot periphery initially have a deficient blood-brain barrier.[5]

Extraaxial hematomas. Clot lysis also occurs in extraaxial collections. In subdural hematomas (SDH), proliferating vessels arise from the dura mater and form an outer membrane along the SDH. An inner membrane of compressed fibrin layers also forms. Vascularization of both layers eventually encloses the hematoma completely.[5]

CT appearance. Between about 1 and 6 weeks subacute ICHs become virtually isodense with adjacent brain parenchyma on CT scans (Fig. 7-9, *A*).[18] Subacute ICHs sometimes show peripheral enhancement after contrast administration because there is blood-brain barrier breakdown in the vascularized capsule that surrounds the hematoma *(see* Fig. 7-12, *B*).[8]

Chronic hemorrhage. Unless rebleeding has occurred, chronic hematomas are hypodense compared to adjacent brain (Fig. 7-10). High attenuation within chronic hematomas is usually secondary to rebleed-

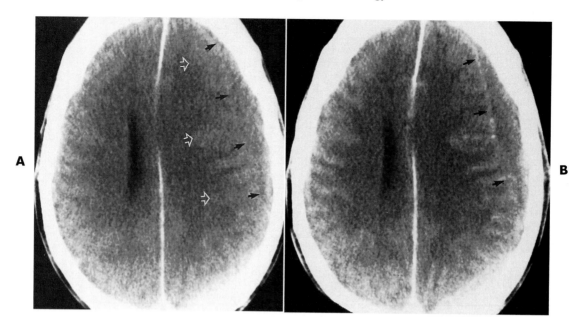

Fig. 7-7. A, Axial precontrast CT scan in a patient with thrombocytopenia and acute onset of left-sided weakness shows displacement of the cortex *(black arrows)* by a nearly isodense subdural hematoma. Inward "buckling" of the gray-white interface *(open arrows)* indicates an extraaxial mass effect. **B,** Postcontrast scan shows displacement of cortical vessels *(arrows)* away from the calvarium and confirms presence of the extraaxial fluid collection.

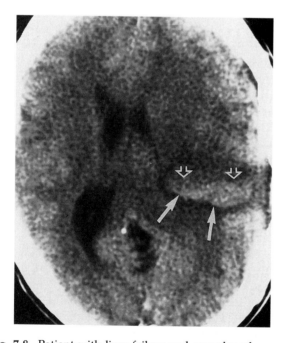

Fig. 7-8. Patient with liver failure and coagulopathy experienced sudden onset of right hemiparesis. Axial NECT shows an intracranial hematoma *(large arrows)* that is nearly isodense with brain. The acute hematoma contains a fluid-fluid level *(open arrows),* a common finding in patients with coagulopathies and intracranial hemorrhage.

ing (Fig. 7-11).[19] A focal hyperdense region within a low density collection (Fig. 7-10) or a fluid-fluid level (Fig. 7-11) can be seen.

Rim enhancement around a resolving parenchymal hematoma typically appears within a few days (Fig. 7-12) and disappears between 2 to 6 months.[20] A "target" sign on postcontrast CT scans can be seen if rehemorrhage takes place within an organizing hematoma; if rebleeding occurs outside an organized hematoma it can resemble tumoral hemorrhage (Fig. 7-13).[8]

Residua of intracerebral hemorrhage include low attenuation foci (37%), slitlike lesions (25%), and calcifications (10%). Twenty-seven per cent of patients surviving ICH have no identifiable residual abnormalities on CT scans.[21]

Magnetic Resonance Imaging: Factors Influencing Hemorrhage Signal

Background. MR imaging of intracerebral hemorrhage is a complex and controversial subject. Much has been learned and debated. Much is still unknown and remains to be elucidated. An exhaustive delineation is well beyond the scope of this text. However, the MR appearance of most intracranial hematomas seems to evolve in a reasonably predictable pattern

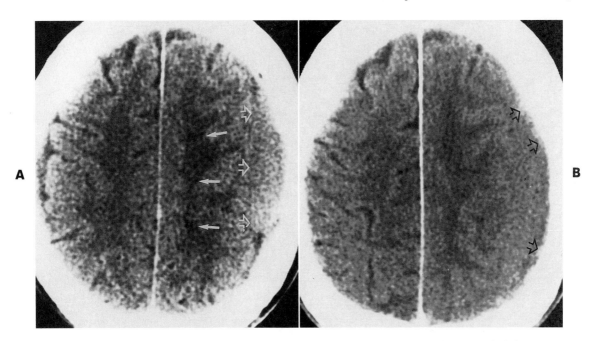

Fig. 7-9. Subacute subdural hematoma. **A,** Precontrast axial CT scan shows medial displacement of the gray-white interface *(white arrows)* by an extraaxial fluid collection *(open arrows)* that is nearly isodense with the underlying cortex. **B,** Postcontrast study shows subtle peripheral enhancement *(arrows).*

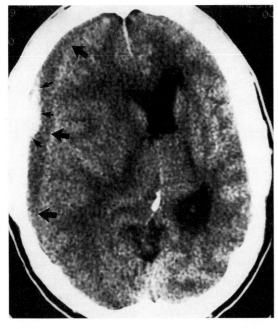

Fig. 7-10. Axial CT scan in a patient with a chronic subdural hematoma. The crescentic, low density extraaxial fluid collection *(large arrows)* is typical. Fresh hemorrhage is seen as a focal high density area *(small arrows)* within the chronic SDH.

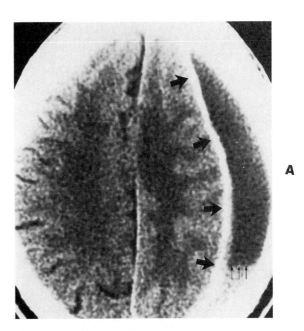

Fig. 7-11. Nonenhanced axial CT scan of a chronic SDH. Acute hemorrhage into the old extraaxial collection forms a fluid-fluid level *(small arrows).* A dense inner membrane is seen *(large arrows).*   *Continued.*

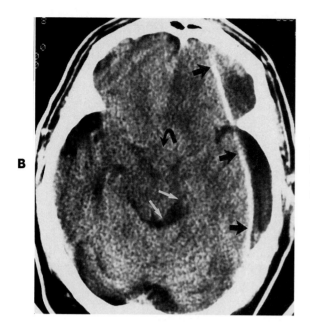

Fig. 7-11, cont'd. Nonenhanced axial CT scan of a chronic SDH. Temporal lobe herniation has effaced the suprasellar cistern (**B,** *curved arrow*) and widened the ipsilateral quadrigeminal plate cistern medial to the tentorial incisura (**B,** *white arrows*).

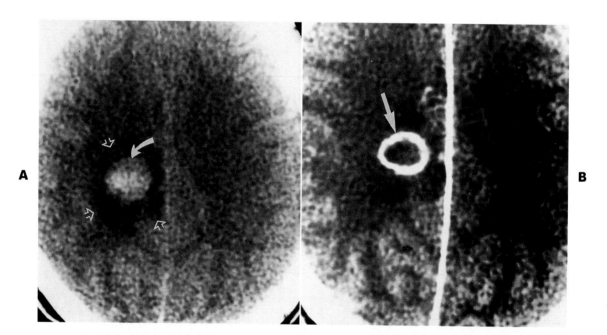

Fig. 7-12. Resolving hematoma secondary to hemorrhagic AVM. **A,** Axial CT scan without contrast enhancement obtained 1 week after hemorrhage shows a slightly hyperdense hematoma *(curved arrow)* surrounded by a rim of edema *(open arrows).* **B,** Postcontrast scan at 3 weeks shows a ringlike enhancement *(arrow)* surrounding the clot that now appears isodense with adjacent white matter. The edema has largely resolved.

over time. This pattern is illustrated by a series of MR scans obtained from a few hours to several months following hematoma formation (Fig. 7-14).

Concepts explaining the MR appearance of intracranial hemorrhage are based on a combination of empirical clinical observations, theoretical explanations, animal models, and in vitro studies of human blood clot composition and evolution.[22] Conclusions regarding hematoma formation and evolutionary changes in intracranial hemorrhage should not be directly extrapolated to the rest of the body.

Intrinsic factors such as gross changes in hematoma structure and the sequential degradation of hemoglobin were initially emphasized as the major factors determining the MR appearance of evolving ICH.[23] Protein concentration,[24] red blood cell hydration status, RBC size and shape,[5,6] hematocrit,[7] and clot formation and retraction, as well as composition

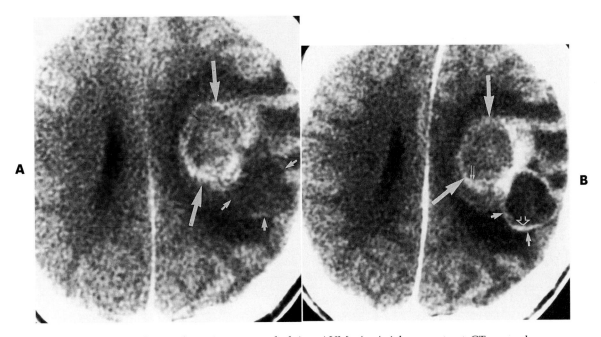

Fig. 7-13. Rehemorrhage into an underlying AVM. **A,** Axial precontrast CT scan obtained 4 days after symptom onset shows a moderately hyperdense acute hematoma *(large arrows)*. The subacute clot *(small arrows)* is virtually invisible. **B,** Postcontrast study shows rim enhancement around the subacute clot *(small arrows)* with contrast accumulation and a fluid-fluid level *(open arrow)* within the hematoma. There is also a fluid-fluid level *(double arrows)* within the more acute clot *(large arrows)*.

Fig. 7-14. A 35-year-old jogger "fell and hit his head" and was brought to the hospital emergency room. Immediate CT scan **(A)** and sequential MR scans obtained from 2 hours to 4 months later are shown. Initial studies show the characteristics of a hyperacute hematoma: **A,** Axial NECT scan shows a small right temporal lobe hematoma *(arrow)*. **B,** Axial T1-weighted MR scan without contrast shows an isointense right temporal lobe mass *(arrows)*. **C,** The lesion shows some patchy enhancement *(arrows)* following contrast administration. (Courtesy B. Hart.)

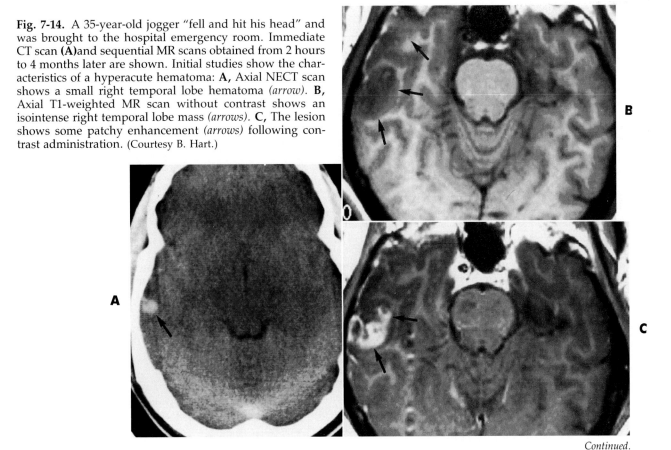

Continued.

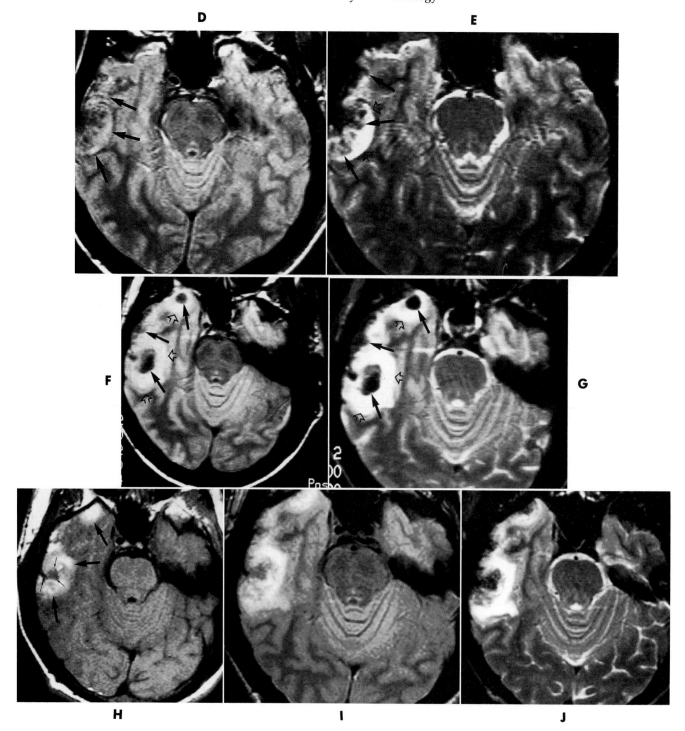

Fig. 7-14, cont'd. D, Long TR/short TE (proton density-weighted) sequence shows the hematoma *(arrows)* is largely isointense with cortex. **E,** T2-weighted study shows the inhomogeneous isointense to moderately hypointense hematoma *(large arrows)* with surrounding edema *(open arrows)*. Follow-up scans were obtained 4 days later. The clot is in the acute stage of evolution: **F,** Axial long TR/short TE sequence shows hypodense clots and contusions *(large arrows)* with significant peripheral edema *(open arrows)*. **G,** T2-weighted sequence shows the clots *(large arrows)* become profoundly hypointense. One week after the initial scan the hematoma shows characteristics of an early subacute clot: **H,** The T1-weighted scan shows the hematoma periphery is hyperintense *(large arrows)* with a smaller isointense core *(small arrows)*. **I,** Long TR/short TE sequence shows the periphery remains hyperintense and the center is isointense to slightly hypointense. Edema is beginning to diminish. **J,** T2WI shows the clot center is mixed iso- to hypointense and the clot periphery is indistinguishable from the remaining peripheral edema. (Courtesy B. Hart.)

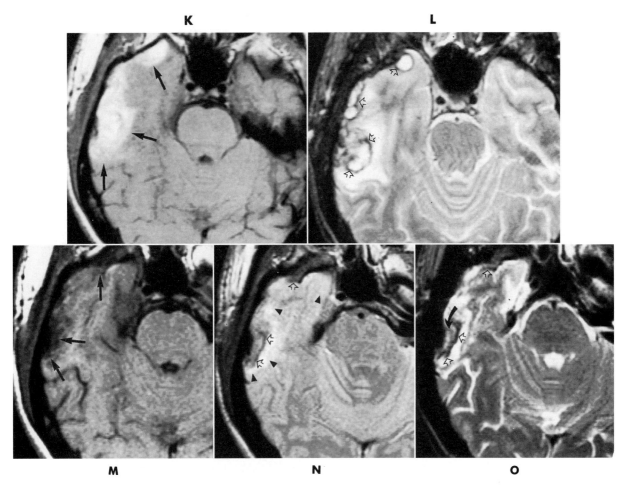

Fig. 7-14 cont'd. Follow-up scans 12 days after the first study show the characteristics of late subacute hematomas: **K,** The clot *(arrows)* is uniformly hyperintense on T1WI. **L,** T2WI shows the clot remains largely hyperintense but beginning to show some hemosiderin deposition, seen as low signal rims *(arrows)* that surround the hyperintense pools of lysed RBCs. Long-term follow-up studies, obtained 4 months later, show the characteristics of early chronic hemorrhage. **M,** T1WI shows the clot *(arrows)* is significantly smaller and is mixed iso- to hypointense with cortex. **N,** Long TR/short TE study shows the hemosiderin rim *(arrows)* is mildly hypointense. Some temporal lobe gliosis with encephalomalacic change is seen as slightly hyperintense parenchyma *(arrowheads)*. **O,** The T2-weighted scan demonstrates "blooming" of the hemosiderin rim *(open arrows)*. The collapsed scar contains a residual high signal pool of lysed RBC debris *(curved arrow)*. (Courtesy B. Hart.)

and structure,[1,2] are now recognized as additional very important intrinsic factors that may influence the MR signal intensity of hemorrhage.

Extrinsic factors such as field strength[11] and pulse sequences[25] have important effects on the MR signals of intracranial hematomas. Known intrinsic and extrinsic factors that contribute to the MR appearance of ICH are summarized in the box. Each of these factors is briefly discussed.

Clot age and blood degradation products. The relaxivity and susceptibility effects of iron-containing hemoglobin are among the many important factors that determine signal intensity of intracranial hemor-

---

Factors That May Influence MR Appearance of Intracranial Hemorrhage

Intrinsic

Macroscopic structure of clot
Hemoglobin oxidation state
Red blood cell morphology
Protein concentration/clot hydration
Size/location of hematoma
Edema

Extrinsic

Pulse sequences
Field strength

rhage. The temporal evolution of hemoglobin degradation products occurs in a predictable fashion. Between 10% to 15% of patients with nontraumatic, nonaneurysmal primary intracranial hemorrhage are on AC therapy.[17] About 1% of patients undergoing thrombolytic therapy for acute myocardial infarction develop ICH. This complication has a grave prognosis, with over 60% of patients dying during hospitalization.[16]

Imaging findings in most coagulopathies are similar. Although bleeding can occur at any location, the common site in these patients is supratentorial and intraparenchymal. Fluid-fluid levels within hematomas are common (Fig. 7-8). Multiple large volume hemorrhages with substantial mass effect can also be seen and are associated with increased mortality.[16]

Hyperacute clots and oxyhemoglobin. Oxyhemoglobin (OxyHb) is initially present in hyperacute clots for a very short period of time (probably from only a few minutes up to a few hours). OxyHb has ferrous iron, lacks unpaired electrons, and is diamagnetic. Therefore OxyHb does not affect either T1 or T2 relaxation times.[26] The MR signal of hyperacute hematomas is due mostly to its protein-rich water content. Hyperacute clots are typically isointense with gray matter on T1-weighted images (T1WI) and hyperintense on T2WI images (Figs. 7-1, *C*; 7-14; and 7-15).

Acute clots and deoxyhemoglobin. Hemoglobin desaturation from OxyHb to deoxyhemoglobin (DeoxyHb) occurs within a few hours of hemorrhage. Like OxyHb, DeoxyHb also has ferrous iron but has

four unpaired electrons in a high-spin state and is therefore strongly paramagnetic.[3]

Subtle alteration in hemoglobin configuration also occurs with oxygen desaturation. The paramagnetic ferrous ion of DeoxyHb is shielded from the close approach of water molecules by the hydrophobic cleft of the globin protein.[26] DeoxyHb therefore cannot cause proton-electron dipole-dipole (PEDD) proton relaxation enhancement, and T1 shortening does not occur. Thus DeoxyHb appears isointense with brain parenchyma on T1WI regardless of whether it is intra- or extracellular (Figs. 7-1, *D*, and 7-16, *B*).[21]

In contrast to its lack of effect on T1 relaxation, the effect of acute clots and DeoxyHb on T2 relaxation is dramatic. The precise reason for this remains controversial. If DeoxyHb is sequestered within intact RBCs, as water diffuses freely across the cell membrane it experiences a substantial magnetic susceptibility gradient. This results in phase dispersion and subsequent preferential T2 proton relaxation enhancement (T2-PRE).

The susceptibility effects seen with acute clots become more pronounced with progressive T2-weighting.[26] Acute clots with DeoxyHb typically appear moderately hypointense on balanced (long TR/short TE) scans and profoundly hypointense on T2WI or gradient-refocussed sequences (Fig. 7-16, *C*). Alteration in RBC morphology also produces T2-PRE.[4,5]

Subacute clots and methemoglobin. As RBC energy status declines, the enzyme systems used to maintain heme iron in the ferrous oxidation state be-

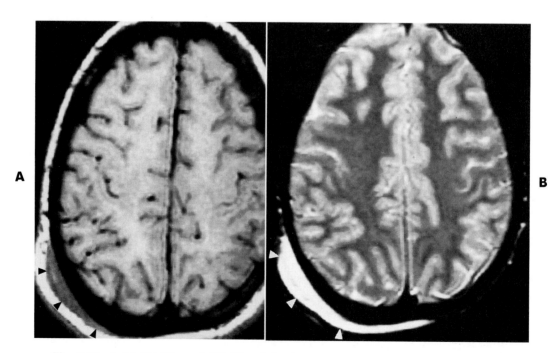

Fig. 7-15. Axial **(A)** T1- and **(B)** T2-weighted MR scans obtained 3 hours after head trauma. The brain is normal. A hyperacute subgaleal hematoma *(arrowheads)* is isointense with gray matter on T1WI but hyperintense on the T2-weighted studies.

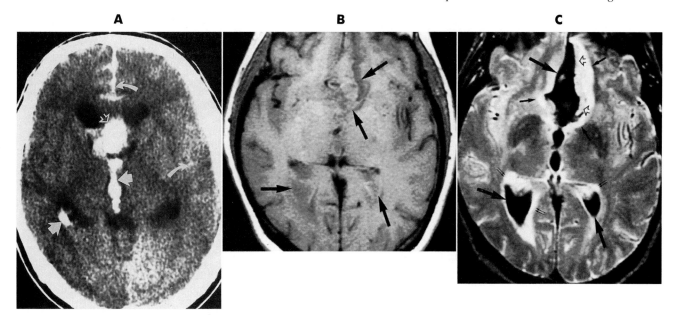

Fig. 7-16. Axial CT scan (**A**) in a patient with an anterior communicating artery aneurysm (not shown) demonstrates extensive intraventricular hemorrhage *(large arrows)*. Some diffuse SAH is seen in the interhemispheric fissure, left sylvian fissure, and cisterna magna *(curved arrows)*. The more focal anterior interhemispheric hematoma *(open arrow)* is characteristic for a ruptured ACoA aneurysm. Axial (**B**) T1- and (**C**) T2-weighted MR scans obtained approximately 12 hours after the initial hemorrhage show the interhemispheric and intraventricular clots are virtually isointense with adjacent brain parenchyma on T1WI (**B,** *arrows*). The clots are profoundly hypointense on T2WI (**B,** *large arrows*). There is some peripheral hyperintensity in the frontal hematoma *(open arrows)*. Note the edema that surrounds the clot *(small arrows)*. Acute obstructive hydrocephalus with some early transependymal extravasation of cerebrospinal fluid is seen as a hyperintense periventricular rim *(double arrows)*.

come nonfunctional and hemoglobin is further oxidized to methemoglobin (MetHb).[26] MetHb is present in subacute hematomas and can be seen from a few days to a few months following hemorrhage. MetHb is ferric, has five unpaired electrons, and is strongly paramagnetic.

In its conversion to MetHB the globin moiety undergoes further structural changes and the ferric ion is no longer contained in a hydrophobic cleft. Exposure of the ion to direct close access of water molecules causes T1 shortening through PEDD interactions. Therefore *early* subacute hematomas have high signal on T1WI. The high signal typically begins at the hematoma periphery and progresses inward. Thus the center of early subacute clots remains relatively isointense on T1WI and the rim becomes hyperintense (Figs. 7-1, *E,* and 7-17, *A*).

In the *early* subacute stage of hematoma formation, MetHb is contained within intact RBCs and preferentially increases T2-PRE. This T2-shortening results in low signal on long TR/short TE (proton density-weighted) scans (Fig. 7-17, *B*). Early subacute clots are profoundly hypointense on T2WI and gradient-refocussed sequences (Fig. 7-17, *C*).

In the *late* subacute stage, hemolysis results in the accumulation of extracellular MetHb within the hematoma cavity.[26] MetHb in free solution is very hyperintense on T1- and T2-weighted images (Figs. 7-1, *F,* and 7-18).

Chronic clots and iron storage. In the *early* chronic stage, a pool of dilute-free methemoglobin is surrounded by the ferritin- and hemosiderin-containing vascularized wall (Fig. 7-1, *G*). At this stage, clots typically are homogeneously hyperintense on both T1- and T2WI and have a pronounced low signal rim on T2WI (Fig. 7-19).[9] Edema and mass effect diminish and then disappear.

The long-term residua of *late* chronic hematomas persist for years following brain hemorrhage because, at least in adults, macrophages laden with iron-storage products remain around the margins of old clots for years. In infants, all the hemosiderin is usually removed (Figs. 7-1, *H,* and 7-20).[5] Heme degradation products are also phagocytosed by glial cells that surround the clot; thus a "brain stain" can also persist indefinitely.

At least two iron-storage substances are present in the late phase of resolving cerebral hematomas: fer-

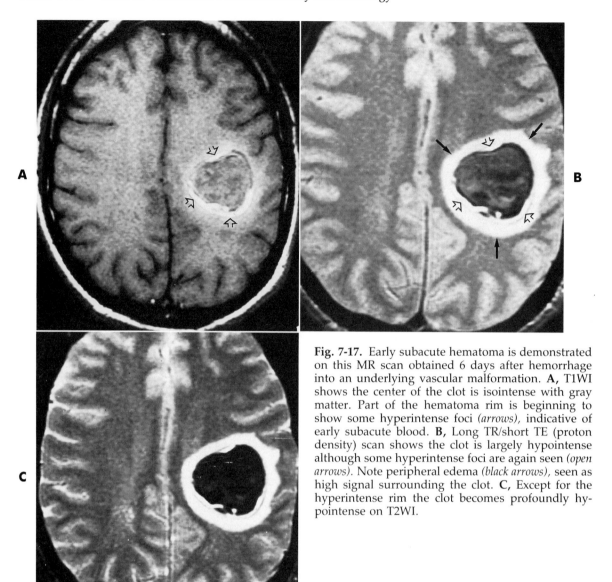

Fig. 7-17. Early subacute hematoma is demonstrated on this MR scan obtained 6 days after hemorrhage into an underlying vascular malformation. **A,** T1WI shows the center of the clot is isointense with gray matter. Part of the hematoma rim is beginning to show some hyperintense foci *(arrows),* indicative of early subacute blood. **B,** Long TR/short TE (proton density) scan shows the clot is largely hypointense although some hyperintense foci are again seen *(open arrows).* Note peripheral edema *(black arrows),* seen as high signal surrounding the clot. **C,** Except for the hyperintense rim the clot becomes profoundly hypointense on T2WI.

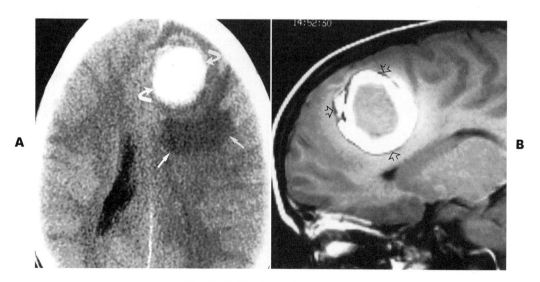

Fig. 7-18. For legend see p. 169.

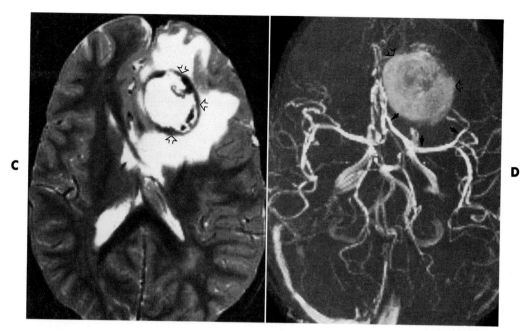

Fig. 7-18, cont'd. Four-year-old boy with intracranial hematoma caused by hemorrhage into a cavernous angioma. **A,** Initial axial CT scan without contrast enhancement shows a left frontal hematoma *(curved arrows)* with adjacent edema *(straight arrows)*. **B,** Sagittal T1-weighted MR scan obtained approximately 10 days after the initial hemorrhage shows the clot is mostly hyperintense with a thin peripheral low signal rim *(arrows)* caused by iron storage products. **C,** Axial T2WI shows "blooming" caused by the ferritin/hemosiderin-containing macrophages in the clot rim *(arrows)*. The center of the clot appears hyperintense. Moderate peripheral edema persists. **D,** MR angiogram shows the hyperintense clot *(open arrows)* has moderate residual mass effect, evidenced by the displaced horizontal anterior and middle cerebral arteries *(black arrows)*.

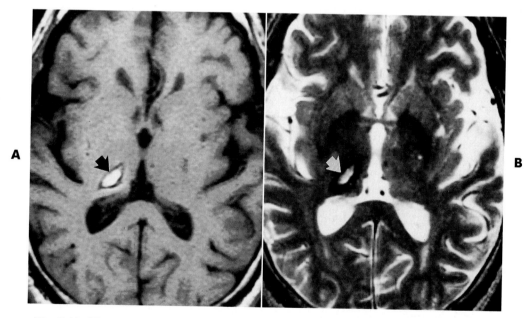

Fig. 7-19. Hypertensive thalamic hemorrhage with classic changes of early chronic hemorrhage. Axial **(A)** T1- and **(B)** T2-weighted sequences show the early chronic hematoma *(arrows)*. The hematoma consists of lysed clot and dilute-free MetHb surrounded by a rim of hemosiderin-containing macrophages.

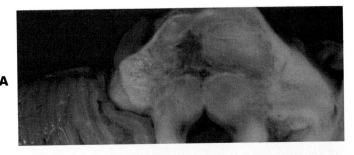

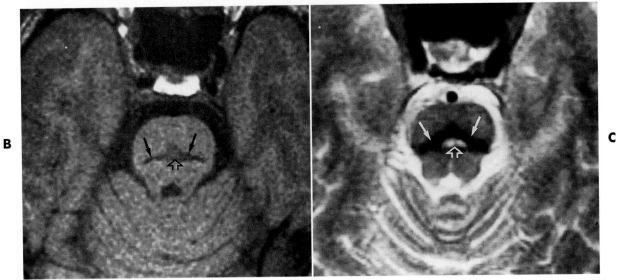

Fig. 7-20. A, Gross specimen shows an old hypertensive hemorrhagic pontine infarct. Iron-containing scar surrounds a small residual collapsed hematoma. Note accompanying atrophy. Axial **(B)** T1- and **(C)** T2-weighted MR scans in another patient with residua of old pontine hemorrhage show the low signal scar *(solid arrows)* surrounding the collapsed hematoma remnant *(open arrows)*. Note "blooming" on the T2WI. (**A,** Courtesy E. Ross.)

ritin and hemosiderin.[9] Hemosiderin is ferric but water insoluble and therefore does not exhibit T1-relaxation enhancement. Hemosiderin preferentially enhances T2-PRE. Therefore hemosiderin is isointense on T1WI and very hypointense on T2WI. Because of strong magnetic susceptibility effects, ferritin and hemosiderin appear profoundly hypointense on gradient-echo studies (*see* Fig. 7-22).

Oxygenation and metabolic effects. As already described, hemoglobin in intracranial hematomas undergoes progressive oxidation. This typically procedes from hematoma periphery toward the center. The clot interior is often profoundly hypoxic with relative delay in hemoglobin denaturation.

Protein concentration effects. Protein concentration in blood clots can be increased by formation and retraction of clot matrix, as well as RBC packing[27] and dehydration.[4] T1 and T2 relaxation times in concentrated protein solutions decrease as concentration increases.[11] At the field strengths currently used in clinical MR imaging, protein concentration has little effect on T1 relaxation. However, T2 relaxation effects are significant. Probably because of protein concentration effects, alterations in hematocrit or RBC hydration alone substantially shorten T2 relaxation even without change in hemoglobin oxygenation status.[4]

Clot structure. Significant macroscopic heterogeneity is present within blood clots.[4] Pools of serum are interspersed with RBC and platelet aggregates. The cellular composition of thrombi also varies greatly. Venous thrombi have an erythrocyte content similar to that of intravascular flowing blood; arterial thrombi have relatively fewer erythrocytes and are composed largely of platelets within a fibrin matrix.[2] Non-RBC cellular components in thrombi such as platelets can also affect the relaxation times of in vitro clotted blood.[28]

Clot inhomogeneity has striking effects on T2-PRE. Gradient-refocussed sequences are even more exquisitely sensitive to the local field inhomogeneities produced by heterogeneous blood clots.

RBC status. T2 relaxation effects of intracellular DeoxyHb and MetHb have already been described. Changes in RBC shape and hydration also affect the MR appearance of blood clots. Loss of membrane integrity with subsequent RBC lysis has a profound effect on the MR appearance of hematomas. Intracellular MetHb is hypointense on T2WI; extracellular MetHb appears very hyperintense (Fig. 7-21). The precise reason for this is unclear, but the very hyperintense appearance of late subacute clots on T2WI may be related to their high free water content.

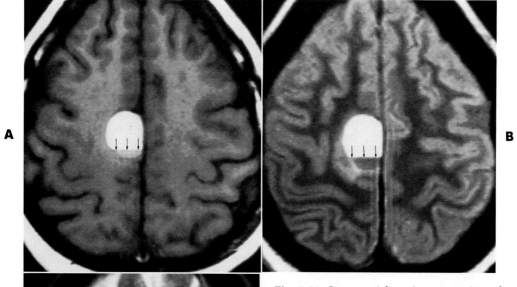

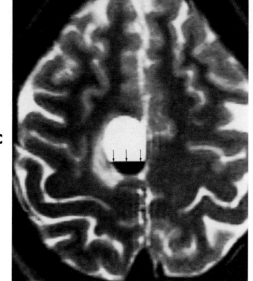

Fig. 7-21. Intracranial cystic metastasis, unknown primary tumor, with hemorrhage and fluid-fluid level demonstrates the effect of RBC status on MR signal intensity. **A,** T1-weighted scan. The top layer consists of lysed RBCs with extracellular dilute-free MetHb. The dependent layer *(arrows)* consists of intact RBCs with intracellular MetHb and is basically isointense with adjacent brain. **B,** Long TR/short TE balanced (proton density) scan shows the upper layer remains hyperintense while the dependent portion *(arrows)* becomes moderately hypointense. **C,** The intracellular MetHb *(arrows)* is profoundly hypointense on this T2WI. (Courtesy D. Meyer.)

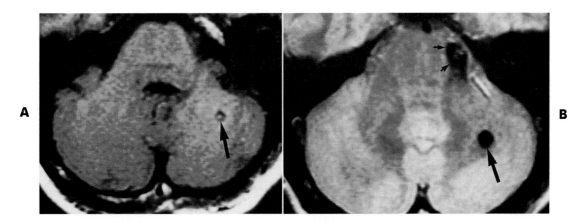

Fig. 7-22. The relative insensitivity of "fast" spin-echo MR sequences to chronic hemorrhage is shown by these studies in a patient with chronic hemorrhagic cavernous angiomas. **A,** Axial T1-weighted scan shows a small left cerebellar hemispheric lesion *(arrow)*. **B,** Long TR/short TE (proton density-weighted) scan shows "blooming" of the cerebellar lesion *(large arrow)*. A second lesion is identified in the pons *(small arrows)*.

Continued.

Fig. 7-22, cont'd. C, Standard T2-weighted spin echo scan shows more extensive "blooming" of the lesions *(arrows)*. **D,** The cerebellar lesion *(arrow)* is barely visible on a T2-weighted "fast" spin-echo sequence. **E,** Gradient-refocussed scan shows the pontine and left cerebellar lesions *(arrows)*. A third lesion is seen in the right cerebellum *(open arrow)*.

Edema. A moderate amount of bulk water is present within acute hematomas. T1 effects are usually minimal, but T2 relaxation times of acute hematomas are prolonged substantially. A typical example is traumatic scalp hematoma in which the clot is usually isointense with cortex on T1WI but appears hyperintense on T2WI (Fig. 7-15).

Size and site of hemorrhage. The temporal evolution of large clots may be retarded compared to smaller lesions. Whether the hemorrhage has occurred in brain parenchyma, cerebrospinal fluid spaces, or in structures outside the blood-brain barrier (e.g., the pituitary or pineal gland) also affects the MR appearance of ICH. For example, when hemorrhage occurs in the subarachnoid space, the formation of DeoxyHb may be retarded because CSF has a higher oxygen tension compared to brain parenchyma.[26] If hemorrhage occurs in areas that are outside the blood-brain barrier, iron-containing macrophages are removed and do not accumulate in the extracellular spaces around these lesions.

Pulse sequences and their effects. On short TR scans (T1-weighted images) acute hematomas of arterial origin are isointense and become hyperintense a few days later. With long TR sequences, acute clots initially demonstrate hyperintensity, then become hypointense within about 5 to 7 days.[25] Gradient-echo studies usually show hypointensity at all time intervals after hemorrhage.

Because of their relative insensitivity to field inhomogeneity, the so-called fast spin-echo sequences may be less sensitive indicators of chronic intracranial hemorrhage (Fig. 7-22). Therefore if ICH is suspected, routine spin-echo or gradient-refocussed scans should be performed.

Field strength effects. Because magnetic susceptibility effects are proportional to the square of the applied magnetic field strength, intracellular deoxyhemoglobin produces very little visible effect on short TR scans obtained with low-field systems. The typical intensity changes observed on long TR scans of acute hematomas can be seen at both intermediate and high-field strengths but are visible sooner and to a greater degree at 1.5T.[25] Lengthening TR and TE theoretically optimizes hematoma visualization at low fields but in practice has relatively little effect.[29]

Gradient-echo studies are helpful and should be performed to improve hematoma detection with low-field MR units.

NONTRAUMATIC INTRACRANIAL HEMORRHAGE

Craniocerebral trauma and traumatic ICH are discussed in Chapter 8. The etiology of nontraumatic hemorrhage is very broad (*see* box).

Perinatal Hemorrhage

Intracranial hemorrhage (ICH) is a major source of morbidity and mortality in the neonate. Although birth trauma was the most common cause of neonatal ICH during the early twentieth century, in the modern era, germinal matrix hemorrhages associated with extreme prematurity have become the common etiology.[30]

Premature infants. Cerebral hemorrhage is the most common acquired structural lesion of the CNS in premature neonates and includes germinal matrix, intraventricular, and intraparenchymal hemorrhages.

Germinal matrix hemorrhage. The germinal matrix is a region of very thin-walled veins and actively proliferating but transient cells located in the subependymal layer of the lateral ventricles. Neuronal precur-

---

Nontraumatic Intracranial Hemorrhage

Very Common

Hypertension
Aneurysm
Vascular malformation (AVM, cavernous angioma)
Prematurity

Common

Embolic stroke with reperfusion
Amyloid angiopathy
Coagulopathies/blood dyscrasias
Drug abuse
Tumor (e.g., pituitary adenoma, anaplastic astrocytoma/glioblastoma multiforme, metastases)

Uncommon

Venous infarction
Eclampsia
Infective endocarditis with septic emboli
Vasculitis (fungal)
Encephalitis (except herpes, which commonly hemorrhages)

Rare

Abscess (unless immunocompromised)
Vasculitis (nonfungal)

---

sors are produced in the germinal matrix, then migrate outward along the radial glial fibers to the cerebral cortex in a highly ordered, predictable pattern (*see* Chapter 3). The germinal matrix involutes by 34 to 36 weeks of gestation; the cells from this zone have almost all migrated by 40 weeks.[31]

Germinal matrix hemorrhage is the most common CNS lesion in high-risk low birth weight infants.[31] Hemorrhage into the germinal matrix is probably caused by hypoxic-ischemic injury to the deep vascular watershed zone in the developing fetus[32,33] (*see* Chapter 11). Matrix zone hemorrhages are unique to the immature brain, rarely occur in utero, and are almost never seen beyond the first 28 days of life.[30]

Germinal matrix hemorrhage is divided into four grades.[34]

Hemorrhage	Definition
Grade I	Hemorrhage confined to one or both germinal matrices
Grade II	Hemorrhage rupture into normal-sized ventricles
Grade III	Intraventricular hemorrhage (IVH) with hydrocephalus
Grade IV	Hemorrhagic extension into the adjacent hemispheric white matter

Although CT accurately depicts acute neonatal hemorrhage, most germinal matrix hemorrhages are currently evaluated by transcranial ultrasound. Regions of hyperechogenicity, particularly in the caudate nuclei, are typical (Fig. 7-23). Intra- and periventricular echogenic material can be identified in more severe acute and subacute hemorrhages (Fig. 7-24). With time, IVH becomes relatively sonolucent.

On MR studies the intensities of hemorrhagic lesions in high-risk neonates undergo evolutionary changes similar to those described in adults, except that subacute signal intensity appears earlier and chronic findings appear later.[32]

Intraventricular and parenchymal hemorrhage. IVH and parenchymal hemorrhages in premature infants are commonly secondary to germinal matrix bleeds.

Term infants. Intracranial hemorrhages in term infants are usually caused by traumatic delivery or hypoxic-ischemic insult.

Traumatic delivery. Although a fetus is occasionally traumatized in utero, isolated mechanical trauma is typically an intrapartum event associated with cephalopelvic disproportion or abnormal presentation.[30]

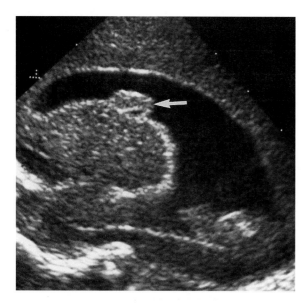

Fig. 7-23. Acute subependymal germinal matrix hemorrhage in a premature infant. Left parasagittal B-mode ultrasound scan obtained through the anterior fontanelle shows a hyperechoic focus *(arrows)* along the left caudothalamic groove. (Courtesy K. Murray.)

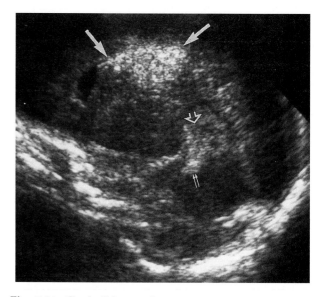

Fig. 7-24. Grade II hemorrhage in a premature infant. Left parasagittal B-mode ultrasound scan demonstrates parenchymal hemorrhage in the caudate nucleus and deep periventricular white matter *(large arrows)*. Increased echogenicity is also seen in the left lateral ventricle *(open arrows)* and choroid plexus *(double arrows)*. (Courtesy K. Murray.)

The following three major types of *extracranial* hemorrhages are caused by birth trauma[35]:

1. Caput succedaneum (cutaneous hemorrhagic edema commonly observed after vaginal delivery)
2. Subgaleal hemorrhage (hemorrhage under the occipito-frontal galea aponeurotica)
3. Cephalohematoma (traumatic subperiosteal hemorrhage)

Cephalohematomas appear as suture-limited, crescent-shaped collections directly adjacent to the calvarium. They are typically parietal in location and often calcify.

Birth trauma can also result in *intracranial* hemorrhage. During passage through the birth canal the head may be subjected to sudden compressive fronto-occipital foreshortening. The tentorium and posterior falx resist this mechanical deformation. Because they are placed under tension and stretched, dural lacerations and vein rupture may result.[30,31] Occasionally, diastatic skull fractures or tearing of bridging superficial cortical veins are responsible for ICH in term infants.[35]

The most common location of ICH with traumatic delivery is the subdural space, followed by the subarachnoid cisterns.[33] Most birth-related SDHs are comparatively small focal collections that are located posteriorly along the interhemispheric fissure and tentorium cerebelli (Fig. 7-25). Sixty percent are unilateral. Posterior fossa SAH in traumatic birth injury is also common.[32] Epidural hemorrhage

is rare.[31] When EDH occurs it is usually venous in origin.

Hypoxic-ischemic injury (HI). Asphyxia and infarction are among the common causes of intracranial hemorrhage in nontraumatized term neonates (*see* Chapter 11). HI can be a prenatal (intrauterine) or perinatal event.[36,37] Globular areas of T1 shortening in the posterolateral lentiform nuclei and ventral thalami are characteristic findings on MR scans (Fig. 7-26). Although the cortex can be involved, in profound asphyxia it is relatively spared compared to the deep gray matter injury.[38]

Hypertension

Hypertension is the most common nontraumatic cause of intracranial hemorrhage in adults.[39] Hypertensive intracerebral hemorrhage (HICH) is a significant cause of mortality and morbidity in elderly patients. A less common manifestation of hypertension, hypertensive encephalopathy, occurs in various settings. HE is a clinical syndrome with particular clinical and imaging manifestations that are distinct from other forms of HICH.

Hypertensive intracerebral hemorrhage.

Incidence and etiology. Most nontraumatic "spontaneous" ICHs in elderly patients are associated with systemic hypertension. In some cases, ruptured microaneurysms (Charcot-Bouchard aneurysms) on deep perforating vessels, particularly the lateral lenticulostriate arteries, have been implicated.[40]

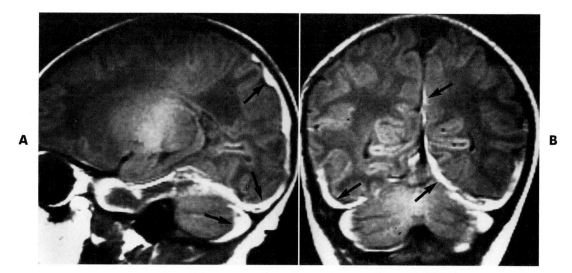

Fig. 7-25. Sagittal **(A)** and coronal **(B)** T1-weighted CT scans in an infant obtained 1 month following traumatic delivery show small bilateral SDHs along the posterior falx cerebri and tentorium *(arrows).*

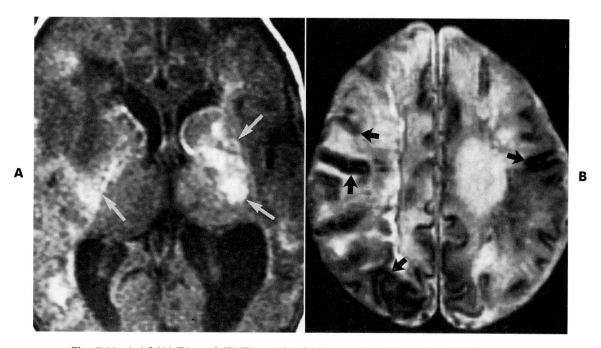

Fig. 7-26. Axial **(A)** T1- and **(B)** T2-weighted MR scans in a 1-month-old child with seizures. The infant had a normal gestation and normal delivery. High-signal hemorrhagic residua are seen in the basal ganglia **(A,** *arrows).* The T2WI shows bilateral very low signal areas in the cortex, particularly in the perirolandic areas **(B,** *arrows),* that are most consistent with hemorrhagic pseudolaminar cortical necrosis. Probably postnatal profound hypoxic-ischemic insult.

Location and clinical course. Hypertensive ICH has a predilection for areas supplied by penetrating branches of the middle cerebral and basilar arteries[41,41] (*see* Fig. 6-26). HICH therefore preferentially involves the external capsule and putamen, thalamus, and pons (Fig. 7-27, *A* and *B)* (Table 7-1).

Nearly two thirds of spontaneous intracerebral hematomas are located in the basal ganglia.[43] Large he-

TABLE 7-1. Location of Hypertensive Hemorrhage

Putamen/external capsule	60% to 65%
Thalamus	15% to 25%
Pons	5% to 10%
Cerebellum	2% to 5%
Subcortical white matter*	1% to 2%

*Excluding amyloid hemorrhages.

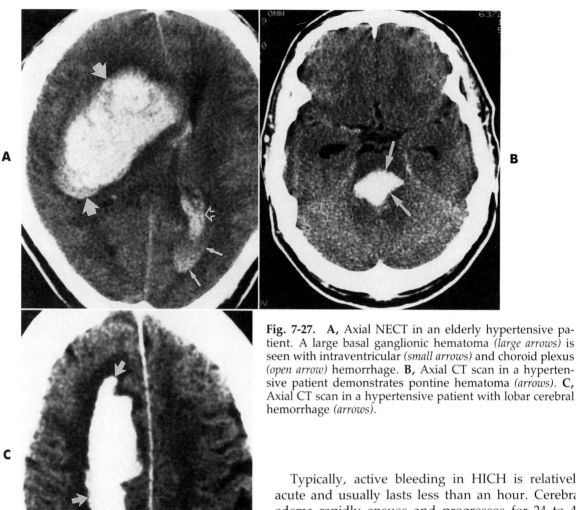

Fig. 7-27. A, Axial NECT in an elderly hypertensive patient. A large basal ganglionic hematoma *(large arrows)* is seen with intraventricular *(small arrows)* and choroid plexus *(open arrow)* hemorrhage. **B,** Axial CT scan in a hypertensive patient demonstrates pontine hematoma *(arrows)*. **C,** Axial CT scan in a hypertensive patient with lobar cerebral hemorrhage *(arrows)*.

Typically, active bleeding in HICH is relatively acute and usually lasts less than an hour. Cerebral edema rapidly ensues and progresses for 24 to 48 hours after ictus.[44] Although the clinical course of HICH is highly variable, about 25% of patients die within the first 48 hours.[45] Delayed neurologic deterioration occurs in a small percentage of cases and is usually due to rapid clot expansion with secondary brain herniation. Delayed hemorrhage usually occurs in patients with persistent hypertension.[44]

Imaging. High-density basal ganglionic hematomas with or without accompanying IVH are the most common CT manifestations of acute HICH, followed by thalamic and pontine hemorrhages (Fig. 7-27). Subacute hematomas may show peripheral "ring" enhancement following contrast administration (*see* Fig. 7-12, *B*). Late CT manifestations in patients who survive hypertensive bleeds include round or slitlike cavities, particularly in the putamen and external capsule. Calcification is uncommon.[47] MR studies reveal typical hemorrhagic residua.

Hypertensive encephalopathy. Hypertensive encephalopathy (HE) is a particular syndrome that occurs in patients with elevated blood pressure. It is characterized by rapidly progressive signs and symptoms, including headache, seizures, visual distur-

matomas often extend beyond the putamen to include the globus pallidus and internal capsule.[44] Clot dissection into the ventricular system occurs in about half the cases of hypertensive ICH and is associated with poor prognosis,[45] particularly when IVH involves the fourth ventricle.[46]

Lobar white matter hemorrhage is seen in 15% to 20% of ICH cases (Fig. 7-27, *C*);[47] some of these "spontaneous" lobar hemorrhages are due to amyloid, but most are hypertensive.[47a] The cerebellum is a relatively common site of HICH; the midbrain, medulla, and spinal cord are rarely involved.[41] Cerebellar hemorrhages typically originate near the dentate nucleus along perforating branches of the superior cerebellar or posterior inferior cerebellar arteries.[48]

bances, altered mental status, and focal neurologic signs.[49] Toxemia is the most common cause of HE, although pregnancy related and nongestational HE occur (*see* box).

The etiology of eclampsia and the other hypertensive encephalopathies is similar. The brain normally is protected by an autoregulation system that ensures constant perfusion over a range of systemic pressures. If these autoregulatory limits are exceeded, passive overdistention of cerebral arterioles may oc-

cur and blood-brain barrier breakdown ensues.[49] Interstitial extravasation of proteins and fluid results in multiple foci of reversible vasogenic edema.

The posterior circulation is particularly prone to develop HE-related lesions. One possible explanation is the significant regional heterogeneity of the sympathetic vascular innervation that normally protects the brain from marked increases in blood pressure. The internal carotid system is much better supplied with sympathetic innervation than the vertebrobasilar system.[49]

Toxemia of pregnancy. Severe preeclampsia and eclampsia represent advanced stages of pregnancy induced hypertension and are associated with considerable morbidity and mortality.[50] CNS involvement is common.

Preeclampsia is defined as the development of hypertension and proteinuria after the 24th week of gestation in a patient without preexisting vascular disease. Preeclampsia affects 5% to 10% of all pregnant patients. Eclampsia is defined as the development of convulsions and/or coma in women with preeclampsia. Eclampsia may occur before, during, or after delivery. Eclampsia affects 0.05% to 0.2% of all pregnancies; it is fatal in 13% of cases.[51]

Reported autopsy findings in fatal cases of eclampsia include cortical petechiae and subcortical hemorrhages, white matter and basal ganglionic hemor-

---

Hypertensive Encephalopathies
Preeclampsia/eclampsia
Chronic renal failure
Thrombotic thrombocytopenic purpura
Hemolytic-uremic syndrome
Systemic lupus erythematosus (rare)

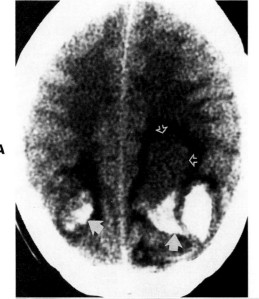

A

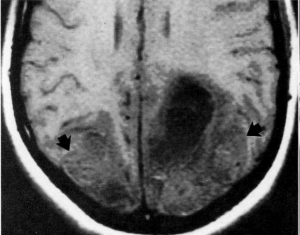

B

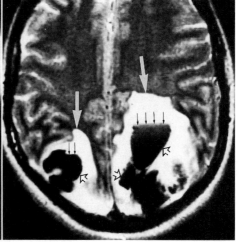

C

Fig. 7-28. **A,** Axial NECT in a patient with eclampsia shows bilateral occipital lobe hemorrhages *(large arrows)*. Note rapidly accumulating isodense unretracted hemorrhage *(open arrows)*. An MR scan was obtained approximately 8 hours later. **B,** Axial T1-weighted scan shows mixed iso- and hypointense cortical and subcortical lesions *(arrows)*. **C,** Axial T2-weighted study shows profoundly hypointense clots *(open arrows)* with striking peripheral edema *(white arrows)*. Note the fluid-fluid levels *(small black arrows)* in the rapidly accumulating hematomas.

rhage, and multifocal nonhemorrhagic white matter lesions.[52] Lesions associated with the hypertensive encephalopathies (including eclampsia) are commonly found at the gray-white matter junction and within the external capsule and basal ganglia. The occipital lobes are a frequent location of cortical and subcortical lesions in HE. This may be related to the higher number of sympathetic synapses on the anterior versus the posterior circulations.

Imaging findings in obstetric and nonobstetric cases of HE are similar.[49] Angiography may show areas of apparent constriction and narrowing of proximal and peripheral vessels.[51] CT scans show multiple low attenuation foci or hemorrhages in the subcortical white matter (Figs. 7-28 and 7-29, *A*) or basal ganglia (Fig. 7-28).

MR scans in women with severe preeclampsia often show nonspecific foci of increased signal in the deep cerebral white matter on T2WI.[50] Studies of women with eclampsia disclose multiple foci of cortical and subcortical white matter edema, primarily in the occipital lobes (Fig. 7-29, *B*).[49] Foci of increased T2 signal in the deep white matter, external capsule, and basal ganglia are also common. In contrast to autopsy studies, frank hemorrhagic lesions on MR scans of patients with preeclampsia and eclampsia are relatively uncommon (Fig. 7-29).[50] Transient contrast enhancement of the cortical and subcortical lesions may occur. Most eclamptic lesions resolve completely on follow-up studies.[50]

Nonobstetric causes of HE. Chronic renal disease, renovascular hypertension, and other systemic disorders such as thrombotic thrombocytopenic purpura (TTP) and the hemolytic-uremic syndrome (HUS) have been reported with CNS complications.[49,53]

In general, imaging findings in nongestational HE are similar to those described in eclampsia (Fig. 7-30).[53,54] In HUS, bilateral basal ganglia infarcts with hemorrhagic foci are seen often and cortical lesions are less common (Fig. 7-31). In TTP, cortical hemorrhages and ischemic infarcts have been reported.[53] Occasionally, other vascular disorders such as systemic lupus erythematosus can present with HE-like symptoms and similar imaging findings, including intracranial hemorrhage[55] (Fig. 7-32).

Hemorrhagic Infarction

Hemorrhagic infarction (HI) comprises a pathologic spectrum that ranges from petechial hemorrhages to frank parenchymal hematomas.[56] HI can be arterial or venous, cortical or deep, microscopic or gross.

Arterial infarction

Pathology and etiology. In contrast to hypertensive intracerebral bleeds, hemorrhage almost never occurs as the primary manifestation of arterial infarction. Nearly all so-called hemorrhagic infarcts occur as hemorrhagic transformation of initially ischemic lesions.[57]

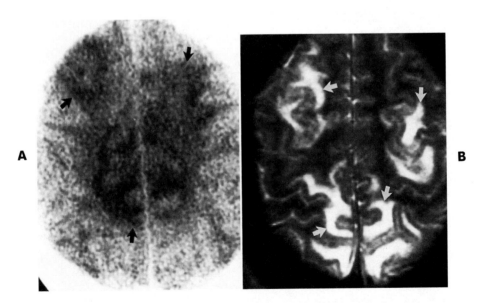

Fig. 7-29. A, Axial NECT scan in a patient with eclampsia shows bilateral low density lesions in the external capsules and subcortical white matter *(arrows).* **B,** Axial T2-weighted MR scan shows multiple high signal foci *(arrows)* in the external capsulel, basal ganglia, caudate nucleus, and subcortical white matter. Note relative sparing of the cortex. (From Digre K, Varner MW, Osborn AG, Crawford S: Cranial magnetic resonance imaging in severe preeclampsia vs. eclampsia, *Arch Neurol* 50:399-406, 1993.)

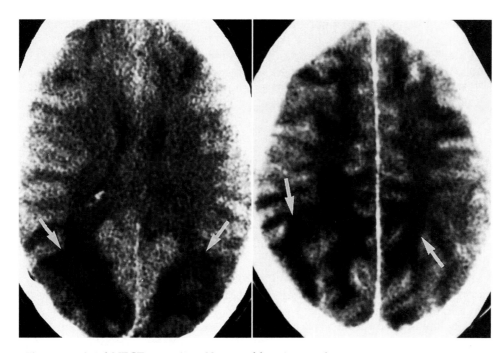

Fig. 7-30. Axial NECT scans in a 32-year-old patient with severe nongestational hypertensive encephalopathy. Bilateral occipital and gray-white matter junction low density lesions are present (*arrows*).

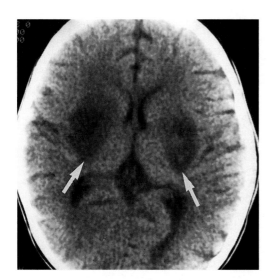

Fig 7-31. Three-year-old boy with hemolytic-uremic syndrome. Axial NECT shows bilateral low density lesions in the putamen and globus pallidus *(arrows)*.

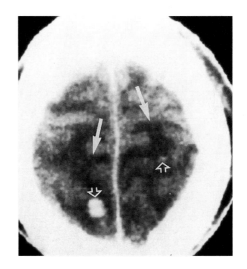

Fig. 7-32. Axial NECT scans in patient with SLE shows multiple low density lesions at the corticomedullary junction *(solid arrows)*. Some petechial hemorrhages are also present *(open arrows)*.

HI probably occurs when ischemically damaged endothelium is reperfused. Cerebral arterial embolism is the initiating lesion in most cases of HI. An embolus initially lodges in a proximal vessel (commonly the middle cerebral artery), producing the early ischemic insult to the brain parenchyma and vascular endothelium. When emboli are subsequently lysed and circulation is restored to the ischemic area, the damaged endothelium permits blood to extravasate into the previously ischemic or infarcted parenchyma.[56] The result is hemorrhagic transformation (HT) of a so-called bland infarct.

Incidence. Autopsy studies demonstrate hemorrhagic foci in 50% to 70% of all arterial infarcts, although the overall incidence of hemorrhagic arterial infarction on imaging studies is significantly lower. CT scans show HI in 5% to 15% of all stroke cases; the incidence of HI on MR studies is somewhat higher.[56] The incidence of HI is also higher in patients with embolic compared to thrombotic occlusions.[58]

Location. Although HI can occur almost anywhere in the brain it has a predilection for two particular areas, the basal ganglia and the cortex (Fig. 7-33). Deep hemorrhagic infarctions are often associated with proximal middle cerebral artery (MCA) occlusion.

Imaging. With the exception of hypertensive and amyloid-related strokes, CT scans obtained within the first 5 hours of cerebral infarction rarely show frank hemorrhage. Because hemorrhage typically occurs when an occluded vessel recanalizes and ischemic areas are reperfused following embolus frag-

mentation and lysis, most HIs are identified 24 to 48 hours following the ischemic event (Fig. 7-33, *B*).[59] Delayed cortical HIs can also develop if collateral blood supply through pial arteries increases after edema and mass effect diminish.[58]

Hemorrhagic transformation occurs in approximately 25% of large infarctions. This is seen as the appearance of high density foci within previously ischemic areas and virtually always associated with mass effect. Hypodensity seen on CT scans obtained within 4 hours after ictus strongly predicts later development of secondary HI in embolic ischemic infarcts. Hypodensity in the lentiform nuclei or cortex is seen initially, with subsequent development of patchy high density foci in the affected areas.[59]

MR findings in hemorrhagic infarction vary (*see* Chapter 11). Temporal evolution in signal changes similar to other parenchymal hematomas occurs. Acute hemorrhagic cortical infarction produces foci of mild cortical low intensity on T2WI that are surrounded by high-signal edema. Subacute infarcts

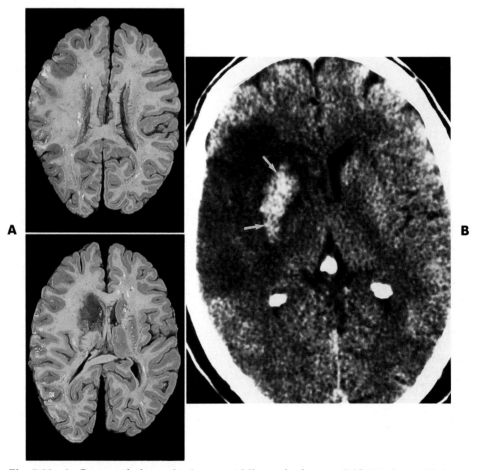

Fig. 7-33. A, Gross pathology of ischemic middle cerebral artery (MCA) infarct with hemorrhagic transformation in the basal ganglia and cortex. **B,** Axial NECT scan of a patient 48 hours after right MCA ischemic infarct. Hemorrhagic transformation in the basal ganglia *(arrows)* has occurred, probably secondary to reperfusion of the ischemic territory. (**A,** Courtesy E. Tessa Hedley-Whyte.)

show high signal on T1- and T2WI (*see* Fig. 11-23), whereas chronic lesions may show markedly low intensity on T2WI.[57] Foci of T1 shortening are identified in about 25% of subacute cerebral infarcts.[60]

Pseudolaminar cortical necrosis. A specific type of cortical infarction, pseudolaminar necrosis, can develop as a result of generalized cerebral hypoxia or anoxia rather than a local vascular abnormality that results in focal cerebral infarction. The middle cortical layers are typically affected and gyriform hemorrhage is common.[61] In some cases, nonhemorrhagic ischemic changes with linear or serpiginous cortical calcifications have been identified.[62] Thus

the high signal on T1WI in pseudolaminar cortical necrosis may be due to frank hemorrhage or relaxivity enhancement from calcification.

Venous infarction. Cerebral venoocclusive disorders are discussed in detail in Chapter 11. Their hemorrhagic manifestations are briefly summarized here.

Pathology and etiology. Although cortical vein thrombosis and venous infarction can occur in isolation, most are associated with occlusion of a major dural sinus (Fig. 7-34, *A* and *B*). In contrast to arterial occlusions, venous infarctions are often hemorrhagic and primarily affect the white matter rather than cortex. Trauma, tumor, infection, and hyperco-

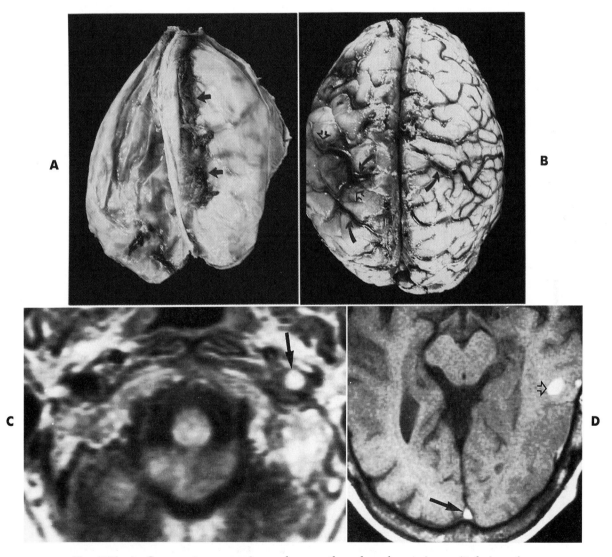

Fig. 7-34. A, Gross autopsy specimen shows a thrombosed superior sagittal sinus *(arrows)*. **B,** Brain specimen in the same case shows cortical vein thrombosis *(curved arrows)* and hemorrhagic venous infarcts *(open arrows)*. **C** and **D,** Axial T1-weighted MR scans in another patient with internal jugular vein thrombosis with occluded superior sagittal and transverse sinuses show subacute clots *(black arrows)* and a hemorrhagic temporal lobe venous infarct in the subcortical white matter *(open arrow)*. (**A** and **B,** From archives of the Armed Forces Institute of Pathology.)

agulable states are frequent etiologies; pregnancy and dehydration are common clinical settings.

Imaging. CT scans without contrast enhancement demonstrate patchy foci of edema and petechial hemorrhage. Signs of dural sinus occlusion may also be present. These include hyperdense clot in a dural sinus, most often the superior sagittal or transverse sinus, and the so-called empty delta sign. Here, dura around the affected sinus enhances intensely and the thrombus inside the sinus appears comparatively hypodense (*see* Figs. 11-78, *C* and 11-79, *B*). MR studies in venous infarction show nonconfluent corticomedullary junction hemorrhagic foci with variable edema. Dural sinus or deep venous thrombi can sometimes be identified (Fig. 7-34, *C* and *D*).

Aneurysms and Vascular Malformations

The pathology and imaging manifestations of intracranial aneurysms and vascular malformations are covered in detail in Chapters 9 and 10, respectively. Their manifestations as causes of nontraumatic intracranial hemorrhage are summarized here.

Aneurysms. In North America, 80% to 90% of nontraumatic subarachnoid hemorrhage (SAH) is caused by rupture of an intracranial aneurysm;[39] conversely, the most common presenting symptom of an intracranial aneurysm is SAH.

Computed tomography. Despite the contributions of magnetic resonance imaging, computed tomography (CT) is still the imaging procedure of choice in the diagnosis of acute SAH.[63,64] Acute SAH appears as high attenuation within the subarachnoid spaces (Fig. 7-35). Because most aneurysms arise from the circle of Willis and middle cerebral artery bifurcation, subarachnoid blood from ruptured saccular aneurysms usually fills the basal cisterns and sylvian fissures first (Fig. 7-35, *A*). When it mixes with cerebrospinal fluid and spreads over the cerebral convexities, subarachnoid blood appears as high density "feathered" collections along the interhemispheric fissure (Fig. 7-35, *B*).

Because CT scans reflect relative electron densities, some conditions with overall low density brain parenchyma may mimic SAH. These include the normal appearance of extremely premature, largely unmyelinated brain and diffuse cerebral edema. Neither should be mistaken for SAH.

Although SAH tends to diffuse quickly throughout the cisterns (Fig. 7-35), more focal cisternal or parenchymal hematomas can be seen with ruptured aneurysms and are helpful in localizing the bleeding source. Blood in the sylvian fissure may be due to an aneurysm on the ipsilateral internal carotid, posterior communicating, or middle cerebral artery (Fig. 7-36), whereas focal interhemispheric blood is usually due to an anterior communicating artery aneurysm (Fig. 7-16).[65] Blood in the fourth ventricle

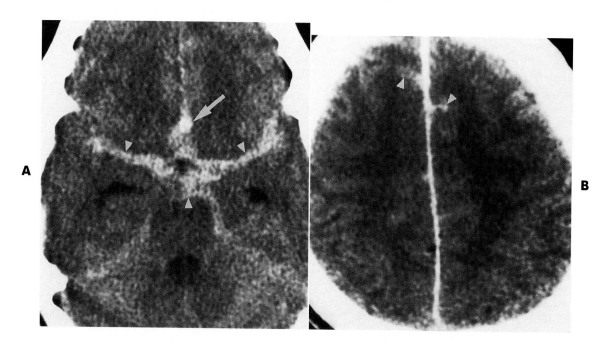

Fig. 7-35. Patient with subarachnoid hemorrhage (SAH) from a ruptured anterior communicating artery aneurysm. **A,** Blood has spread diffusely throughout the basal cisterns (*arrowheads*). A slightly more focal clot in the interhemispheric fissure (*arrow*) suggests the possible location of the ruptured aneurysm. **B,** Blood along the falx cerebri spreads into the paramedian sulci, producing a "feathered" appearance of high density in these spaces (*arrowheads*).

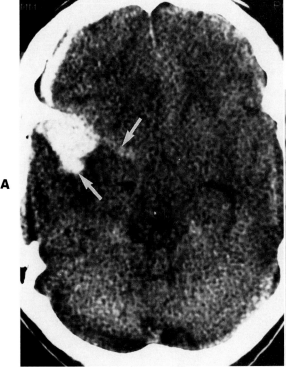

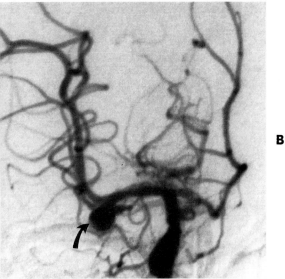

Fig. 7-36. **A,** Axial NECT shows focal SAH in the right sylvian fissure *(arrows)*. **B,** Digital subtraction right internal carotid angiogram, AP view, disclosed a middle cerebral artery bifurcation aneurysm *(arrow)*.

is often caused by a posterior inferior cerebellar artery lesion. "Giant" aneurysms (larger than 2.5 cm) often have spontaneous intramural hemorrhages (Fig. 9-23).

Subacute and chronic SAHs are more difficult to detect on CT scans. Because 90% of extravasated blood is cleared from the CSF within 1 week,[66] only half of all SAHs remain detectable on CT scans.[67] SAH visualized on CT more than 1 week after the initial hemorrhage suggests rebleeding.[68]

Magnetic resonance imaging. Although some au-

thors consider MR a sensitive, specific, and very accurate method for depicting acute SAH,[64] acute SAH can be difficult to detect on MR studies.[63] Blood mixed with cerebrospinal fluid may have a "dirty" appearance on T1-weighted scans and appear slightly higher in signal than clear CSF (Fig. 7-37, *A* and *B*). On long TR/short TE (proton density-weighted) scans, acute SAH is usually somewhat hyperintense to brain parenchyma and CSF (Fig. 7-37, *C* and *D*).[64]

MR is clearly superior to CT in detecting subacute and chronic SAH. Subacute SAH typically appears as

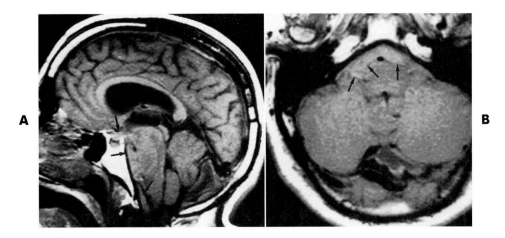

Fig. 7-37. Thirty-year-old woman with acute SAH. Sagittal **(A)** and axial **(B)**T1-weighted MR scans show that blood in the prepontine, medullary, and suprasellar cisterns *(arrows)* is isointense with adjacent brain.

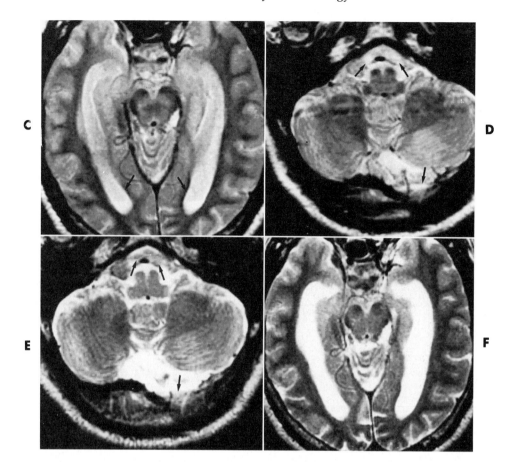

Fig. 7-37, cont'd. **C** and **D,** Axial long TR/short TE (proton density-weighted) scans show that blood in the medullary cisterns, lateral ventricles, and cisterna magna *(arrows)* is slightly hyperintense to CSF. **E** and **F,** On T2-weighted sequences the cisternal blood *(arrows)* appears slightly hypointense. Blood cannot be discerned in the enlarged lateral ventricles on these studies **(F).**

high signal foci within the subarachnoid cisterns on both T1- and T2-weighted studies (Fig. 7-38). Unless rebleeding occurs, blood in parenchymal hematomas associated with ruptured intracranial aneurysms follows the typical evolutionary changes already described on MR scans.

Repeated chronic subarachnoid or intraventricular hemorrhage may cause hemosiderin and ferritin deposition on the leptomeninges over the brain, cerebellum, brainstem, cranial nerves, and spinal cord (Fig. 7-39, *A*).[69] Common clinical presentation includes cerebellar dysfunction, pyramidal tract signs, and hearing loss.[69]

Leptomeningeal hemosiderin deposition is termed *superficial siderosis.* On T2-weighted MR scans, superficial siderosis appears as a very hypointense line along the surface of affected structures, particularly the pons and cerebellar vermis (Fig. 7-39, *B* and *C*).[70] Some MR scan sequences, particularly "fast" spin-echo studies, can cause an artifactual low signal border between the brain and adjacent subarachnoid space that should not be mistaken for this condition (Fig. 7-40).

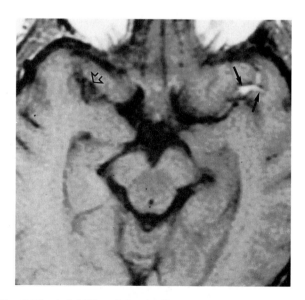

Fig. 7-38. Axial T1-weighted MR scan obtained 1 week after SAH shows subacute hemorrhage in the sylvian fissure as curvilinear hyperintense foci *(solid arrows).* Compare with normal low signal CSF in the right sylvian fissure *(open arrow).*

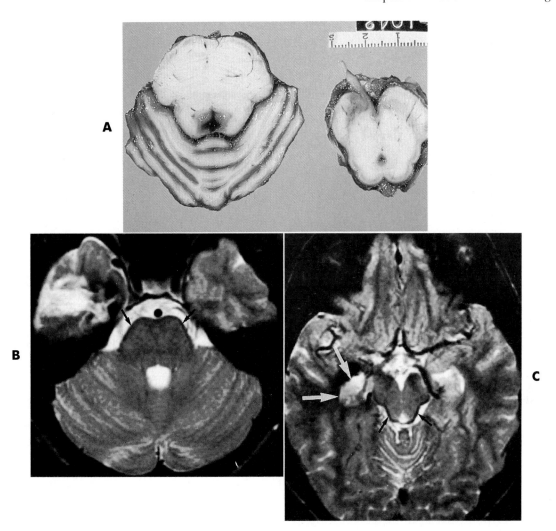

Fig. 7-39. A, Cut specimen through the midbrain and cerebellum shows brain surface and sulci stained from the chronic hemorrhage. **B** and **C,** Axial T2-weighted MR scans in a patient with repeated hemorrhagic episodes caused by a temporal lobe AVM **(C,** *white arrows).* Extensive superficial siderosis is seen as very low signal coating of the brain surface *(black arrows).* (**A,** Courtesy Rubinstein Collection, Armed Forces Institute of Pathology.)

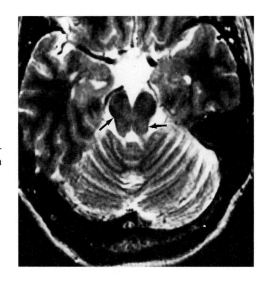

Fig. 7-40. "Fast" spin-echo T2-weighted MR scan has artifactual low signal *(arrows)* at the interface between brain and CSF that can mimic superficial siderosis.

Vascular malformations. Hemorrhage rates and imaging findings vary significantly with the histologic type of malformation. Although four types of intracranial vascular malformations have been identified and any one can bleed, only two, arteriovenous malformations (AVMs) and cavernous angiomas, hemorrhage frequently.

Arteriovenous malformations. The three types of arteriovenous malformations (AVMs) are listed as follows:

1. Pial
2. Dural
3. Mixed pial-dural

Pial AVMs hemorrhage at a cumulative rate of 2% to 3% per year.[71] (*see* Chapter 10). Unexplained intracranial hemorrhage in a child or normotensive young adult is often caused by an AVM (Fig. 7-41).

Nearly 70% of all patients with parenchymal AVMs show evidence of acute or chronic hemorrhage on initial MR examination.[72] Gliosis and encephalomalacic changes are also often present (*see* Fig. 10-15). When repeated hemorrhage into an AVM occurs, it can mimic neoplasm (Fig. 7-42).

Unlike brain AVMs, dural arteriovenous malformations (DAVMs) usually lack a discrete nidus. Instead, DAVMs are composed of numerous microfistulae within the dural wall of a major venous sinus.[71] The transverse and cavernous sinuses are common locations. DAVMs rarely hemorrhage unless drainage is through cortical veins or an intracranial venous varix. Either subarachnoid or parenchymal hemorrhage from a DAVM may occur if this venous drainage pattern is present (*see* Fig. 10-23).

Cavernous angiomas. Cavernous angiomas hem-

orrhage at an estimated rate of 0.5% per year and often show histologic or imaging evidence for repeated bleeds within the same lesion. Cavernous angiomas typically have a popcorn-like appearance with mixed signal foci inside a hemosiderin ring (Fig. 7-43) (*see* Chapter 10).

Venous angiomas. Although hemorrhage has been reported with venous angiomas,[73] it is relatively uncommon (*see* Fig. 10-45). The unusual venous angioma that is complicated by bleeding may appear identical to other hemorrhagic vascular malformations. In the absence of hemorrhage, venous angiomas are seen as a Medusa-like collection of dilated medullary veins near the angle of a cerebral ventricle (*see* Chapter 10).

Capillary telangiectasias. Capillary telangiectasias are usually small and clinically silent, although hemorrhagic residua and adjacent gliosis are frequently observed at autopsy.[41] Capillary telangiectasias' imaging appearances vary. Some have no identifiable imaging abnormalities and others are indistinguishable from cavernous angiomas. Multiple small foci of hemosiderin on T2WI are sometimes seen.

Hemorrhagic Neoplasms and Cysts

Oncologic-associated intracranial hemorrhage can be caused by malignancy induced coagulopathy or bleeding into a CNS tumor.[74]

Malignancy related coagulopathy. Intracranial hemorrhage is common in blood dyscrasias, especially the leukemias (Fig. 7-44). ICH also occurs in patients undergoing chemotherapy. Systemic neoplasms can be associated with terminal coagulopathy.

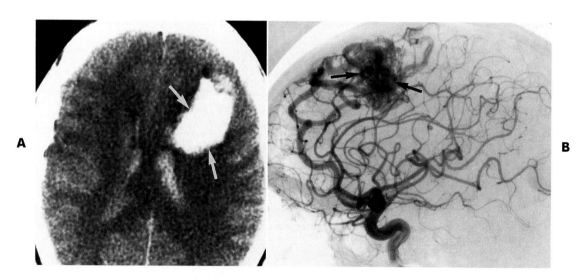

Fig. 7-41. A 25-year-old normotensive man with unexplained intracranial hemorrhage. **A,** Axial NECT scan shows a left frontal lobe hematoma (*arrows*). **B,** Left internal carotid angiogram, midarterial phase, lateral view, disclosed an arteriovenous malformation (*arrows*).

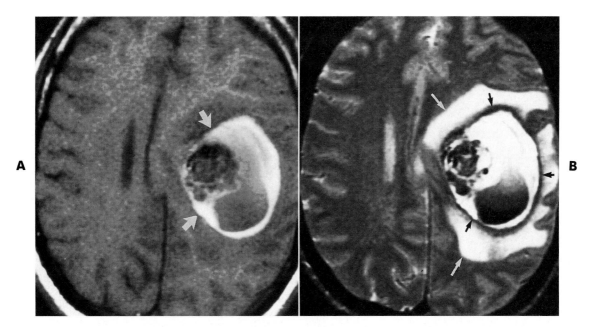

Fig. 7-42. Recurrent hemorrhage into a partially thrombosed AVM produces a complex MR appearance. **A,** Axial T1-weighted scan shows the mixed signal lesion *(arrows)*. T2-weighted **(B)** sequences show the extensive edema that surrounds the lesion as confluent white matter hyperintensity *(white arrows)*. A complete hemosiderin rim from chronic hemorrhage is present *(black arrows)*. These changes suggest hemorrhagic vascular malformation rather than neoplasm. Angiography (not shown) disclosed only an avascular mass effect. Thrombosed AVM was found at surgery.

There are no unique radiologic features that distinguish leukemia- or coagulopathy induced ICH from other intracerebral hematomas.[74]

Intratumoral hematomas

Pathology and etiology. The etiology of tumor-induced ICH is unclear. Factors such as high grade of malignancy, presence of neovascularity, rapid tumor growth with necrosis, plasminogen activators, and direct vascular invasion by neoplasm have been proposed.[74]

Incidence. The reported overall incidence of hemorrhage in intracranial neoplasms is 1% to 15%.[75] Although virtually any tumor in any location can hemorrhage, some tumors commonly bleed and others rarely bleed.

Bleeding varies significantly with histologic type.[76] In general, the more malignant astrocytomas bleed, as do very vascular tumors and necrotic neoplasms such as some pituitary adenomas.[76] Tumors that often show histologic evidence of hemorrhage are listed in the box, p. 188.

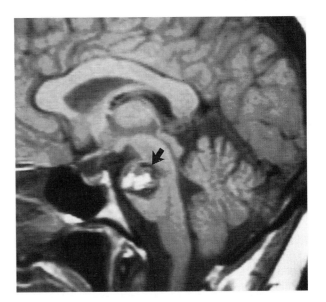

Fig. 7-43. Sagittal T1-weighted MR scan shows the typical popcorn-like appearance of a cavernous angioma. The solitary pontine lesion has a mixed signal reticulated core surrounded by a low signal hemosiderin rim *(arrow)*.

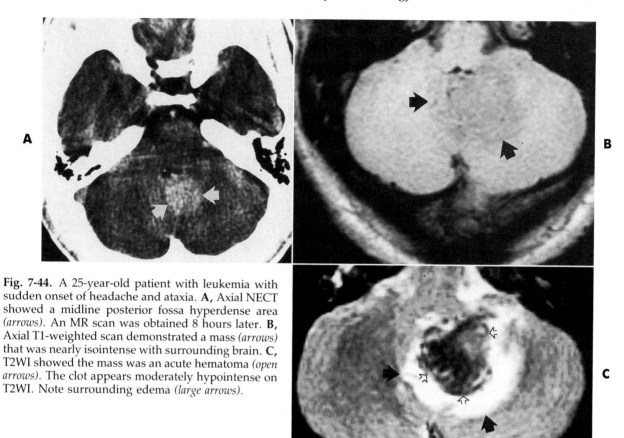

Fig. 7-44. A 25-year-old patient with leukemia with sudden onset of headache and ataxia. **A,** Axial NECT showed a midline posterior fossa hyperdense area *(arrows)*. An MR scan was obtained 8 hours later. **B,** Axial T1-weighted scan demonstrated a mass *(arrows)* that was nearly isointense with surrounding brain. **C,** T2WI showed the mass was an acute hematoma *(open arrows)*. The clot appears moderately hypointense on T2WI. Note surrounding edema *(large arrows)*.

Brain Tumors with Hemorrhage
Pathology Studies

Primary brain tumors

Anaplastic astrocytoma
Glioblastoma multiforme
Oligodendroglioma/mixed glioma
Pituitary adenoma
Hemangioblastoma
Sarcomas
Lymphoma (immunocompromised patients)
Ependymoma
Schwannoma
Epidermoid

Metastatic tumors

Melanoma
Choriocarcinoma
Renal cell carcinoma

Tumors and tumorlike lesions that bleed less frequently are low grade astrocytomas, mesenchymal tumors such as meningioma, nonneoplastic cysts and slowly growing cystic neoplasms such as craniopharyngioma, and ganglioglioma.

Imaging. Because CT and MR depict gross anatomic alterations, only macroscopic hemorrhagic foci are imaged and the frequency of bleeding on radiologic examination *(see box, p. 189)* is somewhat different compared to pathologic data (see previous discussion).

Primary brain tumors that often contain identifiable hemorrhagic foci on MR scans include anaplastic astrocytoma and glioblastoma multiforme (GBM) (Figs. 7-45 and 7-46). Because they often occur in older patients, GBMs are a relatively common cause of unexplained intracranial hemorrhage in a normotensive, nondemented elderly patient. Pilocytic astro-

Brain Tumors With Hemorrhage
Imaging Studies

Common

Pituitary adenoma
Anaplastic astrocytoma/glioblastoma multiforme
Oligodendroglioma
Ependymoma
Primitive neuroectodermal tumor
Epidermoid
Metastases (lung, kidney, choriocarcinoma, melanoma)

Uncommon

Low grade/pilocytic astrocytoma
Meningioma
Schwannoma
Lymphoma (unless immunocompromised)

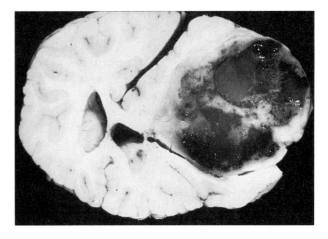

Fig. 7-45. Gross autopsy specimen shows a large necrotic, hemorrhagic glioblastoma multiforme. (Courtesy Rubinstein Collection, Armed Forces Institute of Pathology.)

A

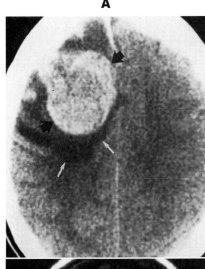

Fig. 7-46. Man, 72 years old, with seizure and left hemiparesis. **A,** Axial precontrast CT scan shows a large hemorrhagic right frontal mass *(black arrow)* with surrounding edema *(white arrows).* Axial T1- **(B)** and T2-weighted **(C)** scans disclosed a very heterogeneous mass *(large arrows)* with multiple cavities that contained blood degradation products *(double arrows).* **D,** Following contrast administration, axial T1-weighted scan shows patchy foci of increased signal in the solid portion of the mass *(arrows).* Glioblastoma multiforme with hemorrhage was found at surgery.

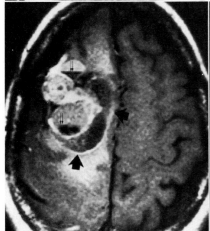

B

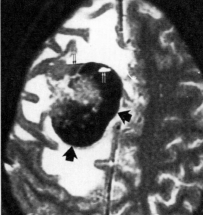

C

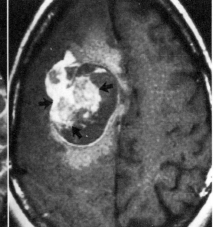

D

cytomas are usually seen in younger patients and only rarely hemorrhage.

Of the nonastrocytic gliomas, oligodendrogliomas commonly show hemorrhagic foci. Mixed gliomas with anaplastic or ependymal elements may also hemorrhage.[74] Ependymomas, particularly those in the spinal cord, sometimes bleed repeatedly and are a classic cause of neoplasm-induced superficial siderosis. Because of their intrinsic vascularity, choroid plexus tumors also often hemorrhage. Repeated episodes of silent hemorrhage may cause intraventricular obstructive hydrocephalus in these cases. Primitive neuroectodermal tumors and teratomas are other tumors occurring in young children that frequently bleed (Fig. 7-47).

The most common nonglial hemorrhagic primary intracranial tumor is pituitary adenoma (Fig. 7-48); in some pathologic series, pituitary adenomas represent the largest group of hemorrhagic brain tumors.[77] Other than pituitary adenoma, nonglial hemorrhagic primary neoplasms are relatively uncommon. Although schwannomas often show microscopic or even macroscopic hemorrhage at pathologic examination, frank hemorrhage is uncommon on imaging studies.[78]

Meningiomas rarely hemorrhage (Fig. 7-49). Germinomas occasionally undergo necrosis and may manifest hemorrhagic changes on MR studies but this is distinctly unusual.

Primary CNS lymphomas in immunocompetent patients rarely have necrosis or hemorrhage, although hemorrhage is common in HIV-infected patients (*see* Chapter 14).[79]

Hemorrhage occurs in up to 15% of brain metastases, with renal cell carcinoma (Fig. 7-50), choriocarcinoma, melanoma, bronchogenic carcinoma, and thyroid carcinoma common primary tumor types. Hemorrhage into metastatic foci can have a complex appearance on MR studies. Marked heterogeneity is common, with blood degradation products of different ages and fluid-fluid levels (Fig. 7-51).[80]

Differential diagnosis. Distinguishing hemorrhagic intracranial neoplasms from nonneoplastic hematomas can be difficult because there is considerable overlap between their imaging findings (*see* box). Multiple lesions and relative lack of edema are sug-

---

Benign Versus Neoplastic Hemorrhage

No absolute criteria

Tumors more complex, heterogeneous

Benign usually has complete hemosiderin rim (tumor doesn't)

Tumor usually has nonhemorrhagic areas that enhance after contrast administration

Benign follows orderly evolution on sequential scans

Hemorrhage evolution in tumors often delayed/disordered

Edema/mass effect resolve with benign; persist with tumor

Hemorrhagic vascular malformations often multiple; tumor usually solitary (unless metastatic)

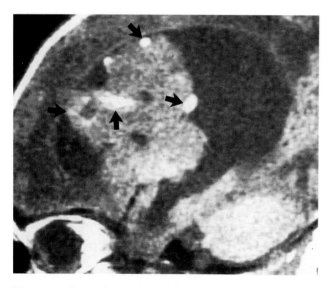

Fig. 7-47. Sagittal T1-weighted MR scan in a 3-month-old child with a left frontal and intraventricular mass. The lesion is mixed signal and contains several hyperintense foci *(arrows)*. Primitive neuroectodermal tumor with hemorrhagic areas was found at surgery.

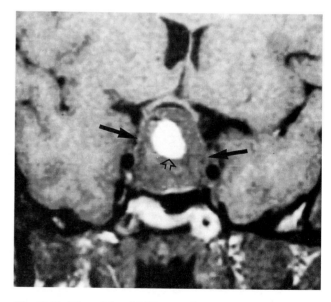

Fig. 7-48. T1-weighted MR scan shows pituitary adenoma *(large arrows)* with intratumoral hemorrhage *(open arrow)*.

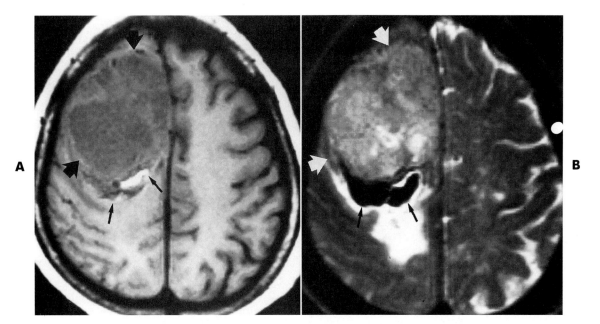

Fig. 7-49. Axial **(A)** T1-weighted plus axial T2-weighted **(B)** MR scans show a large frontal meningioma *(large arrows)* with subacute and early chronic hemorrhage *(small arrows)*. (Courtesy Woo Suk Choi.)

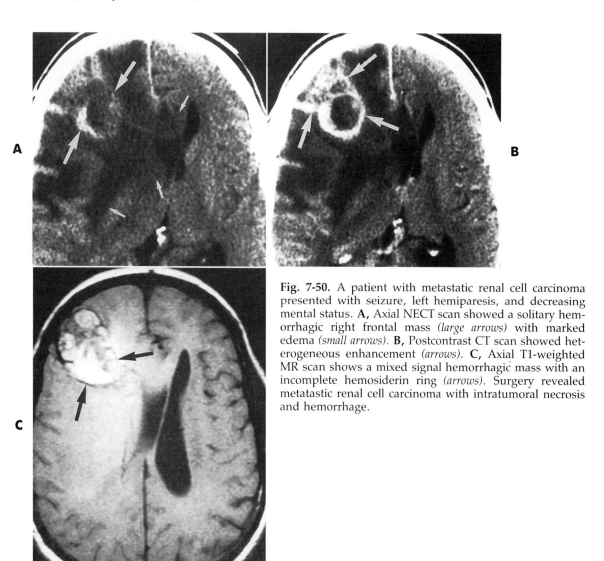

Fig. 7-50. A patient with metastatic renal cell carcinoma presented with seizure, left hemiparesis, and decreasing mental status. **A,** Axial NECT scan showed a solitary hemorrhagic right frontal mass *(large arrows)* with marked edema *(small arrows).* **B,** Postcontrast CT scan showed heterogeneous enhancement *(arrows).* **C,** Axial T1-weighted MR scan shows a mixed signal hemorrhagic mass with an incomplete hemosiderin ring *(arrows).* Surgery revealed metastatic renal cell carcinoma with intratumoral necrosis and hemorrhage.

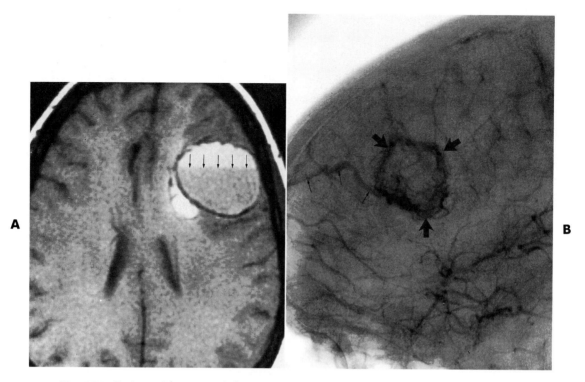

Fig. 7-51. Patient with metastatic breast carcinoma. **A,** Axial T1-weighted MR scan without contrast shows a left frontal lesion with a fluid-fluid level *(arrows)*. **B,** Left internal carotid angiogram, capillary phase, lateral view, shows a vascular mass *(large arrows)* with central necrosis and an early draining vein *(small arrows)*.

gestive of vascular malformation,[81] whereas an incomplete hemosiderin rim may indicate neoplasm.[80] Other reported findings that suggest neoplasm include adjacent nonhemorrhagic tumor foci; diminished, irregular, or absent hemosiderin deposition; delayed hematoma evolution; and pronounced or persistent edema[80] *(see* box, p. 190). Occasionally these guidelines are confounded when a hemorrhagic tumor looks like a vascular malformation or a vascular malformation is so heterogeneous that it mimics neoplasm (Figs. 7-52 and 7-53).

Nonneoplastic hemorrhagic cysts. Hemorrhage into benign, nonneoplastic intracranial cysts may sometimes occur. Colloid cysts almost never bleed, whereas Rathke cleft cysts and arachnoid cysts are occasionally complicated by hemorrhage. Hemorrhage into an arachnoid cyst may be spontaneous or follow minor trauma with rupture of intracystic or bridging vessels.[82] Arachnoid cysts are sometimes associated with subdural hematoma.[83]

Miscellaneous Causes of Intracranial Hemorrhage

Miscellaneous but nevertheless important causes of nontraumatic ICH include amyloid angiopathy, infection, vasculitis, sympathomimetic and recreational drug use, blood dyscrasias, and the coagulopathies. These are discussed in the following section.

Amyloid angiopathy. Cerebral amyloid angiopathy (CAA), also known as congophilic angiopathy, increases with advancing age and may be the most common cause of recurrent ICH in elderly normotensive patients.[84]

Pathology and etiology. Amyloidosis is a disease complex with a common unifying feature: tissue deposition of nonbranching fibrillar proteins that have the crystallographic characteristics of a beta-pleated sheet.[85]

Three forms of amyloid deposits occur in the CNS as follows:

1. The amyloid core of senile plaque
2. Cortical and leptomeningeal vessel wall deposits
3. Extension from small vessels into the surrounding brain parenchyma

The latter two conditions together are termed *amyloid angiopathy.*[86] In CAA the contractile elements of the leptomeningeal and cortical arteries are replaced by noncontractile amyloid beta protein.[87] The arterial walls in CAA stain intensely with Congo red and show birefringence on polarized light.

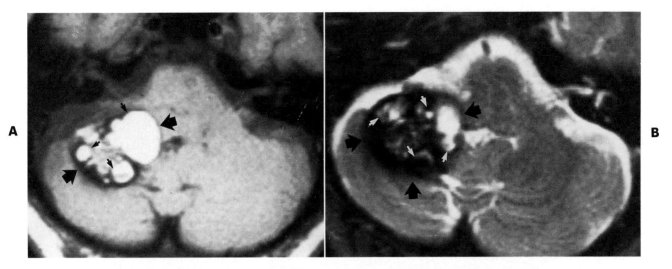

Fig. 7-52. Axial T1- **(A)** and T2-weighted **(B)** MR scans in a 33-year-old woman with a hemorrhagic posterior fossa mass. Multiple septated cysts contain blood degradation products in different stages *(small arrows)*. The lesion is surrounded by a complete hemosiderin rim *(large arrows)*. Pathological diagnosis was hemorrhagic cerebellar hemangioblastoma.

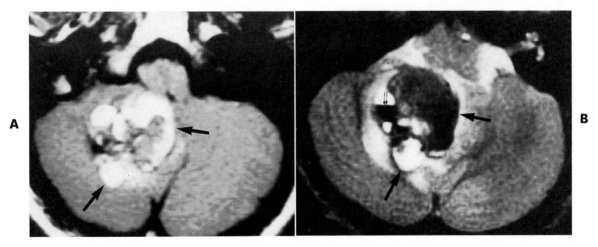

Fig. 7-53. A 35-year-old woman with a hemorrhagic posterior fossa mass and a family history of von Hippel-Lindau syndrome. **A,** Axial T1-weighted MR scan showed a mixed signal mass *(large arrows)* with multiple cysts that contained fluid-fluid levels *(double arrows)*. **B,** Standard T2-weighted scan showed the mass lacked a complete peripheral hemosiderin rim. Preoperative diagnosis was hemorrhagic cerebellar hemangioblastoma. Cavernous angioma was found at surgery.

Location and imaging appearance. In contrast to hypertensive hemorrhage, hemorrhages in CAA are characteristically multiple, spare the basal ganglia and brainstem, and are located at the corticomedullary junction (Fig. 7-54, *A*).[40,86] CT and MR findings of multiple peripherally located hemorrhages of different ages in an elderly normotensive patient strongly suggest CAA (Fig. 7-54, *B* and *C*).

Inflammatory disease and vasculitis. Hemorrhage in brain infections is unusual.[88] Gross hemorrhage is uncommon in uncomplicated pyogenic abscesses, although immunocompromised patients have an increased propensity to develop hemorrhagic lesions. CNS infections and inflammatory processes that have a propensity to bleed include infective endocarditis with septic emboli, fungal vasculitis,

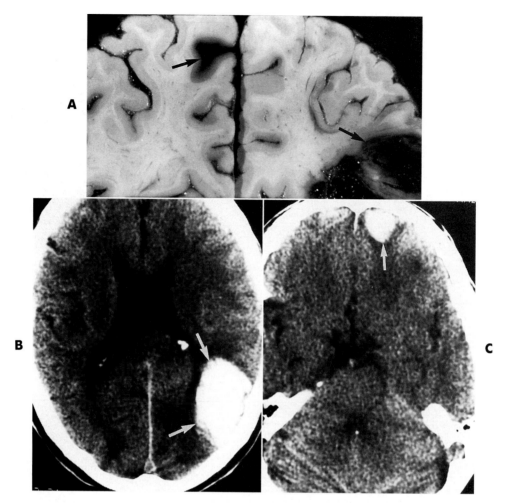

Fig. 7-54. A, Gross autopsy specimen shows bilateral hemorrhages secondary to amyloid angiopathy. A large lobar hemorrhage is seen *(large arrow)*, and a smaller corticomedullary junction lesion *(small arrow)* is identified in the opposite hemisphere. **B** and **C,** Axial NECT scans in an elderly normotensive but demented patient show lobar hemorrhage *(arrows)*, probably due to amyloid angiopathy. (**A,** Courtesy E. Tessa Hedley-Whyte.)

and necrotizing hemorrhagic infections such as herpes encephalitis.

Subarachnoid or parenchymal hemorrhage occurs in 5% to 10% of patients with infective endocarditis and neurologic symptoms (Fig. 7-55).[89] The following three possible etiologies have been proposed[87]:

1. Formation of a mycotic aneurysm (*see* Chapter 9)
2. Hemorrhagic infarction
3. Focal arteritis with septic arterial wall erosion

Aspergillosis and other fungal infections may directly invade vessel walls, resulting in thrombosis, hemorrhage, or cerebral infarction.

With the exception of type II herpes simplex encephalitis, hemorrhage in all types of encephalitis is infrequent.[87] Hemorrhage is especially common with neonatal herpes (*see* Chapter 16).

CNS Complications of Drug Use

Hemorrhage
    50% preexisting abnormality (aneurysm, AVM)
    50% spontaneous
Arterial infarction
Dural sinus/cortical vein occlusion
Abscess
Vasculitis
Mycotic aneurysm

Sympathomimetic and recreational drugs. The spectrum of CNS complications associated with drug abuse is outlined in the box. Most patients have ischemic or hemorrhagic manifestations.

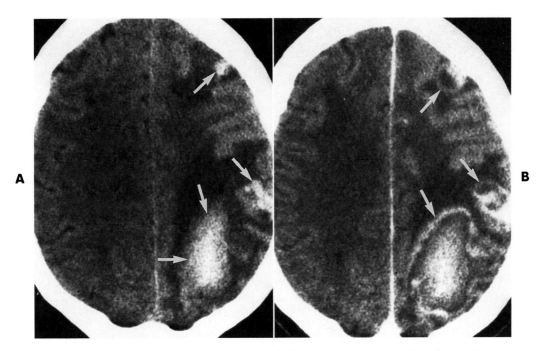

Fig. 7-55. Pre- **(A)** and postcontrast **(B)** axial CT scans in a patient with subacute bacterial endocarditis and multiple hemorrhagic septic emboli. The NECT scan shows three partially resolving hemorrhagic foci **(A,** *arrows).* **B,** The postcontrast studies show a "target" configuration with a thin contrast-enhancing rim *(arrows)* surrounding a peripheral low attenuation ring that in turn surrounds the higher density resolving hematomas.

Drug-related intracranial hemorrhage occurs about twice as frequently as ischemia and can be intraparenchymal or subarachnoid. A preexisting abnormality such as aneurysm or AVM is present in half of these cases.[90] In other cases, street drugs such as cocaine may induce an acute hypertensive episode that results in ICH. Here, the locations are similar to hypertensive hemorrhages seen in older patients, i.e., in the basal ganglia, external capsule, cerebellum, and, occasionally, the lobar white matter.[91]

Cocaine also enhances platelet aggregation and may therefore promote arterial thrombosis. Dural sinus thrombosis with hemorrhagic venous infarction has been reported in some cases of cocaine abuse.[92] Vasospasm and ischemic infarction are common nonhemorrhagic complications of cocaine abuse. Vasculitis occurs but is less common with cocaine use compared to drugs such as amphetamine and phenylpropanolamine.[91]

Other drugs linked to ICH are amphetamine and its derivatives, phenylpropanolamine (PPA), phencyclidine (PCP), ephedrine, and pseudoephedrine.[93] Amphetamines cause endothelial damage and fibrinoid necrosis of vessel walls. Necrotizing cerebral vasculitis is common and the angiographic findings of extensive irregular segmental beading may be striking (Fig. 7-56). Other possible drug-related causes of this angiographic appearance are subarachnoid hemorrhage and vasospasm.[91]

Blood dyscrasias and coagulopathies. Various congenital blood dyscrasias and acquired hemorrhagic diatheses can cause intracranial hemorrhage. A discussion of congenital clotting disorders is beyond the scope of this text. Complications from acquired abnormalities of blood coagulation, particularly iatrogenic bleeding disorders, will be discussed.

There are only four known common causes of acquired noniatrogenic coagulopathy: vitamin K deficiency, hepatocellular disease, antibodies that react with clotting factors, and disseminated intravascular coagulation (DIC), usually with secondary fibrinolysis.[94] Iatrogenic bleeding disorders have been reported with heparin, warfarin, thrombolytic agents such as streptokinase and tissue plasminogen activator (TPA), antiplatelet agents such as aspirin and ibuprofen, alcohol abuse, chemotherapeutic agents, and other drugs such as quinine (reported to cause hemolytic-uremic syndrome) and quinidine.[15]

Bleeding complications are inherent risks of anticoagulant (AC) therapy and most of the fatal bleeds are intracranial.[95] Between 10% to 15% of patients with nontraumatic, nonaneurysmal primary intracranial hemorrhage are on AC therapy.[17] About 1% of patients undergoing thrombolytic therapy for acute myocardial infarction develop ICH. This complication has a grave prognosis, with over 60% of patients dying during hospitalization.[16]

Imaging findings in most coagulopathies are sim-

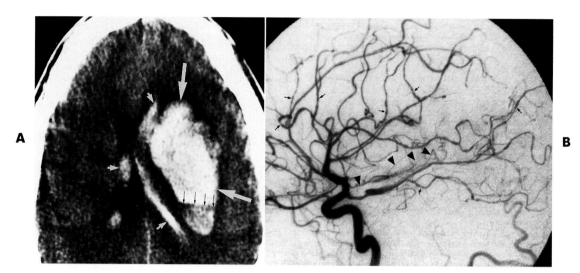

Fig. 7-56. A, Axial NECT scan in a 32-year-old normotensive man with sudden onset of coma showed a basal ganglia hematoma *(large arrows)* with some intraventricular hemorrhage *(small white arrows)*. A fluid-fluid level was seen *(black arrows)*. Cerebral angiography was performed to detect possible underlying vascular malformation. **B,** Digital subtraction common carotid angiogram showed extensive arteritic changes *(small arrows)*. An avascular mass effect is shown by displacement of the choroidal branches *(arrowheads)*. The patient later admitted to sympathomimetic drug abuse.

ilar. Although bleeding can occur at any location, the most common site in these patients is supratentorial and intraparenchymal. Fluid-fluid levels within hematomas are common (Fig. 7-8). Multiple large volume hemorrhages with substantial mass effect can also be seen and are associated with increased mortality.[16]

REFERENCES

1. Hayman LA, Pagani JJ, Kirkpatrick JB, Hincik VB: Pathophysiology of acute intracerebral and subarachnoid hemorrhage: applications to MR imaging, *AJNR* 10:457-461, 1989.
2. Blackmore CC, Francis CW, Bryant RG et al: Magnetic resonance imaging of blood and cells in vitro, *Invest Radiol* 25:1316-1324, 1990.
3. Williams KD, Drayer BP, Bird CR: Magnetic resonance: the diagnosis of intracerebral hematoma, *BNI Quarterly* 5:16-27, 1989.
4. Hayman LA, Taber KH, Ford JJ, Bryan RN: Mechanisms of MR signal alteration by acute intracerebral blood: old concepts and new theories, *AJNR* 12:899-907, 1991.
5. Kirkpatrick JB, Hayman LA: Pathophysiology of intracranial hemmorrhage, *Neuroimaging Clin N Amer* 2:11-23, 1992.
6. Chin HY, Taber KH, Hayman LA et al: Temporal changes in red blood cell hydration: application to MRI of hemorrhage, *Neuroradiol* 33(suppl):79-81, 1991.
7. Clark RA, Watanabe AT, Bradley WG Jr, Roberts JD: Acute hematoma: effects of deoxygenation, hematocit, and fibrin-clot formation and retraction on T2 shortening, *Radiol* 175:201-206, 1990.
8. Lee Y-Y, Moser R, Bruner JM, Van Tassel P: Organized intracerebral hematoma with acute hemorrhage: CT patterns and pathologic correlations, *AJNR* 7:409-416, 1986.
9. Thulborn KR, Sorensen AG, Kowall NW et al: The role of ferritin and hemosiderin in the MR appearance of cerebral hemorrhage: a histopathologic biochemical study in rats, *AJNR* 11:291-297, 1990.
10. Darrow VC, Alvord EC, Mack LA, Hodson WA: Histologic evaluation of the reactions to hemorrhage: the premature human infant's brain, *Am J Pediat* 130:44-58, 1988.
11. Brooks RA, DeChiro G, Patronas N: MR imaging of cerebral hematoma at different field strengths: theory and applications, *J Comp Asst Tomagr* 13:194-206, 1989.
12. Cohen WA, Wayman LA: Computed tomography of intracranial hemmorrhage, *Seuroimaging Clinics N Amer* 2:75-87, 1992.
13. Boyko OB, Cooper DF, Grossman CB: Contrast-enhanced CT of acute isodense subdural hematoma, *AJNR* 12:341-343, 1991.
14. Stein SC, Ross SE: Moderate head injury: a guide to initial management, *J Neurosurg* 77:562-564, 1992.
15. Walenga JM, Marmon JF: Coagulopathies associated with intracranial homorrhage, *Neuroimaging Clin N Amer* 2:137-152, 1992.
15a. Pfleger MJ, Hardee EP, Hayman LA: Fluid/fluid levels in intracerebral hematoma: a sign of coagulopathy. Reported at the 30th Annual Scientific Meeting of the American Society of Neuroradiology, St. Louis, Missouri, May 31–June 5, 1992.
16. Uglietta JP, O'Connor CM, Boyko OB et al: CT patterns of intracranial hemorrhage complicating thrombolytic therapy for acute myocardiac infarction, *Radiol* 181:555-559, 1991.
17. Fogelholm R, Eskola K, Kiminkinen T, Kunnamo I: Anticoagulant treatment as a risk factor for primary intracerebral hemorrhage, *J Neurol Neurosurg Psychiatr* 59:1121-1124, 1992.
18. Triulzi F: Cerebral hemorrhage: CT and MR, *Riv di Neuroradiol* 3(suppl 2):39-44, 1990.
19. Bergstrom M, Ericson K, Levander B, Svendsen P: Computed tomography of cranial subdural and epidural hematoma: variation of attenuation related to time and clinical events such as rebleeding, *J Comp Asst Tomogr* 1:449-455, 1977.
20. Zimmerman RD, Leeds NE, Naidich TP: Ring blush associated with intracerebral hematoma, *Radiol* 122:707-711, 1977.
21. Kreel L, Kay R, Woo J et al: The radiological (CT) and clinical sequelae of primary intracerebral hemorrhage, *Br J Radiol* 64:1096-1100, 1991.

22. Zyed A, Hayman LA, Bryan RN: MR imaging of intracerebral blood: diversity of the temporal pattern at 0.5 and 01.0T, *AJNR* 12:469-474, 1991.

23. Gomori JM, Grossman RI: Mechanisms responsible for the MR appearance and evolution of intracranial hemorrhage, *Radio-Graphics* 8:427-440, 1988.

24. Janick PA, Hackney DB, Grossman RI, Asakura T: MR imaging of various oxidation states of intracellular and extracellular hemoglobin, *AJNR* 12:891-897, 1991.

25. Weingarten K, Zimmerman RD, Deo-Narine V et al: MR imaging of acute intracranial hemorrhage: findings on sequential spin-echo and gradient-echo images in a dog model, *AJNR* 12:457-467, 1991.

26. Thulborn KR, Atlas SW: Intracranial hemorrhage. In SW Atlas, editor: *Magnetic Resonance Imaging of the Brain and Spine,* pp. 175-222, New York, Raven Press, 1991.

27. Stuhlmuller JE, Olson JD, Burns TL, Skorton DJ: Effect of varying fibrinogen and hematocrit concentration on magnetic resonance relaxation times of thrombus, *Invest Radiol* 27:341-345, 1992.

28. Stuhlmuller JE, Scholz TD, Olson JD et al: Magnetic resonance characterization of blood coagulation in vitro: effect of platelet depletion, *Invest Radiol* 26:343-347, 1991.

29. Weingarten K, Zimmerman RD, Cahill PT, Deck MDF: Detection of acute intracerebral hemorrhage on MR imaging: ineffectiveness of prolonged interecho interval pulse sequences, *AJNR* 12:475-479, 1991.

30. Piatt JH Jr, Clunie DA: Intracranial arterial aneurysm due to birth trauma, *J Neurosurg* 77:799-803, 1992.

31. Rorke LB, Zimmerman RA: Prematurity, postmaturity, and destructive lesions in utero, *AJNR* 13:517-536, 1992.

32. Keeney SE, Adcock EW, McArdle CB: Prospective observations of 100 high-risk neonates by high-field (1.5 Tesla) magnetic resonance imaging of the central nervous system: I. Intraventricular and extracerebral lesions, *Pediatr* 87:421-430, 1991.

33. Keeney SE, Adcock EW, McArdle CB: Prospective observations of 100 high-risk neonates by high-field (1.5 Tesla) magnetic resonance imaging of the central nervous system: II. Lesions associated with hypoxic-ischemic encephalopathy, *Pediatr* 87:431-438, 1991.

34. Schellinger D, Grant EG, Manz HJ, Patronas NJ: Intraparenchymal hemorrhage in preterm neonates: a broadening spectrum, *AJNR* 9:327-333, 1988.

35. Barkovich AJ: Intracranial hemorrhage in the newborn. In *Pediatric Neuroimaging,* pp 66-68, New York: Raven Press, 1990.

36. Truwit CL, Barkovich AJ, Koch TK, Ferriero DM: Cerebral palsy: MR findings in 40 patients, *AJNR* 13:67-78, 1992.

37. Volpe JJ: Value of MR in definition of the neuropathology of cerebral palsy in vivo, *AJNR* 13:79-83, 1992.

38. Barkovich AJ: MR and CT evaluation of profound neonatal and infantile asphyxia, *AJNR* 13:959-972, 1992.

39. Bozzola FG, Gorelick PB, Jensen JM: Epidemiology of intracranial hemorrhage, *Neuroimaging Clin N Amer* 2:1-10, 1992.

40. Wakai S, Kumakura N, Nagai M: Lobar intracerebral hemorrhage, *J Neurosurg* 76:231-238, 1992.

41. Okazaki H: Cerebrovascular disease. In *Fundamentals of Neuropathology,* pp 27-93, New York: Szaku-Shoin, 1989.

42. Chung CS, Park CH: Primary pontine hemorrhage, *Neurol* 42:830-834, 1992.

43. Laissy JP, Normand G, Monroc M et al: Spontaneous intracerebral hematomas from vascular causes, *Neuroradiol* 33:291-295, 1991.

44. Bae HG, Lee KS, Yun IG et al: Rapid expansion of hypertensive intracerebral hemorrhage, *Neurosurg* 31:35-40, 1992.

45. Franke CL, van Swieten JC, Algra A, van Gijn J: Prognostic factors in patients with intracerebral hematoma, *J Neurol Neurosurg Psychiat* 55:653-657, 1992

46. Gras P, Giroud M, Dumas R: Intracerebral hemorrhage, *Neurol* 42:1852 (letter), 1992.

47. Loes DJ, Smoker WRK, Biller J, Cornell SH: Nontraumatic lobar intracerebral hemorrhage: CT/angiographic correlation, *AJNR* 8:1027-1030, 1987.

47a. Broderick J, Brott T, Tomsik T et al: Lobar hemorrhage in the elderly: the undiminishing importance of hypertension, *Stroke* 24:49-51, 1993.

48. Gokaslan ZL, Narayan RK: Intracranial hemorrhage in the hypertensive patient, *Neuroimaging Clin N Amer* 2:171-186, 1992.

49. Schwartz RB, Jones KM, Kalina P et al: Hypertensive encephalopathy: findings on CT, MR imaging and SPECT imaging in 14 cases, *AJR* 159:379-383, 1992.

50. Digre KB, Varner MW, Osborn AG, Crawford S: Cranial magnetic resonance imaging in severe pre-eclampsia versus eclampsia, *Arch Neurol,* 50:399-406, 1993.

51. Lewis LK, Hinshaw DB Jr, Will AD et al: CT and angiographic correlations of severe neurological disease in toxemia of pregnancy, *Neuroradiol* 30:59-64, 1988.

52. Sheehan HL, Lynch JB: Cerebral lesions. In *Pathology of toxemia of pregnancy,* pp 525-554, Churchill Livingstone, Edinburgh, London, 1973.

52a. Mantello MT, Schwartz RB, Jones KM et al: Imaging of neurologic complications associated with pregnancy, *AJR* 160:843-847, 1993.

53. Kay AC, Solberg LA Jr, Nichols DA, Petitt RM: Prognostic significance of computed tomography of the brain in thrombotic thrombocytopenic purpura, *Mayo Clin Proc* 66:602-607, 1991.

54. Sherwood JW, Wagle WA: Hemolytic uremic syndrome: MR findings of CNS complications, *AJNR* 12:703-704, 1991.

55. Cunningham S, Conway EE Jr: Systemic lupus erythematosis presenting as an intracranial bleed, *Ann Emer Med* 20:810-812, 1991.

56. Mathews VP, Bryan RN: Intracranial hemorrhage in occlusive vascular disease, *Neuroimaging Clin N Amer* 2:221-233, 1992.

57. Horowitz SH, Zito JL, Donnarumma R et al: Clinical-radiographic correlations within the first five hours of cerebral infarction, *Acta Neurol Scan* 86:207-214, 1992.

58. Bozzao L, Angeloni U, Bastianello S et al: Early angiographic and CT findings in patients with hemorrhagic infarction: the distribution of the middle cerebral artery, *AJNR* 12:1115-1121, 1991.

59. Bozzao L, Angeloni U, Bastianello S: The value of early CT hypodensite in predicting middle cerebral artery hemorrhagic infarction, *Neuroradiol* 33(suppl):42-44, 1991.

60. Nabatame H, Fujimoto N, Nakamura K et al: High intensity areas on noncontrast T1-weighted MR images in cerebral infarction, *J Comp Asst Tomogr* 14:521-526, 1990.

61. Okazaki H: *Fundamentals of Neuropathology,* pp 27-94. Igaju-Shoin, Tokyo, 1989.

62. Boyko OB, Burger PC, Shelburne JD, Ingram P: Non-hememechanisms for T1 shortening: pathologic, CT and MR elucidation, *AJNR* 13:1439-1445, 1992.

63. Atlas SW: MR Imaging is highly sensitive for acute subarachnoid hemorrhage. . .Not! *Radiol* 186:319-332, 1993.

64. Ogawa T, Inugami A, Shimosegawa E et al: Subarachnoid hemorrhage: evaluation with MR imaging, *Radiol* 186:345-351, 1993.

65. Watanabe AT, Mackey JK, Lufkin RB: Imaging diagnosis and temporal appearance of subarachnoid hemorrhage, *Neuroimaging Clin N Amer* 2:53-59, 1992.

66. Wahlgren NG, Lindquist C: Haem derivatives in the cerebrospinal fluid after intracranial hemorrhage, *Eur Neurol* 26:216-221, 1987.

67. Van Gijn J, Van Donger KJ: The time-course of aneurysmal hemorrhage on computed tomography, *Neuroradiol* 23:153, 1982.

68. Scotti G, Ethier R, Melancon D et al: Computed tomography: the evaluation of intracranial aneurysms and subarachnoid hemorrhage, *Radiol* 123:85, 1977.

69. Bourgouin PM, Tampieri D, Melancon D et al: Superficial sederosis of the brain following unexplained subarachnoid hemorrhage: MRI diagnosis and clinical significance, *Neuroradiol* 34:407-410, 1992.

70. Bracchi M, Savoiardo M, Triulzi F et al: Superficial siderosis of the CNS: MR diagnosis and clinical findings, *AJNR* 14:227-236, 1993.

71. Jacobs JM: Angiography in intracranial hemorrhage, *Neuroimaging Clin N Amer* 2:89-106, 1992.

72. Yousem DM, Flamm ES, Grossman RI: Comparison of MR imaging with clinical history in the identification of hemorrhage in patients with cerebral arteriovenous malformations, *AJNR* 10:1151-1154, 1989.

73. Rothfus WE, Albright AL, Casey KF et al: Cerebellar venous angioma: "benign" entity? *AJNR* 61-66, 1984.

74. Leeds NE, Sawaya R, Van Tassel P, Hayman LA: Intracranial hemorrhage in the oncologic patient, *Neuroimaging Clin N Amer* 2:119-136, 1992.

75. Destian S, Sze G, Krol G et al: MR imaging of hemorrhagic intracranial neoplasms, *AJNR* 9:1115-1122, 1988.

76. Kondziolka D, Bernstein M, Resch L et al: Significance of hemorrhage into brain tumors: clinicopathologic study, *J Neurosurg* 67:852-857, 1987.

77. Wakai S, Yamakawa K, Manakas S et al: Spontaneous intracranial hemorrhage caused by brain tumor: its incidence and clinical significance, *Neurosurg* 10:437-444, 1982.

78. Mulkens TH, Parizel PM, Martin JJ et al: Acoustic schwannoma: MR findings in 84 tumors, *AJR* 160:395-398, 1993.

79. Cordoliana Y-S, Derosier C, Pharaboz C et al: Primary cerebral lymphoma in patients with AIDS: MR findings in 17 cases, *AJR* 159:841-847, 1992.

80. Atlas SW, Grossman RI, Gomori JM: Hemorrhagic intracranial malignant neoplasms: spin echo MR imaging, *Radiol* 164:71-77, 1987.

81. Sze G, Krol G, Olson WL et al: Hemorrhagic neoplasms: MR mimics of occult vascular malformations, *AJNR* 8:795-802, 1987.

82. Eustace S, Toland J, Stack J: CT and MRI of arachnoid cyst with complicating intracystic and subdural hemorrhage, *J Comp Asst Tomogr* 16:999-997, 1992.

83. van Burken MMG, Sarioglu AC, O'Donnell HD: Supratentorial arachnoid cyst with intracystic and subdural haematoma, *Neurochir* 35:199-203, 1992.

84. Lee KS, Bae HG, Yun IG: Recurrent intracerebral hemorrhage due to hypertension, *Neurosurg* 26:586-590, 1990.

85. Glenner GG, Murphy MA: Amyloidosis of the nervous system, *J Neurol Sci* 94:1-28, 1989.

86. Awasthi D, Voorhies RM, Eick J, Mitchell WT: Cerebral amyloid angiopathy presenting as multiple intracranial lesions on magnetic resonance imaging, *J Neurosurg* 75:458-469, 1991.

87. Leblanc R, Preul M, Robitaille et al: Surgical considerations in cerebral amyloid angiopathy, *Neurosurg* 29:712-718, 1991.

88. Baker R, Jones HR Jr: Intracranial hemorrhage in infectious diseases, *Neuroimaging Clin N Amer* 2:213-220, 1992.

89. Pruit AA, Rubin RH, Karchmer AW, Duncan GW: Neurologic complications of bacterial endocarditis, *Medicine* 57:329-343, 1978.

90. Brown E, Prager J, Lee H-Y, Ramsey RG: CNS complications of cocaine abuse: prevalence, pathophysiology and neuroradiology, *AJR* 159:137-147, 1992.

91. Landi JL, Spickler EM: Imaging of intracranial hemorrhage associated with drug abuse, *Neuroimaging Clin N Amer* 2:187-194, 1992.

92. Gean-Marton AD et al: Presented at the American Roentgen Ray Society meeting, Boston, Massachusetts, May 1991.

93. Nalls G, Disher A, Daryabagi J et al: Subcortical cerebral hemorrhages associated with cocaine abuse: CT and MR findings, *J Comp Asst Tomogr* 13:1-5, 1989.

94. Rapaport SI: Blood coagulation and its alterations in hemorrhagic and thrombotic disorders, *West J Med* 158:153-161, 1993.

95. Landefild CS, Goldman L: Major bleeding in outpatients treated with warfarin: incidence and prediction by factors known at the start of outpatient therapy, *Am J Med* 87:144-152, 1989.

Craniocerebral Trauma

I n the United States, trauma is the leading cause of death in children and young adults. Head injury is the major contributor to mortality in over half these cases.[1]

Neuroimaging is fundamental to the diagnosis and management of patients with traumatic brain injury. Understanding the mechanisms underlying brain trauma, their basic pathology, and their imaging manifestations is therefore essential for the practicing radiologist.

CLASSIFICATION, ETIOLOGY, AND FREQUENCY OF TRAUMATIC BRAIN INJURY
Classification of Brain Trauma

Brain damage in head-injured patients has been classified in two major ways: focal or diffuse lesions and primary or secondary lesions. We will follow the latter classification.

Primary brain damage. Primary traumatic craniocerebral lesions arise directly from the initial traumatic event (*see* box, p. 200). Skull and scalp lesions are the least important of these and are therefore considered only briefly (see subsequent discussion). The major primary intracranial manifestations of head trauma are extracerebral hemorrhage and a spectrum of intraaxial lesions that includes cortical contusions, diffuse axonal injury, deep cerebral and primary brainstem injury, and intraventricular and choroid plexus hemorrhage.

Secondary brain damage. Secondary manifestations of craniocerebral trauma often develop and are frequently more devastating than the initial injury (*see* box, p. 200). These secondary effects include herniation syndromes, ischemia, diffuse cerebral edema, and secondary infarctions and hemorrhages.

Mechanisms of Traumatic Brain Injury

Projectile or penetrating wounds and nonmissile injury are the two basic mechanisms of traumatic brain damage.

Traumatic Craniocerebral Lesions

Primary lesions

Skull fracture, scalp hematoma/laceration
Extracerebral hemorrhage
   Epidural hematoma
   Subdural hematoma
   Subarachnoid hemorrhage
Intraaxial lesions
   Diffuse axonal injury
   Cortical contusion
   Deep cerebral gray matter injury
   Brainstem injury
   Intraventricular/choroid plexus hemorrhage

Secondary lesions

Cerebral herniations
Traumatic ischemia, infarction
Diffuse cerebral edema
Hypoxic injury

Projectile injuries. Gunshot wounds to the head are the most lethal of all violent injuries.[1a] Wounds are determined by projectile characteristics and the inherent nature of the affected tissues. Some missile characteristics are intrinsic to the projectile itself (e.g., mass, shape, construction) and some are conferred by the weapon that delivers the missile (e.g., longitudinal and rotational velocity).[2]

Severity of a bullet wound is strongly influenced by missile orientation during its path through tissue and whether the projectile fragments or deforms. Wounds are most severe when the missile is large and traveling at high velocities and if it fragments or yaws early in its path through tissue (Fig. 8-1).[2] Tissue crushing and stretching are the major mechanisms of injury in these cases. Elasticity and tissue density, as well as thickness of the affected body part, strongly affect the wound produced.[2]

Imaging analysis in projectile injuries should include the following steps[3]:

1. Assess missile path
2. Determine extent of wound, including bone fragmentation and secondary or ricochet paths
3. Detect presence of missile emboli
4. Localize intraarticular or intraspinal fragments
5. Determine if large vessels or (if abdominal wounds) hollow viscera have been traversed

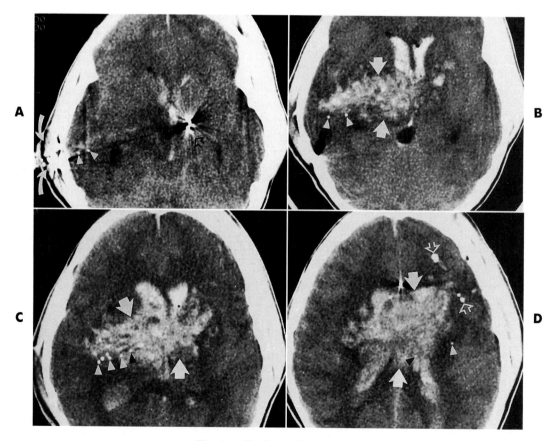

Fig. 8-1. For legend see p. 201.

Plain film radiography and fluoroscopy can be used to determine bullet weight and caliber. CT is best for assessing the extent of soft tissue injury and identifying entrance and exit wounds.[3]

Angiography is the diagnostic procedure of choice for determining the etiology of missile-induced traumatic hemorrhage and delineating underlying vascular abnormalities such as vessel laceration or traumatic pseudoaneurysm (Fig. 8-2). Because half of all patients with gunshot wounds to the head have major vascular lesions, cerebral angiography should be considered in the evaluation and management of these cases.[4]

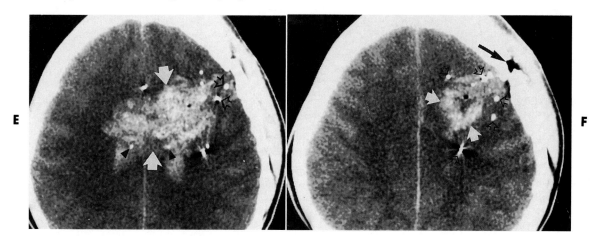

Fig. 8-1, cont'd. Antemortem NECT scans in patient with a gunshot wound show typical abnormalities seen when the missile yaws and fragments early. Entrance wound (*A, curved arrows*). Bullet fragments at entry site and along path (*arrowheads*). Hemorrhagic brain (*large arrows*). Ricochet fragments from striking the inner table opposite entry site (*open arrows*). Skull fracture at exit wound (**F,** *black arrow*).

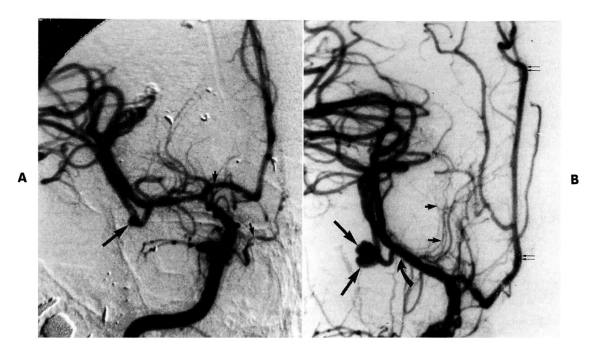

Fig. 8-2. Cranial gunshot wound. **A,** Digital subtraction right internal carotid angiogram, AP view, demonstrates multiple metallic bullet fragments. The small traumatic middle cerebral artery (MCA) aneurysm (*large arrow*) was initially overlooked. Clinical deterioration prompted repeat CT scan (not shown) that disclosed an enlarging middle fossa hematoma. **B,** Repeat angiogram shows the enlarging multilobed traumatic pseudoaneurysm (*large straight arrows*). Note medial displacement of the lenticulostriate arteries (*small arrows*) and elevation of the M1 segment and MCA genu (*curved arrow*) by the expanding hematoma. Also note the accompanying "square"-type anterior cerebral artery shift (*double arrows*).

Nonmissile head injuries. All major traumatic brain lesions can be produced by nonimpact inertial loading of the head.[5] The majority of nonprojectile traumatic brain injury (TBI) is caused by shear-strain forces. These are mechanical stresses on brain tissue that are induced by sudden deceleration or angular acceleration and rotation of the head.[6] Shear-strain injuries may be extensive and severe, are often multiple and bilateral, and frequently occur when there is no direct blow to the head.

Rotationally induced shear-strain forces typically produce intraaxial lesions in the following predictable locations[7]:

1. Brain surface (cortical contusions)
2. Cerebral white matter (so called diffuse axonal injury)
3. Brainstem
4. Along penetrating arteries or veins

Direct impact is significantly less important than shear-strain forces in the genesis of most TBI. With direct blows there is localized skull distortion or fracture and the underlying blood vessels and brain are damaged in a much more focal fashion as the transferred energy dissipates quickly. The typical results are cortical contusions and superficial lacerations localized to the immediate vicinity of the calvarial lesion.[8] Although some extraaxial lesions such as epidural hematoma are frequently associated with skull fracture (see subsequent discussion), significant extracerebral hemorrhage often occurs in the absence of direct blows and is due to shear-strain forces.

Frequency of Traumatic Lesions

Autopsy series. The incidence of head injuries encountered in a recent series of postmortem examinations is shown in Table 8-1.[6] Twenty-five percent of cases with fatal injuries do not demonstrate a skull fracture, although the incidence of intracranial hematomas in patients who have a skull fracture is much higher than in those who do not.[9] Intracranial hematomas, contusions, hypoxic brain damage, and brain swelling are all more frequent in postmortem series compared to surgical series or imaging-based reports.

Surgical and imaging series. The approximate incidence of traumatic injuries in patients who are imaged or operated is listed in Table 8-2. Skull fractures and extraaxial hematomas are less common than in autopsy series, and shear-strain lesions such as diffuse axonal injury are more frequently observed.

PRIMARY TRAUMATIC LESIONS
Skull and Scalp Lesions

Scalp hematomas and lacerations. Scalp lacerations and subgaleal soft tissue swelling commonly accompany head trauma (*see* Fig. 7-15). Other than indicating impact site, these lesions may be cosmetically important but are usually clinically insignificant. Exceptions are penetrating injuries that result in arteriovenous fistula or pseudoaneurysm. These usually involve branches of the superficial temporal or occipital arteries (*see* Fig. 9-30). Important extracalvarial soft tissue lesions are subgaleal extrusion of macerated brain through a comminuted skull fracture with dural laceration (see subsequent discussion).

Table 8-1. Nonmissile Head Injury

Lesion Frequency in the Glasgow Series	
Contusions	94%
Intracranial hematoma*	60%
Epidural	10%
Subdural	18%
Parenchymal	16%
"Burst lobe"	23%
Diffuse axonal injury	29%
Hypoxic brain damage (border zone; diffuse)	55%
Brain swelling (unilateral: bilateral, 2:1)	53%
Brainstem injury	53%

From Adams JH: Pathology of nonmissile head injury, *Neuroimaging Clin N Amer* 1:397-410, 1991.
*More than one hematoma in some cases.

Table 8-2. Craniocerebral Trauma in Operated/Imaged Patients*

Skull fracture	60%
Extraaxial hematoma	
EDH	1% to 4%
SDH	10% to 20%
SAH	60% to 80%
Primary intraaxial lesions	
Diffuse axonal injury	50%
Cortical contusions	45%
Deep cerebral gray matter	5%
Primary brainstem injury	4%
Intraventricular/ choroid plexus hemorrhage	5% to 10%
Secondary effects	
Herniations	60% to 80%
Global/regional ischemia	30% to 50%
Diffuse cerebral edema	10% to 20%

*Approximate; more than one lesion often present.

Skull fracture. Skull fractures are present on CT scans in about two thirds of patients with acute head injury, although 25% to 35% of severely injured patients have no identifiable fracture at all.[10] Therefore plain films obtained solely for the purpose of identifying the presence of a skull fracture have no appropriate role in the current management of the head injured patient.[11,12]

Skull fractures can be linear (Figs. 8-3 and 8-4), depressed, or diastatic and may involve the cranial vault or skull base. Linear fractures are more often associated with epi- and subdural hematomas than are depressed fractures; depressed fractures are typically associated with localized parenchymal injury.[10]

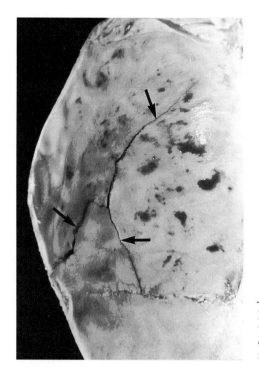

Fig. 8-3. Autopsy specimen of the calvarium in a patient who expired from traumatic brain injury. Endocranial view of the skull shows a nondisplaced linear skull fracture *(arrows)*. (Courtesy E. Tessa Hedley-Whyte.)

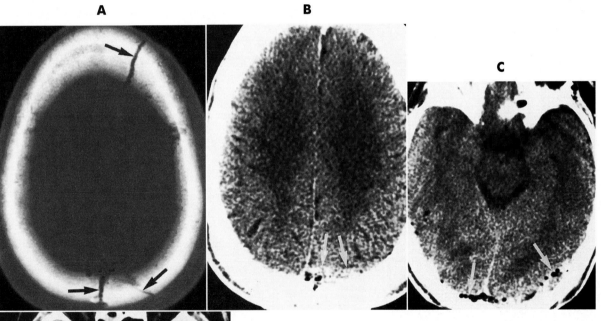

Fig. 8-4. A, Axial nonenhanced CT scan with bone reconstruction demonstrates a nondisplaced comminuted linear calvarial vault fracture *(arrows)*. The fracture crosses the superior sagittal sinus. **B** and **C,** Scans with soft tissue windows show a small epidural hematoma (EDH) *(arrows)* with pneumocephalus, seen as multiple very low density foci mostly within the epidural space. Sudden neurologic deterioration 24 hours later prompted a repeat scan. The repeat CT scan **(D)** shows a large left occipital EDH *(large straight arrows)* with hyperacute unclotted blood seen as low density foci *(black arrows)* within the EDH. Note fluid-fluid levels *(double white arrows)*; also, blood along the tentorium and straight sinus *(open arrows)* and a right temporal pole contusion *(curved white arrows)*. Venous EDH with transverse sinus laceration was found at surgery.

Extraaxial Hemorrhage

There are three types of extracerebral hemorrhage:
1. Epidural hematoma (EDH)
2. Subdural hematoma (SDH)
3. Subarachnoid hemorrhage (SAH)

Epidural hematoma

Incidence and clinical presentation. Epidural hematomas are found in only 1% to 4% of patients imaged for craniocerebral trauma, although EDHs represented 10% of fatal injuries in the Glasgow autopsy series (*see* Table 8-1). A classic "lucid interval" between the traumatic episode and onset of coma or neurologic deterioration is seen in only half the patients with EDH.[13] Delayed development or enlargement is seen in 10% to 30% of EDHs and usually occurs within the first 24 or 48 hours.[14,15] Late hematomas develop in 20% of moderate to severely head-injured patients who do not have signs of cerebral contusions on initial posttrauma CT studies (Fig. 8-4).[16]

Etiology. A fracture that lacerates the middle meningeal artery (MMA) or a dural venous sinus (Fig. 8-4) is present in 85% to 95% of all cases with EDH[16]; venous "oozing" or MMA tear without fracture accounts for the remainder.

Location. Epidural hematomas are located between the skull and dura. As it forcefully strips the dura away from the inner table of the skull an EDH characteristically assumes a focal biconvex or lentiform configuration (Fig. 8-5). EDHs may cross dural attachments but not sutures. Ninety-five percent of EDHs are unilateral and occur above the tentorium. The temporoparietal area is the most common site. Five percent of EDHs are bilateral.[13]

Posterior fossa EDHs are relatively uncommon but have a higher morbidity and mortality rate than their supratentorial counterparts.[17,17a]

Outcome. The overall mortality with EDHs is approximately 5%. Poor outcome is often—but not invariably—related to delayed referral, diagnosis, or operation.[18,19] Occasionally, EDHs resolve spontaneously without surgical intervention, probably by decompression through an open fracture into the extracranial subgaleal soft tissues.[20]

Imaging. (Table 8-3) On CT scans the typical EDH is a biconvex extraaxial mass that displaces the gray-white matter interface away from the calvarium. Two thirds of acute EDHs are uniformly high density; in one third, mixed hyper- and hypodense areas are present and indicate active bleeding (*see* Chapter 7) (Fig. 8-6). The brain adjacent to most EDHs is severely flattened and displaced. Secondary herniations with EDH are very common.

MR scans of hyperacute EDHs demonstrate a lentiform-shaped mass that strips the dura away

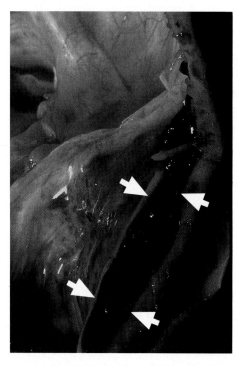

Fig. 8-5. Gross autopsy specimen of acute epidural hematoma. Note dural stripping from the inner table forms a focal biconvex extradural collection (*arrows*) that is filled with "currant jelly" fresh clot. (Courtesy B. Horten.)

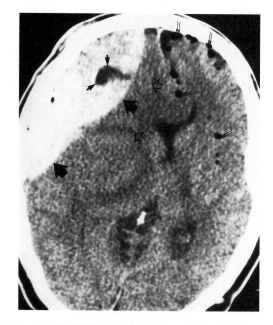

Fig. 8-6. Axial NECT shows a large acute right frontal EDH (*large arrows*). Note the low density area (*small single arrows*) within the EDH. This so-called swirl sign represents active bleeding with unretracted liquid clot. The gray-white matter interface is displaced (*open arrows*) and there is subfalcine herniation of the lateral ventricles. Subarachnoid pneumocephalus (*double arrows*) is present.

from the inner table. The displaced dura appears as a thin very low signal line interposed between the calvarium and brain (Fig. 8-7). Acute EDHs are isointense on T1WI but hyperintense on T2-weighted studies. Late subacute and early chronic EDHs are typically hyperintense on both T1- and T2WI (Fig. 8-13).

Subdural hematoma. Traumatic acute subdural hematoma is among the most lethal of all head injuries. Mortality rates range from 50% to 85% in some reported series.[21]

Incidence and clinical presentation. Subdural hematomas (SDH) are seen in 10% to 20% of all cranio-cerebral trauma cases and occur in up to 30% of fatal injuries (*see* Table 8-2). A definite history of trauma may be lacking, particularly in elderly patients. SDHs are common in abused children (see subsequent discussion). Most patients with acute SDHs have low Glasgow Coma Scores on admission (Table 8-4); 50% are flaccid or decerebrate.[21]

Etiology. Stretching and tearing of bridging cortical veins as they cross the subdural space to drain into an adjacent dural sinus is a common cause of SDH (*see* Fig. 6-37, C). These veins rupture because a sudden change in velocity of the head occurs.[6] The arachnoid may also be torn, creating a mixture of blood and CSF in the subdural space.

Table 8-3. Epidural and Subdural Hematomas Compared

	EDH	SDH
Incidence	1% to 4% overall; 10% injuries fatal	10% to 20% of all cases; 30% of fatal injuries
Etiology	Associated fracture in 85% to 95%; lacerated meningeal artery/dural sinus in 70% to 85%; venous "ooze" or MMA tear without fracture in 15%	Stretching, tearing of bridging cortical veins
Location	Between skull and dura Cross dural attachments but not sutures 95% supratentorial (frontotemporal, frontoparietal) 5% posterior fossa 5% bilateral	Between dura and arachnoid Cross sutures but not dural attachments 95% supratentorial (frontoparietal, convexity, middle fossa most common) Interhemispheric parafalcial, bilateral SDHs common in child abuse 15% bilateral

Imaging	CT
	  Biconvex
	  Displace gray-white interface
	  ⅔ hyperdense; ⅓ mixed hyper/hypodense
	
	MR
	  Biconvex
	  Isointense on T1WI
	  Displaced dura seen as thin, low signal line between hematoma and brain
		CT
		  Acute SDH
		    Crescentic
		    60% hyperdense, 40% mixed hyper/hypodense
		    May be isodense in coagulapathy or severe anemia
		  Subacute SDH
		    May be nearly isodense with underlying cortex
		    Neomembrane, underlying vessels may enhance
		  Chronic SDH
		    Hypodense with enhancing membrane
		    May be loculated
		    Rehemorrhage can cause mixed density
		    5% of chronic SDHs have fluid-blood density levels
		    1% to 2% of very old SDHs may calcify
		MR
		  Hyperacute
		    Iso on T1, iso/hyperintense on T2WI
		  Acute
		    Iso/moderately hypo T1, very hypointense T2WI
		  Subacute
		    Hyperintense on both T1, T2WI
		  Chronic
		    Variable, usually hyperintense on T2WI, 30% iso/hypointense on T1WI

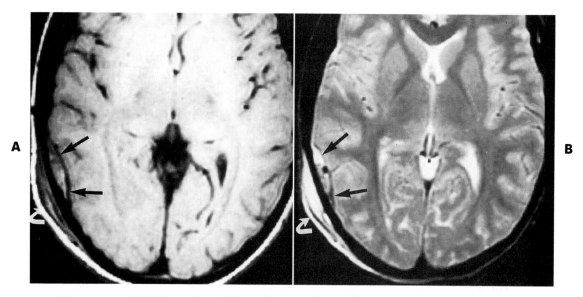

Fig. 8-7. Axial **(A)** T1- and **(B)** T2-weighted MR scans show a small acute right posterior temporal EDH. Note the very low signal displaced dura *(black arrows)*. The acute EDH and overlying subgaleal hematoma *(curved arrows)* are isodense with brain on the T1-weighted study and mostly hyperintense on the T2WI.

Table 8-4. Glasgow Coma Scale

Scoring	
Eye opening	
Spontaneous	4
To sound	3
To pain	2
None	1
Best motor response	
Obeys command	6
Localizes pain	5
Normal flexion (withdrawal)	4
Abnormal flexion	3
Extension	2
None	1
Best verbal response	
Oriented	5
Confused conversation	4
Inappropriate words (e.g., swearing)	3
Incomprehensible	2
None	1
Rating for Total	
Minor head injury	13-15
Moderate head injury	9-12
Severe	8 or less

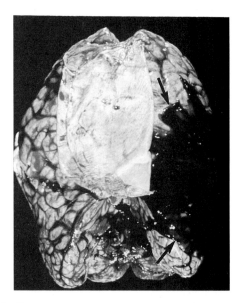

Fig. 8-8. Gross autopsy specimen with acute subdural hematoma *(arrows)*. (Courtesy E. Tessa Hedley-Whyte.)

Ten percent to thirty percent of chronic SDHs show evidence of repeated hemorrhage.[22] Rebleeding usually occurs from rupture of stretched cortical veins as they cross the enlarged fluid-filled subdural space or from the vascularized neomembrane on the calvarial side of the fluid collection.

Location. SDHs are interposed between the dura and arachnoid (Fig. 8-8). Typically crescent-shaped, they are usually more extensive than EDHs and may cross suture lines but not dural attachments. Eighty-five percent are unilateral. Common sites for SDH are over the frontoparietal convexities and in the middle cranial fossa. Isolated interhemispheric and parafalcial SDHs are common in cases of nonaccidental trauma. Bilateral SDHs are also more frequent in child abuse (see subsequent discussion).

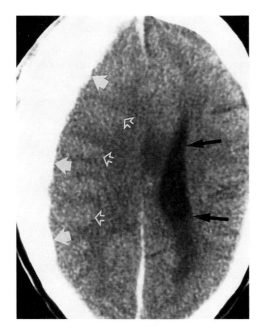

Fig. 8-9. Axial NECT shows a large acute right subdural hematoma (SDH). The high-density crescent-shaped fluid collection *(large white arrows)* spreads diffusely over the underlying hemisphere. Note displacement of the gray-white matter interface *(open arrows)* and the subfalcine herniation of the lateral ventricles. The left lateral ventricle *(black arrows)* is obstructed secondary to foramen of Monro occlusion.

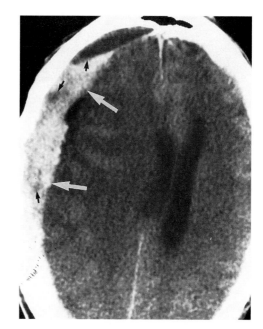

Fig. 8-10. Axial NECT scan in a head-injured patient with rapid clinical deterioration. A large right-sided acute SDH is present *(white arrows)*. Low density areas *(black arrows)* within the SDH could represent unclotted blood, serum extruded during clot retraction, or cerebrospinal fluid from arachnoid tear. Note subfalcine herniation of the lateral ventricles with foramen of Monro obstruction. An actively bleeding SDH with unretracted liquid clots was evacuated surgically.

Imaging. The appearance of SDHs on CT and MR studies varies with clot age and organization *(see* Table 8-3).

The classic CT appearance of an *acute* SDH is a crescent-shaped homogeneously hyperdense extraaxial collection that spreads diffusely over the affected hemisphere (Fig. 8-9). However, up to 40% of acute SDHs have mixed hyper/hypodense areas that reflect unclotted blood, serum extruded during clot retraction, or CSF within the subdural hematoma due to arachnoid laceration (Fig. 8-10).[23] Rarely, acute SDHs may be nearly isodense with the adjacent cerebral cortex. This occurs with coagulopathies or severe anemia when the hemoglobin concentration reaches 8 to 10 g/dl.[24,25]

With time, subdural hematomas undergo clot lysis, organization, and neomembrane formation *(see* Chapter 7). The evolution of an untreated, uncomplicated SDH follows a predictable pattern. *Subacute* SDHs become nearly isodense with the underlying cerebral cortex within a few days to a few weeks after trauma (Fig. 8-11).[26] In such cases the displaced gray-white matter interface, failure of surface sulci to reach the inner calvarial table, and comparison of the subtle extraaxial fluid collection to density of the underlying white matter usually permit detection of a subacute SDH. Contrast administration often delin-

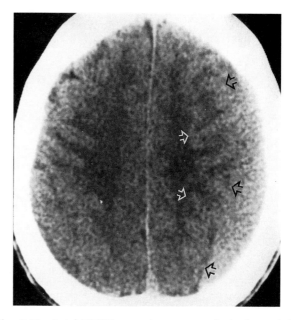

Fig. 8-11. Axial NECT scan shows a nearly isodense left-sided subacute SDH. The border between the extraaxial collection and underlying brain *(black arrows)* is barely discernible. Medially displaced gray-white matter interface *(white arrows)*. Compare to the normal right side.

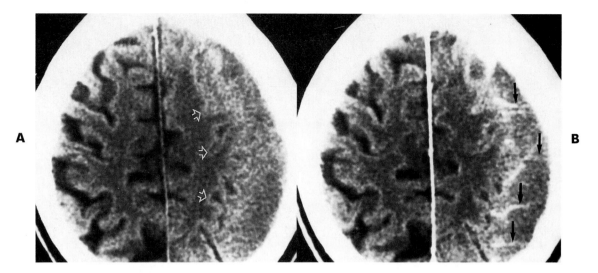

Fig. 8-12. Pre- (**A**) and (**B**) postcontrast axial CT scans of a subacute subdural hematoma show the crescent-shaped extraaxial collection is nearly isodense with the white matter but the corticomedullary interface displacement (**A**, *arrows*) is readily apparent. The postcontrast study shows enhancing cortical veins (**B**, *arrows*) stretched across the subacute SDH. Rupture of these so-called bridging veins can easily occur (compare with Fig. 6-37, C), although recurrent bleeding into subacute or chronic SDHs occurs primarily from the vascularized neomembrane (*see* Fig. 8-13, *A*).

eates an underlying membrane or demonstrates cortical vessel displacement by the nearly isodense extraaxial collection (Fig. 8-12).

Chronic SDHs are encapsulated, often loculated collections of sanguineous or serosanguineous fluid in the subdural space. These may be either crescentic or lentiform (Figs. 8-13 and 8-14). Uncomplicated chronic SDHs are typically low attenuation (Fig. 8-15). Recurrent hemorrhage into a preexisting chronic SDH produces mixed density extraaxial collections, seen in approximately 5% of cases (Figs. 7-10, 7-11, and 8-15).[27]

The capsule of a chronic SDH is a capillary-rich membrane through which active exchange of solutes such as albumin and contrast material can occur.[28] Both the neomembrane and the subdural collection may enhance following contrast administration. Calcification or ossification is seen in 0.3% to 2.7% of chronic SDHs, usually when they have been present for many months to years (Fig. 8-16).[29]

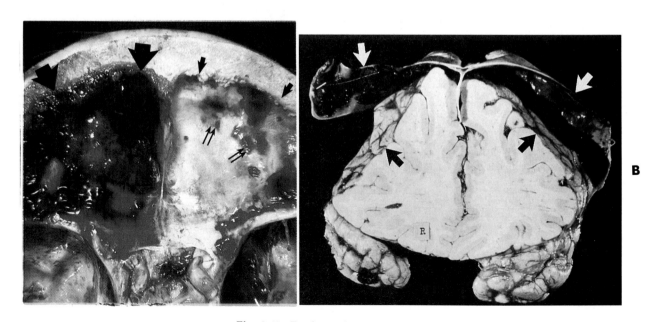

Fig. 8-13. For legend see p. 209.

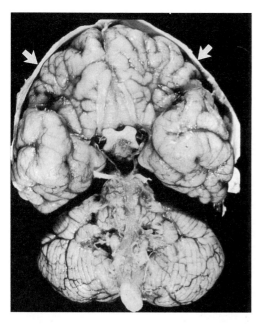

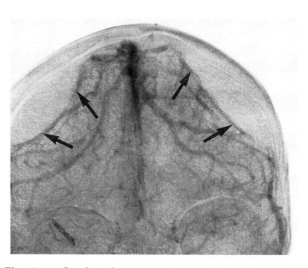

Fig. 8-14. Combined venous phases of the right and left carotid angiograms, AP view, in a patient with bilateral chronic SDHs show the typical lentiform collections outlined by the displaced cortical veins *(arrows).*

Fig. 8-13, cont'd. Three autopsy cases with chronic subdural hematomas (SDHs). **A,** This case demonstrates acute *(left side of photograph, large arrows)* and chronic *(right side of photograph, small arrows)* SDHs. The acute clot has a "currant jelly" consistency and the older SDH consists of an organized membrane. Note the fresh petechial hemorrhages *(double arrows)* oozing from the chronic SDH. **B,** Second case demonstrates the lentiform configuration that these chronic extraaxial collections can assume. Bilateral chronic SDHs are present *(arrows).* **C,** Third case has small bifrontal crescent-shaped organized chronic SDHs *(arrows).* (Courtesy E. Tessa Hedley-Whyte.)

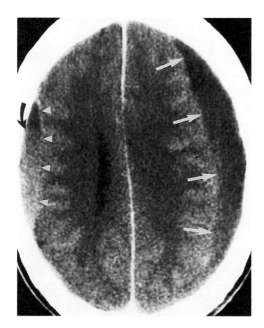

Fig. 8-15. Axial contrast-enhanced CT scan in a patient with bilateral chronic SDHs. The left-sided crescent-shaped low density collection is a classic uncomplicated chronic SDH *(white arrows).* The right-sided lesion is lentiform *(arrowheads)* and has a fluid-fluid level *(black arrow)* that indicates rehemorrhage into the preexisting chronic SDH.

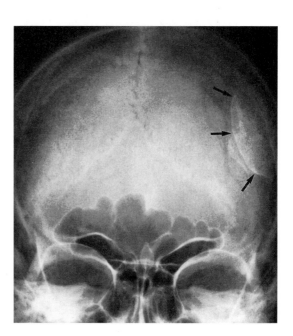

Fig. 8-16. PA plain skull film demonstrates a calcified chronic SDH *(arrows).*

The MR appearance of subdural hematomas and hygromas is quite variable. In general, SDHs evolve in a pattern similar to intracerebral hemorrhage (*see* Chapter 7). The exceptions are chronic subdural hematomas. In these cases the extraaxial collections are often iso- or hypointense on T1WI compared to gray matter, and hemosiderin deposition is rarely observed (Fig. 8-17).[30]

Thirty per cent of chronic SDHs are iso- or hypointense on T1WI but most are hyperintense on T2-weighted studies (Figs. 8-18 and 8-19).[31] If rehemorrhage into subacute or chronic SDHs occurs, MR studies will show mixed signal intensities (Fig. 8-20). Fluid-fluid levels are common with repeated hemorrhages (Fig. 8-21). The neomembranes of subacute and chronic SDHs typically enhance following contrast administration.

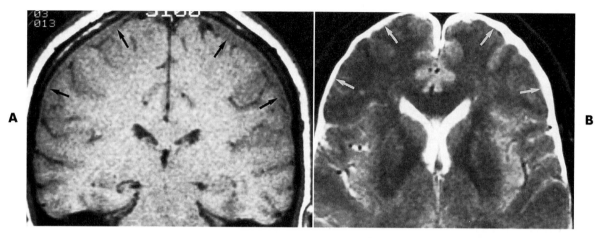

Fig. 8-17. Coronal T1- (**A**) and axial T2-weighted (**B**) MR scans in a patient with small bilateral chronic SDHs. The crescentic extraaxial collections (*arrows*) are isointense with cortex on T1WI and hyperintense on T2-weighted scans (compare with Fig. 8-13, *C*).

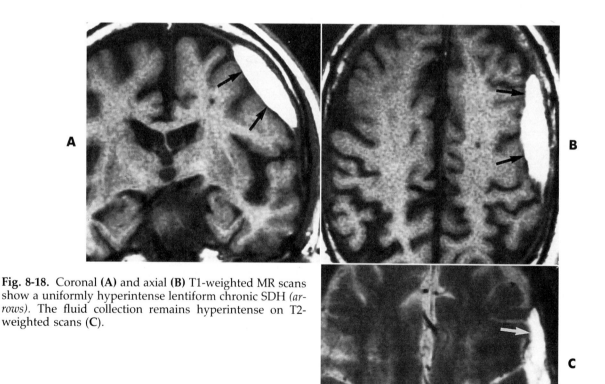

Fig. 8-18. Coronal (**A**) and axial (**B**) T1-weighted MR scans show a uniformly hyperintense lentiform chronic SDH (*arrows*). The fluid collection remains hyperintense on T2-weighted scans (**C**).

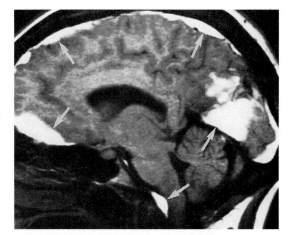

Fig. 8-19. Sagittal T1-weighted MR scan shows diffuse chronic SDHs *(arrows)*.

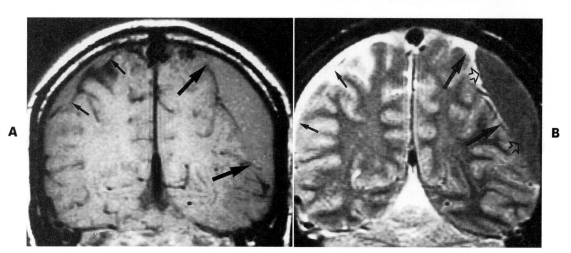

Fig. 8-20. Coronal T1- **(A)** and T2-weighted **(B)** MR scans show bilateral subdural hematomas. The crescentic right-sided collection *(small arrows)* is a chronic SDH. The left-sided chronic SDH *(large arrows)* contains a larger, lentiform subacute collection *(open arrows)*.

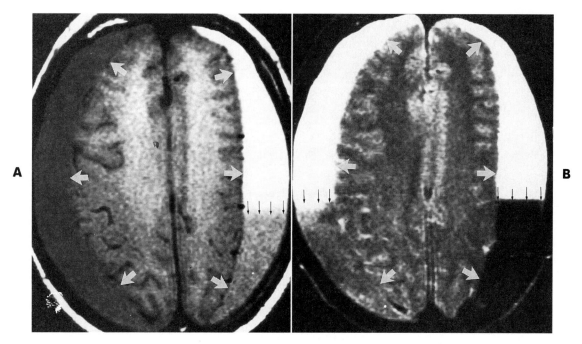

Fig. 8-21. Axial T1- **(A)** and T2-weighted **(B)** MR scans demonstrate large r.ixed-age chronic SDHs *(white arrows)* with fluid-fluid levels *(black arrows)*. (Courtesy L. Blas.)

Traumatic subarachnoid hemorrhage and its "mimics." Subarachnoid hemorrhage (SAH) accompanies most cases of moderate to severe head trauma (Fig. 8-22). On nonenhanced CT scans, acute SAH appears as thin high density fluid collections within the superficial sulci and CSF cisterns (Fig. 8-23).

"Pseudo-subarachnoid hemorrhage" is seen in cases of severe, diffuse cerebral edema when the brain becomes very low in attenuation and dura and circulating blood in the cranial vasculature appear unusually hyperdense compared to adjacent structures. Posterior parafalcine or interhemispheric subarachnoid hemorrhage can mimic the "empty delta sign" of superior sagittal sinus thrombosis and should not be mistaken for dural sinus occlusion (*see* Fig. 8-45, *B*).[32]

Intraaxial Lesions

Diffuse axonal injury. With cortical contusions,[33] diffuse axonal injury (DAI, or "shearing," injury) has been identified as the most important cause of significant morbidity in patients with traumatic brain injuries.[7]

Incidence and clinical presentation. Diffuse axonal injuries represent nearly half of all primary intraaxial traumatic brain lesions[34] (*see* Table 8-2). Patients with DAI typically lose consciousness at the moment of impact[8]; DAI is uncommon in the absence of severe closed head injury.

Etiology and pathology. Axonal shear-strain deformations are induced by sudden acceleration/deceleration or rotational forces on the brain. These injuries tend to be diffuse, bilateral, and occur in very predictable locations (Fig. 8-24). The characteristic shearing injuries are microscopic axonal bulbs or "retraction balls" (Fig. 8-25).[6] Disruption of penetrating blood vessels at the corticomedullary junction, corpus callosum and internal capsule, deep gray matter and upper brainstem produce numerous small hemorrhagic foci that may be the only gross pathologic markers of DAI.

Location. DAI tends to occur in the following three very specific areas (Figs. 8-26 and 8-27)[7]:
1. Lobar white matter, particularly at the gray-white matter interface
2. Corpus callosum
3. Dorsolateral aspect of the upper brainstem

Nearly two thirds of these so-called shearing injuries are seen at the corticomedullary junction, most often in the frontotemporal region; about 20% are found in the corpus callosum (especially the posterior body and splenium).[31] Other less frequent locations include the caudate nuclei and thalamus, internal capsule, and dorsolateral tegmentum.

Imaging. The initial CT scans in DAI are often normal despite profound clinical impairment. Early im-

---

Primary Neuronal Injuries

Diffuse axonal (shearing) injury
Cortical contusions
Deep cerebral/brainstem injury

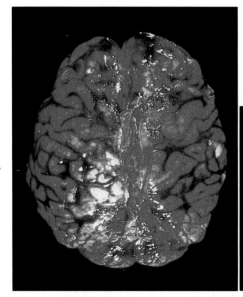
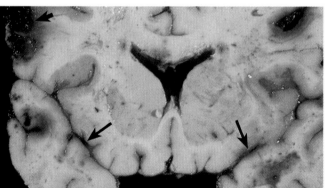

Fig. 8-22. A, Gross autopsy specimen of severe closed head injury shows severe traumatic subarachnoid hemorrhage (SAH). **B,** Coronal cut specimen shows extensive SAH *(large arrows)* plus numerous cortical contusions *(small arrows).* (Courtesy E. Tessa Hedley-Whyte.)

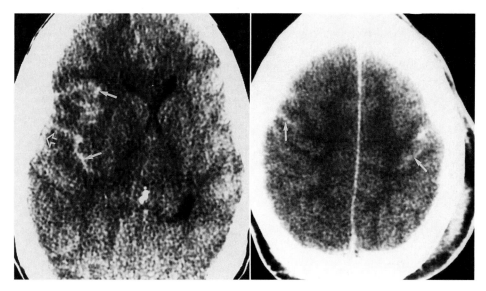

Fig. 8-23. Axial NECT scans in a patient with severe head trauma disclose acute traumatic SAH *(single arrows)*. Right frontotemporal contusion and a small SDH *(open arrows)* are also present.

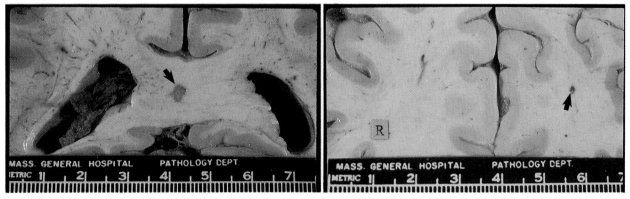

Fig. 8-24. Coronal gross specimen demonstrates multiple small diffuse axonal injuries (DAI), seen as petechial hemorrhages in the deep white matter and corpus callosum *(arrows)*. (Courtesy E. Tessa Hedley-Whyte.)

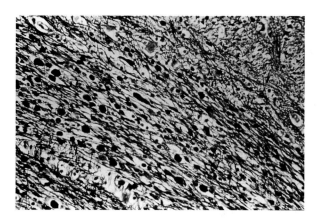

Fig. 8-25. Photomicrograph demonstrates the "axonal retraction balls" characteristically seen in DAI. (Courtesy L. Becker.)

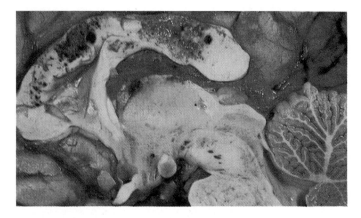

Fig. 8-26. Sagittal gross pathologic specimen demonstrates severe shearing injuries of the corpus callosum (compare with Fig. 8-27, C). (Courtesy E. Ross.)

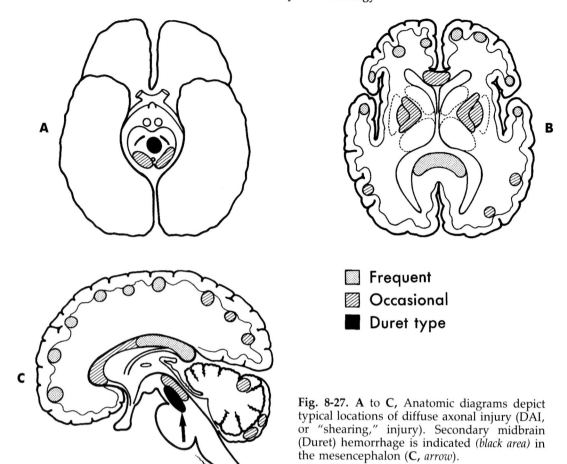

☒ Frequent
▨ Occasional
■ Duret type

Fig. 8-27. A to **C,** Anatomic diagrams depict typical locations of diffuse axonal injury (DAI, or "shearing," injury). Secondary midbrain (Duret) hemorrhage is indicated *(black area)* in the mesencephalon (**C,** *arrow*).

aging evidence for acute DAI may be subtle or nonexistent; only 20% to 50% of patients with DAI have abnormalities on initial CT examination.[35,36] Delayed scans may demonstrate lesions not apparent on initial examination. Acute DAI is seen as small petechial hemorrhages, particularly at the gray-white junction and corpus callosum (Fig. 8-28).[37]

The MR appearance of DAI depends on the presence or absence of hemorrhage and age of the lesions.[8] T1-weighted studies are often unremarkable. On T2WI the most common finding is multifocal hyperintense foci at the gray-white interfaces or in the corpus callosum (Fig. 8-29). The hyperintensity of these lesions tends to diminish with time, although shearing injuries are one of the numerous potential causes of multifocal white matter lesions seen on T2-weighted brain scans (*see* Chapter 17).

If shearing lesions are hemorrhagic, T1-weighted studies may demonstrate blood degradation products. Multiple foci of diminished signal on T2WI and gradient-echo scans can be seen for years after the traumatic event (Fig. 8-30). Occasionally lesions from remote DAI can be identified only on gradient refo-

cussed sequences. Nonspecific atrophic changes can be late sequelae of DAI; on rare occasions they may occur in the absence of other identifiable parenchymal lesions.

Cortical contusions. Cortical contusions are the second most common primary traumatic neuronal injury (*see* box, p. 212).

Incidence and clinical presentation. Cortical contusions represent 45% of primary intraaxial traumatic lesions. Compared to DAI, cortical contusions are less frequently associated with initial loss of consciousness unless they are extensive or occur with other abnormalities such as shearing injury or secondary brainstem trauma.[34]

Etiology and pathology. Contusions are typically superficial foci of punctate or linear hemorrhages that occur along gyral crests[6] (Fig. 8-31). They are induced by brain striking on an osseous ridge, less often a dural fold, and occur when differential acceleration/deceleration forces are applied to the head.[34] Focal contusions may also be associated with a depressed skull fracture. Petechial cortical contusions tend to co-

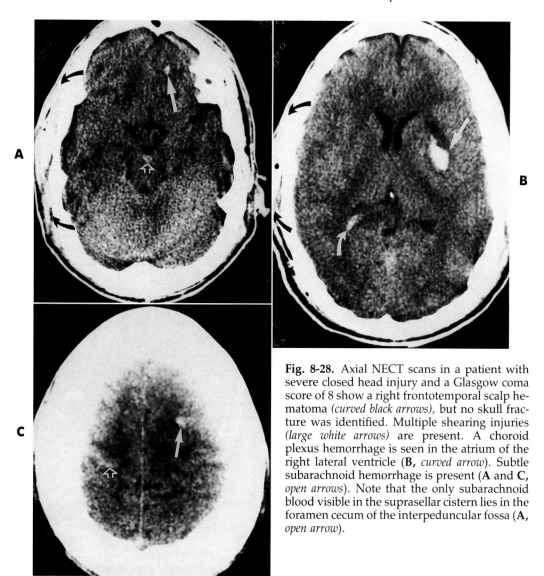

Fig. 8-28. Axial NECT scans in a patient with severe closed head injury and a Glasgow coma score of 8 show a right frontotemporal scalp hematoma *(curved black arrows),* but no skull fracture was identified. Multiple shearing injuries *(large white arrows)* are present. A choroid plexus hemorrhage is seen in the atrium of the right lateral ventricle (**B,** *curved arrow*). Subtle subarachnoid hemorrhage is present (**A** and **C,** *open arrows*). Note that the only subarachnoid blood visible in the suprasellar cistern lies in the foramen cecum of the interpeduncular fossa (**A,** *open arrow*).

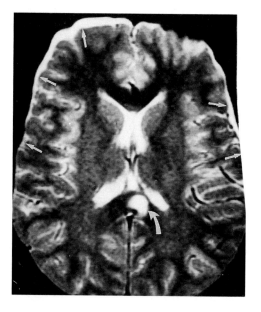

Fig. 8-29. Axial T2-weighted MR scan in a patient with closed head injury 3 weeks before study. Small right frontal and left temporal chronic SDHs are seen as thin crescentic extraaxial fluid collections *(straight arrows).* A high-signal focus in the corpus callosum splenium *(curved arrow)* is a classic shearing injury.

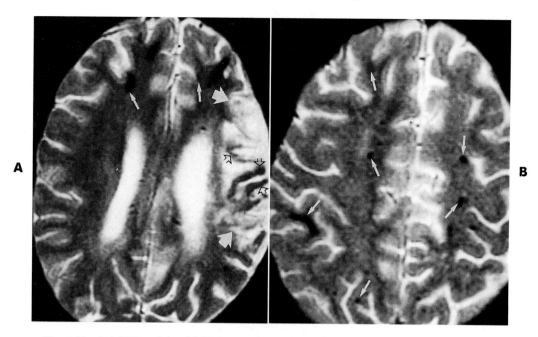

Fig. 8-30. Axial T2-weighted MR scans in a patient with severe closed head injury 2 years before study. Left temporoparietal encephalomalacia is secondary to traumatic MCA infarct (**A,** *large arrows*). Some residua of hemorrhagic transformation are seen as gyriform low signal areas (**A,** *open arrows*). Multiple old hemorrhagic shearing injuries are seen as low signal foci at the corticomedullary junction (*small arrows*). The DAIs are particularly well seen on the higher section (**B**).

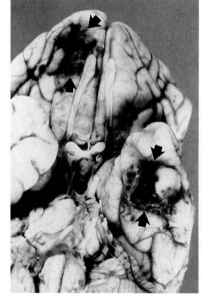

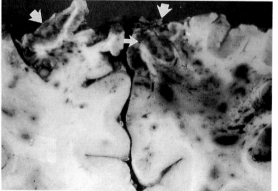

Fig. 8-31. A, Gross autopsy specimen demonstrates the typical frontotemporal contusions (*arrows*) seen with severe closed head injury. **B,** Close-up view of the frontal lobes in another case with fatal closed head injury. Note extensive gyral contusions (*arrows*). (**A,** Courtesy Scott VandenBerg, **B,** Courtesy J. Townsend.)

alesce into larger hemorrhagic foci and often become more evident 24 to 48 hours after the initial trauma.[16]

Location. Because contusions occur when brain contacts a dural ridge or bony protuberance, they occur in very characteristic locations (Figs. 8-31 and 8-32). Nearly half of all cases involve the temporal lobes, most frequently the temporal tip, inferior surface, and cortex around the sylvian fissure. One third occur in the frontal lobes, particularly along the infe-

rior surface and around the frontal poles. Twenty-five per cent are parasagittal or "gliding" contusions (socalled because the convexities of each hemisphere are anchored to the dura by arachnoidal granulations. When the brain abruptly shifts at the time of impact, the subcortical tissue "glides" more than the cortex).[6] The inferior surfaces of the cerebellar hemispheres are less common sites of cortical contusion.

Imaging. Findings are variable because cortical

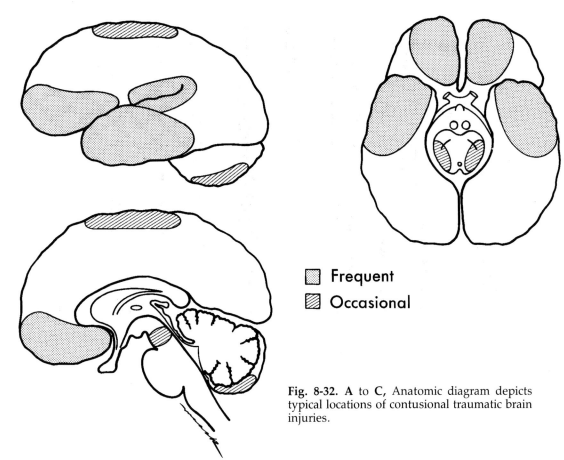

Fig. 8-32. A to **C,** Anatomic diagram depicts typical locations of contusional traumatic brain injuries.

☐ **Frequent**

☐ **Occasional**

contusions tend to evolve with time. Initially, findings on CT scans may be subtle or absent (Fig. 8-33, *A and B*).[33] Early findings include patchy, ill-defined frontal or temporal low density lesions that may be mixed with smaller hyperdense foci of petechial hemorrhage (Fig. 8-34).

CT scans obtained 24 to 48 hours after injury often show more lesions than are identified on initial studies. In 20% of cases, delayed hemorrhages develop in what previously appeared as nonhemorrhagic low density areas.[34] Edema and mass effect typically increase in the first few days after the traumatic insult, then gradually diminish over time. Cortical contusions may enhance following contrast administration (Fig. 8-35; *see* Fig. 7-14, *C*).

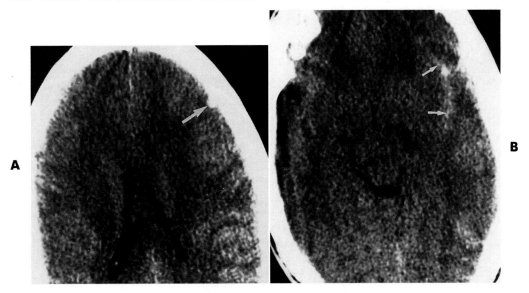

Fig. 8-33. Axial NECT scans in a patient with severe closed head injury. **A** and **B,** Initial scans show a subtle left frontal cortical contusion (**A,** *arrow*) and some traumatic SAH (**B,** *arrows*). Clinical deterioration 12 hours later prompted repeat examination.

Continued.

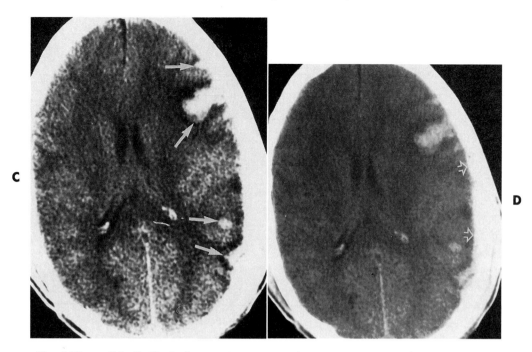

Fig. 8-33, cont'd. **C,** Cortical contusions are much more apparent and seen as patchy hemorrhagic foci mixed with low density edema *(arrows)*. **D,** Wider window also shows a small SDH *(open arrows)* that was difficult to see on the routine study **(C)** because of the high density overlying calvarial vault.

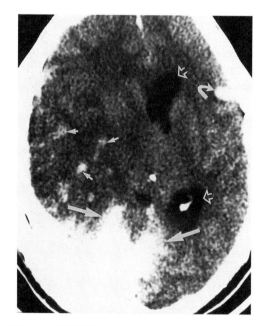

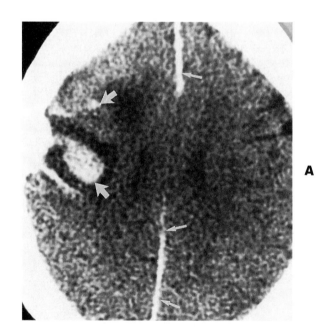

Fig. 8-34. Axial NECT scan in a patient with severe closed head injury. A large tentorial SDH is present *(large arrows)*. The entire right temporal lobe and much of the frontal lobe are severely contused. The contused brain appears as diffuse low density mixed with more focal but patchy hyperdense areas of petechial hemorrhage *(small arrows)*. A small "contre-coup" left frontotemporal contusion is also present *(curved arrow)*. There is subfalcine herniation of the lateral ventricles with foramen of Monro obstruction and enlargement of the entrapped left lateral ventricle *(open arrows)*.

Fig. 8-35. A, Axial NECT scan obtained immediately after trauma shows a high right frontal contusion *(large arrows)* and a small interhemispheric acute SDH *(small arrows)*.

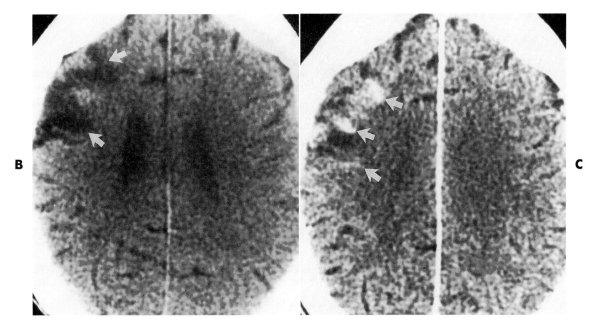

Fig. 8-35, cont'd. B, Follow-up NECT scan 10 weeks later shows the contused brain is now low density *(arrows).* The interhemispheric SDH has resolved. **C,** The contused gyri enhance (arrows) following contrast administration.

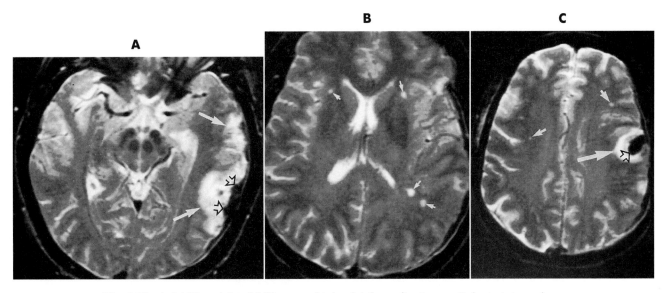

Fig. 8-36. Axial T2-weighted MR scans obtained 4 days after traumatic brain injury show extensive cortical contusions as multifocal low signal areas along the gyral surfaces *(open arrows)* surrounded by high signal edema *(large arrows).* Numerous shearing injuries are also present *(small arrows).*

MR is much more sensitive than CT in detecting cortical contusions, particularly in the subacute stage (Figs. 8-36 and 8-37).[35,36] Multiple superficial areas of poorly delineated, hyperintense signal abnormalities are seen on T2WI (Fig. 7-14). The lesions often appear inhomogeneous on T1- and T2-weighted scans because hemorrhagic foci are present.

Subcortical gray matter (deep cerebral) and brainstem injuries. Less common than DAI and cortical contusions, these lesions nevertheless represent important manifestations of primary intraaxial traumatic injury.

Incidence, etiology, and clinical presentation. Deep gray matter and brainstem lesions represent 5%

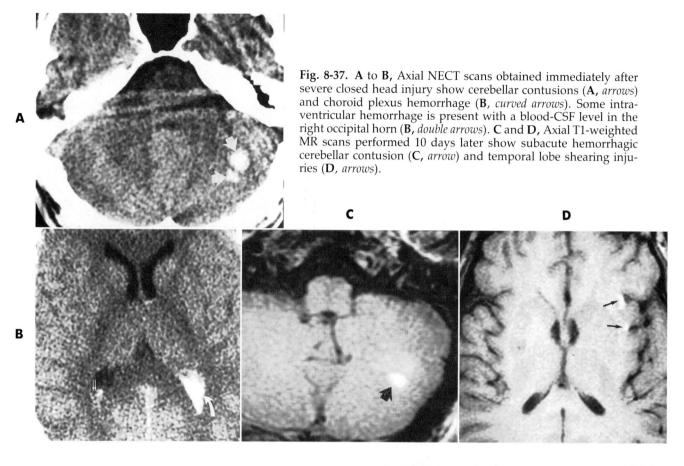

Fig. 8-37. **A** to **B**, Axial NECT scans obtained immediately after severe closed head injury show cerebellar contusions (**A**, *arrows*) and choroid plexus hemorrhage (**B**, *curved arrows*). Some intraventricular hemorrhage is present with a blood-CSF level in the right occipital horn (**B**, *double arrows*). **C** and **D**, Axial T1-weighted MR scans performed 10 days later show subacute hemorrhagic cerebellar contusion (**C**, *arrow*) and temporal lobe shearing injuries (**D**, *arrows*).

to 10% of primary traumatic brain injuries.[7] Most are induced by shearing forces that cause disruption of multiple small perforating blood vessels (Figs. 8-37 and 8-38).[6] Less commonly, the dorsolateral brainstem strikes the tentorial incisura during violent excursions of the brain (Fig. 8-39).[7] Sudden craniocaudal displacement of the brain at impact may also result in anterior rostral midbrain hemorrhage (Fig. 8-40).[38]

Most patients with deep cerebral and brainstem injuries have profound neurologic deficits, low initial Glasgow coma scale scores, and a poor prognosis for neurologic recovery.[39]

Imaging. CT is often normal in these patients. Petechial hemorrhages can sometimes be seen in the dorsolateral brainstem, periaqueductal region, and deep gray matter nuclei (Fig. 8-38). MR depicts these brainstem lesions nicely (Figs. 8-38 and 8-39).

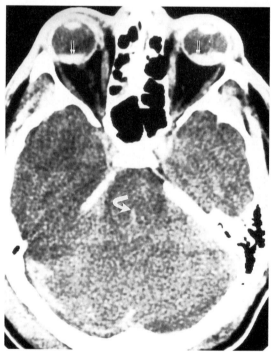

Fig. 8-38. Axial NECT scan in a patient with severe deceleration closed head injury shows bilateral ocular hemorrhages *(double arrows)* and a small hemorrhagic midbrain shearing injury *(curved arrow)*. (From Osborn AG: Secondary effects of intracranial trauma, *Neuroimaging Clin N Amer* 1:461-474, 1991.)

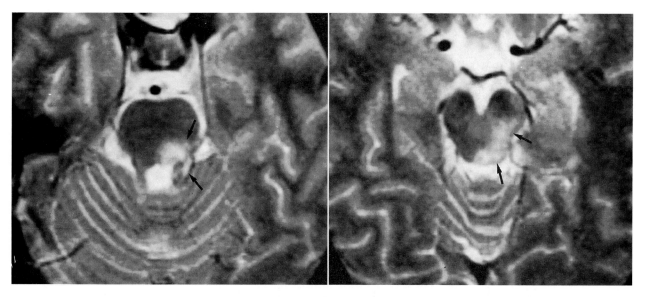

Fig. 8-39. Axial T2-weighted MR scans in a patient with closed head injury shows a left dorsolateral midbrain contusion *(arrows)*. No other abnormalities were identified. The lesion was probably caused by midbrain impaction against the tentorium during the traumatic episode.

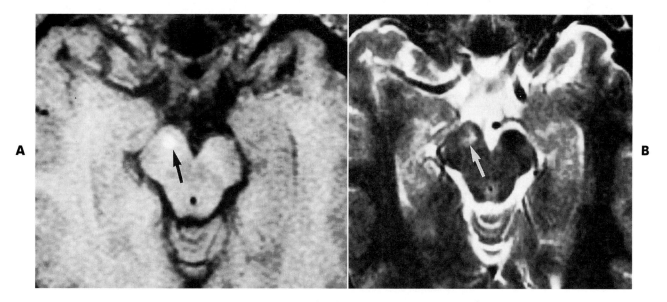

Fig. 8-40. Axial **(A)** T1- and **(B)** T2-weighted MR scans in a patient with traumatic anterior rostral midbrain hemorrhage *(arrows)*, probably from peduncular contusion against the tentorial incisura during sudden craniocaudal displacement at the time of impact.

Intraventricular and choroid plexus hemorrhage

Incidence, etiology and clinical presentation. IVH is identified in 1% to 5% of all patients with closed head injury.[40,41] Traumatic IVH is thus relatively uncommon and usually reflects severe injury.

Most cases of IVH are associated with other manifestations of primary intraaxial brain trauma such as DAI, deep cerebral gray matter, and brainstem lesions. Prognosis is poor, although patients with isolated IVH typically have a somewhat better outcome (Fig. 8-41).[41] Disruption of subependymal veins, shearing injuries, and basal ganglionic hemorrhage with subsequent rupture into the adjacent ventricle are thought to cause most cases of traumatic IVH.[41]

Imaging. CT manifestations of acute IVH are high density intraventricular blood with or without a fluid-fluid level (Fig. 8-41). Occasionally, focal choroid

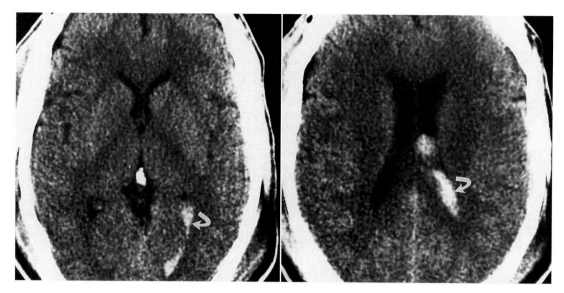

Fig. 8-41. Axial NECT scans in a patient with isolated traumatic intraventricular hemorrhage *(arrows)*. No other lesions were present. The patient recovered with minor neurologic sequelae.

plexus hematomas can be identified in the absence of frank IVH (Fig. 8-42). Most cases of traumatic ICH have hemorrhagic foci in the adjacent deep gray matter nuclei or white matter. Subarachnoid hemorrhage is also commonly associated with IVH.

SECONDARY EFFECTS OF CRANIOCEREBRAL TRAUMA

The secondary effects of craniocerebral trauma are sometimes of greater clinical import than direct manifestations such as focal hematoma, contusion, or DAI. Most secondary injuries are caused by increased intracranial pressure or cerebral herniations. These traumatic sequelae in turn cause compression of brain, nerves, blood vessels, or a combination of all three against the rigid, unyielding bony and dural margins that comprise the cranial cavity.[42]

The major secondary effects of craniocerebral trauma are summarized in the box. Cerebral herniations, traumatic ischemia, infarction and secondary hemorrhage, diffuse cerebral edema, and hypoxic injury are all discussed here. Vascular manifestations and complications of craniocerebral trauma are then specifically addressed.

Cerebral Herniations

Pathology of cerebral herniations. The cranial cavity is functionally divided into compartments by combinations of bony ridges and dural folds (Fig. 8-43, *A* and *B*). Cerebral herniations are caused by mechanical displacement of brain, cerebrospinal fluid, and blood vessels from one cranial compartment to another.

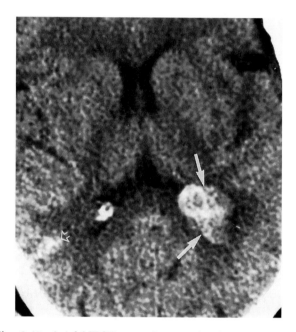

Fig. 8-42. Axial NECT scan shows a localized hematoma in the left choroid plexus glomus *(large arrows)*. Note subtle SAH *(open arrow)*.

Major Secondary Effects of Craniocerebral Trauma

Cerebral herniations
Traumatic ischemia, infarction, secondary
  hemorrhage
Diffuse cerebral edema
Hypoxic injury

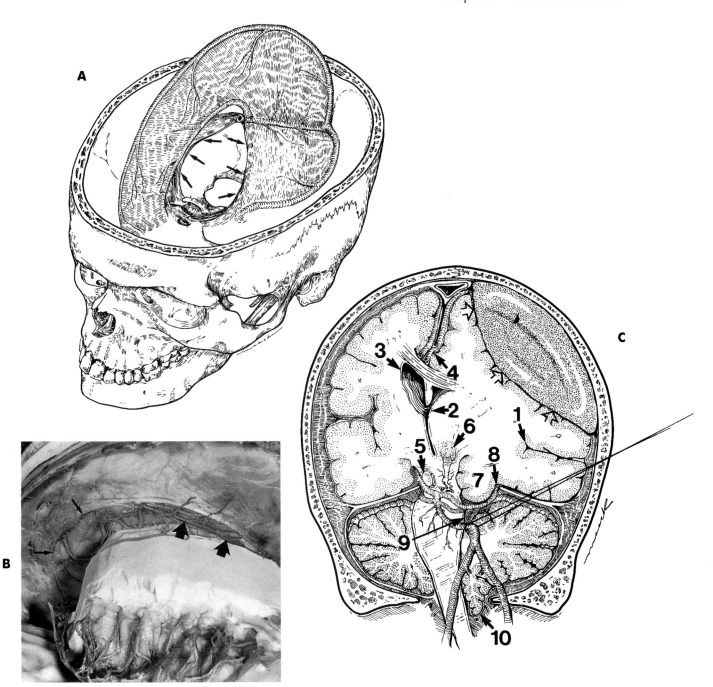

Fig. 8-43. A, Anatomic diagram depicts the falx cerebri and tentorium cerebelli functionally dividing the brain into compartments. The tentorial incisura is indicated by the black arrows. **B,** Anatomic dissection shows relationship of the brain and anterior cerebral artery to the falx cerebri. Note that anteriorly the falx *(small arrows)* is deficient, permitting side-to-side (subfalcine herniation) brain displacement. More posteriorly the ACA *(large arrows)* can be compressed against the inferior falcine edge, with ensuing infarction subsequent to the subfalcine herniation. **C,** Anatomic diagram depicts some potential secondary effects of a large epidural hematoma *(open arrows). 1,* Inferior displacement of sylvian fissure, middle cerebral artery branches. *2,* Subfalcine herniation of lateral ventricles with compression of ipsilateral ventricle. *3,* Contralateral lateral ventricle dilates secondary to functional obstruction at the foramen of Monro. *4,* Anterior cerebral arteries (cut across), shifted across the midline by the mass effect, return to midline under the falx cerebri (may cause secondary ACA infarct). *5,* Midbrain contusion (Kernohan notch) produced by displacement from the mass effect causing the cerebral peduncle to strike the opposite edge of the tentorial incisura. *6,* Midbrain hemorrhage (Duret hemorrhage) caused by downward displacement. *7,* Medial temporal lobe herniates over the tentorial incisura (descending transtentorial herniation). *8,* Ipsilateral posterior cerebral artery (PCA) is compressed against the tentorial incisura (may cause secondary PCA infarct). *9,* Ipsilateral cerebellopontine angle cistern is widened as the brainstem is displaced by the herniating temporal lobe. *10,* Descending tonsillar herniation. (**A,** From Bassett DL: *A Steroscopic Atlas of Human Anatomy*, section 1: *the central nervous system*. Courtesy Bassett Collection, R. Chase (curator), Stanford University.) **B,** Osborn AG: The medial tentorium and incisura: normal and pathological anatomy, *Neuroradiol* 13:109-113, 1977.)

Brain herniations are the most common secondary effect of expanding intracranial masses. The major cerebral herniations are listed in the box. The two most common gross brain displacements are subfalcine and descending transtentorial herniation (Fig. 8-43, C). Transalar, ascending transtentorial, and tonsillar herniations are less frequently encountered.

Subfalcine herniation. Here, the cingulate gyrus is displaced across the midline under the inferior free margin of the falx cerebri (Figs. 8-43, *C,* and 8-44). Initial displacements may be relatively minor. With larger herniations the ipsilateral lateral ventricle is compressed and the contralateral ventricle enlarges as the foramen of Monro becomes obstructed (Figs. 8-44 and 8-45).

Vascular displacements also occur with subfalcine herniation. The ipsilateral anterior cerebral artery (ACA) and deep subependymal veins are shifted across the midline. In severe cases the ACA and its

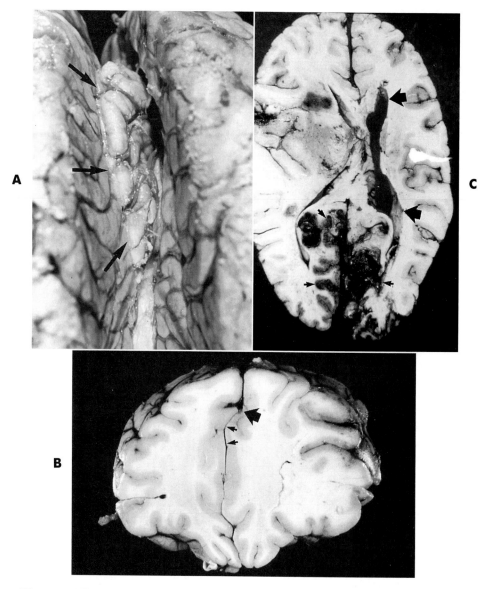

Fig. 8-44. Three gross pathology specimens demonstrate subfalcine (cingulate gyrus) herniation. **A,** Superior view shows the cingulate gyrus herniation *(arrows).* **B,** Coronal specimen in the second case shows sharp angulation of the cingulate gyrus *(small arrows)* against the falx cerebri *(large arrow).* **C,** Axial specimen from a patient with a large hypertensive basal ganglionic hemorrhage. Changes of both subfalcine and descending transtentorial herniation are present. The lateral ventricles are shifted away from the mass and the contralateral ventricle *(large arrows)* is enlarged secondary to foramen of Monro obstruction. Descending transtentorial herniation has resulted in bilateral posterior cerebral artery occlusions with occipital lobe infarcts *(small arrows).* (**A,** Courtesy E. Tessa Hedley-Whyte. **B,** Courtesy J. Townsend and C. Harris.)

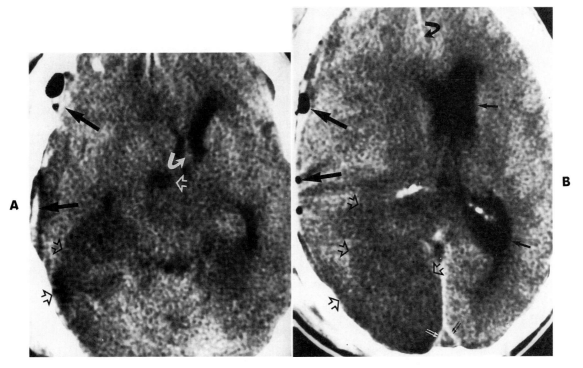

Fig. 8-45. Axial NECT postoperative scans in a patient who had a large acute right SDH evacuated show a small amount of residual subdural blood and air *(large black arrows)*. Subfalcine herniation of the lateral ventricles is present, seen as right-to-left displacement under the anterior falx cerebri *(curved black arrow)*. The left lateral ventricle *(single black arrows)* is enlarged due to foramen of Monro obstruction (**A**, *curved arrow*). Descending transtentorial herniation (not shown) caused by the large SDH has produced secondary infarction of the right posterior cerebral artery territory *(black open arrows)*. Focal infarction in the right internal capsule (**A**, *white open arrow*) was caused by lenticulostriate artery compression from the downward brain displacement. A small amount of blood has collected along the posterior falx cerebri and outlines the straight sinus (**B**, *double arrows*). This appearance of "pseudothrombosis" should not be mistaken for true dural sinus thrombosis on this nonenhanced scan.

Cerebral Herniations
Subfalcine
Transtentorial
Descending
Ascending
Transalar (transsphenoidal)
Descending
Ascending
Tonsillar
Miscellaneous (e.g., transdural/transcranial)

branches may become compressed against the falx. Callosomarginal artery occlusion may result in secondary ischemia and infarction[43] (see subsequent discussion).

Transtentorial herniation. Two types of transtentorial herniations can occur: descending and ascending.

Descending transtentorial herniation. This is by far the most common type of transtentorial herniation. The uncus and parahippocampal gyrus of the temporal lobe are initially displaced medially and protrude over the free tentorial margin (Figs. 8-43, *C*, 8-46, and 8-47). At early stages of descending transtentorial herniation the ipsilateral side of the suprasellar cistern is effaced (Fig. 8-46, *A*). As the brainstem is shifted away from the herniating temporal lobe, the ipsilateral cerebellopontine angle cistern is initially enlarged (Fig. 8-46, *B*).

Progressive obliteration of the suprasellar cistern occurs with increasing supratentorial mass effect until, with severe bilateral descending herniation, the tentorial incisura is completely plugged from displacement of both temporal lobes and the lower diencephalon into the midline basal subarachnoid spaces.

In cases with severe descending transtentorial herniation, CT scans show obliteration of all basal cisterns. The midbrain displacement is nicely delineated

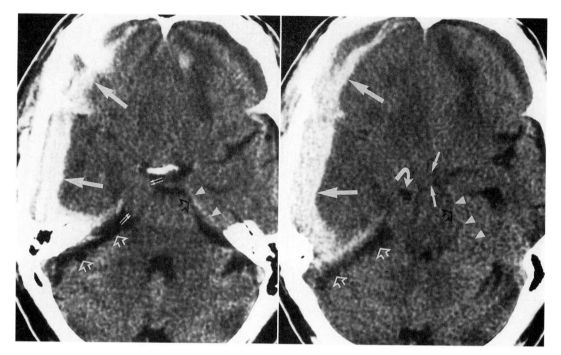

Fig. 8-46. Axial NECT scans show early signs of descending transtentorial herniation caused by a rapidly accumulating right frontotemporal SDH *(large arrows)*. The ipsilateral half of the suprasellar cistern is effaced *(small single arrows)* by the herniating temporal lobe uncus *(double arrows)*. The right temporal horn *(curved arrow)* is displaced almost to the midline. The ipsilateral cerebellopontine angle cistern is widened *(white open arrows)* because the herniating temporal lobe has displaced and rotated the brainstem to the left. The point where the displaced midbrain is compressed against the left side of the tentorial incisura *(arrowheads)* is the point where Kernohan's notch would occur *(black open arrows)*.

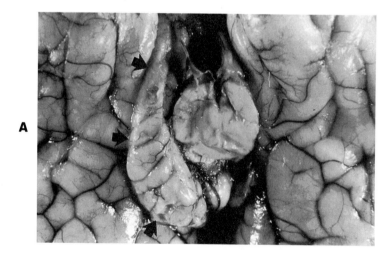

Fig. 8-47. A, Gross pathology of descending transtentorial herniation as seen from below. The uncus and hippocampus are displaced over the medial edge of the tentorial incisura. Note "grooving" produced on the undersurface of the temporal lobe *(arrows)* where the herniating brain has impinged against the tentorium. Axial **(B)** and sagittal **(C)** T1-weighted MR scans in a patient with descending transtentorial herniation secondary to a large chronic SDH (not shown). The axial scan **(B)** shows herniation of the uncus and hippocampus *(large arrows)* over the tentorial edge *(open arrows)* into the suprasellar cistern. Note compression of the right third nerve *(curved arrow)*. The sagittal scan **(C)** shows inferior kinking of the midbrain and tectum *(arrows)* as they are forced below the incisura *(dotted line)*. Note early tonsillar herniation *(small black arrow)*. **(A,** Courtesy B. Horten. **B** and **C,** From Osborn AG: Secondary effects of intracranial trauma, *Neuroimaging Clin N Amer* 1:461-474, 1991.)

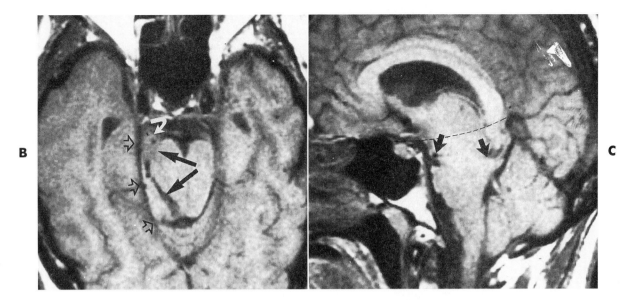

Fig. 8-47, cont'd. For legend see p. 226.

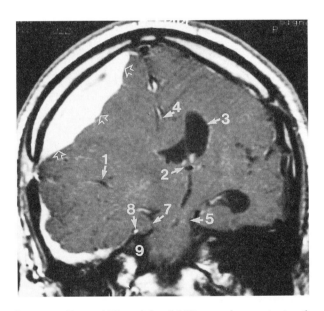

Fig. 8-48. Coronal T1-weighted MR scan demonstrates the secondary effects of a large chronic subdural hematoma *(open arrows)*. Same key as Fig. 8-43, C.

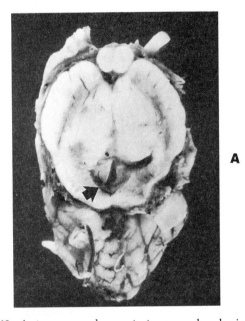

Fig. 8-49. Autopsy case demonstrates secondary brainstem injury caused by descending herniation. **A,** Midbrain periaqueductal necrosis *(arrows)* is shown.   *Continued.*

by multiplanar MR (Figs. 8-47, B and C, and 8-48). The anterior choroidal, posterior communicating, and posterior cerebral arteries (PCA) are all displaced inferomedially in severe descending herniations. The PCA may become compressed against the tentorial incisura, resulting in occipital lobe ischemia or infarction (Fig. 8-43, C). Inferior kinking and occlusion of perforating vessels that arise from the circle of Willis can result in basal ganglia and midbrain infarction (see subsequent discussion).

Other manifestations of descending transtentorial herniation include periaqueductal necrosis (Fig. 8-49,

A), secondary midbrain, or "Duret," hemorrhage (Figs. 8-49, B, and 8-50) and "Kernohan's notch" (Figs. 8-43, C, and 8-51), as well as compressive cranial neuropathies (see subsequent discussion).

Ascending transtentorial herniation. Infratentorial traumatic injuries are less common than their supratentorial counterparts. Trauma-induced upward herniation of the vermis and cerebellar hemispheres through the tentorial incisura is therefore much less common than descending temporal lobe herniation.

With ascending herniations the central lobule, culmen, and superior surface of the cerebellum are dis-

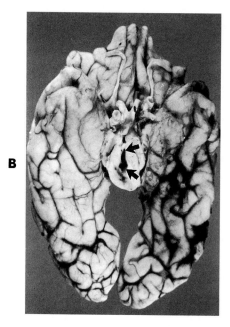

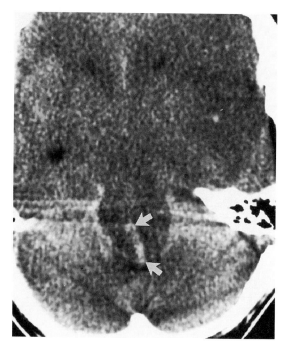

Fig. 8-49, cont'd. B, Closed head injury with contusions and severe brain swelling. A "Duret" midbrain hemorrhage is present *(arrows)*. (Courtesy S. VandenBerg.)

Fig. 8-50. A, Axial NECT scan shows a Duret hemorrhage *(arrows)*. (Courtesy M. Fruin.)

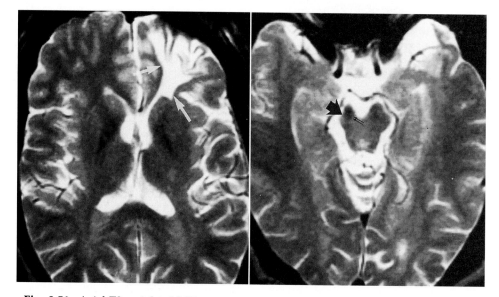

Fig. 8-51. Axial T2-weighted MR scans in a patient who sustained severe head trauma 12 years before the imaging study. A large left frontal subdural hematoma and frontal lobe contusion were present at the time. These follow-up studies show focal encephalomalacic changes *(white arrows)* in the left frontal lobe. The right cerebral peduncle *(large black arrow)* is atrophic and shows an old hemorrhagic contusion *(double black arrows)*. This represents residua of a "Kernohan's notch," i.e., impaction injury of the contralateral cerebral peduncle against the tentorial incisura during descending temporal lobe herniation (compare to Fig. 8-43, *C*).

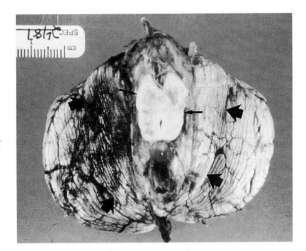

Fig. 8-52. Gross pathology of a massive cerebellar hemorrhage with upward transtentorial herniation. Note midbrain compression *(small arrows)* and grooving of the superior cerebellar surfaces *(large arrows)* by the medial edge of the tentorial incisura. (Courtesy E. Ross.)

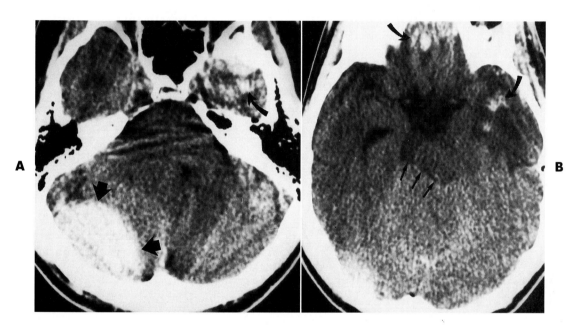

Fig. 8-53. Axial NECT scans show a large posterior fossa EDH (**A,** *large arrows*). The hematoma has displaced the vermis upward through the tentorial incisura, resulting in deformity of the quadrigeminal plate cistern (**B,** *small arrows*). Bifrontal and contralateral temporal lobe contusions are indicated by the curved black arrows. (From Osborn AG: Secondary effects of intracranial trauma, *Neuroimaging Clin N Amer* 1:461-474, 1991.)

placed cephalad through the tentorial incisura (Fig. 8-52; *see* Fig. 9-11, *A, D,* and E). Imaging studies show the superior vermian cistern is effaced and the fourth ventricle is compressed and displaced anteriorly. With increasing upward herniation the quadrigeminal cistern is deformed and the midbrain displaced anteriorly (Fig. 8-53).[42,44] Aqueductal compression may result in obstructive hydrocephalus.

Transalar (transsphenoidal) herniation. This is less common than subfalcine or transtentorial herniations. In descending transalar herniation the frontal lobe is forced posteriorly over the greater sphenoid ala, causing backward displacement of the sylvian fissure, the horizontal middle cerebral artery, and the temporal lobe. In ascending herniations the temporal lobe, sylvian fissure, and middle cerebral artery are displaced up and over the sphenoid ridge.

Tonsillar herniation. Two thirds of patients with upward and one half of those with downward transtentorial shift have concurrent tonsillar herniation.[44a] With large posterior fossa mass effects of any etiology the cerebellar tonsils are displaced inferiorly through the foramen magnum (Fig. 8-54). This is best demonstrated on sagittal MR studies (Fig. 8-47, *C).*

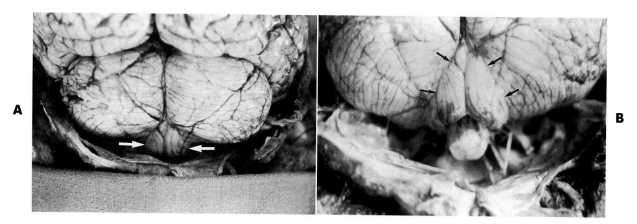

Fig. 8-54. Gross pathology of tonsillar herniation. **A,** In situ specimen shows the cerebellar tonsils *(arrows)* displaced inferiorly through the foramen magnum. **B,** Close-up view of the tonsils as seen from below shows the "grooving" *(arrows)* produced by the foramen magnum. (Courtesy Rubinstein Collection, University of Virginia.)

Cerebral Ischemia, Infarction, and Secondary Hemorrhage

Cerebral ischemia. Some authors believe cerebral ischemia is the single most important cause of secondary brain injury following severe craniocerebral trauma.[45-47] Profound changes in global or regional cerebral blood flow occur in most patients with Glasgow coma scores of 8 or less.[47] Trauma-induced acute and chronic derangements in blood flow can be demonstrated using xenon-enhanced CT; other techniques that may become clinically important include phosphorus-31 magnetic resonance spectroscopy,[48] single photon emission computed tomography,[49] and transcranial doppler sonography.[50] Functional MR imaging may play a major future role as well.

Posttraumatic cerebral infarction. Brain displacements across dural surfaces account for most posttraumatic infarction syndromes. Occipital lobe infarction is the most common and occurs when the posterior cerebral artery is compressed against the tentorial incisura by a herniating temporal lobe[51] (see subsequent discussion). Cingulate gyrus herniation with ACA occlusion, usually caused by callosomarginal compression against the falx cerebri, is next most common (Fig. 8-55). Middle cerebral artery infarction occurs with gross herniation or severe cerebral edema. Less frequently the lenticulostriate, thalamoperforating, or choroidal arteries are occluded against the skull base, resulting in basal ganglionic infarction (Fig. 8-55).

Secondary hemorrhage. Other important secondary effects of craniocerebral trauma include midbrain (Duret) hemorrhages (Figs. 8-49 and 8-50) and "Kernohan's notch" (Fig. 8-51). Caudal displacement of the upper brainstem may compress perforating vessels in the interpeduncular cistern, resulting in single or multiple secondary (Duret) hemorrhages or ischemic foci in the central tegmentum.[39] These secondary central hemorrhages should not be confused with the more uncommon primary brainstem injuries that are typically seen in the dorsolateral region.

"Kernohan's notch" is a secondary feature of descending transtentorial herniation. As the medial temporal lobe herniates over the tentorial edge, the midbrain is displaced away from the expanding mass. The contralateral cerebral peduncle is pinioned against the opposite side of the tentorium. The linear indentation or groove produced by the hard edge of the tentorium is termed *Kernohan's notch*. This compression may result in focal edema, ischemia, or hemorrhagic necrosis of the cerebral peduncle that can be detected on MR studies.[52] This may produce ipsilateral hemiparesis, the so-called false localizing sign,[53] because it is contralateral to the main mass effect.

Diffuse Cerebral Edema

Diffuse brain swelling. Massive cerebral edema with intracranial hypertension is among the most life-threatening of all secondary traumatic lesions.[53a]

Incidence, etiology, and clinical implications. Diffuse cerebral edema is seen in 10% to 20% of severe brain injuries and occurs nearly twice as often in children compared to adults.[54] Unilateral hemispheric swelling is associated with an ipsilateral subdural hematoma in 85% of cases, epidural hematoma in 9%, and occurs as an isolated lesion in 4% to 5% of patients.[55]

Although gross enlargement of one or both hemispheres may occur within hours after the traumatic insult, severe cerebral edema usually takes 24 to 48

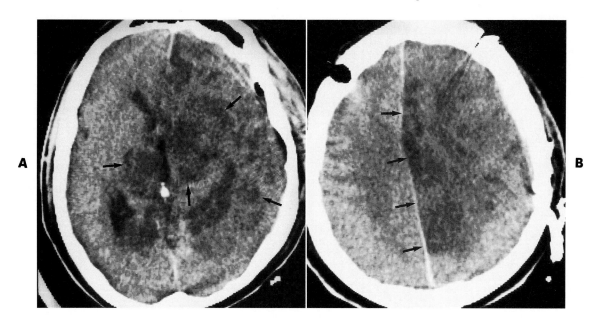

Fig. 8-55. Axial NECT scans show multiple basal ganglionic infarctions (**A,** *arrows*) secondary to severe cerebral edema with compression of numerous perforating arteries against the skull base. A distal ACA infarct is also seen, caused by subfalcine herniation with compression of distal ACA branches against the inferior free edge of the falx cerebri (**B,** *arrows*). (From Osborn AG: Secondary effects of intracranial trauma, *Neuroimaging Clin N Amer* 1:461-474, 1991.)

hours to develop. Diffuse posttraumatic brain swelling is due to increased intravascular blood volume, increased brain water content, or both.[55] Mortality rate in these cases approaches 50%.[54]

Imaging. The most reliable early imaging finding in diffuse cerebral edema is effacement of the surface sulci and basilar subarachnoid spaces, particularly the suprasellar and perimesencephalic (quadrigeminal plate and ambient) cisterns. The cerebral ventricles may appear small or compressed.

The brain in diffuse bilateral cerebral edema typically exhibits homogeneously decreased attenuation on CT scans, with loss of the gray-white matter interface (Fig. 8-56). The cerebellum may appear relatively hyperdense compared to the grossly edematous cerebral hemispheres, the so-called white cerebellum sign (Fig. 8-57). This finding is caused by relative sparing of the cerebellum and brainstem from cerebral hypoxic-ischemic events and is often associated with extracranial trauma such as drowning or strangulation.[56] The "reversal" sign is similar. It is caused by diffuse hypodensity of the cortex and deep white matter compared to the normal density of the thalamus, brainstem, and cerebellum, all of which are perfused by the posterior circulation.[57]

Unilateral or bilateral hemispheric swelling typically is accompanied by signs of cerebral herniation (see previous discussion).

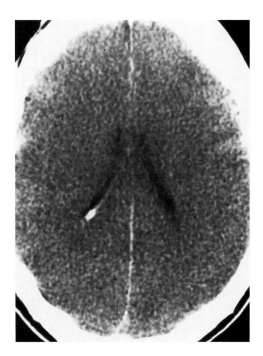

Fig. 8-56. Axial CT scan in a patient with severe cerebral edema shows effacement of superficial sulci, loss of gray-white matter differentiation, and small ventricles.

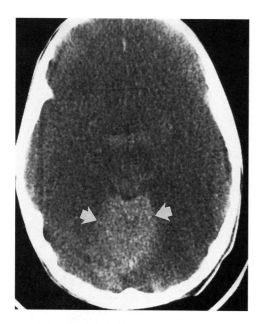

Vascular Manifestation and Complications of Craniocerebral Trauma
Primary injury

Arterial injury

Transection
Laceration
Subintimal tear
Dissection
Pseudoaneurysm
Thrombosis
Arteriovenous fistula

Venous injury

Cortical vein rupture/thrombosis
Dural sinus laceration/thrombosis

Fig. 8-57. A 6-year-old child was resuscitated after drowning. NECT scan obtained 24 hours later demonstrates the so-called white cerebellum sign. Relative sparing of the cerebellum from the hypoxic-ischemic insult makes the vermis *(arrows)* appear high density compared to the abnormally low density edematous cerebral hemispheres.

Brain death. *Brain death* is the colloquial term used when human death is determined by tests showing global brain destruction or irreversible cessation of global brain function.[58] Although the legal definition varies with locality, imaging documentation of brain death is based on demonstrating absent blood flow.

Brain death has been determined by various techniques, including four-vessel cerebral angiography, contrast-enhanced dynamic CT scanning, Xenon CT, transcranial doppler sonography, and radionuclide brain scans.[59] Currently, scintigraphic perfusion studies using 99mTc-HMPAO to demonstrate absent cerebral blood flow are probably the most widely accepted techniques, although MR angiography may prove useful in the future (Fig. 8-58).[60-62]

Vascular Manifestations and Complications of Craniocerebral Trauma

A spectrum of vascular injuries and complications is associated with craniocerebral trauma (*see* box). Some major primary and secondary lesions are discussed next.

Local, regional, and global perfusion disturbances

Primary perfusion disturbances. Primary perfusion disturbances are caused by stab wounds or projectile injuries that transect or occlude vessels. Sometimes the traumatic aneurysms and arteriovenous fis-

tulae that are common angiographic manifestations of penetrating vascular injury[63] also cause perfusion abnormalities. Occasionally intracranial or cervical arterial dissections occlude vessels either directly or by secondary emboli (see subsequent discussion).

Secondary perfusion disturbances. Profound secondary alterations in cerebral blood flow often occur with closed head injury[45-47,49] (see previous discussion). Although the etiology of these perfusion changes is not completely understood, delayed cerebral arterial vasospasm is a frequent complication of closed head injury. In some cases, the severity approaches that seen with aneurysmal SAH.[64] Transcranial doppler ultrasound (TCD) is helpful in managing patients with traumatic brain injury who are at risk for developing secondary ischemia.[64,65] Angiography in severely traumatized patients discloses vasospasm in 5% to 10% of cases.

Although posttraumatic cerebral infarction is a recognized complication, large vessel occlusions with closed head injury are unusual. Most are caused by gross mechanical shifts of the brain, with herniation and occlusion of vessels such as the posterior or anterior cerebral arteries against a relatively unyielding dural fold (Figs. 8-59 and 8-60).[51]

Aneurysm and pseudoaneurysm. Traumatic aneurysms are an uncommon but serious complication of craniocerebral trauma.[4] Traumatic aneurysms due to penetrating and nonpenetrating trauma are discussed in detail in Chapter 9. Most traumatic aneurysms are pseudoaneurysms, i.e., they are secondary to disruption in arterial wall continuity. Typically a periarterial hematoma forms and is contained by adjacent soft tissues. Subsequent encapsulation of the paravascular hematoma results in a pseudoaneurysm (*see* Fig. 9-29).[66,67]

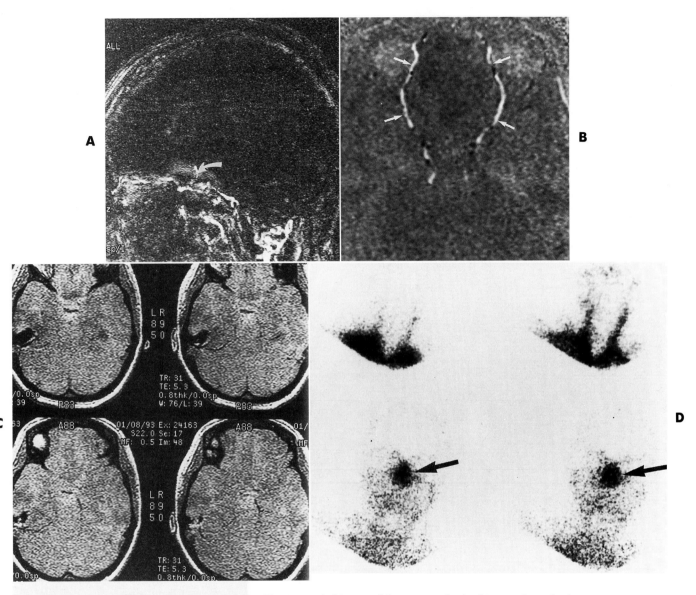

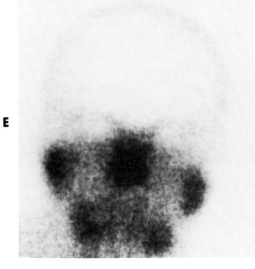

Fig. 8-58. A 28-year-old woman who had internal cerebral vein occlusion, bithalamic infarcts, and massive cerebral edema (*see* Fig. 11-82) was clinically "brain dead." Phase-contrast MR angiography and isotope studies were obtained to evaluate for brain death. Sagittal **(A)** and axial **(B)** 2D-PC MRA studies show no evidence for intracranial blood flow in the intradural ICA (**A,** *arrow*). Some slow venous flow is present in the superior ophthalmic veins (**B,** *arrows*) but no intracranial blood flow is identified. **C,** Source images through the circle of Willis show no intravascular signal. The 99mTc pertechnetate brain flow study obtained shortly after the MR scan was performed shows classic findings of brain death. **D,** Four-view AP flow study shows no perfusion in the anterior or middle cerebral vascular territories. The "hot nose" sign (black arrows) represents vascular shunting to the external carotid system. Delayed AP scan **(E)** obtained 10 minutes after the flow study demonstrates the "light bulb" or "fish-bowl" sign caused by strong mucosal, but no brain, uptake of isotope. (**D,** Courtesy F. Datz and E. Booth.)

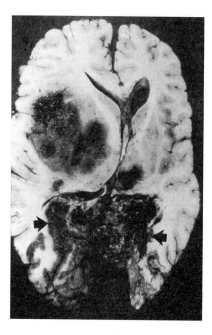

Fig. 8-59. Axial gross specimen with bilateral posterior cerebral artery occlusions secondary to descending transtentorial herniation. Both occipital lobes are infarcted *(arrows)* (same case as Fig. 8-58, *C*).

Arterial dissections and lacerations

Pathology. In arterial dissections, blood penetrates the arterial wall, splitting the media and creating a false lumen that dissects the arterial wall for varying distances; if the intramural hematoma expands toward the adventitia, an aneurysmal dilatation may form a so-called dissecting aneurysm.[68]

Incidence and etiology. Traumatic dissection of the cervicocranial arteries is an increasingly well recognized phenomenon. Besides trauma/cervical manipulation, other factors such as hypertension, migraine, vigorous physical activity, vasculopathy such as fibromuscular dysplasia or Marfan syndrome, drug abuse (principally sympathomimetic drugs), oral contraceptives, pharyngeal infections, and syphilis have also been implicated.[69] Arterial dissections can also occur with minor or no trauma at all.

The precise pathogenesis of traumatic dissections is still unclear. In the case of the cervical internal carotid artery, hyperextension and lateral flexion of the neck may stretch the ICA over the transverse processes of the upper cervical vertebrae.[70]

Clinical presentation. Patients with craniocervical arterial dissections may be normal, have only minor symptoms such as headache or neck pain, or have severe neurologic deficits. A postganglionic Horner syndrome is common with carotid artery dissections[71] (Figs. 8-61 and 8-62).

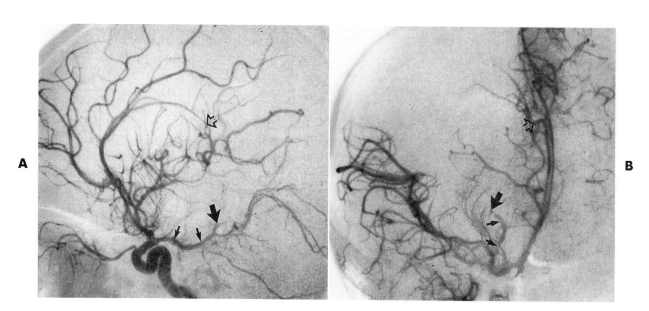

A

B

Fig. 8-60. An 8-year-old child with a large posterior temporoparietal hematoma and severe subfalcine and descending transtentorial herniation. Right internal carotid angiogram with AP **(A)** and lateral **(B)** midarterial phase films show marked displacement of the proximal posterior cerebral artery (PCA) medially and inferiorly through the tentorial incisura *(small arrows)*. The PCA is occluded at the point where it crosses the free margin of the tentorium *(large arrows)*. The anterior cerebral artery is also displaced across the midline and its pericallosal branch is occluded distally where it returns to the midline under the inferior falcine edge *(open arrows)*.

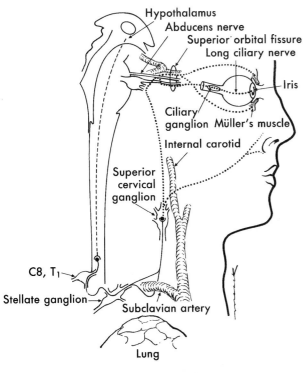

Fig. 8-61. Schematic drawing demonstrates the ocular sympathetic pathway. (From Digre KB: Selective MR imaging approach for evaluation of patients with Horner syndrome, *AJNR* 13:223-227, 1992.)

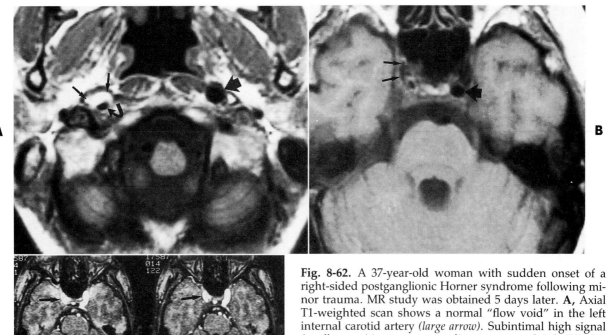

Fig. 8-62. A 37-year-old woman with sudden onset of a right-sided postganglionic Horner syndrome following minor trauma. MR study was obtained 5 days later. **A,** Axial T1-weighted scan shows a normal "flow void" in the left internal carotid artery *(large arrow)*. Subintimal high signal *(small arrows)* is seen surrounding a narrowed right ICA lumen *(curved arrow)*. **B,** Axial T1-weighted scan through the cavernous sinus shows a normal left ICA *(large arrow)*. The right ICA appears abnormally small *(small arrows)* but there is no high signal in its wall. **C,** Four source images from the 3D TOF MR angiogram show the cavernous right ICA *(arrows)* is patent but appears small.

Continued.

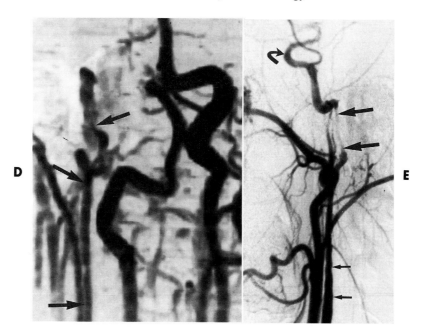

Fig. 8-62, cont'd. D, Reprojected AP oblique image of the multiple overlapping thin slab acquisition MR angiogram (MOTSA sequence) shows a small, irregular right ICA *(arrows)*. **E,** Right digital subtraction common carotid angiogram, midarterial phase, lateral view, shows an ICA dissection with marked narrowing of the distal cervical segment *(large arrows)*. Smooth concentric circular spastic contractions, or arterial "standing waves," are seen in the proximal ICA *(small arrows)*. The ICA distal to the dissection has reduced flow and appears small *(curved arrow)*.

Location. Extracranial carotid artery dissections usually spare the bulb and begin about 2 cm distal to the common carotid bifurcation. The typical dissection extends cephalad for a variable distance, usually terminating at or proximal to the petrous carotid canal (Fig. 8-62).[67]

Less commonly, ICA dissections occur within the petrous canal or the intracavernous carotid segment.[72] These dissections are usually associated with basal skull fracture.[73] Traumatic intradural ICA dissections are rare. When intracranial ICA dissections do occur, the most common site is the midsupraclinoid segment, where the artery is relatively mobile (Fig. 8-63). The ICA is fixed at the anterior clinoid process and relatively fixed at its terminal bifurcation into the anterior and middle cerebral arteries. Supraclinoid ICA dissections may also extend to involve the proximal anterior and middle cerebral arteries (Fig. 8-64).

Traumatic vertebral artery dissections usually involve the distal segment between C2 and the skull base (Fig. 8-65). Occasionally midsegment VA dissections are seen with lateral cervical spine fractures or dislocations.[74,75] (Fig. 8-66). Uncommonly, the first, or proximal, VA segment is involved between its origin from the subclavian artery to its entry into the foramen transversarium of a cervical vertebra (usually C6).[76]

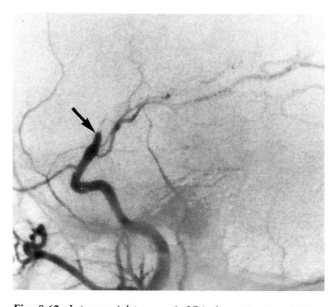

Fig. 8-63. Intracranial traumatic ICA dissection just below the circle of Willis is shown by lateral left common carotid angiogram. The internal carotid artery abruptly terminates below its bifurcation into the ACA and MCA *(arrow)*. The extracranial vessels were normal.

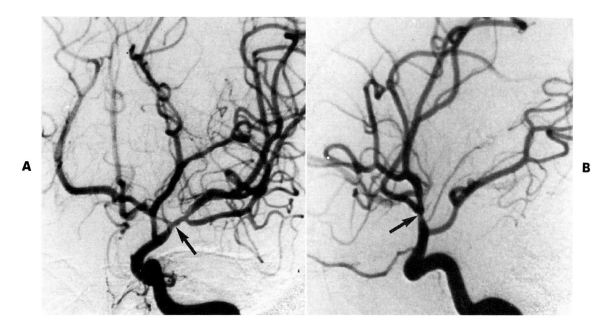

Fig. 8-64. Severe closed head injury with unexplained neurologic deficits prompted cerebral angiography in this 6-year-old child. AP (**A**) and lateral (**B**) digital subtraction left internal carotid angiograms show dissection of the distal ICA extending into the horizontal ACA and MCA segments *(arrows).* The very focal nature of the abnormality plus the absence of any other areas of vascular narrowing is against the other possible diagnosis, that is, posttraumatic vasospasm.

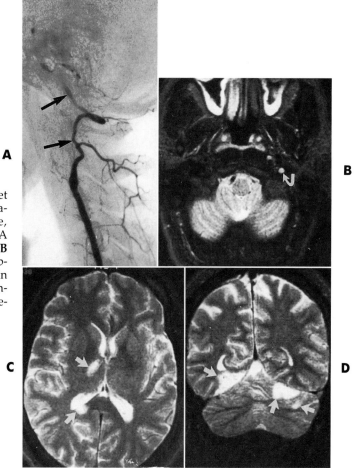

Fig. 8-65. This patient experienced sudden onset of neurologic deficits following neck manipulation. **A,** Left vertebral angiogram, arterial phase, lateral view, shows irregularity of the distal VA between C2 and the skull base *(arrows).* Axial (**B** and **C**) and coronal (**D**) T2-weighted MR scans obtained 5 days later show high signal thrombus in the left VA (**B,** *arrow*) and multifocal embolic infarctions (**C** and **D,** *arrows)* in the distal vertebrobasilar circulation.

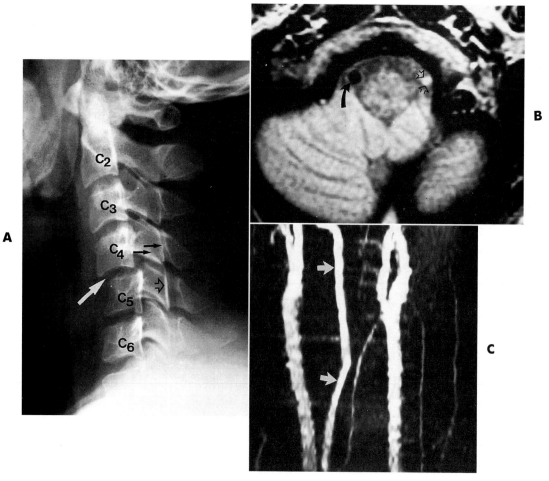

Fig. 8-66. Traumatic vertebral artery injury. **A,** Midcervical fracture subluxation *(white arrow)* is shown on this lateral cervical spine plain film radiograph. Note offset of C4 laminae *(black arrows)* compared to C5 *(open arrow)*, indicating a rotational subluxation also. **B,** Axial proton density-weighted MR scan obtained 5 days later shows the right vertebral artery *(curved arrow)* is patent, but the left vertebral artery (VA) is thrombosed. Note high signal intraluminal thrombus *(open arows)*. **C,** MR angiogram shows the patent right VA *(arrows)*. The thrombosed left VA is not visualized.

Imaging. Angiographic studies typically show a smooth or irregularly tapered vessel (Fig. 8-65, *A*) that is sometimes occluded by the intramural hematoma. Occasionally an intimal tear or intraluminal thrombus can be seen. Routine CT scans are often normal unless distal embolization has resulted in infarction. MR scans may disclose high signal subacute subintimal thrombus (Fig. 8-65, *B*). MR angiography shows focal, segmental, or aneurysmal dilatations (Fig. 8-62).[75]

Cortical vein rupture/thrombosis. Isolated cortical vein rupture with trauma is uncommon. Most cortical vein tears are associated with a preexisting SDH or skull fracture. Posttraumatic cortical vein thrombosis is also rare. Traumatic venous occlusions usually occur with laceration and occlusion of a major dural sinus.

Dural sinus lacerations/thrombosis. Dural sinus lacerations typically occur with skull fracture. Secondary thrombosis with cortical vein infarction can occur (Fig. 8-67).

Traumatic arteriovenous fistulae. Trauma-induced arteriovenous communications occur at several locations. These typically are found where arterial dissections or lacerations occur in close proximity to a vein or dural sinus. Common locations are therefore at the skull base.

The most common traumatic AVF is a carotid-cavernous sinus fistula (CCF) (Fig. 8-68). CCFs can occur spontaneously with closed head injury or basilar skull fracture. Other common posttraumatic AVFs are located near the exocranial opening of the carotid canal or, in the case of the vertebral artery, between C1 and C2 and the foramen magnum (Fig. 8-69). Mid-

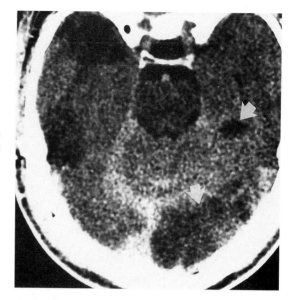

Fig. 8-67. Axial NECT scan in a patient with dural sinus laceration and thrombosis shows multiple venous infarcts *(arrows)* (same case as Fig. 8-4).

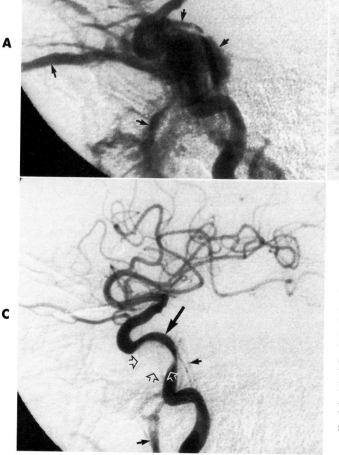

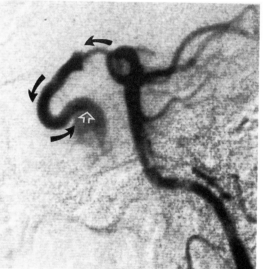

Fig. 8-68. Traumatic carotid-cavernous fistula. **A,** Digital subtraction internal carotid angiogram, early arterial phase, lateral view, shows the cavernous sinus, superior and inferior ophthalmic veins, and pterygoid, deep facial, and clival venous plexuses are all opacified with contrast *(arrows)*. The exact fistula site is obscured. **B,** Injection into the vertebral artery with temporary compression of the ipsilateral carotid artery shows contrast reflux through the posterior communicating artery and internal carotid artery *(curved arrows)* into the cavernous sinus. The exact fistula site is shown by the white arrow. **C,** Post-embolization study shows closure of the fistula by a balloon *(open arrows)* placed in the cavernous sinus. Blood flow to the distal ICA *(large arrow)* is preserved. A small amount of flow into the pterygoid and clival venous plexuses remains *(small arrows)*; this closed spontaneously.

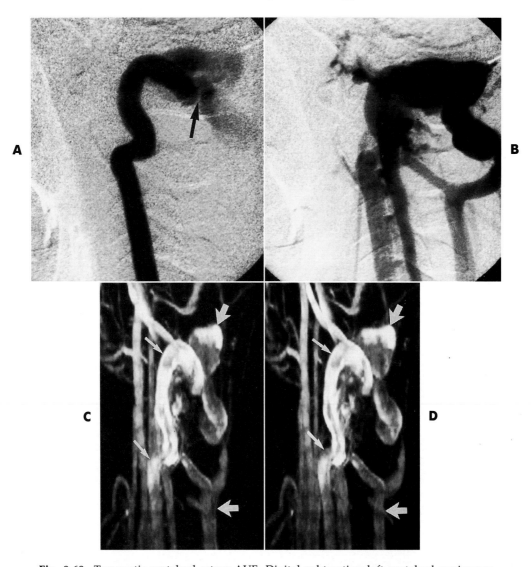

Fig. 8-69. Traumatic vertebral artery AVF. Digital subtraction left vertebral angiogram, lateral view, with early **(A)** and slightly later **(B)** arterial phase frames shows the enlarged VA communicates directly *(arrow)* with markedly enlarged suboccipital veins. **C** and **D,** Two slightly oblique lateral views of a multiple overlapping thin-slab MR angiogram show the prominent VA *(small arrows)* and multiple enlarged draining venous channels *(large arrows)* that include suboccipital, jugular, and vertebral veins.

dle meningeal artery laceration usually results in an epidural hematoma but occasionally can cause a traumatic AVF without an accompanying EDH.

SEQUELAE OF TRAUMA

If patients survive severe head injury, the residual effects may range from mild treatable lesions to devastating permanent neurologic deficits. Some of the more important late sequelae of traumatic brain injury include the following:

1. Encephalomalacia and atrophy
2. Pneumocephalus, pneumatocele formation
3. CSF leaks and fistulae
4. Acquired cephalocele or leptomeningeal cyst
5. Cranial nerve injury
6. Diabetes insipidus

Encephalomalacia

Pathologic residua of closed head injury vary from the microscopic changes associated with DAI (such as axon retraction balls, microglial clusters, and foci of demyelination) to more extensive confluent areas of gross parenchymal loss and deep cerebral or generalized cortical atrophy. Encephalomalacic foci appear as low-density nonenhancing areas on CT scans; MR studies show hypodense areas on T1WI that become hyperintense on T2-weighted scans (Fig. 8-70). Blood degradation products may complicate the im-

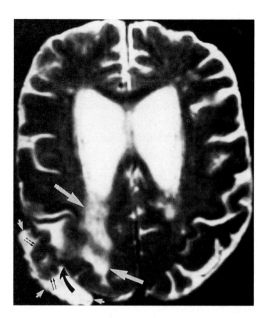

Fig. 8-70. Axial T2-weighted MR scan in a patient with head trauma 1 year before study. Note encephalomalacic changes in the right parietal lobe *(large white arrows)*. A small posttraumatic cephalocele is also present. Brain *(double black arrows)* has herniated through a tear through the dura *(curved arrow)*. Trapped CSF *(small white arrows)* has formed an intraosseous posttraumatic leptomeningeal cyst.

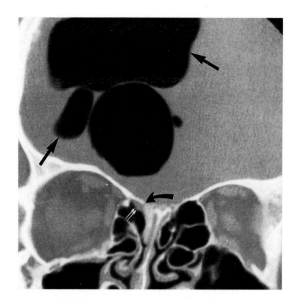

Fig. 8-71. Posttraumatic pneumocephalus and CSF leak in a patient with headache and rhinorrhea. Coronal CT scan shows the pneumatocele *(straight black arrows)*. The cribriform plate fracture *(curved arrow)* was confirmed as the site of CSF leakage at surgery. Note a small amount of fluid or soft tissue in the underlying ethmoid sinus *(white arrows)*. (From Osborn AG: Secondary effects of intracranial trauma, *Neuroimaging Clin N Amer* 1:461-474, 1991.)

aging appearance of encephalomalacia. Secondary changes of volume loss such as ventricular and sulcal enlargement are often present.[77]

Pneumocephalus

Skull base fracture with dural tear and direct communication with an air-containing paranasal sinus may lead to acute and chronic pneumocephalus. Intracranial air can occur in virtually any compartment: extracerebral (epidural, subdural, subarachnoid spaces) or intracerebral (brain parenchyma, cerebral ventricles). Air collections can be diffuse or focal. When they are focal they are often referred to as "pneumatoceles" (Fig. 8-71).

Intracranial air is easily identified as very low attenuation foci on CT scans and areas of absent signal on MR studies. Epidural air tends to remain localized and does not change with alteration in head position. Subdural air often forms an air-fluid level within the subdural space, is confluent, and changes with head position (Fig. 8-72). Subarachnoid air typically is multifocal, nonconfluent, and droplet-shaped, often located within the cerebral sulci (Fig. 8-73; *see* Fig. 8-45, *B*). Intraventricular air, like intraventricular hemorrhage, is typically seen only with severe head trauma. Intraventricular pneumocephalus rarely occurs in isolation and is usually seen with skull base or mastoid fractures that also lacerate the dura. Intravascular air is uncommon and typically only seen with mortal injury.

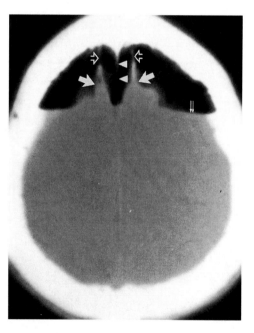

Fig. 8-72. Axial NECT scan with wide windows shows bifrontal subdural air collections. Note air on either side of the falx cerebri *(arrowheads)*. The frontal lobes are tethered anteriorly *(large white arrows)* by cortical veins *(open arrows)* that are stretched as they cross the subdural space. Note air-fluid levels *(double arrows)*.

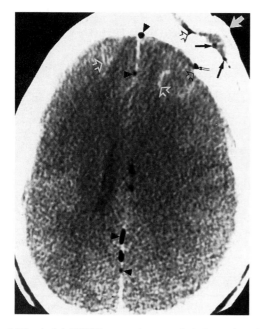

Fig. 8-73. Axial NECT scan shows a left frontal scalp hematoma *(large white arrow)* with subgaleal fluid and air *(single black arrows)*. Open communication with the intracranial space through a comminuted skull fracture *(open black arrows)* and lacerated dura *(double black arrows)* is present. Subarachnoid air droplets are indicated by the arrowheads. Traumatic SAH is also seen *(white open arrows)*.

CSF Leaks and Fistulae

Approximately 80% of CSF fistulas result from skull base fractures.[78] These fistulae are generally basifrontal in location, with drainage into the ethmoid or sphenoid sinuses (Figs. 8-71 and 8-74). Recurrent meningitis complicates 20% of such cases. Although a CSF fistula can develop many years after trauma, 70% occur within 1 week.[78]

High resolution coronal CT, CT cisternography, digital subtraction CT cisternography, isotope tracers, and MR imaging have all been used to localize the precise site of the dural defect in these challenging cases.[78,79]

Cranial Nerve Palsies

Various cranial nerve palsies result from direct craniocerebral trauma. The olfactory nerve and bulbs may be damaged directly by a cribriform plate fracture or indirectly by basifrontal contusion or shearing injuries. The third, fourth, sixth, and ophthalmic division of the fifth cranial nerves can be damaged by complex skull base fractures that extend through the cavernous sinus or orbital apex. The third nerve is also often compressed by the temporal lobe as it herniates over the tentorial incisura *(see* Fig. 8-47, *B)*. The trochlear nerve, having a long, relatively exposed intracranial course after its exit from the dorsal midbrain, can be damaged by the knifelike edge of the tentorium cerebelli during violent cranial excursions. The optic nerve can be lacerated by fractures that extend through the lesser sphenoid wing, optic strut, and optic canal.

Intraaxial damage to cranial nerve nuclei from primary or secondary brainstem traumatic lesions may also produce multiple cranial nerve palsies. Extracra-

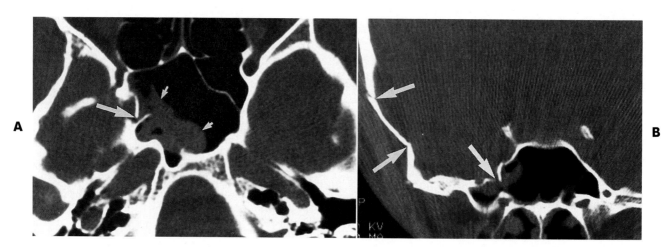

Fig. 8-74. This patient developed CSF rhinorrhea 3 days after head trauma. Axial **(A)** and coronal **(B)** NECT scans show a severely comminuted basilar and right temporal skull fracture *(large arrows)* with CSF leakage *(small arrows)* into the sphenoid sinus, confirmed at surgery and successfully repaired.

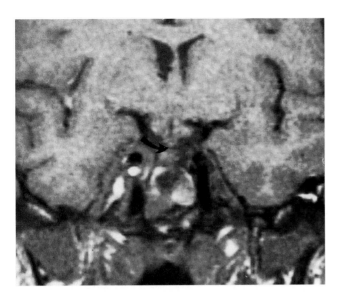

Fig. 8-75. Coronal T1-weighted MR scan in a patient with skull base fracture, thrombosed carotid-cavernous fistula, and diabetes insipidus. The pituitary stalk appears to be transected and retracted *(arrow)*. (From Osborn AG: Secondary effects of intracranial trauma, *Neuroimaging Clin N Amer* 1:461-474, 1991.)

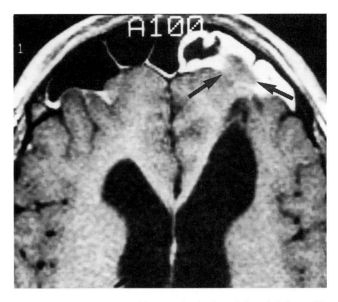

Fig. 8-76. A 34-year-old man had closed head injury 10 years ago. Two weeks before study he developed CSF rhinorrhea. Axial T1-weighted MR scan following contrast administration shows dehiscent posterior wall of the left frontal sinus with brain *(arrows)* herniated through a dural tear into the sinus. Traumatic cephalocele was confirmed at surgery. (From Osborn AG: Secondary effects of intracranial trauma, *Neuroimaging Clin N Amer* 1:461-474, 1991.)

nial lesions such as traumatic or spontaneous internal carotid artery dissection can cause a postganglionic Horner syndrome (see subsequent discussion).

Diabetes Insipidus

Descending transtentorial herniation with secondary hypothalamic ischemia or infarction can result in diabetes insipidus. An absent or transected, retracted infundibular stalk can be seen in some cases with secondary posttraumatic diabetes insipidus (Fig. 8-75).[80] Absence of the usual high intensity signal in the posterior pituitary lobe with an ectopic "bright spot" in the transected, retracted proximal stalk or hypothalamus can occasionally be identified.[81]

Cephaloceles and Leptomeningeal Cysts

Herniation of brain, meninges, CSF, or a combination of all three may occur at the site of a dural laceration and dehiscent skull defect (Figs. 8-70 and 8-76). These acquired cephaloceles can occur at any location but are common in the basifrontal area. Occasionally, acutely increased intracranial pressure combined with surgically or traumatically induced dural and calvarial defects results in extrusion of cerebral tissue and accompanying vessels through the dura into the epidural and subgaleal spaces (Fig. 8-77).

Posttraumatic leptomeningeal cysts or "growing fractures" can occur as a late complication of skull fracture with dural laceration (Fig. 8-78).

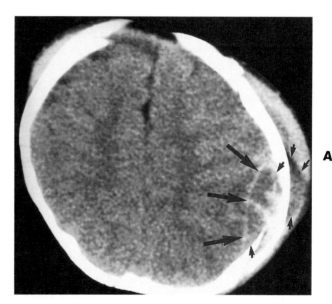

Fig. 8-77. A, Axial CT scan without contrast in a 3-month-old child with nonaccidental trauma. A comminuted skull fracture is present. The dura is seen as a relatively high density curvilinear structure *(large arrows)* outlined by low density brain. Macerated brain has extruded through a tear in the dura, as well as the skull fracture, and is now seen in the epidural and subgaleal spaces *(small arrows)*.

Continued.

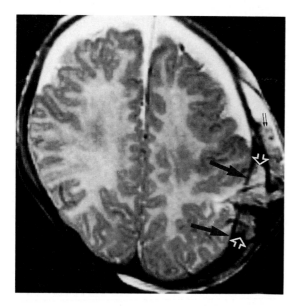

Fig. 8-77, cont'd. B, Axial T2-weighted MR scan shows the dura *(large arrows)* with central tear through which the extruded brain has been squeezed into the epidural *(open arrows)* and subgaleal *(double arrows)* spaces. (From Osborn AG: Secondary effects of intracranial trauma, *Neuroimaging Clin N Amer* 1:461-474, 1991.)

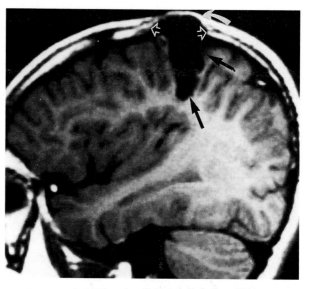

Fig. 8-78. Previous head injury in this 8-year-old child was complicated by an expanding leptomeningeal cyst that presented as a soft subgaleal mass. Sagittal T1-weighted MR scan shows the posttraumatic leptomeningeal cyst *(black arrows)*. The so-called growing fracture is caused by the cyst protruding through the fracture margins *(open arrows)* and under the galea aponeurotica *(curved arrows)*.

HEAD TRAUMA IN CHILDREN: SPECIAL CONSIDERATIONS

Although many manifestations of craniocerebral trauma in children are similar to those seen in adults, the following unique features deserve special attention[56]:

1. The infant skull is extremely malleable and elastic. It can therefore undergo significant deformation and dural laceration without obvious fracture.
2. The combination of a highly flexible spine, disproportionately large head, and comparatively weak cervical musculature permits significant angular excursion and development of substantial shearing forces with relatively minor trauma.
3. Because the sutures are open, intracranial masses in infants and young children may become quite large before neurologic symptoms ensue.
4. The incidence of child abuse appears to be increasing (see subsequent discussion).

CNS Manifestations of Nonaccidental Trauma

Caffey initially identified the presence of multiple long bone fractures and coexisting chronic subdural hematomas in abused children, later describing the prevalence and pathogenesis of CNS damage in the whiplash-shaken infant syndrome.[82,83] Child abuse,

---

Cranial Manifestations of Nonaccidental Trauma
Multiple/complex/bilateral/depressed/unexplained skull fractures
Subdural hematomas in different stages
Cortical contusions/shearing injuries
Retinal hemorrhages
Cerebral ischemia/infarction

---

also known as "nonaccidental trauma" (N.A.T.), is increasing in recognition and incidence worldwide. In the United States, over one million cases of child abuse and neglect are suspected yearly. As Professor Derek Harwood-Nash has emphasized, *"Nobody within the day-to-day environment (of the abused child) is excluded."*[56]

Incidence and clinical presentation. Head trauma is the leading cause of morbidity and mortality in the abused child and occurs in about half of all cases.[84] Nonaccidental trauma may have many manifestations, some of which depend on imaging procedures for identification (see subsequent discussion). Some of the major findings in N.A.T. are listed in the box.

Imaging manifestations of CNS trauma in child abuse. A spectrum of lesions can be identified in the battered child.[85] Only craniocerebral lesions are discussed here.

Skull fractures. The presence of linear skull fracture in a child does not indicate an increased likelihood of significant intracranial injury, nor does its absence lessen the possibility of significant traumatic brain injury. However, the presence of multiple, complex, bilateral, depressed, or unexplained fractures without identifiable significant antecedent trauma should raise the suspicion of N.A.T.[56]

Subdural hematoma. SDHs are the most commonly identified intracranial abnormality in the abused child. Although CT scans can detect the presence of most SDHs (Fig. 8-79), MR studies are more sensitive for delineating small hematomas, identifying SDHs of different ages, and detecting coexisting primary intraaxial lesions such as cortical contusions and shearing injuries (Fig. 8-80).[86] Shaking injuries tear bridging veins along the falx cerebri and may result in interhemispheric (para- and intrafalcial) SDHs. Retinal hemorrhages can sometimes also be identified and are suspicious for N.A.T., particularly if bilateral lesions are present.

Shearing injury and cortical contusions. These were described previously and may presage a poor prognosis,[56] although some children may make a reasonably good functional recovery.[86]

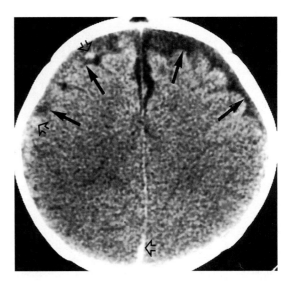

Fig. 8-79. Axial NECT scan shows the classic CNS findings of nonaccidental trauma, SDHs of different ages. The bifrontal extraaxial collections *(large arrows)* are slightly different in density, indicating two separate traumatic episodes. Acute high-density clots *(open arrows)* within the right SDH and along the posterior interhemispheric fissure are imaging evidence for yet a third separate, more recent traumatic event.

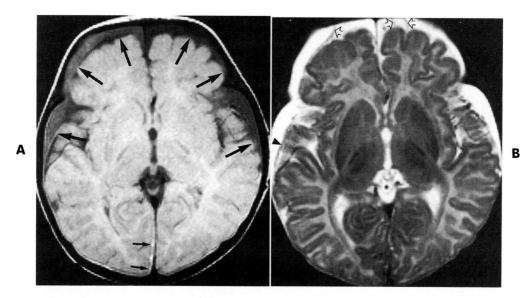

Fig. 8-80. Findings that are strongly indicative of nonaccidental trauma in this child are depicted on MR scans. **A,** Axial T1-weighted scan shows layered bifrontal subacute SDHs of two different signal intensities *(large arrows)*. A small hyperintense SDH is seen posteriorly along the falx cerebri *(small arrows)*. **B,** Axial T2-weighted scan shows a membrane *(arrowhead)* that separates two different SDHs on each side. Note small bridging veins that cross the subdural spaces *(open arrows)*. The small posterior SDH is isointense with adjacent brain and is not visible on the T2WI.

Cerebral edema and ischemic injury. Diffuse cerebral edema with mass effect and herniation is a common manifestation of abuse in newborn to 4-year-old children.[87]

Regional or global cerebral ischemia may also result from child abuse. Imaging findings in hypoxia from smothering or strangling range from selective basal ganglia ischemia, watershed infarction, and laminar cortical necrosis to diffuse cerebral edema and brain death.

REFERENCES

1. Brocker B, Rabin M, Levin A: Clinical and surgical management of head injury, *Neuroimaging Clin N Amer* 1:387-396, 1991.

1a. Kaufman HH: Civilian gunshot wounds to the head, *Neurosurg* 32:962-964, 1993.

2. Hollerman JJ, Fackler ML, Coldwell DM, Ben-Menachem Y: Gunshot wounds: 1. Bullets, ballistics, and mechanisms of injury, *AJR* 155:685-690, 1990.

3. Hollerman JJ, Fackler ML, Coldwell DM, Ben-Menachem Y: Gunshot wounds 2. Radiology, *AJR* 155:691-702, 1990.

4. Jinkins JR, Dadsetan MR, Sener RN et al: Value of acute-phase angiography in the detection of vascular injuries caused by gunshot wounds to the head: analysis of 12 cases, *AJR* 159:365-368, 1992.

5. Gennarelli TA, Thibault LE, Adams JH et al: Diffuse axonal injury and traumatic coma in the primate. In Dacey RG Jr et al: *Trauma of the Central Nervous System,* pp 169-193, New York: Raven Press, 1985.

6. Adams JH: Pathology of nonmissile head injury, *Neuroimaging Clin N Amer* 1:397-410, 1991.

7. Gentry LR: Head trauma. In SW Atlas, editor: *Magnetic Resonance Imaging of the Brain and Spine,* pp 439-466, Raven Press, New York, 1991.

8. Gentry LR: Primary neuronal injuries, *Neuroimaging Clin N Amer* 1:411-432, 1991.

9. Bullock K, Teasdale G: Surgical management of traumatic intracranial hematomas. In Vincken PJ, Bruyn GW, editors: *Handbook of Clinical Neurology,* p 249, New York: Elsevier, 1990.

10. Macpherson BCM, Macpherson P, Jennett B: CT incidence of intracranial contusion and hematoma in relation to the presence, site and type of skull fracture, *Clin Radiology* 42:321-326, 1990.

11. Feuerman T, Wackym PA, Gade GF, Becker DP: Value of skull radiography, head computed tomographic scanning and admission for observation in cases of minor head injury, *Neurosurg* 22:449-453, 1988.

12. Hackney DB: Skull radiography in the evaluation of acute head trauma: a survey of current practice, *Radiology* 181:711-714, 1991.

13. Dharker SR, Bhargava N: Bilateral epidural hematoma, *Acta Neurochir* (Wien) 110:29-32, 1991.

14. Poon WS, Rehman SU, Poon CYF et al: Traumatic extradural hematoma of delayed onset is not a rarity, *Neurosurg* 30:681-686, 1992.

15. Hamilton M, Wallace C: Nonoperative management of acute epidural hematoma diagnosed by CT: the neuroradiologist's role, *AJNR* 13:853-859, 1992.

16. Huneidi AHS, Afshar F: Delayed intracerebral haematomas in moderate to severe head injuries in young adults, *Ann R Coll Surg Engl* 74(5):345-349, 1992.

17. Rivano C, Borzone M, Altomonte M, Capuzzo T: Traumatic posterior fossa extradural hematomas, *Neurochirurgia* 35:43-47, 1992.

17a. Lui T-N, Lee S-T, Chang C-N, Cheng W-C: Epidural hematomas in the posterior cranial fossa, *J Trauma* 34:211-215,1993.

18. Bricolo AP, Pasut LM: Extradural hematoma: toward zero mortality, *Neurosurg* 14:8-12, 1984.

19. Smith HK, Miller JD: The danger of an ultra-early computed tomographic scan in a patient with an evolving acute epidural hematoma, *Neurosurg* 29:258-260, 1991.

20. Kuroiwa T, Tanabe H, Takatsuka H et al: Rapid spontaneous resolution of acute extradural and subdural hematomas, *J Neurosurg* 78:126-128, 1993.

21. Wilberger JE, Harris M, Diamond DL: Auto subdural hematoma: morbidity, mortality, and operative timings, *J Neurosurg* 74:212-218, 1991.

22. Hashimoto N, Sakakibara T, Yamamoto K et al: Two fluid-blood density levels in chronic subdural hematoma, *J Neurosurg* 77:310-311, 1992.

23. Reed D, Robertson WD, Graeb DA et al: Acute subdural hematomas: atypical CT findings, *AJNR* 7:417-421, 1986.

24. Boyko OB, Cooper DF, Grosseman CB: Contrast-enhanced CT of acute isodense subdural hematoma, *AJNR* 12:341-343, 1991.

25. Stein SC, Young GS, Talucci RC et al: Delayed brain injury after head trauma: significance of coagulopathy, *Neurosurg* 30:160-165, 1992.

26. Wilms G, Marchal G, Geusens E: Isodense subdural haematomas on CT: MR findings, *Neuroradiol* 34:497-499, 1992.

27. Hashimoto N, Sakakibara T, Yamamoto K et al: Two fluid-blood density levels in chronic subdural hematoma, *N Neurosurg* 77:310-311, 1992.

28. Karasawa H, Tomita S, Suzuki S: Chronic subdural hematoma, *Neuroradiology* 29:36-39, 1987.

29. Iplikcioglu AC, Akkas O, Sungur R: Ossified chronic subdural hematoma: case report, *J Trauma* 31:272-295, 1991.

30. Fobben ES, Grossman RI, Atlas SW et al: MR characteristics of subdural hematoma and hygromas at 1.5T, *AJNR* 10:687-693, 1989.

31. Hosoda K, Tamaki N, Masumura M et al: Magnetic resonance images of chronic subdural hematomas, *J Neurosurg* 67:677-683, 1987.

32. Yeakley JW, Mayer JS, Patchell CC et al: The pseudodelta sign in acute head trauma, *J Neurosurg* 69:867-868, 1988.

33. Hesselink JR, Dowd CF, Healy ME et al: MR imaging of brain contusions: a comparative study with CT, *AJNR* 9:269-278, 1988.

34. Gentry LR, Gordersky JC, Thompson B: MR imaging of head trauma: review of the distribution and radiopathologic features of traumatic lesions, *AJNR* 9:101-110, 1988.

35. Gentry LR, Gordersky JC, Thompson B, Dunn VD: Prospective comparative study of intermediate-field MR and CT in the evaluation of closed head trauma, *AJNR* 9:91-100, 1988.

36. Kelly AB, Zimmerman RD, Snow RB et al: Head trauma: comparison of MR and CT—experience in 100 patients, *AJNR* 9:699-708, 1988.

37. Besenski N, Jadro-Santel D, Grevic N: Patterns of lesions of corpus callosum in inner cerebral trauma visualized by computed tomography, *Neuroradiol* 34:126-130, 1992.

38. Meyer CA, Mirvis SE, Wolf AL et al: Acute traumatic midbrain hemorrhage: experimental and clinical observation with CT, *Radiology* 179:813-818, 1991.

39. Gentry LR, Gordersky JC, Thompson BH: Traumatic brain stem injury: MR imaging, *Radiology* 171:177-187, 1989.

40. LeRoux PD, Haglund MM, Newell DW et al: Intraventricular hemorrhage in blunt head trauma: an analysis of 43 cases, *Neurosurg* 31:678-685, 1992.

41. Lee J-P, Lui T-N, Change C-N: Acute post-traumatic intraventricular hemorrhage analysis of 25 patients with emphasis on final outcome, *Acta Neurol/Scand* 84:89-90, 1991.

42. Osborn AG: Secondary effects of intracranial trauma, *Neurosurg Clin N Amer* 1:461-474, 1991.

43. Rothfus WE, Goldberg AL, Tabar JE, Deeb ZL: Callosomarginal infarction secondary to transfalcial herniation, *AJNR* 8:1073-1076, 1987.

44. Speigelman R, Hadani M, Ram Z et al: Upward transtentorial herniation: a complication of postoperative edema at the cervicomedullary junction, *Neurosurg* 24:284-288, 1989.

44a. Reich JB, Sierra J, Camp W et al: Magnetic resonance imaging measurements and clinical changes accompanying transtentorial and foramen magnum brain herniation, *Ann Neurol* 33:159-170, 1993.

45. Miller JD: Head injury and brain ischemia—implications for therapy, *B J Anaesth* 47:120-129, 1985.

46. Marion DW, Darby J, Yonas H: Acute regional cerebral blood flow changes caused by severe head injuries, *J Neurosurg* 74:407-414, 1991.

47. Bouma GJ, Muizelaar JP, Stringer WA et al: Ultra-early evaluation of regional cerebral blood flow in severely head-injured patients using xenon-enhanced computerized tomography, *J Neurosurg* 77:360-368, 1992.

48. Kato T, Tokumaru A, O'uchi T et al: Assessment of brain death in children by means of P-31m MR spectroscopy, *Radiol* 179:95-99, 1991.

49. Newton TR, Greenwood RJ, Britton KE et al: A study comparing SPECT with CT and MRI after closed head injury, *J Neurol Neurosurg Psychiat* 55:92-94, 1992.

50. Gorai B, Rifkinson-Mann S, Leslie DR et al: Cerebral blood transfer blow after head injury: transcranial Doppler evaluation, *Radiol* 188:137-141, 1993.

51. Mirvis SE, Wolf AL, Numaguchi Y et al: Post-traumatic cerebral infarction diagnosed by CT: prevalence, origin, and outcome, *AJNR* 12:1238-1239, 1991.

52. Jones KM, Seeger JF, Yoshino MT: Ipsilateral motor deficit resulting from a subdural hematoma and a Kernohan's notch, *AJNR* 12:1238-1239, 1991.

53. Iwama T, Kuroda T, Sugimoto S et al: MRI demonstration of Kernohan's notch: case report, *Neuroradiol* 34:225-226, 1992.

53a. Chan K-H, Dearden NM, Miller JD et al: Multimodality Monitoring as a guide to treatment of intracranial hypertension after severe brain injury, *Neurosurg* 32:547-553, 1993.

54. Aldrich EF, Eisenberg HM, Saydjari C et al: Diffuse brain swelling: severely head-injured children, *J Neurosurg* 76:450-454, 1992.

55. Lobato RD, Sarabia R, Cordobes F et al: Post-traumatic cerebral hemispheric swelling, *J Neurosurg* 68:417-423, 1980.

56. Harwood-Nash DC: Abuse to the pediatric central nervous system, *AJNR* 13:569-575, 1992.

57. Vergote G, Vandeperre H, DeMan R: The reversal sign, *Neuroradiol* 34:215-216, 1992.

58. Bernat JL: Brain death, *Arch Neurol* 49:569-570, 1992.

59. Pistoia F, Johnson DW, Darby JM et al: The role of Xenn CT measurements of cerebral blood flow in the clinical determination of brain death, *AJNR* 12:97-103, 1991.

60. Schlale H-P, Bottger IG, Grotemeyer K-H et al: Determination of cerebral perfusion by means of planar brain scintigraphy and 99mTc-HMPAO in brain death persistent vegetative state and severe coma, *Intensive Care Med* 18:76-81, 1992.

61. de la Riva A, Gonzalez FM, Llamas-Elvira JM et al: Diagnosis of brain death: superiority of perfusion studies with 99mTc-HMPAO over conventional radionuclide cerebral angiography, *Br J Radiol* 65:289-294, 1992.

62. Larar GN, Nagel JS: Technitium-99m-HMPAO cerebral perfusion scintigraphy: considerations for timely brain death declaration, *J Nuc Med* 33:2209-2213, 1992.

63. du Trevou MD, van Dellen JR: Penetrating stab wounds to the brain: the timing of angiography patients presenting with the weapon already removed, *Neurosurg* 31:905-912, 1992.

64. Martin NA, Doberstein C, Zane C et al: Post-traumatic cerebral arterial spasm: transcranial Doppler ultrasound, cerebral blood flow and angiographic fundings, *J Neurosurg* 77:575-583, 1992.

65. Grosset DG, Straiton J, McDonald I et al: Use of transcranial Doppler sonography to predict development of a delayed ischemic deficit after subarachnoid hemorrhage, *J Neurosurg* 25:55-69, 1983.

66. Davis JM, Zimmerman RA: Injury of the carotid and vertebral arteries, *Neuroradiol* 29:55-69, 1983.

67. Anson J, Crowell RM: Craniocervical arterial dissection, *Neurosurg* 29:89-96, 1991.

68. Mokri B: Traumatic and spontaneous extracranial internal carotid artery dissections, *J Neurol* 237:356-361, 1990.

69. Sue DE, Brant-Zawadzki MN, Chana J: Dissection of cranial arteries in the neck: correlation of MRI and arteriography, *Neuroradiol* 34:273-278, 1992.

70. Stringer WL, Kelly DL: Traumatic dissection of the extracranial carotid artery, *Neurosurg* 6:123-130, 1980.

71. Digre KB, Smoker WRK, Johnston P, Tryhus MR, Thompson HS, Cox TA, Yuh WTC: Selective MR imaging approach for evaluation of patients with Horner's syndrome, *AJNR* 13:223-227, 1992.

72. Morgan MK, Besser M, Johnson I, Chaseling R: Intracranial carotid artery injury in closed head trauma, *J Neurosurg* 66:192-197, 1987.

73. O'Sullivan RM, Robertson WD, Nugent RA et al: Supraclinoid carotid artery dissection following unusual trauma, *AJNR* 11:1150-1152, 1990.

74. Bui LN, Brant-Zawadzki M, Verghese P, Gillan G: Magnetic resonance angiography of craniocervical dissection. *Stroke* 24:126-131, 1993.

75. Parent AD, Harkey HL, Touchstone DA et al: Lateral cervical spine dislocation and vertebral artery injury, *Neurosurg* 31:501-509, 1992.

76. Friedman DP, Flanders AE: Unusual dissection of the proximal vertebral artery: description of three cases, *AJNR* 13:283-286, 1992.

77. Reider-Groswasser I, Cohen M, Costeff H, Grosswasser Z: Late CT findings in brain trauma: relationship to cognitive and behavioral sequelae and to vocational outcome, *AJR* 160:147-152, 1993.

78. Creamer MJ, Blendonohy P, Katz R, Russell E: Coronal computerized tomography and cerebrospinal fluid rhinorrhea, *Arch Phys Med Rehab* 73:599-602, 1992.

79. Wakhloo AK, van Velthoven V, Schumacher M, Krauss JK: Evaluation of MR imaging, digital subtraction cisternography and CT cisternography in diagnosing CSF fistulae, *ACTA Neurochir* (Wien) 111:119-127, 1991.

80. Mark AS, Phister SH, Jackson DE Jr, Kolsky MP: Traumatic lesions of the suprasellar region: MR imaging, *Radiol* 182:49-52, 1992.

81. Tien R, Kucharczyk J, Kucharczyk W: MR imaging of the brain in patients with diabetes insipidus, *AJNR* 12:533-542, 1991.

82. Caffey J: On the theory and practice of shaking infants: its potential residual effects of permanent brain damage and mental retardation, *Am J Dis Child* 124:161-169, 1972.

83. Caffey J: The whiplash shaken infant syndrome: manual shaking by the extremities with whiplash induced intracranial and intraarticular bleedings linked with residual permanent brain damage and mental retardation, *Pediatrics* 54:396-403, 1974.

84. Ball WS Jr: Nonaccidental craniocerebral trauma (child abuse): MR imaging, *Radiol* 173:609-610, 1989.

85. Kleinman PK: Diagnostic imaging in infant abuse, *AJR* 155:703-712, 1990.

86. Sato Y, Yuh WTC, Smith WL et al: Head injury in child abuse: evaluation with MR imaging, *Radiol* 173:653-657, 1989.

87. Mendelsohn DB, Levin HS, Harward H, Bruce D: Corpus callosum lesions after closed head-injury in children: MRI clinical features and outcome, *Neuroradiol* 34:384-388, 1992.

88. Levin HS, Aldrich EF, Saydjari C et al: Severe head injury in children: experience of the trauma coma data bank, *Neurosurg* 31:435-444, 1992.

Intracranial Aneurysms

Saccular Aneurysms
    Developmental/Degenerative Aneurysms
    Traumatic Aneurysms
    Mycotic Aneurysms
    Oncotic Aneurysms
    Flow-related Aneurysms
    Vasculopathies, and Drug-related Aneurysms
Fusiform Aneurysms
Dissecting Aneurysms

There are three basic types of intracranial aneurysms: saccular, or "berry," aneurysms; fusiform aneurysms; and dissecting aneurysms.

SACCULAR ANEURYSMS
Developmental/Degenerative Aneurysms

Pathology. Saccular aneurysms are rounded, berrylike outpouchings that arise from arterial bifurcation points (Fig. 9-1). Saccular aneurysms are true aneurysms, i.e., they are dilatations of a vascular lumen due to weakness of all vessel wall layers. The aneurysmal sac itself is usually composed only of intima and adventitia. The intima is typically normal, although subintimal cellular proliferation is common. The internal elastic membrane is reduced or absent and the media ends at the junction of the aneurysm neck with the parent vessel (Fig. 9-2). The adventitia may be infiltrated by lymphocytes and phagocytes. Thrombotic debris is often present in the lumen of

Etiology of Intracranial Aneurysms

Common
Hemodynamically induced degenerative vascular injury
Atherosclerosis (typically causes fusiform aneurysms)
Underlying vasculopathy (e.g., fibromuscular dysplasia)
High flow states (arteriovenous malformations/fistulae)

Uncommon
Trauma
Infection
Drug abuse
Neoplasm (primary or metastatic)

the aneurysmal sac. Atherosclerotic changes in the parent vessel are also common.[1]

Etiology (*see* box, *above*). In the past, most saccular or intracranial "berry" aneurysms were thought to be congenital in origin, arising from focal defects in the media and gradually developing over a period of years as arterial pressure first weakened and then subsequently ballooned out the vessel wall.[1]

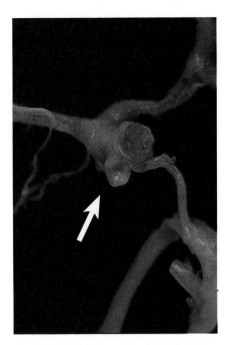

Fig. 9-1. Gross pathology specimen demonstrating saccular aneurysm *(arrow)* that arises from the circle of Willis at the internal carotid-posterior communicating artery (IC-PCoA) junction. (Courtesy B. Horten.)

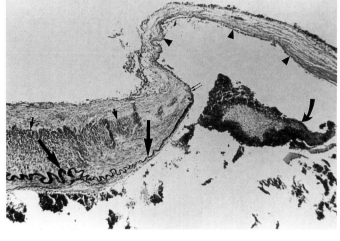

Fig. 9-2. Photomicrograph of an intracranial saccular aneurysm. The intima appears relatively normal but the internal elastic membrane *(large black arrows)* and muscularis *(small black arrows)* are progressively reduced until they disappear at the aneurysm ostium *(double arrows)*. The aneurysm sac *(arrowheads)* is composed primarily of intima and adventitia. Note thrombotic debris *(curved arrow)*.

Recent studies have found no evidence for a congenital, developmental, or inherited weakness of the arterial wall. Instead, most intracranial aneurysms probably result from hemodynamically induced degenerative vascular injury.[2] The occurrence, growth, thrombosis, and even rupture of intracranial saccular aneurysms can be explained by abnormal hemodynamic shear stresses on the walls of large cerebral arteries, particularly at bifurcation points[3a] (see subsequent discussion).

Less common causes of intracranial aneurysms include trauma, infection, tumor, drug abuse, and high flow states associated with arteriovenous malformations or fistulae.

Incidence *(see box, right).* The true incidence of intracranial aneurysm is unknown. Published data vary according to the definition of what constitutes an aneurysm and whether the series is based on autopsy data or angiographic studies. In patients undergoing coronary angiography, incidental intracranial aneurysms were found in 5.6% of cases,[4] and another series found aneurysms in 1% of patients undergoing four-vessel cerebral angiography for indications other than subarachnoid hemorrhage.[5] Familial intracranial aneurysms have been reported but it is unclear if this represents a true increased incidence.[6]

Increased Incidence of Intracranial Aneurysm

Anomalous vessels
Aortic coarctation
Polycystic kidney disease
Fibromuscular dysplasia
Connective tissue disorder (Marfan, Ehlers-Danlos)
High flow states (vascular malformations, fistulae)
With "spontaneous" dissections

Associated conditions. Congenital abnormalities of the intracranial vasculature such as anomalous vessels (Fig. 9-3) are associated with an increased incidence of saccular aneurysms.[7,7a] Arterial fenestrations have been reported with saccular aneurysms both at the fenestration site[7a] and on other nonfenestrated vessels in the same patient (Fig. 9-4). However, recent evidence indicates the incidence of aneurysm at a fenestration site is not different from the typical association of other vessel bifurcations with saccular intracranial aneurysms.[7b]

Vasculopathies such as fibromuscular dysplasia (FMD) (Fig. 9-5), connective tissue disorders, and spontaneous arterial dissection are associated with an increased incidence of intracranial aneurysms.[8,8a] These may be aggravating rather than causal factors in aneurysm development.[2] Conditions that have an increased incidence of cerebral aneurysms are listed in the box, p. 249.

Multiplicity. Intracranial aneurysms are multiple in 15% to 20% of all cases.[9] About 75% of these patients have two aneurysms, 15% have three, and 10% have more than three.[10] There is a strong female pre-

dominance with multiple aneurysms: the overall female:male ratio is 5:1 but rises to 11:1 if more than three aneurysms are present.[10] Multiple aneurysms are also associated with vasculopathies such as FMD and other connective tissue disorders. Polycystic kidney disease has a 10% incidence of associated aneurysms[11]; these aneurysms are also often multiple (Fig. 9-6).

Multiple aneurysms can be bilaterally symmetric (so-called mirror aneurysms) (Fig. 9-6, *C* and *D*) or asymmetrically located on different vessels. Rarely, more than one aneurysm can be present on the same artery.[10]

Age at presentation. Aneurysms typically become symptomatic between the ages of 40 and 60 years. Intracranial aneurysms in children are uncommon, accounting for less than 2% of all cases. When they occur in the pediatric age group they are more often posttraumatic or mycotic than degenerative and have a slight male predominance. Aneurysms in children

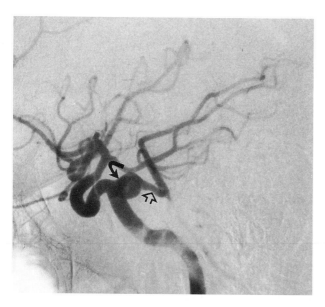

Fig. 9-3. Internal carotid angiogram, arterial phase, lateral view, in a patient with persistent trigeminal artery (PTA) *(open arrow).* A saccular aneurysm *(curved arrow)* arises at the PTA origin from the ICA. (Reprinted with permission from Fortner A et al: Persistent primitive trigeminal artery aneurysm evaluated by MR imaging and angiography, *J Comp Asst Tomogr* 12:847-850, 1988.)

Intracranial Saccular Aneurysms

Incidence: 1% to 5% (incidental angiographic finding)
Location: 90% circle of Willis/middle cerebral artery bifurcation
Multiplicity: 15% to 20% (female predominance)
Age at presentation: usually 40 to 60 years
Symptoms: usually subarachnoid hemorrhage (others: cranial nerve deficit, headache, seizure, TIA, infarction)

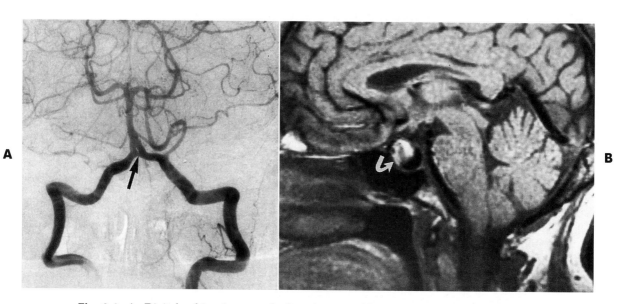

Fig. 9-4. A, Digital subtraction vertebral angiogram, AP view, in a patient with vertebral artery fenestration *(arrow).* **B,** Lateral T1-weighted MR scan shows an aneurysm *(arrow)* that arises from the cavernous internal carotid artery.

are also larger than those found in adults, averaging 17 mm in diameter[12] (*see* box, *right*).

Location. Aneurysms commonly arise at the bifurcations of major arteries (Fig. 9-1). Most saccular aneurysms arise on the circle of Willis or the middle cerebral artery (MCA) bifurcation (Fig. 9-7).

Anterior circulation aneurysms. Approximately 90% of all intracranial aneurysms arise on the ante-

Aneurysms in Children
Rare (<2% of all aneurysms) Average size larger than adults Often associated with trauma, infection Unusual locations common (posterior fossa, peripheral cortical vessels)

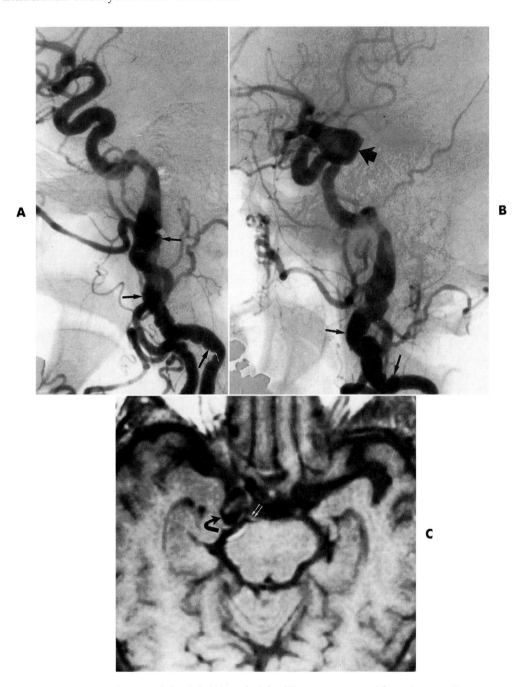

Fig. 9-5. Lateral view of the left **(A)** and right **(B)** common carotid angiograms in a patient with the classic "string-of-beads" appearance of fibromuscular dysplasia *(small arrows)*. A large saccular aneurysm **(B,** *large arrow)* is present. **(C)** Axial T1-weighted MR scan shows the aneurysm *(black arrow)* compressing the third cranial nerve *(white arrows)*. The patient had a right third nerve palsy.

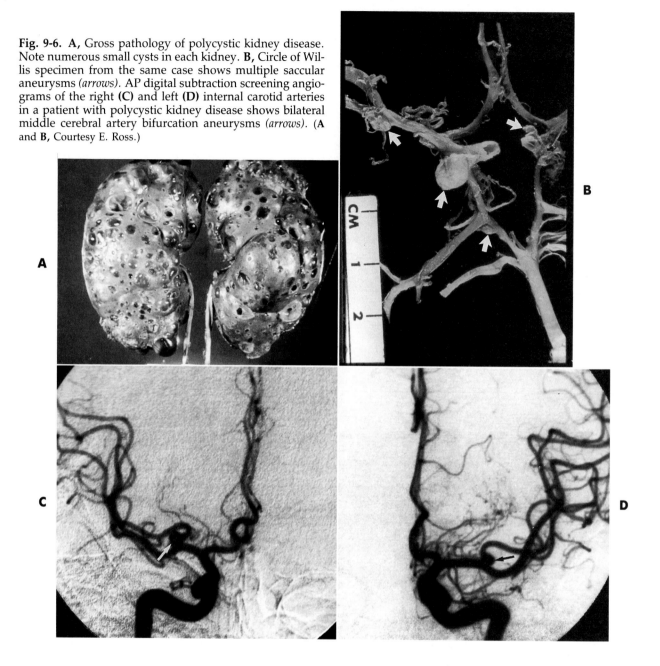

Fig. 9-6. A, Gross pathology of polycystic kidney disease. Note numerous small cysts in each kidney. **B,** Circle of Willis specimen from the same case shows multiple saccular aneurysms *(arrows).* AP digital subtraction screening angiograms of the right **(C)** and left **(D)** internal carotid arteries in a patient with polycystic kidney disease shows bilateral middle cerebral artery bifurcation aneurysms *(arrows).* (**A** and **B,** Courtesy E. Ross.)

rior (carotid) circulation.[1] Common locations are the anterior communicating artery (30% to 35%), the internal carotid artery at the posterior communicating artery origin (30% to 35%), and the middle cerebral artery bifurcation (20%).[13]

Posterior circulation aneurysms. About 10% of all intracranial aneurysms arise on the posterior (vertebrobasilar) circulation.[1] Five per cent arise from the basilar artery bifurcation, and the remaining 1% to 5% arise from other posterior fossa vessels. Very few aneurysms develop on the vertebral artery without involving the VA-PICA junction or the vertebrobasilar union.[14] Common posterior fossa sites include the

superior cerebellar artery and the vertebral artery (VA) at the origin of the posterior inferior cerebellar artery (PICA). Anterior inferior cerebellar artery (AICA) aneurysms are rare.

Miscellaneous locations. Saccular aneurysms are uncommon in locations other than the circle of Willis or middle cerebral artery bifurcation. When aneurysms occur at distal sites in the intracranial circulation they are often due to trauma or infection (see subsequent discussion). Nontraumatic distal aneurysms, particularly along the ACA, have a high frequency of multiplicity and spontaneous hemorrhage.[15]

Intracranial aneurysms

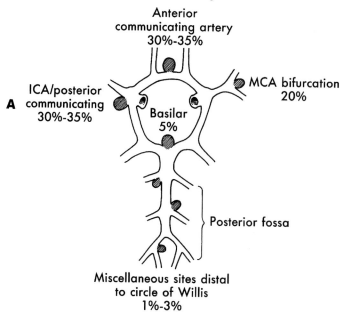

Anterior
communicating artery
30%-35%

MCA bifurcation
20%

ICA/posterior
communicating
30%-35%

Basilar
5%

A

Posterior fossa

Miscellaneous sites distal
to circle of Willis
1%-3%

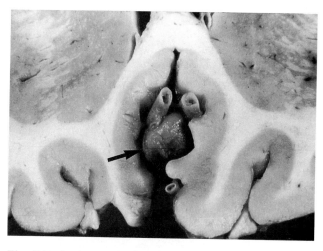

B

Fig. 9-7. A, Anatomic diagram depicts common locations of intracranial saccular aneurysms. **B,** Gross pathology of a saccular anterior communicating artery aneurysm (*arrow*). (**A,** Reprinted from Osborn AG: *Handbook of Neuroradiology,* Mosby-Yearbook 1991. **B,** Courtesy J. Townsend.)

Clinical presentation. Most aneurysms are asymptomatic until they rupture; when they do so, they are associated with significant morbidity and mortality.

Subarachnoid hemorrhage. The most common presentation of intracranial aneurysm is subarachnoid hemorrhage (SAH) (Fig. 9-8, *A*). In North America, 80% to 90% of nontraumatic SAH is caused by rupture of an intracranial aneurysm.[16] Another 15% is associated with bleeding from an arteriovenous malformation, and the remaining 5% is caused by various other lesions such as carotid artery dissection.[17]

The widely used clinical method for grading SAH is the Hunt and Hess scale:

Status	Signs and Symptoms
Grade I	Patients who are basically asymptomatic or have minimal headache
Grade II	Moderate to severe headache, nuchal rigidity, oculomotor palsy but with normal level of consciousness
Grade III	Confusion, drowsiness, mild focal neurologic deficits
Grade IV	Stupor or hemiparesis
Grade V	Patients are comatose or moribund with decerebrate posturing

Another grading system for SAH is the Cooperative Aneurysm Study Neurological Status Scale[18]:

Status	Signs and Symptoms
Status 1	Symptom free
Status 2	Minor symptoms
Status 3	Major neurologic deficit, but fully responsive
Status 4	Impaired state of alertness, but capable of protective or adaptive responses to noxious stimuli
Status 5	Poorly responsive, but with vital signs
Status 6	No response to shaking, nonadaptive responses to stimuli, and progressive instability of vital signs

Other symptoms. Signs and symptoms of aneurysm other than those associated with SAH are relatively uncommon. Some intracranial aneurysms produce cranial neuropathies. A common example is third nerve palsy secondary to posterior communicating artery aneurysm (Fig. 9-5, *C*). Cavernous ICA aneurysms can compress nerves III to VI. Other less common symptoms include seizures, headaches, and transient ischemic attacks or cerebral infarction secondary to emboli.[18a] The so-called giant aneurysms (diameter greater than 2.5 cm) are more often symptomatic because of their mass effect.

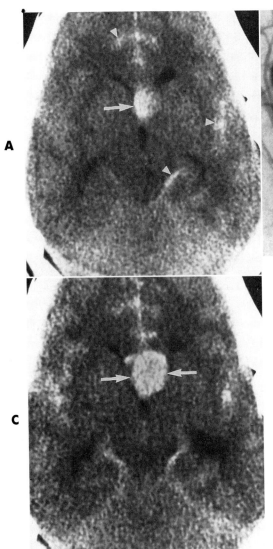

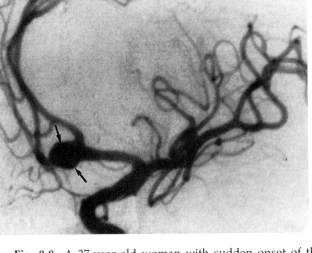

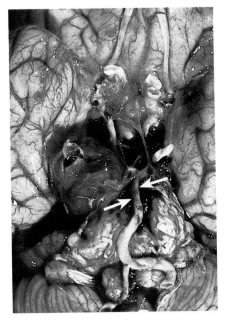

Fig. 9-8. A 37-year-old woman with sudden onset of the "worst headache of my life." Physical examination placed the patient at Hunt-Hess grade II. **A,** Initial axial CT scans showed diffuse subarachnoid hemorrhage *(arrowheads)* with more focal clot in the interhemispheric fissure *(arrow)*. **B,** Oblique view of digital left internal carotid angiogram demonstrated an ACoA aneurysm *(arrows)*. Surgery was delayed; 24 hours later the patient experienced sudden deterioration, progressing to clinical grade IV. **C,** Repeat CT scan showed increased size of the interhemispheric hematoma *(arrows)*, indicating repeat hemorrhage.

Clinical outcome. Vasospasm is the leading cause of disability and death from aneurysm rupture[19] (Figs. 9-9 to 9-11). Up to one third of all patients with aneurysmal SAH die, and a significant percentage of survivors have residual neurologic deficits. Ruptured aneurysms have their highest rebleeding rate within the first day (Fig. 9-8, *C*); if untreated, at least 50% will rebleed during the 6 months after the initial hemorrhage.[18] Ultra-early referral, earliest possible surgery, and aggressive antiischemic treatment (antivasospastic drugs, intravascular volume expansion, and transcranial doppler monitoring) are gradually improving the outcome.[21,22]

Natural history (*see* box, p. 256). The risk of aneurysm rupture is difficult to determine precisely but is estimated at 1% to 2% per year, cumulative, for asymptomatic as-yet-unruptured lesions.[23] With the combined operative mortality and major morbidity risk of about 3.5% for aneurysm surgery in skilled

Fig. 9-9. Gross pathologic specimen of a large saccular aneurysm with subarachnoid hemorrhage and severe vasospasm. Note marked narrowing of the distal basilar artery *(arrows)*.

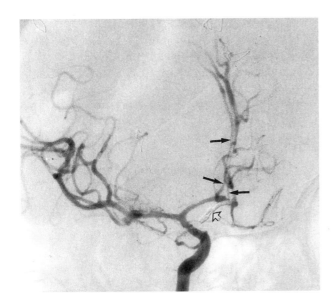

Fig. 9-10. AP view, right internal carotid artery angiogram, of a patient with severe vasospasm following surgical occlusion of an ACoA aneurysm. Note marked narrowing of both proximal ACAs *(black arrows)* and surgical clip *(open arrows).*

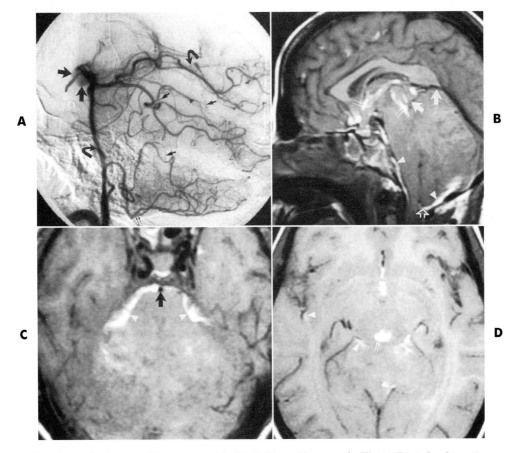

Fig. 9-11. A 25-year-old woman with SAH, Hunt-Hess grade III. **A,** Digital subtraction left vertebral angiogram, lateral view, disclosed a large basilar bifurcation aneurysm *(large arrows).* Moderate vasospasm is already present *(curved arrows)* on the initial angiogram. Also seen are several occluded posterior fossa vessels *(small arrows)* and descending tonsillar herniation, shown by displacement of the PICA tonsillar branches below the foramen magnum *(double arrows).* An MR scan obtained 5 days later after continued clinical deterioration. Sagittal **(B)** and axial **(C** and **D)** T1-weighted studies show multiple high signal foci in the subarachnoid spaces consistent with subacute hemorrhage *(arrowheads).* Some blood is also present in the third ventricle and aqueduct *(double arrows).* Ascending transtentorial herniation of the superior vermis *(large arrows)* and descending tonsillar herniation *(open arrow)* are present.   *Continued.*

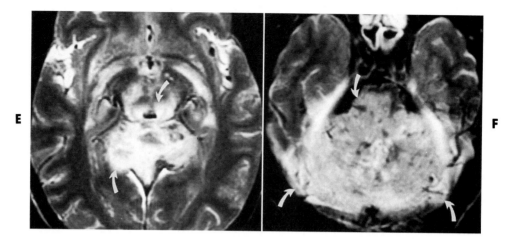

Fig. 9-11, cont'd. E and **F,** Axial T2-weighted scans show diffuse midbrain, brainstem, and cerebellar infarction *(arrows)* secondary to severe vertebrobasilar artery vasospasm (**C,** *arrow*).

Natural History of Saccular Aneurysms
Risk of rupture: 1% to 2% per year, cumulative
Rebleed risk from ruptured, unclipped aneurysm: 20% to 50% (highest in first week)
Large size correlates with increased rupture risk but no "critical" size below which rupture does not occur
Irregular, lobulated configuration, or "tit," correlates with increased rupture risk

hands, recent conclusions are that any patient with a life expectancy of greater than 3 years would benefit from surgical obliteration of an unruptured asymptomatic aneurysm.[22]

Ruptured but unoperated aneurysms have a very high risk of rebleeding after the initial hemorrhage has occurred; the risk is estimated at 20% to 50% in the first 2 weeks and carries a mortality rate of nearly 50%.[10,20]

There is no consensus about the risks associated with aneurysms. The size of an intact saccular aneurysm as seen on cerebral angiography is the most important (but not absolute) determinant of the risk of aneurysmal rupture.[22] In one long-term study, all aneurysms that subsequently ruptured were larger than 10 mm in diameter,[23] although a follow-up study reported hemorrhage from several previously documented small asymptomatic saccular aneurysms.[24]

Although some authors suggest that the critical size for saccular aneurysm rupture is between 4 and 7 mm in diameter, they also caution that there appears to be no "critical size" below which SAH does not occur. When an aneurysm is discovered inciden-

tally or at the time of investigation of SAH from another source, definitive repair of the unruptured lesion should be considered because small asymptomatic aneurysms clearly are not innocuous.[22,24]

Other risk factors such as age, sex, hypertension, or multiple aneurysms seem to have comparatively little relationship to the risk of aneurysm rupture.[2,23]

Flow dynamics and aneurysm growth. The apex of vessel bifurcations is the site of maximum hemodynamic stress in a vascular network.[24a] Vascular and internal flow hemodynamics have a crucial effect on the origin, growth, and configuration of intracranial aneurysms.[2,2a] Wall shear stress caused by the rapid changes of blood flow direction in the aneurysm that occur with systole and diastole produce continuing damage to the intima at an aneurysm cavity neck. These augmented hemodynamic stresses probably cause the initiation and subsequent progression of most saccular aneurysms. Thrombosis and rupture are also explained by intraaneurysmal hemodynamic stresses.[2,25]

Recent studies demonstrate that the geometric relationship between an aneurysm and its parent artery is the principal factor determining intraaneurysmal flow patterns.[26] In lateral aneurysms such as those arising directly from the internal carotid artery, blood typically moves into the aneurysm at the distal aspect of its ostium and exits at its proximal aspect, producing a slow flow vortex in the aneurysm center.[27] Opacification of the lumen then proceeds in a cranial-to-caudal fashion (Fig. 9-12). Contrast stagnation within these aneurysms is often pronounced.[25,26]

In contrast to the lateral aneurysms, when aneurysms arise at the origin of branching vessels or a terminal bifurcation, intraaneurysmal circulation is rapid and vortex formation with contrast stasis is rare.[26] These patterns of intraaneurysmal flow are im-

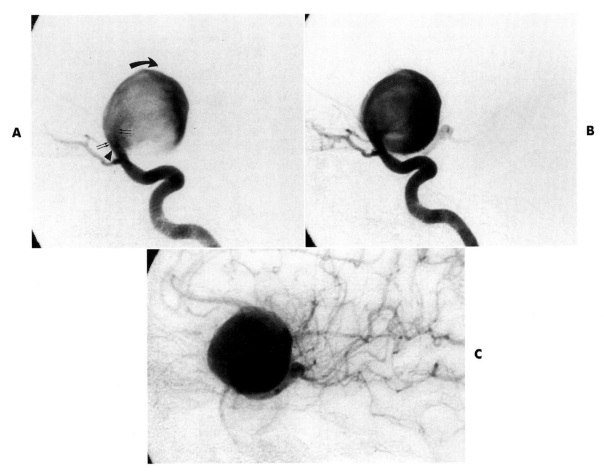

Fig. 9-12. Digital subtraction internal carotid angiogram, lateral view, with serial frames depicting intraaneurysmal flow dynamics. **A,** Early arterial phase shows the contrast "jet" *(double arrows)*. Opacified blood enters the aneurysm ostium at its distal aspect *(arrowhead)*. Intraaneurysmal circulation occurs in the cranial-caudal direction *(curved arrow)* and opacifies the aneurysm lumen. **B,** The slow flow vortex in the center of the aneurysm appears as an area of slightly lesser opacification. **C,** Contrast stagnation is shown by aneurysm opacification that persists into the late arterial phase.

portant not only for the formation and progression of an aneurysm itself but also because they influence the selection and placement of endovascular treatment devices.[27]

In "giant" saccular aneurysms (larger than 2.5 cm), slow growth can occur by recurrent hemorrhages into the lesion. The highly vascularized membranous wall of giant intracranial aneurysms is the most likely source of these intraaneurysmal hemorrhages (Fig. 9-13).[28] Giant sacs commonly contain multilayered laminated clots of varying ages and consistency (Fig. 9-14).[29] The outer wall is fibrous and thick; these multilaminated giant aneurysms seldom rupture into the subarachnoid space and typically produce symptoms related to their mass effect.[30]

Imaging of Intracranial Aneurysms

Angiography. Although MR angiography appears promising (see subsequent discussion), the definitive

diagnosis and preoperative delineation of intracranial aneurysms remains the domain of catheter angiography.

Technical considerations. The role of diagnostic cerebral angiography in the patient with nontraumatic subarachnoid hemorrhage is to identify the presence of any and all aneurysms, delineate the relationship of a given aneurysm to its parent vessel and adjacent penetrating branches, define the potential for collateral circulation to the brain, and assess for vasospasm (Fig. 9-15).[13]

Technically adequate cerebral angiography in the assessment of nontraumatic SAH is essential. This requires visualizing the entire intracranial circulation, including the anterior and posterior communicating arteries and both posterior inferior cerebellar arteries.[30a] Injections with cross-compression, multiple oblique plus submentovertex views and the standard AP and lateral projections, and subtraction (whether cut film

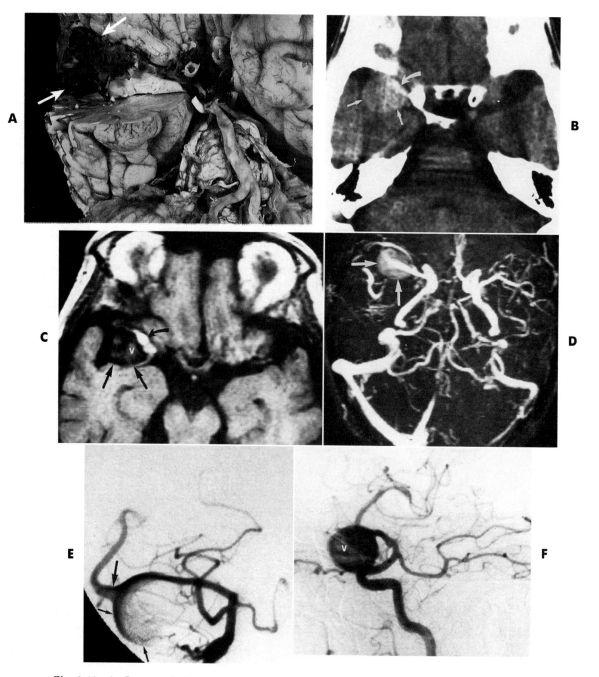

Fig. 9-13. **A,** Gross pathology of a partially thrombosed middle cerebral artery aneurysm. Note fresh clot in the vessel wall *(arrows)*. **B** to **F,** Imaging studies in a 64-year-old woman with a right middle cerebral artery aneurysm. **B,** Axial CT scan without contrast enhancement shows a well-delineated, slightly hyperdense mass *(straight arrows)* in the right sylvian fissure. A hyperdense rim of hemorrhage is seen in the anterior aneurysm wall *(curved arrow)*. **C,** Axial T1-weighted MR scan shows most of the aneurysm is patent with high-velocity signal loss *(straight arrows)* with some intermediate signal from turbulent flow in the vortex *(v)*. *Subacute mural thrombus is seen as a layer of high signal clot (curved arrow)* in the periphery of the aneurysm. **D,** MR angiogram shows flow in the aneurysm lumen *(arrows)*. **E,** Digital subtraction of the right internal carotid angiogram, AP view, shows the broad-based aneurysm *(small arrows)*. Note that the distal MCA arises from the aneurysm *(large arrow)*. Midarterial phase **(F)** lateral view of the right ICA angiogram shows the typical cranial-caudal filling of the aneurysm with a central vortex *(v)*.

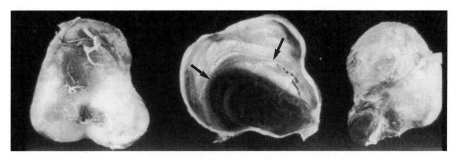

Fig. 9-14. Gross pathologic specimen of a giant aneurysm. Note the multilayered, laminated clot of varying ages within the sac *(arrows)*. (Courtesy E. Ross.)

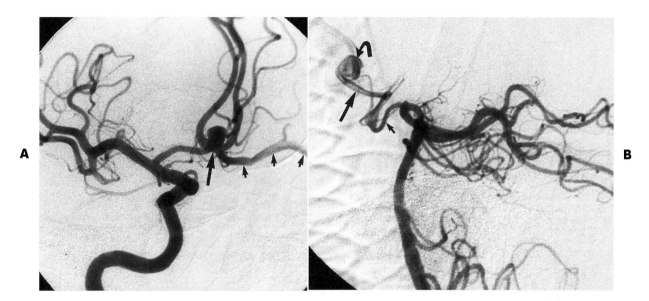

Fig. 9-15. A, High resolution (1024 × 1024) digital subtraction right ICA angiogram, oblique view, demonstrates an ACoA aneurysm *(large arrow)*. The study was performed with temporary compression of the cervical left common carotid artery to reflux contrast across the ACoA and left A1 and M1 segments *(small arrows)*. **B,** Left vertebral angiogram, lateral view, demonstrates contrast reflex through the left PCoA *(small arrow)* and A1 segment *(large arrow)* into the aneurysm *(curved arrow)*.

or high-resolution digital) studies are all integral parts of the complete angiographic evaluation.

Angiographic findings. A patent intracranial aneurysm is seen as a contrast-filled outpouching that commonly arises from an arterial wall or bifurcation (Fig. 9-16). The circle of Willis and the middle cerebral artery bifurcation are common locations. Thrombosed aneurysms usually have normal angiographic studies. Large thrombosed aneurysms can cause an avascular mass effect.

Aneurysms must be distinguished from vascular loops and infundibuli. Infundibuli are smooth funnel-shaped dilatations that are caused by incomplete regression of a vessel present in the developing fetus. Their most common location is at the origin of the posterior communicating artery from the

internal carotid artery. Less commonly an infundibulum arises from the anterior choroidal artery origin. Infundibuli are 2 mm or less in diameter, regular in shape, and the distal vessel exits from their apices (Fig. 9-16, *D*).

Vascular "loops" are caused by overlapping projections of a three-dimensional vessel onto a two-dimensional image. They typically appear more dense than an aneurysm and can be identified using multiple oblique views.

When cerebral angiography demonstrates more than one aneurysm it is important to determine which lesion is the most likely rupture site.[30a] Clinical signs alone localize a ruptured aneurysm in only about one third of these patients.[10] Imaging findings of aneurysm rupture are listed in the box, p. 260. Ac-

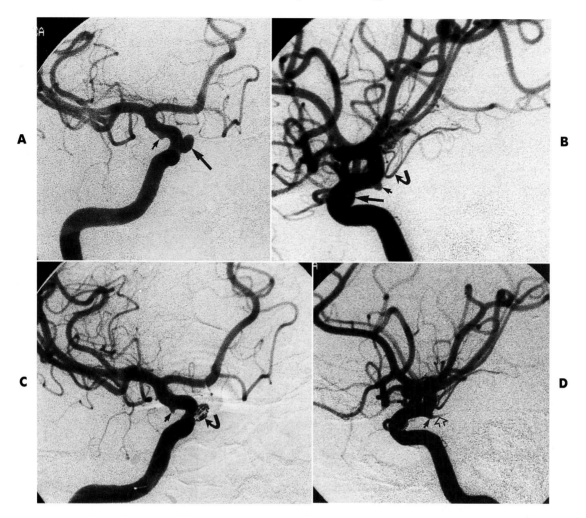

Fig. 9-16. A, High resolution digital subtraction right ICA angiogram, oblique view, demonstrates a small aneurysm *(large arrow)* arising from the cavernous ICA. A small funnel-shaped outpouching from the posterolateral ICA is seen *(small arrow)*. **B,** Lateral view shows the ICA aneurysm *(large arrow)* is mostly hidden from view by the carotid siphon. The small outpouching *(small arrow)* is again seen arising just below the anterior choroidal artery *(curved arrow)*. Repeat oblique **(C)** and lateral **(D)** angiograms following endovascular occlusion of the aneurysm *(curved arrow)* again show the outpouching *(small arrows)*. The lateral view shows transient reflux of contrast from the dome of the outpouching into a small posterior communicating artery **(D,** *open arrow)*. This is a PCoA "infundibulum."

Which Aneurysm Ruptured?
Pathognomonic sign
Contrast extravasation (rare)
Very helpful signs
Surrounding clot seen on CT/MR
Size (larger: more likely)
Configuration (irregular, lobulated, "tit")
Helpful
Localized subarachnoid hemorrhage
Localized vasospasm
Unhelpful
Location (exception: cavernous ICA aneurysms rarely rupture and cause SAH)

tual contrast extravasation during angiography is, of course, pathognomonic but extremely rare; rapid hemorrhage within the closed intracranial space is usually fatal.

A focal parenchymal or cisternal hematoma surrounding an aneurysm is diagnostic of rupture (Fig. 9-17, *A*).[10] Larger aneurysms are also more likely to rupture. Lobulation (Fig. 9-17, *B* to *D*) or irregularly shaped dome, or "tit," indicates possible rupture. Although focal vasospasm is a helpful finding, subarachnoid blood quickly spreads along the basal cisterns, making this a somewhat less reliable sign of aneurysm rupture.

In approximately 15% of patients with nontrau-

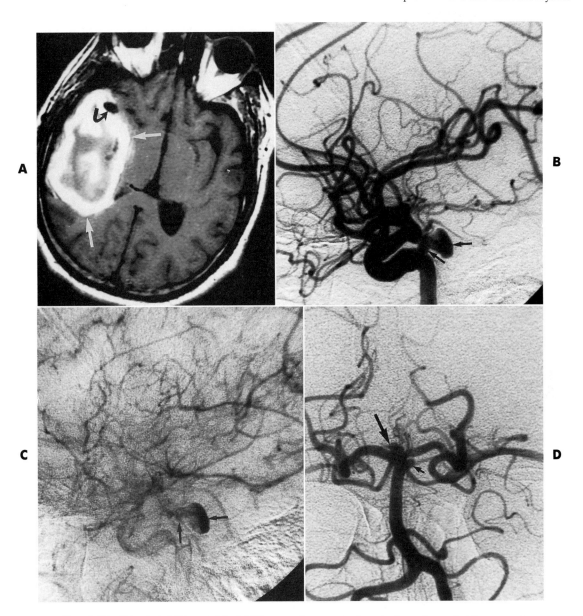

Fig. 9-17. (A), Axial T1-weighted MR scan shows a subacute hematoma *(white arrows)* surrounding a ruptured right MCA aneurysm *(curved black arrow).* **B** to **D**, Another case demonstrates angiographic determination of aneurysm rupture. Early **(B)** and late arterial **(C)** phase, left internal carotid angiogram, lateral view, in a 32-year-old woman with multiple saccular aneurysms and diffuse SAH on CT scan (not shown). A large bi-lobed aneurysm **(B,** *arrows)* arises from the distal internal carotid artery. Note contrast stasis **(C,** *arrows).* **D,** Left vertebral angiogram, AP view, shows small aneurysms arising from the basilar bifurcation *(large arrow)* and superior cerebellar artery origin *(small arrow).* Of these three aneurysms, the ICA aneurysm is the largest and most irregular of the lesions and therefore the most likely to have ruptured. Surgery confirmed the diagnosis of ruptured ICA aneurysm.

matic subarachnoid hemorrhage, no aneurysm is found despite a complete, high-quality four vessel cerebral angiogram.[31] Two distinct subsets of these patients have been recognized. The first group consists of those with so-called nonaneurysmal perimesencephalic subarachnoid hemorrhage in which bleeding on CT or MR scans is localized immediately anterior

to the brainstem and adjacent areas such as the interpeduncular fossa and ambient cisterns (Fig. 9-18). Initial and follow-up angiography is almost always negative in these patients and their prognosis is excellent.[32] In these cases, SAH probably results from spontaneous rupture of small pontine or perimesencephalic veins.

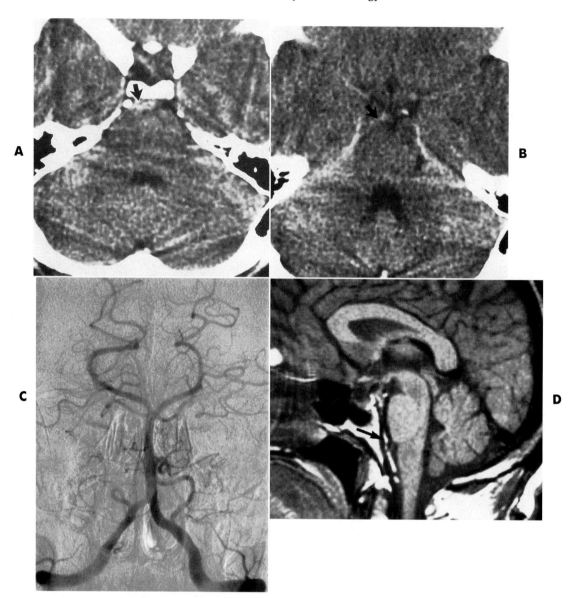

Fig. 9-18. Characteristic CT findings of nonaneurysmal SAH are demonstrated by this case of a 28-year-old man with sudden onset of severe headache. **A** and **B,** Axial NECT scans show isolated prepontine and perimesencephalic subarachnoid blood *(arrows)* without significant hemorrhage in the suprasellar cistern or the sylvian fissures. **C,** Cerebral angiography, including this AP view of the vertebrobasilar study, was normal. **D,** Follow-up MR scan 1 week later shows subacute SAH isolated to the prepontine cistern *(arrow).* In this case, hemorrhage was probably from ruptured perimesencephalic veins. The prognosis is excellent and repeat angiography is unnecessary.

The second group with angiogram-negative SAH has CT scans with an "aneurysmal" pattern of hemorrhage, i.e., blood fills the suprasellar cistern and extends completely into the lateral sylvian or anterior interhemispheric fissures. The risk of rebleeding, cerebral ischemia, and neurologic deficit is high in this group and warrants repeat angiography to identify an occult aneurysm.[32,33] Repeat four-vessel cerebral angiography demonstrates a lesion in 10% to 20% of these cases (Fig. 9-19).

Computed tomography. Bone erosion can be seen in long-standing lesions that arise near the skull base (Fig. 9-20). Mural calcification is common (Fig. 9-20), with both punctate and curvilinear types identified. The attenuation characteristics of a saccular aneurysm vary, depending on whether the lesion is patent and partially or completely thrombosed.

Patent aneurysms. On noncontrast CT the typical nonthrombosed aneurysm appears as a well delineated isodense to slightly hyperdense (Fig. 9-21) mass located somewhat eccentrically in the suprasellar subarachnoid space or sylvian fissure.[35] Patent aneu-

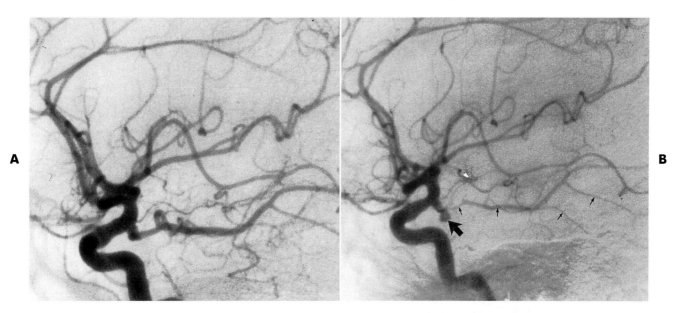

Fig. 9-19. A 31-year-old man had diffuse basilar SAH on CT (not shown). Initial complete four-vessel cerebral arteriogram was normal. **A,** The left common carotid angiogram is shown. **(B)** Repeat angiogram 3 weeks later disclosed a saccular aneurysm *(large arrow)* that arises from the left PCoA. Note narrowing of the PCoA and PCA from vasospasm *(small arrows).*

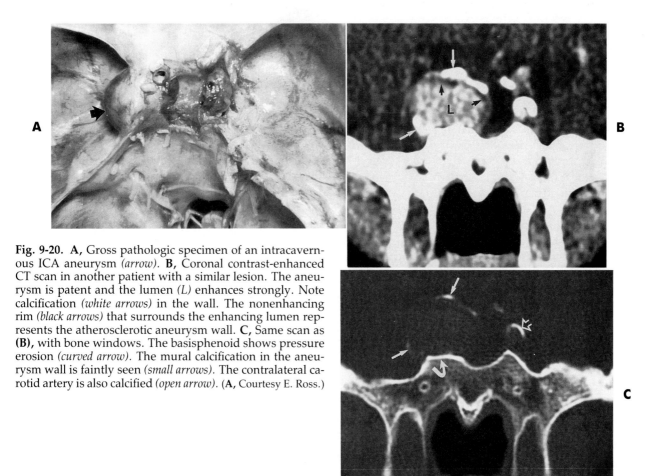

Fig. 9-20. A, Gross pathologic specimen of an intracavernous ICA aneurysm *(arrow).* **B,** Coronal contrast-enhanced CT scan in another patient with a similar lesion. The aneurysm is patent and the lumen *(L)* enhances strongly. Note calcification *(white arrows)* in the wall. The nonenhancing rim *(black arrows)* that surrounds the enhancing lumen represents the atherosclerotic aneurysm wall. **C,** Same scan as **(B),** with bone windows. The basisphenoid shows pressure erosion *(curved arrow).* The mural calcification in the aneurysm wall is faintly seen *(small arrows).* The contralateral carotid artery is also calcified *(open arrow).* (**A,** Courtesy E. Ross.)

Continued.

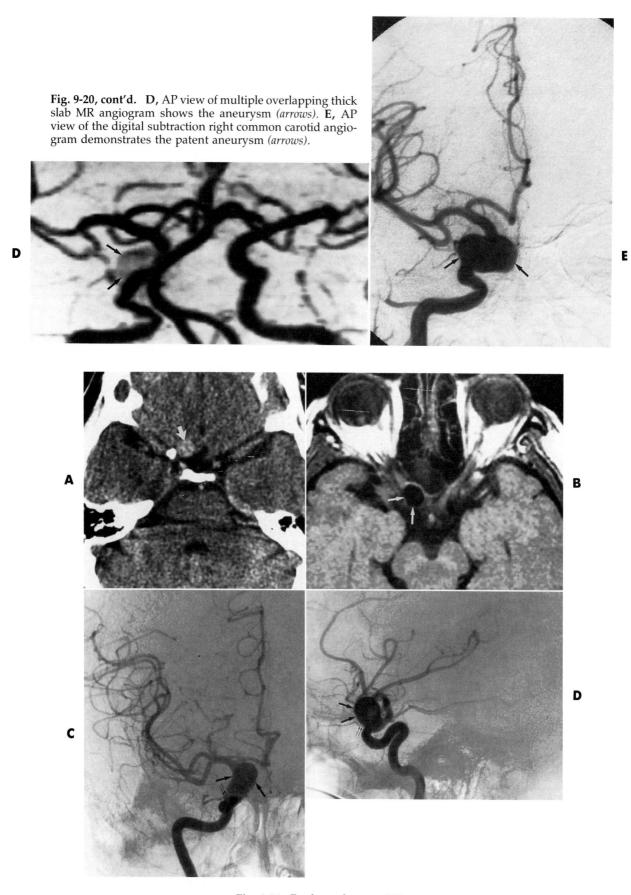

Fig. 9-20, cont'd. D, AP view of multiple overlapping thick slab MR angiogram shows the aneurysm *(arrows).* **E,** AP view of the digital subtraction right common carotid angiogram demonstrates the patent aneurysm *(arrows).*

Fig. 9-21. For legend see p. 265.

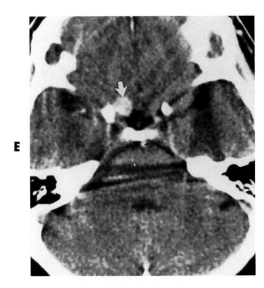

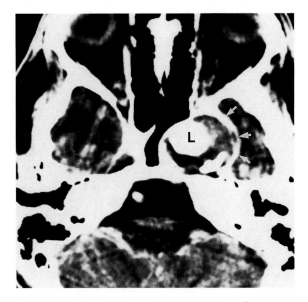

Fig. 9-21, cont'd. A, CT scan without contrast enhancement shows a well-delineated mass *(arrow)* somewhat eccentrically located in the suprasellar cistern. **B,** Axial T1-weighted MR scan shows a "flow void" from high-velocity signal loss *(arrows)*. AP **(C)** and lateral **(D)** views of the right internal carotid angiogram show an aneurysm *(single arrows)* that arises from the ICA near the ophthalmic artery origin *(double arrows)*. **E,** Postangiogram CT scan shows the aneurysm enhances uniformly *(arrow)*.

Fig. 9-22. Contrast-enhanced axial CT scan shows a partially thrombosed left cavernous ICA aneurysm. Note the enhancing outer wall *(arrows)* and the intensely enhancing residual lumen *(L)*.

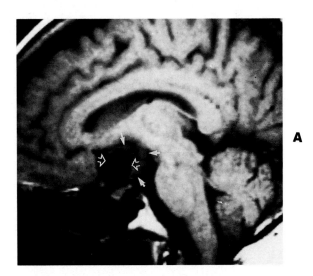

Fig. 9-23. Two cases demonstrate MR findings in partially **(A** and **B)** and completely thrombosed **(C** to **F)** aneurysms. **A,** Sagittal T1-weighted MR scan shows a suprasellar mass *(solid arrows)* that is barely discernible because it is nearly isointense with CSF. The center of the mass shows high-velocity signal loss *(open arrows)*.

Continued.

rysms enhance intensely and quite uniformly following administration of intravenous contrast material.[36]

Angiographic-like images of the cerebral vasculature can be obtained using rapid contrast infusion and thin-section dynamic CT scanning. Various three-dimensional display techniques, including shaded surface display, volume rendering, and maximal intensity projection, are used to complement the conventional transaxial images.[37] Such studies provide multiple projections of anatomically complex vascular lesions such as giant aneurysms and delineate their relationships to adjacent structures.[37,38]

The accuracy of high-resolution axial CT in the diagnosis of cerebral aneurysms 3 mm and larger has been reported at about 97%.[39]

Thrombosed aneurysms. Partially thrombosed aneurysms have a patent lumen inside a thickened, often partially calcified wall that is lined with laminated clot *(see* Fig. 9-13). The residual lumen and outer rim of the aneurysm may enhance strongly following contrast administration (Fig. 9-22). Rarely, atherosclerotic debris in the wall (Fig. 9-20, *B*) or sac of an aneurysm may appear hypodense on CT scans.

Completely thrombosed aneurysms are variably hyperintense on NECT and usually show no increase in attenuation on CECT (Fig. 9-23, *C*).

Subarachnoid hemorrhage. The presence of SAH

may complicate the CT appearance of aneurysms. The reported CT detectability of SAH due to ruptured cerebral aneurysms in the acute phase is from 60% to 100%.[40] Acute SAH appears as high attenuation within the subarachnoid cisterns. SAH may quickly spread diffusely throughout the CSF spaces, giving little clue to its site of origin. Suprasellar cistern blood from many sites is common with SAH *(see* Fig. 9-8, *A).* However, some bleeding patterns have been as-

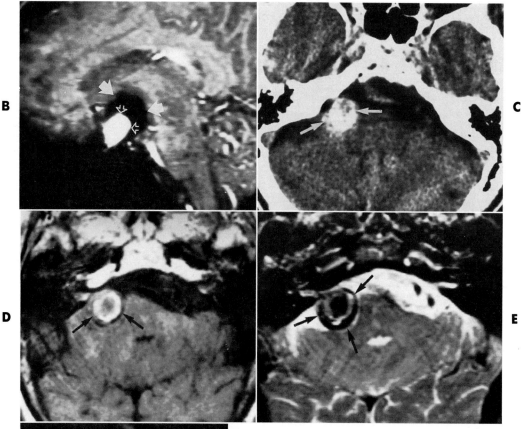

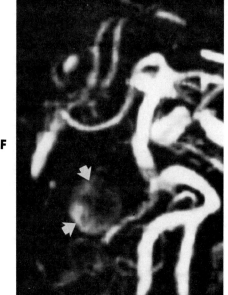

Fig. 9-23, cont'd.   B, Gradient-refocussed sagittal scan shows flow in the patent lumen *(open arrows)* and "blooming" of the acute thrombus in the vessel wall *(solid arrows).* **C,** CT scan of a completely thrombosed right PICA aneurysm *(arrows).* The clot is hyperdense to brain (this is a contrast-enhanced scan; however, the density on NECT was identical). Axial **(D)** T1-weighted MR scan shows the aneurysm is completely filled with subacute thrombus *(arrows).* **E,** The axial T2-weighted scan shows the hypointense center and rim of the thrombosed PICA aneurysm. **F,** 3D TOF MR angiogram shows high signal from subacute clot in the thrombosed aneurysm *(arrows).*

sociated with particular aneurysm locations.

Hemorrhage located predominately within the interhemispheric fissure is common with anterior communicating artery aneurysms *(see* Fig. 9-8, *B*), and sylvian fissure blood is often seen with middle cerebral artery lesions (Fig. 9-17, *A*). Intraventricular blood can be helpful in localizing ruptured aneu-

rysms. Fourth ventricle hemorrhage is common with posterior fossa aneurysms, and frontal horn blood typically occurs with ACoA lesions (Fig. 9-17, *A*).

Magnetic resonance imaging. Aneurysm appearance on MR scans is highly variable and may be quite complex. Signal on routine spin-echo sequences depends on the presence, direction, and rate of flow, as well as the presence of clot, fibrosis, and calcification within the aneurysm itself.

Patent aneurysms. Flowing spins can produce hyper- or hypointense signals on routine spin-echo MR studies, depending on specific flow characteris-

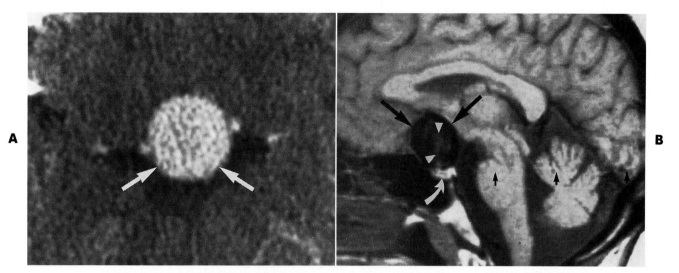

Fig. 9-24. A, Axial postcontrast CT scan in a 41-year-old woman with bitemporal hemianopsia. A well-delineated, strongly enhancing noncalcified suprasellar mass is present *(arrows)*. The diagnostic considerations are suprasellar extension of a pituitary adenoma, diaphragma sellae meningioma, or aneurysm. **B,** Sagittal T1-weighted MR scan shows the lesion has high-velocity signal loss, characteristic of a patent aneurysm *(large black arrows)*. Some turbulent flow with spin dephasing is present in the lumen *(arrowheads)*, producing foci that are isointense with brain. Note the phase-encoding artifact *(small arrows)*, indicating flow within the lesion. The pituitary gland *(curved arrow)* is compressed but otherwise normal. Angiography (not shown) demonstrated a supraclinoid ICA aneurysm.

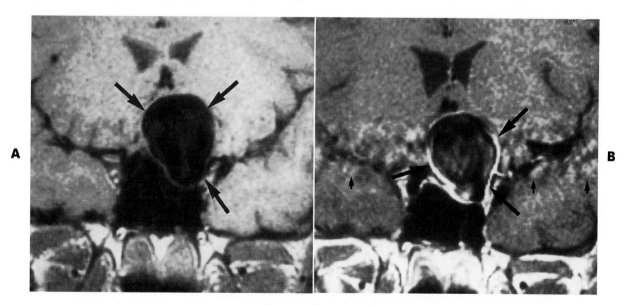

Fig. 9-25. Coronal T1-weighted MR scans obtained before **(A)** and after **(B)** contrast administration. A large patent aneurysm is seen **(A,** *arrows)*. The postcontrast study demonstrates aneurysm wall enhancement **(B,** *large arrows)* and striking phase-encoding flow artifact *(small arrows)*. (Courtesy W. Gibby.)

tics and pulse sequences used.[41] The typical patent aneurysm lumen with rapid flow is seen as a well delineated suprasellar mass that shows high-velocity signal loss (flow void) on T1- and T2-weighted images (Figs. 9-23, *A,* and 9-21, *B*). Some signal heterogeneity may be seen if turbulent flow in the aneurysm is present *(see* Fig. 9-13, *E*). Pulsation artifacts are common if flow compensation techniques are not used (Figs. 9-24, *B,* and 9-25). Gradient-refocused scans delineate the patent lumen of aneurysms (Fig.

9-23, *A* and *B*) and are particularly helpful when acute thrombus makes the aneurysm difficult to identify.

Intravenous contrast typically does not enhance patent aneurysms with high flow rates, but wall enhancement may occur (Fig. 9-25, *B*). Contrast in the intravascular space also often increases phase-encoding artifacts seen with rapid intraluminal flow (Fig. 9-25, *B*). Aneurysms that are patent but have slow or turbulent flow may appear iso- or even hyperintense on MR scans and show variable enhancement following contrast administration.

Thrombosed aneurysms. Partially thrombosed aneurysms often have complex signal on MR scans. An area of high-velocity signal loss in the patent lumen with surrounding concentric layers of multilaminated clot and variable signal intensities can be seen (Fig. 9-23, *A*). Larger aneurysms may have a thick signal void rim caused by nonhemosiderin-containing mural thrombus and a hemosiderin laden fibrous capsule.[42] If intraluminal flow is slow or turbulent, the residual lumen may be isointense with the remainder of the aneurysm and difficult to detect without contrast enhancement.

Completely thrombosed aneurysms also frequently have variable MR findings. Subacute thrombus is predominately hyperintense on T1- and T2-weighted studies (Fig. 9-26). Multilayered clots can be seen in thrombosed aneurysms that have undergone repeated episodes of intramural hemorrhage (Fig. 9-27). On occasion, acutely thrombosed aneurysms may be isointense with brain parenchyma and difficult to distinguish from other intracranial masses.

Magnetic resonance angiography. The macroscopic motion of the moving spins in flowing blood together with background suppression of stationary tissue can be used to create images of the cerebral vasculature. The images can be viewed as individual thin sections (source images) or reprojected in the form of flow maps or MR "angiograms" (MRA).[43]

Two standard techniques currently used for MRA are phase-contrast (PC) studies and time-of-flight (TOF) acquisitions. PC creates projection angiographic images by using bipolar pulse sequences to detect the phase shifts that are caused by blood flowing through magnetic field gradients. PC imaging has excellent background suppression, allows for variable velocity encoding, and can provide directional flow information.[44]

TOF uses the inflow of fully magnetized spins into saturated stationary tissue to create angiographic images. TOF methods use two-dimensional projection and direct three-dimensional acquisitions.[44] 3D TOF images are useful in depicting small and medium-sized aneurysms. However, the sensitivity of TOF techniques to signal loss from flow saturation limits its use. In addition, short T1 substances such as subacute blood may simulate flow.[44]

A recently developed multislab 3D-TOF technique, MOTSA, combines the advantages of two-dimensional multiple section and direct three-dimensional TOF techniques (Fig. 9-28).[45] This sequence successfully delineates the parent artery and depicts the size and orientation of an aneurysm dome and neck.[45] Multislab techniques are less affected by flow saturation and have substantially improved ves-

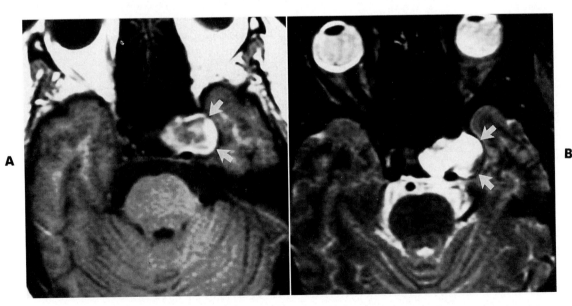

Fig. 9-26. Axial **(A)** T1- and **(B)** T2-weighted MR scans of a completely thrombosed cavernous ICA aneurysm *(arrows).* The subacute intraluminal clot is hyperintense on both pulse sequences.

sel visualization.[46] Other sequences and future technical refinements will undoubtedly improve the MRA delineation of the intracranial vasculature and its lesions.

Traumatic Aneurysms

Traumatic aneurysms account for less than 1% of all aneurysms.[47] Two general types of traumatic aneurysms are identified: (1) aneurysms secondary to penetrating trauma and (2) aneurysms secondary to nonpenetrating trauma.

Penetrating trauma. Intracerebral aneurysms secondary to penetrating injuries are commonly due to high velocity missile head wounds.[47,48] A recent study demonstrated a 50% overall prevalence of major vascular lesions in civilian patients with penetrating missile injuries examined in the acute stage.[49] Nearly half of these patients had traumatic aneurysms. The diagnosis of posttraumatic aneurysm may be delayed or overlooked on CT because the lesion is often obscured by the presence of an accompanying hemorrhagic intraparenchymal contusion[49] (*see* Chapter 8).

Penetrating injuries to extracranial vessels can cause lacerations, arteriovenous fistulae, dissection, or traumatic pseudoaneurysm[50] (*see* Chapter 8). The carotid artery is the most frequently involved vessel.

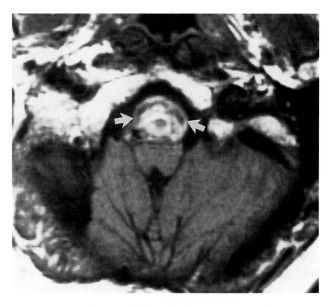

Fig. 9-27. Axial T1-weighted MR scan shows a thrombosed posterior inferior cerebellar artery (PICA) aneurysm *(large arrows)* with laminated thrombus. No patent lumen is seen.

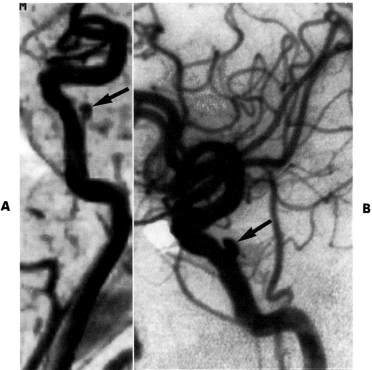

Fig. 9-28. **A,** 3D TOF MRA in a 56-year-old man with transient ischemic attacks. Lateral view shows a small distal ICA aneurysm *(arrow).* **B,** Conventional left common carotid angiogram, lateral view, confirms presence of the aneurysm *(arrow).*

A **B** **C**

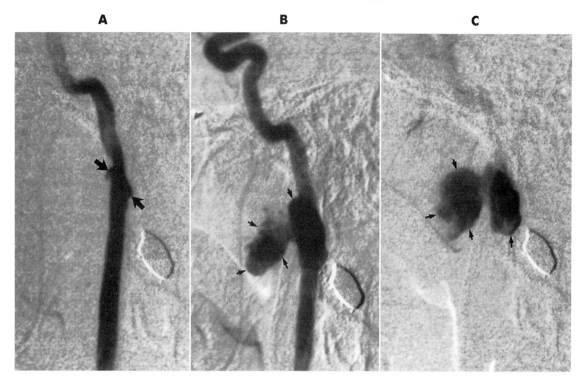

Fig. 9-29. Cervical gunshot wound with early **(A)**, mid- **(B)**, and late arterial phase studies of the left ICA angiogram, lateral view. Vessel laceration is seen in the early frame **(A,** *arrows*). Blood mixed with contrast extravasates through the laceration into the cervical soft tissues, forming a pseudoaneurysm **(B,** *arrows*). Late frame shows persistent contrast accumulation in the pseudoaneurysm **(C,** *arrows*).

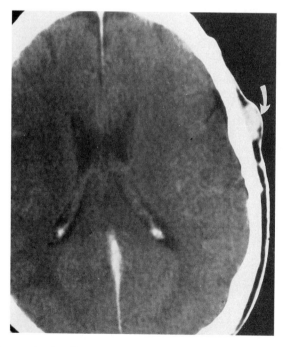

Fig. 9-30. Axial postcontrast CT scan in a patient with a traumatic pseudoaneurysm of the superficial temporal artery *(arrow)*.

Pathologically, a false aneurysm lacks any components of a vessel wall. These false, or "pseudoaneurysms," are really just cavities, typically within adjacent blood clots, that communicate with a vessel lumen. Radiographically, a false aneurysm projects beyond the vessel margin into the adjacent soft tissues (Fig. 9-29). The periadventitial hematoma can be delineated on CT or MR studies.

A particular type of carotid injury occurs with intraoral trauma and is common in children. This so-called pencil injury may have a significant delay between the time of injury and onset of neurologic sequelae.[50]

Occasionally the external carotid artery is a site of traumatic injury. The superficial temporal artery (STA) is the most commonly affected vessel (Fig. 9-30). STA traumatic pseudoaneurysm occurs as a complication of scalp trauma and may result from penetrating injury or blunt trauma.[51]

Meningeal vessels are uncommon sites of traumatic pseudoaneurysm development; most occur on branches of the middle meningeal artery. When hemorrhage from a meningeal pseudoaneurysm occurs it is usually into the epidural space.[52]

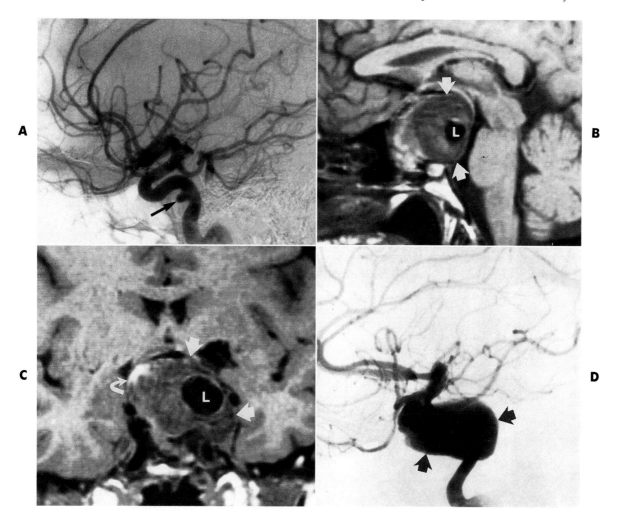

Fig. 9-31. A patient sustained a comminuted skull base fracture. A traumatic carotid-cavernous fistula formed and then closed spontaneously. **A,** Follow-up internal carotid angiogram, lateral view, disclosed a small posttraumatic aneurysm *(arrow).* Another patient also had a severely comminuted skull base fracture and developed a very large aneurysm of the internal carotid artery. Sagittal **(B)** and coronal **(C)** T1-weighted MR scans show a giant aneurysm with a small patent lumen, *(L),* surrounded by clot *(large arrows)* that is largely isointense to gray matter. A small more subacute mural thrombus is seen as a high signal focus in the outer wall (**C,** *curved arrow*). **D,** Internal carotid angiogram, midarterial phase, lateral view, shows the aneurysm *(arrows).* (**B** to **D,** Courtesy L. Gentry.)

Direct penetrating injury to the vertebral artery (VA) is uncommon. Occasionally, cervical spine fracture-dislocations will damage the VA. These typically produce dissection or occlusion (*see* Chapter 8); pseudoaneurysms are rare.[53]

Nonpenetrating trauma. Intracranial aneurysms secondary to nonpenetrating trauma usually occur at the skull base (where they involve the petrous, cavernous, or supraclinoid internal carotid artery) or along the peripheral intracranial vessels.[54] ICA aneurysms at the skull base can be caused by blunt trauma or skull fracture (Fig. 9-31). Hyperextension and head rotation may stretch the ICA over the lateral mass of C1 or shear the artery at its intracranial entrance.[55]

Peripheral intracranial aneurysms can be caused by closed head injury. The distal anterior cerebral artery and peripheral cortical branches are commonly involved sites distal to the circle of Willis.[54] Frontolateral impacts produce shearing forces between the inferior free margin of the falx cerebri and the distal ACA. This can cause a common type of nonpenetrating traumatic intracranial aneurysm: a traumatic aneurysm of the pericallosal artery.[56] The presence of a traumatic distal ACA aneurysm should be suspected if a juxtafalcine hematoma is seen at CT scanning (Fig. 9-32).

Traumatic cortical artery aneurysm should be suspected if a delayed hematoma near the brain periphery develops adjacent to the site of a skull fracture.

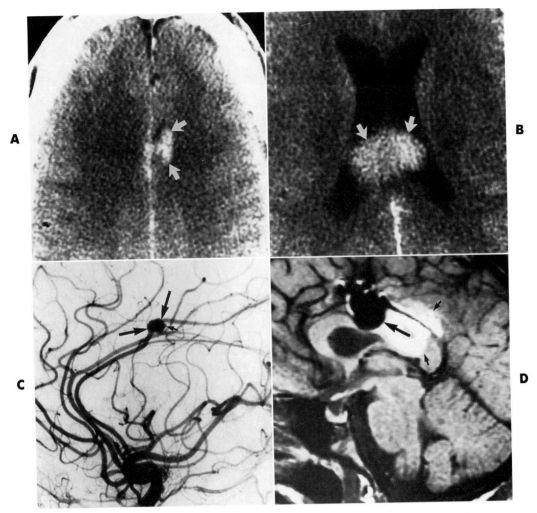

Fig. 9-32. A, Axial CT without contrast enhancement in a patient with closed head injury. A small parafalcine hematoma *(arrows)* was identified. The patient did well but had sudden neurologic deterioration 2 weeks after the initial injury. **B,** Repeat CT scan shows a large hematoma of the corpus callosum *(arrows)*. **C,** Right internal carotid angiogram, lateral view, shows a distal pericallosal artery aneurysm *(large arrows)*. Note the small "tit" *(small arrow)*. The traumatic pseudoaneurysm was clipped. **D,** Postoperative sagittal T1-weighted MR scan shows metallic artifact from the clips and acute clot in the residual lumen *(large arrow)*. The subacute hematoma in the corpus callosum and cingulate gyrus is indicated by the *small arrows*. (Courtesy L. Cromwell.)

Mycotic Aneurysms

The term *mycotic* aneurysm is used to describe any aneurysm that is the result of an infectious process that involves the arterial wall. These aneurysms may be caused by a septic cerebral embolus that results in inflammatory destruction of the arterial wall beginning with the endothelial surface.[56a] A more likely explanation is that infected embolic material reaches the adventitia through the vasa vasorum. Inflammation then disrupts the adventitia and muscularis, resulting in aneurysmal dilatation.[57]

In the past, mycotic aneurysms were estimated to account for 2% to 3% of all intracranial aneurysms but were described as decreasing in the antibiotic era.[58] However, with the increased incidence of drug abuse

and immunocompromised states from various causes, mycotic aneurysms may increase in frequency.

The thoracic aorta has been described as the most common site of mycotic aneurysm.[58] Intracranial mycotic aneurysms are less common. They occur with greater frequency in children and are often found on vessels distal to the circle of Willis (Fig. 9-33).[59] Rarely, deep neck space infections are complicated by pseudoaneurysm of the cervical internal carotid artery.[59a]

Oncotic Aneurysms

Extracranial oncotic pseudoaneurysms with exsanguinating epistaxis are a common terminal event

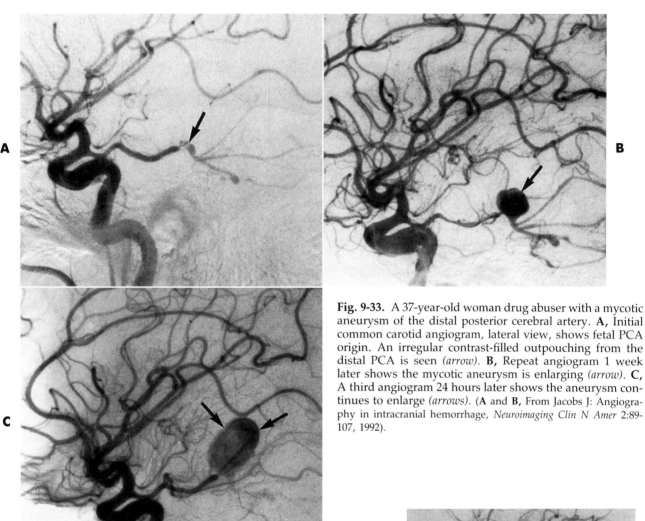

Fig. 9-33. A 37-year-old woman drug abuser with a mycotic aneurysm of the distal posterior cerebral artery. **A,** Initial common carotid angiogram, lateral view, shows fetal PCA origin. An irregular contrast-filled outpouching from the distal PCA is seen *(arrow).* **B,** Repeat angiogram 1 week later shows the mycotic aneurysm is enlarging *(arrow).* **C,** A third angiogram 24 hours later shows the aneurysm continues to enlarge *(arrows).* (**A** and **B,** From Jacobs J: Angiography in intracranial hemorrhage, *Neuroimaging Clin N Amer* 2:89-107, 1992).

Fig. 9-34. Elderly patient with extensive nasopharyngeal squamous cell carcinoma and severe epistaxis caused by tumor erosion into the ICA. Left common carotid angiogram, lateral view, shows an oncotic distal ICA pseudoaneurysm *(large arrow)* with contrast extravasation *(curved arrow)* indicating active hemorrhage. Note displacement, stretching, and draping of small external carotid artery branches secondary to intratumoral hemorrhage *(small arrows).*

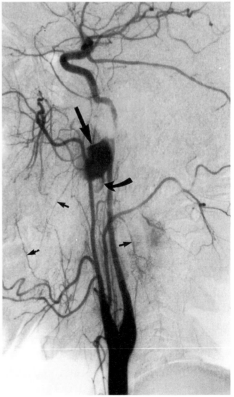

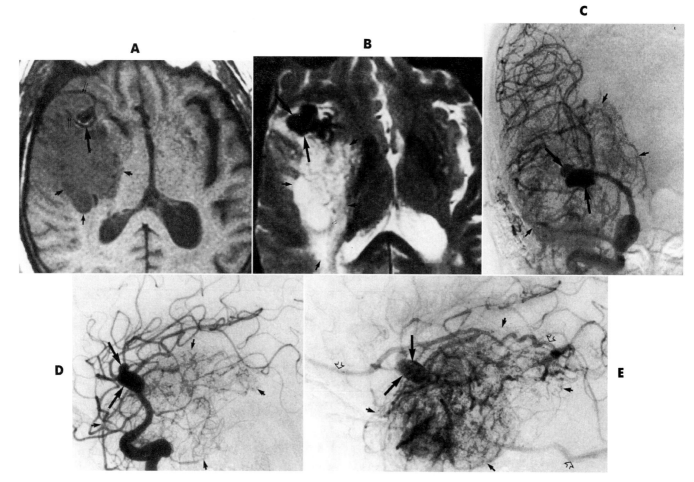

Fig. 9-35. A 52-year-old man with a large right temporal lobe glioblastoma multiforme. **A,** Axial T1-weighted MR scan shows the low signal tumor *(small single arrows).* A partially thrombosed MCA aneurysm *(large arrow)* is present. Acute clot in part of the aneurysm *(double arrows)* is isointense with cortex. **B,** Axial T2-weighted study shows the tumor *(small arrows)* and the large, multilobed aneurysm *(large arrows).* The profoundly hypointense signal from the acute thrombus cannot be distinguished from the high-velocity signal loss (flow void) in the patent lumen. **C,** Left common carotid angiogram, arterial phase, AP view, shows the extensive neovascularity of the tumor *(small arrows)* and the lobulated aneurysm *(large arrows).* Early **(D)** and late **(E)** arterial phase films, lateral view, again show the tumor blush *(small arrows)* and the lobulated aneurysm *(large arrows).* Arteriovenous shunting causes early filling of cerebral veins *(open arrows).* At surgery, the glioblastoma had invaded the middle cerebral artery, producing this oncotic aneurysm.

with malignant head and neck tumors (Fig. 9-34). Intracranial oncotic aneurysms are less common. They may be associated with either primary or metastatic tumors. Neoplastic aneurysms result from direct vascular invasion by a tumor or implantation of metastatic emboli that infiltrate and disrupt the vessel wall.[60,61]

Primary tumors. Intracranial aneurysms associated with primary brain tumors are less common than those caused by metastases.[62] The incidence of saccular aneurysms in patients with primary cerebral neoplasms does not appear to be significantly higher than the incidence of aneurysms in the general population, although some authors report a slightly higher incidence with meningiomas.[63] High-grade gliomas (Fig. 9-35)[62] and pituitary adenomas have been reported associated with focal saccular aneurysm. Glioblastoma multiforme and pituitary adenoma are also common primary CNS neoplasms that demonstrate intratumoral hemorrhage *(see* Chapter 7).

Metastatic tumors. Some metastatic tumors that have been implicated in the development of an intracranial aneurysm are left atrial myxoma[60] and cho-

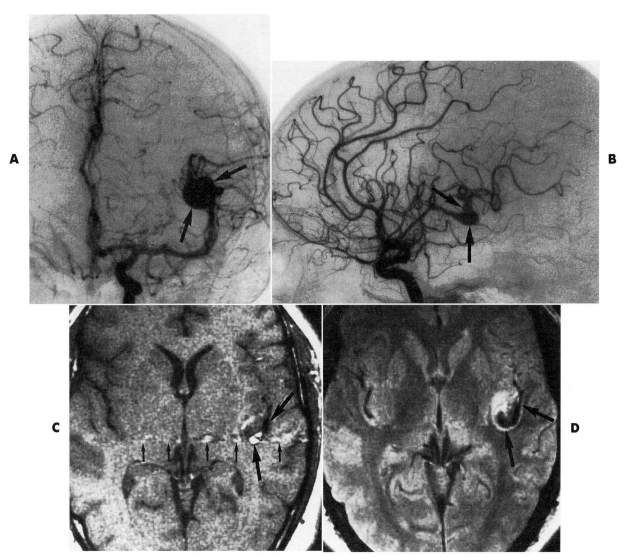

Fig. 9-36. A 40-year-old-male with temporal lobe seizures and an intracardiac mass in the left atrium. AP **(A)** and lateral **(B)** views of the left carotid angiogram show a distal MCA aneurysm *(arrows)*, presumed secondary to atrial myxoma. Axial T1-weighted **(C)** and long TR/short TE **(D)** MR scans show the aneurysm *(large arrows)*. Note phase-encoding artifact **(C,** *small arrows).*

riocarcinoma[61,65] (Fig. 9-36). Because metastatic tumors are common at the gray-white junction, aneurysms from metastatic implants often involve peripheral cerebral vessels.

Flow-Related Aneurysms

The coexistence of arteriovenous malformations (AVMs) and aneurysm is well known. The frequency of aneurysm with AVM has been reported from 2.7% to 30%.[66-69] Flow-related aneurysms occur along proximal and distal feeding vessels. Proximal lesions arise in the circle of Willis or on vessels feeding the AVM[70] and are probably related to increased hemodynamic stress.[71] There is no reported increased frequency of hemorrhage in patients with proximal feeding-artery aneurysms.[72]

Distal flow-related aneurysms are located within the AVM nidus (Fig. 9-37). Intranidal aneurysms have been reported in 8% to 12% of AVMs.[70,70a] These lesions are thin-walled vascular structures without the elastic or muscular layers that characterize arteries (Fig. 9-38). It is unclear whether intranidal aneurysms arise from venous ectasias or from the flow-weakened walls of arterial vessels. Nevertheless, these thin-walled structures are exposed to arterial pressure and are considered a likely site for AVM hemorrhage.[70]

Vasculopathies, Vasculitis, and Drug-Related Aneurysms

There is an increased incidence of cephalocervical aneurysms with some vasculopathies such as FMD

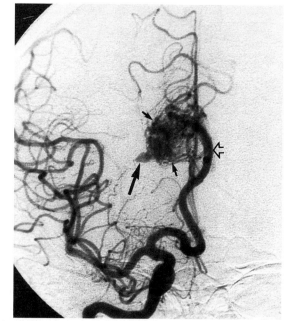

Fig. 9-37. High-resolution (1024 × 1024) digital subtraction internal carotid angiogram, AP view, in a patient with an AVM *(small arrows)* fed by an enlarged anterior cerebral artery *(open arrow)*. A flow-related nidal aneurysm *(large arrow)* is present.

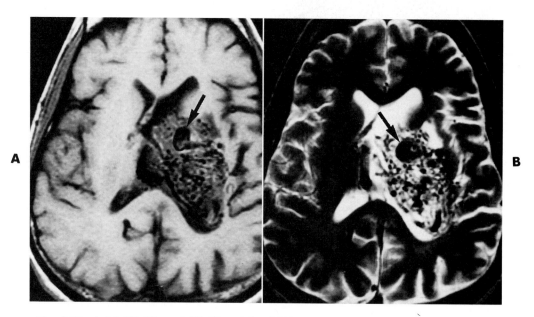

Fig. 9-38. Axial **(A)** T1- and **(B)** T2-weighted MR scans in a patient with a large deep thalamic AVM. A thin-walled intranidal aneurysm is indicated by the arrows.

(see previous discussion). Some vasculitides such as systemic lupus erythematosus and even Takayasu's arteritis have been associated with aneurysms. Substance abuse can cause certain forms of vasculitis, thus contributing to aneurysm formation, or cause hemorrhage from preexisting vascular abnormalities such as arteriovenous malformations or saccular aneurysms.

Vasculopathies

Systemic lupus erythematosus (SLE). Commonly reported CNS vascular lesions with SLE are infarcts and transient ischemic attacks. Intracranial hemorrhages are present in approximately 10% of patients with CNS symptoms.[73] Although uncommon, arteritic and nonvasculitic aneurysms occur in SLE. These can be saccular, fusiform, or a bizarre-appearing mixture of both (Fig. 9-39).

Takayasu's arteritis. Although the characteristic vascular lesions are occlusion, stenosis, and luminal irregularities, ectasia and aneurysm formation have been described in Takayasu's arteritis.[74]

Fibromuscular dysplasia (FMD). Some investigators report a 20% to 50% incidence of aneurysms in

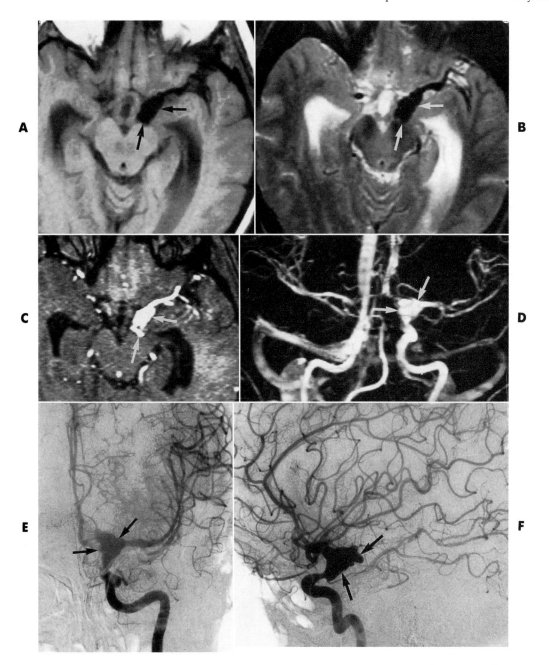

Fig. 9-39. A 37-year-old woman with long-standing SLE. Transient ischemic attacks prompted MR examination. Axial **(A)** T1- and **(B)** T2-weighted scans show a large multilobulated aneurysm at the distal ICA bifurcation *(arrows)*. **C,** Axial gradient-refocussed scan shows the lesion has flow *(arrows)*. **D,** Coronal multiple overlapping thin slab acquisition (MOTSA) MR angiogram shows the lesion *(arrows)*. AP **(E)** and lateral **(F)** views of the conventional left carotid angiogram demonstrate the aneurysm *(arrows)*.

patients with cervical FMD.[75] Other abnormalities associated with FMD include spontaneous dissection, dissecting aneurysm (see subsequent discussion), and arteriovenous fistulae.[76]

Dissections. (see subsequent discussion) Pseudo-aneurysm formation occurs in approximately one third of nontraumatic internal carotid dissections and 7% of vertebral artery dissections.[77]

Drug abuse. Various intracranial vascular lesions have been reported with substance abuse.

Cocaine. Cocaine abuse is associated with various CNS complications, including subarachnoid hemorrhage, cerebral ischemia or infarction, intraparenchymal hemorrhage, seizures, vasculitis, vasospasm, and death.[78,79] Approximately 50% of drug-abusing patients with CNS symptoms have SAH; of these,

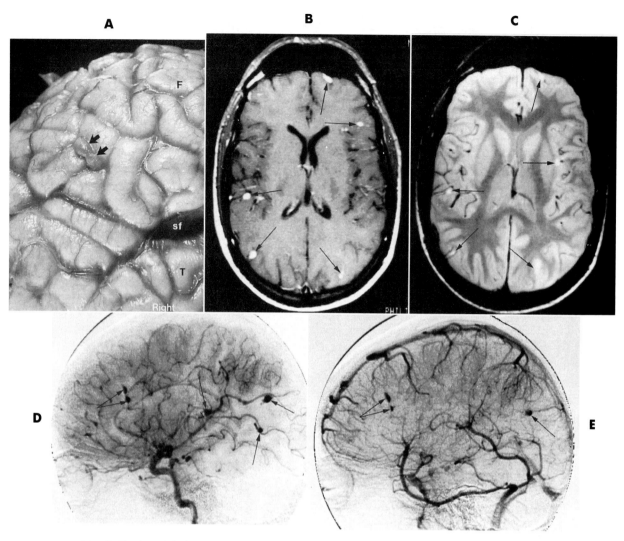

Fig. 9-40. Arterial changes with methamphetamine abuse. **A,** Gross pathologic specimen shows saccular enlargement of a cortical artery *(arrows)*. *sf,* Sylvian fissure; *T,* temporal lobe; *F,* frontal lobe. **B,** Axial postcontrast T1-weighted MR scan shows multiple bilateral peripheral saccular aneurysms *(arrows)*. **C,** Long TR/short TE scan shows the lesions are slightly hyperintense *(arrows)*. **D,** Right internal carotid angiogram, lateral view. Late arterial phase shows the saccular enlargements of numerous peripheral arteries *(arrows)*. **E,** Stasis in the aneurysms is seen as contrast persisting into the venous phase *(arrows)*. (Courtesy E. J. Russell; from Lazar EB, Russell EJ at al: Contrast-enhanced MR of cerebral arteritis: intravascular enhancement related to flow stasis within areas of focal arterial ectasia, *AJNR* 13:271-276, 1992.)

about half have an underlying abnormality such as aneurysm or vascular malformation.[80,81] Hemorrhage may also be related to the acute hypertensive response that occurs with cocaine use[80,80a] (*see* Chapter 7).

Other drugs. Heroin, ephedrine, methamphetamine, and cocaine can cause cerebral vasculitis.[82] Necrotizing angiitis, histologically similar to periarteritis nodosa, has been identified in methamphetamine abusers. Focal arterial ectasias, aneurysms, and sacculations have been reported in this form of drug-induced cerebral arteritis[83] (Fig. 9-40).

FUSIFORM ANEURYSMS

Pathology. "Fusiform" aneurysms are also known as atherosclerotic aneurysms. These lesions are exaggerated arterial ectasias due to a severe and unusual form of atherosclerosis.[2] Damage to the media results in arterial stretching and elongation that may extend over a considerable length. These ectatic vessels may have more focal areas of fusiform or even saccular enlargement (Fig. 9-41). Intraluminal clots are common, and perforating branches often arise from the entire length of the involved parent vessel.[29]

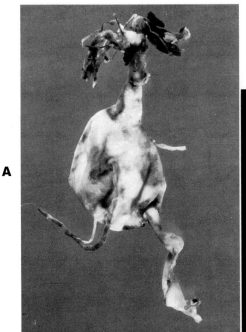
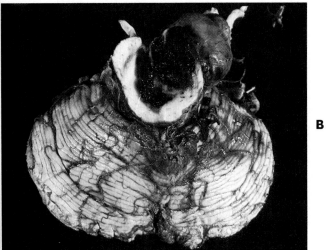

Fig. 9-41. **A,** Gross pathologic specimen of atherosclerotic verte-brobasilar dolichoectasia with a fusiform aneurysm. **B,** Specimen from another case shows a fusiform aneurysm with acute thrombosis and hemorrhagic brainstem infarction. (**A,** Courtesy Rubinstein Collection, University of Virginia.)

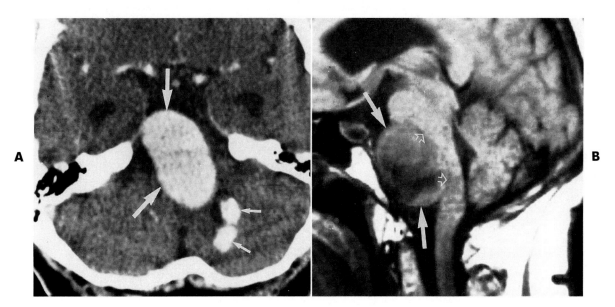

Fig. 9-42. **A,** Axial contrast-enhanced CT scan in an elderly patient with striking verte-brobasilar dolichoectasia *(small arrows)* and a large patent fusiform aneurysm *(large arrows)*. **B,** Sagittal T1-weighted MR scan shows the aneurysm *(large arrows)*. Slow, turbulent flow produces mixed iso/hypointense signal within the lumen. Note the marked brainstem compression by the aneurysm *(open arrows)*.

Clinical presentation. Fusiform aneurysms usually occur in older patients. The vertebrobasilar system is commonly affected. Fusiform aneurysms may thrombose, producing brainstem infarction (Fig. 9-41, *B*). They can also compress the adjacent brain or cause cranial nerve palsies.

Imaging. Fusiform atherosclerotic aneurysms usually arise from elongated, tortuous arteries. Patent aneurysms enhance strongly after contrast administration (Fig. 9-42); thrombosed aneurysms are hyperintense on NECT scans (*see* Fig. 9-23, *C*). Tubular calcification with intraluminal and mural thrombi in the ectatic parent vessels and aneurysm wall are frequent. Occasionally fusiform aneurysms cause skull base erosion.

At angiography, fusiform aneurysms often have bizarre shapes with serpentine or giant configurations.[84] Intraluminal flow is often slow and turbulent. These aneurysms typically do not have an identifiable neck. MR is helpful in delineating the relationship between vessels and adjacent structures such as the brainstem and cranial nerves (Fig. 9-42, *B*).[85]

DISSECTING ANEURYSMS

Pathology. In arterial dissections, blood accumulates within the vessel wall through a tear in the intima and internal elastic lamina.[1] The consequences of this intramural hemorrhage vary. If blood dissects subintimally it causes luminal narrowing or even occlusion. If the intramural hematoma extends into the subadventitial plane, a saclike outpouching may be formed.[86,87] These focal aneurysmal dilatations should not be confused with the so-called pseudoaneurysms that result from arterial rupture and subsequent encapsulation of the perivascular hematoma.[86,87] Thus uncomplicated dissections do not project beyond the lumen of the parent vessel, and dissections with saclike outpouchings are termed *dissecting aneurysms*. The term *false saccular aneurysm,* or *pseudoaneurysm,* should be used for encapsulated,

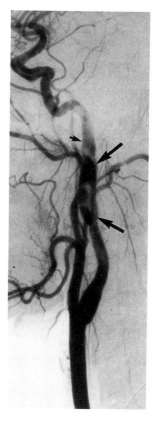

Fig. 9-43. Patient with a dissecting aneurysm *(large arrows)* and fibromuscular dysplasia of the cervical ICA *(small arrow).*

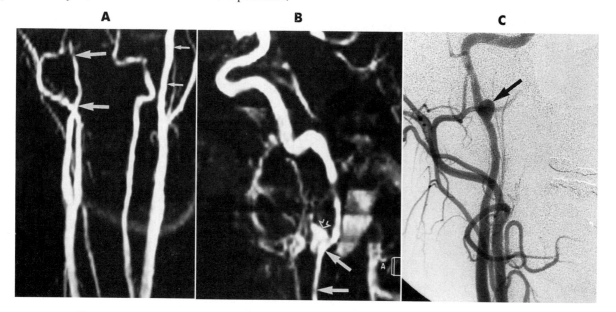

Fig. 9-44. A 21-year-old woman with spontaneous onset of diminished left-sided sensation. **A,** 3D time-of-flight MR angiogram, oblique view, shows a normal left ICA *(small arrows)* and gradual tapering of the right ICA *(large arrows).* Because of slow flow and saturation effects, the intrapetrous ICA is not visualized. **B,** Lateral projection of the multiple overlapping thin slab acquisition (MOTSA) sequence shows the ICA narrowing *(large arrows).* A possible dissecting aneurysm at the skull base is indicated by the *open arrow.* **C,** Digital subtraction right common angiogram, early arterial phase, obtained 6 weeks later shows persistent dissecting aneurysm *(arrow).* This oblique projection has same orientation as **A.**

cavitated, paravascular hematomas that communicate with the arterial lumen.[48]

Etiology. Dissecting aneurysms may arise spontaneously. More commonly, trauma[88] or an underlying vasculopathy such as FMD is implicated[89,90] (Fig. 9-43).

Location. Most dissecting aneurysms that involve the craniocerebral vessels affect the extracranial segments; intracranial dissections are rare and usually occur only with severe head trauma (*see* Chapter 8). Although the common carotid artery (CCA) can be involved by cephalad extension of an aortic arch dissection, the CCA and carotid bulb are usually spared. The ICA is commonly affected. Most dissections involve the midcervical ICA segment and terminate at the exocranial opening of the petrous carotid canal.[50,86]

The vertebral artery is also a common site of arterial dissection. The common location is between the VA exit from C2 and the skull base.[91] Involvement of the first segment, which extends from the VA origin to its entry into the foramen transversarium (usually at the C6 level), is relatively rare.[92]

Imaging. Dissecting aneurysms are elongated, ovoid (Fig. 9-43) or saccular contrast collections that extend beyond the vessel lumen.[86] MR delineates an intra- or perivascular hematoma associated with dissections, particularly during the subacute stage (*see* Chapter 11). MR angiography is a helpful screening procedure (Fig. 9-44, *A* and *B*), but catheter angiography is the procedure of choice for imaging vessel details such as dissection site (Fig. 9-44, *C* and *D*).

REFERENCES

1. Okazaki H: Malformative vascular lesions. In *Fundamentals of Neuropathology*, ed 2, pp 70-74, New York, Igaku-Schoin, 1989.
2. Stehbens WE: Etiology of intracranial berry aneurysms, *J Neurosurg* 70:823-831, 1989.
2a. Meyer FB, Huston J III, Reiderer SS: Pulsatile increases in aneurysm size determined by cine phase-contrast MR angiography, *J Neurosurg* 78:879-883, 1993.
3. Strother CM, Graves VB, Rappe A: Aneurysm hemodynamics: an experimental study, *AJNR* 13:1089-1095, 1992.
3a. Sakaki T, Tominaga M, Miyamoto K et al: Clinical studies of *de novo* aneurysms, *Neurosurg* 32:512-517, 1993.
4. Iwata K, Misu N, Terada K et al: Screening for unruptured asymptomatic intracranial aneurysms in patients undergoing coronary angiography, *J Neurosurg* 75:52-55, 1991.
5. Atkinson JLD, Sundt TM Jr, Houser OW et al: Angiographic frequency of anterior circulation intercranial aneurysms, *J Neurosurg* 70:551-555, 1989.
6. Schievink WI, Limburg M, Dreissen J Jr et al: Screening for unruptured familiar aneurysms: subarachnoid hemorrhage 2 years after angiography negative for aneurysms, *Neurosurg* 29:434-438, 1991.
7. San-Galli F, Leman C, Kein P et al: Cerebral arterial fenestrations associated with intracranial saccular aneurysms, *Neurosurgery* 30:279-283, 1992.
7a. Picard L, Roy D, Bracard S et al: Aneurysm associated with a fenestrated basilar artery: report of two cases treated by endovascular detachable balloon embolization, *AJNR* 14:591-594, 1993.
7b. Sanders WP, Sorek PA, Mehta BA: Fenestration of intracranial ateries with special attention to associated aneurysms and other anomalies, *AJNR* 14:675-680, 1993.
8. Schievink WI, Mokri B, Piepgras DG: Angiographic frequency of saccular intracranial aneurysms in patients with spontaneous cervical arterial dissection, *J Neurosurg* 76:62-66, 1992.
8a. Camarata PJ, Latchaw RE Jr, Rüffenacht DA, Heros RC: Intracranial aneurysms, *Invest Radiol* 28:373-382, 1993.
9. Vajda J: Multiple intracranial aneurysms: a high risk condition, *Acta Neurochir* (Wien) 118:59-75, 1992.
10. Stone JL, Crowell RM, Gandhi YN, Jafar JJ: Multiple intracranial aneurysms: magnetic resonance imaging for determination of the site of rupture, *Neurosurg* 23:97-100, 1988.
11. Ruggieri PM: Presented at the 78th Annual Scientific Assembly of the Radiological Society of North America, Chicago, Nov. 29-Dec. 4, 1992.
12. Armstrong DC: Presented at the 29th Annual Scientific Meeting of the American Society of Neuroradiology, Washington, May 1991.
13. Osborn AG: Intracranial aneurysms. In *Handbook of Neuroradiology*, pp. 79-84, Mosby-Yearbook Co, St.Louis 1991.
14. Andoh T, Shirakami S, Nakashima T et al: Clinical analysis of a series of vertebral aneurysm cases, *Neurosurg* 31:987-993, 1992.
15. Herneshiemi J, Tapaninaho A, Vapalahti M et al: Saccular aneurysms of the distal anterior cerebral artery and its branches, *Neurosurg* 31:994-999, 1992.
16. Suzuki S, Kayama T, Sakurai Y et al: Subarachnoid hemorrhage of unknown origin, *Neurosurg* 21:310-313, 1987.
17. Massoud TF, Anslow P, Molyneux AJ: Subarachnoid hemorrhage following spontaneous intracranial carotid artery dissection, *Neuroradiol* 34:33-35, 1992.
18. Brott T, Mandybur TI: Case-control study of clinical outcome after aneurysmal subarachnoid hemorrhage, *Neurosurg* 19:891-895, 1986.
18a. Raps EC, Rogers JD, Galeta SL et al: The clinical spectrum of unruptured intracranial aneurysms, *Arch Neurol* 50:265-268, 1993.
19. McCormick PW, McCormick J, Zimmerman R et al: The pathophysiology of acute subarachnoid hemorrhage, *BNI Quarterly* 7:18-26, 1991.
20. Jane JA, Kassell NF, Torner JC, Winn HR: The natural history of aneurysms and arteriovenous malformations, *J Neurosurg* 62:321-323, 1985.
21. Saveland H, Hillman J, Brandt et al: Overall outcome in aneurysmal subarachnoid hemorrhage, *J Neurosurg* 76:729-734, 1992.
22. Wascher TM, Golfinos J, Zabramski JM, Spetzler RF: Management of unruptured intracranial aneurysms, *BNI Quarterly* 8:2-7, 1992.
22a. Juvela S, Porras M, Heiskanen O: Natural history of unruptured intracranial aneurysms: a long-term follow-up study, *J Neurosurg* 79:174-182, 1993.
23. Weibers DO, Whisnant JP, Sundt T et al: The significance of unruptured intracranial aneurysms, *J Neurosurg* 66:23-29, 1987.
24. Schievink WI, Piepgras DG, Wirth FP: Rupture of previously documented small asymptomatic saccular intracranial aneurysms, *J Neurosurg* 76:1019-1024, 1992.
24a. Rossitti S, Löfgren K: Optimality principles and flow orderliness at the branching points of cerebral arteries, *Stroke* 24:1029-1032, 1993.
25. Gonzales CF, Cho YI, Ortega HV, Moret J: Intracranial aneurysms: flow analysis of their origin and progression, *AJNR* 13:181-1888, 1992.

26. Strother CM, Graves VB, Rappe A: Aneurysm hemodynamics: an experimental study, *AJNR* 13:1089-1095, 1992.

27. Graves VB, Stother CM Partington CR, Rappi A: Flow dynamics of lateral carotid artery aneurysms and their effect on coils and balloons: an experimental study in dogs, *AJNR* 13:189-196, 1992.

28. Schubiger O, Valavanis A, Wichmann W: Growth-mechanism of giant intracranial aneurysms: demonstration by CT and MR imaging, *Neuroradiol* 29:266-271, 1987.

29. Symon L: Surgical experiences with giant intracranial aneurysms, *Acta Neurochir* (Wien) 118:53-58, 1992.

30. Kassel NJ, Torner JC: Size of intracranial aneurysms, *Neurosurg* 12:291-297, 1983.

30a. Rosenorn J, Eskesen V, Madsen F, Schmidt K: Importance of cerebral pan-angiography for detection of multiple aneurysms in patients with aneurysmal subarachnoid haemorhage, *Acta Neural Scan* 87:215-218, 1993.

31. Kassell NF, Torner JC, Jane JA et al: The international cooperative study on the timing of aneurysm surgery. Part 2: Surgical results, *J Neurosurg* 73:37-47, 1990.

32. Rinkel GJE, Wijdicks EFM, Vermeulen M et al: Nonaneurysmal perimesencephalic subarachnoid hemorrhage: CT and MR patterns that differ from aneurysmal rupture, *AJNR* 12:829-834, 1991.

33. Rinkle GJE, Wijdicks EFM, Hasan D et al: Outcome in patients with subarachnoid haemorrhage and negative angiography according to pattern of haemorrhage on computed tomography, *Lancet* 338:964-968, 1991.

34. Farres MT, Ferraz-Leite H, Schindler E, Muhlbauer M: Spontaneous subarachnoid hemorrhage with negative angiography: CT findings, *J Comput Assist Tomogr* 16:534-537, 1992.

35. Yamamoto Y, Asari S, Sunami N et al: Computed angiotomography of unruptured cerebral aneurysms, *J Comp Assist Tomogr* 10:21-27, 1986.

36. Newell DW, LeRoux PD, Dacey RG Jr et al: CT infusion scanning for the detection of cerebral aneurysms, *J Neurosurg* 71:175-179, 1989.

37. Napel S, Marks MP, Rubin GP et al: CT angiography with spiral CT and maximum intensity projection, *Radiol* 185:607-610, 1992.

38. Aoki S, Sasaki Y, Machida T et al: Cerebral aneurysms: detection and delineation using 3-D-CT angiography, *AJNR* 13:1115-1120, 1992.

39. Schmid UD, Steiger HJ, Huber P: Accuracy of high resolution computed tomography in direct diagnosis of cerebral aneurysms, *Neuroradiol* 29:152-159, 1987.

40. Sadato N, Numaguchi T, Rigamonti D et al: Bleeding patterns in ruptured posterior fossa aneurysms: a CT study, *J Comp Asst Tomogr* 15:612-617, 1991.

41. Bosmans H, Marchal G, Van Hecke P, Vanhoenacker P: MRA review, *Clin Imaging* 16:152-167, 1992.

42. Hahn FJ, Cng E, McComb R, Leibrock L: Peripheral signal void ring in giant vertebral aneurysm: MR and pathology findings, *J Comp Asst Tomogr* 10:1036-1038, 1986.

43. Tsuruda J, Saloner D, Norman D: Artifacts associated with MR neuroangiography, *AJNR* 13:1411-1422, 1992.

44. Huston J III, Ehman RL: Comparison of time-of-flight and phase-contrast MR neuroangiographic techniques, *Radio-Graphics* 13:5-19, 1993.

45. Blatter DD, Parker DL, Ahn SS et al: Cerebral MR angiography with multiple overlapping thin slab acquisition. Part II: Early clinical experience, *Radiol* 183:379-389, 1992.

46. Davis WL, Warnock SH, Harnsberger HR et al: Intracranial MRA: single volume vs. multiple thin slab 3D time-of-flight acquisition, *J Comput Assist Tomogr* 17:15-21, 1993.

47. Nakstad P, Nornes H, Hauge HN: Traumatic aneurysms of the pericallosal arteries, *Neuroradiol* 28:335-338, 1986.

48. Arabi B: Traumatic aneurysms of brain due to high velocity missile head wounds, *Neurosurg* 22:1056-1063, 1988.

49. Jinkins JR, Dadsetan MR, Sener RN et al: Value of acute-phase angiography in the detection of vascular injuries caused by gunshot wounds to the head: analysis of 12 cases, *AJR* 169:365-368, 1992.

50. Davis JM, Zimmerman RA: Injury of the cortical and vertebral arteries, *Neuroradiol* 25:55-69, 1983.

51. Sharma A, Tyagi G, Sahai A, Baijal SS: Traumatic aneurysm of superficial temporal artery: CT demonstration, *Neuroradiol* 33:510-512, 1991.

52. Toro VE, Fravel JF, Weidman TA: Posttraumatic pseudoaneurysm of the posterior meningeal artery associated with intraventricular hemorrhage, *AJNR* 14:264-266, 1993.

53. Parent AD, Harkey HL, Touchstone DA et al: Lateral cervical spine dislocation and vertebral artery injury, *Neurosurg* 31:501-509, 1992.

54. Senegor M: Traumatic pericallosal aneurysm in a patient with no major trauma, *J Neurosurg* 75:475-477, 1991.

55. Magnan P-E, Branchereau A, Cannoni M: Traumatic aneurysms of the internal carotid artery at the base of the skull, *J Cardiovasc Surg* 33:372-379, 1992.

56. Nov AA, Cromwell LD: Traumatic pericallosal artery aneurysm, *J Neuroradiol* 11:3-8, 1984.

57. Lawrence-Friedl D, Bauer KM: Bilateral cortical blindness: an unusual presentation of bacterial endocarditis, *Ann Emer Med* 21:1502-1504, 1992.

58. Kaufman SL, White RI Jr, Harrington DP et al: Protean manifestations of mycotic aneurysms, *Am J Roentgenol* 131:1019-1025, 1978.

59. Lee KS, Liu SS, Spetzler RF, Rekate HL: Intracranial mycotic aneurysm in an infant: report of a case, *Neurosurg* 26:129-133, 1990.

59a. Krysl J, de Tilly LN, Armstrong D: Pseudoaneurysm of the internal carotid artery: comparison of deep neck space infection, *AJNR* 14:696-698, 1993.

60. Hofmann E, Becker T, Romberg-Hahnloser R et al: Cranial MRI and CT in patients with left atrial myxoma, *Neuroradiol* 34:57-61, 1992.

61. Giannakapoulos G, Nair S, Snider C, Amenta DS: Implications for the pathogenesis of aneurysm formation: metastasis choroicarcinoma with spontaneous splenic rupture, *Surg Neurol* 38:236-240, 1992.

62. Barker CS: Peripheral cerebral aneurysm associated with a glioma, *Neuroradiol* 34:30-32, 1992.

63. Licata C, Pasqualin A, Freschini A et al: Management of associated primary cerebral neoplasms and vascular malformations: 1. Intracranial aneurysms, *Acxta Neurochir* (Wien) 82:28-38, 1986.

64. Weir B: Pituitary tumors and aneurysms: case report and review of the literature, *Neurosurg* 30:585-591, 1992.

65. Fujiwara T, Mino S, Nagao S, Ohmoto T: Metastasis choricarcinoma with neoplastic aneurysms cured by aneurysm resection and chemotherapy, *J Neurosurg* 76:148-151, 1992.

66. Kondziolka D, Nixon BJ, Lasjaunias P et al: Cerebral arteriovenous malformations with associated arterial aneurysms: hemodynamic and therapeutic considerations, *Can J Neurol Sci* 15:130-134, 1988.

67. Brown RD, Wiebers DO, Forbes GS: Unruptured intracranial aneurysms and arteriovenous malformations: frequency of intracranial hemorrhage and relationship of lesions, *J Neurosurg* 73:859-863, 1990.

68. Monaco RG, Alvarez H, Goulas A et al: Posterior fossa arteriovenous malformations: angioarchitecture in relation to their hemorrhagic episodes, *Neuroradiol* 31:471-475, 1990.

69. Cunha e Sa MJ, Stein BM, Solomon RA, McCormic PC: The treatment of associated intracranial aneurysms and arteriovenous malformations, *J Neurosurg* 77:853-859, 1992.

70. Marks MP, Lane B, Steinberg GK, Snipes GJ: Intranidal aneurysms in cerebral arteriovenous malformations: evaluation and endovascular treatment, *Radiol* 183:355-360, 1992.

70a. Garcia-Monaco R, Rodesch G, Alvarez H et al: Pseudoaneurysms within ruptured intracranial arteriovenous malformations: diagnosis and early endovascular management, *AJNR* 14:315-321, 1993

71. Mabuchi S, Kamiyama H, Abe H: Distal aneurysms of the superior cerebellar artery and posterior inferior cerebellar artery feeding an associated arteriovenous malformation: case report, *Neurosurg* 30:284-287, 1992.

72. Marks MP, Lane B, Steinberg GK, Chang PJ: Hemorrhage in intracerebral aneurysms and arteriovenous malformations: frequency of intracranial hemorrhage and relationship of lesions, *J Neurosurg* 73:859-863, 1990.

73. Eustace S, Hutchinson M, Bresnihan B: Acute cerebrovascular episodes in systemic lupus erythematosus, *Quart J Med* 81:739-750, 1991.

74. Hargraves RW, Spetzler RF: Takayasu's arteritis: case report, *BNI Quarterly* 7:20-23, 1991.

75. Healton EB: Fibromuscular dysplasia. In Barnett HJM, editor, *Stroke* Vol 2, pp 831-843, New York, Livingstone, 1986.

76. Heiserman JE, Drayer BP, Fram EK, Keller PJ: MR angiography of cervical fibromuscular dysplasia, *AJNR* 13:1454-1457, 1992.

77. Sorek PA, Silbergleit R: Multiple asymptomatic cervical cephalic aneurysms, *AJNR* 14:31-33, 1993.

78. Yapor WY, Gutierrez FA: Cocaine-induced intratumoral hemorrhage: case report and review of the literature, *Neurosurg* 30:288-291, 1992.

79. Brown E, Prager J, Lee H-Y, RamseyRG: CNS complications of cocaine abuse: prevalence, pathophysiology, and neuroradiology, *AJR* 159-137-147,1992.

80. Jacobs IG, Roszler MH, Kelly JK et al: Cocaine abuse: neurovascular complications, *Radio* 170-223-227, 1989.

80a. Oyesiku N, Colohan ART, Barow DL, Reisner A: Cocaine-induced aneurysmal rupture: an emergent negative factor in the natural history of intracranial aneurysms? *Neurosurg* 32:518-526, 1993.

81. Leavine SR, Brust JCM, Futrell N et al: A comparative study of the cerebrovascular complication of cocaine: alkaloidal versus hydrochloride—a review, *Neuroradiol* 41:1173-1177, 1991.

82. Nalls G, Disher A, Darybagi J et al: Subortical cerebral hemorrhages associated with cocaine abuse: CT and MR findings, *J Comp asst Tomor* 13:1-5, 1989.

83. Lazar EB, Russell EJ, Cohen BA et al: Contrast-enhanced MR of cerebral arteritis: intravascular enhancement related to flow stasis within areas of focal arterial ectaisa, *AJNR* 13:271-276, 1992.

84. Sugita K, Kobayashi S, Takemae T et al: Giant aneurysm of the vertebral artery, *J Neurosurg* 68:960-966, 1988.

85. Tien RD, Wilkins RH: MRA delineation of the vertebrovascular system in patients with hemifacial spasm and trigeminal neuralgia, *AJNR* 14:34-36, 1993.

86. Mokri B: Traumatic and spontaneous extracranial internal carotid artery dissection, *J Neurol* 237:356-361, 1990.

87. Anson J, Cromwell RM: Craniocervical arterial dissection, *Neurosurg* 29:89-96, 1991.

88. Mann CI, Dietrick RB, Schrader MT et al: Posttraumatic carotid artery dissection in children: evaluation with MR imaging, *AJR* 160:134-136, 1993.

Intracranial Vascular Malformations

Arteriovenous Malformations (AVMs)
    Parenchymal (Pial) Malformations
    Dural AVMs and Fistula
    Mixed Pial-Dural AVMs
Capillary Telangiectasias
Cavernous Angiomas
Venous Malformations
    Venous Angioma
    Vein of Galen Malformations
    Venous Varix

The Four Basic Types of Intracranial Vascular Malformations

Arteriovenous malformations
Capillary telangiectasias
Cavernous angiomas
Venous vascular malformations (angiomas)

Intracranial vascular malformations traditionally are divided into the following four basic types (*see* box):

1. Arteriovenous malformations
2. Capillary telangiectasias
3. Cavernous angiomas
4. Venous malformations

Some investigators treat capillary telangiectasias and cavernous angiomas as a spectrum within a single pathologic entity.[1,2] Others regard venous vascular malformations, or "angiomas," as extreme but otherwise normal variants of venous drainage, classifying them as developmental venous anomalies (DVAs) rather than true vascular malformations.

Some add a fifth category of vascular malformations, venous varix.[3-5]

Although histopathologically heterogeneous vascular malformations with varying mixtures of cavernous and capillary elements, AVMs, and venous anomalies have been reported,[2,6,6a] we will follow the traditional division of vascular malformations in the four basic categories.

ARTERIOVENOUS MALFORMATIONS

Intracranial arteriovenous malformations (AVMs) are subdivided into two basic types, brain parenchymal (pial) malformations and dural malformations. A third type, mixed pial-dural AVM, occurs when a parenchymal malformation recruits vascular supply from dural sources.

Parenchymal (Pial) AVMs

Pathology (*see* box, p. 286)

Gross pathology. AVMs are a complex network of abnormal vascular channels that consists of arterial feeders, arterial collaterals, the AVM nidus, and enlarged venous outflow channels[7] (Fig. 10-1, *A*). Grossly, AVMs appear as tightly packed masses of abnormal vascular channels without intervening normal brain parenchyma (Fig. 10-1, *B*). AVMs sometimes contain small amounts of gliotic, nonfunctional brain. Residua of previous hemorrhagic episodes such as dystrophic calcification and blood in different stages of degradation are common.

Secondary changes occur within and around AVMs. The overlying leptomeninges are often thickened and sometimes hemosiderin stained.[8] Flow-related aneurysms on feeding vessels or within the AVM nidus itself are seen in 8% to 12% of all cases[9] (*see* Chapter 9). Degenerative angiopathic changes such as thrombosis or stenosis of feeding arteries and draining veins are common (Fig. 10-1, *A*). Vascular steal phenomena may cause ischemic and atrophic changes in the brain adjacent to the malformation.[1]

Microscopic pathology. There is no intervening capillary bed in AVMs. Thus blood is shunted directly from enlarged feeding arteries to dilated draining veins.[1] Some vessels within an AVM have the thin collagenous walls of veins; others possess the muscular and elastic laminae of arteries.[8] There is an abrupt, direct transition from these thick-walled feeding arteries to thin venous-type channels that lack smooth muscle in their walls and have a reduced internal elastic lamina.

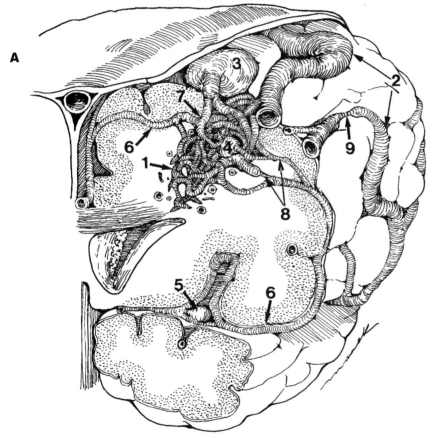
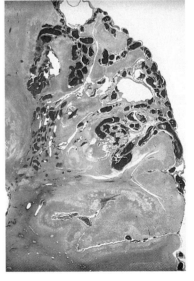
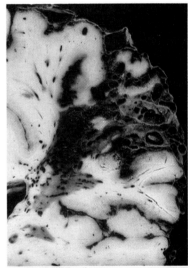
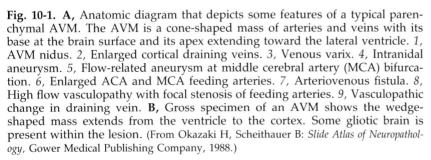

Fig. 10-1. A, Anatomic diagram that depicts some features of a typical parenchymal AVM. The AVM is a cone-shaped mass of arteries and veins with its base at the brain surface and its apex extending toward the lateral ventricle. *1,* AVM nidus. *2,* Enlarged cortical draining veins. *3,* Venous varix. *4,* Intranidal aneurysm. *5,* Flow-related aneurysm at middle cerebral artery (MCA) bifurcation. *6,* Enlarged ACA and MCA feeding arteries. *7,* Arteriovenous fistula. *8,* High flow vasculopathy with focal stenosis of feeding arteries. *9,* Vasculopathic change in draining vein. **B,** Gross specimen of an AVM shows the wedge-shaped mass extends from the ventricle to the cortex. Some gliotic brain is present within the lesion. (From Okazaki H, Scheithauer B: *Slide Atlas of Neuropathology,* Gower Medical Publishing Company, 1988.)

Parenchymal (Pial) AVMs

Pathology

Congenital

98% solitary (multiple in Wyburn-Mason and Rendu-Osler-Weber syndromes)

Dilated arteries and veins without capillary bed

May contain gliotic brain, hemorrhagic residua

Flow-related aneurysm in 10% to 12% (intranidal or on feeding vessel)

Vasculopathic changes in feeding arteries are common

Location

85% supratentorial, 15% posterior fossa

Age at presentation

Peak between 20 and 40 years

25% in childhood/adolescence

Symptoms

Hemorrhage 50% with 2% to 3%/year cumulative risk

Seizures 25%

Neurologic deficit 20% to 25%

Imaging (see Table 10-1)

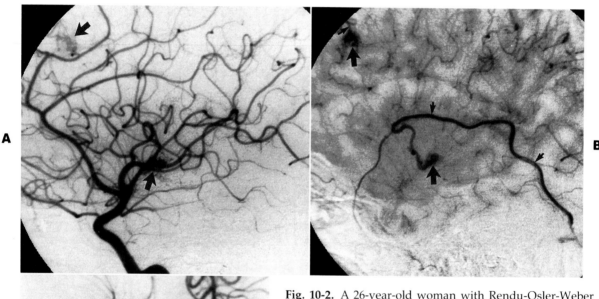

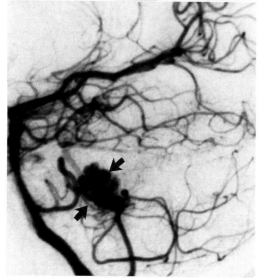

Fig. 10-2. A 26-year-old woman with Rendu-Osler-Weber syndrome presented with posterior fossa hemorrhage. Four-vessel digital subtraction cerebral angiogram disclosed seven intracranial AVMs; three are shown here. **A,** Left internal carotid angiogram, arterial phase, lateral view, shows tangles of abnormal vessels in the frontal and temporal lobes *(arrows)*. **B,** Same study, capillary phase. The two AVMs *(large arrows)* are clearly seen. Note prominent early draining veins *(small arrows)*. **C,** Left vertebral angiogram, arterial phase, lateral view, shows another AVM *(arrows)* fed by branches of the anterior and posterior inferior cerebellar arteries.

Location. Eighty-five percent of all pial AVMs are found in the cerebral hemispheres, and 15% occur in the posterior fossa. Although they can be found in virtually any location, the typical parenchymal AVM extends from the subpial surface of the brain through the cortex and underlying white matter. AVMs are often shaped like a cone with its base on the cortex and apex pointing toward the ventricle (Fig. 10-1, *B*).[1]

Incidence and clinical presentation

Incidence. Parenchymal AVMs are the common symptomatic vascular malformation. Both sexes are affected equally. AVMs are usually solitary lesions, although approximately 2% are multiple. Although multiple AVMs can occur spontaneously,[10] they are usually associated with extracerebral cutaneous or vascular anomalies.

Multiple AVMs are seen in Rendu-Osler-Weber (ROW) and Wyburn-Mason syndromes[11-12] (*see* Chapter 5). ROW is characterized by multiple capillary telangiectasias of the skin and mucosa plus pulmonary arteriovenous fistulae and brain AVMs (Fig. 10-2). Wyburn-Mason is characterized by retinal and brain AVMs with multiple cutaneous nevi[12] (Fig. 10-3). Other than these two neurocutaneous syndromes, there is no known genetic predisposition for developing brain AVMs.

Age. AVMs are congenital lesions. Although about one quarter of all AVMs hemorrhage within the first 15 years of life, the common age at presentation is between 20 and 40 years.[13-15] The majority of AVMs become symptomatic by age 50.

Symptoms. About half of all AVMs hemorrhage, and 25% have seizures as the presenting symptom.[16] The remainder have symptoms of mass effect, headaches, vascular steal phenomena, or focal neurologic deficit.[8,16]

Risk. The cumulative risk of hemorrhage from a parenchymal AVM is estimated at 2% to 4% per year.[13,14] Each hemorrhagic episode carries a 30% risk of death and about 25% risk of significant long-term morbidity.[13-15] There is no difference in hemorrhage rates between supra- and infratentorial lesions.[17]

Although some authors state that the size of an AVM and the presence of treated or untreated hypertension are of little or no value in predicting AVM rupture,[15] others have found that small AVMs are more likely to bleed than large lesions.[17,18] Smaller AVMs also have significantly higher feeding artery pressures.[18]

Other characteristics that have been correlated with hemorrhage are central (deep) venous drainage pattern, peri- or intraventricular location, and presence of an intranidal aneurysm[9,19] (see subsequent discussion). Factors that correlate with decreased risk of hemorrhage are a peripheral or mixed venous drainage pattern and the presence of angiomatous change (i.e., presence of dilated cortical vessels derived from arteries not usually expected to supply the territory occupied by an AVM).[19]

Imaging. Comparative imaging findings of intracranial vascular malformations are summarized in Table 10-1.

Cerebral angiography. Parenchymal AVMs appear as tightly packed masses of enlarged feeding arteries

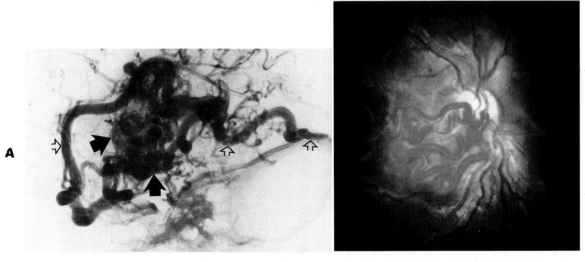

Fig. 10-3. Patient with Wyburn-Mason syndrome. Late arterial phase film, **(A)** lateral view, of the left internal carotid angiogram shows extensive basal ganglionic and midbrain AVMs *(black arrows)* with early draining veins *(open arrows)*. Funduscopic examination **(B)** shows an extensive retinal AVM. (Courtesy K. Kikuchi; reprinted from *CT: The Journal of Computed Tomography*, 12:111-115, 1988.)

Table 10-1. Imaging of Intracranial Vascular Malformations

Malformation	Angiography	Computed tomography	Magnetic resonance imaging
AVMs *Parenchymal (pial)* Patent	Enlarged arteries, veins AV shunting, "early" draining veins Minimal mass effect	Iso/hyperdense on NECT Strong serpentine enhancement on CECT ± hematoma, edema, mass effect Calcification 25% to 30%	Tightly packed flow voids Gliosis (hyperintense on T2WI) Hemorrhage (variable signal) MRA shows vessels, nidus
Thrombosed	May be normal + mass effect "stagnant" flow Subtle AV shunting	Calcification frequent Variable enhancement	Mixed signal lesion
Dural	Enlarged dural arteries AV shunting Stenotic/occluded dural sinus common	May be normal + enlarged dural sinus, venous varix	May be normal PC MRA can show flow direction in fistulae
Capillary telangiectasias	Often normal Racemose type may show faint blush ROW has vascular "nests" in nasopharyngeal mucosa	Normal/hyperdense on NECT Variable calcification Variable enhancement Usually no mass effect, edema	Racemose type may show curvilinear faint enhancement Cavernous type often hypointense, like cavernous angiomas
Cavernous angiomas	Usually normal	Iso/hyperdense on NECT Variable calcification Minimal/no enhancement on CECT Edema, mass effect usually absent	Mixed signal reticulated core, hemosiderin/ferritin rim "Blooms" on T2WI, GRE 50% to 80% multiple

---

Etiology of "Early Draining" Veins on Angiograms
Common Arteriovenous malformation Cerebral infarction (with "luxury perfusion") Neoplasm 　Primary (e.g., glioblastoma multiforme) 　Metastatic (e.g., renal cell carcinoma) **Uncommon** Contusion, resolving hematoma Post-ictal Infection (abscess, encephalitis)

and dilated, tortuous draining veins with little or no intervening brain parenchyma within the AVM nidus itself (Fig. 10-4). On the arterial phase of cerebral angiograms a parenchymal AVM often appears wedge-shaped with a broad cortically based mass of tangled, snarled vessels that extends toward the subependymal surface (Figs. 10-1 and 10-5).

Uncomplicated AVMs have minimal or no mass effect unless a hematoma or venous varix is present. Arteriovenous shunting with abnormally early filling of veins that drain the lesion is characteristic of, but not pathognomonic for, AVM. Other causes of so-called early draining veins are shown in the box.[20]

With the increasing use of superselective angiography in the diagnosis and the treatment of AVMs, subtle angiographic findings that may be overlooked on routine studies can be seen. Superselective studies delineate the internal angioarchitecture in detail (Fig. 10-5). The presence or absence of dysplastic an-

Malformation	Angiography	Computed tomography	Magnetic resonance imaging
Venous malformations Venous angioma (developmental venous anomaly)	Arterial phase normal ± blush in capillary phase "Medusa head" of enlarged medullary veins Enlarged transcortical or subependymal draining vein	NECT normal CECT shows tuft of vessels near ventricle, dilated draining vein	Tubular and stellate vessels, variable signal Strong enhancement 10% to 15% have gliotic, hemorrhagic changes in adjacent brain
Vein of Galen malformation	Enlarged choroidal/thalamoperformating arteries Aneurysmal enlargement of vein of Galen Accessory/falcine sinus common May have atretic straight sinus, slow flow, and thrombosis	Iso/hyperdense posterior third ventricular mass on NECT Strong enhancement on CECT Obstructive hydrocephalus, encephalomalacia common	Mixed signal from turbulent flow common along with areas of high-velocity signal loss
Venous varices	Coexisting high-flow AVM or AVF, less often venous angioma Saccular or fusiform enlargement of cortical/deep veins May have sinus pericranii	Iso/hyperdense serpentine or saccular vessels on NECT Strong uniform enhancement on CECT	Ovoid/fusiform vessels often with high-velocity signal loss

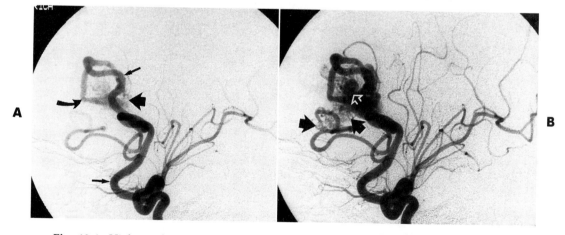

Fig. 10-4. High resolution (1024 × 1024) digital subtraction left internal carotid angiogram, lateral view, shows the typical findings of a pial AVM. **A,** Early arterial phase frame shows enlarged MCA branches *(small arrows)* feeding the AVM nidus *(large arrow)*. Flow-related angiopathic change is illustrated by the stenosis *(curved arrow)* of a feeding artery. Note the relative absence of mass effect. **B,** Slightly later frame shows the nidus *(black arrows)* more clearly. An enlarged vascular channel within the AVM could represent an intranidal aneurysm or venous ectasia *(open arrow).*   *Continued.*

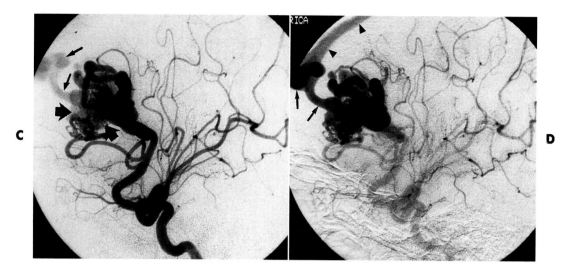

Fig. 10-4, cont'd. C, Midarterial frame again shows the nidus *(large arrows).* Arteriovenous shunting is seen as early appearance of contrast in an enlarged cortical draining vein *(small arrows).* **D,** Late arterial phase study shows drainage into dilated cortical veins *(arrows)* and the superior sagittal sinus *(arrowheads).*

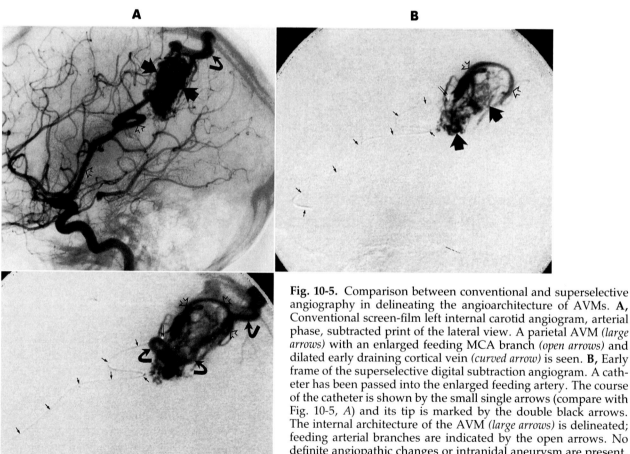

Fig. 10-5. Comparison between conventional and superselective angiography in delineating the angioarchitecture of AVMs. **A,** Conventional screen-film left internal carotid angiogram, arterial phase, subtracted print of the lateral view. A parietal AVM *(large arrows)* with an enlarged feeding MCA branch *(open arrows)* and dilated early draining cortical vein *(curved arrow)* is seen. **B,** Early frame of the superselective digital subtraction angiogram. A catheter has been passed into the enlarged feeding artery. The course of the catheter is shown by the small single arrows (compare with Fig. 10-5, *A*) and its tip is marked by the double black arrows. The internal architecture of the AVM *(large arrows)* is delineated; feeding arterial branches are indicated by the open arrows. No definite angiopathic changes or intranidal aneurysm are present. **C,** Later frame shows contrast in enlarged cortical draining veins *(curved arrows).* Slightly different digital masking allows the catheter *(single small arrows)* to be seen more clearly; its tip is again indicated by the double black arrows. Feeding arteries *(open arrows)* can be distinguished from draining veins *(curved arrows)* on this superselective study.

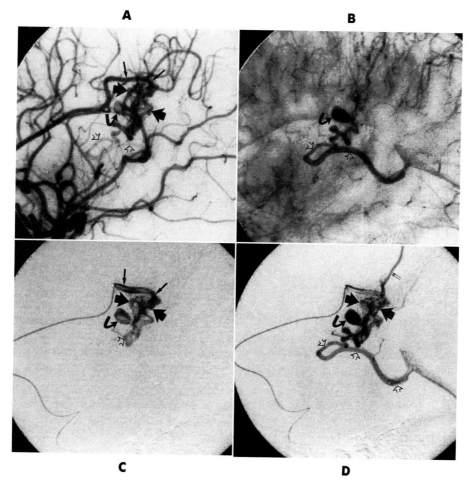

Fig. 10-6. Early **(A)** and late **(B)** arterial frames of the lateral projection show the AVM *(large arrows),* enlarged ACA feeding branches *(small arrows),* early draining veins *(open arrows),* and intranidal lesion *(curved arrow).* Early **(C)** and later **(D)** frames of the superselective distal ACA angiogram, lateral view, show the AVM nidus *(large arrows)* and feeding ACA branch *(small arrows).* An intranidal aneurysm *(curved arrow)* is present. Arteriovenous shunting into deep subependymal *(open arrows)* and cortical veins *(double arrows)* is seen.

eurysms on feeding vessels can be determined, intralesional aneurysms differentiated from venous ectasias (Fig. 10-6), and arteriovenous fistulae within the lesion nidus demonstrated.[21]

A flow-related aneurysm on the circle of Willis or within the AVM nidus (Fig. 10-6, *E* and *F*) is seen in 10% to 12% of all cases.[9] In some cases, stenosis or occlusion of feeding arteries or draining veins is also present, probably representing flow-induced angiopathic vascular disease (Figs. 10-1, 10-4, *A*).

Occasionally an AVM is diffuse and appears to involve an entire lobe. Unlike most AVMs (compare Fig. 10-5, *A*), an identifiable compact nidus is not present and the AVM seems to be a diffuse collection of multiple tortuous vessels with multiple arterial feeders and numerous draining veins (Fig. 10-7). Deep venous drainage is common. Histopathology in

these unusual cases shows AVM vessels interspersed among some normal-appearing neurons and white matter.[22]

Completely thrombosed AVMs may have a normal angiogram, show only a minimal avascular mass effect, or demonstrate very subtle arteriovenous shunting, seen as an early draining vein without dilated feeding vessels or an identifiable vascular nidus.[22a] Occasionally arteries with slow blood flow visible into the late arterial or capillary phases can be seen. These abnormal vessels have been termed *stagnating arteries* (Fig. 10-8). Stagnating arteries are also sometimes present on the postoperative angiograms of excised AVMs.[23]

The angiographic differential diagnosis of a patent AVM is limited. Occasionally, highly vascular anaplastic astrocytomas or glioblastoma multiforme can mimic AVM (see subsequent discussion).

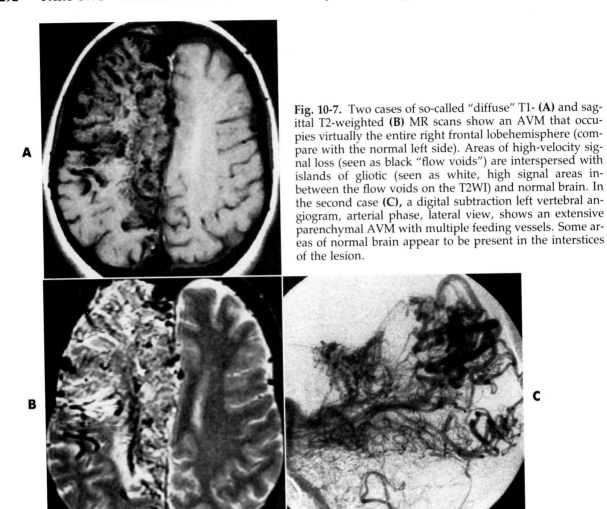

Fig. 10-7. Two cases of so-called "diffuse" T1- (A) and sagittal T2-weighted (B) MR scans show an AVM that occupies virtually the entire right frontal lobehemisphere (compare with the normal left side). Areas of high-velocity signal loss (seen as black "flow voids") are interspersed with islands of gliotic (seen as white, high signal areas inbetween the flow voids on the T2WI) and normal brain. In the second case (C), a digital subtraction left vertebral angiogram, arterial phase, lateral view, shows an extensive parenchymal AVM with multiple feeding vessels. Some areas of normal brain appear to be present in the interstices of the lesion.

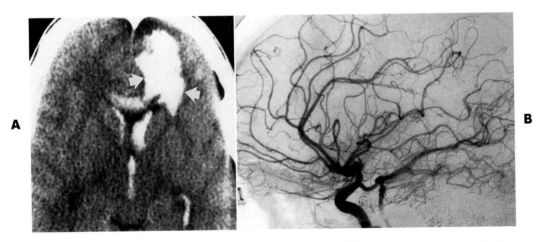

Fig. 10-8. A 16-year-old male had a seizure. A, Initial NECT scan disclosed a small left frontal lobe hematoma (arrows) with some peri- and intraventricular hemorrhage. B, Left internal carotid angiogram, midarterial phase, lateral view, appears normal.

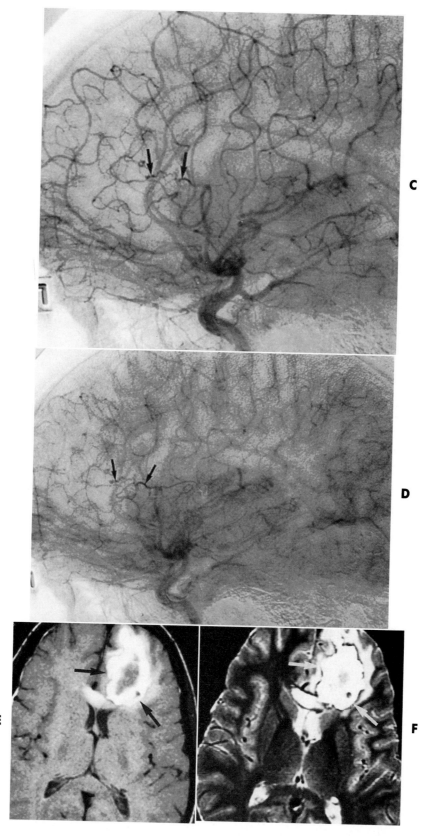

Fig. 10-8, cont'd. C, Late arterial phase film shows some small abnormal vessels that have an irregular, beaded appearance *(arrows)*. **D,** Capillary phase film shows contrast stagnation in these abnormal vessels *(arrows)*. No early draining veins were identified. Axial T1- **(E)** and T2-weighted **(F)** MR scans obtained 10 days later show subacute blood *(arrows)*. A completely thrombosed AVM was found at surgery.

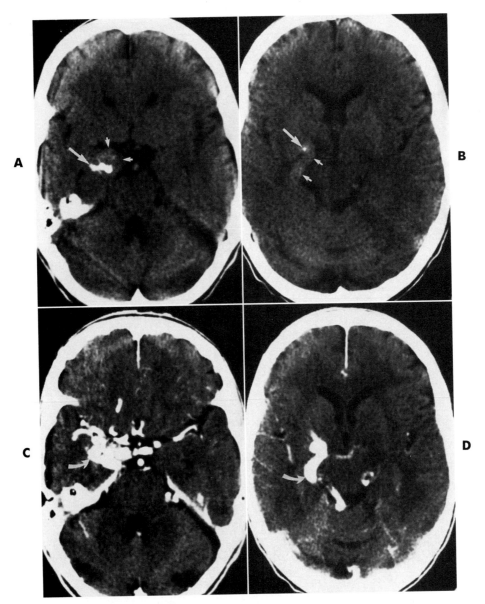

Fig. 10-9. Patient with seizures and a classic temporal lobe AVM. **A** and **B,** Precontrast CT scans show slightly hyperdense areas *(small arrows)* in the medial right temporal lobe with calcific foci *(large arrows).* **C** and **D,** Postcontrast studies show multiple intensely enhancing round and serpentine lesions *(arrows).*

Computed tomography (CT). CT findings of patent AVMs include serpiginous isointense or slightly hyperintense vessels that enhance strongly following contrast administration. Calcification is identified in 25% to 30% of cases (Fig. 10-9). Sometimes an AVM has a small nidus but very prominent enlarged draining veins (Fig. 10-10). Occasionally even large AVMs are identified only after contrast administration (Fig. 10-11). Angiographic-like images can be obtained using spiral CT and maximum intensity reprojection of the axial data set (Fig. 10-15).

CT scans are useful for demonstrating acute hemorrhage from AVMs[24] (*see* Chapter 7). CT also may show subtle changes that are not evident at angiography. These include local and distant mass effects, the presence of surrounding edema and focal compression, and distortion and displacement of normal anatomic structures by the AVM or its afferent and efferent vessels.[25] MRI is superior for delineating subacute or chronic hemorrhage, as well as secondary changes such as mass effect, edema, and ischemic changes in the adjacent brain[8,26] (see subsequent discussion).

Magnetic resonance imaging (MRI). The MR findings in patent parenchymal AVMs are variable and depend on the flow rate and direction in feeding

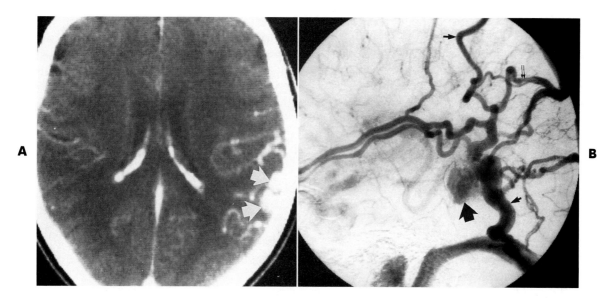

Fig. 10-10. A, Axial postcontrast CT scan in a patient with seizures shows prominent superficial cortical vessels *(arrows).* **B,** Digital subtraction left internal carotid angiogram, late arterial phase, lateral view. A small AVM nidus is seen *(large arrow)* but the most striking abnormalities are the numerous enlarged draining veins *(small single arrows).* Note venous angiopathic changes of focal stenosis *(double arrows).*

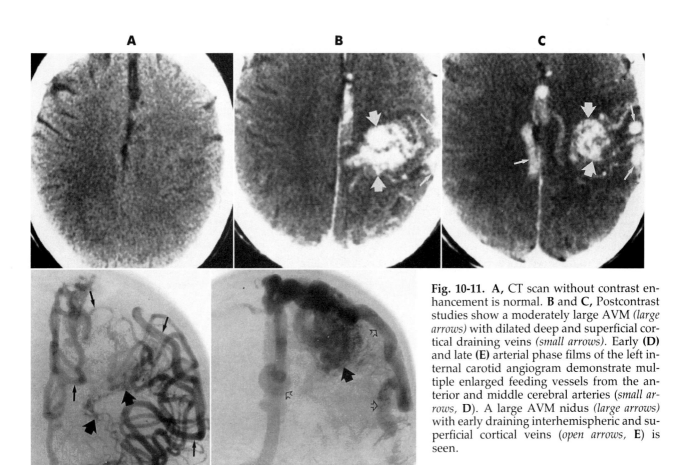

A   **B**   **C**

Fig. 10-11. A, CT scan without contrast enhancement is normal. **B** and **C,** Postcontrast studies show a moderately large AVM *(large arrows)* with dilated deep and superficial cortical draining veins *(small arrows).* Early **(D)** and late **(E)** arterial phase films of the left internal carotid angiogram demonstrate multiple enlarged feeding vessels from the anterior and middle cerebral arteries *(small arrows,* **D**). A large AVM nidus *(large arrows)* with early draining interhemispheric and superficial cortical veins *(open arrows,* **E**) is seen.

D   **E**

and draining vessels, presence of hemorrhage, and secondary changes in the brain. On standard spin-echo images the typical unruptured AVM appears as a tightly packed "honeycomb" of "flow voids" caused by high-velocity signal loss (Fig. 10-12, *A*). Areas of increased signal may be seen in thrombosed vessels or vessels with slow or turbulent flow (Fig. 10-12, *B*).

Hemorrhage in different stages of evolution is commonly present in AVMs. Patent AVMs with hyperacute clot show areas of high-velocity signal loss with adjacent hemorrhage that is typically isointense to brain on T1WI, hyperintense on T2-weighted sequences, and low signal on gradient-refocussed studies (Fig. 10-13). Because hemorrhage in AVMs evolves as the clot matures (*see* Chapter 7), associated

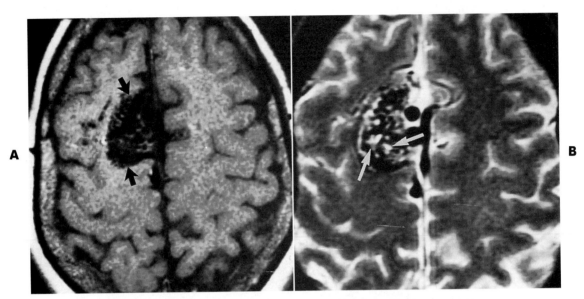

Fig. 10-12. Axial **(A)** T1-weighted MR scan of an unruptured AVM shows the nidus as a tightly packed "honeycomb" of enlarged vessels *(arrows)*. Note absence of mass effect. Axial T2-weighted scan **(B)** shows some round high signal foci *(arrows)* within the nidus that probably represent thrombosed vessels.

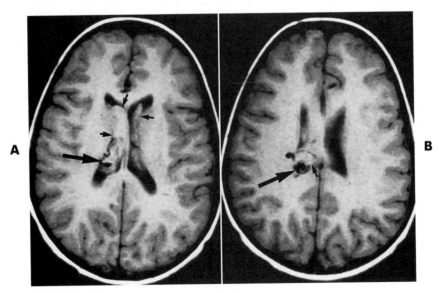

Fig. 10-13. A 6-year-old boy had a seizure. NECT scan (not shown) disclosed intraventricular hemorrhage. An MR scan was performed 4 hours after the first seizure. Axial **(A** and **B)** T1-weighted sequences without contrast enhancement show a deep AVM *(large arrows)* with hyperacute IVH, seen as fluid in the right lateral ventricle *(small black arrows)* that appears isointense with adjacent brain.

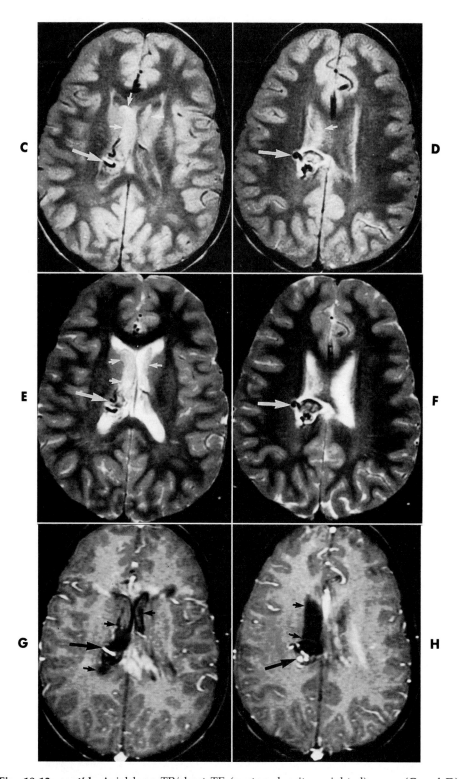

Fig. 10-13, cont'd. Axial long TR/short TE (proton density-weighted) scans **(C** and **D)** show the AVM *(large arrows)*. The IVH *(small arrows)* is hyperintense to white matter and cerebrospinal fluid (CSF). Axial T2-weighted scans **(E** and **F)** show the AVM *(large arrows)*. The IVH *(small arrows)* is hyperintense to brain but nearly isointense with high signal CSF, rendering the hyperacute blood nearly invisible. Axial gradient-refocussed scans **(G** and **H)** show the AVM has some patent flow, seen as serpentine high signal areas *(large arrows)*. The hyperacute IVH is profoundly hyperintense *(small arrows)*.

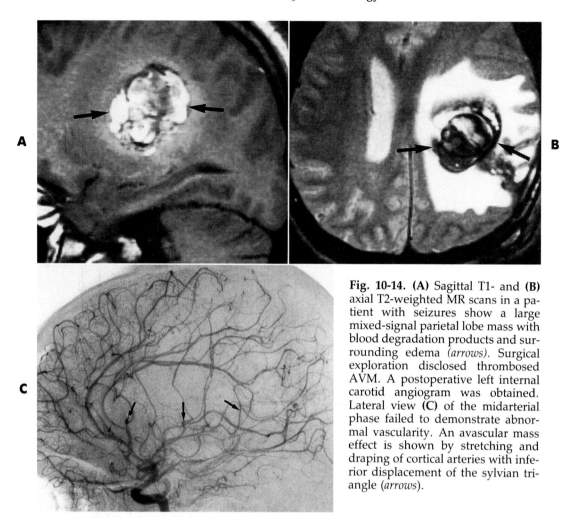

Fig. 10-14. (A) Sagittal T1- and **(B)** axial T2-weighted MR scans in a patient with seizures show a large mixed-signal parietal lobe mass with blood degradation products and surrounding edema *(arrows)*. Surgical exploration disclosed thrombosed AVM. A postoperative left internal carotid angiogram was obtained. Lateral view **(C)** of the midarterial phase failed to demonstrate abnormal vascularity. An avascular mass effect is shown by stretching and draping of cortical arteries with inferior displacement of the sylvian triangle *(arrows)*.

subacute hematomas usually display mixed signal intensities (Fig. 10-14, *A* and *B*). Chronic hemorrhages with hemosiderin or ferritin appear as areas of hypointense signal within and around the AVM on T2-weighted and gradient-echo scans.[27]

Hypoperfusion of brain adjacent to an AVM, the so-called steal phenomenon, occurs when arterial blood is shunted through the relatively low-resistance arteriovenous fistulae of the AVM and away from the higher-resistence capillary bed in adjacent normal brain.[28] This may cause atrophy and gliosis of brain tissue that is not directly part of the AVM (Fig. 10-15). These changes are best delineated on MR and appear as areas of increased T2 signal within shrunken, atrophic brain. Secondary hemorrhagic laminar cortical necrosis is occasionally seen as hyperintense gyriform foci on T1WI (Fig. 10-15, *A*) and linear low signal areas on T2-weighted studies (Fig. 10-15, *B*).

As with cerebral angiography, the MR differential diagnosis of uncomplicated AVM is limited. Occa-

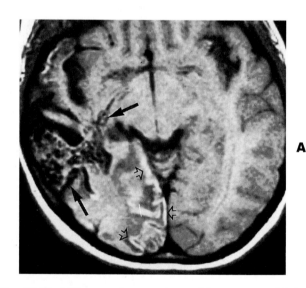

Fig. 10-15. MR scans in a patient with a temporal lobe AVM. Axial T1- **(A)** and T2-weighted scans **(B)** show the AVM *(large arrows)*. Extensive atrophy and gliosis are also present. Note occipital lobe hemorrhagic cortical infarction *(open arrows)* caused by "steal" from the posterior cerebral artery territory to supply the AVM. Gradient-refocussed study **(C)** shows flow in the AVM *(arrows)*.

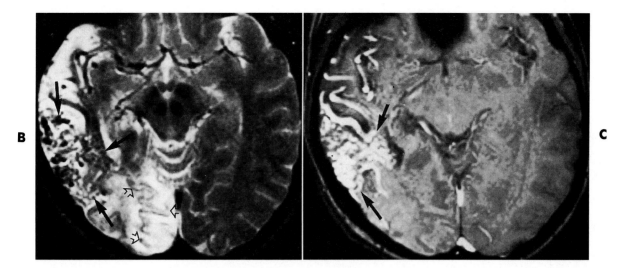

Fig. 10-15, cont'd. For legend see p. 298.

sionally a very vascular neoplasm can mimic AVM at angiography, although MR typically demonstrates more tissue between vessels than is seen with AVMs (Fig. 10-16). Thrombosed AVMs with hemorrhage usually have a complete hemosiderin rim (Fig. 10-8). Occasionally an AVM with repeated bleeds may have a very complex appearance and be difficult to distinguish from hemorrhagic neoplasm (Fig. 10-14) (*see* box, p. 190).

Magnetic resonance angiography (MRA). The sensitivity of MR to flow phenomena can be used to provide projection angiographic images of flowing blood. Numerous MRA pulse sequences have been

devised, and each has its own unique advantages and disadvantages.[29] Single pedicle AVMs are delineated well with most techniques, although complete definition of complex lesions and their internal angioarchitecture requires cerebral angiography.[30]

The two major MRA techniques that are currently used are time-of-flight (TOF) and phase-contrast (PC) MRA. A modified TOF MRA technique, multiple overlapping thin slab acquisition (MOTSA), combines the advantages of two- and three-dimensional time-of-flight techniques and detects most AVMs (Fig. 10-17).[30] PC MRA allows velocity determination and yields directional flow information in the vessels

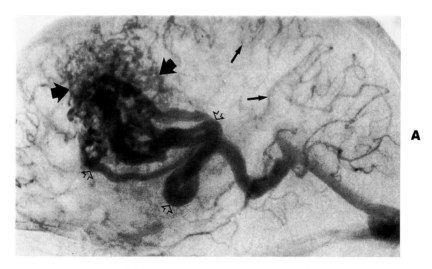

Fig. 10-16. A, Right internal carotid angiogram, late arterial phase, lateral view, shows a highly vascular posterior frontal lobe lesion *(large arrows).* Arteriovenous shunting with early draining veins *(open arrows)* is seen. Angiographically the lesion somewhat resembles an AVM, although the amount of edema and mass effect *(small black arrows)* would be unusual for an uncomplicated vascular malformation.   *Continued.*

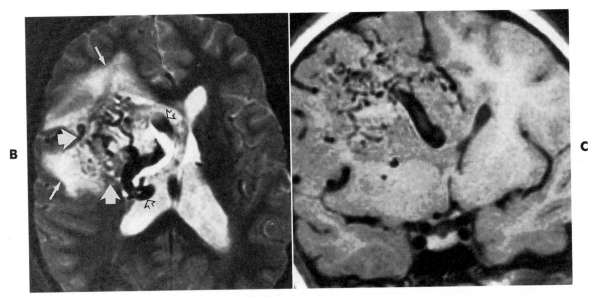

Fig. 10-16, cont'd. B, Axial T2-weighted MR scan shows the lesion *(large arrows)* has significant edema *(small arrows)*. Some areas of brain parenchyma are present within the lesion. Note prominent draining veins (open arrows). **C,** Coronal T1-weighted MR scan shows multiple foci of high-velocity signal loss are interspersed with significant amounts of brain parenchyma, making malignant brain tumor more likely than AVM. Anaplastic astrocytoma was found at surgery.

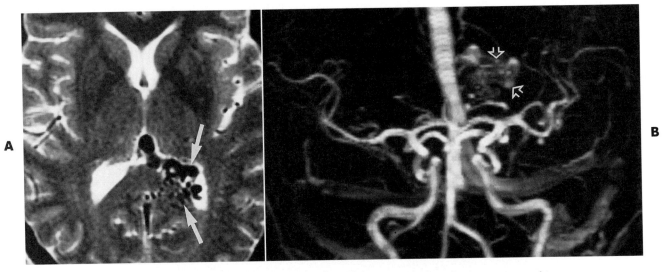

Fig. 10-17. Small para- and intraventricular AVM is nicely delineated using a combination of standard spin-echo images and MRA. Axial T2-weighted scan **(A)** shows the lesion as multiple foci of high-velocity signal loss in the corpus callosum splenium and choroid plexus *(arrows)*. Coronal 3D TOF MRA with multiple overlapping thin-slab technique (MOTSA) **(B)** demonstrates the lesion nidus *(arrows)*.

feeding an AVM, as well as those supplying adjacent brain.[31] PC MRA is also helpful in delineating very small AVMs (Fig. 10-18).

Treatment. With a mortality rate of 1.3% and morbidity as low as 7.8% in experienced hands, elective surgical resection is recommended for unruptured AVMs, particularly in young patients with lesions that have a favorable location, size, and venous drainage pattern.[16] Because the risk of hemorrhage is high, complete obliteration of an AVM nidus is the goal regardless of treatment modality. Surgical resection, endovascular occlusion, stereotactic radiation, or a combination of these modalities are all currently

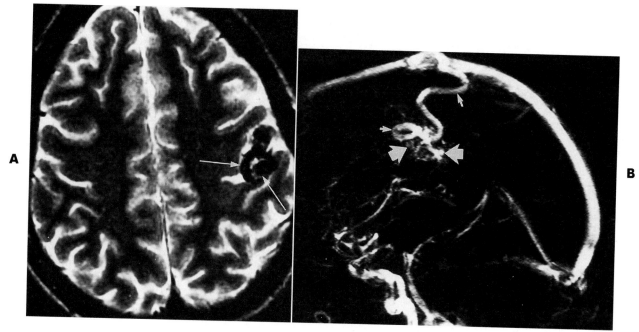

Fig. 10-18. A, Very small cortical AVM is barely visible on this T2-weighted scan. A few foci of high-velocity signal loss are seen *(arrows)*. **B,** Phase-contrast MRA shows the lesion nidus *(large arrows)* and cortical draining vein *(small arrows)*.

used. Stereotaxic angiography is a useful diagnostic and targeting adjunct for the treatment of AVMs, particularly small lesions.[32]

Endovascular techniques are commonly used as an adjunct to reduce the size of larger AVMs prior to treatment. Preoperative embolization with nidus-occluding substances such as *N*-butyl cyanoacrylate makes larger, higher grade AVMs the surgical equivalent of smaller, lower grade lesions by reducing operative time and intraoperative blood loss.[33]

Dural AVMs and Fistulae *(see box)*

Dural vascular malformations consist of arteriovenous malformations (DAVMs) and arteriovenous fistulae (DAVFs).

Pathology and etiology

Gross pathology. Thickened dural arteries and dilated dural veins form an abnormal vascular network within the wall of a venous sinus. Unlike brain AVMs, DAVMs seldom have a discrete nidus. Instead, the malformation is composed of numerous arteriovenous microfistulae.[34] Stenosis or occlusion of the sinus lumen is often but not invariably present in DAVMs[35] (Fig. 10-19).

Etiology. Although parenchymal AVMs are congenital lesions, most dural vascular malformations are acquired abnormalities. Some authors postulate that DAVMs arise following sinus thrombosis or occlusion. With subsequent recanalization, numerous

---

Dural AVMs
Pathology: network of microfistulae with thickened dural arteries, dilated draining veins in wall of dural sinus
Etiology: sinus thrombosis and recanalization
Location: posterior fossa, skull base
Age at presentation: between 40 and 60 years
Symptoms: bruit, proptosis, cranial nerve palsies common
Hemorrhage: uncommon unless intracranial venous varices
Imaging: *see* Table 10-1

small direct artery-to-sinus communications, or "microfistulae," are formed.[34] Others theorize that a single arteriovenous fistula initially forms in the dura near a venous sinus and, as blood flow increases, adjacent dural arteries are subsequently recruited and form a DAVM.

The vessels that supply a DAVM gradually become thickened and tortuous. Dural draining veins also dilate and thicken. This is followed by dilatation and thickening of the fistula within the sinus wall itself. Thrombogenesis and intimal injury secondary to turbulent flow produce regional thrombus formation, eventually resulting in stenosis or occlusion of the sinus lumen.[35]

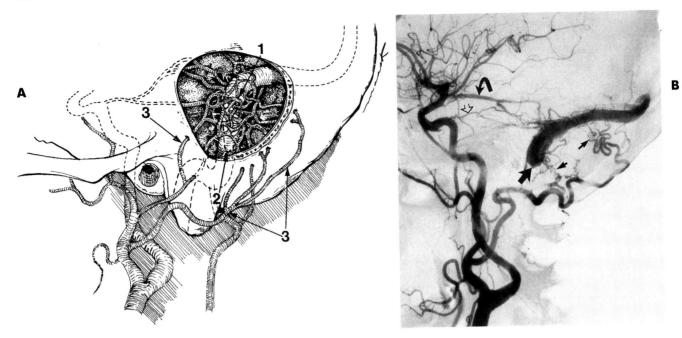

Fig. 10-19. A, Anatomic diagram of a transverse sinus AVM. The calvarium over the transverse and sigmoid sinuses has been removed to show the vascular malformation. *1,* Tangle of dural arteries and draining veins in the transverse and sigmoid sinus wall forms the dural AVM. *2,* Dotted line shows the sinus lumen is occluded. *3,* Transosseous feeders arise from the occipital, posterior auricular, and vertebral arteries to supply the AVM. **B,** Common carotid angiogram, arterial phase, lateral view, of a dural AVM. The transverse sinus is occluded *(large arrow)* and multiple transosseous feeders from the occipital artery *(small arrows)* supply the lesion. Note enlarged meningohypophyseal trunk *(open arrow)* and posterior division of the middle meningeal artery *(curved arrow)* also contribute vascular supply to the dural AVM.

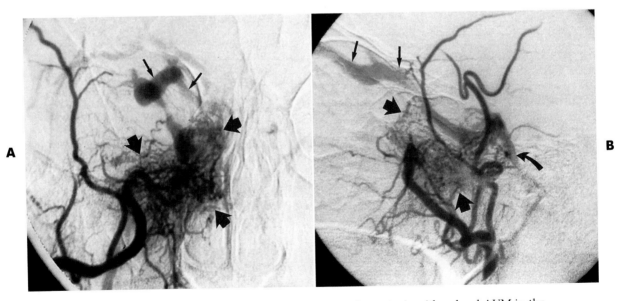

Fig. 10-20. Elderly woman with bruit, chemosis, and proptosis with a dural AVM in the cavernous sinus. AP **(A)** and lateral **(B)** views of the selective right external carotid angiogram show numerous enlarged dural vessels that comprise the lesion *(large arrows).* Arteriovenous shunting into the superior ophthalmic vein *(small arrows)* and clival venous plexus *(curved arrow)* is present.

Location. Most dural vascular malformations involve the venous sinuses along the base of the brain; the transverse or sigmoid sinus is most frequently affected (Fig. 10-19, *B*). The cavernous sinus is also a common site (Fig. 10-20).[36] The superior sagittal sinus and straight sinus are uncommon sites.[36]

DAVFs are usually solitary. With the exception of bilateral cavernous sinus DAVFs, multiple dural fistulae are uncommon and account for only 7% of all DAVFs (Fig. 10-21). No known predisposing conditions for multiplicity are known, although hypercoagulable states could conceivably lead to thrombosis and subsequent fistulization at several sites.[37]

Incidence and clinical presentation

Incidence. Dural vascular malformations account for 10% to 15% of all intracranial arteriovenous malformations. One third of posterior fossa AVMs are purely dural. These most often involve the transverse or sigmoid sinuses.[38]

Age. Most dural vascular malformations become symptomatic between the ages of 40 and 60 years.[39]

Clinical presentation. Clinical signs of DAVMs and DAVFs vary according to their location and type of venous drainage.[40] Bruit and headache are the most common symptoms of DAVF involving the transverse or sigmoid sinuses, whereas proptosis,

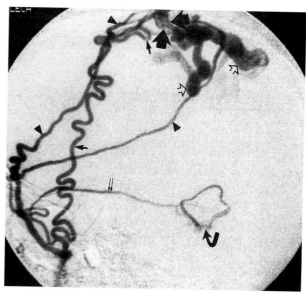

Fig. 10-21. Digital subtraction external carotid angiogram, early arterial phase, lateral view, of a 40-year-old man with multiple dural AVFs. Transosseous branches of an enlarged superficial temporal artery *(small single arrows)* and anterior branches of the middle meningeal artery *(arrowheads)* supply a dural AVF *(large arrows)* near the superior sagittal sinus. Drainage is primarily via dilated cortical veins *(open arrows)*. Posterior branches of the middle meningeal artery *(double arrows)* supply a second AVF that involves the transverse sinus *(curved arrow)*.

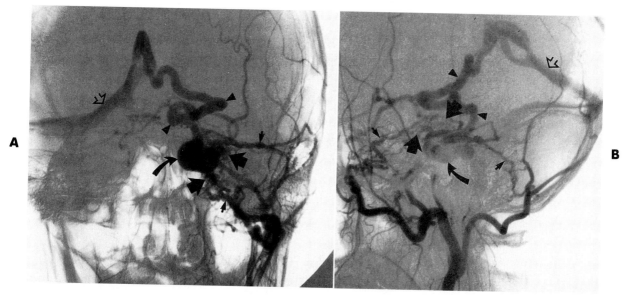

Fig. 10-22. A 27-year-old man with tinnitus and left-sided trigeminal neuralgia. AP **(A)** and lateral **(B)** views of the selective distal left external carotid angiogram, arterial phase, show a dural AVM *(large arrows)* at the petrous apex. Numerous enlarged branches from the internal maxillary and external occipital arteries *(small arrows)* supply the lesion. Venous drainage from this dural vascular malformation is almost exclusively intracranial. A large venous varix *(curved arrow)* drains into prominent lateral mesencephalic veins *(arrowheads)* and from there into the straight and contralateral transverse sinuses *(open arrows)*.

chemosis, retroorbital pain, bruit, and ophthalmoplegia are associated with cavernous sinus lesions[41] (Fig. 10-24). If the DAVF involves a dural sinus that contacts the petrous pyramid, pulse-synchronous tinnitus may result.[36] Cavernous sinus lesions, as well as DAVMs with intracranial venous varices, can have cranial nerve palsies as their most prominent or sole clinical manifestation (Fig. 10-22).

Venous drainage patterns are important determinants of clinical presentation. If venous drainage is unobstructed and drainage occurs directly into a sinus with normal flow direction, collateral cortical venous pathways usually do not develop, and hemorrhagic complications are uncommon. However, if reflux into cortical veins is present or if there is direct drainage into cortical veins with retrograde flow, subarachnoid or intracerebral hemorrhage is common (Fig. 10-23).[38]

Risk and complications. DAVMs rarely cause intracranial hemorrhage. However, the presence of intracranial venous varices carries an increased risk of hemorrhage and intracranial mass effect with subsequent symptoms such as cranial nerve palsy (Fig. 10-22). Retrograde venous flow accompanied by increased venous pressure may also lead to hemorrhagic venous infarction and focal neurologic deficit (Fig. 10-23). Obstructive hydrocephalus from direct mechanical cerebral aqueduct compression or communicating hydrocephalus with decreased CSF absorption caused by chronic passive venous congestion and elevated venous pressure can also occur.[36]

Imaging of DAVMs and DAVFs (*see* Table 10-1)
Cerebral angiography. Any dural vessel is a potential supply source to dural vascular malformations (Fig. 10-24). Most DAVMs have multiple feeders. Be-

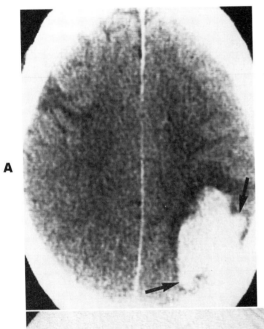

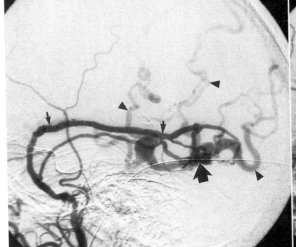

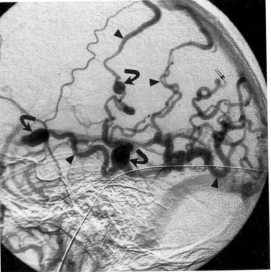

Fig. 10-23. A 40-year-old normotensive man with intracranial hemorrhage demonstrated on CT scan (**A,** *arrows*). Digital left external carotid angiogram, early (**B**) and late (**C**) arterial phase frames, shows a large dural AVF *(large arrow)* fed by enlarged posterior branches of the middle meningeal artery *(small single arrows)*. Drainage is primarily via numerous enlarged cortical draining veins *(arrowheads)* into the superior sasgittal sinus. Variceal enlargement of several veins *(curved arrows)* is present. One of the parietal draining veins appears to be occluded *(double arrows)* and may have caused hemorrhagic venous infarction. Cortical venous drainage from a dural AVM or AVF is often associated with intracranial hemorrhage. (**A** and **C**, From Jacobs J: Angiography in intracranial hemorrhage, *Neuroimaging Clin N Amer* 2:89-106, 1992.)

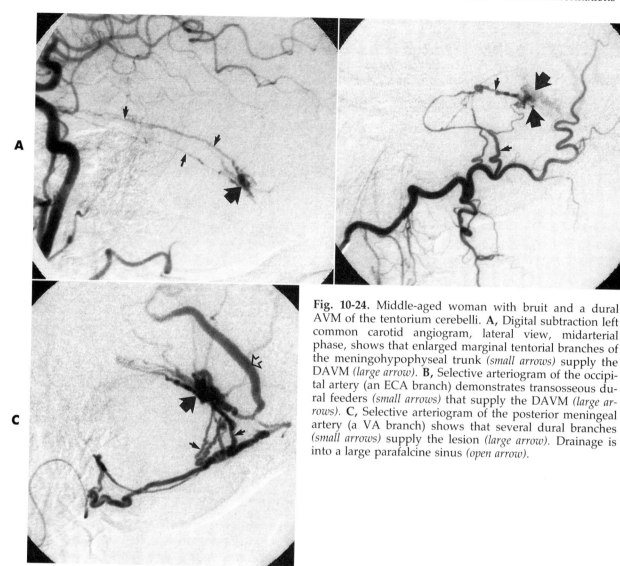

Fig. 10-24. Middle-aged woman with bruit and a dural AVM of the tentorium cerebelli. **A,** Digital subtraction left common carotid angiogram, lateral view, midarterial phase, shows that enlarged marginal tentorial branches of the meningohypophyseal trunk *(small arrows)* supply the DAVM *(large arrow).* **B,** Selective arteriogram of the occipital artery (an ECA branch) demonstrates transosseous dural feeders *(small arrows)* that supply the DAVM *(large arrows).* **C,** Selective arteriogram of the posterior meningeal artery (a VA branch) shows that several dural branches *(small arrows)* supply the lesion *(large arrow).* Drainage is into a large parafalcine sinus *(open arrow).*

cause these lesions usually occur in the posterior fossa, the common vessels that supply DAVMs are the occipital artery and meningeal branches of the external carotid artery. Tentorial and small dural ICA or VA branches are also frequent sources of supply.[42] Dural sinus occlusion is common.

Fistulae between a single dural artery and sinus occasionally occur (Fig. 10-25). A particular kind of DAVF, traumatic carotid-cavernous fistula (CCF), often has a single direct communication between the ICA and cavernous sinus (Fig. 10-26). In these cases, rapid flow can obscure the exact site of fistulous communication unless the vertebral artery is injected during compression of the ipsilateral carotid artery *(see Fig. 8-68).*

A less common type of CCF is seen primarily in middle-aged women with proptosis, bruit, and chemosis. These lesions are often spontaneous and un-

related to trauma. Multiple dural feeders are the rule. Numerous microfistulae within the cavernous sinus wall comprise this type of DAVM (Fig. 10-20).

Computed tomography. CT scans in dural vascular malformations are often normal. Sometimes enlargement of a dural sinus or draining vein can be identified. In CCFs, an enlarged cavernous sinus is seen in half of all cases, and a dilated superior ophthalmic vein can be identified on most contrast-enhanced scans (Fig. 10-24, *A*).

Magnetic resonance imaging. On MR scans the finding of dilated cortical veins without an identifiable parenchymal nidus suggests the presence of a DAVF with associated venoocclusive disease.[36] Routine spin-echo MR is the procedure of choice for demonstrating the complications of DAVF, including infarction and hemorrhage. Conventional MR imaging is less successful at direct visualization of the exact

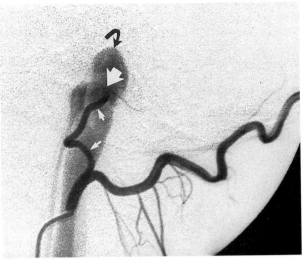

Fig. 10-25. Digital subtraction superselective occipital artery angiogram, early arterial frame, lateral view, of a dural AVF. A single enlarged occipital artery branch *(small arrows)* was the sole source of flow to this DAVF. The fistulous site between the occipital artery and jugular bulb *(curved arrow)* is indicated by the *large arrow*.

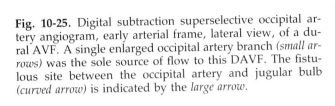

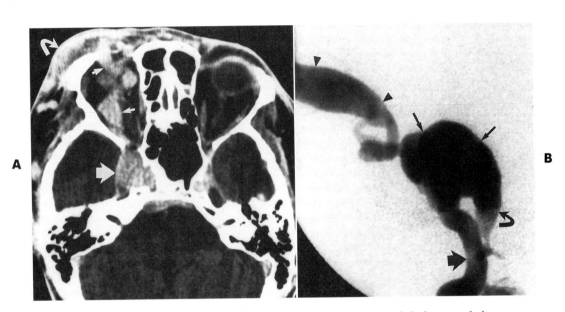

Fig. 10-26. Middle-aged woman with onset of pulsatile right exophthalmos and chemosis 3 months after head trauma. **A,** Postcontrast axial CT scan shows the right cavernous sinus *(large arrow)* and superior ophthalmic vein (SOV) *(small arrows)* are enlarged. Note enlarged eyelid *(curved arrow)*. **B,** Digital subtraction right internal carotid angiogram, lateral view, early arterial phase, shows the ICA *(large arrow)* communicates directly with the massively enlarged cavernous sinus *(small arrows)*. The SOV *(arrowheads)* and clival plexus *(curved arrow)* are enlarged collateral venous drainage channels. No intracranial ICA flow is present. The exact fistulous site is obscured.

fistula site, although dural engorgement can sometimes be seen on postcontrast studies. Enlarged superior ophthalmic veins with CCFs are readily identified (Fig. 10-27, *B*).

The arterial feeders that supply DAVMs are poorly seen on MR unless MRA is used.[43] Phase-contrast MRA can demonstrate flow direction in draining veins and dural sinuses (Fig. 10-27, *C*).

Miscellaneous techniques. Color flow doppler ultrasound studies have been used recently to demonstrate flow reversal in the superior ophthalmic vein caused by CCFs (Fig. 10-27, *D*).

Mixed Pial-Dural AVMs

If a parenchymal (pial) AVM attains sufficient size, it can recruit vascular supply from dural arterial branches. In such cases the malformation has the imaging characteristics of both pial and dural AVMs (Fig. 10-28). Meningeal artery contribution to pial AVMs occurs in 15% to 50% of cases.[43a]

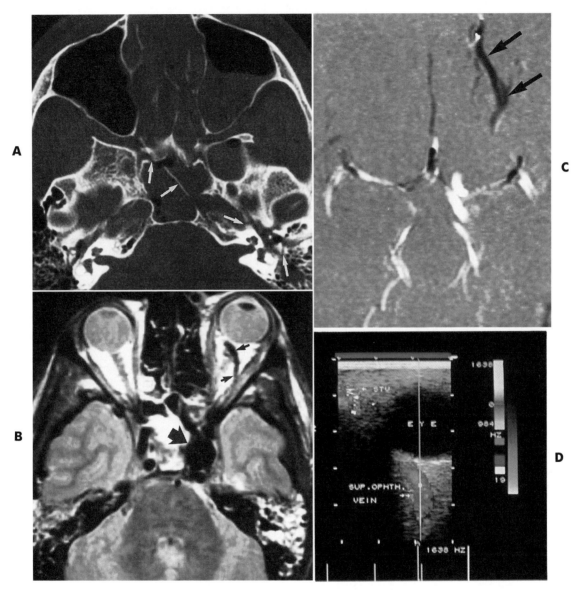

Fig. 10-27. Posttraumatic carotid-cavernous fistula (CCF). **A,** Axial CT scan immediately following the traumatic episode disclosed a comminuted skull base fracture *(arrows).* Ten days later the patient developed left pulsatile exophthalmos. **B,** Axial long TR/short TE (proton density) MR scan shows the left cavernous sinus is enlarged and a prominent area of high-velocity signal loss *(large arrow)* is present. The superior ophthalmic vein (SOV) is enlarged *(small arrows)* and the left globe is mildly proptotic. **C,** Directional-encoded (A/P) PC MRA with flow reversal in the SOV *(arrows)* shows black (normal SOV is extra- to intracranial, i.e., anterior to posterior and would appear white). A CCF was demonstrated on conventional angiographic studies (not shown). **D,** Color flow doppler ultrasound in another case with a dural cavernous sinus fistula shows flow reversal in the SOV (normal SOV flow is blue, not red). (**A** to **C,** Courtesy D. Blatter. **D,** Courtesy P. Flaherty, reprinted from Flaherty P et al: *Arch Ophthal* 109:522-526, 1991.)

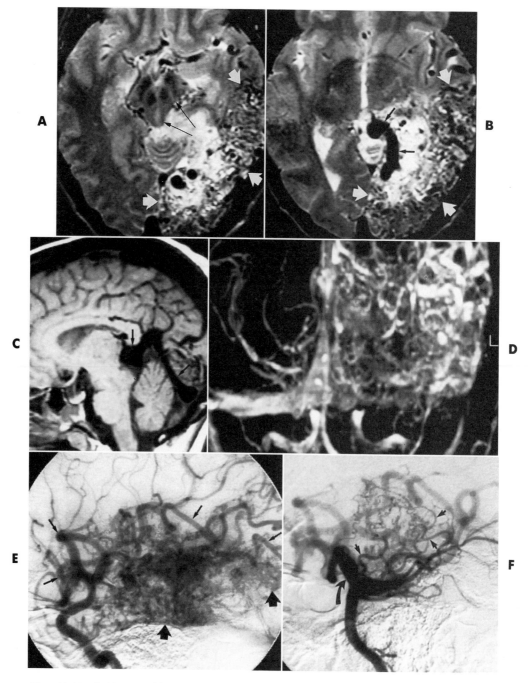

Fig. 10-28. A 28-year-old woman with a huge mixed pial-dural AVM. **A** and **B,** Axial T2-weighted MR scans show the extensive AVM *(large arrows)* involves the entire occipital and part of the parietal lobes. Note variceal enlargement of the vein of Galen (**B,** *black arrows).* Some mass effect is present as shown by midbrain compression (**A,** *black arrows).* **C,** Sagittal T1-weighted scan shows the massively enlarged vein of Galen and straight sinus *(arrows).* **D,** 3D TOF MRA with multiple overlapping thin slab technique shows the huge AVM, but its internal angioarchitecture cannot be determined accurately. **E,** Digital subtraction left internal carotid angiogram, arterial phase, lateral view, shows that the extensive supratentorial AVM *(large arrows)* is supplied by multiple enlarged MCA and PCA branches *(small arrows).* **F,** Digital subtraction left vertebral angiogram, arterial phase, lateral view, shows that a massively enlarged posterior communicating artery *(curved arrow)* and numerous enlarged thalamoperforating and posterior choroidal branches *(small arrows)* supply the AVM.

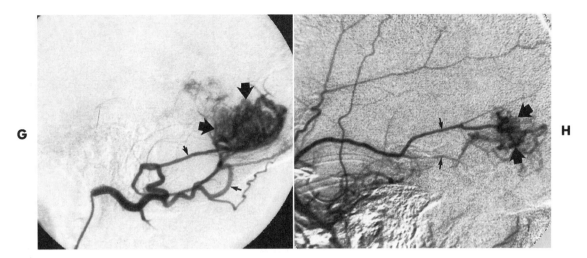

Fig. 10-28, cont'd. G, Digital subtraction superselective occipital artery angiogram, arterial phase, lateral view, shows that multiple enlarged transosseous dural feeders *(small arrows)* have been recruited to supply part of the AVM *(large arrows).* **H,** Digital subtraction distal external carotid angiogram shows that enlarged posterior branches of the middle meningeal artery *(small arrows)* also supply the lesion *(large arrows).*

CAPILLARY TELANGIECTASIAS

Pathology

Gross pathology. Capillary telangiectasias appear as multiple small brown or pink lesions. They most often occur in the pons or cerebellum and are usually incidental findings at autopsy (Fig. 10-29).

Microscopic pathology. Capillary telangiectasias are nests of dilated capillaries whose walls lack smooth muscle and elastic fibers. Racemose capillary telangiectasias have normal brain parenchyma interposed between the dilated, thin-walled vessels that compose the malformation (Fig. 10-30). Gliosis in the surrounding brain is occasionally identified, as is hemosiderin staining from previous hemorrhage.[1]

Capillary telangiectasias also often coexist with cavernous angiomas.[6a] Some authors suggest the two are not separate entities but represent extremes within the same histopathologic spectrum of vascular malformations.[1,2] The "cavernous" form of capillary telangiectasia may be pathologically and radiographically indistinguishable from cavernous angiomas.

Location *(see* box, p. 310). Although capillary telangiectasias may be found in virtually any part of the brain or spinal cord, they have a predilection for the pons. The cerebral cortex and spinal cord are also commonly involved.

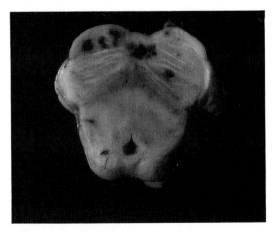

Fig. 10-29. Gross pathology specimen shows multiple small midbrain lesions with brown discoloration. Microscopic examination disclosed capillary telangiectasias. (Courtesy E. Ross.)

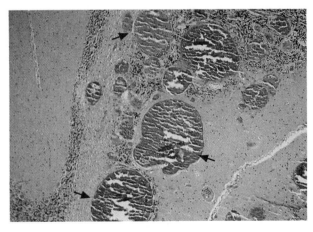

Fig. 10-30. Photomicrograph of a racemose capillary telangiectasia shows multiple dilated vascular channels *(arrows)* that are separated by normal brain parenchyma.

Visceral angiodysplasia with scalp and mucocutaneous telangiectasias is a feature of Rendu-Osler-Weber disease (hereditary hemorrhagic telangiectasia). Twenty-eight percent of patients with Rendu-Osler-Weber syndrome have associated brain vascular malformations; these are typically true AVMs, not capillary telangiectasias (see Fig. 10-2).[44,45]

Incidence and clinical presentation. Capillary telangiectasias are common lesions that are often found at autopsy; they are second only to venous angioma as the most common vascular malformation identified at postmortem examination. Multiple lesions are the rule.[1] Most lesions are small and clinically silent, discovered incidentally at MR scan or autopsy in middle-aged and elderly patients. If they occur in association with cavernous elements, capillary telangiectasias may hemorrhage and become symptomatic.[2]

Capillary Telangiectasias

Pathology: nests of dilated capillaries with interposed normal brain

Location: multiple lesions in pons, spinal cord, and cerebellum but can be anywhere; mucocutaneous lesions with Rendu-Osler-Weber syndrome

Age at presentation: most often found incidentally at autopsy

Symptoms: often none

Imaging: *see* Table 10-1; if seen, multiple "black spots" on T2WI

Imaging findings (*see* Table 10-1)
Cerebral angiography. Intracranial capillary telangiectasias are usually occult to cerebral angiography, although a faint vascular stain can sometimes be identified with racemose telangiectasias. On selective external carotid angiograms the mucocutaneous lesions seen in Rendu-Osler-Weber disease appear as multiple small nests of capillary-like vessels with vascular staining. Because severe epistaxis is common in these cases, active hemorrhage can sometimes be

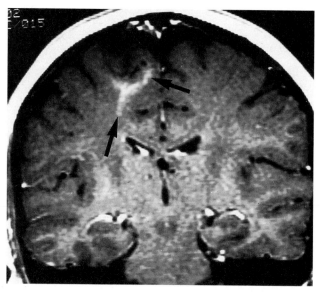

Fig. 10-31. Postcontrast coronal T1-weighted MR scan shows a parietal lobe racemose capillary telangiectasia (*arrows*) in this patient with left temporal lobe seizures. Other sections (not shown) disclosed a smaller lesion in the subcortical white matter of the left temporal lobe.

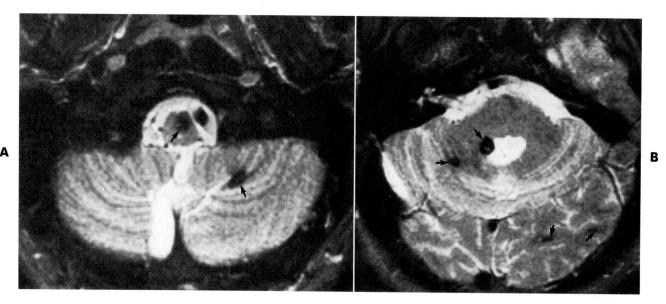

Fig. 10-32. Axial T2-weighted MR scans through the medulla (**A**) and pons (**B**) show multiple capillary telangiectasias in the medulla, pons, cerebellum, and left occipital lobe (*arrows*).

seen as contrast extravasation on mid- and late arterial phase studies.

Computed tomography. CT scans are also often normal, although faint areas of increased density can sometimes be seen following contrast administration.

Magnetic resonance imaging. Racemose telangiectasias appear as poorly delineated foci of increased signal on contrast-enhanced studies (Fig. 10-31). If hemorrhage has occurred, capillary telangiectasias can be seen as multiple hypointense foci on T2-weighted and gradient refocussed MR studies (Fig. 10-32).

CAVERNOUS ANGIOMAS

Pathology

Gross pathology. Cavernous angiomas are typically discrete multilobulated berrylike lesions that contain hemorrhage in various stages of evolution (Fig. 10-33, *A* and *B*).

Microscopic pathology. Histologic heterogeneity and overlap with other vascular malformations such as capillary telangiectasia is common.[2,6a] Cavernous angiomas are composed of closely approximated endothelial-lined sinusoidal spaces not separated by significant amounts of neural tissue (Fig. 10-33, *C*). Hemorrhagic residua are common. Clots at different stages of evolution within the lesion and hemosiderin staining of the surrounding brain are seen (Fig. 10-33, *B*). Re-endothelialization of hemorrhagic cavities, growth of new blood vessels, and the proliferation of granulation tissue may account for the apparent growth of some cavernous hemangiomas.[46]

Location (*see* box, p. 312). Cavernous malformations can be found in any part of the brain. About 80% are supratentorial, with the frontal and temporal lobes the most frequent sites.[47] The deep cerebral white matter, corticomedullary junction, and basal ganglia are common supratentorial locations, whereas the pons and cerebellar hemispheres are common posterior fossa sites.[48] Cavernous angiomas also occur in the spinal cord, where they frequently coexist with multiple brain lesions.[49]

Extracerebral cavernous angiomas also occur but are less common. Subarachnoid, intraventricular, subdural, dural sinus, and even extradural lesions have been described[50-52] (see subsequent discussion).

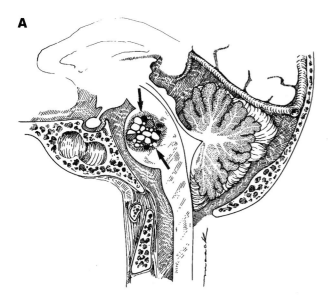

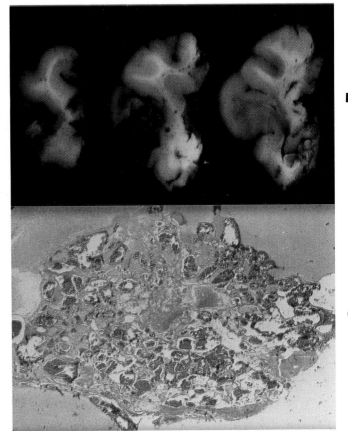

Fig. 10-33. A, Anatomic diagram of pontine cavernous angioma. The lesion has a reticulated core with multiple cavities containing blood degradation products. The angioma is surrounded by a hemosiderin/ferritin rim *(arrows).* **B,** Gross pathologic specimen of cavernous angioma shows a hemorrhagic lesion with blood in different stages of degradation. Note hemosiderin staining of surrounding brain. **C,** Photomicrography of cavernous angioma shows a well-delineated lesion with multiple enlarged endothelial-lined vascular channels. No normal brain is present within the lesion. (**B** and **C,** From Okazaki H, Scheithauer B: *Slide Atlas of Neuropathology,* vol 1, Gower Medical Publishing, 1988.)

Cavernous Angiomas

Pathology

Lobulated collection of dilated endothelial-lined spaces

No normal brain in lesion

Hemorrhage in various stages within lesion; hemosiderin-stained brain around lesion

Location

80% supratentorial but occur in any location
50% to 80% multiple

Age at presentation

Between 20 and 40 years

Symptoms

Seizure, focal neurologic deficit, headache

Hemorrhage risk

Estimated 0.5% to 1%/year (note: occult bleeds common)

Imaging

See Table 10-1; reticulated "popcorn-like" lesion on MR (note importance of gradient-refocussed scans to detect multiple occult lesions)

Incidence and clinical presentation

Incidence. With the advent of MR scanning, cavernous angiomas are the most commonly identified brain vascular malformation. These lesions occur in all age groups without a predilection for either sex. In a recent series, 0.4% of unselected patients had a presumed cavernous angioma.[53] Multiple lesions are seen in approximately half of spontaneously occurring cases, and they occur in 80% of familial cases.

Age and symptoms. The typical age at presentation is 20 to 40 years. Common clinical symptoms are seizure, focal neurologic deficit, and headache.[47,54]

Risk. Repeated, often occult hemorrhagic episodes are common,[55] although the reported overt annualized bleeding rate is slightly less than 1%.[47] Infratentorial location and previous gross hemorrhage are associated with increased risk of subsequent neurological disability.[55a]

Imaging findings (see Table 10-1)

Cerebral angiography. Because most cavernous angiomas are angiographically occult, the common finding is a normal study. If the lesion has hemorrhaged, an avascular area with moderate mass effect can sometimes be identified. Occasionally a faint blush on the late capillary or early venous phase of high-quality cerebral angiograms can be seen.[56]

Computed tomography. Cavernous angiomas are usually isodense to moderately hyperdense on nonenhanced CTs. Calcification is common (Fig. 10-34, *A*). Enhancement following contrast administration

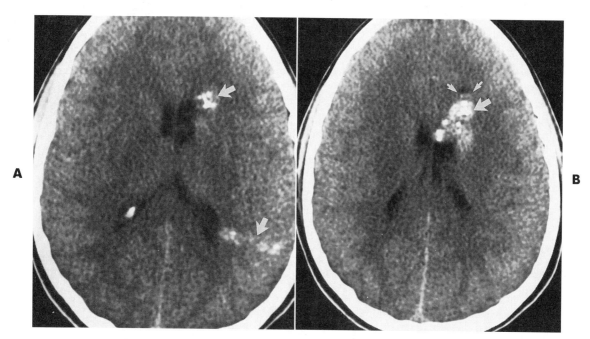

Fig. 10-34. A and **B,** Axial CT scans without contrast enhancement show multiple calcified lesions in the deep cerebral white matter *(large arrows).* One of the lesions has a fluid-fluid level *(small arrows).*

varies from none or minimal to striking (Fig. 10-34, *B*).[56]

Magnetic resonance imaging. MR scans of parenchymal cavernous angiomas show a typical "popcorn-like" lesion with a well-delineated complex reticulated core of mixed signal intensities represent-

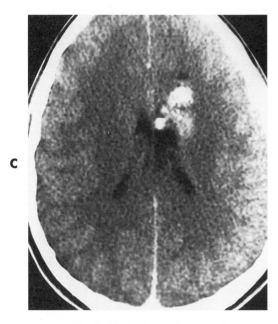

Fig. 10-34, cont'd. C, Little change is seen after contrast administration. Stereotaxic biopsy disclosed cavernous angiomas.

ing hemorrhage in different stages of evolution (Fig. 10-35).[57] Multiple lesions are seen in at least half of all cases with cavernous angiomas (Fig. 10-36). Solitary cavernous angiomas with acute hemorrhage can sometimes be difficult to distinguish from hemorrhagic neoplasm (*see* Figs. 7-52 and 7-53) (*see* box, p. 190).

A low signal hemosiderin rim that completely surrounds the lesion is typical with cavernous angiomas (Figs. 10-35 and 10-36). The low signal becomes more prominent, or "blooms" on T2-weighted and gradient refocussed studies occur because of magnetic susceptibility effects[57] (Fig. 10-37). Gradient echo studies should always be performed when a solitary intracranial hemorrhagic lesion is identified to look for multiple lesions that may not be visible on standard spin-echo studies (Fig. 10-37). Gradient echo studies should also be obtained if T2-weighted pulse sequences that are less sensitive to chronic hemorrhage are routinely used (*see* Chapter 7). So-called fast spin-echo techniques are an example (*see* Fig. 7-22).

Extraaxial cavernous angiomas may have somewhat different imaging features compared to their intraparenchymal counterparts. Although some extracerebral lesions have the classic inhomogeneous reticulated or "popcorn-like" appearance, others closely resemble meningioma. Hyperintense signal on T2-weighted scans and strong, homogeneous enhancement after contrast administration are characteristic.[50-52]

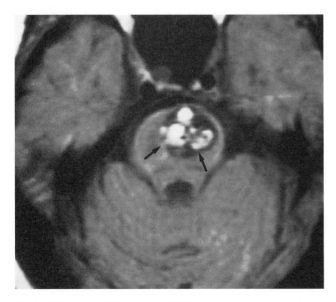

Fig. 10-35. Axial T1-weighted MR scan shows a classic pontine cavernous angioma *(arrows)*. The lesion has a mixed-signal reticulated, or "popcorn-like," core that is surrounded by a low signal hemosiderin/ferritin rim.

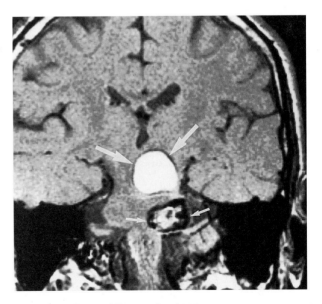

Fig. 10-36. Coronal T1-weighted MR scan in a patient with sensorineural hearing loss demonstrates two separate cavernous angiomas with hemorrhage in different stages of evolution. The midbrain lesion *(large arrows)* shows subacute hemorrhage with a uniform cystlike cavity that contains lysed red blood cells. The cerebellopontine angle lesion *(small arrows)* shows mixed age hemorrhagic debris.

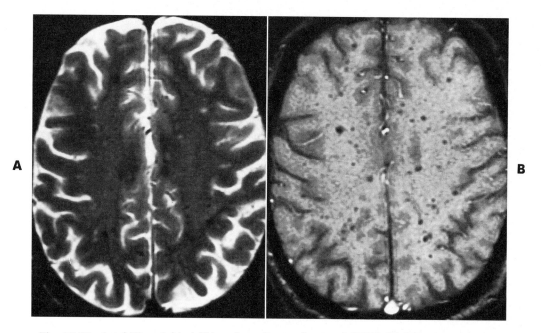

Fig. 10-37. Axial T2-weighted **(A)** and gradient-refocussed (GRE) **(B)** MR scans in a patient with multiple cavernous angiomas. The lesions are difficult to identify on the T2-weighted study but are readily apparent on the GRE sequence. (Courtesy M. Fruin.)

VENOUS MALFORMATIONS
Venous Angioma

Pathology and etiology

Gross pathology. Venous angiomas are composed of radially arranged, dilated anomalous veins that converge in an enlarged transcortical draining vein (Figs. 10-38 and 10-39).[58]

Microscopic pathology. Venous angiomas consist of dilated, thin-walled venous channels separated by intervening normal brain. Hemorrhage is uncommon.

Etiology. Although the precise etiology of venous angioma is unknown, these lesions are probably not true vascular malformations but instead represent extreme anatomic variants or developmental venous anomalies (DVAs) (Fig. 10-40).[59] Arrested venous development after the brain arterial system has been formed could result in retention of primitive embryologic medullary veins that drain into a single, large draining vein and form a "venous angioma."[59] The reported association of focal neuronal migrational anomalies with anomalies of cortical venous drainage supports this concept (*see* Chapter 4).[59] Up to one third of DVAs are associated with cavernous angiomas.[59a]

Location (*see* box, p. 316).   Venous angiomas are located in the deep cerebral or cerebellar white matter, most often near the margin of the adjacent ventricle. The most common site is adjacent to the frontal horn of the lateral ventricle[60]; the next most frequent location is the cerebellum.[61,62]

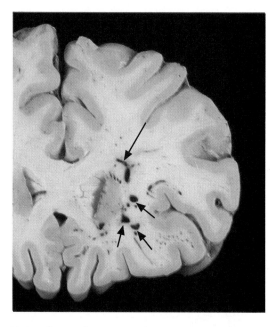

Fig. 10-38. Coronal gross pathologic specimen of a venous vascular malformation. Numerous dilated venous channels *(small arrows)* are seen in the deep white matter adjacent to the caudate nucleus and frontal horn of the lateral ventricle. A segment of the "collector" vein *(large arrow)* is seen. Note normal brain in between the enlarged venous channels. (Courtesy P. Burger, reprinted from Burger PC et al: *Surgical Pathology of the Nervous System and Its Coverings*, edition 3, Churchill Livingstone, New York, 1991.)

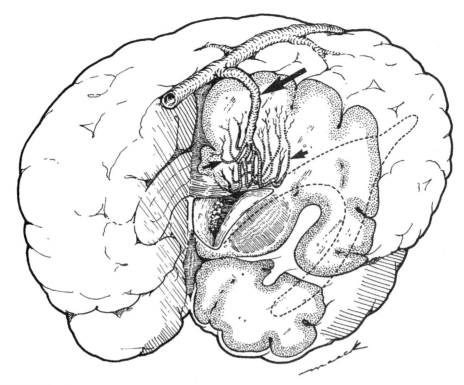

Fig. 10-39. Anatomic diagram depicting a venous angioma. Numerous enlarged medullary veins *(small arrows)* within the deep white matter converge near the ventricular angle and drain into an enlarged transcortical "collector vein" *(large arrow)*. The collector vein then empties into the superior sagittal sinus. The brain parenchyma in-between the enlarged venous channels is normal. The prominent medullary veins form the familiar "Medusa head" that is seen on cerebral angiograms of venous angiomas.

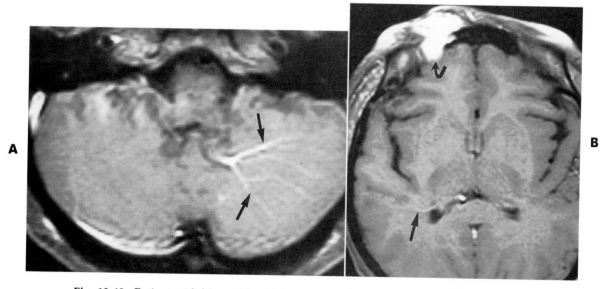

Fig. 10-40. Patient with blue rubber bleb nevus syndrome. **A** and **B,** Contrast-enhanced T1-weighted MR scans show multiple venous angiomas or developmental venous anomalies (DVAs) in the cerebrum and cerebellum *(straight arrows)*. The deep cerebral DVAs drain into strikingly enlarged subependymal veins *(open arrows)*. A right frontal sinus pericranii *(curved arrow)* is also present. (Courtesy D. Blatter.)

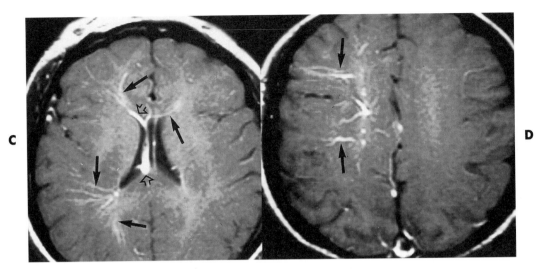

Fig. 10-40, cont'd. Patient with blue rubber bleb nevus syndrome. **C** and **D,** Contrast-enhanced T1-weighted MR scans show multiple venous angiomas or developmental venous anomalies (DVAs) in the cerebrum and cerebellum *(straight arrows)*. The deep cerebral DVAs drain into strikingly enlarged subependymal veins *(open arrows)*. A right frontal sinus pericranii *(curved arrow)* is also present. (Courtesy D. Blatter.)

Venous Angiomas

Pathology

Dilated medullary tributaries, enlarged "collector" vein
Normal brain interposed

Etiology

Probably developmental venous anomaly (DVA) rather
    than true vascular malformation

Location

Deep cerebral/cerebellar white matter
Near ventricular angle
Usually solitary (multiple in blue rubber bleb nevus syndrome)

Age at presentation

Any age; often incidental finding on imaging studies

Symptoms

Often asymptomatic; occasionally hemorrhage, cause
    seizures

Imaging

See Table 10-1; "Medusa head" is classic

Incidence and clinical presentation

Incidence. Venous angioma is the most common brain vascular malformation found at autopsy.[1] Most venous angiomas are solitary, although multiple lesions can occur in the blue rubber bleb nevus syndrome (Fig. 10-40) (*see* Chapter 5).

Symptoms. Most cerebral venous angiomas are asymptomatic and discovered incidentally at autopsy or on imaging studies. Headache, seizure, and focal neurologic deficit are less common.[60] Hemorrhagic complications occur but are rare and are often secondary to a coexisting cavernous angioma.[6a,63,63a]

Imaging (*see* Table 10-1)

Cerebral angiography. The angiographic appearance of venous angiomas is diagnostic. Cerebral angiograms always have a normal arterial phase (Fig. 10-41, *A*). Although a late capillary blush may be present the pathognomonic angiographic appearance of venous angioma is seen on venous phase images. A collection of dilated medullary veins (the so-called Medusa head) converges in an enlarged transcortical "collector" draining vein (Fig. 10-41, *B*).[62,64] In 70% of cases, drainage is into the superficial venous system (Fig. 10-41, *B*); subependymal drainage occurs in

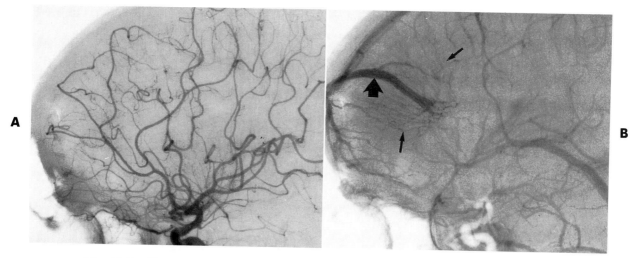

Fig. 10-41. Classic angiographic findings of venous angioma are illustrated by this case. Midarterial **(A)** and venous phase **(B)** films. The arterial phase is normal. The venous phase study shows that multiple enlarged medullary veins *(small arrows)* converge near the frontal horn into a dilated transcortical "collector" vein *(large arrow)*. The hairlike appearance of the enlarged deep white matter veins gives rise to the appellation, "Medusa head" (named after the mythical Greek goddess whose hair was turned into a mass of hissing snakes).

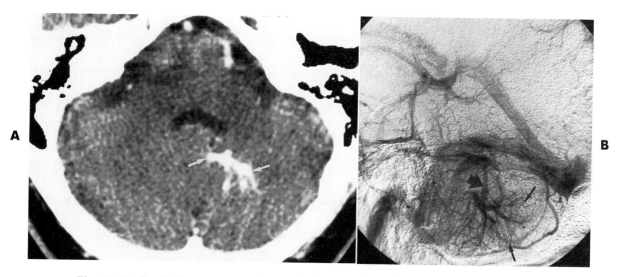

Fig. 10-42. Cerebellar venous angioma. Axial postcontrast CT scan shows a tuft of enhancing vessels *(arrows)* in the deep cerebellar white matter adjacent to the fourth ventricle. Digital subtraction left vertebral angiogram, midarterial frame, lateral view **(B)**, shows the "Medusa head" *(small arrows)* and the dilated collector vein *(large arrow).*

22%.[62] Occasionally there is focal stenosis of the terminal draining vein where it enters the dural sinus. Venous restrictive disease may be associated with an increased propensity for hemorrhage.[65]

Computed tomography. Nonenhanced CT scans are typically normal or show an ill-defined slightly hyperdense area. Following contrast administration, an enhancing tuft of rounded or linear vessels near the angle of a ventricle is identified (Fig. 10-42). These enlarged medullary veins become continuous, with a dilated transcortical draining vein that in turn empties into an adjacent dural sinus, cortical, or subependymal vein.[63] If the section includes the entire length of the "collector" vein a well-delineated linear contrast-enhancing area that extends from the ventricular wall to the cortex is seen (*see* Fig. 10-44, *A*). If the collector vein courses obliquely, serial sections show ovoid areas of contrast enhancement (Fig. 10-43).

Edema and mass effect are typically absent with venous angiomas.[62]

Magnetic resonance imaging. On MR scans a stellate tangle of venous tributaries drains into a larger, sharply delineated vein that often shows high-velocity signal loss (Fig. 10-44, *A* and *D*). Flow-related enhancement can occasionally be seen (Figs. 10-44, *B*, and 10-45, *C*). After contrast administration, the enlarged medullary tributaries and the transcerebral or subependymal draining veins are typically well seen, (Figs. 10-39 and 10-45, *A*).[66, 59a] Evidence of gliosis or hemorrhage is present in 10% to 15% of venous angiomas (Fig. 10-45, *B* and *C*).[60]

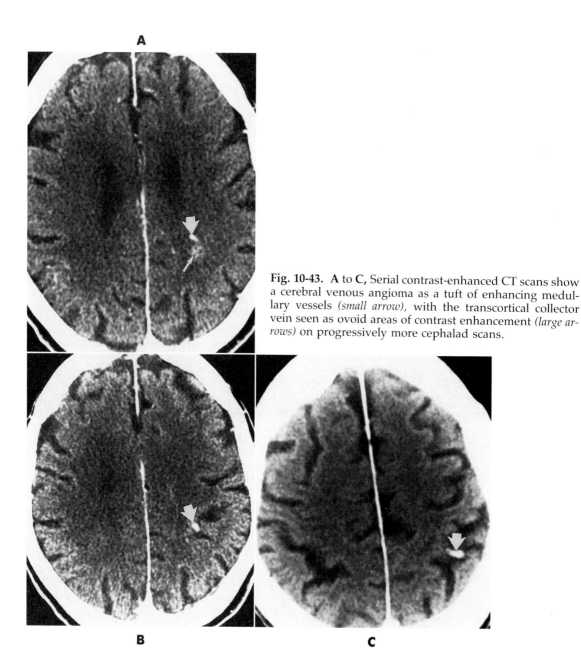

Fig. 10-43. **A** to **C,** Serial contrast-enhanced CT scans show a cerebral venous angioma as a tuft of enhancing medullary vessels *(small arrow),* with the transcortical collector vein seen as ovoid areas of contrast enhancement *(large arrows)* on progressively more cephalad scans.

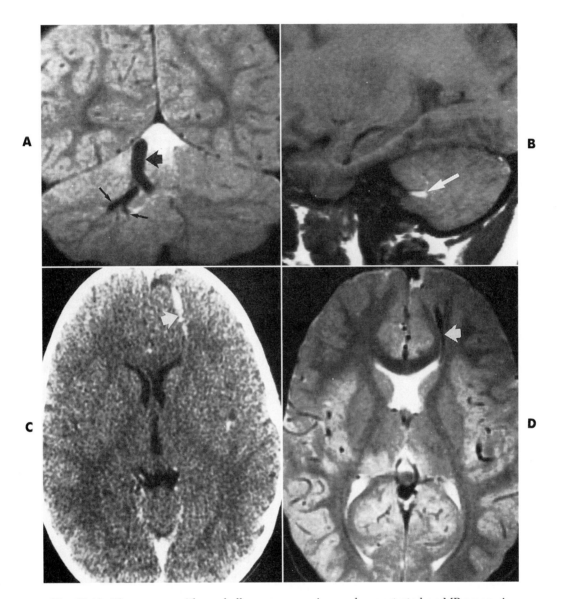

Fig. 10-44. Three cases with cerebellar venous angiomas demonstrated on MR scans. **A,** Coronal T2-weighted study in the first case shows a stellate collection of venous tributaries *(small arrows)* that drains into a prominent collector vein *(large arrow).* High-velocity signal loss is present in the angioma. **B,** Precontrast sagittal T1-weighted MR scan in another case shows a cerebellar venous angioma with flow related enhancement *(arrow).* In the third case, axial postcontrast CT scan **(C)** shows a frontal lobe venous angioma *(arrow)* that is seen on the T2-weighted MR scan **(D)** as a linear area of high-velocity signal loss *(arrow).*

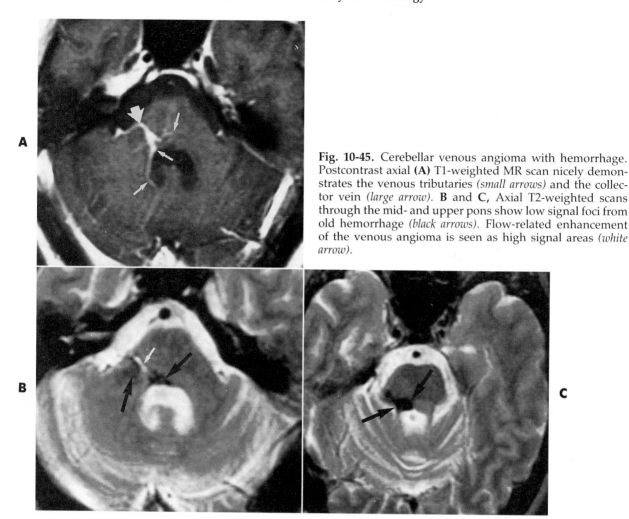

Fig. 10-45. Cerebellar venous angioma with hemorrhage. Postcontrast axial **(A)** T1-weighted MR scan nicely demonstrates the venous tributaries *(small arrows)* and the collector vein *(large arrow)*. **B** and **C,** Axial T2-weighted scans through the mid- and upper pons show low signal foci from old hemorrhage *(black arrows)*. Flow-related enhancement of the venous angioma is seen as high signal areas *(white arrow)*.

Vein of Galen Malformations

Vein of Galen malformation (VOGM) is used to describe a heterogeneous group of anomalies with enlarged deep venous structures of the galenic system that are fed by abnormal midline arteriovenous communications.[67]

Pathology. "Aneurysmal" dilatation of the vein of Galen is the pathologic finding most common to the heterogeneous group of vascular malformations that involve the Galenic system (Fig. 10-46).

Etiology *(see* box). There are two basic types of VOGM. In the first type, single or multiple arteries drain directly into enlarged deep venous structures of the Galenic system. The most common abnormality is single or multiple direct arteriovenous fistulae between choroidal or quadrigeminal arteries and a median venous sac. The sac probably represents persistence of a primitive venous channel that is the embryonic precursor of the vein of Galen.[68] Some type of venous outflow restriction typically coexists with this type of VOGM.[67,69]

In the second type of VOGM, a parenchymal AVM is present. The AVM is usually in the thalamus or midbrain and its nidus has deep Galenic drainage. Venous outflow constraint is also common in this group.[67]

Clinical presentation. Presenting symptoms and age of onset vary with VOGM type. Patients with fistulae present early in life, often at birth. High-output congestive heart failure and macrocephaly with hydrocephalus are the common symptoms. Developmental delay and ocular symptoms are more common in VOGMs with a true AVM nidus in the thalamus or brainstem.[70] Cranial bruit, focal neurologic deficit, seizure, and hemorrhage can occur in both groups.[71]

Imaging findings *(see* Table 10-1)
Ultrasound. Transcranial B-mode ultrasound shows a sonolucent posterior third ventricular mass and obstructive hydrocephalus (Fig. 10-47, *A*). Color-flow doppler imaging often discloses turbulent bidirectional flow within the enlarged vein of Galen (Fig. 10-47, *B*).[71a]

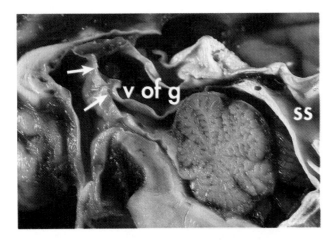

Fig. 10-46. Autopsy specimen of a newborn infant with high-output congestive heart failure (CHF) shows a massively enlarged vein of Galen *(v of g)* and straight sinus *(ss)*. The enlarged vein of Galen compresses the posterior third ventricle *(arrows)*. (From archives of the Armed Forces Institute of Pathology.)

Vein of Galen Malformations

Pathology

Massively enlarged galenic system from thalamic AVM or choroidal AVF

Clinical

Usually newborn with congestive heart failure (direct arteriovenous fistula without nidus)

Older infants in AVM with nidus

Imaging

See Table 10-1

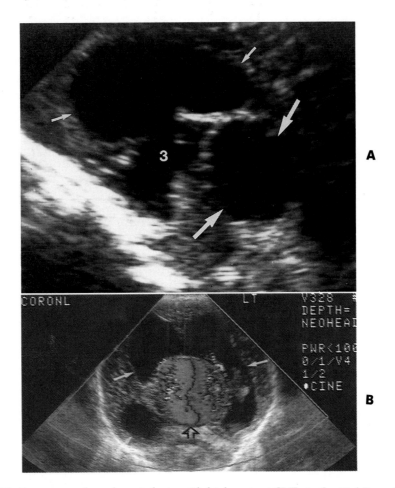

Fig. 10-47. Two cases of newborn infants with high-output CHF. **A,** Sagittal B-mode ultrasound in the first case shows a sonolucent mass *(large arrows)* that compresses the posterior third ventricle *(3)*. Note enlargement of the lateral ventricle *(small arrows)*. **B,** Coronal color flow doppler ultrasound scan in the second case shows turbulent bidirectional flow in the massively enlarged vein of Galen *(open arrow)*. Note severe obstructive hydrocephalus *(white arrows)* (**B,** Courtesy C. Rumack.)

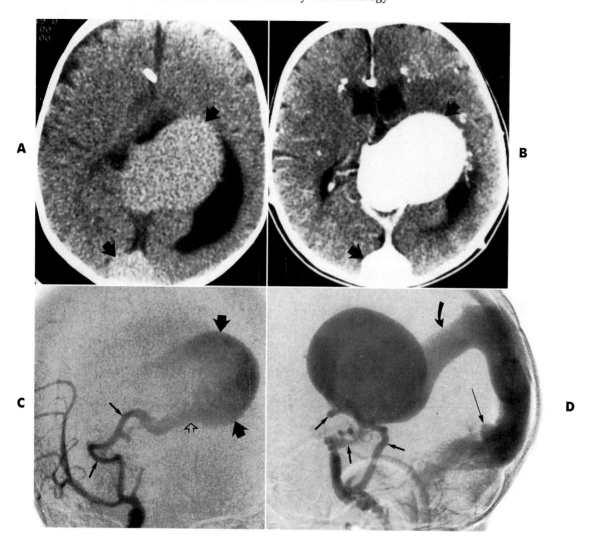

Fig. 10-48. A, Axial CT scan without contrast enhancement in an infant with a massive vein of Galen malformation shows the hyperdense dilated vein of Galen and sinus confluence *(arrows).* **B,** Contrast-enhanced scan in the same patient obtained earlier shows strong, uniform enhancement *(arrows).* **C,** Right internal carotid angiogram, early arterial phase, AP view, shows an enlarged choroidal artery *(small arrows)* that has a direct fistulous communication *(open arrow)* with a massively enlarged vein of Galen *(large arrows).* **D,** Left vertebral angiogram, late arterial phase, lateral view, shows that prominent posterior choroidal and thalamoperforating arteries *(small arrows)* feed the massively enlarged vein of Galen *(large arrows).* This may represent a combination of vein of Galen fistulae and thalamic AVM. Note the presence of a large falcine sinus *(curved arrow).* The straight sinus is not opacified and may have thrombosed *(long arrow).*

Cerebral angiography. Arterial supply to VOGMs is usually via enlarged choroidal and thalamoperforating arteries. In the fistula group, the posterior choroidal vessels are the dominant supply (Fig. 10-48), followed by anterior choroidal (Fig. 10-49), thalamoperforating, and anterior cerebral artery branches. In the nidus type, thalamoperforating vessels are the common arterial feeders.[70]

Venous drainage patterns include aneurysmal dilatation of the vein of Galen (venous varix), with or without distal stenosis. Drainage into an accessory or inferior falcine sinus with absence of the vein of Galen is also common.[72]

Slow arteriovenous shunts with contrast stagnation in the venous sac secondary to severe outflow restriction (Fig. 10-48) may eventually thrombose spontaneously. These cases often have comparatively good clinical outcome.[73]

Computed tomography. An iso- or hyperdense midline mass posterior to the third ventricle is seen on nonenhanced studies (Figs. 10-48, *A,* and 10-49, *A*). Mass effect with hydrocephalus and secondary encephalomalacic changes are common (Fig. 10-49). Patent VOGMs enhance strongly following contrast administration (Figs. 10-48, *B,* and 10-49, *B*).[74]

Magnetic resonance imaging. MR improves depic-

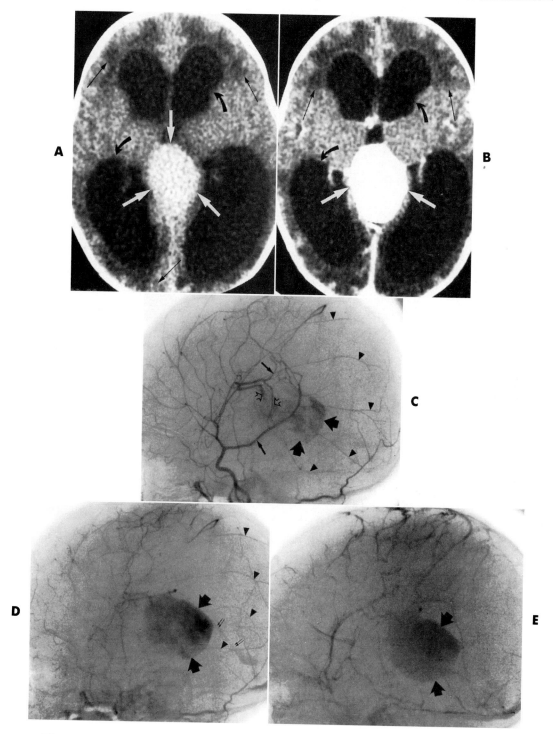

Fig. 10-49. A 3-month-old infant with enlarging head and partially thrombosed, aneurysmally dilated vein of Galen. Axial CT scans without **(A)** and with **(B)** contrast enhancement show a hyperdense mass **(A,** *white arrows)* at the posterior third ventricle. Strong, uniform enhancement is present **(B,** *white arrows)*. Note severe ventricular enlargement *(curved arrows)* and secondary encephalomalacic changes in the deep periventricular white matter *(long arrows)*. **C** to **E,** Left common carotid angiogram, lateral view, with midarterial **(C),** capillary **(D),** and venous phase **(E)** films shows a multisite slow flow fistula *(open arrows)* between enlarged choroidal arteries *(small single arrows)* and a dilated vein of Galen *(large arrows)*. The massively enlarged lateral ventricles cause avascular mass effect with stretching and draping of smaller choroidal artery branches *(arrowheads)*. Severe outflow obstruction caused by a hypoplastic straight sinus *(double arrows)* is present. Contrast stagnation within the enlarged vein of Galen is present **(E,** *arrows)* and persists into the venous phase. The malformation eventually thrombosed spontaneously.

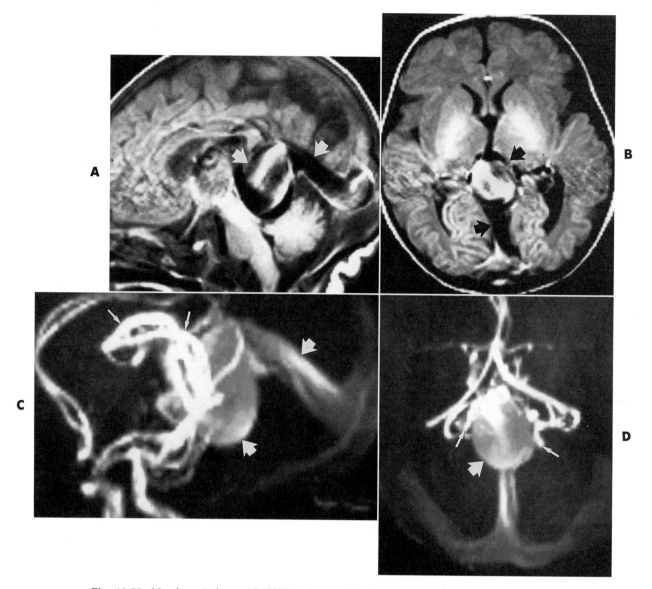

Fig. 10-50. Newborn infant with CHF and vein of Galen malformation. Sagittal **(A)** and axial **(B)** T1-weighted MR scans without contrast enhancement show marked enlargement of the vein of Galen and falcine sinus *(arrows)*. Turbulent flow within the dilated vein of Galen produces mixed signal (compare with Fig. 10-47, *B*). 3D TOF MRA with lateral **(C)** and submentovertex **(D)** projections shows the enlarged vein of Galen and falcine sinus *(large arrows)*. Prominent choroidal arteries are present *(small arrows)*.

tion of both arterial and venous anatomy (Fig. 10-50).[67] Thrombosis, as well as secondary hemorrhage and brain parenchymal changes, are well delineated. MRA can depict the arterial feeders and venous drainage pattern and delineate venous outflow restrictions.

Venous Varix

Varicose dilatation of cerebral veins can be seen in association with several types of intracranial vascular abnormalities.

Pathology and etiology. Varices are enlarged thin-walled veins that may become thrombosed or rupture and produce subarachnoid hemorrhage. Giant intracranial varices are rare and are seen mostly with vein of Galen malformations. High-flow arteriovenous malformations or fistulae may also cause varicose dilatation of their draining veins.[75] Rarely, venous angioma may cause a venous varix.[76]

Occasionally an abnormally large communication between the intracranial and extracranial venous circulations can be found, the so-called sinus pericra-

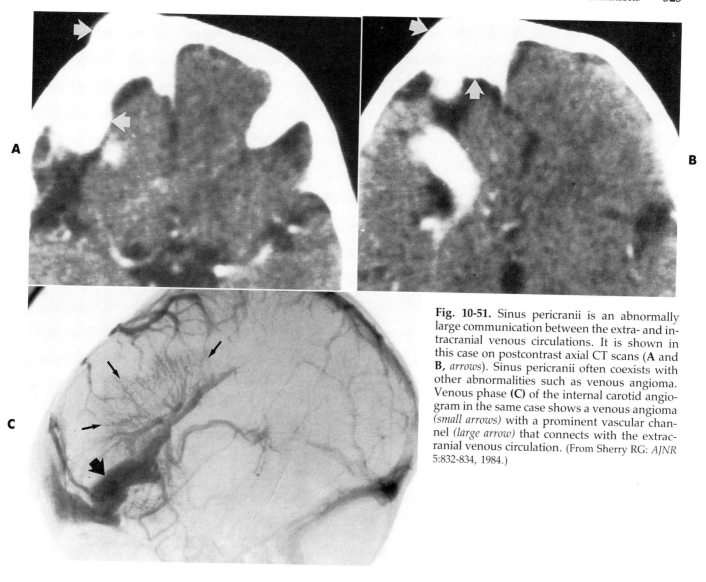

Fig. 10-51. Sinus pericranii is an abnormally large communication between the extra- and intracranial venous circulations. It is shown in this case on postcontrast axial CT scans (**A** and **B**, *arrows*). Sinus pericranii often coexists with other abnormalities such as venous angioma. Venous phase (**C**) of the internal carotid angiogram in the same case shows a venous angioma (*small arrows*) with a prominent vascular channel (*large arrow*) that connects with the extracranial venous circulation. (From Sherry RG: *AJNR* 5:832-834, 1984.)

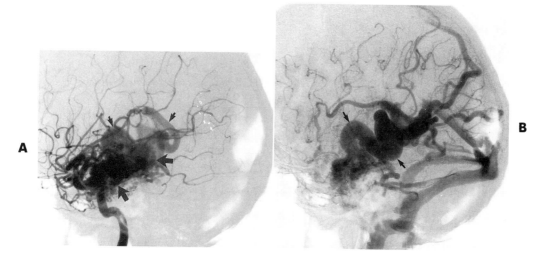

Fig. 10-52. A and **B,** Serial films from a right internal carotid angiogram, lateral view, show a large temporal lobe AVM (*large arrows*). Arteriovenous shunting with fusiform enlargement of the draining veins (*small arrows*) is present.

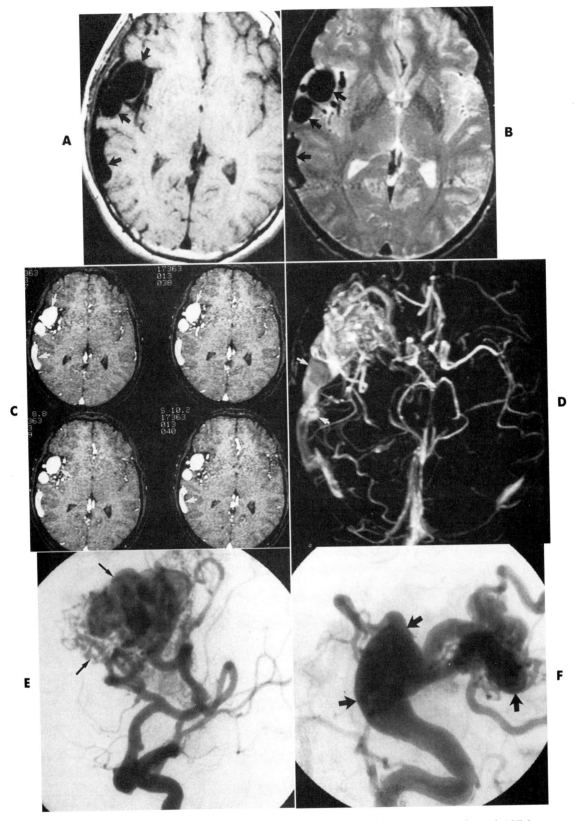

Fig. 10-53. Axial T1- **(A)** and T2-weighted **(B)** MR scans show a posterior frontal AVM with variceal enlargement of multiple cortical draining veins *(arrows)*. 3D TOF MRA with source images **(C)** and submentovertex view **(D)** show the venous varices *(arrows)*. Digital subtraction right internal carotid angiogram: lateral views of the midarterial **(E)** and venous **(F)** phase frames show the AVM **(E,** *arrows)* and the venous varices **(F,** *arrows)*.

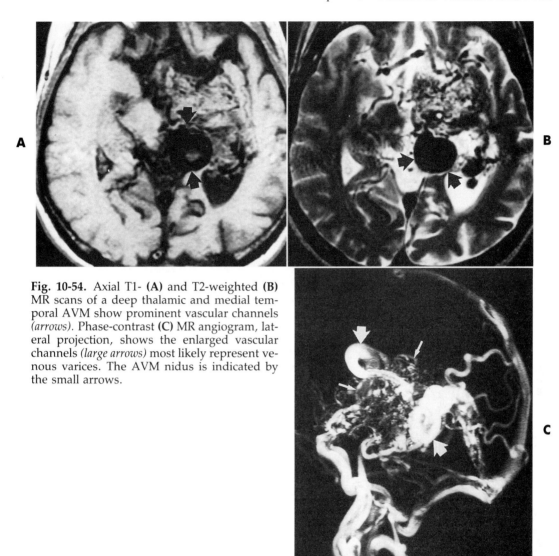

Fig. 10-54. Axial T1- **(A)** and T2-weighted **(B)** MR scans of a deep thalamic and medial temporal AVM show prominent vascular channels *(arrows)*. Phase-contrast **(C)** MR angiogram, lateral projection, shows the enlarged vascular channels *(large arrows)* most likely represent venous varices. The AVM nidus is indicated by the small arrows.

nii.[77] Sinus pericranii can occur as an acquired lesion, often secondary to trauma. It may also be a congenital malformation that coexists with other developmental vascular anomalies such as venous angiomas (Fig. 10-51).[78] Sinus pericranii has been reported with blue rubber bleb nevus syndrome.[79]

Location. Cerebral varices are located in the brain parenchyma or leptomeninges and may be found with pial and dural vascular malformations.

Clinical presentation. Patients with deep cerebral or galenic intracranial varices often have hydrocephalus and increased intracranial pressure. Occasionally an intracranial varix may cause symptoms of mass effect such as seizure or cranial nerve deficit.[75] The di-

agnosis of sinus pericranii is suggested by a soft, fluctuant bulging mass that varies in size and tension with changes in head position or intrathoracic pressure.[77]

Imaging findings
Cerebral angiography. Saccular aneurysmal dilatation is common in the veins that lie in the subarachnoid space. Fusiform enlargement of draining veins located within the brain parenchyma and the subarachnoid cisterns also occurs.[80] Coexisting congenital vascular malformations such as AVM are usually identified (Fig. 10-52). Venous varices with high flow AVMs are readily visualized; lesions with extremely slow flow such as sinus pericranii may require delayed imaging with digital or film subtraction.[77]

Computed tomography. Venous varices are usually slightly hyperdense to brain on nonenhanced studies and show strong, uniform enhancement following contrast administration.[80]

Magnetic resonance imaging. Well-delineated ovoid or fusiform areas with variable signal are characteristic. If flow is sufficiently rapid, areas of high-velocity signal loss are present (Figs. 10-53 and 10-54). Phase-contrast MRA is helpful in demonstrating venous varices with slow flow.

REFERENCES

1. Okazaki H: Cerebrovascular disease. In *Fundamentals of Neuropathology*, pp 27-94, New York: Igaku-Shoin, 1989.
2. Rigamonti D, Johnson PC, Spetzler RF et al: Cavernous malformations and capillary telangiectasia: a spectrum within a single pathological entity, *Neurosurg* 28:60-64, 1991.
3. Goulao A, Alvarez H, Monaco RG et al: Venous anomalies and abnormalities of the posterior fossa, *Neuroradiol* 31:476-482, 1990.
4. Scazzeri F, Prosetti D, Nenci R et al: Angioma venoso, *Riv di Neuroradiol* 4:201-208, 1991.
5. Fukusumi A, Okudera T, Huang YP et al: Neuroradiological analysis of medullary venous malformations in the cerebellar hemisphere, *Neuroradiol* 33:359, 1991.
6. Ebeling JD, Tranmer BI, Davis KA et al: Thrombosed arteriovenous malformations: a type of occult vascular malformation, *Neurosurg* 23:605-610, 1988.
6a. Awad IA, Robinson JR Jr, Mohanty S, Estes ML: Mixed vascular malformations of the brain: clinical and pathogenetic considerations, *Neurosurg* 33:179-188, 1993.
7. Graves VB, Duff TA: Intracranial arteriovenous malformations: current imaging and treatment, *Invest Radiol* 25:952-960, 1990.
8. Burger PC, Schuthaver BW, Vogel FS: *Surgical Pathology of the Nervous System and its Coverings*, edition 3, pp 439 and 443, Churchill Livingston, 1991.
9. Marks MP, Lane B, Steinberg GK, Snipes GJ: Intracranial aneurysms in cerebral arteriovenous malformations: evaluation and endovascular treatment, *Radiol* 183:355-360, 1992.
10. Salcman M, Scholtz H, Numaguchi Y: Multiple intracerebral arteriovenous malformations: report of three cases and review of the literature, *Surg Neurol* 38:121-128, 1992.
11. Iizuka Y, Lasjaunias P, Garcia-Monaco R et al: Multiple cerebral arteriovenous malformations in children (15 patients), *Neuroradiol* 33:538, 1991.
12. Mizutani T, Tanaka H, Aruza T: Multiple arteriovenous malformations located in the cerebellum, posterior fossa, spinal cord, dura, and scalp with associated port wine stain and supratentorial venous anomaly, *Neurosurg* 31:137-141, 1992.
13. Brown RD Jr, Wiebers DO, Forbes G et al: The natural history of unruptured intracranial arteriovenous malformations, *J Neurosurg* 68:352-357, 1988.
14. Auger RG, Wiebers DO: Management of unruptured intracranial arteriovenous malformations: a decision analysis, *Neurosurg* 30:561-569, 1992.
15. Golfinos JG, Wascher TM, Zabramski JM, Spetzler RF: The management of unruptured intracranial vascular malformations, *BNI Quarterly* 8:2-11, 1992.
16. Piepgras DG, Sundt TM Jr, Ragoowansi AT, Stevens L: Seizure outcome in patients with surgically treated cerebral arteriovenous malformations, *J Neurosurg* 78:5-11, 1993.
17. Monaco RG, Alvarez H, Goulao A et al: Posterior fossa arteriovenous malformations: angio architecture in relation to their hemorrhagic episodes, *Neuroradiol* 31:471-475, 1990.
18. Spetzler RF, Hargraves RW, McCormick PW et al: Relationship of perfusion pressure and size to risk of hemorrhage from arteriovenous malformations, *J Neurosurg* 76:918-923, 1992.
19. Marks MP, Lane B, Steinberg GK, Chang PJ: Hemorrhage in intracerebral arteriovenous malformations: angiographic determinants, *Radiol* 176:807-813, 1990.
20. Toffol GJ, Gruener G, Naheedy MH: Early-filling cerebral veins, *J of AOA* 88:1007-1009, 1988.
21. Willinsky R, TerBrugge K, Montanera W et al: Microarteriovenous malformations of the brain: superselective angiography in diagnosis and treatment, *AJNR* 13:325-330, 1992.
22. Chin LS, Raffel C, Gonzalez-Gomez I et al: Diffuse arteriovenous malformations: a clinical, radiological, and pathological discription, *Neurosurg* 31:863-868, 1992.
22a. Willinsky RA, Fitzgerald M, TerBrugge K et al: Delayed angiography in the investigation of intracranial intracerebral hematomas caused by small arteriovenous malformations, *Neuroradiol* 35:307-311, 1993.
23. Miyasaka Y, Yada K, Ohwada T et al: Pathophysiologic assessment of stagnating arteries after removal of arteriovenous malformations, *AJNR* 14:15-18, 1993.
24. Prayer L, Wimberger D, Kramer J et al: MRI—a noninvasive tool for evaluating therapeutic embolization of cerebral arteriovenous malformations, *Eur Radiol* 1:51-57, 1991.
25. Kumar AJ, Vinuela F, Fox AJ, Rosenbaum AE: Unruptured intracranial arteriovenous malformations do cause mass effect, *AJNR* 6:29-32, 1985.
26. Smith HJ, Strother CM, Kikuchi Y et al: MR imaging in the management of supratentorial intracranial AVMs, *AJNR* 9:225-235, 1988.
27. Chappell PM, Steinberg GK, Marks MP: Clinically documented hemorrhage in cerebral arteriovenous malformations: MR characteristics, *Radiol* 183:719-724, 1992.
28. Marks MP, Lane B, Steinberg G, Chang P: Vascular characteristics of intracerebral arteriovenous malformations in patients with clinical steal, *AJNR* 12:489-496, 1991.
29. Huston J III, Rufenacht DA, Ehman RL, Wiebers DO: Intracranial aneurysms and vascular malformations: comparison of time-of-flight and phase-contrast MR angiography, *Radiol* 181:721-730, 1991.
30. Blatter DB, Parker DL, Ahn SS et al: Cerebral MR angiography with multiple overlapping thin slab acquisition, *Radiol* 183:379-389, 1992.
31. Marks MP, Pelc MJ, Ross MR, Enzmann DR: Determination of cerebral blood flow with a phase-contrast cine MR imaging technique: evaluation of normal subjects and patients with arteriovenous malformation, *Radiol* 182:467-476, 1992.
32. Guo W-Y, Lindquist M, Lindquist C et al: Sterotaxic angiography in gamma knife radiosurgery of intracranial arteriovenous malformations, *AJNR* 13:1107-1114, 1992.
33. Jafar JJ, Davis AJ, Berenstein A et al: The effect of embolization with N-butyl cyanoacrylate prior to surgical resection of cerebral arteriovenous malformations, *J Neurosurg* 78:60-69, 1993.
34. Jacobs J: Angiography in intracranial hemorrhage, *Neuroimaging clin N Amer* 2:89-106, 1992.
35. Nishijima M, Takaku A, Endo S et al: Etiological evaluation of dural arteriovenous malformations of the lateral and sigmoid sinuses based on histopathological examinations, *J Neurosurg* 76:600-606, 1992.
36. DeMarco JK, Dillon WP, Halback VV, Tsuruda JS: Dural arteriovenous fistulas: evaluation with MR imaging, *Radiol* 175:193-199, 1990.
37. Barnwell SL, Halbach VV, Dowd CF et al: Multiple dural arteriovenous fistulas of the cranium and spine, *AJNR* 12:441-445, 1991.
38. Pierot L, Chiras J, Meder J-F et al: Dural arteriovenous fistulas of the posterior fossa draining into subarachnoid veins, *AJNR* 13:315-323, 1992.

39. Osborn AG: Intracranial vascular malformations. In *Introduction to Cerebral Angiography*, pp 85-91, St. Louis: Mosby-Year Book, 1991.

40. Rodesch G, Lasjaunias P: Physiopathology and semeiology of dural arteriovenous shunts, *Riv di Neuroradiol* 5:11-21, 1992.

41. Komiyama M, Fu Y, Yagura H et al: MR imaging of dural AV fistulas at the cavernous sinus, *J Comp Asst Tomogr* 14:397-401, 1990.

42. Osborn AG: *Introduction to Cerebral Angiography*, pp 49-86, Harper and Row, 1980.

43. Chen JC, Tsuruda JS, Halbach VV: Suspected dural arteriovenous fistula: results with screening MR angiography in seven patients, *Radiol* 183:265-271, 1992.

43a. Miyachi S, Negoro M, Harda T, Sugita K: Contribution of meningeal arteries to cerebral arteriovenous malformations, *Neuroradiol* 35:205-209, 1993.

44. Aesch B, Lioret E, de Toffol B, Jan M: Multiple cerebral angiomas and Rendu-Osler-Weber disease: case report, *Neurosurg* 29:599-602, 1991.

45. deTilly LN, Willinsky R, Ter Brugge K et al: Cerebral arteriovenous malformation causing epitaxis, *AJNR* 13:333-334, 1992.

46. Scott RM, Branes P, Kupski W, Adelman LS: Cavernous angiomas of the central nervous system in children, *J Neurosurg* 76:38-46, 1992.

47. Robinson JR, Awad IA, Little JR: Natural history of the cavernous angioma, *J Neurosurg* 75:709-714, 1991.

48. Huk WJ: Vascular malformations. In Huk WJ, Gademann G, Friedmann G, editors: *MRI of the Central Nervous System*, pp 325-346, Berlin, Springer-Verlag, 1990.

49. Bourgouin PM, Tampieri D, Johnston W et al: Multiple occult vascular malformations of the brain and spinal cord: MRI diagnosis, *Neuroradiol* 34:110-111, 1992.

50. Krief O, Sichez JP, Chedid G et al: Extraaxial cavernous hemangioma with hemorrhage, *AJNR* 12:988-990, 1990.

51. Katayama Y, Tsubokawa T, Miyazaki S et al: Magnetic resonance imaging of cavernous sinus cavernous hemangioma, *Neuroradiol* 33:118-122, 1991.

52. Linsky ME, Sekhar LN: Cavernous sinus hemangioma: a series, a review, and an hypothesis, *Neurosurg* 3:101-108, 1992.

53. Curling OP, Kelly DL, Elster AD, Craven TE: An analysis of the natural history of cavernous hemangiomas, *J Neurosurg* 75:702-708, 1991.

54. Churchyard A, Khangure M, Grainger K: Cerebral cavernous angioma: a potentially benign condition? Successful treatment in 16 cases, *J Neurol Neurosurg Psychiah* 55:1040-1045, 1992.

55. Sigal R, Krief O, Houtteville JP et al: Occult cerebrovascular malformations: follow-up with MR imaging, *Radiol* 176:815-819, 1990.

55a. Robinson JR Jr, Awad IA, Magdinec M, Paranandi L: Factors predisposing to clinical disability in patients with cavernous malformations of the brain, *Neurosurg* 32:730-736, 1993.

56. Savoiardo M, Strada L, Passerini A: Intracranial cavernous hemangioma: neuroradiologic review of 36 operated cases, *AJNR* 4:945-950, 1983.

57. Gomori JM, Grossman RI, Goldberg HI et al: Occult cerebral vascular malformations: high-field MR imaging, *Radiol* 158:707-713, 1986.

58. Rigamonti D, Spetzler D: The association of venous and cavernous malformations: report of form cases and discussions of the pathophysiological, diagnostic and therapeutic implications, *Acta Neurochir* (Wien) 92:100-105, 1988.

59. Lasjaunias P, Burrows P, Planet C: Developmental venous anomalies (DVA): the so-called venous angioma, *Neurosurg Rev* 9:233-244, 1986.

59a. Osterton B, Solymosi L: Magnetic resonance angiography of cerebral developmental anomalies: its role in differential diagnosis, *Neuroradiol* 35:97-104, 1993.

60. Wilms G, Demaerel P, Marchi G et al: Gadolinium-enhanced MR imaging of cerebral venous angiomas with emphasis on their drainage, *J Comput Assist Tomogr* 15:199-206, 1991.

61. Wilms G, Goffin J, VanDriessche J, Demaerel P: Posterior fossa venous anomaly and ipsilateral acoustic neuroma: two cases, *Neuroradiol* 34:337-339, 1992.

62. Valavanis A, Wellauer J, Yasargil MG: The radiological diagnosis of cerebral venous angioma: cerebral angiography and computed tomography, *Neuroradiol* 24:193-199, 1983.

63. Truwit CL: Venous angioma of the brain: History, significance and imaging findings, *AJR* 159:1299-1307, 1992.

63a. Lindquist C, Guo W-Y, Karlsson B, Steiner L: Radiosurgery for venous angiomas, *J Neurosurg* 78:531-536, 1993.

64. Uchino A, Imador H, Ohno M: Magnetic resonance imaging of intracranial venous angioma, *Clinical Imaging* 14:309-314, 1990.

65. Dillon WP: Venous angiomas. Presented at the 29th Annual Meeting of the American Society of Neuroradiology, Washington, June 9-14, 1991.

66. Wilms G, Marchal G, Vas Hecke P et al: Cerebral venous angioma: MR imaging at 1.5 tesla, *Neuroradiol* 32:81-85, 1990.

67. Seidenwurm D, Berenstein A, Hyman A, Kowalsla H: Vein of Galen malformation: correlation of clinical presentation, arteriography, and MR imaging, *AJNR* 12:347-345, 1991.

68. Raybaud CA, Strother CM, Hald JK: Aneurysms of the vein of Galen: embryonic considerations and anatomical features relating to the pathogenesis of the malformations, *Neuroradiol* 31:109-128, 1989.

69. Lasjaunias P, TerBrugge, Ibor LL et al: The role of dural anomalies in vein of Galen aneurysms: report of six cases and review of the literature, *AJNR* 8:185-192, 1987.

70. Seidenwurm D, Berensteis A: Vein of Galen malformation: clinical relevance of angiographic classification, and utility of MRI in treatment planning, *Neuroradiol* 33(suppl):153-155, 1991.

71. Johnston IH, Whittle IR, Besser M et al: Vein of Galen malformation: diagnosis and management, *Neurosurg* 20:747-758, 1987.

71a. Westra SJ, Curran JG, Duckwiler GR et al: Pediatric intracranial vascular malformations: evaluation of treatment results with color doppler US, *Radiol* 186:775-783, 1993.

72. Lasjaunias P, Garcia-Monaco R, Rodesch G, Terbrugge K: Deep venous drainage in great cerebral veins (vein of Galen) absence and malformations, *Neuroradiol* 33:234-238, 1991.

73. Hurst RW, Kagetser NJ, Berenstein A: Angiographic findings in two cases of aneurysmal malformation of vein of Galen prior to spontaneous thrombosis: therapeutic implications, *AJNR* 13:1446-1450, 1992.

73a. Baenziger O, Martin E, Willi V et al: Prenatal brain atrophy due to a giant vein of Galen malformation, *Neuroradiol* 35:105-106, 1993.

74. Martelli A, Scotti G, Harwood-Nash DC et al: Aneurysm of the vein of Galen in children: CT and angiographic correlations, *Neuroradiol* 20:123-133, 1980.

75. Viñuela F, Drake CG, Fox AJ, Pelz DM: Giant intracranial varices secondary to high-flow arteriovenous fistulae, *J Neurosurg* 66:198-203, 1987.

76. Dross P, Raji MR, Dastur KJ: Cerebral varix associated with a venous angioma, *ANJR* 8:373-374, 1987.

77. Sadler LR, Tarr RW, Jungreis CA, Sekhar L: Sinus pericranii: CT and MR findings, *J Comp Asst Tomogr* 14:124-127, 1990.

78. Bollar A, Allut AG, Prieto A et al: Sinus pericranii: radiological and etiopathological considerations, *J Neurosurg* 77:469-472, 1992.

79. Sherry RG, Walker ML, Olds MV: Sinus pericranii and venous angioma in the blue-rubber bleb nevus syndrome, *AJNR* 5:832-834, 1984.

80. Rao KCVG, Chiantella NM, Arora S, Gellad F: Intracranial venous aneurysms: vein of Galen and other similar vascular anomalies, *CT: J Comp Tomogr* 7:345-350, 1983.

11

Stroke

I n the United States, education about stroke risk factors combined with hypertension control has reduced stroke and stroke-related deaths by 50% over the last three decades. Nevertheless, stroke remains the major cause of disability among adult Americans and the third leading cause of death after noncerebral cardiovascular disease and cancer.[1,2] With aggressive but promising new therapies for treating stroke, early recognition of ischemic-related disease places diagnostic neuroimaging at the forefront of stroke management.

ATHEROSCLEROSIS
Pathology and Pathogenesis

The principal cause of cerebral infarction is atherosclerosis and its sequelae. In industrialized nations, atherosclerosis is the underlying basis for cerebral thromboembolism in over 90% of all cases.[3] Atherosclerosis is also the most common cause of craniocerebral vascular stenosis in adults. First, the pathology and pathogenesis of atherosclerosis will be reviewed; second, the imaging manifestations of atherosclerotic vascular disease (ASVD) will be discussed.

Pathology. Atherosclerotic plaques are eccentric focal fibrofatty intimal thickenings (Fig. 11-1, *A* to *E*). Atherosclerosis affects large, medium, and small arteries and arterioles (Fig. 11-1, *F* to *H*). Craniocerebral ASVD occurs commonly and most severely at the internal carotid artery origin and the distal basilar artery (Fig. 11-1, *G*).[3-5]

Etiology. The pathogenesis of atherosclerosis remains controversial. There is probably no single cause, no single initiating event, and no exclusive pathogenetic mechanism.[7] Two major theories are that ASVD is a reaction to injury or a cellular prolif-

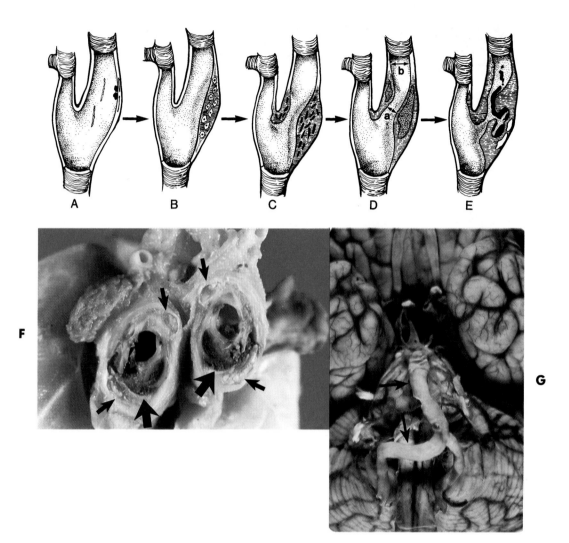

Fig. 11-1. Anatomic diagrams and gross pathology specimens depict craniocerebral atherosclerotic vascular disease (ASVD). **A** to **E,** Development of atherosclerotic plaque at the common carotid artery (CCA) bifurcation and internal carotid artery (ICA) origin is shown schematically. **F** to **H,** Gross pathology specimens illustrate a spectrum of ASVD that extends from the aortic arch and its branches **(F)** to large **(G)** and medium-sized **(H)** intracranial vessels. **A,** Intimal fatty streaks are present. Some platelet adhesion to the intima is noted but the carotid artery is otherwise normal. **B,** Monocyte-derived macrophages and smooth muscle cells proliferate under the intima, becoming lipid-filled foam cells. **C,** Foam cell necrosis produces a thickened plaque with cellular debris and cholesterol crystals. **D,** Intraplaque subintimal hemorrhage occurs, further narrowing the vessel lumen. Stenosis calculation is performed by measuring the narrowest diameter of the diseased artery *(a)* and subtracting from the normal ICA diameter *(b)* distal to the bulb beyond the angiographically recognizable diseased segment. This gives the calculated stenosis diameter. To obtain the percentage stenosis, stenosis is divided by the normal lumen diameter and multiplied by 100. For example, if the normal ICA is 8 mm at *b* and the residual lumen is 2 mm at *a,* the stenosis diameter is 6 mm (6 ÷ 8 × 100 = 75% stenosis). According to the North American Symptomatic Carotid Endarterectomy Trial (NASCET), symptomatic lesions with 70% to 99% stenosis are clinically significant.[16] **E,** Plaque rupture produces intimal ulceration with platelet thrombi that may embolize distally. **F,** Gross specimen shows atherosclerotic plaque with circumferential luminal narrowing of the brachiocephalic and right common carotid arteries. Note cholesterol clefts *(small arrows)* and subintimal hemorrhage *(large arrows)*. **G,** Atheroma of distal vertebral and basilar arteries *(arrows)*.

Continued.

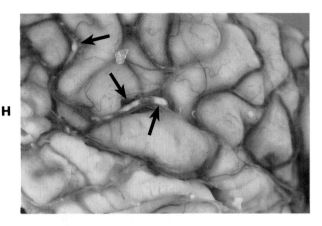

Fig. 11-1, cont'd. H, Atherosclerotic plaques *(arrows)* in cortical branches of the middle cerebral artery. (**F** to **H,** Courtesy Rubinstein Collection, University of Virginia.)

eration disorder with underlying mechanisms similar to neoplastic transformation. Aspects of both may be involved in the complex events associated with ASVD.

Atherogenesis is probably initiated by focal endothelial change or subtle intimal injury that leads to platelet aggregation. The flow reversal that is normally seen in the posterior carotid bulb may also be a contributing factor to platelet adhesion and initial plaque formation. Endothelial injury permits increased permeability to macromolecules such as low density lipoproteins. Monocyte-derived macrophages and smooth muscle cells are recruited to the intima where they proliferate and accumulate fatty esters, becoming lipid-filled foam cells. As these cells die, their detritus produces the extracellular cholesterol deposits that form the atherosclerotic plaque.[7]

Intimal fatty streaks are the earliest macroscopically visible lesions in atherosclerosis (Fig. 11-1, *A*). As the disease progresses a fibrotic cap is formed that covers a core of foam cells, necrotic debris, and cholesterol crystals (Fig. 11-1, *B* and *C*).[6] Underlying secondary inflammatory changes ensue with formation of granulation tissue and neovascularity. Eventually, intraplaque subintimal hemorrhage and necrosis occur (Fig. 11-1, *D*). As the plaque ruptures, endothelial integrity is lost. The ulcerated intimal plaque may serve as a nidus for thrombi (Fig. 11-1, *E*) that embolize distally.

Imaging of Atherosclerotic Vascular Disease

Numerous imaging modalities have been used to evaluate atherosclerosis. Conventional film-screen and high-resolution digital subtraction angiography remain the standards by which other diagnostic techniques are judged. However, noninvasive modalities such as ultrasound, CT, and MR angiography have an increasingly important role in the evaluation of craniocerebral atherosclerosis and occlusive vascular disease.[6]

Ultrasound (US) (with Derek Priest, R.V.T.). The techniques that evaluate blood flow in the orbital and ophthalmic vessels can be used as an indirect means of assessing internal carotid artery disease. These include oculoplethysmography, periorbital bidirectional doppler US, and color flow doppler sonography (CFDS).[8]

Until recently, morphologic changes in the carotid artery wall could not be detected accurately. However, refinements in duplex sonography now permit noninvasive detection of atherosclerotic plaque and vascular stenosis.[9,10,10a] Direct examination of the cervical vasculature can be achieved using high definition gray-scale US, doppler spectral analysis, and CFDS.[11] In recent years, color doppler has rapidly become the preferred US technique.[9] A comprehensive discussion of duplex sonography is beyond the scope of this text. However, other excellent texts are available that address this subject.[9] Here, we briefly cover some basic principles and then focus on the current use of CFDS in the diagnosis of carotid stenosis.

Arterial stenosis is assessed by determining flow velocities in the narrowed vessel lumen (Fig. 11-2). In CFDS, color saturation is directly related to flow velocity and velocity is proportional to severity of obstruction. Elevated flow velocity is indicated by color shift areas (dark red to light pink) on CFDS (Fig. 11-3, *A*). Spectral analysis measures flow velocity in cm/sec. Morphologic changes in waveforms also occur

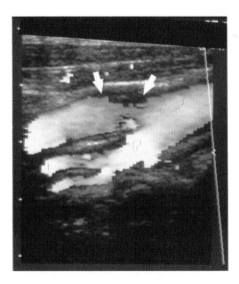

Fig. 11-2. Color flow doppler sonogram (CFDS) depicts the common carotid artery bifurcation. A nonshadowing fibrofatty plaque *(arrows)* at the carotid bulb produces slight increase in intraluminal flow velocity, shown as color change from dark red to light pink.

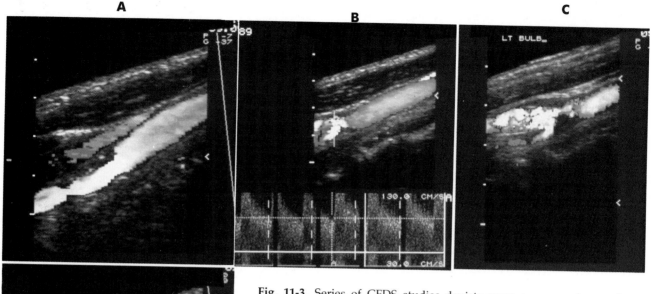

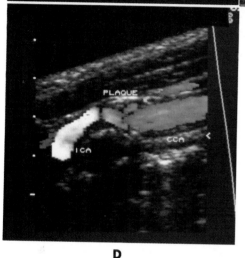

Fig. 11-3. Series of CFDS studies depicts some common abnormalities produced by atherosclerotic disease at the carotid bifurcation. **A,** Narrowed common carotid artery (CCA) with decreased lumen diameter and increased flow velocity is shown as color shift to brighter hues. **B,** Moderately severe stenosis is seen as forward and reversed flow in the post-stenotic zone. The severe stenosis produces broadening of the spectral waveform, as well as color shift from red to light pink. **C,** High-grade stenosis at the ICA origin with disturbed flow pattern is seen. **D,** Flow pattern, red-blue-red, is produced by vessel tortuosity that causes changes in flow direction relative to the transducer. Note velocity change *(light pink)* in the ICA distal to the stenotic plaque (compare to CCA, which is deep red).

with increasing stenosis (Fig. 11-3, *B* and *C*). Peak systolic velocity in the internal carotid artery (ICA) is the best single velocity parameter for quantifying a stenosis.[11]

Flowing blood has phase and frequency shift that permits directional-dependent color assignment. By convention, in most units, flow toward the probe is red; flow away from the probe is blue (Fig. 11-3, *D*). Nonlaminar flow distal to a stenosis is indicated by a mixture of red and blue colors (Fig. 11-3, *C* and *D*). Flow reversal in the posterior carotid bulb is normal. (*see* Fig. 6-6, *C*).

Calcification within an atherosclerotic plaque appears as acoustic shadowing behind the plaque. Sometimes a loud bruit is produced by a hemodynamically significant stenosis. This can be seen as a dramatic "burst" of color on CFDS. CFDS can also be used to detect surface irregularities in atherosclerotic plaques.

Arterial occlusion is diagnosed by absent arterial pulsations, lumen occlusion by echogenic material,

absent doppler flow signal, and subnormal vessel size (chronic occlusion) (Fig. 11-4).[9] Because US tends to overestimate stenosis, extremely high-grade stenosis may mimic occlusion on duplex sonography. Occasionally a very low flow lesion can be distinguished from an occluded one by an antegrade "trickle" of color within the narrowed lumen (Fig. 11-5).

The efficacy of doppler sonography and other noninvasive techniques such as MR angiography in the preoperative evaluation of patients with carotid artery stenosis is controversial.[12,13] Under optimum circumstances, some MRA techniques that are sensitive to low flow (such as 2D TOF MRA) in combination with carotid sonography may be helpful in detecting—and possibly grading—the severity of carotid artery stenosis.[14]

Angiography. Intraarterial contrast angiography is still the most precise technique for evaluating intrinsic abnormalities of the cervicocranial vasculature. Atherosclerotic vascular disease (ASVD) is seen at an-

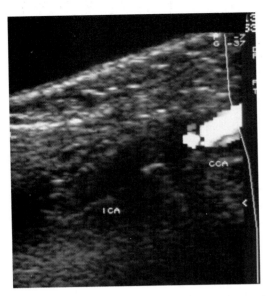

Fig. 11-4. ICA occlusion is indicated by the absence of color on this CFDS study.

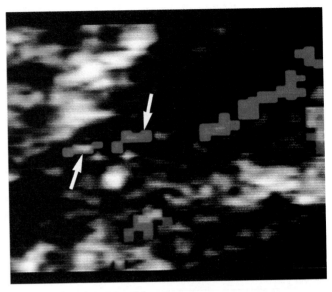

Fig. 11-5. CFDS enhances identification of high-grade stenosis because even minimal flow stream is easily detected in color. "String" stenosis of the ICA is shown here with a "trickle" of color *(arrows)*. A doppler spectral waveform would show the typical diminished velocity that is present with a long-segment stenosis.

giography as vessel irregularity, elongation or tortuosity, and narrowing or frank occlusion. Although these morphologic changes can be identified readily, the three most important goals of cervicocranial angiography in ASVD are as follows[15]:

1. Determine degree of carotid stenosis
2. Identify "tandem" lesions in the carotid siphon or intracranial circulation
3. Evaluate existing and potential collateral circulation

Some authors add a fourth, more controversial goal: assess for possible plaque ulceration.[15]

Carotid origin stenosis. Currently the major goal of cerebral angiography in a patient with extracranial ASVD is to place the arterial lesion into one of the following three groups[15]:

1. Occluded vessel
2. Clinically significant stenosis (see subsequent discussion)
3. Normal or minor stenosis

Because the North American Symptomatic Carotid Endarterectomy Trial (NASCET) and the European Carotid Surgery Trial demonstrated definite benefit of carotid endarterectomy in symptomatic patients with narrowing of the internal carotid artery lumen diameter by 70% to 99%,[16] accurate determination of maximum stenosis on cerebral angiograms is extremely important. At least two projections are required to profile the plaque adequately and measure maximum stenosis (Fig. 11-6). Percentage stenosis is calculated by determining the ratio between the stenosis and normal distal internal carotid artery (ICA) lumen (*not* the carotid bulb or an area with poststenotic dilatation) and multiplying by 100 (Fig. 11-1, *D*)[13].

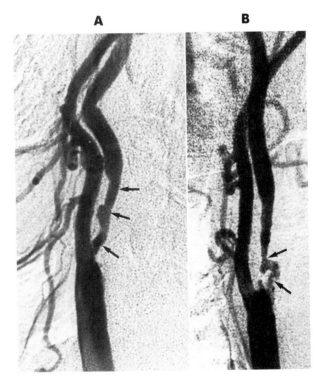

A   **B**

Fig. 11-6. The importance of imaging the carotid bifurcation in multiple projections is shown in this case. **A,** Digital subtraction CCA angiogram, lateral view, shows 60% ICA narrowing *(arrows)*. **B,** Oblique AP view shows the stenosis *(arrows)* is much more severe than is apparent on the lateral view. By the NASCET criteria[16] this symptomatic patient would benefit from carotid endarterectomy.

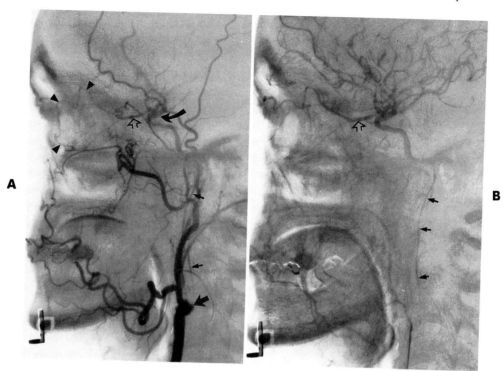

Fig. 11-7. A 45-year-old man had left cerebral hemisphere transient ischemic attacks (TIAs). **A,** Left CCA angiogram, lateral view, midarterial phase, shows what at first glance appears to be occlusion at the carotid bifurcation (*large straight arrow*). However, a small "trickle" of antegrade flow is present (*small black arrows*). Note external-to-internal collateral flow through the orbit (*arrowheads*) to the ophthalmic artery (*open arrow*) and ICA (*curved arrow*). **B,** Late arterial phase study shows the "string sign" of slow but antegrade flow through the nearly occluded ICA (*black arrows*). Note filling of the intracranial ICA and its branches via the ECA orbital to ophthalmic artery (*open arrow*) collaterals.

Occasionally, cervical ICA stenosis is so severe that at first inspection the vessel appears occluded (Fig. 11-7). Close examination of slow contrast injection with prolonged image acquisition may disclose a thin "trickle" of delayed antegrade flow. Correctly distinguishing between true occlusion and this "pseudoocclusion," or *string sign*, is important because patients with very high grade stenosis are still endarterectomy candidates. MR angiography and duplex sonography may fail to show slow antegrade flow in some severely stenotic vessels (see subsequent discussion).[15]

Distal stenosis. So-called *tandem lesions*, or distal stenoses, are present in approximately 2% of patients with significant cervical ICA lesions.[16] The hemodynamic effect of sequential stenoses is additive if both lesions are severe enough to reduce flow separately; if only one is critical, flow is governed by the more severe lesion.[17]

The most common site for a tandem lesion is the carotid siphon, followed by the horizontal middle cerebral artery segment. Because some of these patients may be excluded from cervical carotid endarterectomy or require balloon angioplasty, adequate angiographic evaluation of the patient with craniocervical ASVD should also include the carotid siphon and intracranial circulation.[18]

Plaque ulcerations. Identification of plaque ulceration may be important in some cervical ICA lesions without significant stenosis (Fig. 11-8).[10a,19] Because atherosclerotic subintimal hematomas with intact endothelium can resemble ulcerated plaque the accuracy for diagnosing plaque ulcerations on conventional angiograms is only 60%.[20] However, the availability of ultra-high resolution digital subtraction angiography may improve detection of surface ulcerations in atherosclerotic plaques (Fig. 11-8, *B*).

Intravascular thrombi. Intraplaque and intraluminal thrombi are present in some cases and are seen as filling defects within the opacified vessel.

Collateral circulation. In the event of cervical or intracranial vascular occlusion or hemodynamically significant stenosis, the adequacy of collateral circulation becomes critical. Because the common carotid artery is clamped during endarterectomy, preoperative determination of collateral blood flow is also helpful in determining whether a shunt across the bifurcation will be necessary.[21]

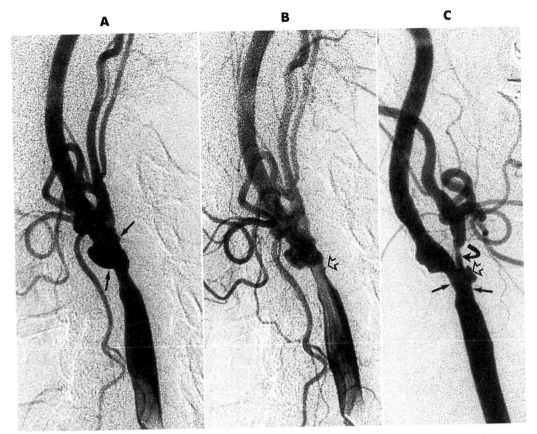

Fig. 11-8. A 62-year-old woman with left hemispheric TIAs and a right carotid bruit. **A,** Digital subtraction left common carotid angiogram, midarterial phase, oblique view, shows a smooth-appearing distal CCA and proximal ICA plaque *(arrows)*. **B,** Late arterial phase study shows a tiny contrast-filled ulcer *(open arrow)* within the atherosclerotic plaque. Endarterectomy confirmed the angiographic findings. **C,** Right CCA angiogram, midarterial phase, oblique view, in the same patient shows an atherosclerotic plaque *(small arrows)* at the CCA bifurcation with only minimal ICA narrowing. A high-grade ECA stenosis *(curved arrow)* is seen with poststenotic dilatation. The ECA stenosis accounts for the audible bruit. The "collar-button" outpouching of contrast *(open arrow)* is not pathognomonic for ulceration.

Various potential collateral pathways exist *(see Chapter 6)*. The most important potential pathway is through the circle of Willis, the large anastomotic vascular ring at the base of the brain (Fig. 11-9, *E*). A so-called complete circle of Willis in which no component is hypoplastic or absent is present in only 15% to 25% of individuals *(see Chapter 6)*. If both proximal segments of the anterior cerebral arteries and the anterior communicating artery are visualized at angiography or if filling and washout of the ipsilateral PCA is seen, collateral flow is usually adequate and most patients do not require shunting during endarterectomy.[21]

Extra- to intracranial pathways from external carotid branches to the ophthalmic artery or cavernous ICA are also important (Figs. 11-7 and 11-9, *B*). Intracranial pial and leptomeningeal collaterals may develop (Fig. 11-9, *C* to *E*) but are often inadequate to prevent neurologic deficit.

Aortic arch and proximal great vessel disease. ASVD also occurs more proximally at the aortic arch. The proximal subclavian (SCA), innominate artery (IA), and vertebral artery (VA) origins are commonly affected. So-called *subclavian steal phenomenon* (SSP) occurs if an SCA is occluded and flow is reversed in the vertebral artery to supply the shoulder and arm distal to the obstruction.[22,22a] Symptoms are due to ipsilateral arm ischemia and episodic neurologic symptoms from posterior fossa ischemia (steal). Diminished or absent pulse in the affected arm may be present. Although standard angiography has been used in the past, duplex ultrasound and MR angiography with flow direction encoding are effective noninvasive methods for diagnosis SSP (Fig. 11-10).[22,23,23a]

Intracranial ASVD. Manifestations of intracranial ASVD include luminal irregularities and stenoses, elongated tortuous vessels, and fusiform aneurysms

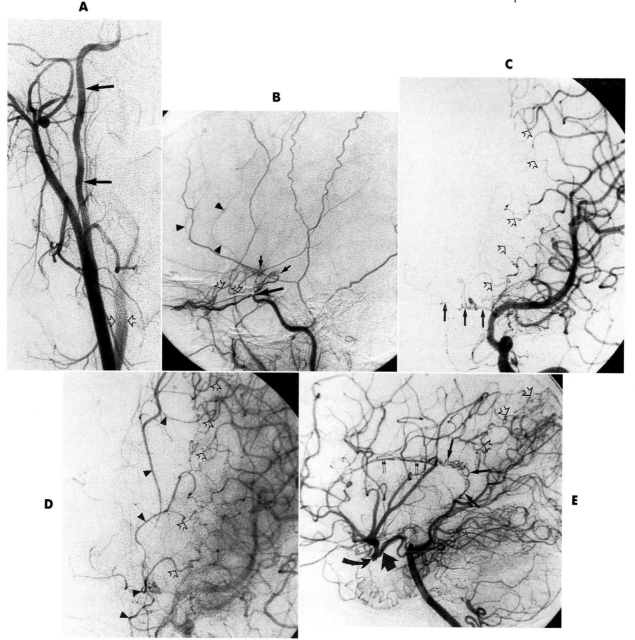

Fig. 11-9. An 11-year-old boy with severe head trauma at age 6 had worsening symptoms of right hemisphere ischemia. **A,** Digital subtraction right CCA angiogram, midarterial phase, oblique view, shows a small ICA *(large arrows)* secondary to reduced intracranial flow. Compare size of the ICA to the right VA *(open arrows)*, which is transiently filled with contrast. **B,** Lateral view of the distal right ICA shows occlusion of the supraclinoid segment *(large arrow),* probably secondary to previous traumatic dissection. Enlarged basal leptomeningeal collaterals are indicated by the small arrows. Minimal dural-to-leptomeningeal collateral circulation via recurrent meningeal branches *(open arrows)* of the ophthalmic artery is present. Very faint opacification of the ACA *(arrowheads)* is seen. **C,** Left ICA angiogram, early arterial phase, AP view, shows bilateral hypoplastic A1 ACA segments *(solid arrows)* and a small anterior communicating artery. This allows only minimal collateral flow through the anterior circle of Willis to the right hemisphere. Note some early flow across the middle-to-anterior cerebral watershed zone *(open arrows)*. **D,** Late arterial phase shows these artery-to-artery collaterals *(open arrows)* across the watershed zone opacify ACA branches *(arrowheads)*. **E,** Left vertebral angiogram, midarterial phase, lateral view, shows extensive collateral circulation through the posterior communicating artery *(large arrow)* to the supraclinoid ICA *(curved arrow)*. Arterial-to-arterial anastomoses are seen from posterior splenial PCA branches *(small single arrows)* to the pericallosal artery *(double arrows)*. The angular MCA branch is not visualized. Leptomeningeal collateral circulation from the PCA to angular artery territory *(open arrows)*.

Continued.

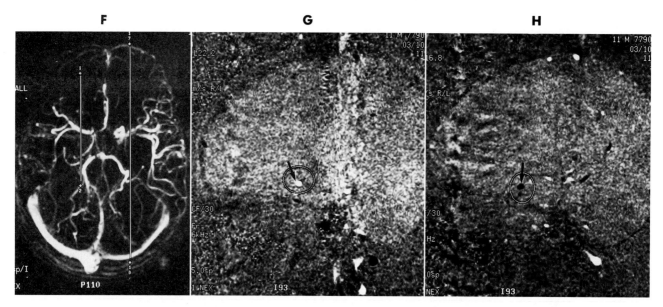

Fig. 11-9, cont'd. F, 2D PC MRA was performed for flow analysis. The scan was interrogated for right and left MCA flow. **G,** Directional encoding is from right to left. The left MCA is seen within the circled region of interest as a white area *(arrow)*. Measured flow was 162 ml/minute. **H,** The right MCA shows normal flow direction *(left-to-right)*, so this vessel is seen within the ROI as the black area *(arrow)*. However, the right MCA flow is markedly reduced (93 ml/minute). Note that flow can be very abnormal even when angiography shows robust collateral circulation (**E**).

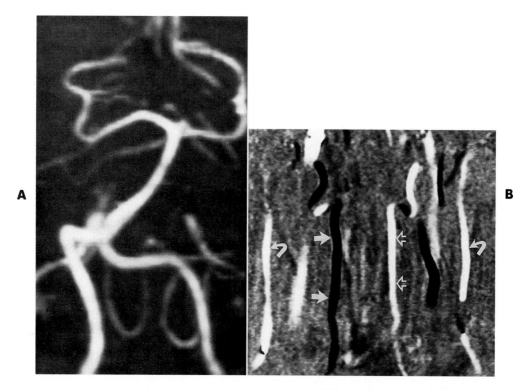

Fig. 11-10. This 62-year-old patient had bihemispheric TIAs and symptoms of posterior fossa ischemia. **A,** MOTSA MR angiogram, AP view, shows normal appearing posterior fossa circulation, **B,** Phase-contrast MR angiogram of the cervical vasculature shows normal (cephalad) blood flow in the right vertebral artery *(solid straight arrows)*. Flow direction in the left vertebral artery *(open arrows)* is reversed and from cranial to caudal (compare with flow in the jugular veins, *curved arrows*). Subclavian steal phenomena.

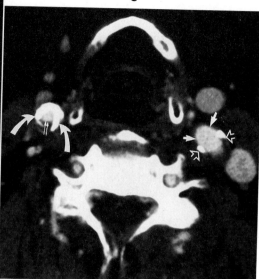

Fig. 11-11. A, Right CCA angiogram, arterial phase, lateral view, in a 76-year-old man with TIAs shows severe stenosis of the right ICA *(straight arrow).* Tapering of the distal CCA *(between curved arrows)* suggests presence of atherosclerotic plaque extending from the distal portion of the common carotid artery into the bifurcation. **B,** Spiral CT angiogram with maximum intensity projection of the right CCA demonstrates the region of severe stenosis *(arrow).* The area of narrowing in the distal CCA noted on the angiogram **(A,** *curved arrows)* is obscured on this view due to calcification. **C,** Axial slice through the distal common carotid arteries. The right CCA shows nearly circumferential calcification *(curved arrows).* Note the small right CCA lumen *(double arrows)* seen clearly filled with contrast as compared to the larger left CCA lumen *(small solid arrows).* The left CCA has punctate mural calcifications *(open arrows).* (Reprinted from Marks MP et al: *AJR* 160:1267-1271, 1993.)

(see Figs. 9-41 and 9-42). ASVD in medium-sized vessels is the most common cause of an "arteritic-like" pattern on angiography. Focal vascular stenoses alternate with normal or slightly dilated segments (Figs. 11-1, *H,* and 11-53).

Computed tomography. Because contrast-enhanced CT (CECT) allows visualization of a vessel wall and its lumen, degenerative atheromatous changes in the extracranial vasculature can be easily identified. Findings of ASVD on CECT include mural calcifications (Fig. 11-11, *C*) and intimal plaques. Atherosclerotic plaques with subintimal hemorrhage and necrosis are seen as circumferential or eccentric lucent areas surrounding the strongly enhancing vessel lumen.[4] With CCA or ICA occlusion, intraluminal thrombus appears as a rounded or ovoid low density area surrounded by an enhancing rim.

Three-dimensional spiral computed tomographic angiography can be used to image intraluminal vessel contrast directly. These CT "angiograms" are obtained using multiple thin sections acquired rapidly during bolus contrast administration. Maximum intensity three-dimensional reprojection of the data set is used to profile the carotid bifurcation (Fig. 11-11, *B*).[24]

Common manifestations of intracranial ASVD that are identified on CT scans are vessel ectasias and mural calcifications. Atherosclerotic vascular calcification beyond the circle of Willis or horizontal M1 segment is uncommon. Occasionally, debris from extracranial atherosclerotic plaque embolizes to the distal intracranial circulation. ASVD also causes arterial elongation and tortuousity, especially in the posterior circulation. The basilar artery (BA) may become markedly ectatic and elongated. In extreme cases, vertebrobasilar dolichoectasia (VBD) causes a mass effect at the posterior third ventricle or foramen of Monro.

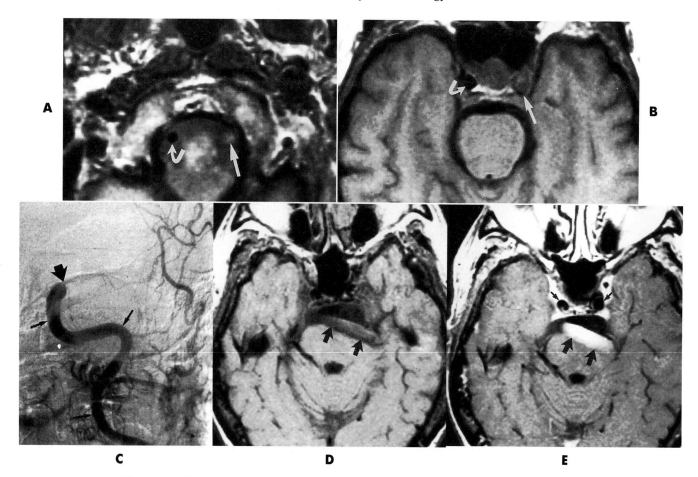

Fig. 11-12. Three cases illustrate the difficulties encountered in assessing arterial patency on standard spin-echo MR imaging. **A,** Axial long TR/short TE scan in a case of posterior fossa stroke following chiropractic manipulation shows a patent right VA, seen as the typical "flow void" of high-velocity signal loss *(curved arrow)*. The left VA is filled with clot *(straight arrow)* that appears isointense with brain. **B,** Axial T1WI in a patient with left hemisphere TIAs shows a normal right ICA "flow void" *(curved arrow)*; the normal left ICA high-velocity signal loss is not seen. Instead the cavernous left ICA *(straight arrow)* appears isointense with cortex. **C,** Left CCA angiogram, late arterial phase, AP view, shows the ICA *(small arrows)* is actually patent but has very slow flow with an extremely high-grade stenosis at its supraclinoid segment *(large arrow)*. **D** and **E,** A 70-year-old man has severe vertebrobasilar dolichoectasia. **D,** Axial T1-weighted MR scan shows an elongated basilar artery (BA) with intraluminal signal *(arrows)* that is isointense with brain. **E,** Postcontrast T1WI shows the lumen is patent but has very slow flow *(large arrows)*. Compare with the cavernous ICA "flow voids" *(small arrows)*. The intraluminal BA signal is caused by slow in-plane flow.

Magnetic resonance imaging. Arterial patency may be difficult to assess with standard spin-echo MR imaging. If intraluminal signal that is isointense with brain on long TR/short TE or long TR/long TE is observed, vessel occlusion with intraluminal thrombus is usually present (Fig. 11-12, *A*).[25] However, in-flow phenomena, as well as slow (Fig. 11-12, *B* and *C*) or in-plane flow, in tortuous, ectatic vessels (Fig. 11-12, *D* and *E*), can mimic intraluminal thrombi. Presence of a normal "flow void" also does not exclude significant extracranial carotid stenosis.[25]

Magnetic resonance angiography (MRA). In MRA the sensitivity of MR imaging to flow is used to produce angiographic-like images of the cervicocranial vasculature. Pulse sequences based on contrast differences between moving blood and stationary tissues have been described. The two basic techniques are time-of-flight (TOF) and phase-contrast (PC) MRA.

Three-dimensional TOF MRA studies are based on flow-related enhancement. 3D TOF MRA depicts normal and occluded vessels well but is less useful for

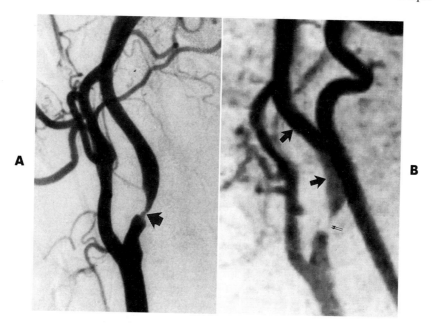

Fig. 11-13. A 67-year-old man had a left carotid bruit and amaurosis fugax. **A,** Digital subtraction left CCA angiogram, midarterial phase, lateral view, shows a high-grade ICA stenosis *(arrow)*. **B,** Multiple overlapping thin slab (MOTSA) MR angiogram, lateral view, depicts the distal ICA *(large arrows)* but overestimates the stenosis, where slow flow makes the residual lumen *(double arrows)* difficult to identify.

slow-flow lesions because spin saturation may cause overestimation of stenosis.[26]

In *two-dimensional TOF MRA* sequences (2D TOF) the relative contrast between flowing blood and stationary tissues is increased by the high signal of maximally magnetized spins as they flow into the individually imaged slice.[27] Although 2D TOF MRA is better than 3D sequences in slow flow situations, significant "stepladder" artifacts often occur and may obscure vessel detail. In addition, the echo time with 2D TOF MRA is longer than with three-dimensional sequences due to greater gradient requirements. This leads to more signal loss from intravoxel dephasing secondary to turbulent or complex flow. 2D TOF MRA correlates well with contrast arteriography in evaluating cervical carotid bifurcation disease.[28,28a] Surgically significant stenosis is seen as a focal area of signal loss at the stenotic level with reappearance of the signal distally. If the distal signal intensity does not reappear the artery is probably occluded.[28,28b]

A modified time-of-flight MR angiographic technique that uses multiple overlapping thin slab acquisitions (MOTSA) combines the advantages of two-dimensional multiple section and direct 3D TOF techniques.[28] Severe stenoses with slow flow are depicted well with this technique, although the degree of stenosis is often slightly overestimated (Fig. 11-13).[29,29a]

Two-dimensional phase-contrast (PC) MRA is helpful in differentiating abnormally slow flow or absent flow from normal flow.[30] PC MRA can also be used to pro-

vide directional information and quantify flow velocities (Fig. 11-9, *F* to *H*). Because only the true patent lumen is depicted by PC MRA, standard spin-echo or gradient-echo sequences should be used to demonstrate other abnormalities such as paravascular hematoma. A relative disadvantage of 2D PC MRA compared to TOF techniques is increased signal loss from intravoxel phase dispersion resulting from complex or turbulent flow in tortuous vessels.

CEREBRAL ISCHEMIA AND INFARCTION
Pathophysiology

Cerebral ischemia is significantly diminished blood flow to all parts (global ischemia) or selected areas (regional or focal ischemia) of the brain.[31] Stroke is a dynamic process in which the location and degree of cerebral ischemia and resultant infarction change over time.[32] Ischemic manifestations are predicated by the clinically important parameters of flow decrement, location, duration, and tissue volume involved.[31] The pathophysiology of cerebral ischemia and infarction will be addressed first, followed by a discussion of various imaging manifestations.

Physiology of cerebral ischemia and infarction. Stroke progresses in stages from ischemia to actual infarction. This process involves many simultaneous, as well as sequential, events.[2] In the most common situation, i.e., ischemia due to middle cerebral artery occlusion, there is a densely ischemic central focus and a less densely ischemic "penumbra." Cells within the densely ischemic area are usually damaged irretrievably unless reperfusion is quickly established, whereas cells within the penumbra may remain viable but at risk for several hours.[33] Current salvage therapies attempt to rescue these "at risk" cells.[34]

Ischemia produces energy depletion in the affected cells. Loss of ion homeostasis, accumulation of Ca^{++}, Na^+, and Cl^- along with osmotically obligated water, and anaerobic glucolysis with production of intra- and extracellular metabolic acidosis occur.[33] Hypoxic-ischemic injury also leads to the accumulation of extracellular glutamate and free radicals. These changes are part of the so-called ischemic cascade, a complex series of biochemical reactions that leads to lost cell membrane function and cytoskeletal integrity with subsequent cell death. Macroscopic secondary manifestations such as edema and mass effect eventually ensue and can be observed on standard imaging studies.[2]

Neuropathology of ischemic brain damage. The results of brain ischemia vary with the sensitivity of individual cell types to ischemia. The adequacy of collateral blood supply and the degree, the duration, and the distribution of flow reduction are also important factors.

Selective vulnerability. Sensitivity to ischemic damage varies with different cell types. There is a well-defined hierarchy of sensitivity to ischemic damage among different cell types that constitute the neuropil. The neurons are most vulnerable and are followed in descending order of susceptibility by astrocytes, oligodendroglia, microglia, and endothelial cells. Among neurons there also is a regional hierarchy of sensitivity with the CA_1 hippocampal pyramidal cells; neurons in neocortex layers III, V, and VI; cerebellar Purkinje cells; and small and medium-sized neurons in the neostriatum the most vulnerable.[35]

Collateral supply. The consequences of cerebral arterial occlusion vary because alterations in cerebral blood flow change with time, location, and potentially available collateral circulation.

Large arterial-to-arterial anastomoses through the circle of Willis (Fig. 11-9, *E*) and the external to internal carotid distributions (Figs. 11-7, *A*, and 11-9, *B*) have already been illustrated. The cerebral microvasculature also offers relative protection to some regions while leaving others comparatively vulnerable. Some areas such as the subcortical white matter U-fibers, extreme and external capsule, and claustrum have dual or even triple interdigitating supply. Others such as the cortex have short arterioles from a single source. The thalamus, basal ganglia, and centrum semiovale have large, long, single source vessels that are not only more susceptible to hypoten-

sion but are also affected by aging, hypertension, diabetes, and atherosclerosis.[36] These areas are thus relatively vulnerable to anoxia or hypoperfusion.

In adults and term infants, so-called border zones exist between the terminal capillary beds of the major cerebral arteries in the cortex and cerebellum. Arterial perfusion pressure is lowest in these zones because of arteriolar arborization. These peripheral zones receive the lowest CBF and are the first to suffer ischemia and infarction during generalized systemic hypotension[31] (see subsequent discussion).

In the fetus and in premature infants the vascular watershed is in the deep periventricular region (*see* Fig. 11-30, *B*).[37,38]

Degree and duration of cerebral ischemia. Neuropathologists have identified several morphologically distinct patterns of ischemic brain damage. Frank *cerebral infarction* is characterized by irreversible damage to all cell types within the infarcted zone. This includes neurons, glia, and, sometimes, endothelial cells as well. Histologic findings range from coagulative necrosis, typically in the central ischemic focus, to astrocytic swelling near the periphery of the lesion.

Within the surrounding ischemic penumbral zone the neurons may be injured but supporting cell types

TABLE 11-1. Stroke etiologies

Type of stroke	Percent (%)
Cerebral infarction (80%)	
Large vessel occlusions (ICA, MCA, PCA)	40-50
Small vessel (lacunar) infarcts	25
Cardiac emboli (myocardial infarction, valvular disease, cardiomyopathy, etc)	15
Blood disorders	5
Nonatheromatous occlusions (e.g., vasculitis, vasculopathy)	5
Primary intracranial hemorrhage (15%)	
Hypertensive bleeds	40-60
Amyloid angiopathy	15-25
Vascular malformation	10-15
Drugs (anticoagulants, sympathomimetics)	1-2
Bleeding diathesis	<1
Nontraumatic subarachnoid hemorrhage (5%)	
Aneurysm	75-80
Vascular malformation	10-15
"Nonaneurysmal" SAH	5-15
Miscellaneous	
Dural sinus/cerebral vein occlusion	1

Adapted from Bradac GB: Angiography in cerebral ischemia, *Riv di Neuoradiol* 3 [suppl 2]: 57-66, 1990, and Hankey GJ, Warlow CP: The role of imaging in the management of cerebral and ocular ischemia, *Neuroradiol* 33:381-390, 1991.

are preserved. This pattern of brain injury is termed *generalized* or *partial neuronal necrosis.*[35] So-called selective neuronal necrosis involves only certain populations of highly vulnerable neurons (see previous discussion). This type of ischemic damage typically occurs in patients who suffer cardiac arrest and are successfully resuscitated.[35]

Imaging of Cerebral Ischemia and Infarction: Overview

Stroke is a lay term that encompasses a heterogeneous group of cerebrovascular disorders with widely different clinical presentations, pathology, etiology, prognosis, and treatment.[39] The four major types of stroke are cerebral infarction, primary intracerebral hemorrhage (ICH), subarachnoid hemorrhage (SAH), and venous occlusions (Table 11-1). Arterial infarction and venoocclusive disorders are included in this chapter; nontraumatic ICH is discussed in Chapter 7 and aneurysmal SAH is covered in Chapter 9.

The imaging manifestations of cerebral ischemia vary significantly with time. Therefore acute, subacute, and chronic infarctions will be considered separately. Then lacunar infarction, hypoxic-ischemic

damage, and strokes in specific vascular distributions will be discussed. Finally, special consideration is given to strokes in children and the imaging differential diagnosis of stroke and its "mimics."

Acute Infarcts

Cerebral angiography. Angiography is often not performed during the hyperacute stage of cerebral infarction unless fibrolytic therapy is being considered or other causes of stroke besides ASVD are entertained. The angiographic signs of acute cerebral infarction are summarized in Table 11-2. The most

TABLE 11-2. Angiographic signs of acute cerebral infarction

Angiographic sign	Percent (%)
Vessel occlusion (with or without meniscus)	45-50
Slow antegrade flow with delayed arterial emptying	15
Collateral, retrograde filling	15-25
"Bare" (nonperfused) areas	5-10
Vascular blush (luxury perfusion)	15-25
Arteriovenous shunting with early appearing draining vein	10-15
Mass effect (variable)	25-50

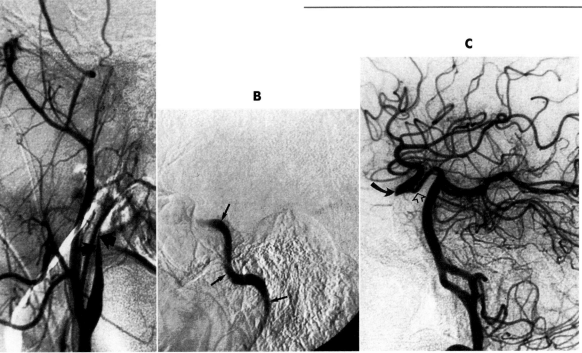

Fig. 11-14. Spontaneous ICA dissection with distal embolus occluding the supraclinoid ICA. Common carotid angiogram with mid- **(A)** and late **(B)** arterial phase films, lateral view, shows the dissection severely narrows the cervical ICA **(A,** *arrows).* Contrast stasis in the distal ICA is shown **(B,** *arrows).* **C,** Left vertebral angiogram, midarterial phase, lateral view, shows collateral circulation through the posterior communicating artery *(open arrow).* Retrograde filling of the supraclinoid ICA shows an abrupt cut-off caused by a distal embolus *(curved arrow).*

specific finding is vessel occlusion, seen in about half of all angiograms performed within the first few hours after cerebral infarction.[40] Embolic obstruction may appear as a persistent contrast column in the affected artery (Fig. 11-14, *B*), a distal meniscal filling defect (Fig. 11-14, *C*), or both.[19]

Other angiographic abnormalities observed in acute cerebral infarction include slow antegrade flow with prolonged circulation time and delayed arterial emptying in the affected area, seen in about 15% of acute strokes.[40] Collateral filling with retrograde flow, "bare" or nonperfused areas, hyperemia or vascular blush in the ischemic penumbra (so-called luxury perfusion), arteriovenous shunting with early appearance of contrast in draining veins, and mass effect are other angiographic manifestations of acute cerebral infarction that can be identified in some cases (Fig. 11-15).[41]

Computed tomography. Although "stroke" is a clinical diagnosis, the clinical diagnosis of stroke is inaccurate in approximately 13% of patients admitted to stroke units.[42] Therefore the role of immediate CT

in the management of acute cerebral infarction is twofold: (1) diagnose or exclude intracerebral hemorrhage (ICH) because the causes, treatment, and prognosis of primary ICH differ from those of cerebral ischemia and (2) identify the presence of an underlying structural lesion such as tumor, vascular malformation, or subdural hematoma that can mimic stroke clinically. Nonvascular lesions cause 1% to 2% of stroke syndromes.[39]

The CT findings in acute cerebral infarction evolve with time. Although almost 60% of CT scans obtained within the first few hours after cerebral infarction are normal,[43] several early signs of acute stroke can often be identified in strokes less than 4 to 6 hours old (*see* box, p. 347). These include a hyperattenuating artery (usually the middle cerebral artery, the so-called dense MCA sign),[44] obscuration of the lentiform nucleus,[45] gray-white interface loss along the lateral insula (insular ribbon sign)[46] (Fig. 11-16), and effacement of the gray-white junction along the cortex (Fig. 11-17).

A hyperdense MCA is caused by acute intraluminal thrombus (Fig. 11-18). The hyperdense MCA sign

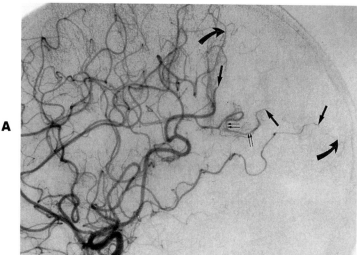

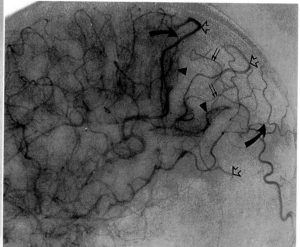

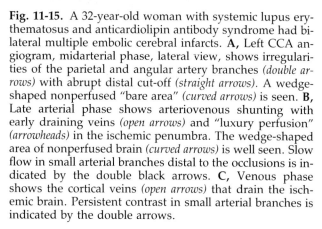

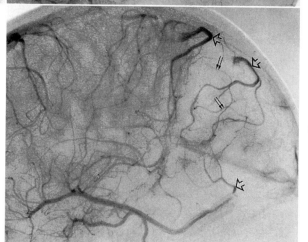

Fig. 11-15. A 32-year-old woman with systemic lupus erythematosus and anticardiolipin antibody syndrome had bilateral multiple embolic cerebral infarcts. **A,** Left CCA angiogram, midarterial phase, lateral view, shows irregularities of the parietal and angular artery branches (*double arrows*) with abrupt distal cut-off (*straight arrows*). A wedge-shaped nonperfused "bare area" (*curved arrows*) is seen. **B,** Late arterial phase shows arteriovenous shunting with early draining veins (*open arrows*) and "luxury perfusion" (*arrowheads*) in the ischemic penumbra. The wedge-shaped area of nonperfused brain (*curved arrows*) is well seen. Slow flow in small arterial branches distal to the occlusions is indicated by the double black arrows. **C,** Venous phase shows the cortical veins (*open arrows*) that drain the ischemic brain. Persistent contrast in small arterial branches is indicated by the double arrows.

Cerebral Infarction
CT Findings

Hyperacute infarct (<12 hours)

Normal (50% to 60%)
Hyperdense artery (25% to 50%)
Obscuration of lentiform nuclei

Acute (12 to 24 hours)

Low density basal ganglia
Loss of gray-white interfaces (insular ribbon sign,
  obscuration of cortex-medullary white matter border)
Sulcal effacement

1 to 3 days

Increasing mass effect
Wedge-shaped low density area that involves both
  gray and white matter
Hemorrhagic transformation may occur (basal ganglia
  and cortex are common sites)

4 to 7 days

Gyral enhancement
Mass effect, edema persist

1 to 8 weeks

Contrast enhancement persists
Mass effect resolves
Transient calcification can occur (pediatric strokes)

Months to years

Encephalomalacic change, volume loss
Calcification rare

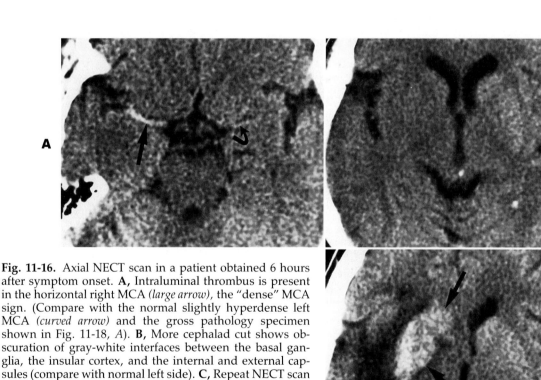

Fig. 11-16. Axial NECT scan in a patient obtained 6 hours after symptom onset. **A,** Intraluminal thrombus is present in the horizontal right MCA *(large arrow)*, the "dense" MCA sign. (Compare with the normal slightly hyperdense left MCA *(curved arrow)* and the gross pathology specimen shown in Fig. 11-18, *A*). **B,** More cephalad cut shows obscuration of gray-white interfaces between the basal ganglia, the insular cortex, and the internal and external capsules (compare with normal left side). **C,** Repeat NECT scan obtained 4 days later shows hemorrhagic transformation *(arrows)* of the basal ganglia ischemic infarction. The frontal horn of the right lateral ventricle is compressed, indicating mass effect.

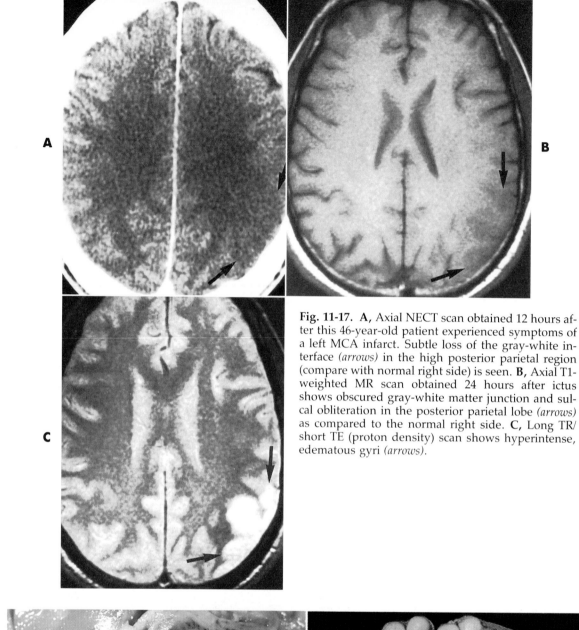

Fig. 11-17. **A,** Axial NECT scan obtained 12 hours after this 46-year-old patient experienced symptoms of a left MCA infarct. Subtle loss of the gray-white interface *(arrows)* in the high posterior parietal region (compare with normal right side) is seen. **B,** Axial T1-weighted MR scan obtained 24 hours after ictus shows obscured gray-white matter junction and sulcal obliteration in the posterior parietal lobe *(arrows)* as compared to the normal right side. **C,** Long TR/short TE (proton density) scan shows hyperintense, edematous gyri *(arrows)*.

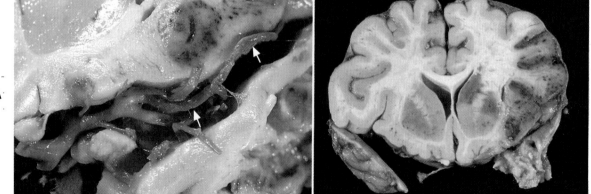

Fig. 11-18. Gross specimen of MCA infarct. **A,** Close-up view of the sylvian fissure shows extensive thrombus *(arrows)* is present in the horizontal (M1) and insular MCA segments. **B,** Coronal whole brain section shows hemorrhagic cortical and basal ganglionic infarction *(arrows)*. (Case courtesy E. Tessa Hedley-Whyte.)

Cerebral Infarction
MR Findings

Immediate

Absence of normal "flow void"
Intravascular contrast enhancement
Low apparent diffusion coefficient (ADCs)
Perfusion alterations

<12 hours

Anatomic alterations on T1WI
   Sulcal effacement
   Gyral edema
   Loss of gray-white interfaces

12 to 24 hours

Hyperintensity on T2WI develops
Meningeal enhancement adjacent to infarct
Mass effect

1 to 3 days

Intravascular, meningeal enhancement begin
  decreasing
Early parenchymal contrast enhancement
Signal abnormalities striking on T1WI, T2WI
Hemorrhagic transformation may become evident

4 to 7 days

Striking parenchymal contrast enhancement
Hemorrhage apparent in 25%
Mass effect, edema begin diminishing
Intravascular, meningeal enhancement disappear

1 to 8 weeks

Contrast enhancement often persists
Mass effect resolves
Decrease in abnormal signal on T2WI sometimes noted
  (fogging effect)
Hemorrhagic changes evolve, become chronic

Months to years

Encephalomalacic changes, volume loss in affected
  vasular distribution
Hemorrhagic residua (hemosiderin/ferritin)

---

has been reported in 25% of all unselected acute infarcts and is seen in 35% to 50% of patients who have stroke symptoms in the MCA territory.[44,47,48] The hyperdense MCA sign typically occurs with cortical and large, deep MCA infarcts.[47] Conventional or MR angiography in such cases discloses an occluded MCA. Because unclotted circulating intravascular blood is normally somewhat hyperdense to brain, caution should be exercised in calling a mildly hyperattenuating MCA a thrombosed vessel (Fig. 11-16, *A*).[48a]

Frank hypodensity of the lentiform nuclei on early CT studies is strongly associated with later hemorrhagic transformation of the initially ischemic infarction.[49] With the exception of hypertensive ICH and amyloid angiopathy, hemorrhagic "strokes" are uncommon within the first 24 to 48 hours after ictus (*see* Chapter 7). In normotensive patients most hemorrhagic strokes occur with reperfusion of a previously ischemic infarct (Fig. 11-16, *C*). In these cases, hemorrhage occurs from injured capillaries after emboli lyse and flow is reestablished.[50]

Magnetic resonance imaging. Acute infarcts are identified more often and localized more accurately on MR compared to CT scans.[42] Eighty percent are visible on standard spin-echo MR scans obtained within 24 hours of the ictus (Fig. 11-17).[43] The earliest MR findings are vascular flow-related abnormalities (*see* box). These include absence of normal flow void and slow flow with intravascular arterial enhancement (Fig. 11-19).[50a] These signs can be detected within minutes of symptom onset.[51,52] Intravascular enhancement is seen in nearly three quarters of acute cortical infarcts.[51]

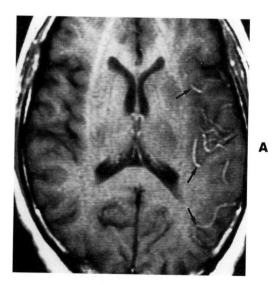

Fig. 11-19. A, Contrast-enhanced axial T1-weighted MR scan obtained 4 hours after symptoms of left MCA infarct shows extensive intravascular enhancement (*small arrows*).

Continued.

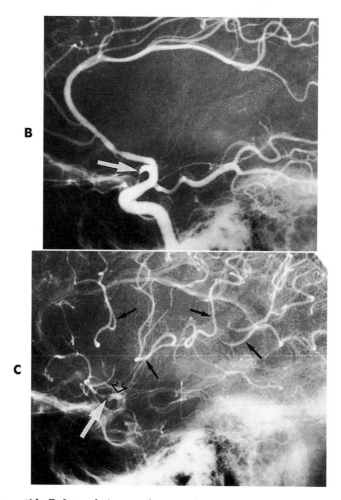

Fig. 11-19, cont'd. B, Lateral view, early arterial phase, shows abrupt cut-off of the MCA *(arrow)*. The anterior and posterior cerebral arteries are opacified but the insula is devoid of contrast. **C,** Late arterial phase shows slow retrograde filling of MCA branches *(black arrows)*, accounting for the intravascular contrast observed on the enhanced MR scans. The junction between the MCA distal to the clot, filled by retrograde flow, and the MCA proximal to the embolus, seen as persistent opacification in the horizontal MCA *(open arrow)*, represents the location of the embolus *(white arrow)*. (Courtesy L. Cromwell.)

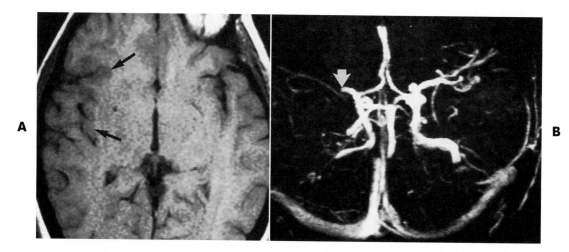

Fig. 11-20. A 44-year-old man experienced sudden onset of left hemiparesis. CT scan (not shown) was normal. **A,** Axial T1-weighted MR scan obtained 12 hours after ictus shows subtle insular cortical swelling *(arrows)* with compression of the adjacent sylvian fissure (compare to normal left side). **B,** MR angiogram shows MCA occlusion *(arrow)*.

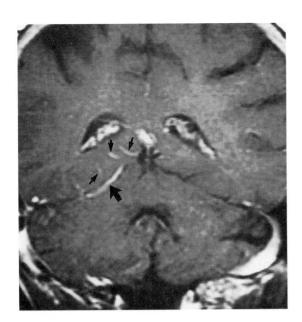

Fig. 11-21. Coronal postcontrast T1-weighted MR scan obtained 24 hours after PCA infarct shows intravascular enhancement *(small arrows)*. The adjacent tentorium shows abnormal meningeal enhancement *(large arrow)*.

Other early MR findings include morphologic changes (particularly brain swelling) on T1-weighted images (Figs. 11-17, *B*, and 11-20, *A*). These anatomic changes may precede the development of increased signal on proton density- or T2-weighted sequences. T2 hyperintensity occurs but is usually not observed before 8 hours.[52] Abnormal meningeal enhancement adjacent to cortical infarcts aged 1 to 3 days is seen in about one third of cases (Fig. 11-21).[51] Standard MRI sequences may fail to detect acute stroke in 10% to 20% of patients.[53]

Magnetic resonance angiography. MRA can demonstrate vascular occlusion or severe stenosis in many patients with major vessel disease (Fig. 11-20, *B*). Spin saturation reduces sensitivity for small or distal lesions.[54]

Miscellaneous techniques. Ultra-early evaluation of stroke and ischemia-induced changes in cerebral metabolism is now possible using powerful new morphologic and functional clinical imaging techniques. These include transcranial doppler ultrasound, proton MR spectroscopy, diffusion imaging, and perfusion studies.

Transcranial doppler ultrasonography (TCD). TCD is sensitive to vascular anatomy and blood flow. Although it has primarily been used to monitor post-SAH and posttraumatic vasospasm, TCD can be used in acute MCA occlusion. Abnormal TCD findings include an unobtainable MCA flow signal or significantly depressed MCA flow velocity.[55]

Proton magnetic resonance spectroscopy (MRS). MRS can be used to observe ischemia-induced changes in cerebral metabolism. Acute ischemic infarctions are characterized by decreased *N*-acetylaspartate resonances and elevated lactate (lac); the highest lac levels are observed in complete MCA territory infarcts.[56,57] Creatine and phosphocreatine are also reduced in infarcted areas, but no significant change has been reported in the choline content.[58]

Diffusion-weighted imaging. Diffusion-weighted MR imaging is sensitive to the microscopic motion of water protons. In the presence of a magnetic field gradient, protons carried by moving water molecules undergo phase shift of their transverse magnetization. In a diffusion-weighted MR image, structures with fast diffusion are dark because they are subject to greater signal attenuation. Structures with slower diffusion are bright.[59]

Cytotoxic edema is initiated within minutes of ischemia onset and can produce an increase in brain tissue water of 3% to 5%. Using diffusion-weighted MR imaging, signal intensity changes can be detected within minutes of arterial occlusion.[60] Acute infarcts have lower apparent diffusion coefficients (ADCs) compared to noninfarcted brain[61] and may be a very sensitive indicator of early cytotoxic brain edema.[62] The early detection of stroke, at a stage when tissue damage may still be reversible, could potentially justify more aggressive salvage therapies with acute cerebral ischemia.[59,63]

Echo-planar imaging (EPI) can be used to visualize physiologic parameters in addition to measuring diffusion coefficients of ischemic brain. Deoxygenated blood behaves as an effective susceptibility contrast agent. Changes in brain oxygenation can be monitored using gradient-echo echo-planar MR imaging.[64]

EPI and fast gradient echo techniques can also be used in conjunction with bolus injection of intravascular paramagnetic agents to assess cerebral perfusion and image functional changes in cerebral blood volume.[65,65a] In normal brain with an intact blood-brain barrier, lanthanide chelates such as dysprosium DTPA-BMA are confined to the intravascular space. Field gradients induced between the capillary spaces and the surrounding perfused tissue result in transient but substantial signal loss in regions with normal blood flow. Nonperfused or hypoperfused tissues devoid of contrast consequently appear relatively hyperintense.[66,67]

Subacute Infarcts

Because cerebral infarction is a dynamic process, its imaging manifestations continue to evolve with time.

Computed tomography (*see* box, p. 345). After the first 24 to 48 hours, most large vessel infarcts are visible on NECT as wedge-shaped areas of decreased attenuation that involve both the gray and white matter in a typical vascular distribution (Fig. 11-22). Mass effect initially increases, then begins to diminish after 7 to 10 days. Frank hemorrhagic transformation (HT) of an initially ischemic infarction occurs in 15% to 20% of MCA occlusions. Common locations of HT are the basal ganglia and cortex (Figs. 11-16, *C*, and 11-23, *E*).[49] Some hemorrhagic foci can be detected in the majority of medium and large size subacute infarcts.[67a]

Because of blood-brain barrier disruption, enhancement following contrast administration can often be seen in subacute infarcts (Fig. 11-23, *A* to *D*).

Enhancement patterns are typically patchy or gyral, may appear as early as 3 or 4 days after ictus, and persist up to 8 to 10 weeks.[41,68]

Magnetic resonance imaging. The two earliest signs of acute infarction—intravascular and meningeal enhancement—begin to diminish within 2 to 4 days after the ictus.[51] Parenchymal contrast enhancement then ensues and can persist for weeks (Figs. 11-24, *A*, and 11-25, *B*). Edema becomes more prominent and appears hypointense to cortex on T1WI and hyperintense on T2WI (Fig. 11-24, *B*). Mass effect increases, then gradually diminishes.

During the second post-ictal week, a noticeable decrease in signal intensity is sometimes observed on T2WI. The initial high-signal changes may largely re-

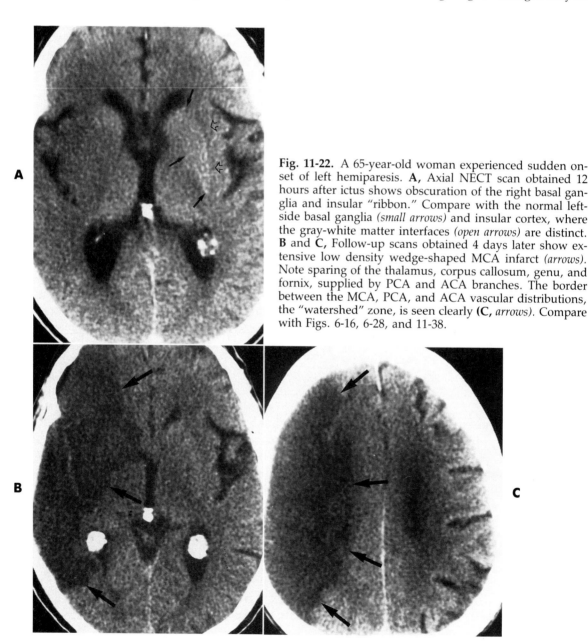

Fig. 11-22. A 65-year-old woman experienced sudden onset of left hemiparesis. **A,** Axial NECT scan obtained 12 hours after ictus shows obscuration of the right basal ganglia and insular "ribbon." Compare with the normal left-side basal ganglia *(small arrows)* and insular cortex, where the gray-white matter interfaces *(open arrows)* are distinct. **B** and **C,** Follow-up scans obtained 4 days later show extensive low density wedge-shaped MCA infarct *(arrows)*. Note sparing of the thalamus, corpus callosum, genu, and fornix, supplied by PCA and ACA branches. The border between the MCA, PCA, and ACA vascular distributions, the "watershed" zone, is seen clearly **(C,** *arrows)*. Compare with Figs. 6-16, 6-28, and 11-38.

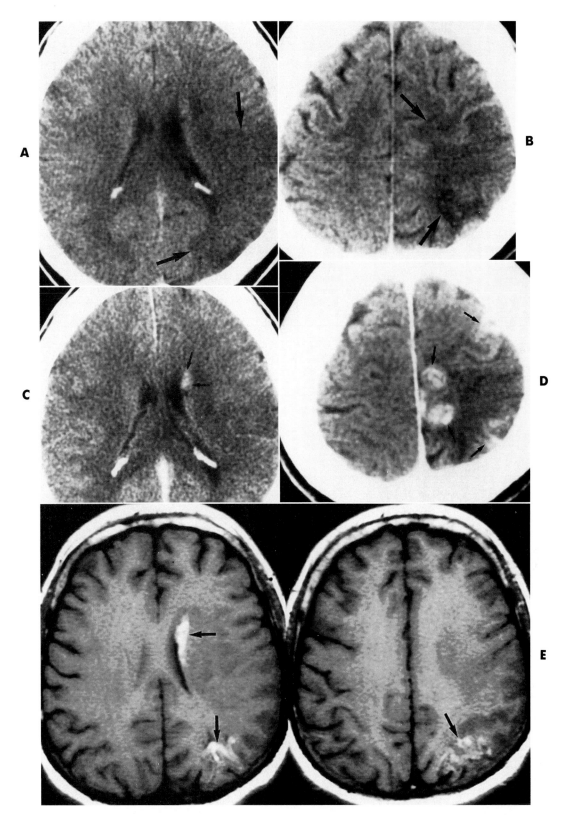

Fig. 11-23. A and **B,** Axial NECT scans obtained 1 week after ictus show a left-sided wedge-shaped low density area in the posterior MCA distribution *(arrows).* **C** and **D,** Postcontrast studies show patchy enhancement in the caudate nucleus and cortex along the ischemic penumbra *(arrows).* **E,** Axial T1-weighted MR scans without contrast enhancement show partial hemorrhagic transformation *(arrows).*

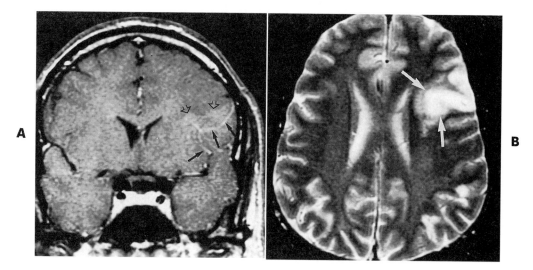

Fig. 11-24. **A,** Coronal postcontrast T1-weighted MR scan obtained 3 days after left MCA branch occlusion shows intravascular contrast *(solid arrows)* and a faint gyral blush *(open arrows).* **B,** Axial T2-weighted scan shows focal gyral hyperintensity *(arrows)* with mass effect and obliteration of adjacent sulci.

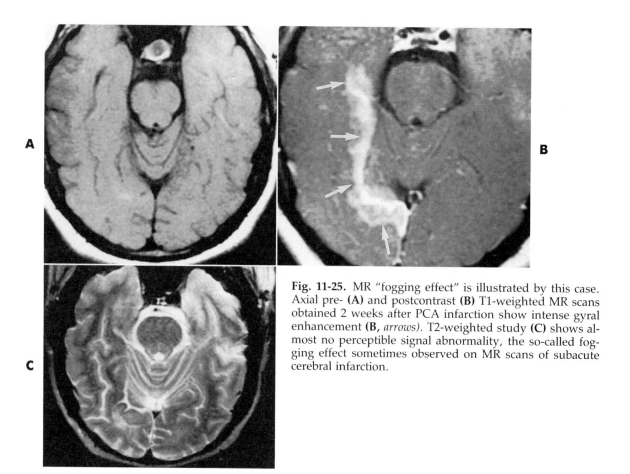

Fig. 11-25. MR "fogging effect" is illustrated by this case. Axial pre- **(A)** and postcontrast **(B)** T1-weighted MR scans obtained 2 weeks after PCA infarction show intense gyral enhancement **(B,** *arrows).* T2-weighted study **(C)** shows almost no perceptible signal abnormality, the so-called fogging effect sometimes observed on MR scans of subacute cerebral infarction.

gress or even disappear. This so-called fogging effect is probably due to a reduction in edema and leakage of proteins from cell lysis.[68,69] Scans performed 1 to 2 weeks after cerebral infarction in these cases may show striking enhancement on postcontrast T1-weighted sequences yet have a virtually normal-appearing T2WI (Fig. 11-25).

If HT occurs, signal changes of evolving hemorrhage are observed (Fig. 11-23, *E* and *F*) (*see also* Chapter 7). Early wallerian degeneration can occur and is seen as a well-defined hypointense band in the corticospinal tract on T2-weighted sequences.[70]

Chronic Infarcts

Prolonged ischemia causes irreversible brain damage. Chronic infarction represents the end result of this destructive process.

Pathology.   Gross specimens of chronic infarcts reflect the volume loss and gliosis that are the pathologic hallmarks of stroke residua (Fig. 11-26).

Imaging.   Focal well-delineated low-attenuation or encephalomalacic areas are seen in the affected vascular distribution on both CT and MR studies (Fig. 11-27). Adjacent sulci become prominent and the ipsilateral ventricle enlarges, reflecting loss of cerebral tissue volume. Enhancement disappears after 8 to 10 weeks. Dystrophic calcification may occur in infarcted brain but is very rare (Fig. 11-28).[71]

The MR differentiation of subacute from chronic (>2 weeks) infarction on standard spin-echo sequences may be difficult because relaxation times are prolonged in both.[72] In old infarcts (>8-10 weeks), mass effect and contrast enhancement are absent. Wallerian degeneration of axons and their myelin sheaths may result in ipsilateral brain stem atrophy.[70] If cortical hemorrhage or secondary calcification has occurred, gyriform signal changes can sometimes be identified on T1WI. Depending on age of the hemorrhage these are either hypo- or hyperintense. With old infarcts, ribbonlike very hypointense foci are present on T2WI.[73]

A

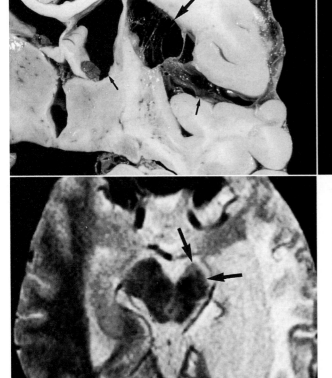

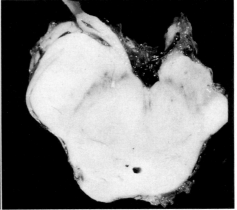

B

C

Fig. 11-26. **A,** Coronal gross pathology specimen demonstrates typical residua of old cerebral infarction. Encephalomalacic changes are striking *(large arrow).* The lateral ventricle and sylvian fissure are enlarged *(small arrows).* **B,** Axial midbrain section in another case with a large left MCA infarct (not shown) demonstrates striking wallerian degeneration of the ipsilateral cerebral peduncle. **C,** Axial T2-weighted MR scan in another patient with extensive left hemisphere encephalomalacia shows the cerebral peduncles are markedly asymmetric. The left peduncle *(arrows)* demonstrates striking changes of Wallerian degeneration. Compare with **B.** (**B,** Courtesy E. Tessa Hedley-Whyte.)

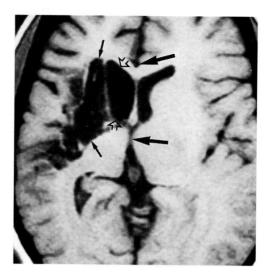

Fig. 11-27. Axial T1-weighted MR scan in another case demonstrates typical residua of old cerebral infarct. Well-delineated encephalomalacic areas are seen *(small black arrows;* compare with Fig. 11-26, *A.)* The ipsilateral ventricle is enlarged *(open arrows).* Note shift of the midline toward the atrophic changes as seen by left-to-right displacement of the third ventricle and interhemispheric fissure *(large arrows).*

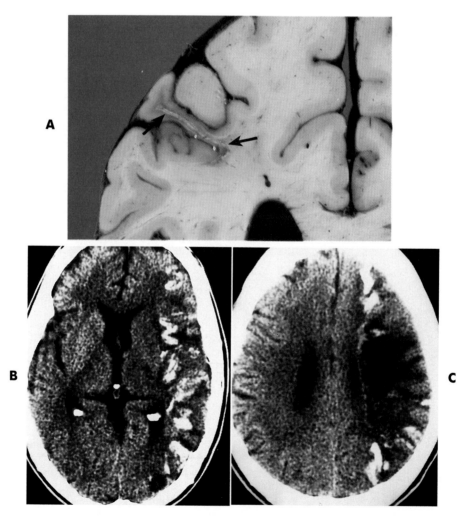

Fig. 11-28. **A,** Gross pathology of an old calcified right frontal hemorrhagic infarction. **B** and **C,** Axial NECT scans show an old calcified left middle cerebral artery infarct *(arrows).* (**A,** Courtesy Rubinstein Collection, University of Virginia.)

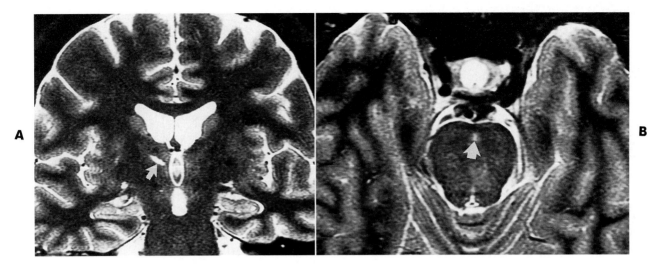

Fig. 11-29. Coronal **(A)** and axial **(B)** T2-weighted MR scans show thalamic and brainstem lacunar infarcts *(arrows)*.

Lacunar Infarcts

Lacunar infarcts account for 15% to 25% of all strokes.[74]

Pathology. "Lacunar" infarcts are small deep cerebral infarcts that are typically located in the basal ganglia and thalamus. These small infarcts are often multiple and are due to embolic, atheromatous, or thrombotic lesions in the long single penetrating end arterioles that supply the deep cerebral gray matter.

Imaging. Because of their small size, most true lacunar infarcts are not seen on CT scans. When present they are usually seen as part of more extensive white matter disease.

On MR scans lacunar infarcts are seen as rounded or slitlike lesions that are hypointense to brain on T1WI. Well-delineated hyperintense areas are identified on T2-weighted sequences (Fig. 11-29, A and B).[74] The MR differential diagnosis includes enlarged perivascular (Virchow-Robin) spaces and subependymal myelin pallor[75] *(see* Chapter 17). Some late acute or early subacute lacunar infarcts may enhance following contrast administration.[74]

Hypoxic-ischemic Encephalopathy

Etiology. Hypoxic-ischemic encephalopathy (HIE) is the result of global rather than focal brain injury. Whereas cerebral infarction results from abnormalities in local vascular circulation, HIE is the consequence of global perfusion or oxygenation disturbance. Some common causes of HIE are severe prolonged hypotension, cardiac arrest with successful resuscitation, profound neonatal asphyxia, and carbon monoxide inhalation.

Cerebral blood flow (CBF) is maintained over moderate decreases in perfusion pressure by vasodilatation and reduction in cerebral vascular resistance. When this autoregulatory process fails, CBF falls. Although most HIE is caused by global perfusion disturbances, occasionally perfusion is normal but red blood cell oxygenation is faulty.

Pathology. Two basic patterns are seen in HIE: arterial or *"border zone" infarcts* and *generalized cortical (pseudolaminar) necrosis.* Ischemic changes in HIE are concentrated primarily along the arterial border zones between the major cerebral and cerebellar artery territories (Fig. 11-30, C). The most frequently and severely affected area is the parietooccipital region at the confluence between the ACA, MCA, and PCA territories[3] *(see* Chapter 6). The basal ganglia are also common sites for HIE. In premature infants the border zone is in the deep periventricular white matter and HIE manifestations are those of periventricular leukomalacia *(see* Chapter 17).[37,38]

In generalized cortical laminar necrosis, the third, fifth, and sixth cortical layers are affected (Fig. 11-31). The caudate nucleus and putamen are also often involved.[3]

Imaging. The most common abnormality observed on NECT scans in HIE is a low density band at the interface between major vascular territories. The basal ganglia (Fig. 11-32, A) and parasagittal areas (Fig. 11-32, B) are the most frequent sites. MR studies show border zone area hyperintensities on T2WI (Fig. 11-33). Enhancement after contrast administration can be striking (Fig. 11-34). Because cortical laminar necrosis is often hemorrhagic, MR scans in

Text continued on p. 360.

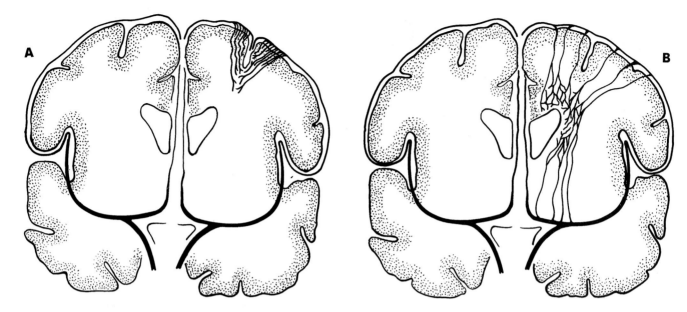

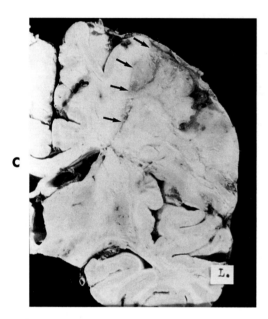

Fig. 11-30. Anatomic drawing depicts location of the adult **(A)** and fetal **(B)** vascular watershed, or "border zone," areas. Note that in the adult the watershed is peripheral and parasagittal; in the fetus it lies in the deep periventricular white matter. Coronal gross pathology specimen **(C)** demonstrates a typical adult-type watershed infarct *(arrows)* in the ACA-MCA border zone. (**C,** Courtesy E. Tessa Hedley-Whyte.)

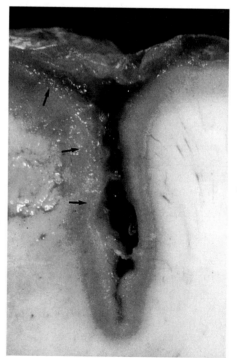

Fig. 11-31. A, Gross pathology demonstrates laminar necrosis of the middle cortical layers *(arrows).* (Courtesy J. Townsend.)

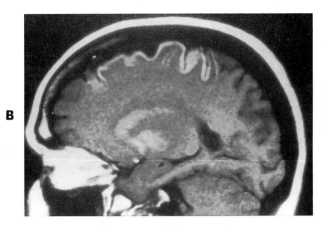

B

Fig. 11-31, cont'd. B, Sagittal T1-weighted MR scan in a patient with laminar cortical necrosis following an hypoxic-ischemic episode. Subacute hemorrhage is seen in the cortex and basal ganglia.

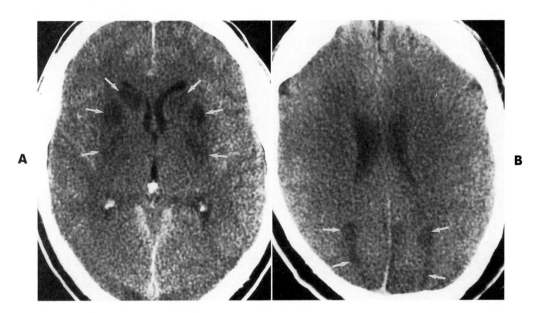

A

B

Fig. 11-32. Hypotension with changes of hypoxic encephalopathy are demonstrated on axial CECT scans. Note selective infarction in the basal ganglia (**A,** *arrows*) and in both parietooccipital areas along the MCA-PCA watershed zone (**B,** *arrows*) seen as low density foci.

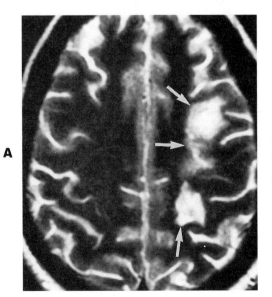

A

Fig. 11-33. Axial T2-weighted MR scan in a patient with cardiac arrest and prolonged resuscitation. **A** and **B** show multiple cerebral and cerebellar border zone infarcts (*arrows*). *Continued.*

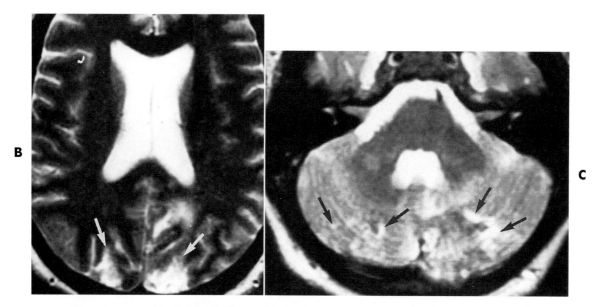

Fig. 11-33, cont'd. Axial **(C)** T2-weighted MR scan in a patient with cardiac arrest and prolonged resuscitation shows multiple cerebral and cerebellar border zone infarcts *(arrows)*.

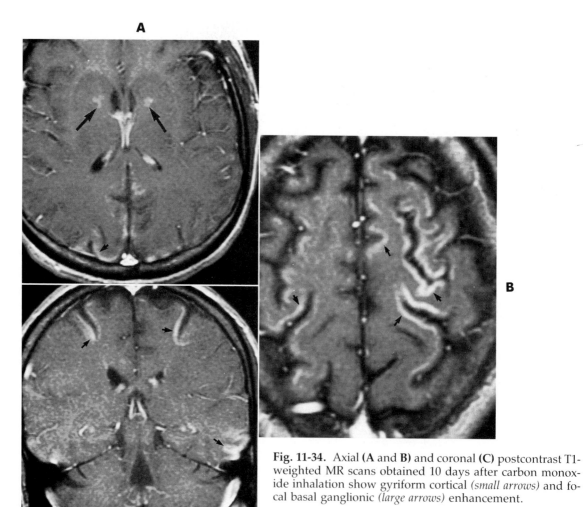

Fig. 11-34. Axial **(A and B)** and coronal **(C)** postcontrast T1-weighted MR scans obtained 10 days after carbon monoxide inhalation show gyriform cortical *(small arrows)* and focal basal ganglionic *(large arrows)* enhancement.

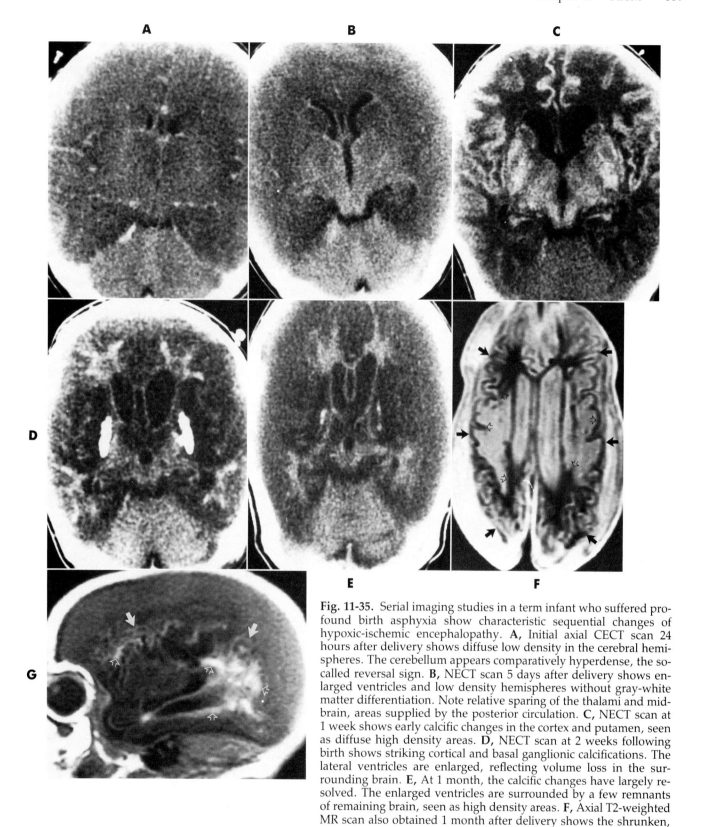

A   **B**   **C**

D   **E**   **F**

G

Fig. 11-35. Serial imaging studies in a term infant who suffered profound birth asphyxia show characteristic sequential changes of hypoxic-ischemic encephalopathy. **A,** Initial axial CECT scan 24 hours after delivery shows diffuse low density in the cerebral hemispheres. The cerebellum appears comparatively hyperdense, the so-called reversal sign. **B,** NECT scan 5 days after delivery shows enlarged ventricles and low density hemispheres without gray-white matter differentiation. Note relative sparing of the thalami and midbrain, areas supplied by the posterior circulation. **C,** NECT scan at 1 week shows early calcific changes in the cortex and putamen, seen as diffuse high density areas. **D,** NECT scan at 2 weeks following birth shows striking cortical and basal ganglionic calcifications. The lateral ventricles are enlarged, reflecting volume loss in the surrounding brain. **E,** At 1 month, the calcific changes have largely resolved. The enlarged ventricles are surrounded by a few remnants of remaining brain, seen as high density areas. **F,** Axial T2-weighted MR scan also obtained 1 month after delivery shows the shrunken, severely encephalomalacic brain *(large arrows)* with diffuse gyriform and white matter low signal foci *(open arrows)*. **G,** Sagittal T1-weighted MR scan obtained 1 month after delivery shows shrunken, severely encephalomalacic brain *(large arrows)* surrounding enlarged lateral ventricles. Residual calcification is seen as high signal changes *(open arrows)*. (Imaging studies courtesy of the patient's family.)

subacute cases may show serpentine, gyriform foci that are typically high signal on T1WI. Basal ganglia hyperintensities are also common (Fig. 11-31, B).

Term infants suffering profound perinatal asphyxia show a characteristic sequence of imaging findings (Fig. 11-35). Initial CT scans may be normal or minimally abnormal. Severe generalized cerebral edema ensues over 24 to 48 hours and is seen as diffusely low density brain, often with a "reversal" sign (*see* Chapter 8). Here, the cerebellum appears hyperdense compared to the abnormally low density cerebral hemispheres (Fig. 11-35, A). Gray-white matter differentiation is lost (Fig. 11-35, B). Hemorrhagic cortical necrosis with secondary calcifications can often be observed within a few days after the hypoxic-ischemic insult (Fig. 11-35, C and D).[76] Severe atrophic changes are common in surviving infants (Fig. 11-35, E).

MR scans show high signal on T1WI in the basal ganglia, particularly the posterior lateral lentiform nuclei and ventrolateral thalamus. The midbrain tegmentum and the lateral geniculate nuclei are commonly affected.[77] Thinning of the perirolandic gyri can be seen in surviving infants. Low signal serpiginous perirolandic cortical lesions on T2-weighted sequences reflect hemorrhagic or calcific residua (Fig. 11-35, G).[73] Multicystic encephalomalacia is seen in severe cases (Fig. 11-35, F).[37]

Postnatal hypoxic-ischemic insults such as nonaccidental trauma with strangulation can produce CT and MR findings that are somewhat similar to those of profound birth asphyxia. Most of these patients have T1 and T2 prolongation involving the corpus striatum and much of the cerebral cortex, although the thalami and suprasylvian/perirolandic cortex are relatively spared.[77]

Strokes in Specific Vascular Distributions

Imaging manifestations of strokes in specific vascular distributions are considered here. The old con-

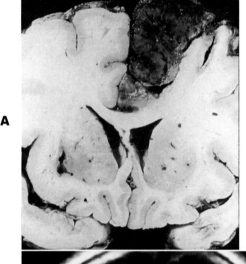

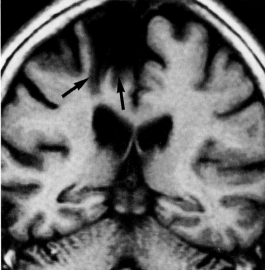

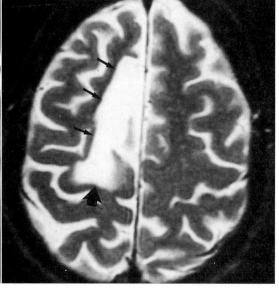

Fig. 11-36. A, Coronal gross pathology specimen depicts a hemorrhagic distal ACA infarct. Note wedge-shaped lesion extends from the interhemispheric fissure over the convexity. The border between ACA and MCA territories in this case is typical. The corpus callosum and septum pellucidum are spared. **B,** Coronal T1-weighted MR scan shows a typical old distal right ACA infarct *(arrows)*. Compare with **A. C,** The T2-weighted axial scan shows the posterior ACA-PCA watershed lies in the superior parietal lobule *(large arrow)*. The ACA-MCA border zone is indicated by small black arrows. Compare with Fig. 6-16. (**A,** Courtesy E. Tessa Hedley-Whyte.)

cept that vascular distribution patterns are relatively constant has been replaced by the recognition that boundaries between vascular territories are dynamic rather than static.[78] The location of these boundaries is determined by hemodynamic conditions that govern flow in leptomeningeal anastomoses connecting two larger arterial territories.[78] The usual, maximum, and minimum territories that are supplied by the three major cerebral arteries are depicted in Chapter 6 (*see* Figs. 6-23, 6-28, and 6-32).

Anterior cerebral artery (ACA). Variation in the ACA territory is large, especially on the superior lateral and medial hemisphere surfaces.[78] In over two thirds of all cases the anterior-posterior cerebral artery boundary is found on the convexity in the external parietooccipital sulcus or along the superior parietal lobule. The middle of the orbitofrontal gyrus usually demarcates the inferior border between the anterior and middle cerebral arteries.

The ACA supplies a variable amount of the lateral hemispheric surface, usually just a thin strip over the anterior two thirds of the convexity (Fig. 11-36, *A; see* Figs. 6-16 and 6-23, *C*). Pericallosal branches supply the septum pellucidum and the anterior two thirds of the corpus callosum. ACA supply to the deep frontal white matter and basal ganglia is quite variable, although some supply to the caudate nucleus and an-

terior limb of the internal capsule is typical.

Isolated ACA infarcts are rare (0.6% of all infarcts).[78a] When present, they typically involve a strip of cortex along the anterior aspect of the interhemispheric fissure (Fig. 11-36, *B* and *C*). Both conventional and MR angiography in ACA occlusion often disclose collateral circulation through splenial posterior cerebral artery (PCA) branches (Fig. 11-37, *D*) and leptomeningeal MCA branches over the cortical watershed area (Fig. 11-37, *A* to *C*).

Middle cerebral artery (MCA). The MCA typically supplies most of the lateral hemisphere and the anterior temporal lobe (Fig. 11-38; *see* Fig. 6-28). MCA supply to the deep white matter and basal ganglia is highly variable.[78] Anteriorly it is completely complementary to the ACA contribution. In most all cases the MCA irrigates the lentiform nucleus and participates in supplying the caudate nucleus (Fig. 6-16).

Over 75% of all strokes occur in the MCA territory. Imaging manifestations vary with time and occlusion site. If the entire MCA distribution is affected, the basal ganglia, deep cerebral white matter, and much of the hemispheric cortex are involved. A wedge-shaped area that extends from the lateral ventricle to the brain surface is typical in such cases. Sometimes MCA infarcts involve only the anterior or posterior MCA division. Distal emboli may affect just a single

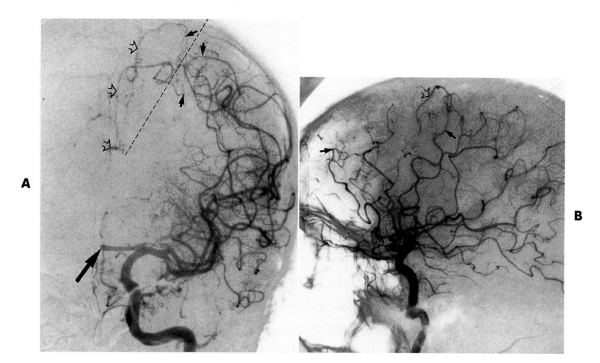

Fig. 11-37. ACA embolic infarct. **A,** Left ICA angiogram, midarterial phase, AP view, shows the left ACA is occluded at the A1-A2-ACoA junction *(large arrow)*. Pial collaterals from the MCA *(small black arrows)* fill the distal ACA *(open arrows)*. ACA-MCA watershed area *(dotted line)*. **B,** Lateral view of the midarterial phase shows the MCA pial collaterals *(black arrows)* begin to opacify some ACA branches *(open arrow)*.

Continued.

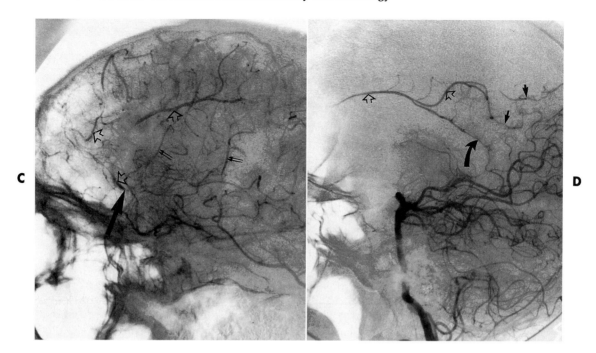

Fig. 11-37, cont'd. **C,** Capillary phase shows partial opacification of the ACA and its branches *(open arrows).* Site of embolic occlusion *(large arrow).* Slow flow in some MCA branches *(double arrows)* indicates smaller emboli in this vascular distribution as well. **D,** Left vertebral angiogram, midarterial phase, lateral view, shows artery-to-artery collaterals from splenial PCA branches *(curved arrow)* to the pericallosal artery *(open arrows).* PCA-ACA pial collaterals *(small black arrows).*

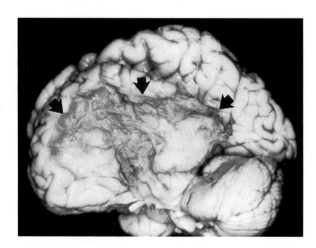

Fig. 11-38. Lateral view of gross pathology specimen with an old MCA infarct. The MCA-ACA and MCA-PCA watershed zones *(arrows)* are clearly apparent. Compare with Fig. 6-26. (Courtesy E. Ross.)

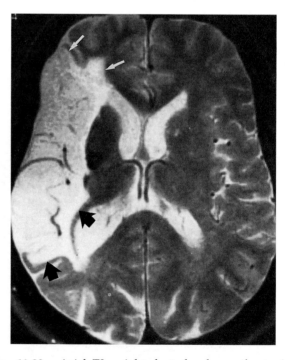

Fig. 11-39. Axial T2-weighted study shows the typical wedge-shaped encephalomalacic area of an old infarct. The MCA-ACA *(white arrows)* and MCA-PCA *(black arrows)* watershed zones are indicated. The infarct involved the external capsule, claustrum, and insular cortex but spared the basal ganglia.

branch. The lenticular nucleus can be spared if occlusion occurs distal to the MCA bifurcation (Fig. 11-39).

Posterior cerebral artery (PCA). The PCA-ACA and PCA-MCA boundaries are quite variable. Particularly in the basal regions, many different locations and orientations of the PCA-MCA boundary occur.[78] In the most common situation the PCA supplies the posterior one third of the convexity and most of the inferior temporal lobe (Fig. 11-40; *see* Fig. 6-32). It also usually supplies the occipital lobe and participates in supplying the posterior limb of the internal capsule and other deep structures (*see* Fig. 6-16).

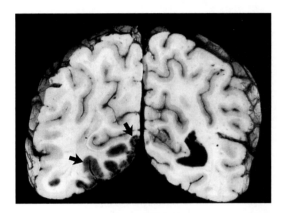

Fig. 11-40. Coronal gross specimen shows a hemorrhagic cortical PCA infarct that involves the inferior temporal and medial occipital lobes *(arrows)*. (Courtesy E. Tessa Hedley-Whyte.)

Hemispheric PCA infarcts are second in frequency to MCA occlusions. Common sites are the calcarine cortex (Fig. 11-41) and deep penetrating branches to the thalami, midbrain, and posterior limb of the internal capsule.

Anterior (AChA) and posterior choroidal (PChA) arteries. The AChA usually arises from the distal internal carotid artery above the posterior communicating artery (PCoA) origin. The medial (MPChA) and lateral (LPChA) posterior choroidal arteries arise from the PCA.

The three choroidal arteries are in hemodynamic balance with each other and their vascular territories are complementary (*see* Fig. 6-11). The AChA typically supplies part of the posterior limb and genu of the internal capsule, medial globus pallidus, optic tract, temporal lobe uncus, and amygdaloid nucleus and choroid plexus of the lateral ventricle (*see* Fig. 6-16).[79] Isolated choroidal artery infarcts are rarely identified on imaging studies.

Perforating branches. Perforating branches arise from the circle of Willis and the choroidal arteries to supply the basal structures. These include ACoA perforators, medial and lateral lenticulostriate arteries (branches of the ACA and MCA), anterior and posterior thalamoperforating arteries (branches of the PCoA, basilar bifurcation, and proximal PCA) and thalamogeniculate arteries (*see* Fig. 6-16). Occlusion of these vessels typically produces small focal (lacunar) infarcts in the basal ganglia, internal capsule, mesencephalon, or diencephalon (Fig. 11-35, *B*).

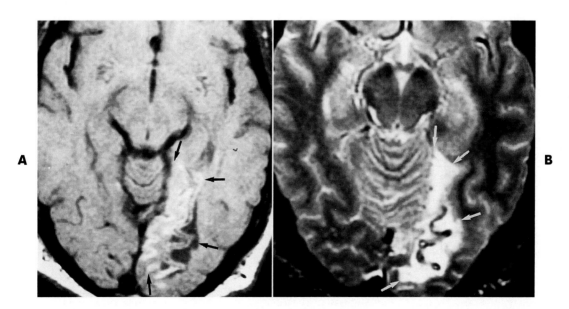

A   B

Fig. 11-41. Axial T1- **(A)** and T2-weighted **(B)** MR scans show a subacute hemorrhagic PCA infarct *(arrows)* that involves the occipital and medial temporal lobes. Compare with Fig. 11-40.

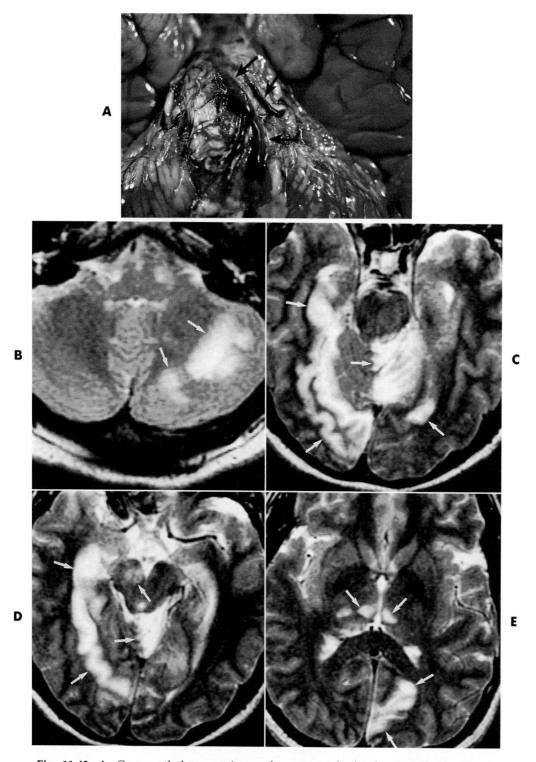

Fig. 11-42. A, Gross pathology specimen of acute vertebrobasilar thrombosis. Clot is present in both vertebral arteries, the basilar artery, and their major branches *(arrows)*. **B** to **E,** Axial T2-weighted MR scans in another case with acute basilar thrombosis show multiple infarcts in both PCAs, the left superior cerebellar artery (SCA), and areas supplied by posterior thalamoperforating branches *(arrows)*. **B** to **E,** Axial T2-weighted MR scans in a patient with vertebrobasilar thrombosis show multifocal infarcts *(arrows)*. **(A,** Courtesy Rubinstein Collection, University of Virginia.)

Basilar artery (BA). Small BA penetrating branches supply the pons, part of the mesencephalon, and posteroinferior thalami. Penetrating branch occlusion results in pontine infarcts. MR scans in such cases typically show well-delineated lesions that are hypointense on T1WI and hyperintense on T2-weighted sequences (Figs. 11-29, *B,*).

Major BA branches are the anterior inferior and superior cerebellar arteries and PCAs. Basilar artery thrombosis typically results in patchy multifocal lesions that involve all these vascular distributions (Fig. 11-42). When only the distal BA is occluded, the result is the so-called *top of the basilar syndrome.* Here, the predominant lesions are found in the thalami, posterior limb of the internal capsule, mesencephalon, pons, and posterior temporal and occipital lobes (Fig. 11-43). *Locked-in syndrome,* i.e., loss of all voluntary movements (except vertical eye movements) with maintained consciousness, is usually caused by large ventral pontine infarcts.[79a]

Superior cerebellar artery (SCA). Two or more SCAs arise from the distal basilar artery prior to its terminal bifurcation into the posterior cerebral arteries. The SCAs supply the entire superior aspect of the cerebellar hemispheres, superior vermis, and most of the deep cerebellar white matter.[80] SCA infarcts affect the superior cerebellum, the ipsilateral half of the vermis, and various amounts of the white matter (Fig. 11-44). Vermian or paravermian branch occlusions have a quadrangular shape, medial location, and sagittal orientation (Fig. 11-42, *C* and *D*); hemispheric branch occlusions are oriented more obliquely and laterally (Fig. 11-45).[80]

Anterior inferior cerebellar artery (AICA). The AICA course and vascular territory are quite variable. AICA usually has the smallest territory of all the cerebellar arteries and a reciprocal supply with the posterior inferior cerebellar artery. AICA typically supplies the flocculus, the anterior (petrosal) surface of

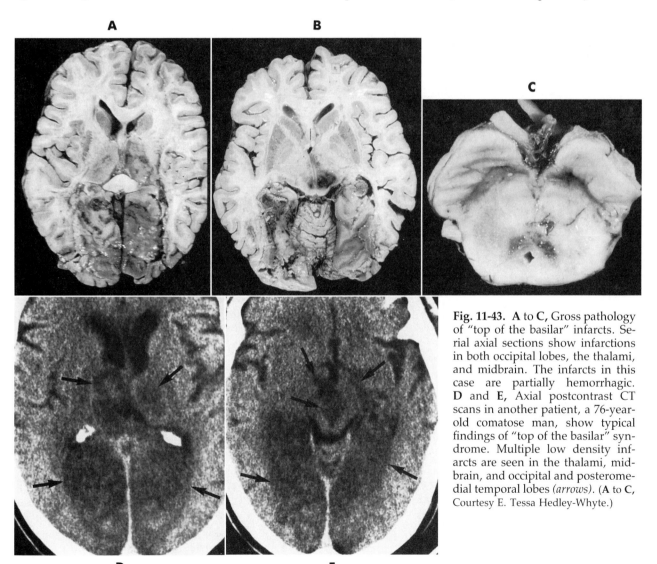

Fig. 11-43. A to **C,** Gross pathology of "top of the basilar" infarcts. Serial axial sections show infarctions in both occipital lobes, the thalami, and midbrain. The infarcts in this case are partially hemorrhagic. **D** and **E,** Axial postcontrast CT scans in another patient, a 76-year-old comatose man, show typical findings of "top of the basilar" syndrome. Multiple low density infarcts are seen in the thalami, midbrain, and occipital and posteromedial temporal lobes *(arrows).* (**A** to **C,** Courtesy E. Tessa Hedley-Whyte.)

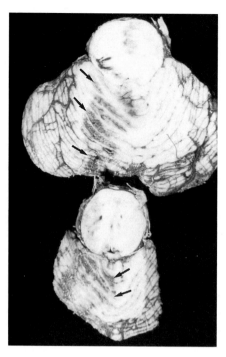

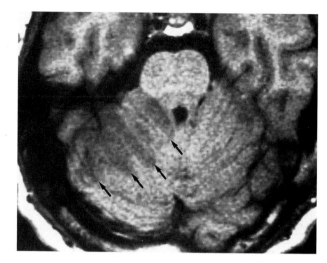

Fig. 11-45. Axial T1-weighted MR scan shows a hemispheric SCA infarct *(arrows)*. The vermis is spared.

Fig. 11-44. Axial sections of gross pathology specimen demonstrate right superior cerebellar artery infarct *(arrows)*. (Courtesy E. Tessa Hedley-Whyte.)

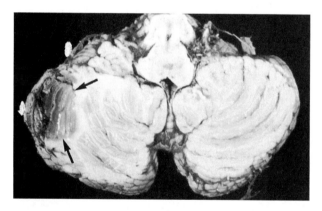

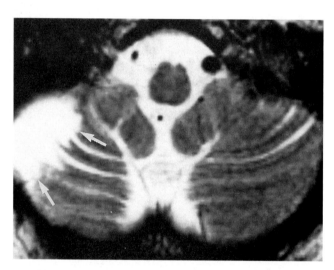

Fig. 11-46. Axial gross pathology specimen of anterior inferior cerebellar artery (AICA) infarct *(arrows)* secondary to meningitis. (Courtesy E. Tessa Hedley-Whyte.)

Fig. 11-47. Axial T2-weighted MR scan shows an AICA infarct *(arrows)*. The location along the lateral angle and petrosal surface of the cerebellum is typical.

the cerebellum (Fig. 11-46), the middle cerebellar peduncle, and part of the pons.[81] It may also supply part of the medulla.

Isolated AICA infarcts are uncommon and typically occur in diabetic, hypertensive patients with ASVD.[82] They are seen as focal lesions in the brachium pontis or a more extensive curvilinear infarct along the petrosal surface of the cerebellum (Fig. 11-47).[80] If AICA supplies part of the PICA territory, more extensive involvement of the inferior cerebellar hemisphere and vermis may be present. More widespread infarcts that include the BA territory typically

are due to basilar artery occlusive disease with secondary AICA involvement.[82] Small "border zone" cerebellar infarcts are often found on CT or MR studies and usually result from large or pial artery disease rather than from systemic hypotension.[82a]

Posterior inferior cerebellar artery (PICA). The usual PICA territory includes the entire posteroinferior cerebellum, tonsil, and ipsilateral inferior vermis. PICA also often supplies the posterolateral medulla (Fig. 11-48). The variability in vascular supply of the cerebellum and medulla is reflected by PICA infarcts.

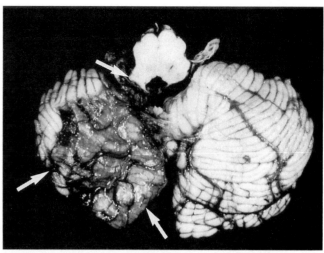

Fig. 11-48. Axial gross pathology specimen of posterior inferior cerebellar artery (PICA) infarct. The posterolateral medulla and most of the cerebellar hemisphere are involved *(large arrows)*. The AICA territory is not affected. (Reproduced with permission from Okazaki H, Scheithauer B: *Slide Atlas of Neuropathology*, Gower Medical Publishing, 1988).

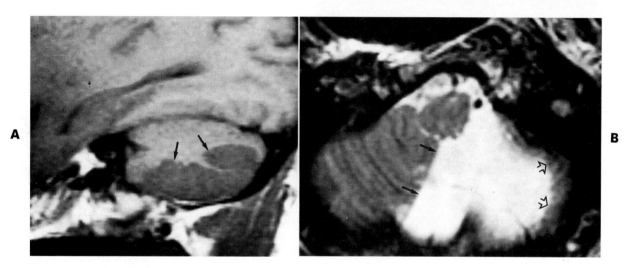

Fig. 11-49. Sagittal T1- **(A)** and axial T2-weighted **(B)** MR scans of a PICA infarct *(solid black arrows)* that spares the medulla. The border zone between the PICA and AICA distributions is shown (**B,** *open arrows.*)

Sometimes a PICA infarct produces a classic Wallenberg syndrome *(see box, p. 368, left)*, although vertebral artery occlusion is a more common cause of this syndrome.[82b] Other PICA infarcts may spare the medulla (Fig. 11-49). Single PICA branch occlusions can affect a very small area (Fig. 11-50).

If PICA supplies part or all of the AICA territory, infarcts may be very extensive (Fig. 11-51, *A*). Because the deep cerebellar white matter is supplied primarily by SCA branches, PICA infarcts tend to spare this region and the dentate nuclei (Fig. 11-51, *B*).[80]

Strokes in Children

About 3% of cerebral infarcts occur in young individuals,[83] and pediatric stroke is even less common. Cerebral infarcts in children have different etiologies compared to adults. Common causes of pediatric strokes are listed in the box, p. 368, *right*.

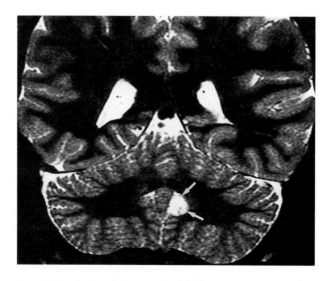

Fig. 11-50. Coronal T2-weighted MR scan shows a focal infarct *(arrows)* that involves only the left tonsillar PICA branch.

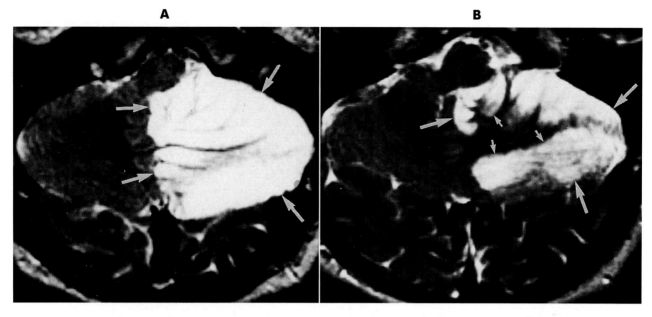

Fig. 11-51. Embolic occlusion of a common PICA-AICA trunk distal to the medullary segment. **A** and **B,** Axial T2-weighted scans show the infarct *(large arrows)*. The PICA-SCA watershed zone is indicated (**B,** *small arrows*.) (Courtesy M. Fruin.)

Lateral Medullary (Wallenberg) Syndrome
Clinical manifestations and structures affected*

Ipsilateral

Preganglionic Horner syndrome (miosis, ptosis, decreased sweating) (descending reticulospinal tracts to cord sympathetics)

Ataxia (cerebellum, inferior peduncle)

Facial pain, numbness, impaired sensation (CNV nucleus, spinal tract)

Dysphagia, hoarseness, diminished gag reflex (CNs IX, X)

Diminished taste (CN IX nucleus and solitary tract)

Vertigo, nausea, vomiting (vestibular nuclei and connections)

Nystagmus, diplopia, oscillopsia (restiform body, inferior and medial vestibular nuclei)

Hiccups

Contralateral

Numbness, decreased pain and temperature in trunk and extremities (spinothalamic tract)

Adapted from Adams RD, Victor M: *Principles of Neurology,* ed 3, p. 589, New York: McGraw-Hill, 1985.
*Usually caused by PICA occlusion but can also occur with AICA or medullary branch infarcts.

Strokes in Children

Most common

Congenital heart disease with cerebral thromboembolism

Common

Dissection (traumatic, spontaneous)
Infection (tonsillitis, abscess, meningitis, sinusitis)
Drug abuse (sympathomimetics, cocaine)
Blood dyscrasias, clotting disorders

Uncommon

Fibromuscular dysplasia
Marfan disease
Collagen-vascular diseases
Idiopathic progressive arteriopathy of childhood (moyamoya)
Neurofibromatosis type 1
Vasculitis

Rare

Atherosclerosis (e.g., progeria)
Radiation angiopathy
Tuberous sclerosis
Tumor

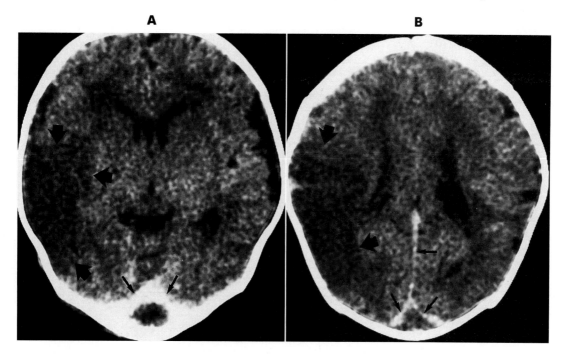

Fig. 11-52. A term infant with normal delivery had sudden onset of left hemiparesis 5 days after delivery. Axial NECT scans show a right MCA embolic infarct *(large arrows)*, probably from a patent foramen of ovale and right-to-left intracardiac shunt. Note the high density falx cerebri and tentorium cerebelli *(small arrows),* a normal finding. This creates a "pseudo-thrombosis" appearance that should not be mistaken for dural sinus occlusion.

Cerebral emboli from congenital heart disease with right-to-left shunts are probably the most common cause of cerebral infarcts in children (Fig. 11-52). Traumatic or spontaneous dissection of the cervical internal carotid or vertebral arteries is also comparatively common (Fig. 11-9). Because aneurysmal SAH is uncommon in this age group, vasospasm is usually secondary to meningitis or nonaneurysmal ICH from trauma or vascular malformations.

Congenital vascular stenoses such as those associated with neurofibromatosis type 1 (*see* Fig. 5-16, *A* and *B*) or tuberous sclerosis are rare. Idiopathic progressive arteriopathy of childhood (so-called moyamoya) is also uncommon (see subsequent discussion).

NONATHEROMATOUS CAUSES OF ARTERIAL NARROWING AND OCCLUSION

Although atherosclerosis is by far the most common cause of intracranial arterial narrowing and occlusion in adults (Figs. 11-1, *H,* and 11-53), several nonatheromatous disorders also produce vascular stenoses in children and older individuals (*see* box). This heterogeneous group is composed both of congenital and acquired abnormalities.

Vascular Narrowing
Common Nonatheromatous Causes

Dissection (traumatic, spontaneous, underlying vasculopathy)
Vasospasm (SAH, trauma, infection)
Vasculopathy (FMD)
Drug abuse
Tumor encasement (pituitary adenoma, nasopharyngeal squamous cell carcinoma)

Congenital Abnormalities

Aplasia/hypoplasia. Aortic arch anomalies are discussed in detail in Chapter 6. Congenital absence of an internal carotid artery (ICA) is an uncommon occurrence and should be diagnosed only if the bony carotid canal is absent. In such cases, collateral circulation to the distal ICA distribution is via the contralateral ICA or vertebrobasilar system via the circle of Willis.[84]

True ICA hypoplasia is also uncommon (*see* box, p. 370). Although a small ICA can occur as an isolated phenomenon, most narrow ICAs result from ASVD, dissection (Fig. 11-14, *A*), vasospasm (Fig. 11-

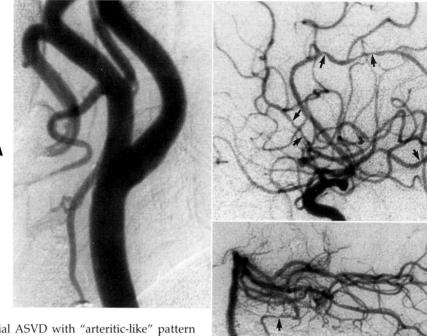

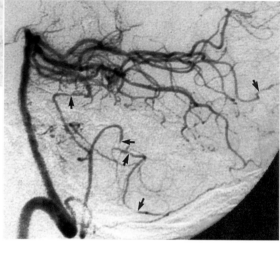

Fig. 11-53. Intracranial ASVD with "arteritic-like" pattern is demonstrated on the angiogram of this 76-year-old man. Digital subtraction left CCA angiogram **(A)**, lateral view, shows a normal bifurcation free of atherosclerotic plaque. Lateral **(B)** view of the intracranial right ICA distribution shows multiple segmental areas of vascular narrowings and poststenotic dilatations *(arrows)*. Left vertebral angiogram **(C)**, midarterial phase, lateral view, shows similar but somewhat more mild disease *(arrows)*.

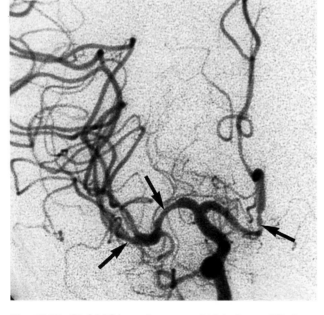

Fig. 11-54. Right ICA angiogram, arterial phase, AP view, with multiple narrowings *(arrows)* secondary to vasospasm from subarachnoid hemorrhage.

The "Small" Internal Carotid Artery

Common

Dissection (traumatic, spontaneous, underlying vasculopathy)

Catheter spasm

Vasospasm (SAH, trauma, infection)

Reduced distal run-off (e.g., severe vasospasm, increased intracranial pressure)

Tumor encasement (pituitary adenoma, nasopharyngeal squamous cell carcinoma)

Uncommon

Tubular form of FMD

Migraine headaches

Congenital hypoplasia

54), reduced intracranial runoff (Fig. 11-9, *A*), fibromuscular dysplasia, and other abnormalities (see subsequent discussion). In contrast, absence or hypoplasia of a vertebral artery is a common normal variant.

Neurocutaneous syndromes. Craniocerebral vascular lesions are uncommon but striking manifestations of the phakomatosis.

Neurofibromatosis type 1 (NF-1). NF-1 (von Recklinghausen disease) is the most common of the neurocutaneous syndromes and the one most frequently associated with vascular abnormalities. The association of NF-1 with aortic, celiac, mesenteric, and renal vascular stenoses is well documented; craniocerebral lesions are less common.[85] Nearly 90% are occlusive or stenotic (*see* Fig. 5-16, *A* and *B*)[86]; the remainder primarily consists of aneurysms, arteriovenous malformations, and extracranial arteriovenous fistulae (*see* Fig. 5-16, *C* to *E*).[87,88]

Occasionally NF-1 causes progressive intracranial arterial occlusive disease with development of a moyamoya pattern of collateral circulation (*see* Fig. 5-16, *A* and *B*).[89] The vascular lesions in NF-1 are probably manifestations of the generalized mesenchymal dysplasia that occurs in this disorder.

Neurofibromatosis type 2 (NF-2). Vascular disease is not a recognized manifestation of NF-2 (bilateral acoustic schwannomas).[88]

Tuberous sclerosis (TS). A few reports have described vascular abnormalities in TS. Arterial dysplasia with progressive degenerative changes and aneurysm formation are occasionally seen with TS, commonly in the thoracic or abdominal aorta.[90] A few cases of progressive vascular stenosis involving the internal carotid arteries have been reported.[91]

Miscellaneous neurocutaneous syndromes. Carotid aplasia, circle of Willis ectasias, and intracranial aneurysms have been reported with Klippel-Trenaunay-Weber syndrome.[92] Vascular abnormalities such as infarcts, aneurysms, and blood vessel dysplasia are associated with epidermal nevi.[93]

Idiopathic progressive arteriopathy of childhood (moyamoya)

Pathology and etiology. So-called moyamoya disease is an idiopathic progressive occlusive cerebrovascular disorder of unknown etiology. It is commonly seen in Japan but has been reported elsewhere as well.[94]

Clinical manifestations. Symptom onset is typically in childhood or adolescence, although adult cases have been reported.[95,95a] Repeated ischemic episodes are common.[96] The clinical course ultimately depends on the rapidity and extent of the vascular occlusion and the effectiveness of collateral circulation. Progressive stenosis or frank occlusion involving the distal ICAs and proximal aspects of the anterior and middle cerebral arteries occurs. Multiple, extensive parenchymal, leptomeningeal, and transdural collateral vascular channels develop.[96a]

Imaging findings. At angiography, contrast fills numerous enlarged lenticulostriate and thalamoperforating arteries, as well as dural, leptomeningeal, and pial collateral vessels (Fig. 11-55), leading to the

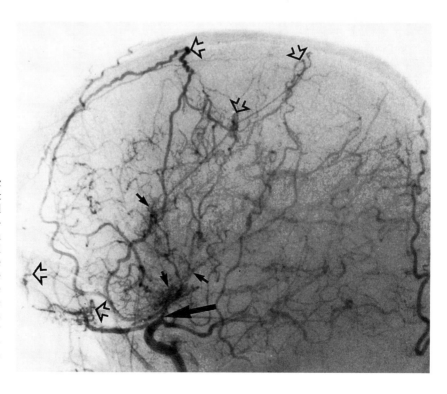

Fig. 11-55. A 10-year-old girl with idiopathic progressive arteriopathy of childhood. Left CCA angiogram, late arterial phase, lateral view, shows the typical "moyamoya" patterns of collateral circulation associated with this occlusive disorder. The supraclinoid ICA is occluded *(large arrow)*, and multiple small basal telangiectatic collaterals are present *(small black arrows)*. This gives the "puff of smoke" appearance for which the pattern is named. Prominent transosseous collaterals from superficial temporal artery and transdural collaterals from the ophthalmic and middle meningeal arteries are also present *(open arrows)*.

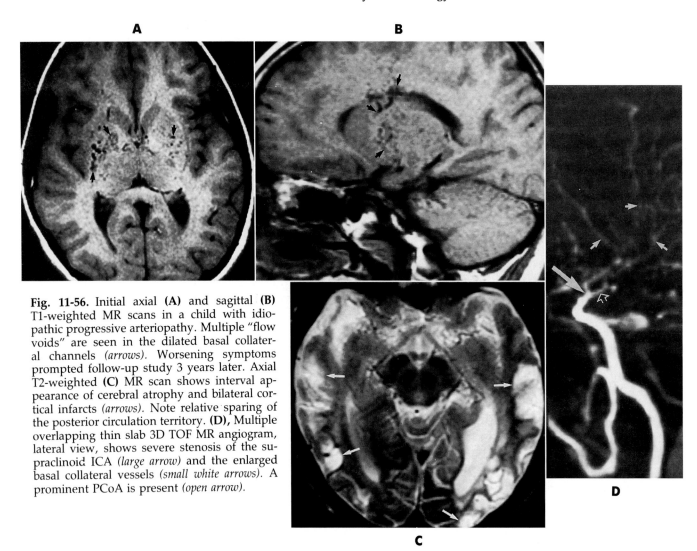

Fig. 11-56. Initial axial **(A)** and sagittal **(B)** T1-weighted MR scans in a child with idiopathic progressive arteriopathy. Multiple "flow voids" are seen in the dilated basal collateral channels *(arrows)*. Worsening symptoms prompted follow-up study 3 years later. Axial T2-weighted **(C)** MR scan shows interval appearance of cerebral atrophy and bilateral cortical infarcts *(arrows)*. Note relative sparing of the posterior circulation territory. **(D),** Multiple overlapping thin slab 3D TOF MR angiogram, lateral view, shows severe stenosis of the supraclinoid ICA *(large arrow)* and the enlarged basal collateral vessels *(small white arrows)*. A prominent PCoA is present *(open arrow)*.

"puff of smoke" appearance for which the disease is named. CT scans disclose multiple infarcts in over 80% of all patients with abnormal enhancement, and cerebral atrophy is identified in 50% to 60%. The anterior circulation is most frequently affected,[97] although the posterior cerebral artery is also often involved.[98] MR scans demonstrate collateral channels (Fig. 11-56) and ischemic changes.[99] MR angiography depicts most large vessel occlusions and major collateral flow patterns.[100]

It should be noted that the moyamoya pattern of collateral blood flow is nonspecific and can be seen in any slowly progressive intracranial occlusive vascular disorder such as atherosclerosis, radiation-induced angiopathy, and sickle-cell disease.[101]

Menkes' kinky hair disease. Menkes' kinky hair disease is an X-linked neurodegenerative syndrome associated with a defect in copper metabolism. Mental retardation, seizures, and light stubbly coarse hair (pili torti) are characteristic.[102] Imaging studies disclose severely elongated, tortuous abdominal, visceral, and cranial arteries (Fig. 11-57).[102]

Sickle-cell anemia. Stroke is a devastating complication of sickle cell disease (SCD) and occurs in 6% to 9% of affected individuals. Most infarcts in SCD are ischemic; hemorrhagic complications are uncommon.[103] Both small- and large-vessel occlusions occur. Multiple intracranial aneurysms, often in atypical locations, have also been reported in SCD.[104]

The pathology of sickle-cell cerebrovascular disease is controversial. Initially, small vessel thrombi of sickled cells were thought to result in cerebral infarction and hemorrhage. Vasa vasorum occlusion by sickled erythrocytes leading to progressive intimal and medial proliferation with eventual obliteration of the lumen was also proposed.[103] More recent evidence indicates that the degenerative insult is initiated by endothelial injury from adhesions of sickled erythrocytes to endothelial cells.[104] This results in internal elastic lamina fragmentation and degeneration

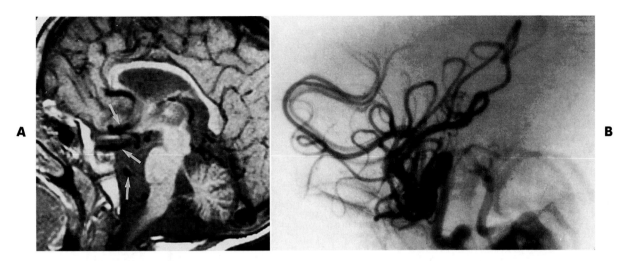

Fig. 11-57. Two cases demonstrate imaging findings of Menke's kinky hair syndrome. Sagittal T1-weighted **(A)** MR scan shows enlarged, elongated tortuous vessels *(arrows).* Common carotid angiogram **(B)**, arterial phase, lateral view, of another case shows severe vessel tortuosity.

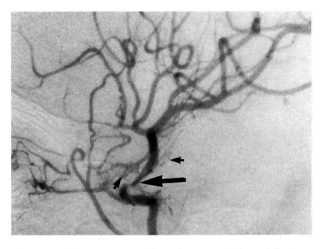

Fig. 11-58. Common carotid angiogram, midarterial phase, lateral view, in a 5-year-old African-American child with sickle cell disease and TIAs. Note severe narrowing of the distal intracavernous and supraclinoid ICA segments *(large arrow).* Some basal leptomeningeal collaterals are beginning to develop *(small arrows).*

of the muscularis, resulting in the large vessel vasculopathy and aneurysm formation observed in sickle cell patients (Fig. 11-58).

Miscellaneous. Miscellaneous congenital causes of arterial narrowing and occlusion include connective tissue disorders such as *Ehlers-Danlos syndrome, Marfan disease,* and *homocystinuria.* Marfan disease and homocystinuria have large vessel vasculopathy, clotting abnormalities, and subluxed lenses (classically downward in homocystinuria, up and inward

in Marfan disease). In addition to intimal irregularities and vascular stenosis, arterial and venous thrombi with intraluminal filling defects have been identified on cerebral angiography in these patients.[105]

Acquired Disorders: Vasculitis, Vasculopathy, and Miscellaneous Lesions

The vasculitides are a heterogeneous group of uncommon CNS disorders that are characterized by inflammation and necrosis of blood vessel walls.[106] Cerebral vasculitis can be infectious or noninfectious and primary (e.g., polyarteritis nodosa) or secondary (e.g., systemic lupus erythematosus).[107]

Several different classifications of cerebral vasculitis have been proposed. One system divides the vasculitides into the following three general categories[108]:

1. Those due to immune complex deposition
2. Those that appear to be cell-mediated disorders
3. A miscellaneous group

More traditional systems divide arteritis into bacterial, mycotic, necrotizing, and collagen-vascular disorders. We will use a combination of these classifications that initially subdivides the arteritides into infectious and noninfectious disorders (*see* box, p. 374).

Infectious arteritides. Infectious causes of arteritis include purulent bacterial meningitis, tuberculosis, fungal and viral infections, and syphilis.

Bacterial meningitis. CNS infection is a common cause of acquired cerebrovascular disease in children. Usually due to *Haemophilus influenzae* infection, cere-

Cerebral Vasculitis

Infectious vasculitis
Bacterial arteritis
Tuberculous arteritis
Fungal arteritis
Viral arteritis
Syphilitic arteritis

Noninfectious vasculitis

Immune complex deposition diseases
Necrotizing systemic vasculitides
   Polyarteritis nodosa
   Allergic angiitis
Hypersensitivity vasculitis
   Serum sickness
   Collagen vascular disease
Cell-mediated disorders
Giant cell and primary arteritides
   Temporal arteritis
   Takayasu arteritis
   Granulomatous arteritis
Wegener granulomatosis
Lymphomatoid granulomatosis
Chemical vasculitis
Ergot derivatives
Drug abuse
Miscellaneous disorders
Kawasaki disease
Buerger disease
Behcet disease
Neoplastic angiitis
Sarcoid

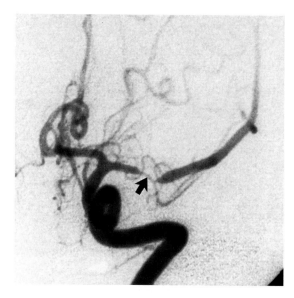

Fig. 11-59. Digital subtraction ICA angiogram, arterial phase, AP view, shows severe narrowing of the horizontal MCA *(arrow)* in this patient with possible tuberculous meningitis.

bral infarctions develop in up to one quarter of children with complicated bacterial meningitis.[109] The pathophysiology of stroke in these patients is unclear but may be secondary to vasculitis, coagulopathy, vasospasm, or a combination of factors. The most common angiographic finding is narrowing of the vessels at the base of the brain, although more peripheral involvement can also occur.[110] Multiple infarctions, particularly in the lenticulostriate distributions, are often seen on MR studies.

Tuberculous meningitis. Vascular effects of CNS tuberculosis are manifested as tuberculous meningitis with arteritis or tuberculoma with adjacent focal arteritis. The generalized arteritis associated with tuberculosis tends to involve the basilar vessels, particularly the supraclinoid internal carotid arteries and M1 segments of the middle cerebral arteries (Fig. 11-59).[111] Angiographic and CT/MR findings are nonspecific and include vascular stenoses and frank occlusions.

Mycotic arteritis. Fungal arteritides include actinomycosis, aspergillosis, coccidioidomycosis, and other disorders. Some fungi, particularly *Actinomyces*, have a predilection to invade vessel walls directly and may produce multiple hemorrhagic infarctions (*see* Chapter 16). Angiographic findings are nonspecific, i.e., narrowing of the basal cerebral or cortical vessels.

Viral arteritis. Several viruses involve the CNS. Herpes encephalitis is the most common nonepidemic viral meningitis in North America. Herpes encephalitis is discussed in detail in Chapter 16. It is a hemorrhagic, necrotizing encephalitis that may affect any part of the brain but has a predilection for the temporal and parietal lobes.

Syphilitic arteritis. Cerebrovascular lues is typically diffuse, affecting cortical veins and arteries. Gummous arteritis commonly affects branches of the middle cerebral artery.[112]

Noninfectious vasculitides. A spectrum of noninfectious disorders affects the intracranial vasculature. Some of these vasculitides such as polyarteritis nodosa and the collagen vascular diseases are probably related to immune complex deposition disorders. Others such as giant cell arteritis, Wegener granulomatosis, and primary (isolated) angiitis are probably cell mediated. Finally, a diverse group of miscellaneous disorders causing vasculitis-like CNS lesions includes Kawasaki disease, Behcet disease, and drug-abuse arteritis, among others.

Immune complex diseases. The vasculitides that are probably related to immune complex deposition include polyarteritis nodosa and collagen vascular diseases such as systemic lupus erythematosus.

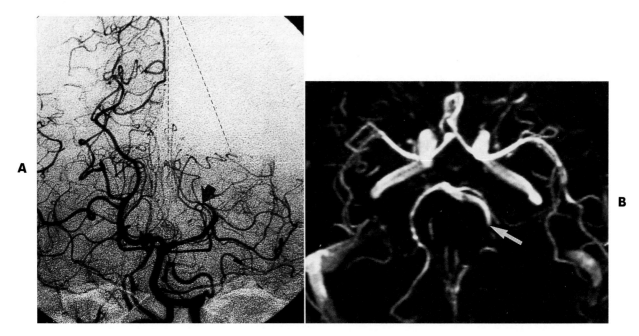

Fig. 11-60. A 32-year-old woman with SLE and antiphospholipid antibody syndrome presented with sudden onset of right homonymous hemianopsia. **A,** Vertebrobasilar angiogram, midarterial phase, AP view, shows occlusion of the left P2 PCA segment *(arrow)*. Posterior parietal and occipital lobe infarction *(dotted lines)*. **B,** 3D TOF MR angiogram, basal view, shows the occlusion *(arrow)*.

Polyarteritis nodosa (PAN) is the most common systemic necrotizing vasculitis with CNS manifestations.[113] The ubiquitous nature of this vasculitis commonly leads to widespread multiorgan dysfunction.[107] PAN primarily affects small and medium-sized muscular arteries. Microaneurysms resulting from internal elastic lamina necrosis are the diagnostic hallmark of PAN and are seen in 60% to 75% of patients in the acute phase of the disease. Later manifestations are nonspecific and include vascular thrombosis, luminal irregularities, and segmental stenoses. CNS involvement is typically a late manifestation of PAN.[107]

Systemic lupus erythematosus (SLE) is a complex multisystem disease that often has both central and peripheral nervous system manifestations. CNS lupus produces a diverse spectrum of neurologic dysfunction via multiple mechanisms that may or may not involve an immune-mediated mechanism.[114] Stroke occurs in up to half of these patients and most likely results from cardiac valvular disease, coagulopathy, antiphospholipid antibody syndrome (Figs. 11-15 and 11-60), or a combination of these factors.

True CNS lupus "vasculitis" is uncommon.[110] The angiographic spectrum ranges from normal or subtle small vessel disease (Fig. 11-61) to large vessel arteriopathy with bizarre fusiform aneurysms *(see Fig. 9-39)*. MR findings in patients with nonfocal symptoms include multifocal areas of increased signal in-

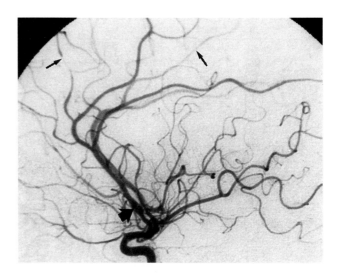

Fig. 11-61. Digital subtraction ICA angiogram, arterial phase, lateral view, in a patient with long-standing SLE. Segmental dilatation and narrowing is seen in the proximal ACA *(large arrow)*. More peripheral irregularities and stenoses are also present *(small arrows)*.

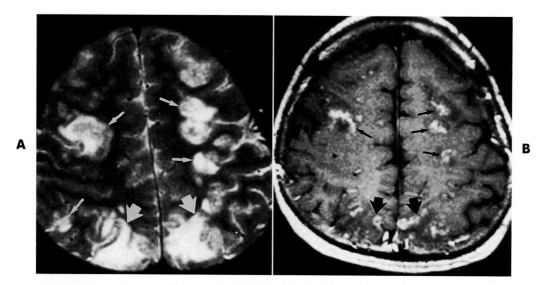

Fig. 11-62. Axial T2WI **(A)** in a 14-year-old girl with SLE shows multifocal high signal areas at the corticomedullary junctions *(small arrows)*. **(B)** Axial T1WI with contrast enhancement shows the lesions have produced blood-brain barrier dysfunction, demonstrated by the patchy multifocal enhancing areas *(small arrows.)* Because this patient also had renal involvement, it is unclear whether the CNS lesions are due to true SLE vasculitis or renovascular hypertensive encephalopathy. The more focal parietooccipital lesions **(A** and **B,** *large arrows)* favor the latter.

tensity in the subcortical white matter on T2WI (Fig. 11-62, *A*). Some lesions may enhance following contrast administration (Fig. 11-62).

Patients with SLE and symptoms of focal intracranial disease may have areas of increased signal intensity and atrophic changes in regions corresponding to major cerebral vascular distributions.[114] Multifocal subcortical hemorrhages have also been identified[115] (*see* Fig. 7-32). Marked intracranial calcification in the basal ganglia and dentate nuclei has been reported with SLE.[116]

A close relationship between antiphospholipid antibodies (APLA) and neurologic disease has been documented. APLA occurs most frequently in patients with SLE and lupus-like disease but also has been reported with infections, neoplasms (particularly lung cancer), certain drugs that induce lupus-like phenomena, oral contraceptives, hematologic disorders (idiopathic thrombocytopenic purpura, hemolytic anemias, and hairy cell leukemia), primary immunodeficiency disorders, and in a subgroup of patients with idiopathic APLA.[117,118]

Venous or arterial thrombotic occlusions are characteristic abnormalities in APLA and occur in 25% to 30% of these patients (Fig. 11-60). CNS symptoms range from dementia to transient cerebral infarction and stroke. MR scans show nonspecific findings of diffuse cerebral atrophy and multiple high signal foci in the periventricular and subcortical white matter on

T2WI. The differential diagnosis includes multiple sclerosis, SLE, Behcet disease, Sneddon syndrome, migraine, degenerative microangiopathy, and multifocal infarcts.[117] Angiographic findings are multiple progressive arterial thromboses.[118]

Cell-mediated disorders. Cell-mediated disorders include the spectrum of giant cell arteritides (temporal arteritis, Takayasu arteritis), granulomatous arteritis (idiopathic, neurosarcoid), primary (isolated) angiitis, Wegener granulomatosis, and lymphomatoid granulomatosis.[113]

Takayasu arteritis and temporal arteritis are different forms of giant cell arteritis that are characterized by a granulomatous infiltration in the arterial wall. Variable cellular infiltration with lymphocytes, histiocytes, plasma cells, giant cells, or a combination are present, with intimal and subintimal proliferative changes.[107] *Temporal arteritis* is a systemic vasculitic syndrome characterized by inflammation and multifocal stenoses of the temporal and other extracranial arteries.[107]

Takayasu arteritis involves the aorta, its branches, and, occasionally, the pulmonary arteries. The following four types of characteristic lesions are identified at angiography[119]:

1. Occlusions
2. Stenoses (Fig. 11-63)
3. Luminal irregularities
4. Ectasia or aneurysmal dilatations

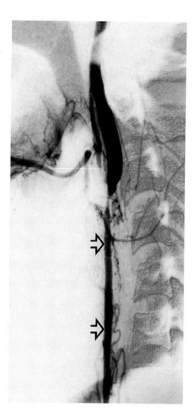

Fig. 11-63. Left CCA angiogram, arterial phase, lateral view, in a patient with Takayasu arteritis. Severe stenosis of the CCA is present *(arrows)*.

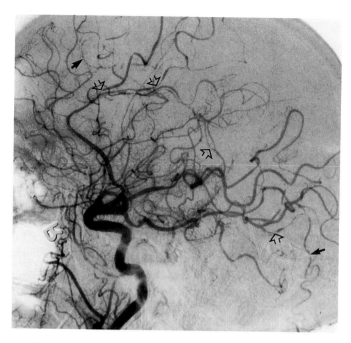

Fig. 11-64. Lateral right CCA angiogram in a patient with granulomatous angiitis shows nonspecific multifocal segmental vascular stenoses *(open arrows)* affecting all three major vascular territories. Note "beaded" appearance in some of the affected vessels *(black arrows)*.

Granulomatous angiitis is an uncommon small vessel vasculitis of unknown etiology that has been reported in association with CNS tumors and infections.[120] An idiopathic, isolated form of CNS angiitis also occurs.[121] Imaging findings are nonspecific.MR scans may show nonspecific multifocal whitematter hyperintensities on T2WI. Angiographic findings are those of multiple intracranial segmental stenoses (Fig. 11-64). Although parenchymal-leptomeningeal biopsy is the diagnostic procedure of choice, the yield from open biopsy is only about 50%.[122]

Sarcoidosis affects the CNS in 3% to 5% of all cases.[113] In neurosarcoid the vessels at the base of the brain are infiltrated with nonnecrotizing periepithelial granulomas. Meningeal and systemic involvement are also common. Imaging studies in these patients show enhancing, thickened leptomeninges *(see* Chapter 12). Nonspecific vascular stenoses can sometimes be identified on cerebral angiograms in these cases.

Wegener granulomatosis is a chronic systemic disorder characterized by granulomatous and focal arteritis in the respiratory tract, kidneys, and other organs. CNS involvement occurs in 15% to 30% of cases.[123] The following three types of lesions have been identified[123]:

1. Direct granulomatous invasion from contiguous lesions in the nose and paranasal sinuses
2. Remote (i.e., meningeal and intracerebral granulomas) lesions from the nose and paranasal sinuses
3. Vasculitis of the nervous system

Angiographic findings are nonspecific and include arterial wall irregularities and vessel occlusions.

Miscellaneous vasculitides. Various miscellaneous noninfectious inflammatory disorders affect the craniocerebral vessels. These include mucocutaneous lymph node syndrome (Kawasaki disease), thromboangiitis obliterans (Buerger disease), Behcet disease, and chemical arteritis.

Mucocutaneous lymph node syndrome can have dilated, fusiform ectasias and aneurysmal dilatations of multiple arteries. *Thromboangiitis obliterans* is an idiopathic, recurrent segmental obliterative vasculopathy that involves small and medium-sized arteries and veins of the extremities.[107] There is a strong association with cigarette smoking. Craniocerebral involvement in Buerger disease is controversial; if it occurs, cortical venous occlusions predominate.[112]

Behcet disease is a rare multisystem immune-related vasculitis that involves both arteries and veins.[124] It is prevalent in Japan, the Middle East, and many Mediterranean countries. The syndrome consists of recurrent oral and genital aphthous ulcerations, uveitis, skin lesions, and arthritis.[125]

Behcet disease has neurologic manifestations in 10% to 45% of patients. The following three clinical patterns of CNS involvement have been observed[126]:

1. A brainstem syndrome
2. A meningoencephalitic syndrome
3. An organic confusion syndrome

CT is usually unhelpful; MR studies show high signal foci in the brainstem, diencephalon, and the cerebral hemispheres on T2-weighted images.[124] Vascular lesions range from arterial occlusions and aneurysms to superficial thrombophlebitis, occlusion of the superior and inferior vena cava, and cerebral venous thrombosis.[127,128]

Drug-induced arteritis is becoming increasingly widespread. It results from direct toxic injury to the vessel wall or hypersensitivity to impurities in the diluent.[129] Different legitimate and nonprescriptive pharmaceutical agents (such as pseudoephedrine), as well as illegal drugs (e.g., cocaine), have been reported as causes of cerebral vasculitis. Ergot derivates may cause peripheral, visceral, and CNS arteriopathy.[130] Oral contraceptives and concomitant cigarette smoking appear to accelerate intracranial occlusive disease.[131]

Amphetamines can cause a necrotizing cerebral angiitis, resulting in arterial aneurysms and sacculations (*see* Fig. 9-40).[129] Methamphetamine also causes vasospasm and stroke, particularly when coadministered with cocaine (Fig. 11-65).[132] Adverse CNS effects reported with heroin and phenylpropanolamine include cerebral vasculitis, vasospasm, and congenital malformations caused by prenatal exposure to these vasoactive drugs.[133]

Cocaine is a potent sympathomimetic drug that blocks presynaptic reuptake of norepinephrine and dopamine. The resultant postsynaptic receptor stimulation produces various acute cardiovascular and systemic pressor effects. Cocaine abuse is also associated with various CNS complications that include intracranial hemorrhage, ischemia and infarction, seizures, vasospasm, and death (*see* Chapter 7). True cocaine-induced vasculitis is uncommon; the vessel narrowing sometimes observed in cases of cocaine abuse (Fig. 11-66) may be due to vasospasm.[134]

Miscellaneous vasculopathies. Several nontraumatic, noninflammatory, nonatherosclerotic disorders can produce craniocerebral vascular stenoses and occlusions. These include fibromuscular dysplasia, flow-related vasculopathy, extrinsic compression from neoplasms or cervical spondylosis, and radiation-induced vascular changes.

Fibromuscular dysplasia. Fibromuscular dysplasia (FMD) is a vasculopathy of unknown etiology that causes intimal or medial proliferative changes in the cervical internal carotid (ICA) and vertebral (VA) arteries. The common carotid bifurcation and proximal ICA are typically spared, with a characteristic segmental "string of beads" appearance at around the C2 level. Occasionally, long-segment

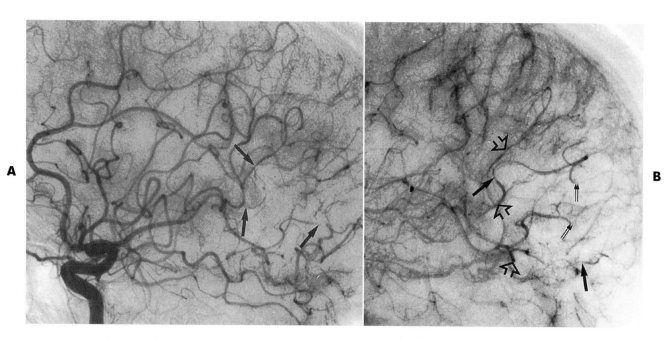

Fig. 11-65. A 20-year-old with amphetamine abuse. Left ICA angiogram, lateral view, with arterial **(A)** and early venous **(B)** studies shows vasculitic changes (*single black arrows*) with slow flow, seen as arterial contrast that persists into the venous phase (*open arrows*). Some occluded vessels can be identified (*double arrows*).

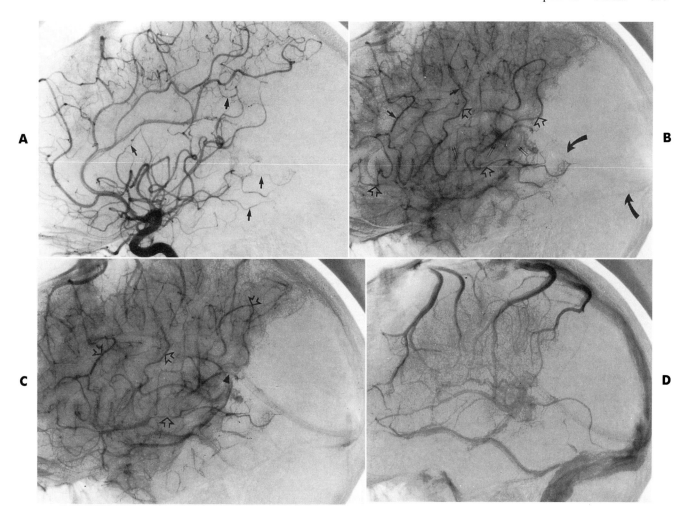

Fig. 11-66. Serial views of the left ICA angiogram in a patient with cocaine abuse show findings of frank cerebral infarction. Midarterial phase **(A)** shows some vessel irregularities *(arrows)* and a large area of nonperfused brain in the posterior parietal region. Late arterial phase **(B)** shows slow flow in numerous MCA branches *(open arrows)* with some irregular stenosis and "beading" *(single small arrows)*. Arteriovenous shunting with early appearance of contrast in the internal cerebral vein and vein of Galen *(double arrows),* as well as the straight and transverse sinuses *(curved arrows)* is present. Midvenous phase **(C)** film shows persistent intraarterial contrast *(open arrows)*. Intraluminal clot in the angular artery *(arrowhead)* is present. Late venous phase **(D)** shows no cortical vein opacification in the unperfused parietooccipital area.

tubular stenosis or asymmetric saccular dilatations can be identified (Fig. 11-67). The ICA is affected in about three quarters of all cases, with the VA involved in 15% to 25%. Bilateral involvement is present in 60% to 75%.[19]

FMD is associated with an increased incidence of intracranial aneurysms. Complications of FMD include dissection (Fig. 11-67), SAH secondary to aneurysm rupture or intracranial emboli (Fig. 11-68).

Flow-related vasculopathy. Cerebral arteriovenous malformations (AVMs) are associated with various alterations in the angioarchitecture of feeding arteries and draining veins. Histologic examination of

the vessel walls in these cases shows irregular intimal thickening with destructive changes in the internal elastic membrane and media, as well as desquamated epithelium.[135] Observed angiographic changes in the afferent vessels include ectasia and tortuosity, aneurysm formation, thrombosis, and stenosis (*see* Figs. 10-1 and 10-5).[136,137]

Extrinsic compressive lesions. Compressive lesions that involve the craniocerebral vasculature include tumors, cervical osteophytes, fibrous bands, and infection.[138] The cervical carotid artery and its branches can be encased by nasopharyngeal tumors that compress or invade the carotid space. Intracranial narrowing or vessel occlusion secondary to neo-

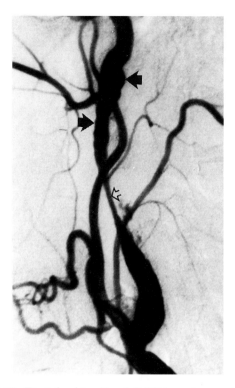

Fig. 11-67. Digital subtraction left CCA angiogram in a patient with known FMD and sudden onset of right-sided weakness shows the typical "string-of-beads" appearance of FMD in the ICA *(large arrows)*. Midcervical dissection *(open arrow)* is present.

plasm is uncommon. Meningiomas, pituitary adenomas, and gliomas are often implicated. The intracranial vessels at or near the skull base are narrowed and encased.[139]

Infection can cause narrowing of the craniocerebral vessels. Tonsillar abscess in children and sphenoid sinusitis in adults are rare but potentially serious causes of ICA narrowing. Raeder syndrome is an uncommon disorder that consists of unilateral headache and facial pain in the first and second divisions of the trigeminal nerve, typically accompanied by an incomplete postganglionic Horner syndrome. Severe narrowing of the ICA secondary to sinusitis, arteritis, or dissection has been implicated.[140]

Radiation vasculopathy. Late injury to the brain is the major hazard of CNS exposure to therapeutic radiation doses.[141] The reported spectrum of radiation-induced vascular lesions includes accelerated focal arteriosclerosis, mineralizing microangiopathy, progressive occlusion of large intracranial vessels (Fig. 11-69), and embolic stroke from thrombus forming on denuded ulcerated endothelium.[142,143,143a]

Endothelial or elastica degeneration, intimal fibrosis, media fibroplasia, accelerated atherosclerosis, and angiomatous malformations can be seen. These secondary vascular changes can occur many months to years after treatment.[141,143b] Associated brain parenchymal necrosis and gliosis are often identified. The combination of some chemotherapeutic agents plus radiation therapy may increase late toxicity by inhibiting DNA repair processes.[144]

Spontaneous dissection. Dissection of the cervical

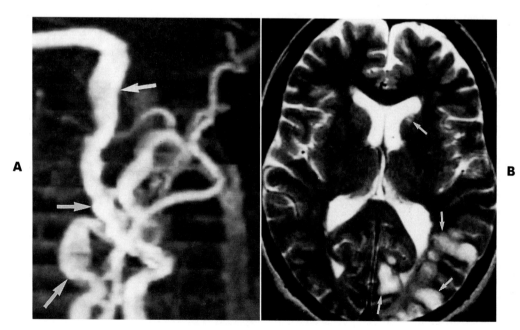

Fig. 11-68. A, MR angiogram shows FMD involving the left internal carotid and vertebral arteries *(arrows).* **B,** Axial T2-weighted MR scan shows embolic infarcts in both the carotid and the vertebral basilar territories *(arrows).*

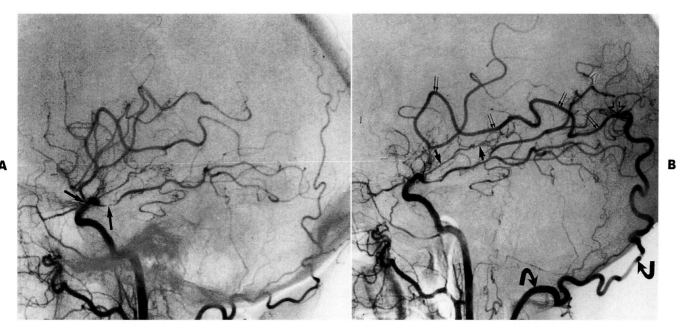

Fig. 11-69. Radiation vasculopathy with progressive arterial stenosis is illustrated by this case. **A,** Right CCA angiogram, early arterial phase, lateral view, in a patient who had been operated and then radiated for pituitary adenoma. The patient suffered from right hemisphere TIAs. Moderately severe stenoses of the supraclinoid ICA, PCA, and MCA are seen *(arrows)*. An occipital artery to MCA bypass was performed. Increasing symptoms prompted repeat examination 18 months later. **B,** Follow-up right CCA study shows the anastomosis *(open arrow)* between the enlarged occipital artery *(curved arrows)* and the angular artery *(double arrows)* is patent. However, the supraclinoid ICA is now even more stenotic and fills only a few lenticulostriate branches, the anterior choroidal artery *(small single arrows)*, and the PCA.

internal carotid and vertebral arteries is a recognized cause of stroke, particularly in young individuals. In addition to trauma (*see* Chapter 8), reported predisposing conditions for dissection include hypertension, migraine headaches (Fig. 11-70), vigorous physical activity, sympathomimetic drugs, oral contraceptives, pharyngeal infections, and underlying vasculopathies such as fibromuscular dysplasia and Marfan syndrome (*see* box).

The angiographic appearance of extracranial internal carotid dissection is that of a long midcervical narrowing that spares the carotid bulb and terminates near the skull base (Fig. 11-70, *A*). Angiographic demonstration of an intimal flap or false lumen is relatively uncommon (Fig. 11-70, *C* and *D*). Vertebral dissections are most commonly located between the skull base and second cervical vertebra (Fig. 11-70, *C*).

MR is a useful screening modality for patients suspected of harboring a dissection. Standard spin-echo images disclose a paravascular hematoma with narrowed vessel lumen (Fig. 11-70, *B*). MR angiography is often helpful, although the high signal of subacute clot may simulate flow in images that are reconstructed with maximum intensity projection algorithms. Occasionally, dissections are subadventitial instead of subintimal. Angiography may be normal in such cases but MR usually discloses the paravascular hematoma.[144a]

Causes of Arterial Dissection

Trauma

Direct penetrating injury
Blunt injury
Stretching, impaction against cervical vertebrae
Chiropractic manipulation
Cervical spine fracture (vertebral artery injury)
Vigorous physical activity

Underlying vasculopathy

Fibromuscular dysplasia
Cystic medial necrosis
Ehlers-Danlos
Homocystinuria

Migraine headache

Hypertension

Oral contraceptives

Drug abuse

Spontaneous

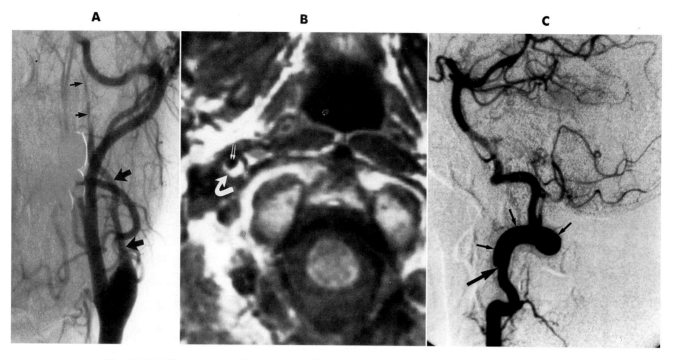

Fig. 11-70. Three cases of imaging findings in spontaneous craniocerebral arterial dissections are illustrated. A 26-year-old woman with migraine headaches for several years had a 2 week history of right arm and leg weakness with visual difficulty in the left eye. **A,** Left CCA angiogram, arterial phase, AP view, shows a spontaneous dissection of the cervical ICA. The lumen is severely narrowed *(large arrows)* just distal to the carotid bulb, then tapers to a "string sign" *(small arrows).* **B,** Another young woman had spontaneous onset of a right-sided Horner's syndrome 5 days before MR imaging. Axial T1-weighted MR scan shows a narrowed ICA with a small "flow void" *(double arrows)* surrounded by a subacute paravascular hematoma *(curved arrow).* **C,** A third young woman had sudden onset of visual field defect due to spontaneous vertebral artery dissection at the C1-C2 level with embolic occlusion of the right PCA. A digital subtraction left VA angiogram, arterial phase, lateral view, was obtained within a few hours. VA dissection beginning between C1 and C2 *(large arrow)* and ending at the craniocervical junction is seen. Both the true and false lumens are opacified, accounting for the enlarged appearance of the dissected VA segment *(small black arrows).*

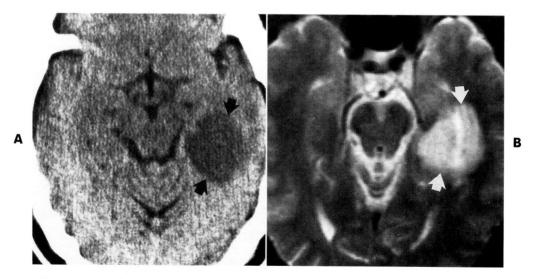

Fig. 11-71. Stroke or tumor? **A,** NECT scan in a patient with first-time seizure shows a round low density mass *(arrows)* in the posterior temporal lobe. **B,** Axial T2-weighted MR scan shows a hyperintense mass *(arrows)* that suggests neoplasm.

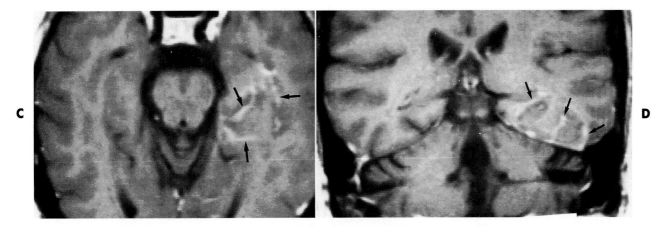

Fig. 11-71 cont'd.   C, Axial and, **D,** coronal postcontrast T1-weighted studies show gyriform enhancement *(arrows)* in the PCA distribution. Cerebral angiography (not shown) disclosed PCA infarct.

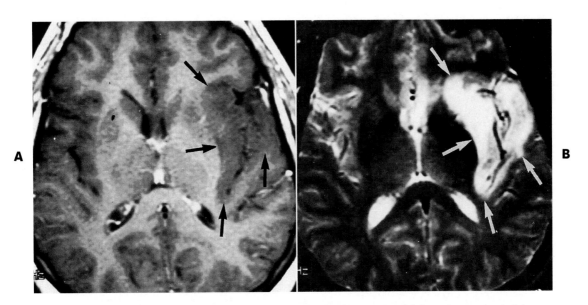

Fig. 11-72. Stroke or tumor? A 26-year-old man had a temporal lobe seizure. **A,** Axial postcontrast T1-weighted MR scan shows a nonenhancing mass that involves the insular and temporal lobe cortex *(arrows)*. **B,** T2-weighted study shows the mass *(arrows)* is uniformly hyperintense. The differential diagnostic considerations were infiltrating neoplasm, encephalitis, and infarct. The absence of other abnormalities in the MCA territory mitigate against infarct; the lack of contrast enhancement or hemorrhage would be somewhat unusual for herpes encephalitis, although encephalitis remains a diagnostic possibility. Biopsy disclosed grade II infiltrating astrocytoma.

Stroke "Mimics"

The clinical and imaging diagnoses of stroke are sometimes challenging. The clinical diagnosis of stroke may be inaccurate in up to 10% to 15% of cases. Occasionally, lesions such as tumor and subdural hematoma present with sudden onset of focal neurologic deficits similar to those produced by cerebral infarction. Imaging findings that suggest stroke include a full thickness lesion that affects gray and white matter and follows a typical vascular distribution (*see* box, p. 385, *left*). Strokes often affect the cortex and spare the underlying white matter, and tumors tend to involve the white matter and spare the cortex.

Strokes tend to be wedge-shaped or serpentine; tumors are usually round, lobulated, or infiltrating. However, sometimes strokes look like tumors (Fig. 11-71) and neoplasms can resemble strokes (Fig. 11-72) on imaging studies.

Gyriform enhancement following contrast admin-

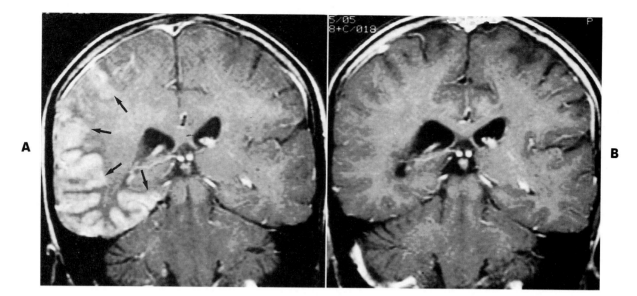

Fig. 11-73. A 22-year-old man had a contrast-enhanced scan performed 12 hours after temporal lobe seizure. Coronal **(A)** postcontrast T1-weighted MR scan shows striking cortical enhancement *(arrows)*. Follow-up scan **(B)** obtained 3 months later is normal. The gyriform enhancement was probably secondary to transient blood-brain barrier disruption caused by the seizure.

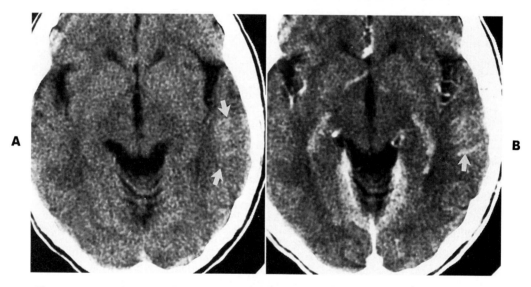

Fig. 11-74. Axial pre- **(A)** and postcontrast **(B)** CT scans obtained almost immediately after a left temporal lobe seizure in this patient show focal gyriform hyperdensities *(arrows,* **A)** with some intravascular contrast enhancement **(B,** *arrow)*. MR scan without and with contrast enhancement performed 24 hours later (not shown) was normal. These changes may represent transient post-ictal hyperemia.

istration is a nonspecific finding (*see* box, p. 385, *top right*). It can occur with cerebral infarction (Fig. 11-25, *B*), encephalitis, infiltrating neoplasm, cortical contusions (*see* Fig. 8-35, *C*), or with hypermetabolic states such as epilepsy.[145] Post-ictal enhancement may be striking and is probably caused by transient blood-brain barrier disruption (Fig. 11-73). In addition to MR abnormalities, reversible focal abnormalities on CT scans also occur with prolonged seizure activity (Fig. 11-74).[146] Gyriform enhancement of cortical hamartomas in tuberous sclerosis has also been reported.[147]

Stroke or Tumor?*
Stroke
Sudden onset
Gray and white matter involved
Wedge-shaped or gyriform
Typical vascular distribution
Tumor
Gradual onset
Tends to spare cortex, preferentially involves white matter
Round or infiltrating
Not confined to a specific vascular territory

*No absolutes; these are helpful but not pathognomonic findings.

Gyriform Enhancement
Differential Diagnosis
Common
Stroke
Encephalitis
Contusion
Uncommon
Post-ictal
Gliomatosis cerebri
Infiltrating primary tumor
Subpial metastases
Rare
Tuberous sclerosis

VENOUS OCCLUSIONS

Cerebral venoocclusive disease is an elusive, often underdiagnosed cause of acute neurologic deterioration.[148] Because clinical signs and symptoms are often nonspecific, imaging is critical to the diagnosis of this disorder.

Pathology. Sinus-vein thrombosis is a multistep process that probably begins when thrombus incompletely occludes a dural sinus, usually the superior sagittal sinus. The thrombus progresses, obstructing first the sinus and then extending to involve bridging veins anterior to the obstruction. Once the tributary cortical veins are occluded, petechial perivascular hemorrhages and cortical venous infarctions occur (Fig. 11-75, *see* Fig. 7-34).[149]

Etiology. Several different disease processes can cause cerebral venous thrombosis (CVT) (*see* box, *right*). Local disease processes such as sinusitis or mastoiditis, trauma, and tumor can occlude dural sinuses. Common systemic disorders that cause dural sinus and cortical vein thrombosis in children include dehydration, infection, trauma, and hematologic diseases.[150,150a] In adults, infection, oral contraceptives, puerperium, pregnancy,[150b] malignancy, dehydration, collagen vascular diseases, antiphospholipid antibody syndrome,[150c,d] inflammatory bowel disease (ulcerative colitis and Crohn's disease),[151] miscellaneous other hypercoagulable states, Behcet disease,[152] and hematologic disorders can cause cerebral venous or dural sinus thrombosis.[153] No cause for CVT is identified in one quarter of all cases.[154]

Location. The superior sagittal sinus (SSS) is the

Dural Sinus/Cerebral Venous Occlusions
Predisposing Conditions
Common
Pregnancy/puerperium
Infection
Dehydration
Oral contraceptives
Blood dyscrasias, coagulopathies
Tumor (local invasion, e.g., meningioma)
Trauma
High-flow vasculopathic changes secondary to AVM, AVF
Uncommon
Inflammatory bowel disease (ulcerative colitis, Crohn's disease)
Behcet syndrome
Lupus anticoagulant
Paroxysmal nocturnal hemoglobinuria
Drug abuse
Systemic malignancy; paraneoplastic syndromes

most commonly occluded dural sinus, followed by the transverse, sigmoid, and cavernous sinuses. Commonly occluded veins are the superficial cortical veins that drain into the SSS. Cortical vein occlusion usually occurs with dural sinus thrombosis and is rare in its absence.

Internal cerebral vein (ICV) thrombosis is a less common but clinically devastating event. ICV clots may extend to involve the vein of Galen or straight

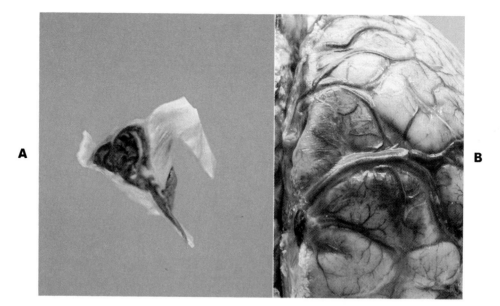

Fig. 11-75. Gross autopsy specimen shows typical findings in dural sinus and cortical vein occlusion. **A,** The superior sagittal sinus (SSS) is filled with fresh thrombus. **B,** The brain shows thrombosed cortical veins and multifocal hemorrhagic venous infarcts.

sinus. ICV thrombus causes bilateral venous infarcts in the deep gray matter nuclei, upper midbrain, and adjacent matter.[154b]

Imaging

Cerebral angiography. Dural sinus occlusion and cortical vein thrombosis can be diagnosed using conventional film-screen or digital subtraction techniques. Aortic arch injection with the head filmed in a slightly oblique position is the best approach because this technique opacifies all the craniocerebral vessels and their draining veins. Inflow of unopacified blood into cortical veins and dural sinuses will not be mistaken for clot. ICV thrombosis causes bilateral venous infarcts in the deep grey matter nuclei, upper midbrain, and adjacent white matter.[154b]

At angiography a thrombosed sinus appears as an empty channel devoid of contrast and surrounded by dilated collateral venous channels in the dural leaves (Fig. 11-76, *A* and *B*). Enlarged medullary veins and other collateral draining channels are often present. Thrombosed cortical veins are seen as cordlike contrast collections that seem to "hang in space," persisting into the late venous phase (Fig. 11-77). Intraluminal thrombi may produce linear or meniscoid filling defects (Fig. 11-76, *B*).

Deep cerebral vein thrombosis is seen as nonfilling of the internal cerebral veins or vein of Galen with enlarged collateral channels (*see* Fig. 11-82, *G* and *H*).

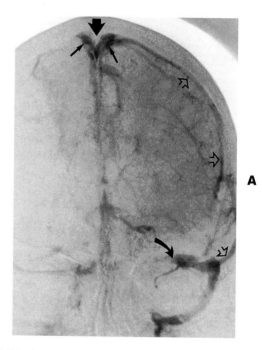

Fig. 11-76. Angiographic findings of dural sinus occlusion. **A,** A 24-year-old man had severe headache and confusion following a flu-like episode. A left ICA angiogram, venous phase, AP view, shows nonfilling of the superior sagittal sinus (SSS), seen as a triangular area devoid of contrast (*large arrow*) surrounded by parasagittal collateral venous channels (*small black arrows*). The transverse sinus is also occluded and is reconstituted distally (*curved arrow*) by prominent superficial cortical veins (*open arrows*).

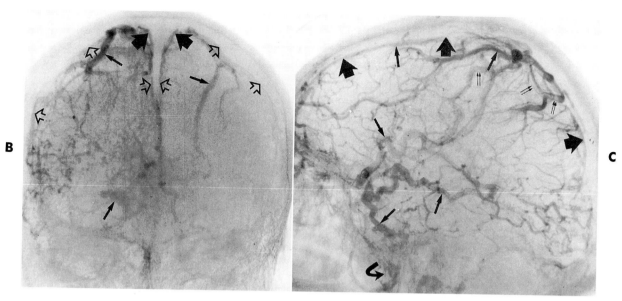

Fig. 11-76, cont'd. Angiographic findings of dural sinus occlusion. **B** and **C,** A 65-year-old man abruptly terminated his anticoagulant therapy. Several days later he experienced confusion, decreasing mental status, and coma. AP **(B)** and lateral **(C)** venous phase films from his cerebral angiogram show an occluded SSS, seen as a triangular **(B,** *large arrows)* or crescentic **(C,** *large arrows)* area that is devoid of contrast. Numerous prominent parasagittal, superficial, and deep collateral venous channels are seen *(small, single arrows)*. Cortical vein thrombi are seen as intraluminal filling defects *(double arrows)* in some of the veins adjacent to the occluded SSS. The torcular herophili, straight and transverse sinuses, and internal cerebral veins (ICVs) are not opacified and are probably occluded. Extracranial drainage is primarily via the pterygoid venous plexus *(curved arrow)*. Bilateral extraaxial fluid collections are seen as displacement of venous channels away from the inner calvarial vault and falx cerebri *(open arrows)*. Autopsy confirmed extensive dural sinus and ICV occlusion, cortical vein thrombosis with venous infarcts, and bilateral subdural hematomas.

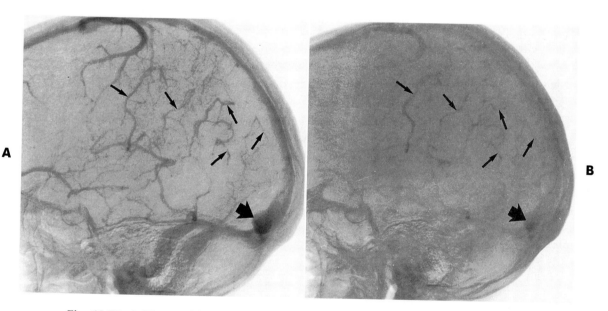

Fig. 11-77. A 28-year-old pregnant woman had onset of severe headaches 1 day after parturition. Five days later she had a seizure followed by precipitous decline in mental status. Right CCA angiogram with mid- **(A)** and late **(B)** venous phase films, lateral view, show the SSS and deep cerebral veins are patent. The straight sinus (SS) is not visualized, and only a residual "stump" *(large arrow)* is seen at its entrance into the torcular herophili. Several cortical veins appear to "hang in space" **(A,** *small arrows)* with contrast persisting into the very late venous phase **(B,** *small arrows)* after contrast in nearly all the other veins and dural sinuses has disappeared. Note contrast remaining in the residual SS stump **(B,** *large arrow)*. Postmortem examination confirmed straight sinus thrombosis and multiple occluded cortical veins.

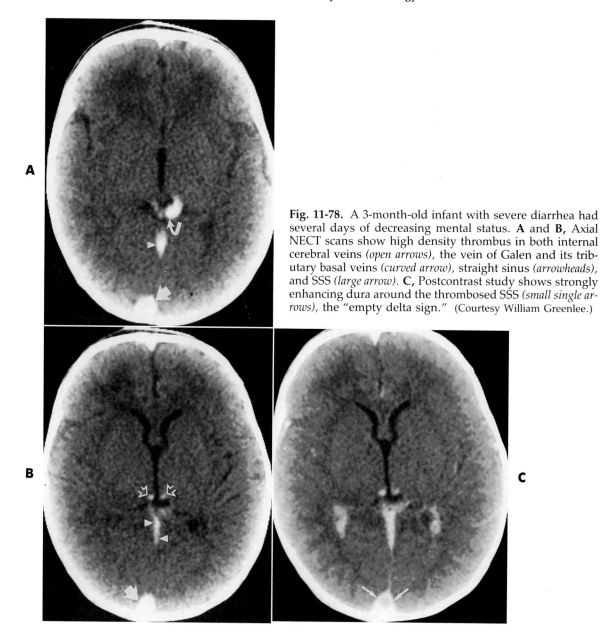

Fig. 11-78. A 3-month-old infant with severe diarrhea had several days of decreasing mental status. **A** and **B,** Axial NECT scans show high density thrombus in both internal cerebral veins *(open arrows),* the vein of Galen and its tributary basal veins *(curved arrow),* straight sinus *(arrowheads),* and SSS *(large arrow).* **C,** Postcontrast study shows strongly enhancing dura around the thrombosed SSS *(small single arrows),* the "empty delta sign." (Courtesy William Greenlee.)

Computed tomography. NECT scans may disclose hyperdense thrombus in the thrombosed dural sinus or veins (Figs. 11-78, *A* to *B,* and 11-79, *A*). Occasionally, thrombosed cortical veins are seen as linear high density areas (cord sign). Cortical and subcortical hemorrhages can sometimes be identified adjacent to an occluded sinus. On CECT scans the engorged dural cavernous spaces, meningeal venous tributaries, and collateral venous channels that surround a relatively hypodense occluded sinus may enhance around the thrombus, producing the so-called empty delta sign (Figs. 11-78, *C*; 11-79, *B*; and 11-84, *A*).[155] In subacute or chronic cases of dural sinus thrombosis, the tentorium and falx appear strikingly thickened, engorged, and somewhat ill-defined or shaggy (Fig. 11-80).

The differential diagnosis of dural sinus thrombo-

sis on CT scans is relatively limited (*see* box). In premature and in term newborn infants the combination of low density unmyelinated brain and physiologic polycythemia normally makes the falx and dural sinuses appear quite dense (*see* Fig. 7-81, *A*). A "pseudodelta" sign can sometimes be seen on nonenhanced scans in patients with head trauma or subarachnoid hemorrhage. Unclotted circulating blood in the SSS or torcular herophili creates a low density area that is surrounded by hyperdense acute subarachnoid or subdural hemorrhage layered along the falx and tentorium (Fig. 11-81, *B*; see Fig. 8-45, *B*).[156] This should not be mistaken for dural sinus thrombosis. Occasionally, a high-splitting tentorium can also mimic SSS thrombosis on CECT scans (Figs. 11-81, *C*).

Deep cerebral vein thrombosis is seen as hyper-

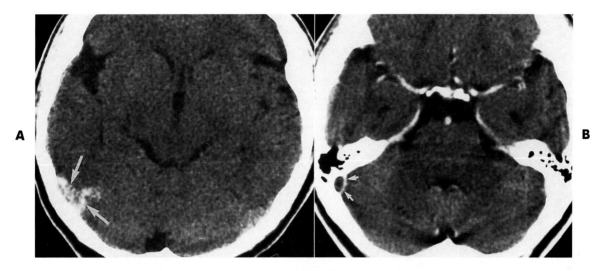

Fig. 11-79. Axial pre- **(A)** and postcontrast **(B)** CT scans in a pregnant woman with severe headaches shows focal parenchymal hemorrhage in the right posterior temporal lobe (**A**, *arrows*.) The enhanced study shows a thrombosed sigmoid sinus (**B**, *arrows*) seen as an "empty delta sign." This appearance is caused by enhancing dura surrounding intraluminal clot.

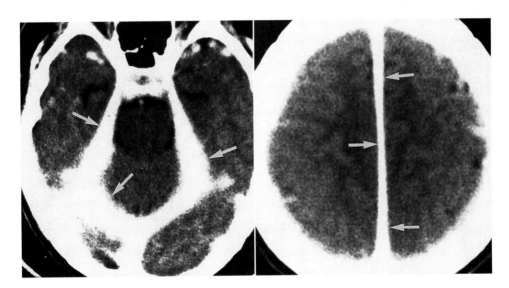

Fig. 11-80. Axial CECT scans in a patient with SSS thrombosis show a thickened falx and a "shaggy" appearing tentorium *(arrows)*.

Dural Sinus Thrombosis
Differential Diagnosis

CT	MR
Normal	*Normal high signal on T1WI with:*
Neonates: low density unmyelinated brain, high hematocrit make sinuses relatively dense on NECT	Inflow of fully magnetized spins (flow-related enhancement or "entry" phenomena)
Others: high-splitting tentorium on CECT	In-plane flow/slow flow
Abnormal	Flow-compensated postcontrast scan
SAH/SDH along tentorium, falx	*Normal high signal on T2WI with:*
	Even-echo rephasing
	Cardiac pseudogating
	Very slow in-plane flow (theoretically could allow spins to receive both 90° and 180° pulses)

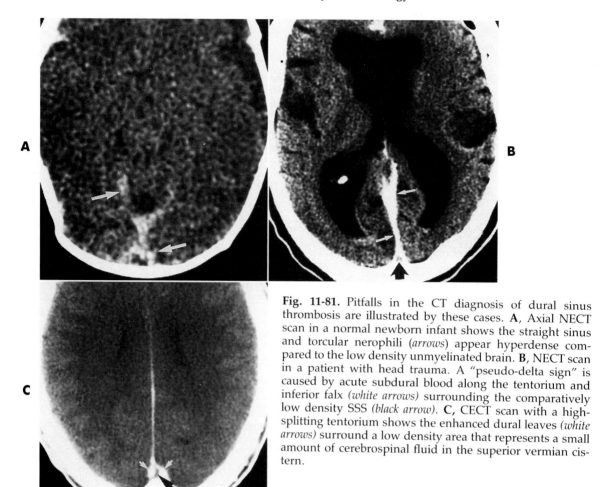

Fig. 11-81. Pitfalls in the CT diagnosis of dural sinus thrombosis are illustrated by these cases. **A,** Axial NECT scan in a normal newborn infant shows the straight sinus and torcular nerophili *(arrows)* appear hyperdense compared to the low density unmyelinated brain. **B,** NECT scan in a patient with head trauma. A "pseudo-delta sign" is caused by acute subdural blood along the tentorium and inferior falx *(white arrows)* surrounding the comparatively low density SSS *(black arrow).* **C,** CECT scan with a high-splitting tentorium shows the enhanced dural leaves *(white arrows)* surround a low density area that represents a small amount of cerebrospinal fluid in the superior vermian cistern.

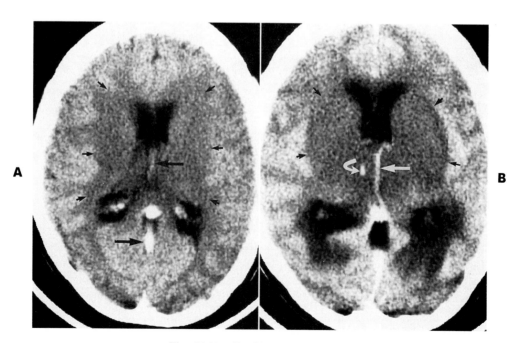

Fig. 11-82 . For legend see p. 391.

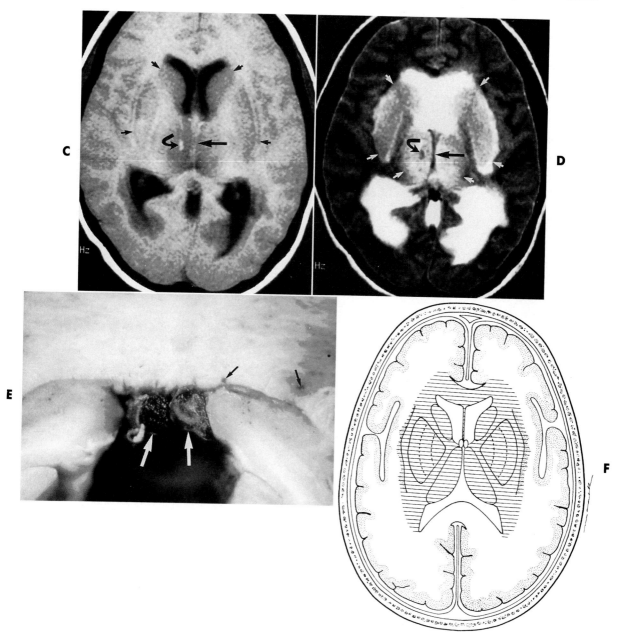

Fig. 11-82 cont'd. A 28-year-old woman had a flu-like episode followed by several days of headache and confusion. Decreasing mental status prompted CT scan. **A,** First NECT scan, initially interpreted as normal, shows high density in the ICVs and SS *(large arrows)*. Bilateral low density changes in the basal ganglia with obscuration of the borders between lenticular nuclei, thalami, and internal capsules are present *(small arrows)*. **B,** Repeat study 24 hours later after the patient became unresponsive shows striking low density basal ganglia *(black arrows)* and ICV thrombosis *(large arrow)*. A petechial hemorrhage *(curved arrow)* is seen in the right thalamus, and severe obstructive hydrocephalus is present. An MR scan was obtained after the patient was transferred. Axial T1- **(C)** and T2-weighted **(D)** studies show late acute thrombus in both ICVs *(large straight arrows)*, the thalamic clot *(curved arrows)*, and venous infarcts of the basal ganglia *(small arrows)*. Mass effect from the edematous thalami has caused severe obstructive hydrocephalus with transependymal CSF flow. Clinical brain death prompted isotope flow study a few hours later *(see* Fig. 8-58*)*. **E,** Close-up coronal view of autopsied brain in another patient who died of deep cerebral vein thrombosis shows clots occluding both internal cerebral veins *(large arrows)*. The basal ganglia and thalami are severely edematous and show multifocal petechial hemorrhages *(small arrows)*. **F,** Anatomic diagram illustrates deep cerebral venous infarction territory. (**E,** Courtesy J. Townsend.)

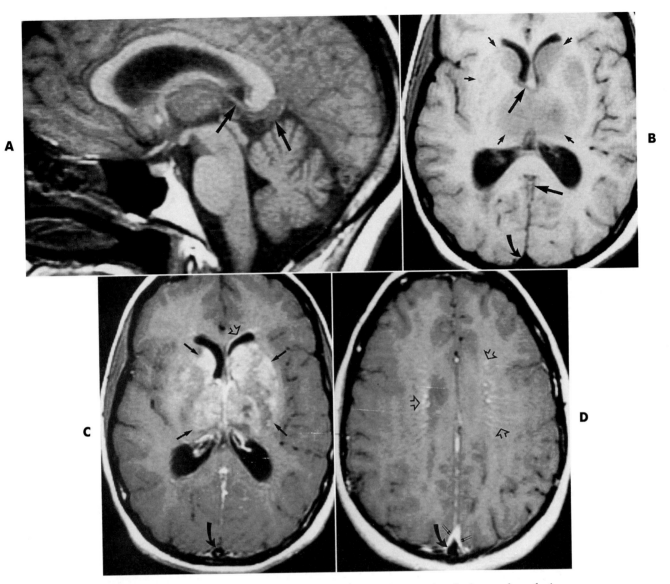

Fig. 11-83. A patient with Crohn's disease developed severe headaches and confusion. Sagittal **(A)** and axial **(B)** precontrast T1-weighted axial MR scans show acute thrombus *(large arrows)* in the ICV, vein of Galen, and SS that is isodense to gray matter. The basal ganglia and thalami appear edematous with ill-defined gray-white matter interfaces *(small arrows)*. The SSS *(curved arrow)* is patent.

dense thrombus in the deep veins, vein of Galen, or straight sinus (Figs. 11-78, *A* and *B;* 11-82, *A* and *B,* and 11-83, *A*). Secondary changes include bilateral low density basal ganglia with or without associated petechial hemorrhages (Figs. 11-82, *A* and *B*).[157] Autopsy in these cases typically discloses severely edematous thalami with multifocal hemorrhagic venous infarcts (Fig. 11-83, *C* and *D*).

Magnetic resonance imaging. MR findings in dural sinus thrombosis and cortical vein occlusion vary with clot age. Acute thrombus is isointense with cortex on T1WI (Fig. 11-83, *A* and *B*), whereas late acute clots are hyperintense on T1-weighted scans and hypointense on T2WI (Fig. 11-82, *C* and *D*). Subacute thrombi are typically hyperintense on all pulse sequences (Fig. 11-84, *B* to *D*). On gradient-refocussed scans the high signal intensity that is usually noted in normal dural sinuses and large veins is replaced by a signal void. Chronically thrombosed sinuses often undergo fibrosis and may develop prominent collateral venous channels within and around the clotted sinus (Fig. 11-85).

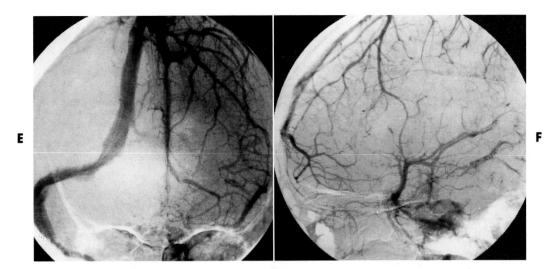

Fig. 11-83, cont'd.   Postcontrast T1WIs (**C** and **D**, see previous page) show striking enhancement of the subependymal and deep medullary veins *(open arrows)*. The venous infarcts of the basal ganglia show patchy enhancement *(single, straight black arrows)*. Note high-velocity signal loss in the patent SSS *(curved arrows)* surrounded by enhancing dural leaves *(double arrows)*, a normal finding. Digital subtraction left ICA angiogram with AP **(E)** and lateral **(F)** venous phase frames shows no contrast in the ICVs, vein of Galen, or straight sinus. The SSS is patent. (Courtesy S. Crawford.)

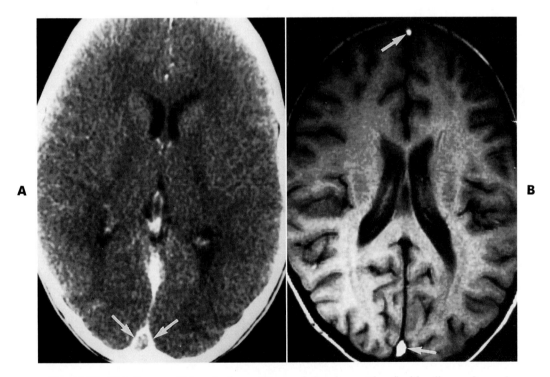

Fig. 11-84.   This 5-year-old boy had vomiting and diarrhea with a flu-like illness. Several days of headache and increasing drowsiness prompted imaging examination. CECT scan **(A)** shows the classic "empty delta" sign *(arrows)* of SSS thrombosis caused by enhancing dura around a dural sinus filled with clot. Axial **(B)** and sagittal **(C)** T1-weighted MR scans show high signal SSS thrombus *(arrows)*.   *Continued.*

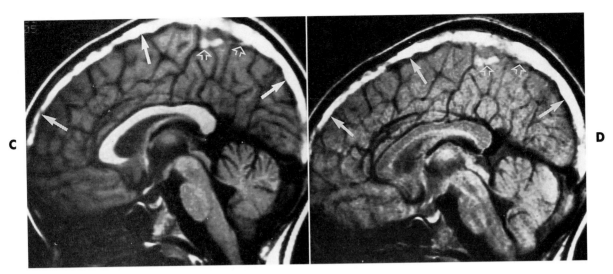

Fig. 11-84, cont'd. Long TR/short TE **(D)** sequence shows the subacute clot remains hyperintense *(large arrows)*. A thrombosed cortical vein is also present, seen as a cordlike area of increased signal intensity **(C** and **D,** *open arrows)*.

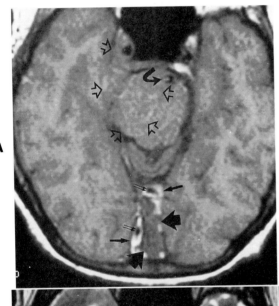

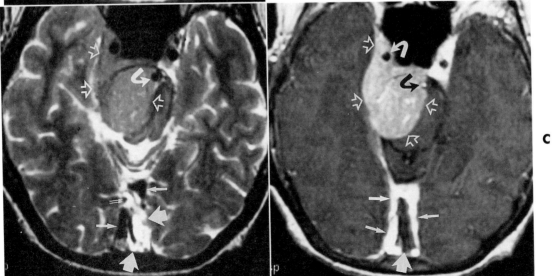

Fig. 11-85. Middle-aged woman with a cavernous sinus and tentorial incisura meningioma *(open arrows)* with chronic dural sinus thrombosis had sudden neurologic deterioration. Axial precontrast T1- **(A)** and T2-weighted **(B)** MR scans show an enlarged straight sinus filled with soft tissue *(large arrows)* that appears isointense to gray matter on T1WI and hyperintense on T2WI. Prominent vascular channels around the SS are partially filled with late acute clot *(small single arrows)* alternating with patent channels, seen as flow voids *(double arrows)*. The internal carotid artery *(curved white arrow)* and the basilar artery *(curved black arrow)* are encased by the tumor *(open arrows)*. Post-contrast T1WI **(C)** shows the enhancing, thickened dura *(small white arrows)* surrounding the fibrosed, nonenhancing SS *(large arrow)*.

MR angiography can replace conventional angiography in the diagnosis of dural sinus occlusion. Because of their sensitivity to slow flow, 2D time-of-flight (2D TOF) and phase contrast (2D PC) sequences are the studies frequently used for screening the cerebral venous circulation. Sagittal 2D PC or coronal 2D TOF MRA is best used to evaluate the SSS.

The MR differential diagnosis of dural sinus thrombosis is primarily imaging artifacts that can mimic intravascular clot. These include contrast-enhanced scans with flow compensation techniques, unenhanced scans with inflow of fully unsaturated spins into the imaged slice (flow-related enhancement or "entry" phenomena), incorrect pulse sequence selection or misplaced pre-saturation bands, and incorporation of hyperintense clot in the maximal intensity projected image on TOF MRA. 2D PC MRA with low velocity encoding obviates most of these difficulties.[158]

REFERENCES

1. Goldstein M: Decade of the brain: National Institute of Neurological Disorders and Stroke, *Neurosurg* 32:297, 1993.
2. Bryan RN: Imaging of acute stroke, *Radiol* 177:615-616, 1990.
3. Okazaki H: *Fundamentals of Neuropathology*, ed 2, pp 27-70, Tokyo: Igaku-Shoin, 1989.
4. Cacayorin ED, Hochhauser L, Hodge CJ et al: Comprehensive experience on intraplaque hemorrhage of the carotid artery, *Neuroradiol* 33[suppl]:75-78, 1991.
5. Yasake M, Yamaguchi T, Shichiri M: Distribution of atherosclerosis and risk factors in atherothrombotic occlusion, *Stroke* 24:206-211, 1993.
6. Vinitski S, Consigny PM, Shapiro MJ et al: Magnetic resonance chemical shift imaging and spectroscopy of atherosclerotic plaque, *Invest Radiol* 26:703-714, 1991.
7. Davies PF: Atherosclerosis. Presented at the second basic sciences course of the American Society of Neuroradiology, Chicago, August 1990.
8. Wolfgang EL, Flaharty PM, Sergott RC: Color Doppler imaging provides accurate assessment of orbital blood flow in occlusive carotid artery disease, *Ophthal* 98:548-552, 1991.
9. Zwiebel WJ: *Introduction to Vascular Sonography*, ed 3, Philadelphia, WB Saunders, 1992.
10. Fürst H, Harti WH, Jansen I et al: Color-flow Doppler sonography in the identification of ulcerative plaques in patients with high-grade carotid artery stenosis, *AJNR* 13:1581-1581, 1992.
10a. Polak JF, O'Leary DH, Kronmal RA et al: Sonographic evaluation of carotid artery atherosclerosis in the elderly: relationship of disease severity to stroke and transient ischemic attack, *Radiol* 188:363-370, 1993.
11. Hunink MGM, Polak JF, Barlan MM, O'Leary DH: Detection and quantification of carotid artery stenosis: efficacy of various Doppler velocity parameters, *AJR* 160:610-625, 1993.
12. Polak JF, Kalena P, Donaldson MC et al: Carotid endarterectomy: preoperative evaluation of candidates with combined Doppler sonography and MR angiography. Work in progress. *Radiol* 186:333-338, 1993.
13. Masaryk TJ, Obuchowski NA: Noninvasive carotid imaging: caveat emptor, *Radiol* 186:325-331, 1993.
14. Polak JF, Bajakian RL, O'Leary DH et al: Detection of internal carotid artery stenosis: comparison of MR angiography, color Doppler sonography, and arteriography, *Radiol* 182:35-40, 1992.
15. Wolpert SM, Caplan LR: Current role of cerebral angiography in the diagnosis of cerebrovascular disease, *AJR* 159:191-197, 1992.
16. North American Symptomatic Carotid Endarterectomy Trial Collaborators: Beneficial effect of carotid endarterectomy in symptomatic patients with high-grade stenosis, *N Engl J Med* 325:445-453, 1991.
17. Beckmann CF, Levin DC, Kubicka RA, Henschke CI: The effect of sequential arterial stenoses on flow and pressure, *Radiol* 140:655-658, 1981.
18. Bradac GB: Angiography in cerebral ischemia, *Riv di Neuroradiol* 3[suppl 2]:57-66, 1990.
19. Goldberg HI: Angiography of extra- and intracranial occlusive cerebrovascular disease, *Neuroimaging Clin N Amer* 2:487-507, 1992.
20. Edwards JH, Kricheff II, Riles T, Imparato A: Angiographically undetected ulceration of the carotid bifurcation as a cause of embolic stroke, *Radiol* 132:369-373, 1979.
21. Schwartz RB, Jones KM, LeClerq GT et al: The value of cerebral angiography in predicting cerebral ischemia during carotid endarterectomy, *AJR* 159:1057-1061, 1992.
22. Turjman F, Tournut P, Baldy-Porcher C et al: Demonstration of subclavian steal by MR angiography, *J Comp Asst Tomogr* 16:756-759, 1992.
23. Yip PK, Liuh M, Hwang BS, Chen RC: Subclavian steal phenomenon: a correlation between sonographic and angiographic findings, *Neuroradiol* 34:279-282, 1992.
23a. Trattnig S, Karnel F, Kautzky A et al: Color doppler imaging of partial subclavian steal syndrome, *Neuroradiol* 35:293-295, 1993.
24. Marks MP, Napel S, Jordan JE, Enzmann DR: Diagnosis of carotid artery disease: preliminary experience with maximum-intensity-projection spiral CT angiography, *AJR* 160:1267-1271, 1993.
25. Lane JI, Flanders AE, Doan HT, Bell RD: Assessment of carotid artery patency in routine spin-echo MR imaging of the brain, *AJNR* 12:819-826, 1991.
26. Heiserman JE, Drayer BP, Keller PJ, Fram EK: Intracranial vascular occlusions: evaluation with three dimensional time-of-flight MR angiography, *Radiol* 185:667-673, 1992.
27. Litt AW, Eidelman EM, Pinto RS et al: Diagnosis of carotid artery stenosis: comparison of 2DFT time-of-flight MR angiography with contrast angiography in 50 patients, *AJNR* 12:149-154, 1991.
28. Blatter DD, Parker DL, Ahn SS et al: Cerebral MR angiography with multiple overlapping thin slab acquisition. Part II. Early clinical experience, *Radiol* 183:379-389, 1992.
28a. Laster RE Jr, Acker JD, Halford HH III, Navert TC: Assessment of MR angiography versus arteriography for evaluation of cervical carotid bifurcation disease, *AJR* 14:681-688, 1993.
28b. Anson JA, Heiserman JE, Drayer BP, Spetzler RF: Surgical decisions on the basis of magnetic resonance angiography of the carotid arteries, *Neurosurg* 32:335-343, 1993.
29. Davis WL, Warnock SH, Harnsberger HR et al: Intracranial MRA: single volume vs. multiple thin slab 3D time-of-flight acquisition, *J Comp Asst Tomogr* 17:15-21, 1993.
29a. Evans AJ, Richardson DB, Tien R et al: Poststenotic signal loss in MR angiography: effects of echo time, flow compensation, and fractional echo, *AJNR* 14:721-729, 1993.
30. Huston J III, Ehrman RL: Comparison of time-of-flight and phase-contrast MR neuroangiographic technique, *RadioGraphics* 13:9-19, 1993.
31. terPenning B: Pathophysiology of stroke, *Neuroimaging Clin N Amer* 2:389-408, 1992.
32. Price TR: Progressing ischemic stroke. In Barnet R et al, editor: *Stroke*, vol 2, pp 1059-1068, New York: Churchill Livingstone, 1986.

33. Siesjö BK: Pathophysiology and treatment of focal cerebral ischemia, *J Neurosurg* 77:169-184, 1992.

34. Marshall RS, Mohr JP: Current management of ischaemic stroke, *J Neurol Neurosurg Psychiatr* 56:6-46, 1993.

35. Plum F, Pulsinelli W: Cerebral metabolism and hypoxic-ischemic brain injury. In Asbury A et al, editor: *Diseases of the Nervous System*, pp 1086-1100, Philadelphia, WB Saunders, 1986.

36. Moody DM, Bell MA, Challa VR: Features of the cerebral vascular patterns that predict vulnerability to perfusion or oxygenation deficiency: an anatomic study, *AJNR* 11:431-439, 1990.

37. Truwit CL, Barkovich AJ, Koch TK, Ferriero DM: Cerebral palsy: MR findings in 40 patients, *AJNR* 13:67-78, 1992.

38. Volpe JJ: Value of MR in definition of the neuropathology of cerebral palsy in vivo, *AJNR* 13:79-83, 1992.

39. Hankey GJ, Warlow CP: The role of imaging in the management of cerebral and ocular ischaemia, *Neuroradiol* 33:381-390, 1991.

40. Horowitz SH, Zito JL, Donnarumma R et al: Computed tomographic-angiographic findings within the first five hours of cerebral infarction, *Stroke* 22:1245-1253, 1991.

41. Osborn AG: *Handbook of Neuroradiology*, pp 92-101, St. Louis: Mosby Yearbook, 1991.

42. Shuaib A, Lee D, Pelz D et al: The impact of magnetic resonance imaging on the management of acute ischemic stroke, *Neurol* 42:816-818, 1992.

43. Bryan RN, Levy LM, Whitlow WD et al: Diagnosis of acute cerebral infarction: comparison of CT and MR imaging, *AJNR* 12:611-620, 1991.

44. Bastianello S, Pierallini A, Colonnese C et al: Hyperdense middle cerebral artery CT sign, *Neuroradiol* 33:207-211, 1991.

45. Tomura N, Uemura K, Inugami A et al: Early CT finding in cerebral infarction: obscuration of the lentiform nucleus, *Radiol* 168:463-467, 1988.

46. Truwit CL, Barkovich AJ, Gean A et al: Loss of the insular ribbon: another CT sign of acute middle cerebral artery infarction, *Radiol* 176:801-806, 1990.

47. Leys D, Pruvo JP, Godefroy O et al: Prevalence and significance of hyperdense middle cerebral artery in acute stroke, *Stroke* 23:317-324, 1992.

48. Tomsick T, Brott T, Barsan W et al: Thrombus localization with emergency cerebral CT, *AJNR* 13:257-263, 1992.

48a. Rauch RA, Bazan C III, Larsson E-M, Jinkins JR: Hyperdense middle cerebral arteries as identified on CT as a false sign of vascular occlusion, *AJNR* 14:669-674, 1993.

49. Bozzao L, Angeloni U, Bastianello S et al: Early angiographic and CT findings in patients with hemorrhagic infarction in the distribution of the middle cerebral artery, *AJNR* 12:1115-1121, 1991.

50. Pessin MS, Teal PA, Caplan LR: Hemorrhagic infarction: guilt by association? *AJNR* 12:1123-1126, 1991.

50a. Mueller DP, Yuh WTC, Fisher DJ et al: Arterial enhancement in acute cerebral ischemia: clinical and angiographic correlation, *AJNR* 14:661-668, 1993.

51. Elster AD, Moody DM: Early cerebral infarction: gadopentetate dimeglumine enhancement, *Radiol* 177:627-632, 1990.

52. Yuh WTC, Crain MR, Loes DJ et al: MR imaging of cerebral ischemia: findings in the first 24 hours, *AJNR* 12:621-629, 1991.

53. Alberts MJ, Faulstich ME, Gray L: Stroke with negative brain magnetic resonance imaging, *Stroke* 23:663-667, 1992.

54. Warach S, Li W, Ronthal M, Edelman RR: Acute cerebral ischemia: evaluation with dynamic contrast-enhanced MR imaging and MR angiography, *Radiol* 182:41-47, 1992.

55. Kushner MJ, Zanette EM, Biastianello S et al: Transcranial Doppler in acute hemispheric brain infarction, *Neurol* 41:109-113, 1991.

56. Felber SR, Aichner FT, Sauter R, Gerstenbrand F: Combined magnetic resonance imaging and proton magnetic resonance spectroscopy of patients with acute stroke, *Stroke* 23:1106-1110, 1992.

57. Petroff OAC, Graham GD, Blamire AM et al: Spectroscopic imaging of stroke in humans: histopathology correlates of spectral changes, *Neuro* 42:1349-1354, 1992.

58. Gideon P, Henriksen O, Sperling B et al: Early time course of N-acetylaspartate, creatine and phosphocreatine, and compounds containing choline in the brain after acute stroke, *Stroke* 23:1566-1572, 1992.

59. LeBihan D, Turner R, Douek P, Patronas N: Diffusion MR imaging: clinical applications, *AJR* 159:591-599, 1992.

60. Chien D, Kwong KK, Gress DR et al: MR diffusion imaging of cerebral infarction in humans, *AJNR* 13:1097-1102, 1992.

61. Warach S, Chien D, Li W et al: Fast magnetic resonance diffusion-weighted imaging of acute human stroke, *Neurol* 42:1717-1723, 1992.

62. Sevick RJ, Kanda F, Mintorovich J et al: Cytotoxic brain edema: assessment with diffusion-weighted MR imaging, *Radiol* 185:687-690, 1992.

63. Wolpert SM, Bruckmann H, Greenlee R et al: Neuroradiologic evaluation of patients with acute stroke treated with recombinant tissue plasminogen activator, *AJNR* 14:3-13, 1993.

64. Turner R, LeBihan D, Moonen CTW et al: Echo-planar time course MRI of cat brain oxygenation changes, *Magnetic Resonance in Medicine* 22:159-166, 1991.

65. Conturo TE, Barker PB, Mathews VP et al: MR imaging of cerebral perfusion by phase-angle reconstruction of bolus paramagnetic-induced frequency shifts, *Magnetic Resonance in Medicine* 27:375-390, 1992.

65a. Kucharczyk J, Asgari H, Mintorovich J et al: Cerebrovascular transit characteristics of DyDTPA-BMA and Gd DTPA-BMA in normal and ischemic cat brain, *AJNR* 14:289-296, 1993.

66. Truwit CL, Kucharczyk J: Reversible cerebral ischemia, *Neuroimaging Clin N Amer* 2:577-595, 1992.

67. Runge VM, Kirsch JE, Wells JW, Woolfolk CE: Assessment of cerebral perfusion by first-pass dynamic, contrast-enhanced, steady-state-free-precession MR imaging: an animal study, *AJR* 160:593-600, 1993.

67a. Hornig CR, Bauer T, Simon C et al: Hemorrhagic transformation in cardioembolic cerebral infarction, *Stroke* 24:465-468, 1993.

68. Elster AD: Enhancement patterns in cerebral infarction, *MRI Decisions*, pp 30-33, Sept/Oct 1992.

69. Asato R, Okumura R, Konishi J: "Fogging effect" in MR of cerebral infarct, *J Comp Asst Tomogr* 15:160-162, 1991.

70. Kuhn MJ, Mikulis DJ, Ayoub DM et al: Wallerian degeneration after cerebral infarction: evaluation with sequential MR imaging, *Radiol* 172:170-182, 1989.

71. Parisi J, Place C, Nag S: Calcification in a recent cerebral infarct: radiologic and pathologic correlation, *Can J Neurol Sci* 15:192-195, 1988.

72. Lundblom N, Katevuo K, Kumo M et al: T1 in subacute and chronic brain infarctions: time-dependent development, *Invest Radiol* 27:673-680, 1992.

73. Boyko OB, Burger PC, Shelburne JD, Ingram P: Non-heme mechanisms for T1 shortening: pathologic, CT, and MR elucidation, *AJNR* 13:1439-1445, 1992.

74. Regli L, Regli F, Maeder P, Bogousslavski J: Magnetic resonance imaging with gadolinium contrast in small deep (lacunar) cerebral infarcts, *Arch Neurol* 50:175-180, 1993.

75. Heier L: White matter disease in the elderly: vascular etiologies, *Neuroimaging Clin N Amer* 2:441-461, 1992.

76. Close PJ, Carty HM: Transient gyriform brightness on non-contrast enhanced computed tomography (CT) brain scan of seven infants, *Pediatr Radiol* 21:189-192, 1991.

77. Barkovich AJ: MR and CT evaluation of profound neonatal and infantile asphyxia, *AJNR* 13:79-83, 1992.

78. van der Zwan A, Hillen B, Tulleken CAF et al: Variability of the major cerebral arteries, *J Neurosurg* 77:927-940, 1992.

78a. Kazui S, Sawada T, Naritomi H et al: Angiographic evaluation of brain infarction limited to the anterior cerebral artery territory, *Stroke* 24:549-553, 1993.

79. Naidich TP: Brain vascular distribution: classical patterns of stroke: categorical course on cerebrovascular disease, pp. 63-77, American Society of Neuroradiology, 1989.

79a. Latronico N, Tansini A, Gualandi GF et al: Ischaemic pontomedullary transection with incomplete locked-in syndrome, *Neuroradiol* 35:332-334, 1993.

80. Cormier PJ, Long ER, Russell EJ: MR imaging of posterior fossa infarctions: vascular territories and clinical correlates, *RadioGraphics* 12:1079-1096, 1992.

81. Milandre L, Rumeau C, Sangla I et al: Infarction in the territory of the anterior inferior cerebellar artery: report of five cases, *Neuroradiol* 34:500-503, 1992.

82. Amarenco P, Rosengart A, DeWitt et al: Anterior inferior cerebellar artery territory infarcts: mechanisms and clinical features, *Arch Neurol* 50:154-161, 1993.

82a. Amarenco P, Kase CS, Rosengart A et al: Very small (border zone) cerebellar infarcts, *Brain* 116:161-186, 1993.

82b. Sacco RL, Freddo L, Bello JA: Wallenberg's lateral medullary syndrome, *Arch Neurol* 50:609-614, 1993.

83. Lisovoski F, Rosseaux P: Cerebral infarction in young people: a study of 148 patients with early cerebral angiography, *J Neurol Neurosurg Psuchiatr* 34:576-579, 1991.

84. Cali RL, Berg R, Rama K: Bilateral internal carotid artery agenesis: a case study and review of the literature, *Surgery* 113:227-233, 1993.

85. Gomori JM, Weinberger G, Schachar E, Freilich G: Multiple intracranial aneurysms and neurofibromatosis: a case report, *Australas Radiol* 35:271-273, 1991.

86. Sobota E, Ohkuma H, Suzuki S. Cerebrovascular disorders associated with von Recklinghausen's neurofibromatosis: a case report, *Neurosurg* 22:544-549, 1988.

87. Frank E, Brown BM, Wilson DF: Asymptomatic fusiform aneurysm of the petrous carotid artery in a patient with von Recklinghausen neurofibromatosis, *Surg Neurol* 32:75-78, 1989.

88. Schievink WI, Piepgras DG: Cervical vertebral artery aneurysms and arteriovenous fistulae in neurofibromatosis type 1: case reports, *Neurosurg* 29:760-765, 1991.

89. Battistella PA, Monciotti C, Carra S et al: Neurofibromatosis di von Recklinghausen e vasculopatia arteriosa cerebrale, *Riv di Neuroradiol* 5(suppl 1):147-150, 1992.

90. Ng S-H, Ng K-K, Pai S-C, Tsai C-C: Tuberous sclerosis with aortic aneurysm and rib changes: CT demonstration, *J Comput Asst Tomogr* 12:666-668, 1988.

91. Towbin RB, Ball WS, Kaufman RA: Pediatric case of the day, *RadioGraphics* 7:818-821, 1987.

92. Taira T, Tamura Y, Kawamura H: Intracranial aneurysms in a child with Klippel-Trenaunay-Weber syndrome: case report, *Surg Neurol* 36:303-306, 1991.

93. Dobyns WB, Garg BP: Vascular abnormalities in epidural nevus syndrome, *Neurol* 41:276-278, 1991.

94. Yamada I, Matsushima Y, Suzuki S: Childhood moyamoya disease before and after encephalo-duro-arterio-syanangiosis: an angiographic study, *Neuroradiol* 34:318-322, 1992.

95. Matsushima Y, Aoyagi M, Suzuki R et al: Perioperative complications of encephalo-duro-arterio-synangiosis: prevention and treatment, *Surg Neurol* 36:343-353, 1991.

95a. Takanashi J, Sugita K, Ishii M et al: Moyamoya syndrome in young children: MR comparison with adult onset, *AJNR* 14:1139-1143, 1993.

96. Karasawa J, Touho H, Onishi H et al: Long-term follow-up study after extracranial-intracranial bypass surgery for anterior circulation ischemia in childhood moyamoya disease, *J Neurosurg* 77:84-89, 1992.

96a. Kinugasa K, Mandai S, Kamata I et al: Surgical treatment of moyamoya disease: operative technique for encephalo-duro-arterio-myo-synangiosis, its follow-up, clinical results, and angiograms, *Neurosurg* 32:527-531, 1993.

97. Jayakumar PN, Arya BYT, Vasudev MK et al: Moyamoya disease: computed tomographic and angiographic correlation in 10 caucasoid patients, *Acta Neurol Scan* 84:339-343, 1991.

98. Satoh S, Shibuya H, Matsushima Y, Suzuki S: Analysis of the angiographic findings in cases of childhood moyamoya disease, *Neuroradiol* 30:111-119, 1988.

99. Demaerel P, Casaer P, Casteels-Van Daele M et al: Moyamoya disease: MRI and MR angiography, *Neuroradiol* 33(suppl): 50-52, 1991.

100. Yamada I, Matsushima Y, Suzuki S: Moyamoya disease: diagnosis with three-dimensional time-of-flight MR angiography, *Radiol* 184:773-778, 1992.

101. Debrun G, Sauvegrain J, Aicardi J, Goutieres F: Moyamoya, a nonspecific radiological syndrome, *Neuroradiol* 8:241-244, 1975.

102. Jacobs DS, Smith AS, Finelli DA et al: Menkes kinky hair disease: characteristic MR angiographic findings, *AJNR* 14: 1160-1163, 1993.

103. Wang Z, Bogdan AR, Zimmerman RA et al: Investigation of stroke in sickle cell disease by ^{1}H nuclear magnetic resonance spectroscopy, *Neuroradiol* 35:57-65, 1992.

104. Oyesiku N, Barrow DL, Eckman JR et al: Intracranial aneurysms in sickle-cell anemia: clinical features and pathogenesis, *J Neurosurg* 75:356-363, 1991.

105. Zimmerman R, Sherry RG, Elwood JC et al: Vascular thrombosis and homocytinuria, *AJR* 148:953-957, 1987.

106. Fauci AS: NIH Conference. The spectrum of vasculitis: clinical, pathologic, immunologic, and therapeutic considerations, *Ann Intern Med* 89(part 1):660-676, 1978.

107. Chopra PS, Kandarpa K: Arteritides: an angiographic perspective, *Appl Radiol* 20:13-21, 1991.

108. Ledford DK: Immunologic aspects of cardiovascular disease, *JAMA* 258:2974-2982, 1987.

109. Kerr L, Filloux FM: Cerebral infarction as a remote complication of childhood *Haemophilus influenzae* meningitis, *West J Med* 157:179-182, 1992.

110. Greenan TJ, Grossman RI, Goldbert HI: Cerebral vasculitis: MR imaging and angiographic correlation, *Radiol* 182:65-72, 1992.

111. Ferris EJ, Levine HL: Cerebral arteritis: classification, *Radiol* 109:327-341, 1973.

112. Solé-Lienas J, Pons-Tortella E: Cerebral angiitis, *Neuroradiol* 15:1-11, 1978.

113. Sigal LH: The neurologic presentation of vasculitic and rheumatologic syndromes, *Medicine* 66:157-180, 1987.

114. Bell CL, Partington C, Robbins M et al: Magnetic resonance imaging of central nervous system lesions in patients with lupus erythematosus, *Arthritis and Rheumatism* 34:437-441, 1991.

115. Eustace S, Hutchinson M, Breshnihan B: Acute cerebrovascular episodes in systemic lupus erythematosus, *Quart J Med* 293:739-750, 1991.

116. Yamamoto K, Nogaki H, Takase Y, Morimatsu M: Systemic lupus erythematosus associated with marked intracranial calcification, *AJNR* 13:1340-1342, 1992.

117. Pulpeiro JR, Cortes JA, Macarron J et al: MR findings in primary antiphospholipid syndrome, *AJNR* 12:452-453, 1991.

118. Castillo M: Angiographic findings in a patient with primary antiphospholipid syndrome: case report, *Cardiovasc Intervent Radiol* 15:244-246, 1992.

119. Hargraves RW, Spetzler RF: Takayasu's arteritis: case report, *BNI Quarterly* 7:20-23, 1991.

120. Koo EH, Massey EW: Granulomatous angiitis of the central nervous system: protean manifestations and response to treatment, *J Neurol Neurosurg Psychiatr* 51:1126-1133, 1988.

121. Crane R, Kerr LD, Spiera H: Clinical analysis of isolated angiitis of the central nervous system, *Arch Int Med* 151:2290-2294, 1991.

122. Stübgen P, Lotz BP: Isolated angitis of the central nervous system: involvement of penetrating vessels at the base of the brain, *J Neurol* 238:235-238, 1991.

123. Yamashita Y, Takahashi M, Brussaka H et al: Cerebral vasculitis secondary to Wegener's granulomatosis: computed tomography and angiographic findings, CT. *J Comp Tomogr* 10:119-120, 1986.

124. Erdem E, Carlier R, Idir ABC et al: Gadolinium-enhanced MRI in central nervous system Behcet's disease, *Neuroradiol* 35:142-144, 1993.

125. Kazui S, Naritomi H, Imakita S et al: Sequential gadolinium-DTPA enhanced MRI studies in neuro-Behcet's disease, *Neuroradiol* 33:136-139, 1991.

126. Serdaroglu P, Yazici H, Ozdemir C et al: Neurologic involvement in Behcet's syndrome: a prospective study, *Arch Neurol* 46:265-269, 1989.

127. Nishimura M, Satoh K-I, Suga M, Oda M: Cerebral angio-and neuro-Behcet's syndrome: neuroradiological and pathological study of one case, *J Neurol Sci* 106:19-24, 1991.

128. Tacal T, Cekirge S, Balkanci F, Besim A: Saccular extracranial carotid artery aneurysm secondary to Behcet's disease, *Clin Imaging* 17:70-72, 1993.

129. Lazar EB, Russel EJ, Cohen BA et al: Contrast-enhanced MR of cerebral arteritis: intravascular enhancement related to flow stasis within areas of focal arterial ectasia, *AJNR* 13:271-276, 1992.

130. Barinagarrementeria F, Cantú C, Balderrama J: Postpartum cerebral angiopathy with cerebral infarction due to ergonnine use, *Stroke* 23:1364-1366, 1992.

131. Levine SR, Fagan SC, Pessin MS et al: Accelerated intracranial occlusive disease, oral contraceptives, and cigarette use, *Neurol* 41:1893-1901, 1991.

132. Wang A-M, Suojanen JN, Colucci VM et al: Cocaine- and methamphetamine-induced acute cerebral vasospasm: an angiographic study in rabbits, *AJNR* 11:1141-1146, 1990.

133. Dominguez R, Vila-Coro AA, Slopis JM, Bohan TP: Brain and ocular abnormalities in infants with in utero exposure to cocaine and other street drugs, *AJDC* 145:688-695, 1991.

134. Brown E, Prager J, Lee H-Y, Ramsey RG: CNS complications of cocaine abuse: prevalence, pathophysiology, and neuroradiology, *AJR* 159:137-147, 1992.

135. Montanera W, Marotta TR, terBrugge KG et al: Cerebral arteriovenous malformations associated with moyamoya phenomenon, *AJNR* 11:1153-1156, 1990.

136. Pile-Spellman JMD, Baker KF, Liszczak TM et al: High-flow angiopathy: cerebral blood vessel changes in experimental chronic arteriovenous fistula, *AJNR* 7:811-815, 1986.

137. Omojola MF, Fox AJ, Viñuela F, Debrun G: Stenosis of afferent vessels of intracranial arteriovenous malformations, *AJNR* 6:791-793, 1985.

138. George B, Laurian C: Impairment of vertebral artery flow caused by extrinsic lesions, *Neurosurg* 24:206-214, 1989.

139. Launay M, Fredy D, Merland J-J, Bories J: Narrowing and occlusion of arteries by intracranial tumors, *Neuroradiol* 14:117-126, 1977.

140. Castillo M, Kramer L: Raeder syndrome: MR appearance, *AJNR* 13:1121-1123, 1992.

141. Epstein MA, Packer RJ, Rorke LB et al: Vascular malformations with radiation induced angiopathy after treatment of chiasmatic/hypothalamic gloma, *Cancer* 70:887-893, 1992.

142. Brant-Zawadzki M, Anderson M, DeArmond SJ et al: Radiation-induced large intracranial vessel occlusive vasculopathy, *AJR* 134:51-55, 1980.

143. Hayashida K, Nishimura T, Imakita S et al: Embolic stroke following carotid radiation angiography demonstrated with I-213 IMP brain SPECT, *Clin Nuc Med* 16:580-582, 1991.

143a. Kestle JRW, Koffman HJ, Mock AR: Moyamoya phenomenon after radiation for optic glioma, *J Neurosurg* 79:32-35, 1993.

143b. Bowen J, Paulsen CA: Stroke after pituitary irradiation, *Stroke* 23:908-911, 1992.

144. Trott KR: Radiation-chemotherapy interactions, *Int J Radiat Oncol Biol Phys* 12:1409-1413, 1986.

144a. Assaf M, Sweeny PJ, Kosmorsky G, Masaryk T: Horner's syndrome secondary to angiogram negative subadventitial carotid artery dissection, *Can J Neurol Sci* 20:62-64, 1993.

145. Horowitz SW, Merchut M, Fine M, Azar-Kia B: Complex partial seizure-induced transient MR enhancement, *J Comput Assist Tomogr* 16:814-816, 1992.

146. Lee BI, Lee BC, Hwang YM et al: Prolonged ictal amnesia with transient focal abnormalities on magnetic resonance imaging, *Epilepsia* 33:1042-1046, 1992.

147. Castillo M, Whaley RA: Gyriform enhancement in tuberous sclerosis simulating infarction, *Radiol* 185:613, 1992.

148. Zimmerman RD, Ernst RJ: Neuroimaging of cerebrovenous thrombosis, *Neuroimaging Clin N Amer* 2:463-485, 1992.

149. Fries G, Wallenberg T, Henner J et al: Occlusion of the pre-superior sagittal sinus, bridging and cortical veins: multistep evolution of sinus-vein thrombosis, *J Neurosurg* 77:127-133, 1992.

150. Medlock MD, Olivero WC, Hanigan WC et al: Children with cerebral venous thrombosis diagnosed with magnetic resonance imaging and magnetic resonance angiography, *Neurosurg* 31:870-876, 1992.

150a. Taha JM, Crone KR, Berger TS et al: Sigmoid sinus thrombosis after closed head injury in children. *Neurosurg* 32:544-546, 1993.

150b. Mantello MT, Schwartz RB, Jones KM et al: Imaging of neurological complications associated with pregnancy, *AJR* 160:843-847, 1993.

150c. Mokri B, Jack CR Jr, Petty GW: Pseudotumor syndrome associated with cerebral venous sinus occlusion and antiphospholipid antibodies, *Stroke* 24:469-472, 1993.

150d. Bacharach JM, Stanson AW, Lie JT, Nichols DA: Imaging spectrum of thrombo-occlusive vascular disease associated with antiphospholipid antibodies, *RadioGraphics* 13:417-423, 1993.

151. Musio F, Older SA, Jenkins T, Gregorie EM: Case Report: cerebral venous thrombosis as manifestation of acute ulcerative colitis, *Am J Med Sci* 305:28-35, 1993.

152. Wechsler B, Vidailhet M, Piette JC et al: Cerebral venous thrombosis in Behcet's disease, *Neurol* 42:614-618, 1992.

153. Diaz JM, Schiffman JS, Urban ES, Maccario M: Superior sagittal sinus thrombosis and pulmonary embolism: a syndrome rediscovered, *Acta Neurol Scand* 86:390-396, 1992.

154. Kristensen B, Malm J, Markgren P, Ekstedt J: CSF hydrodynamics in superior sagittal sinus thrombosis.

154b. Ur-Rahman N, Al-Tahan AR: Computed tomographic evidence of an extensive thrombosis and infarction of the deep venous system, *Stroke* 24:744-746, 1993.

155. Virapongse C, Cazenave C, Quisling R et al: The empty delta sign: frequency and significance in 76 cases of dural sinus thrombosis, *Radiol* 162:779-785, 1987.

156. Khandelwal N, Malik N: Head injury: pseudodelta sign on CT, *Australas Radiol* 36:303-304, 1992.

157. Sandhu AS, Johns D, Albertyn LE: Deep cerebral vein thrombosis, *Neuroradiol* 33(suppl):241-243, 1991.

158. Tsuruda JS, Shimakawa A, Pelc JN, Saloner D: Dural sinus occlusion: evaluation with phase-sensitive gradient-echo MR imaging, *AJNR* 12:481-488, 1991.

PART THREE

Brain Tumors and Tumorlike Processes

Brain Tumors and Tumorlike Masses: Classification and Differential Diagnosis

with
Wolfgang Rauschning

The crude incidence rate of brain tumors in the United States is estimated at 4.5 persons per 100,000 population. Brain neoplasms are found in approximately 2% of autopsy series and account for 1% of all hospital admissions.[1] Therefore understanding the classification, pathology, imaging appearance, and differential diagnosis of brain tumors by anatomic location is an essential component of modern neuroimaging.

Brain tumefactions comprise a remarkably diverse group of neoplastic and nonneoplastic conditions that occur at any age and in virtually every location.[2] Brain tumors can be any of the following:

1. Primary neoplasms derived from normal cellular constituents
2. Primary neoplasms that arise from embryologically misplaced tissues
3. Secondary neoplasms from extracranial primary sites that metastasize to the CNS
4. Nonneoplastic conditions that can mimic tumors.

Any classification system that addresses this multitude of entities is prone to complexity, redundancy, and controversy.[2] As the eminent neuropathologist Lucy B. Rorke has wryly noted, "Pathologists are neither genealogists nor prophets!"

Although the value of classifying CNS neoplasms and tumorlike lesions is obvious, the conceptual basis for such a scheme remains controversial and a source of continual differences among neuropathologists.[3] Despite numerous attempts, no universally acceptable general classification system has been devised, and some specific tumors remain unclassifiable (or at least create considerable disagreement among recognized authorities).[1]

Using clinical and imaging data rather than biopsy

or autopsy specimens to establish an appropriate differential diagnosis is the domain of radiologists. We will address the complex issue of brain tumor classification by using an approach that combines pathologic and imaging appearances.

First, we consider brain tumors as they are traditionally classified, i.e., by their histologic characteristics. We then categorize these lesions by age and general location on imaging studies. The normal and pathologic anatomy, classification, and differential diagnosis of tumors and nonneoplastic tumorlike processes in seven specific intracranial locations is then considered. These seven areas are selected for particular attention because their anatomic complexity and broad pathologic spectrum present special diagnostic challenges.

CLASSIFICATION BY HISTOLOGY

Despite numerous efforts, no universally acceptable pathologic classification of brain tumors has been proposed. Traditionally, the putative histogenetic, or "cell of origin," approach proposed by Bailey and Cushing has been the most widely used, although its many shortcomings have long been recognized.[3] The classification system subsequently developed by Russell and Rubinstein has been expanded and is in widespread use.[4] More recently, modifications and revisions of the original World Health Organization (WHO) classification have been proposed by several authors.[1-6a]

We will use a modification of the 1993 WHO and Russell and Rubinstein classifications (see box) and begin by dividing brain tumors into primary and metastatic lesions.

Primary Brain Tumors

The term *primary brain tumor* encompasses neoplasms and related mass lesions that arise from the brain and its linings. Nonneoplastic intracranial cysts and tumorlike lesions are also included, with pituitary tumors and local extensions from regional tumors (e.g., craniopharyngioma and chordoma) that arise from adjacent structures such as the skull base.[6]

Primary neoplasms account for approximately two thirds of all brain tumors (Fig. 12-1, *A*). Primary brain tumors are subdivided into two basic groups: (1) tumors of neuroglial origin (so-called gliomas) and (2) nonglial tumors that are specified by a combination of putative cell origin and specific location.[1] Some pathologists include all so-called neuroectodermal tumors (neoplasms that theoretically arise from the embryonic medullary epithelium) in a single large category that includes both gliomas and nonglial neoplasms such as primitive neuroectodermal tumors.[6] Because the latter approach is somewhat unwieldy,

---

Brain Tumors
Histologic classification

Primary brain tumors

Glial tumors (gliomas)
Astrocytomas
   Fibrillary astrocytomas
      Benign astrocytoma
      Anaplastic astrocytoma
      Glioblastoma multiforme
   Pilocytic astrocytoma
   Pleomorphic xanthoastrocytoma
   Subependymal giant cell astrocytoma
Oligodendroglioma
Ependymal tumors
   Ependymoma (cellular, papillary)
   Anaplastic (malignant) ependymoma
   Myxopapillary ependymoma
   Subependymoma
Choroid plexus tumors
   Choroid plexus papilloma
   Choroid plexus carcinoma
   Choroid plexus xanthogranulomas

Nonglial tumors
Neuronal and mixed neuronal-glial tumors
   Ganglioglioma
   Gangliocytoma
   Lhermitte-Duclos disease
   Dysembryoplastic neuroepithelial tumors (DNETs)
   Central neurocytoma
   Olfactory neuroblastoma (esthesioneuroblastoma)
Meningeal and mesenchymal tumors
   Meningioma
   Osteocartilagenous tumors
   Fibrous histiocytoma
   Malignant mesenchymal tumors (e.g., rhabdomyosarcoma)
   Hemangiopericytoma
   Hemangioblastoma
Pineal region tumors
   Germ cell tumors
      Germinoma
      Embryonal carcinoma
      Yolk sac (endodermal sinus) tumors
      Choriocarcinoma
      Teratoma
      Mixed tumors

---

we will use the system that divides primary brain tumors into glial and nonglial neoplasms.

Neuroglial tumors (gliomas). These tumors are the largest group of primary CNS neoplasms (Fig. 12-1, *B*). Gliomas are named for their supposed cell of origin (*see* box). The three most common gliomas are astrocytoma, oligodendroglioma, and ependy-

---

Brain Tumors, cont'd
Histologic classification

Pineal region tumors, cont'd
  Pineal cell tumors
    Pineoblastoma
    Pineocytoma
  Other cell tumors
    Astrocytoma
    Meningioma
    Benign pineal cysts
Embryonal tumors
  Neuroblastoma
  Retinoblastoma
  Primitive neuroectodermal tumors (PNET)
    Medulloblastoma (posterior fossa PNET or
      PNET-MB)
    Cerebral/spinal PNET
Cranial and spinal nerve tumors
  Schwannoma ("neurinoma" or "neurilemoma")
  Neurofibroma
  Malignant peripheral nerve sheath tumors (MP-
    NSTs)
Hemopoetic neoplasms
  Lymphoma
  Leukemia (granulocytic sarcoma or "chloroma")
  Plasmacytoma
Pituitary tumors
Cysts and tumorlike lesions
  Rathke cleft cyst
  Dermoid cyst
  Epidermoid cyst
  Colloid cyst
  Enterogenous cyst
  Neuroglial cyst
  Lipoma
  Hamartoma
Local extensions from regional tumors
  Craniopharyngioma
  Paraganglioma
  Chordoma

Metastatic tumors

---

moma. Because the choroid epithelium is derived from modified ependymal cells, some authors include choroid plexus papillomas and carcinomas within the neuroglial tumors.[1] A so-called mixed glioma that contains two or more different cell types also occurs.

Astrocytomas. Astrocytic neoplasms are subdivided into several different types (*see* Chapter 13).

Fibrillary (diffuse) astrocytomas range from the rare low-grade "benign" astrocytoma to the more common anaplastic astrocytoma and glioblastoma multiforme. Fibrillary astrocytomas are primarily supratentorial neoplasms.

Pilocytic (hair-like) astrocytomas occur primarily in childhood and adolescence. These tumors are generally—but not invariably—slow growing and occur predominately in the hypothalamus and visual pathways, brainstem, and cerebellum.

Less common astrocytoma subtypes are *pleomorphic xanthoastrocytoma*, and *subependymal giant cell astrocytoma* (*see* Chapter 13). The rare "protoplasmic" and "gemistocytic" astrocytomas are included with anaplastic astrocytoma (see subsequent discussion).

Oligodendroglioma. These tumors arise from oligodendrocytes and occur mainly in middle-aged adults. They are primarily supratentorial masses and occur mostly in the cerebral hemispheres. Cortical involvement is common. *Oligodendrogliomas* are usually relatively well defined and slow growing, although a more malignant anaplastic variety is occasionally encountered.

So-called mixed gliomas are relatively rare tumors and histologically heterogeneous neoplasms that consist of at least two different glial cell lines. The most common mixed glioma is an *oligoastrocytoma*. Occasionally, ependymal elements are also present. Patients with mixed tumors have a slightly better prognosis than those with tumors of pure astrocytic lineage.[7]

Ependymal tumors. Several different cell types have been described. The most common variety, *cellular ependymoma,* is predominately an infratentorial tumor that occurs mainly in children and adolescents. It typically fills the fourth ventricle and extrudes through natural passageways such as the lateral recesses and foramen of Magendie into the adjacent CSF cisterns.

Myxopapillary ependymomas occur exclusively in the spinal cord and are typically found in the conus medullaris or filum terminale (*see* Chapter 21). *Subependymomas* are small nodular or lobulated tumors that are located at the caudal fourth ventricle or foramen of Monro. Most occur in middle-aged patients and are usually discovered incidentally or at autopsy.

Choroid plexus tumors. These uncommon tumors consist of *choroid plexus papilloma* (CPP) and *choroid plexus carcinoma.* Over 90% of primary choroid plexus tumors are papillomas; carcinomas are very rare. CPPs typically affect children under the age of 5 years. Most are found in the atrium of the lateral ventricle. Fourth ventricular CPPs are more common in adults. The third ventricle is an uncommon location at any age (*see* Chapter 13).

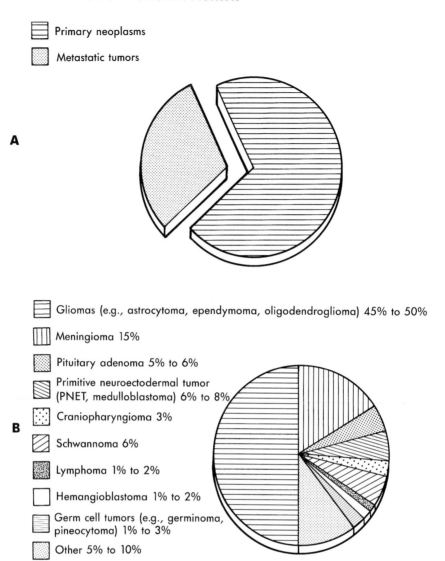

Fig. 12-1. Graphic depiction of brain tumors and their relative incidence. **A,** Primary neoplasms account for approximately two thirds of all brain tumors; metastases from extracranial primary malignancies account for the remainder. **B,** Incidence of common primary brain tumors. Gliomas are the largest single group of primary brain tumors, and astrocytomas are the most frequently encountered glioma. High-grade astrocytomas (anaplastic astrocytoma and glioblastoma multiforme) are the most common of all primary cerebral neoplasms.

Neuronal and mixed neuronal-glial tumors. In adults, glial tumors outnumber neuronal neoplasms by approximately 100:1.[8] Neuronal and mixed neuronal-glial tumors include *gangliocytoma* and *ganglioglioma, Lhermitte-Duclos disease, dysembryoplastic neuroepithelial tumors (DNETs), central neurocytoma,* and *olfactory neuroblastoma (esthesioneuroblastoma)* (*see* Chapter 14).

Tumors of the mesenchyme and meninges. Most primary intracranial mesenchymal tumors arise from meningothelial cells. Meningiomas are the most common of these mesenchymal neoplasms (*see* Chapter 14) and the second most common primary CNS neoplasm after glioblastoma multiforme. Nonmeningothelial tumors are rare.

Meningioma. Meningiomas are typically well-circumscribed slow-growing tumors that arise from meningothelial arachnoid cap cells. More than 90% of meningiomas are supratentorial and occur in certain specific locations, typically around arachnoid villi. With the general exception of children who have neurofibromatosis type 2 (NF-2), meningiomas are usually tumors of adults.

Miscellaneous mesenchymal tumors. These mesenchymal, non-meningothelial tumors include benign neoplasms such as *osteocartilagenous tumors* and *fibrous histiocytoma.* Malignant mesenchymal neoplasms are *chondrosarcoma, rhabdomyosarcoma,* and *meningeal sarcomatosis,* among others. A combined glial-mesenchymal tumor, *gliosarcoma,* is usually classified with malignant astrocytomas.

Hemangiopericytoma is a mesenchymal tumor that was formerly classified as angioblastic meningioma. There is increasing evidence that these tumors arise from modified smooth muscle cells and not meningothelial cells (*see* Chapter 14). Some authors include *hemangioblastoma* with meningeal and mesenchymal tumors.[1] Others regard hemangioblastoma and hemangiopericytoma as tumors of blood vessel origin.

Pineal region tumors. A regional approach to tumors of the pineal region is justified by the common symptomatology and distinctive histologic appearance of these tumors.[2] Pineal region tumors include germ cell tumors, pineal cell tumors, and other cell tumors.

Germ cell tumors. Most primary pineal tumors originate from displaced embryonic tissue.[2] The most common intracranial germ cell tumor is *germinoma,* and the typical germinoma location is in the pineal gland. Less common germ cell neoplasms include *embryonal carcinoma, yolk sac (endodermal sinus) tumors, choroicarcinoma, teratoma,* and *mixed tumors.*

Pineal cell tumors. Tumors that arise from the pineal gland parenchyma are much less common than germ cell tumors. The two major pineal parenchymal tumors are pineoblastoma and pineocytoma.

Pineoblastomas usually occur within the first three decades of life. These tumors are composed of primitive cells that are histologically similar to medulloblastoma (primitive neuroectodermal tumor) and retinoblastoma. Pineoblastomas disseminate within the cerebrospinal fluid (CSF) pathways.

In contrast to pineoblastoma, *pineocytomas* occur mostly in adolescents and adults. The distinction between pineocytoma and normal pineal parenchyma or a benign pineal cyst is sometimes difficult on both imaging and pathologic studies.

Other cell tumors. A spectrum of other neoplasms and nonneoplastic masses are found in the pineal region. Examples are *benign pineal cysts, astrocytoma* (usually in the tectum, although sometimes primary pineal gliomas do occur) and *meningioma* (see subsequent discussion).

Embryonal tumors. These primitive tumors include neuroblastoma, ependymoblastoma, and primitive neuroectodermal tumors (PNET). PNETs are multipotential neoplasms. They can differentiate along neuronal, astrocytic, ependymal, melanotic, or miscellaneous cell lines. The WHO recognizes two subtypes of PNET: *medulloblastoma (posterior fossa PNET or PNET-MB)* and *cerebral or spinal PNETs.*

Cranial and spinal nerve tumors. Three types of nerve sheath tumors occur, as follows:
1. Schwannoma (neurinoma or neurilemoma)
2. Neurofibroma
3. Malignant peripheral nerve sheath tumor

Schwannoma. Intracranial schwannomas constitute 5% to 10% of all intracranial tumors and occur primarily in middle-aged adults.[1] They show a definite predilection for sensory nerves; the vestibular division of CN VIII is by far the most common site, followed by the trigeminal nerve. Bilateral acoustic schwannomas occur in NF-2 (*see* Chapter 5).

Neurofibroma. Neurofibromas do not arise from intracranial nerves. They are found along posterior ganglia as central extensions of more peripheral tumors.[1] Exiting spinal nerves and nerve plexuses are common sites. The plexiform type of neurofibroma is part of the NF-1 spectrum (von Recklinghausen neurofibromatosis) (*see* Chapter 5).

Malignant peripheral nerve sheath tumor (MPNSTs). MPNSTs arise de novo or from degeneration of neurofibromas. Malignant transformation of schwannoma is extremely rare, although primary malignant melanotic schwannomas do occur.[1]

Hemopoetic neoplasms. Hemopoetic neoplasms include malignant lymphoma, leukemia (granulocytic sarcoma), and plasmacytoma.

Lymphoma. *Primary cerebral lymphoma* accounts for approximately 50% of intracranial malignant lymphomas. Once considered uncommon, the incidence of primary CNS lymphoma is rapidly rising with the worldwide increase in immunocompromised patients.

Leukemia. CNS leukemic infiltrates or so-called *granulocytic sarcomas* are almost always secondary to systemic acute myelogenous leukemia. A discrete tumefaction or granulocytic sarcoma sometimes occurs, usually in the subdural space or infundibular region. The greenish hue of this disorder gives rise to the descriptive term *chloroma.*[2]

Plasmacytoma. Disseminated vertebral and epidural tumor is the most common CNS manifestation of multiple myeloma. *Solitary plasmacytomas* are uncommon, although diffuse skull involvement occurs in up to 70% of patients with disseminated multiple myelomatosis.[1] Focal dural masses are occasionally observed. Cerebral parenchymal and spinal cord lesions are rare.

Pituitary tumors. Tumors of the anterior pituitary gland, or adenohypophysis, are technically not brain tumors. They are considered in detail in Chapter 15. The differential diagnosis of sellar and parasellar masses is considered next.

Cysts and tumorlike lesions. These cysts and tumorlike masses include a spectrum of largely unrelated lesions that are all grouped together (*see* box, p. 403). This broad category includes *Rathke's cleft cyst, dermoid* and *epidermoid cysts, colloid cysts, enterogenous* and *neuroglial cysts, lipomas,* and *hamartomas.* These lesions are discussed in Chapter 15.

Local extensions from regional tumors. Also discussed in Chapter 15, this group of lesions includes neoplasms that extend intracranially from adjacent structures in or near the skull base. *Craniopharyngioma, paraganglioma,* and *chordoma* are examples.

Metastatic Tumors

These neoplasms arise from sources outside the CNS and account for approximately one third of all brain tumors (see Fig. 12-1, *A*). CNS metastatic disease has numerous different manifestations and is considered in detail in Chapter 15.

CLASSIFICATION BY AGE AND GENERAL LOCATION

Between 15% to 20% of all intracranial tumors occur in children under 15 years of age.[4] CNS tumors are second only to lymphoreticular malignancies in frequency of childhood cancers and account for 15% of all neoplasms occurring in this age group.[9] Because the histologic spectrum and general locations of primary brain tumors are quite different in children compared to adults, it is useful to consider these two age groups separately.

Primary Brain Tumors in Children

Incidence. The incidence of brain tumors in children is approximately 2.5 per 100,000 per year.[10] Most pediatric brain tumors are primary neoplasms; CNS metastases are rare in children.

Age and presentation. Primary brain tumors are more common in the first decade than in the second; the peak occurrence is between 4 and 8 years of age.[9] Neoplasms in children under 2 years of age are uncommon. These are considered congenital tumors and represent a distinctly different histologic spectrum compared to older children.

Brain tumors in neonates and infants. (*see* box, *above*). Only 1% to 2% of all brain tumors occur in children under 2 years of age.[11] Tumors of neonates and infants have a different topographic and pathologic distribution compared to those found in older children.[12] Tumors in very young children are often large and highly malignant. Two thirds occur in the supratentorial compartment. Obstruction of CSF pathways with hydrocephalus, split sutures, and macrocrania are common first signs.[9]

Common brain tumors in children under 2 years of age are *primitive neuroectodermal tumor* (PNET or "peanut" tumor), *teratoma, astrocytoma* (often anaplastic astrocytoma or glioblastoma multiforme), and *choroid plexus papilloma.* Teratoma is the most common intracranial tumor in the neonatal period.[13] Less common neoplasms in this age group include *angiosarcoma, malignant rhabdoid tumor, medulloepithelioma,* and *meningioma.*[11,14,15] Regardless of histology, the dominant imaging appearance is that of a large heterogeneous lesion with associated hydrocephalus. Overall prognosis is poor.[11]

Brain tumors in older children (*see* box, *right*). Approximately half of all intracranial neoplasms in children are gliomas; 15% are PNETs (including medulloblastoma). Ependymoma and craniopharyngioma account for about 10% each, whereas pineal region neoplasms cause 3% of tumors in this age group.[9]

General location and histology. Slightly more primary intracranial neoplasms in children are supratentorial (52%) compared to infratentorial (48%) in location[9]; the proportion of supra- to infratentorial lesions varies significantly with age (Fig. 12-2).

Supratentorial neoplasms. Slightly less than half of all supratentorial childhood neoplasms are astrocytomas; most are *pilocytic or low-grade astrocytomas,* and the opticochiasmatic-hypothalamic area is the

---

Brain Tumors In Children Less Than Two Years of Age

Etiology
Probably congenital

Presentation
Large, bulky masses (bulging fontanelles)
Hydrocephalus, macrocrania
Seizure, focal neurologic deficit

Location
Two thirds are supratentorial
Most common tumors
  Primitive neuroectodermal tumor (PNET)
  Astrocytoma (often anaplastic, glioblastoma multiforme)
  Teratoma
  Choroid plexus papilloma

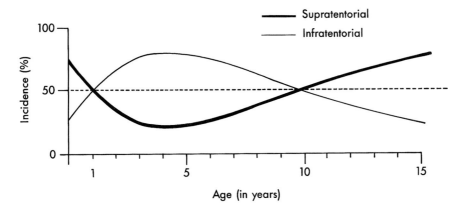

Fig. 12-2. Relative incidence of supra- and infratentorial primary brain tumors in children related to age. Supratentorial neoplasms are more common in neonates and young children, and posterior fossa tumors are more common in older children.

Brain Tumors in Children

Incidence

15% of all neoplasms in infants and children are intracranial

Presentation

Seizure
Hydrocephalus, macrocrania
Nausea, vomiting (posterior fossa)
Focal neurological deficit (e.g., visual abnormalities with chiasmatic glioma)

Age

Occurrence in first decade more common than in second decade
Peak age between 4 and 8 years

Location and histology

52% supratentorial
   Just under half are cerebral hemisphere astrocytomas (mostly low grade)
   One eighth craniopharyngiomas
   One eighth opticochiasmatic-hypothalamic gliomas
   Remainder
      Pineal region tumors (germinoma, pineal parenchymal cell tumors)
      PNET
      Choroid plexus papilloma
      Miscellaneous (ganglioglioma, oligodendroglioma are rare)
48% infratentorial
   One third cerebellar astrocytomas
   One quarter brainstem gliomas
   One quarter medulloblastomas (PNET-MB)
   One eighth ependymomas

Data from Harwood-Nash DC: Primary neoplasms of the central nervous system in children, *Cancer* 67:1223-1228, 1991.

---

most common location. *Craniopharyngiomas* represent another one eighth of supratentorial neoplasms in children.[9] *Ganglioglioma, ependymoma, oligodendroglioma, meningioma,* and miscellaneous other uncommon tumors account for the remainder.[16] Metastases from extracerebral primary sites are uncommon in children.

Infratentorial neoplasms. About one third of posterior fossa neoplasms in children are *cerebellar astrocytomas,* and one third to one quarter are *PNET/medulloblastomas. Brainstem glioma* represents another one fourth, whereas one eighth of pediatric infratentorial neoplasms are *ependymomas.*[9,17] Other posterior fossa tumors such as choroid plexus papilloma are unusual in children.

Most cerebellar astrocytomas are pilocytic astrocytomas; intrinsic pontine gliomas are infiltrative, and all are malignant regardless of their histology at the time of biopsy.[18] Medullary gliomas behave more benignly.[18-20]

More than 90% of medulloblastomas (posterior fossa PNET) arise in the vermis. Occasionally, medulloblastomas occur off-axis; about 7% are found in the cerebellar hemispheres.[21]

Adult Primary Brain Tumors

Incidence. Approximately 80% to 85% of all intracranial tumors occur in adults.[22] Most occur in the supratentorial compartment (*see* box, p. 408). Adult primary infratentorial tumors are uncommon; most are extraaxial lesions.[23]

Age and clinical presentation. The peak incidence of gliomas, the most common group of adult primary brain tumors, is in the seventh decade. Clinical manifestations include seizure, focal neurologic deficit, or symptoms of increased intracranial pressure such as

---

Brain Tumors in Adults

Supratentorial

Common
Astrocytoma
   Anaplastic astrocytoma
   Glioblastoma multiforme
Meningioma
Pituitary adenoma
Oligodendroglioma
Metastases
Uncommon
Lymphoma
Rare
Ependymoma

Infratentorial

Common
Schwannoma
Meningioma
Epidermoid
Metastases
Uncommon
Hemangioblastoma
Brainstem glioma
Rare
Choroid plexus papilloma

---

headache, nausea, vomiting, and visual symptoms.[22] One to two percent of intracranial tumors present with strokelike symptoms (*see* Chapter 11).

General location and histology. Primary brain tumors comprise about one half to two thirds of all intracranial tumors in adults, and metastases account for the remainder.

Supratentorial tumors. Most primary brain tumors in adults occur above the tentorium.[22] Approximately one half are gliomas. About 70% of gliomas are astrocytomas; more than half of all astrocytomas are *anaplastic astrocytoma* or *glioblastoma multiforme*.[1] Increasing age generally correlates with increasing malignancy.

The second most common primary brain tumor in adults is *meningioma*, representing 15% to 20% of these neoplasms. More than three quarters of meningiomas are supratentorial.[24]

Eight percent of primary intracranial tumors in adults occur in the sellar/paraseIlar region. *Pituitary adenoma* is by far the most common neoplasm in this area.

Oligodendrogliomas represent about 5% of all primary brain tumors. Most oligodendrogliomas occur in adults, and almost all are found in the supratentorial compartment. Other gliomas such as ependy-

moma and CPP occasionally occur in adults. They are often in unusual or atypical locations (e.g., supratentorial or extraaxial ependymoma, or fourth ventricular CPP).

Lymphomas cause 1% to 2% of adult primary CNS tumors, but their incidence is rising rapidly with the increase in immunocompromised patients.

Infratentorial tumors. Posterior fossa tumors in adults are subdivided into intra- and extraaxial processes. The three most common primary posterior fossa neoplasms in adults are all extraaxial: *schwannoma, meningioma,* and *epidermoid tumors.*[21]

In contrast to children, intraaxial posterior fossa tumors in adults are rare. *Hemangioblastoma* and *brainstem glioma* are the two most common adult primary neoplasms in this location. *Metastasis* from extracranial primary tumors is by far the most common intraaxial posterior fossa tumor in adults.[21a] Fifteen to twenty percent of all intracranial metastases are found in the posterior fossa.[21]

CLASSIFICATION AND DIFFERENTIAL DIAGNOSIS BY SPECIFIC ANATOMIC LOCATION

The most important factor in establishing an appropriate differential diagnosis for an intracranial mass is location (age is second).[25] This section considers the diagnosis of intracranial neoplasms in seven specific, anatomic locations. These areas are listed as follows:

1. Pineal
2. Intraventricular
3. Cerebellopontine angle
4. Foramen magnum
5. Sellar/suprasellar
6. Skull base and cavernous sinus
7. Scalp, calvarium, and meninges

In each region, we briefly discuss normal gross and imaging anatomy, then review the tumors and nonneoplastic lesions such as vascular malformations and benign cysts that occur in these specific locations.

Pineal Region Masses

Normal anatomy. The pineal region is a histologically heterogeneous area that includes the pineal gland itself, the posterior third ventricle and aqueduct, the subarachnoid cisterns (quadrigeminal plate and ambient cisterns plus the velum interpositum), brain (tectum and brainstem, thalami, corpus callosum splenium), dura (tentorial apex), and vessels (internal cerebral veins and vein of Galen, and posterior choroidal and posterior cerebral arteries) (Fig. 12-3).

The pineal gland lies behind the third ventricle, above the posterior commissure, cerebral aqueduct, and tectal plate, and anterioinferior to the corpus cal-

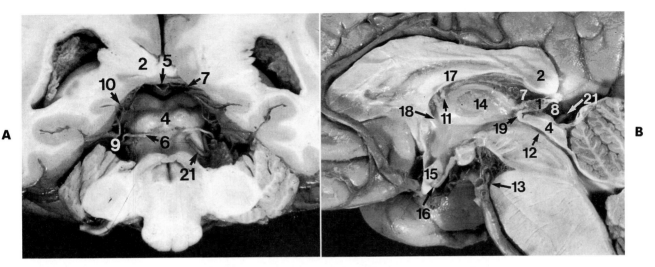

Fig. 12-3. A, Gross anatomy of the pineal region and tectal plate, posterior view. The vein of Galen has been removed. **B,** Midsagittal section through the third ventricle and pineal gland showing relationships with adjacent structures: *1,* Pineal gland. *2,* Splenium of corpus callosum. *3,* Internal cerebral vein. *4,* Tectum (collicular plate). *5,* Vein of Galen. *6,* Trochlear nerve (CN IV). *7,* Velum interpositum. *8,* Quadrigeminal plate cistern. *9,* Ambient cistern. *10,* Posterior choroidal arteries. *11,* Choroid plexus of third ventricle. *12,* Cerebral aqueduct. *13,* Basilar bifurcation with midbrain perforating branches. *14,* Thalamus (with massa intemedia). *15,* Optic chiasm. *16,* Hypothalamus with infundibular stalk. *17,* Fornix. *18,* Foramen of Monro. *19,* Posterior commissure. *20,* Basal veins of Rosenthal. *21,* Posterior cerebral artery. *22,* Tentorium cerebelli. (From Basset DL: *A Stereoscopic Atlas of Human Anatomy: the Central Nervous System,* Section 1. Courtesy Bassett Collection, R. Chase (curator), Stanford University.)

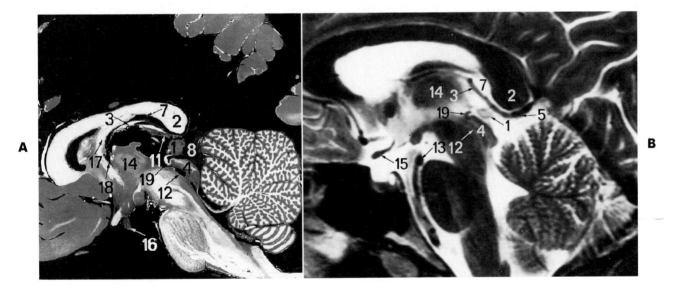

Fig. 12-4. A, Midsagittal cut brain section and, **B,** sagittal T2-weighted MR scan depict the pineal gland and its adjacent structures. Same key as Fig. 12-3. (Brain section courtesy Yakovlev Collection, Armed Forces Institute of Pathology.)

losum splenium (Fig. 12-4). The suprapineal recess of the third ventricle extends posteriorly immediately above the pineal gland. The quadrigeminal plate cistern lies behind the pineal gland. An anterior extension of this cistern, the velum interpositum, lies above the pineal gland and extends anteriorly under the fornix.

Important vascular, dural, and neural structures are adjacent to the pineal gland. The tentorial apex arches above and behind the pineal gland, and the internal cerebral veins and vein of Galen lie in close proximity (Figs. 12-4 and 12-5). Branches of the medial and lateral posterior choroidal arteries are also present (*see* Fig. 6-19). The two CN IVs exit dorsally

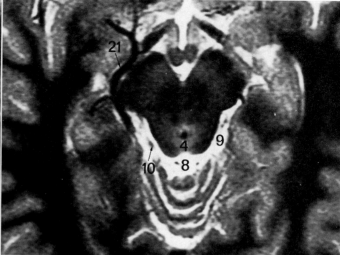

Fig. 12-5. Axial (**A** and **B**) and coronal (**C**) T2-weighted MR scans show the pineal region anatomy in detail. Same key as Fig. 12-3.

Common Pineal Region Masses

Germ cell tumors
Germinoma
Teratoma

Pineal parenchymal cell tumors
Pineocytoma
Pineoblastoma

Other cell tumors and neoplastic-like masses
Pineal cysts
Astrocytoma (thalamus, midbrain, tectum, corpus callosum)
Meningioma
Metastases
Vascular malformation (with or without enlarged vein of Galen)
Miscellaneous (lipoma, epidermoid, arachnoid cyst)

---

from the midbrain, decussate, and then course anteriorly in the ambient cisterns adjacent to the tentorial incisura.

Pathology: overview. The list of possible pineal region masses is extensive and includes germ cell tumors, pineal cell tumors, "other" cell tumors, and nonneoplastic masses (*see* box). Together these lesions represent about 1% to 3% of all intracranial masses.[26,27]

It is very helpful to subdivide pineal region masses into more specific locations (Fig. 12-6). We first consider lesions that arise within the pineal gland itself, then discuss posterior third ventricle and quadrigeminal cistern masses. Adjacent brain parenchyma areas such as the tectum, midbrain, and corpus callosum have a different spectrum of abnormalities that may cause a pineal region mass. Finally, we consider lesions that arise in the pineal region from adjacent vascular and dural structures.

Pineal gland lesions. Pineal region masses account for 1% to 2% of all brain tumors but constitute 3% to 8% of intracranial tumors in children.[4,28-30]

Pineal gland neoplasms. Pineal tumors are commonly but mistakenly referred to as "pinealomas." The correct terminology of pineal region masses is listed in the box.

Common pineal gland tumors are neoplastic derivatives of multipotential embryonic germ cells.[27] These tumors account for more than two thirds of all pineal region masses. Germ cell tumors have a peak incidence during the second decade.[30]

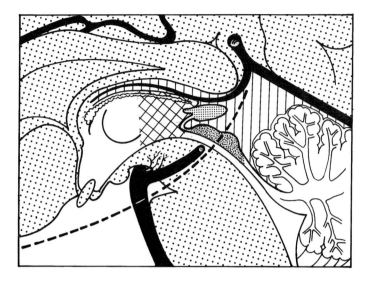

Pineal gland
  Germinoma
  Teratoma
  Pineoblastoma/pineocytoma
  Benign cyst

Tectum
  Chiari II (beaking)
  Astrocytoma
  Multiple sclerosis
  Contusion

Vessels, dura
  Tortuous vessels
  Enlarged vein of Galen
  Meningioma
  Tentorial subdural hematoma

Posterior third ventricle
  Astrocytoma
  Dilated suprapineal recess
  Ependymal/inflammatory cyst
  Choroid plexus papilloma

Quadrigeminal cistern/
velum interpositum
  Cavum velum interpositum
  Arachnoid cyst
  Metastases
  Meningitis
  Subarachnoid hemorrhage

Brain
  Astrocytoma
  Vascular malformation
  Stroke
  Demyelinating disease
  Metastasis
  Herniations

Fig. 12-6. Anatomic diagram depicts the pineal region and its common lesions. The approximate course of the tentorial incisura is shown by the dotted line.

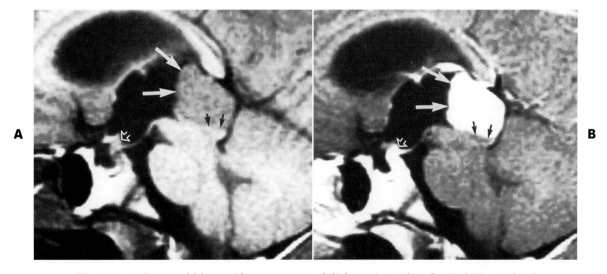

A   B

Fig. 12-7. A 7-year-old boy with acute onset of diabetes insipidus. Sagittal T1-weighted MR scans without **(A)** and with **(B)** contrast enhancement show a large uniformly enhancing pineal region mass *(white arrows)*. The mass depresses the tectal plate *(black arrows)*. The infundibular recess appears slightly thickened and enhances following contrast administration *(open arrows)*. *Continued.*

Germinoma is by far the most common of the germ cell neoplasms (Fig. 12-7) (*see* Chapter 14). Synchronous lesions in the pineal and suprasellar regions account for 5% to 10% of all intracranial germ cell tumors.[31] The second most common germ cell tumor is teratoma, accounting for approximately 15% of all pineal masses (Fig. 12-8).[27] *Teratomas* arise from multipotential cells that produce tissues representing a mixture of two or more embryologic layers.[27] Terato-

mas can be benign (typical, or mature or immature) or malignant (formerly called teratocarcinoma).

Less common germ cell tumors include *choriocarcinoma, endodermal sinus (yolk sac) tumor,* and *embryonal carcinoma.* Mixed cell types also occur.[32]

Tumors that arise from pineal parenchymal cells account for less than 15% of all pineal region neoplasms. Unlike germinomas these tumors may be found in patients beyond the second decade of life.[27] There are two types of pineal cell neoplasms: pineocytoma and pineoblastoma. *Pineocytomas* are benign, well-delineated tumors with mature cells that are histologically—and often radiologically—almost indistinguishable from normal pineal parenchyma (Fig. 12-9). *Pineoblastomas* are malignant neoplasms that are composed of undifferentiated or immature pineal cells. Pineoblastomas are considered a type of PNET similar to medulloblastoma.[27]

Pineal parenchymal neoplasms other than pineocytoma or pineoblastoma are rare. Occasionally, metastases or gliomas with ganglionic or astrocytic differentiation are identified.[27]

Nonneoplastic pineal gland masses. Nonneoplastic *pineal cysts* are benign cystic lesions that are lined by collagenous fibers, glial cells, and normal pineal parenchymal cells.[33,34] Theories on the origin of pineal cysts include degenerative change, coalescence of smaller cysts, sequestration of the pineal diverticulum, and failure of normal pineal development.[35]

Small asymptomatic nonneoplastic pineal gland cysts are common incidental findings, seen in up to

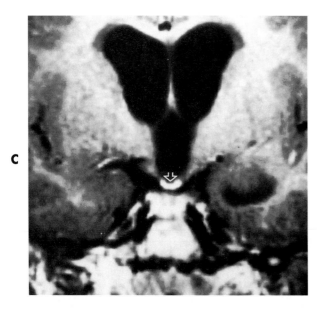

Fig. 12-7, cont'd. Coronal postcontrast study (**C**) confirms a second lesion in the inferior third ventricle *(arrow).* Note hydrocephalus secondary to aqueductal stenosis. Synchronous pineal-suprasellar germinomas.

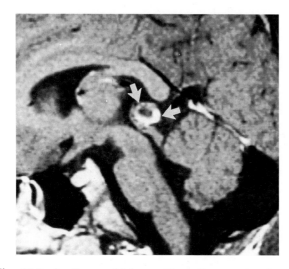

Fig. 12-8. An 8-year-old boy with malignant pineal teratoma. Postcontrast sagittal T1-weighted MR scan shows a partially enhancing mixed signal pineal gland mass *(arrows).*

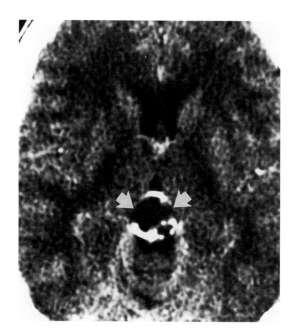

Fig. 12-9. A 24-year-old woman with headaches and normal neurologic examination. Axial postcontrast CT scan shows a partially calcified cystic-appearing pineal gland mass *(arrows).* Pineocytoma.

40% of routine autopsies (Fig. 12-10, *A* and *B*) and 1% to 5% of unselected MR scans (Fig. 12-10, *C* to *F*).[36,37] Occasionally, the imaging appearance of benign pineal cyst is indistinguishable from small cystic pineal neoplasms such as pineocytomas.[33] CT or MR-guided stereotactic biopsy has been recommended for the evaluation and management of symptomatic cases.[38]

Other than glial cysts, benign pineal masses are uncommon. Sarcoidosis has been reported as causing a focal pineal mass.[39]

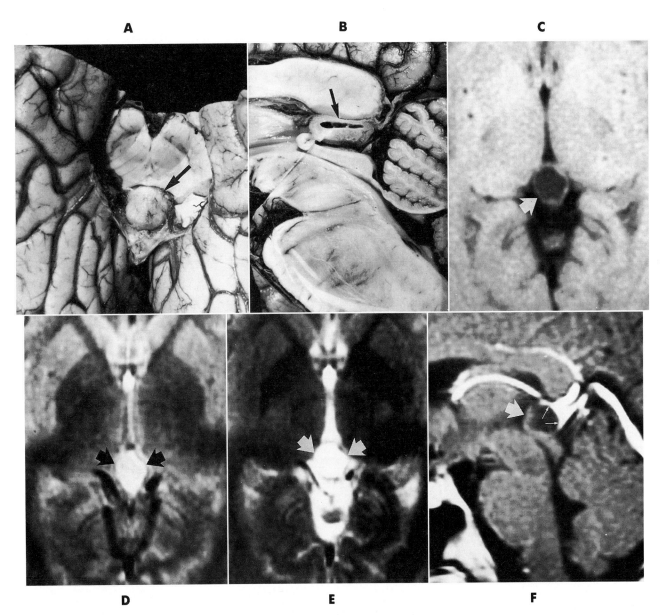

Fig. 12-10. Gross pathology of benign pineal cyst incidentally found at autopsy. **A,** View from below shows the cyst *(arrow)* compresses and flattens the midbrain. **B,** Midsagittal section shows the cyst *(arrow)* and compressed tectal plate. Axial T1- **(C),** proton density **(D),** and T2-weighted **(E)** MR scans without contrast in a 34-year-old woman with headaches disclosed a cystic pineal mass *(arrows)* that is slightly hyperintense to CSF on all sequences. Sagittal postcontrast T1WI **(F)** shows partial rim enhancement *(small arrows).* The lesion was followed for 3 years and did not show interval change on serial imaging studies. Presumed nonneoplastic benign pineal cyst. (**A** and **B,** Courtesy E. Tessa Hedley-Whyte.)

Posterior third ventricle lesions

Nonneoplastic masses. A markedly *dilated suprapineal recess* may occur with longstanding aqueductal stenosis (Fig. 12-11). Occasionally, *ependymal or inflammatory cysts* can be found in the posterior third ventricle. Colloid cysts are typically located more an-teriorly near the foramen of Monro (see subsequent discussion). The third ventricle can be elevated and extrinsically compressed by an ectatic, elongated basilar artery or basilar bifurcation aneurysm (Fig. 12-12).

Neoplasms. Masses located entirely within the posterior third ventricle are rare; most arise from the choroid plexus. *Meningioma, choroid plexus papilloma,* and *metastases* are the most common neoplasms that occur in this location (Fig. 12-13). Tumors that involve the posterior third ventricle usually arise from the thalamus or pineal gland and extend into the ventricle secondarily.[40]

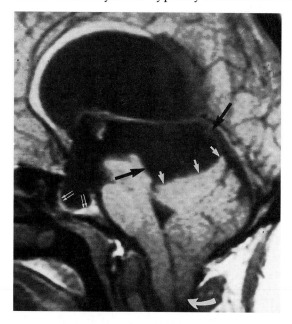

Fig. 12-11. Sagittal T1-weighted MR scan in a patient with long-standing aqueductal stenosis and severe hydrocephalus shows a massively enlarged suprapineal recess of the third ventricle *(black arrows)*. Note flattening and inferior displacement of the vermis *(single white arrows)*, descending tonsillar herniation *(curved arrow)*, and "partially empty" sella *(double arrows)* caused by inferior herniation of the anterior third ventricular recesses into the sella turcica.

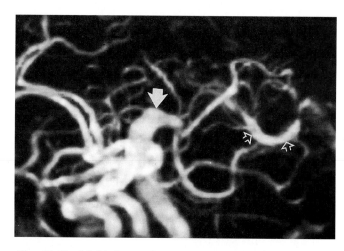

Fig. 12-12. Multiple overlapping thin-slab MR angiogram shows an extremely ectatic, tortuous basilar artery *(large arrow)*. Vein of Galen is seen *(open arrows)*.

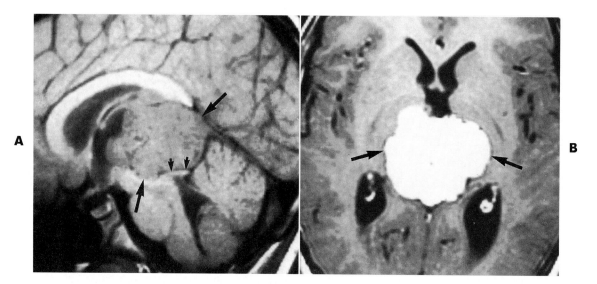

Fig. 12-13. A, Sagittal precontrast T1-weighted MR scan in a 2-year-old child with Parinaud syndrome shows a large posterior third ventricular mass *(large arrows)* with severe compression of the tectum *(small arrows)*. **B,** Axial postcontrast T1WI shows the mass *(arrows)* enhances intensely. Choroid plexus papilloma was found at surgery.

Tectum. The lamina quadrigemina (paired superior and inferior colliculi) forms the midbrain roof. Although a diverse group of lesions may affect the tectum, intrinsic tectal lesions have a comparatively limited differential diagnosis.[41]

Normal variations and congenital anomalies. There is little variation in tectal size, although the inferior colliculus may be slightly larger than the superior colliculus. A superior colliculus that is larger than its inferior counterpart is usually abnormal. Most patients with *Chiari II malformation* have mesencephalic abnormalities. These range from slight loss of the normal intercollicular groove through collicular fusion to a markedly elongated beak-shaped tectum[42] (*see* Chapter 2). Mesencephalic beaking is seen in nearly 90%.[43]

Neoplasms. *Tectal gliomas* are usually low-grade astrocytomas that enlarge the tectum (Fig. 12-14). The aqueduct may be engulfed and occluded (Fig. 12-15), resulting in obstructive hydrocephalus. *Lymphoma* occasionally involves the tectum.[41]

Nonneoplastic masses and miscellaneous lesions. Vascular malformations that involve the tectum include *cavernous angiomas* (Fig. 12-16, *A*), *pial AVMs*, and mesencephalic AVMs with *aneurysmal dilatation of the vein of Galen* (Fig. 12-16, *B*)[44] (*see* Chapter 10). Thalamoperforating artery occlusions may result in midbrain and tectal *infarcts*. Other abnormalities of the dorsolateral midbrain include *trauma* (Fig. 12-17), *demyelinating disease*, and *progressive supranuclear palsy*.[41]

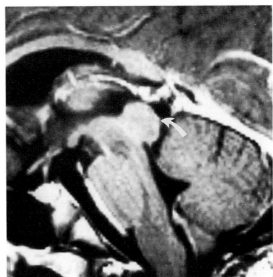

Fig. 12-14. Sagittal postcontrast T1-weighted MR scan shows a tectal plate glioma *(arrow)*.

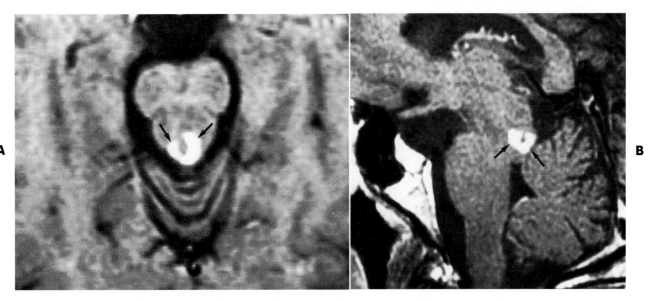

Fig. 12-15. Axial **(A)** and sagittal **(B)** postcontrast T1-weighted MR scans show an enhancing mass in the periaqueductal region *(arrows)*. Presumed glioma (not biopsied).

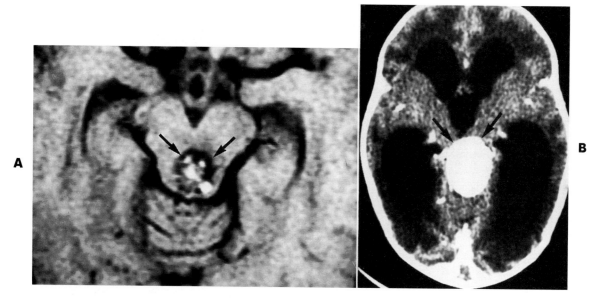

Fig. 12-16. Two cases illustrate vascular malformations in the pineal region. **A,** Axial T1-weighted MR scan shows a cavernous angioma *(arrows).* **B,** Axial postcontrast CT scan in a newborn with high-output congestive heart failure shows an enlarged vein of Galen *(arrows)* secondary to mesencephalic AVM (not shown).

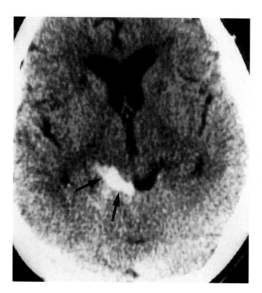

Fig. 12-17. Axial NECT scan in a patient with severe head trauma. Initial CT scan obtained 2 days earlier showed only minor abnormalities. Dorsolateral midbrain contusion with hemorrhage in the quadrigeminal cistern and tectum is now apparent *(arrows).* (Courtesy Ivan Robinson.)

Quadrigeminal cistern and velum interpositum. Various lesions occur in the subarachnoid spaces that surround the pineal gland.

Normal variations and congenital anomalies. A common normal variation is a *cavum velum interpositum* (CVI) (Fig. 12-18, *A*). CVI is a triangular-shaped, CSF-filled anterior extension of the quadrigeminal plate cistern that lies above the pineal gland and dorsal third ventricle. CVIs and masses within and above the velum interpositum (e.g., arachnoid cyst and corpus callosum gliomas) typically displace the internal

cerebral veins and pineal gland inferiorly (Fig. 12-18, *B*).

Dorsal mesencephalic *lipomas* are occasionally identified incidentally on MR scans (Fig. 12-19).[41] Intracranial lipomas are congenital malformations that result from persistence and maldifferentiation of the meninx primitiva, an embryologic structure that normally differentiates into the leptomeninges[45] (*see* Chapter 15). Quadrigeminal plate lipomas usually occur in isolation, but up to one third are associated with other congenital anomalies.[27]

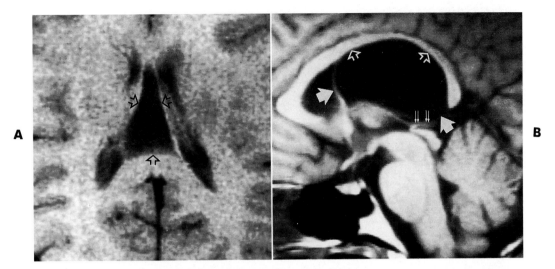

Fig. 12-18. A, Axial T1-weighted MR scan shows a cavum velum interpositum (CVI) *(arrows).* The pyramidal-shaped CSF collection that lies between the two lateral ventricles is characteristic. **B,** Sagittal T1-weighted MR scan in another patient shows an arachnoid cyst within the CVI *(large arrows).* Note inferior displacement of the pineal gland *(double arrows)* and elevation of the corpus callosum *(open arrows),* indicating the mass is located in the CVI.

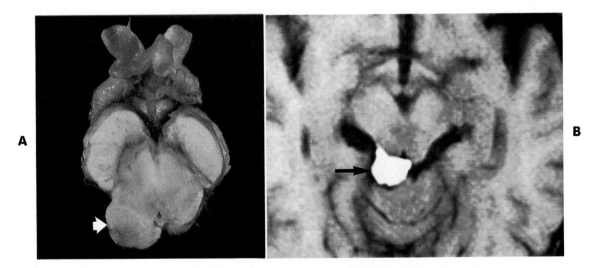

Fig. 12-19. A, Gross pathology specimen shows a quadrigeminal plate lipoma *(arrow)* found incidentally at autopsy. **B,** Axial T1-weighted MR scan shows an incidental lipoma, seen as the hyperintense lesion *(arrow).* (**A,** Courtesy E. Tessa Hedley-Whyte.)

Nonneoplastic masses and miscellaneous lesions. Quadrigeminal cistern *arachnoid cysts* are congenital cystic CSF collections located between the tectum and tentorial incisura (Fig. 12-20).[46] They represent about 8% of all intracranial arachnoid cysts.[47] Occasionally, an arachnoid cyst occurs within the velum interpositum (Fig. 12-18, *B*). *Meningitis* and *subarachnoid hemorrhage* (SAH) can affect the quadrigeminal cistern (Fig. 12-21). *Nonaneurysmal perimesencepha-*

lic SAH typically involves the pontine and ambient cisterns but may extend dorsally into the quadrigeminal cistern *(see* Chapter 7).

Neoplasms. Primary neoplasms of the quadrigeminal cistern are rare. Occasionally, *epidermoid* or *dermoid tumors* occur in this location (Fig. 12-22). Leptomeningeal *metastases* from numerous primary brain tumors and extracerebral sources most often affect the basilar CSF subarachnoid spaces, but diffuse tu-

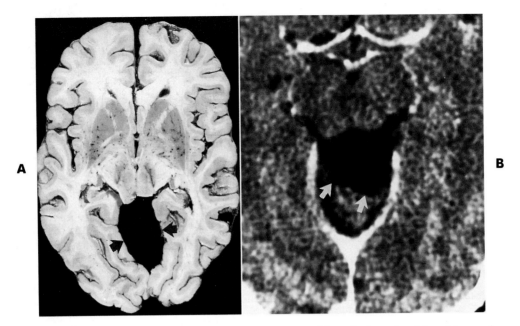

Fig. 12-20. A, Gross pathology specimen shows a quadrigeminal arachnoid cyst *(arrows)* found incidentally at autopsy. **B,** Axial CECT scan shows a quadrigeminal arachnoid cyst *(arrows),* seen as the low-density CSF collection immediately posterior to the tectum. **(A,** Courtesy E. Tessa Hedley-Whyte.)

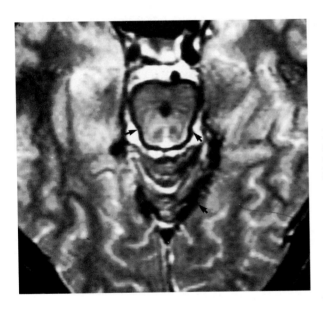

Fig. 12-21. Striking changes of superficial siderosis are seen on the axial T2-weighted MR scan of a patient with repeated subarachnoid hemorrhages. Note pial hemosiderin staining of all the pineal region structures *(arrows).*

mor spread can involve the ambient, superior vermian, and quadrigeminal plate cisterns and even the velum interpositum (Fig. 12-23).

Vascular and dural lesions. The most common vascular mass in the pineal region is an elongated, tortuous basilar artery that elevates and compresses the third ventricle. Occasionally, *aneurysms* of the P2 or P3 posterior cerebral artery segments occur here (Fig. 12-24). A choroidal artery fistula or mesence-

phalic *AVM with an aneurysmally dilated vein of Galen* is a rare but important vascular lesion that causes a pineal region mass (Fig. 12-16, *B*). Common tentorial apex masses include *meningioma* (Fig. 12-25) and *subdural hematoma.*

Brain parenchyma. Brain parenchymal structures that lie in close proximity to the pineal gland are the corpus callosum splenium, tectum, posterior commissure, and midbrain. Therefore the full spectrum

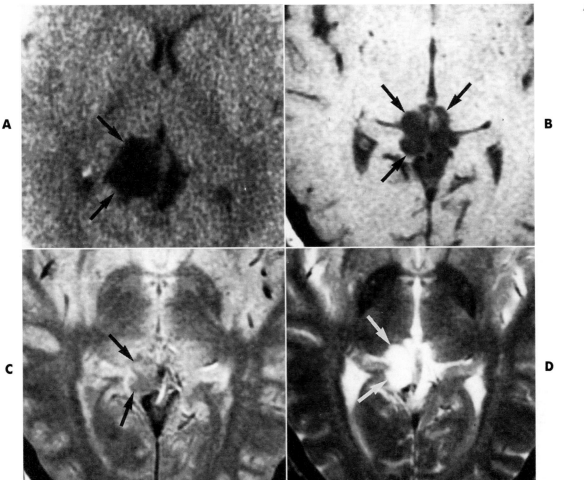

Fig. 12-22. Quadrigeminal and ambient cistern epidermoid tumor is shown in these studies. **A,** Axial NECT scan shows a very low density, slightly lobulated mass in the right ambient cistern *(arrows).* Axial T1- **(B),** proton density- **(C)** and T2-weighted **(D)** MR scans show the mass *(arrows)* has the same signal intensity as CSF.

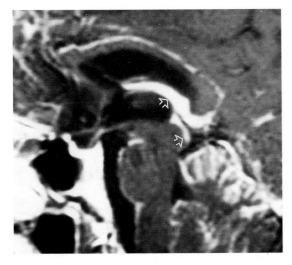

Fig. 12-23. Sagittal postcontrast T1-weighted MR scan in a patient with diffuse leptomeningeal metastases from breast carcinoma shows extensive tumor covering nearly all pial surfaces. Note thick, enhancing rind of tumor that covers the quadrigeminal plate and extends anteriorly into the velum interpositum *(arrows).*

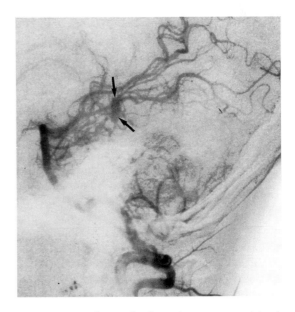

Fig. 12-24. Lateral vertebral angiogram, arterial phase, shows a distal posterior cerebral artery aneurysm *(arrows).* The patient had systemic fungal infection.

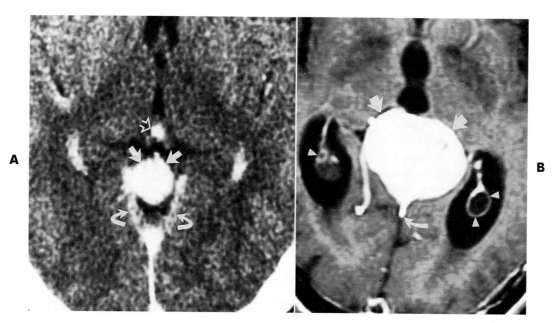

Fig. 12-25. Two cases of tentorial apex meningioma causing a pineal region mass. **A,** Axial CECT scan shows a round, uniformly enhancing mass *(large arrows)* that lies between the tentorial leaves *(curved arrows)*. Note the calcified pineal gland *(open arrow)* is *anterior* to the mass. **B,** A 73-year-old woman with ataxia, gait abnormalities, and urinary incontinence had a CT scan (not shown) that showed a "pineal tumor." Axial postcontrast T1-weighted MR scan shows a large intensely enhancing mass *(large arrows)* at the tentorial apex. Note the dural "tail" *(curved arrow)*. Incidentally noted are bilateral choroid plexus cysts *(arrowheads)*. (**A,** Courtesy J. Jones.)

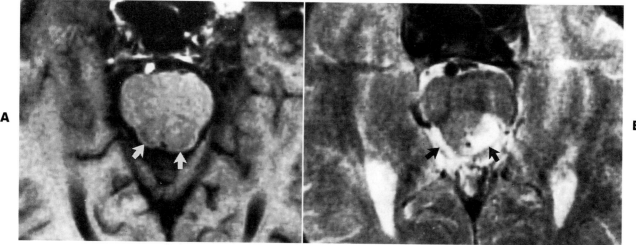

Fig. 12-26. Autopsy-proven multiple sclerosis in this patient is seen as a tectal mass. **A,** Axial T1WI shows the low signal mass enlarges and distorts the tectum *(arrows)*. **B,** The T2-weighted study shows the hyperintense midbrain lesions *(arrows)*.

of brain *demyelinating* (Fig. 12-26) and *metabolic diseases, vascular malformations* and *infarcts* (Fig. 12-27), and *primary* (Fig. 12-28) *and metastatic tumors* (Fig. 12-29) may involve the brain around the pineal region.

Displacement of otherwise normal brain structures into the quadrigeminal cistern occurs with some brain herniations. Upward herniation of the cerebellar vermis through the tentorial incisura obliterates the quadrigeminal plate cistern and compresses the tectum (Fig. 12-30). Descending temporal lobe herniation may cause medial displacement of the hippocampus over the incisura, compressing the midbrain and adjacent ambient cistern.

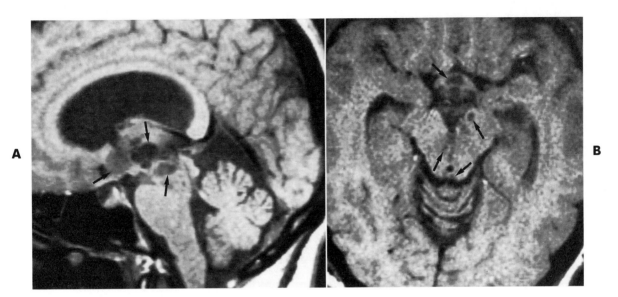

Fig. 12-27. Sagittal **(A)** and axial **(B)** T1-weighted MR scans in a patient with "top of the basilar" infarctions secondary to multiple thalamoperforating artery embolic occlusions. Note multiple lacunar infarcts in the thalami, hypothalamus, midbrain, and tectum *(arrows)*.

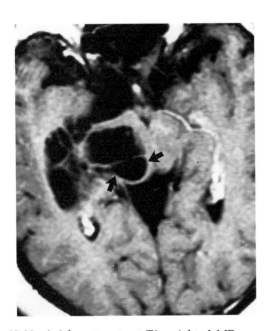

Fig. 12-28. Axial postcontrast T1-weighted MR scan in a patient with an extensive cystic midbrain astrocytoma that involves the tectum *(arrows)*.

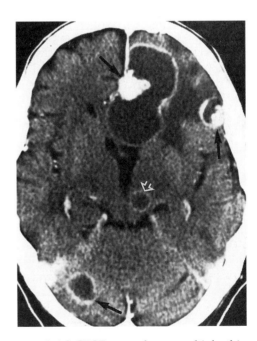

Fig. 12-29. Axial CECT scan shows multiple thin-walled metastases, some with mural nodules *(black arrows)*. A midbrain metastasis is indicated *(open arrow)*. Carcinoma of the lung.

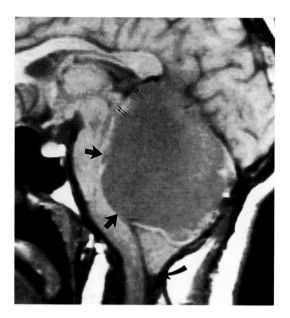

Fig. 12-30. Sagittal T1-weighted MR scan shows a huge cystic cerebellar astrocytoma *(large arrows)* fills most of the posterior fossa. The enlarged vermis herniates upward through the tentorial incisura, compressing the tectum *(double arrows)*. Note downward tonsillar displacement through the foramen magnum *(curved arrow).*

Intraventricular Masses

One tenth of all CNS neoplasms involve the ventricles. Imaging characteristics are usually nonspecific; exact location of the mass and the patient's age are the most helpful information in the differential diagnosis of these lesions (*see* boxes).[49]

Lateral ventricles. The lateral ventricles are paired C-shaped structures (Fig. 12-31). Each is subdivided into frontal horn, body, atrium (trigone), occipital horn, and temporal horn. The lateral ventricles curve around the thalami and diverge from the midline as they pass posteriorly. The superior surface of each lateral ventricle is formed by the corpus callosum. The caudate nucleus, thalamus, and hippocampus form the lateral and inferior borders.

Half the intraventricular tumors in adults and one quarter of the intraventricular masses in children are found in the lateral ventricles.[50] The diagnosis of these lesions varies significantly with age and location within the ventricle itself (Fig. 12-32).[25]

Frontal horn. The frontal horns of the lateral ventricles are separated by the septum pellucidum (Fig. 12-33). The septum pellucidum is a thin translucent triangular membrane that consists of two glial laminae with a potential space (cavum) in between.[51] The septum pellucidum extends anteriorly and superiorly from the fornix to the corpus callosum.[52]

Intraventricular Masses In Children

Lateral ventricles

Frontal horn
Cavum septi pellucidi and cavum vergae
Astrocytoma (usually low grade)
Giant cell astrocytoma
Body
PNET
Astrocytoma
Atrium
Choroid plexus papilloma
Ependymoma (rare)
Occipital and temporal horns (rare)
Meningioma
Enlarged calcified choroid plexus with NF-2

Foramen of Monro/third ventricle

Foramen of Monro
Subependymal giant cell astrocytoma
Astrocytoma
(N.B.—colloid cysts are *rare* in children; when they occur they are usually in older children and adolescents)
Third ventricle
Extrinsic mass (e.g., craniopharyngioma)
Astrocytoma (low grade, pilocytic)
Histiocytosis (anterior recesses/hypothalamus/infundibular stalk)
Germinoma

Fourth ventricle

Astrocytoma (usually pilocytic type)
Medulloblastoma
Ependymoma
Exophytic brainstem glioma

Several congenital anomalies affect the septum pellucidum and frontal horns. An *absent septum pellucidum* almost always indicates substantial neurologic disease (Fig. 12-34, *A* and *B*).[52] The septum is absent in *holoprosencephaly, septooptic dysplasia,* and *corpus callosum dysgenesis.*

Cavum septi pellucidi (CSP) and *cavum vergae* (CV) are common developmental anomalies that represent persistence of normal fetal cavities. Eighty percent of normal neonates have CSPs; a CV is seen in 30% of term infants. Both CSP and CVs shrink and eventually disappear after birth. A persistent CSP is present in 2% to 4% of normal adults[51] and is seen on imaging studies as a CSF-filled collection that is contained between the two septal leaves (Fig. 12-33, *B*). A CV appears as a posterior extension of a CSP. CV never occurs without a CSP. On imaging studies a CV is seen as a fingerlike CSF collection that lies in the mid-

Intraventricular Masses in Adults

Lateral ventricles

Frontal horn
Astrocytoma (anaplastic, glioblastoma)
Giant cell astrocytoma
Central neurocytoma
Subependymoma
Cavum septi pellucidi and cavum vergae
Body
Astrocytoma
Central neurocytoma
Oligodendroglioma
Subependymoma
Atrium
Choroid plexus cysts/xanthogranulomas
Meningioma
Metastases
Occipital and temporal horns (rare)
Meningioma
Enlarged calcified choroid plexus with NF-2

Foramen of Monro/third ventricle

Foramen of Monro
Astrocytoma (anaplastic, glioblastoma)
Central neurocytoma
Oligodendroglioma
Subependymal giant cell astrocytoma
Third ventricle
Colloid cyst
Extrinsic mass (pituitary adenoma, aneurysm, glioma)
Sarcoid, germinoma (anterior recesses/hypothalamus/
    infundibular stalk)

Aqueduct/fourth ventricle

Aqueduct
Hemorrhage
Midbrain glioma
Metastasis
Fourth ventricle
Metastasis
Hemangioblastoma
Exophytic brainstem glioma
Subependymoma

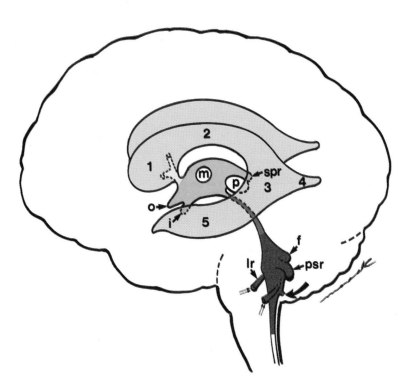

Fig. 12-31. Anatomic diagram depicts the brain ventricular system: *Green,* Lateral ventricles. *1,* Frontal horn. *2,* Body. *3,* Atrium. *4,* Occipital horn. *5,* Temporal horn. *Yellow,* Foramen of Monro. *Blue,* Third ventricle with pineal gland *(p),* massa intermedia *(m),* suprapineal recess *(spr),* and optic *(o)* and infundibular recesses *(i). Orange,* Aqueduct. *Red,* Fourth ventricle with fastigium *(f),* posterosuperior recesses *(psr),* and lateral recesses *(lr).* Foramen of Magendie *(curved arrow).* Foramina of Luschka *(double arrows).*

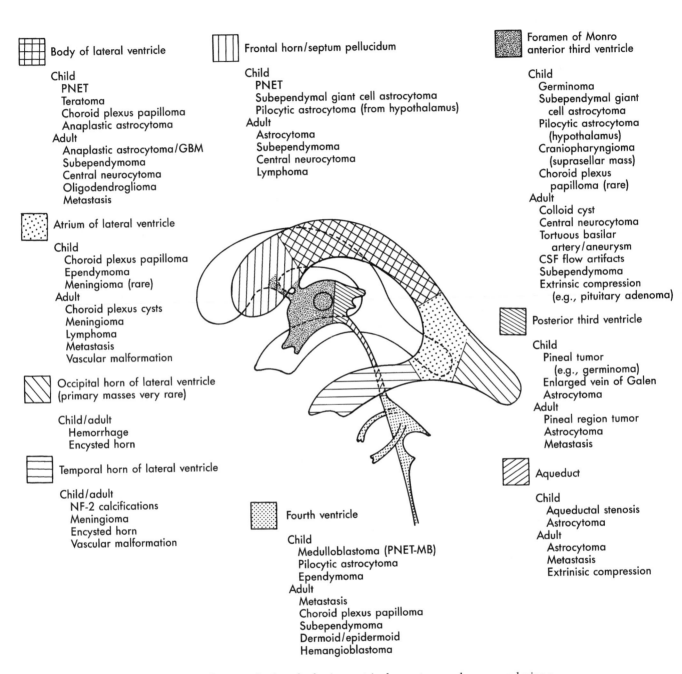

Body of lateral ventricle

Child
  PNET
  Teratoma
  Choroid plexus papilloma
  Anaplastic astrocytoma
Adult
  Anaplastic astrocytoma/GBM
  Subependymoma
  Central neurocytoma
  Oligodendroglioma
  Metastasis

Atrium of lateral ventricle

Child
  Choroid plexus papilloma
  Ependymoma
  Meningioma (rare)
Adult
  Choroid plexus cysts
  Meningioma
  Lymphoma
  Metastasis
  Vascular malformation

Occipital horn of lateral ventricle
(primary masses very rare)

Child/adult
  Hemorrhage
  Encysted horn

Temporal horn of lateral ventricle

Child/adult
  NF-2 calcifications
  Meningioma
  Encysted horn
  Vascular malformation

Frontal horn/septum pellucidum

Child
  PNET
  Subependymal giant cell astrocytoma
  Pilocytic astrocytoma (from hypothalamus)
Adult
  Astrocytoma
  Subependymoma
  Central neurocytoma
  Lymphoma

Fourth ventricle

Child
  Medulloblastoma (PNET-MB)
  Pilocytic astrocytoma
  Ependymoma
Adult
  Metastasis
  Choroid plexus papilloma
  Subependymoma
  Dermoid/epidermoid
  Hemangioblastoma

Foramen of Monro
anterior third ventricle

Child
  Germinoma
  Subependymal giant
    cell astrocytoma
  Pilocytic astrocytoma
    (hypothalamus)
  Craniopharyngioma
    (suprasellar mass)
  Choroid plexus
    papilloma (rare)
Adult
  Colloid cyst
  Central neurocytoma
  Tortuous basilar
    artery/aneurysm
  CSF flow artifacts
  Subependymoma
  Extrinsic compression
    (e.g., pituitary adenoma)

Posterior third ventricle

Child
  Pineal tumor
    (e.g., germinoma)
  Enlarged vein of Galen
  Astrocytoma
Adult
  Pineal region tumor
  Astrocytoma
  Metastasis

Aqueduct

Child
  Aqueductal stenosis
  Astrocytoma
Adult
  Astrocytoma
  Metastasis
  Extrinisic compression

Fig. 12-32. Anatomic diagram depicts the brain ventricular system and common lesions encountered in each specific location.

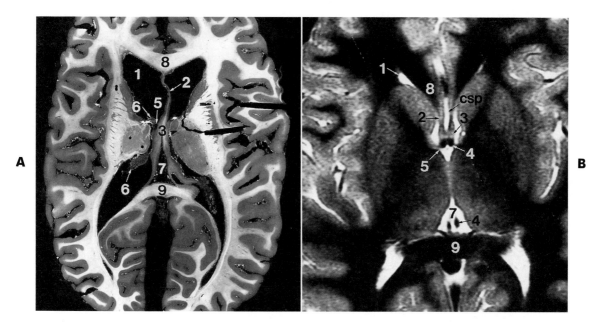

Fig. 12-33. A, Axial cut brain section through the lateral ventricles and foramen of Monro. **B,** Axial T2-weighted MR scan through the frontal horns shows foramen of Monro anatomy: *1,* Frontal horns. *2,* Septum pellucidum. *3,* Pillars of fornix. *4,* Internal cerebral veins. *5,* Foramen of Monro. *6,* Choroid plexus. *7,* Velum interpositum. *8,* Corpus callosum genu. *9,* Corpus callosum splenium. B, A small cavum septi pellucidi (csp) is shown. (**A,** Courtesy Yakovlev Collection, Armed Forces Institute of Pathology.)

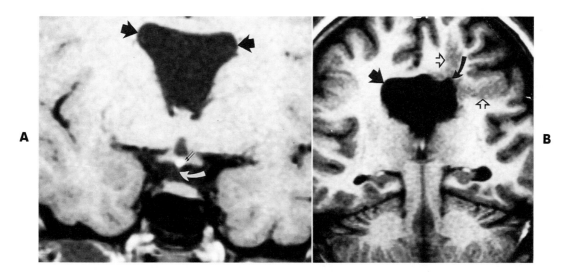

Fig. 12-34. Congenital anomalies of the septum pellucidum are illustrated in three cases. **A,** An 8-year-old child who has had panhypopituitarism since birth. Coronal T1-weighted MR scan shows absent septum pellucidum. The frontal horns of the lateral ventricle have a "squared-off" appearance *(large black arrows).* The posterior pituitary gland is ectopically located in the hypothalamus *(double arrows),* and the infundibular stalk is extremely small *(curved, white arrow).* **B,** A 20-year-old patient with seizures. Coronal T1-weighted MR scan shows absent septum pellucidum, the "nipple" of a schizencephalic cleft *(curved arrow)* and heterotopic gray matter *(open arrows).* Note "squared-off" appearance of the frontal horns *(large black arrow).*   *Continued.*

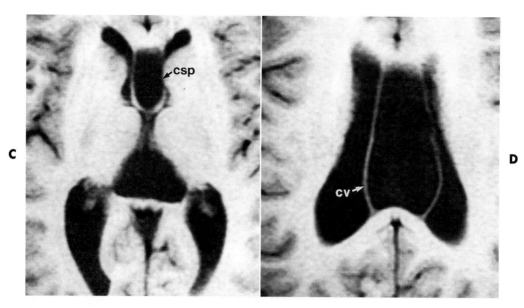

Fig.12-34, cont'd. C and **D,** Axial T1-weighted MR scans show a cavum septi pellucidi *(csp)* and vergae *(cv).*

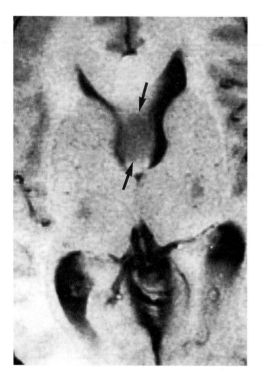

Fig. 12-35. Axial T1-weighted MR scan shows a slightly hypointense mass in the septum pellucidum *(arrows).* Infiltrating low-grade astrocytoma.

line below the corpus callosum and between the fornices (Fig. 12-34, *C* and *D*).

Primary septal neoplasms are uncommon. In the absence of a CSP, a septum pellucidum that is thicker than 3 mm is suspicious for infiltrating neoplasm. The most common primary septal tumor is *astrocytoma* (Fig. 12-35). Other neoplasms in this region include *lymphoma* (Fig. 12-36) and *germinoma* (Fig. 12-37). Dysplastic thickening can sometimes be seen in NF-1.

Most frontal horn masses actually arise from adjacent structures, i.e., the head of the caudate nucleus, septum pellucidum, or foramen of Monro (see subsequent discussion). Intraventricular extension of anaplastic astrocytoma is an example. Other tumors with a strong predilection for the septum pellucidum or frontal horn include *central neurocytoma, subependymoma,* and *giant cell astrocytoma* (Fig. 12-38).[53]

Body. In children younger than 5 or 6 years of age,

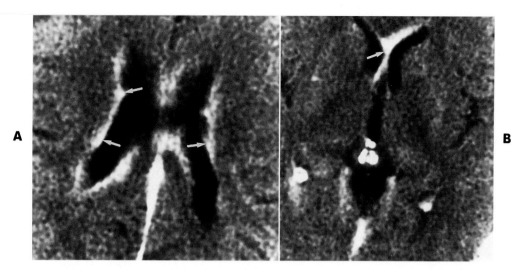

Fig. 12-36. CNS lymphoma. Axial CECT scans show extensive subependymal enhancing tumor along the lateral ventricular walls and septum pellucidum *(arrows)*.

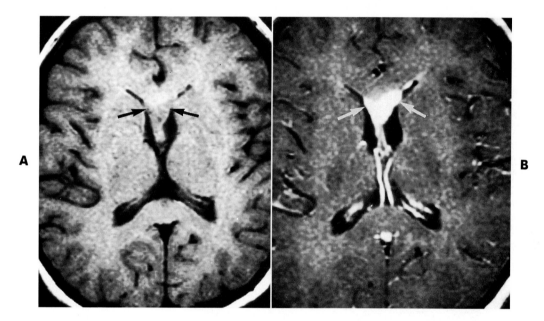

Fig. 12-37. Axial pre- **(A)** and postcontrast **(B)** T1-weighted MR scans show thickened, enhancing septum pellucidum *(arrows)*. Germinoma.

Fig. 12-38. Tumors at the foramen of Monro, septum pellucidum, and frontal horns are illustrated. **A,** Coronal gross pathology specimen of incidental subependymoma found at autopsy. (**A,** Courtesy Rubenstein Collection, University of Virginia.)

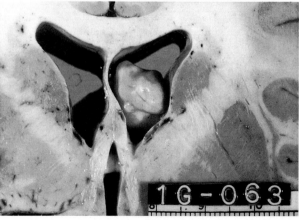

Continued.

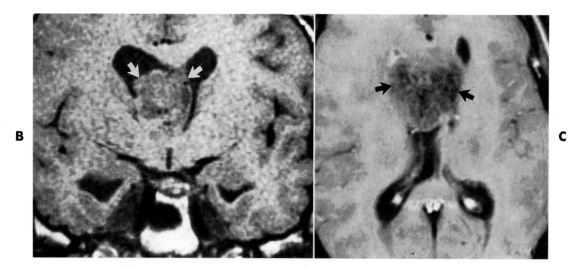

Fig. 12-38, cont'd.   **B,** Coronal T1-weighted MR scan in a patient with tuberous sclerosis shows a mixed iso- and hypointense mass at the foramen of Monro *(arrows).* Subependymal giant cell astrocytoma. **C,** Axial postcontrast T1-weighted MR scan in another patient with a central neurocytoma *(arrows).* (**C,** Courtesy D. Baleriaux.)

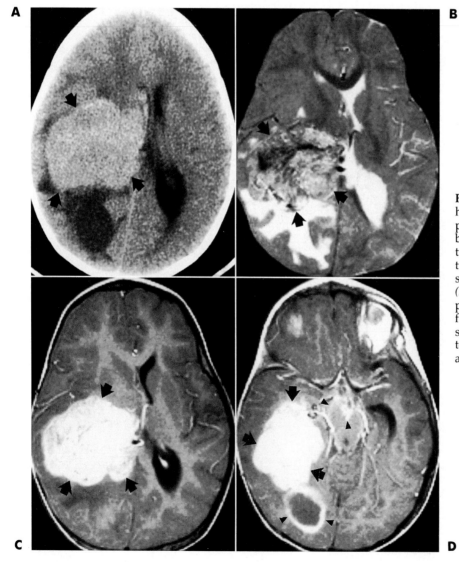

Fig. 12-39. Newborn infant with large head. **A,** Axial NECT shows a large hyperdense mass *(arrows)* that occupies the body and atrium of the right lateral ventricle. Axial T2-weighted (**B**) and postcontrast T1WI (**C** and **D**) MR scans show a strongly enhancing mixed signal mass *(large arrows)* that has trapped the temporal and occipital horns. Note diffuse ependymal and subarachnoid tumor spread *(arrowheads).* Anaplastic astrocytoma with widespread leptomeningeal and ependymal metastases.

lateral ventricular masses that are located primarily in the body include *primitive neuroectodermal tumor (PNET), teratoma,* and *astrocytoma* (usually anaplastic astrocytoma or glioblastoma multiforme) (Fig. 12-39). In older children and young adults, astrocytoma is the most common neoplasm in this location.

Two tumors that are often found in the lateral ventricle body are *central neurocytoma* and *oligodendroglioma.* They are usually seen in patients between 20 and 40 years of age.[53] *Ependymomas* occasionally oc-

cur in this location, although most supratentorial ependymomas are extraventricular (*see* Chapter 13). Lateral ventricular masses in older patients are *astrocytoma* (usually higher-grade tumors), *oligodendroglioma, meningioma, lymphoma, metastases,* and *subependymoma.*

Atrium. *Choroid plexus papilloma* (CPP) is the most common trigone mass in young children (Fig. 12-40). *Ependymomas* and *astrocytomas* occur in older children (Fig. 12-41). *Meningioma, metastasis* (Fig. 12-42), and

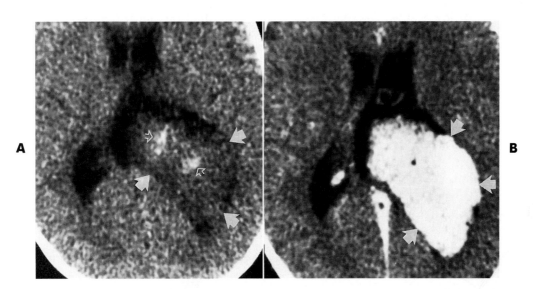

Fig. 12-40. Axial pre- **(A)** and postcontrast **(B)** CT scans in a 1-year-old child with delayed development show a large soft tissue mass in the atrium of the left lateral ventricle. **A,** The mostly isodense mass *(large arrows)* has some internal calcifications *(open arrows).* **B,** The mass *(arrows)* enhances strongly and uniformly after contrast administration. Some slight surface lobulation is apparent, caused by CSF trapped between the fronds of this classic choroid plexus papilloma.

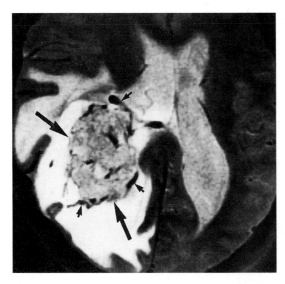

Fig. 12-41. Axial T2-weighted MR scan of an ependymoma in the atrium of the right lateral ventricle shows a large mixed signal mass *(large arrows)* with prominent foci of high-velocity signal loss *(small arrows)* caused by tumor vascularity.

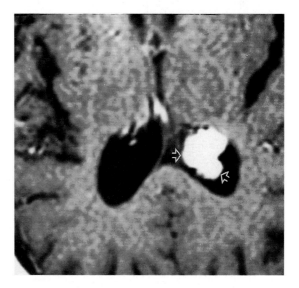

Fig. 12-42. Axial CECT scan in a 74-year-old man with renal carcinoma shows an enhancing mass in the choroid glomus *(arrows).* Metastatic carcinoma was found at surgery.

lymphoma are typical lesions in older adults.[54] Vascular malformations can be seen at any age.[55]

Choroid plexus cysts are nonneoplastic epithelial-lined cysts that usually occur within the glomus (Fig. 12-43, *A*). Most are bilateral and are found incidentally in neonates and older adults.[56,57] Most appear isointense with CSF on T1-weighted MR scans but slightly hyperintense on long TR/short TE sequences (Fig. 12-43, *B* to *D*). *Xanthogranulomas* are benign choroid plexus masses composed of large foam-filled cells with clusters of lymphocytes and macrophages. They are usually bilateral and typically occur in older adults. Occasionally, they can be seen in children and may attain strikingly large size.[58]

Occipital and temporal horns. Primary intraventricular masses are very uncommon in the occipital horn. Occasionally, meningiomas occur here (*see* Chapter 14). The temporal horn choroid plexus is sometimes enlarged and calcified in patients with neurofibromatosis type 2 (Fig. 12-44). The temporal and occipital horns may become trapped and encysted by neoplasms in the atrium or adjacent brain parenchyma (Fig. 12-45).

Foramen of Monro and anterior third ventricle. The foramen of Monro (FM) is a Y-shaped structure that connects the two lateral ventricles with the third ventricle (Fig. 12-46). The FM is bordered rostrally and anteriorly by the columns of the fornix. Its posterolateral margins are demarcated by choroid plexus and confluence of the septal, anterior caudate, terminal, and choroidal veins. The roof of the anterior third ventricle is formed by the fornix, tela choroidea, and internal cerebral veins. It normally has a smooth, upwardly convex configuration.[59]

FM masses are uncommon in young children. *Subependymal giant cell astrocytoma* (SGCA) occurs in older children and young adults with tuberous scle-

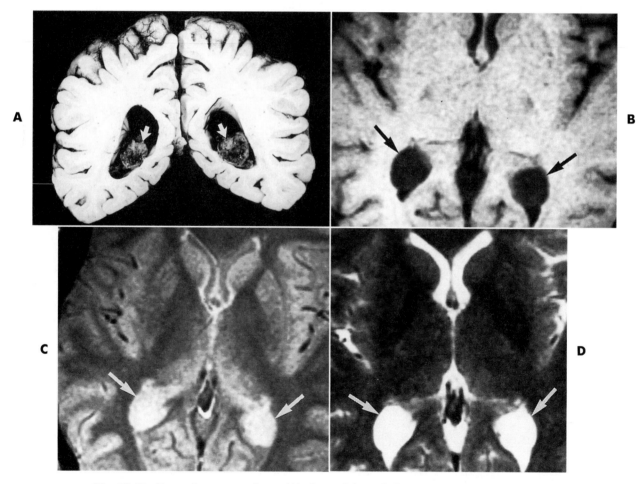

Fig. 12-43. Coronal gross specimen **(A)** shows bilateral choroid plexus xanthogranulomatous cysts *(arrows)*, found incidentally at autopsy. Axial T1- **(B)**, proton density **(C)**, and T2-weighted **(D)** MR scans in another patient show bilateral choroid plexus cysts *(arrows).* The cysts are slightly hyperintense to CSF on all sequences. (**A**, From Okazaki H, Scheithauer B: *Slide Atlas of Neuropathology,* Gower Medical Publishing, 1988. With permission.)

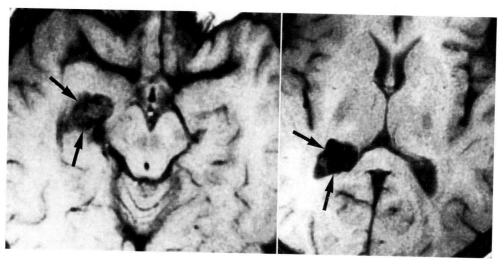

Fig. 12-44. Axial T1-weighted MR scans in a patient with neurofibromatosis type 2 (NF-2) show enlarged, partially calcified choroid *(arrows)* in the temporal horn and atrium of the right lateral ventricle.

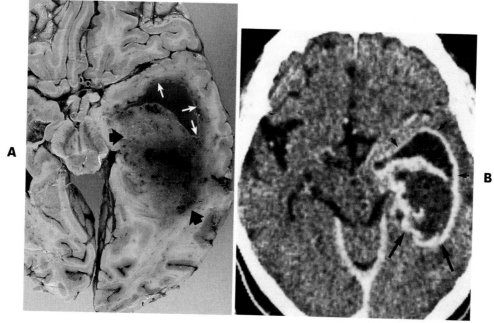

Fig. 12-45. A, Gross autopsy specimen of a glioblastoma multiforme shows a large, necrotic, hemorrhage mass *(large arrows)* has trapped the temporal horn. The enlarged temporal horn shows abnormally thickened ependyma *(small arrows).* **B,** Axial CECT shows the tumor mass *(large arrows)* with ependymal enhancement *(small arrows)* around the encysted temporal horn. (Courtesy D. Baleriaux and J. Flament-Durand.)

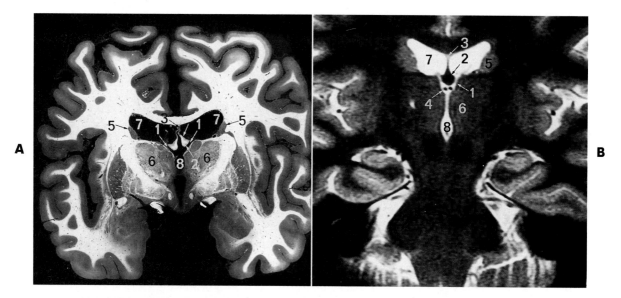

Fig. 12-46. A, Coronal gross specimen shows the foramen of Monro and adjacent structures. **B,** Coronal T2-weighted MR scan shows normal foramen of Monro anatomy: *1,* Foramen of Monro. *2,* Pillars of fornix. *3,* Septum pellucidum. *4,* Internal cerebral veins. *5,* Caudate nuclei. *6,* Thalami. *7,* Frontal horns of lateral ventricles. *8,* Third ventricle. (**A,** Courtesy Yakovlev Collection, Armed Forces Institute of Pathology.)

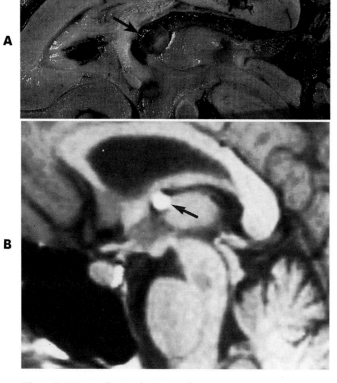

Fig. 12-47. A, Sagittal view of gross autopsy specimen with an incidental colloid cyst *(arrow)* at the foramen of Monro. **B,** Sagittal T1-weighted MR scan in a patient with headaches shows a focal high signal mass *(arrow)* at the foramen of Monro. A small colloid cyst was surgically removed. (**A,** Courtesy E. Tessa Hedley-Whyte.)

rosis. *Pilocytic astrocytoma* also occurs in this age group. *Subependymoma* and *central neurocytoma* occur in adults (see preceding discussion).

Anterior third ventricle. *Colloid cysts* are the most common mass in this location (Fig. 12-47).[59] These lesions are common in adults but rare in children. Colloid cysts have a variable imaging appearance that depends on their contents (*see* Chapter 15).[60] Turbulent CSF flow can produce a "pseudotumor" in this location (Fig. 12-48). Occasionally an extremely elongated, ectatic basilar artery or basilar tip aneurysm is seen as a foramen of Monro mass (Fig. 12-49).

Primary third ventricular neoplasms are rare at any age; most are *astrocytomas* that arise from the floor (Fig. 12-50), or tela choroidea, of the third ventricle. The vast majority of neoplasms that involve the third ventricle originate in adjacent structures and affect the third ventricle by direct extension. In children, craniopharyngioma and hypothalamic astrocytoma are the two most common tumors in this location.[61] *Germinoma* may involve the anterior third ventricular recesses. Suprasellar germinomas usually—but not always—occur with a synchronous pineal tumor (Fig. 12-7) and often involve the infundibular stalk as well.[31] Ten percent of *choroid plexus papillomas* are located within the third ventricle; almost all occur in children under 5 years of age (Fig. 12-13).

In adults, third ventricular masses are also usually secondary to extraventricular lesions. The third ventricle is often elevated and compressed by suprasel-

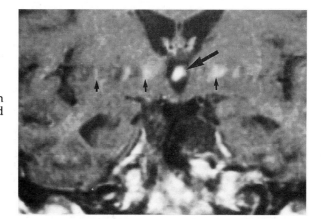

Fig. 12-48. Coronal postcontrast T1-weighted MR scan shows a foramen of Monro pseudomass *(large arrow)* caused by pulsatile flow (note phase artifact *[small arrows]*).

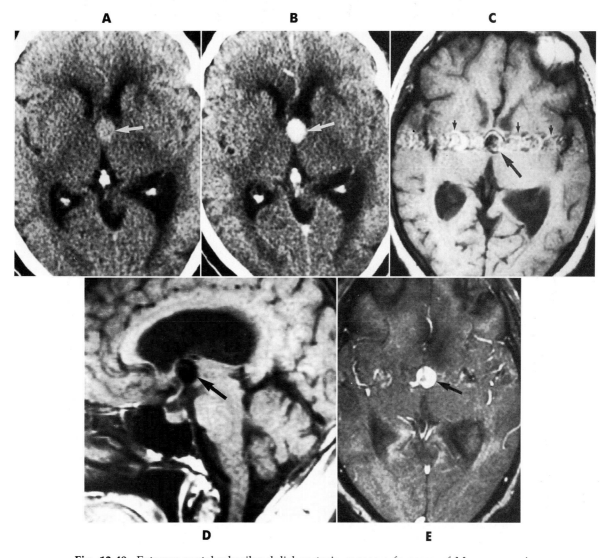

Fig. 12-49. Extreme vertebrobasilar dolichoectasia causes a foramen of Monro mass in this elderly patient. Axial CT scan **(A)** without contrast enhancement shows a hyperdense mass *(arrow)* at the foramen of Monro. CECT scan **(B)** shows a sharply delineated, strongly enhancing mass *(arrows)*. Axial **(C)** and sagittal **(D)** T1-weighted MR scans show the high-velocity signal loss (flow void) *(large arrow)* in the ectatic basilar artery. Note phase artifact **(C,** *small arrows)*. Gradient-refocussed study **(E)** confirms flow in the mass *(arrow)*. **(A** and **B,** Courtesy E. Fulton.)

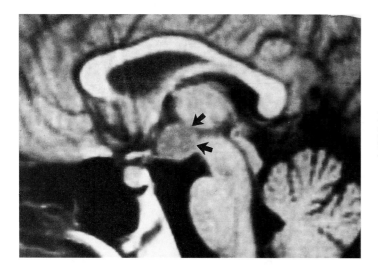

Fig. 12-50. Sagittal T1-weighted MR scan in this 12-year-old girl shows a mass *(arrows)* on the inferior floor of the third ventricle. Low-grade astrocytoma was found at surgery.

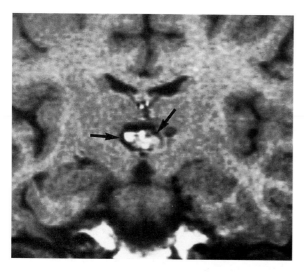

Fig. 12-51. Coronal T1-weighted MR scan shows a mixed signal mass *(arrows)* within the third ventricle. This "popcornlike" appearance is typical for cavernous angioma.

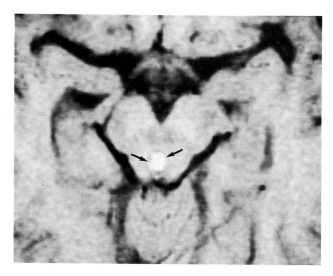

Fig. 12-52. Axial T1-weighted MR scan shows subacute hemorrhage *(arrows)* within the cerebral aqueduct.

lar extension of a *pituitary adenoma,* diaphragma sellae *meningioma,* giant *aneurysm,* or *craniopharyngioma.* Other masses that involve the third ventricule include thalamic anaplastic *astrocytoma* or glioblastoma multiforme. *Metastases* and *lymphoma* involve the anterior recesses, hypothalamus, and, often, the infundibular stalk.

Primary third ventricle tumors in adults are rare. A third ventricle meningioma can arise either from choroid plexus stromal cells or from the tela choroidea. Very rarely a pituitary adenoma is found entirely within the third ventricle.

Examples of nonneoplastic masses in the anteroinferior third ventricle are *histiocytosis* in children and *sarcoidosis* in adults (see subsequent discussion). *Vascular malformations* (Fig. 12-51) and *cysts* (glioependymal, choroid, or inflammatory cysts) are also sometimes found in the third ventricle.[62]

Aqueduct. The cerebral aqueduct (of Sylvius) communicates anterosuperiorly with the third ventricle and posteroinferiorly with the fourth ventricle. It is bordered posteriorly by the tectum (quadrigeminal plate) and anteriorly by the periaqueductal gray matter of the midbrain (tegmentum).

Stenosis is the most common intrinsic aqueductal abnormality. *Congenital stenosis* often results in severe obstructive hydrocephalus. Acquired aqueductal stenosis is caused by midbrain tumors such as *astrocytoma* or *metastasis.* *Ependymitis* and *intraventricular hemorrhage* sometimes obstruct the aqueduct[47] (Fig. 12-52).

Fourth ventricle. Primary fourth ventricular neoplasms are common in children but rare in adults.

Pediatric tumors. *Cerebellar astrocytomas* are the most common posterior fossa tumor in children[63] and

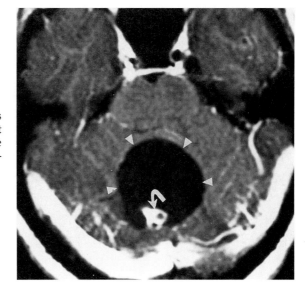

Fig. 12-53. Axial postcontrast T1-weighted MR scan shows a cystic astrocytoma of the vermis. The nonneoplastic cyst wall *(arrowheads)* does not enhance; the mural nodule *(curved arrow)* shows strong but heterogeneous enhancement.

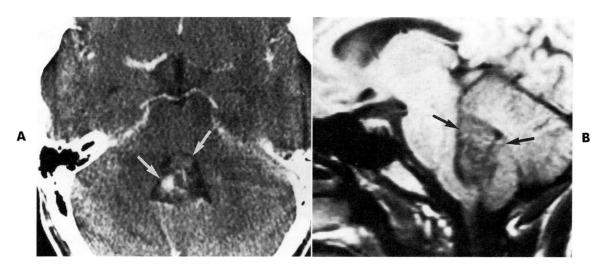

Fig. 12-54. Pilocytic astrocytoma of the fourth ventricle *(arrows)* is shown on **(A)** axial CECT and **(B)** sagittal T1-weighted MR scans.

account for about one quarter of all fourth ventricular tumors in this age group.[64] Most cerebellar astrocytomas are the pilocytic type. The most common appearance is that of a large cystic mass with a mural nodule.[21] Cerebellar astrocytomas usually originate from the vermis and extend anteriorly into the fourth ventricle (Fig. 12-53), although occasionally entirely intraventricular tumors are seen (Fig. 12-54).

Medulloblastoma (posterior fossa primitive neuroectodermal tumor or PNET-MB) is the second most common posterior fossa tumor in children, accounting for 25% of all intracranial tumors in this age group.[21] Ninety percent of PNET-MBs are midline posterior fossa tumors that originate in the inferior vermis and fill the fourth ventricle (Fig. 12-55).[10] Subarachnoid dissemination is common (*see* Chapter 14).

Ependymomas account for about 10% of all pediatric brain tumors and are the third most common fourth ventricular neoplasm in children.[64] Ependymomas arise in the ependymal lining of the fourth ventricle and extend into the lateral recesses and through the foramina of Luschka into the cerebellopontine angle cisterns (*see* Fig. 13-51, *A*). Posteroinferior extension through the foramen of Magendie into the cisterna magna is also common (*see* Fig. 12-95).

The fourth most common posterior fossa mass in children is *brainstem glioma*.[63] About one quarter are low-grade medullary astrocytomas with a dorsal exophytic component that grows posteriorly into the fourth ventricle.[20]

Other than medulloblastoma, ependymoma, and astrocytoma, fourth ventricular tumors in children

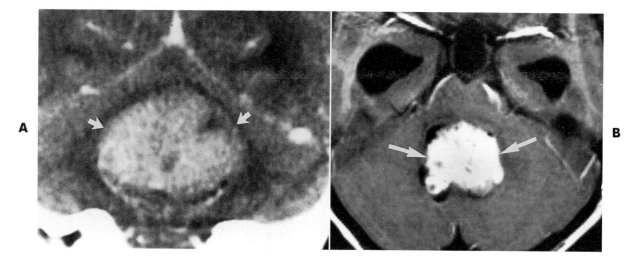

Fig. 12-55. A, Coronal postcontrast CT scan shows a classic medulloblastoma *(arrows)*. The midline posterior fossa mass enhances strongly but somewhat inhomogeneously. **B,** Axial postcontrast T1-weighted MR scan in this 4-year-old child shows a lobulated, strongly enhancing mass in the fourth ventricle *(arrows)*. Ependymoma.

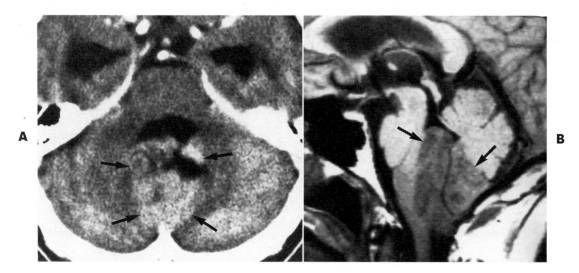

Fig. 12-56. A 54-year-old man with known oat cell carcinoma had headaches, nausea, and vomiting. **A,** CECT scan shows a mildly enhancing lobulated mass in the fourth ventricle *(arrows)*. **B,** Sagittal T1-weighted MR scan shows the mass fills the fourth ventricle and extends posteriorly into the cisterna magna. No other CNS lesions were identified. Surgery disclosed metastatic oat cell carcinoma.

are rare. *Choroid plexus papilloma, ganglioglioma,* and *dermoid cyst* are uncommon tumors that can occur in this location.

Adult tumors. The most common fourth ventricular neoplasm in an adult is *metastasis* (Fig. 12-56). Primary intraaxial posterior fossa neoplasms in adults are rare.[23] *Hemangioblastoma* is the most frequent of these uncommon lesions. Most hemangioblastomas are located in the paramedian cerebellum, but large tumors can compress or distort the fourth ventricle.

Primary fourth ventricular tumors such as *choroid plexus papilloma, epidermoid,* or *dermoid* tumors are rare (Fig. 12-57). *Subependymomas* occur in the inferior fourth ventricle near the obex and are usually found incidentally in older patients *(see* Chapter 13).

Nonneoplastic masses. Inflammatory cysts, vascular malformations, and other benign lesions are occasionally seen within the fourth ventricle (Fig. 12-58).

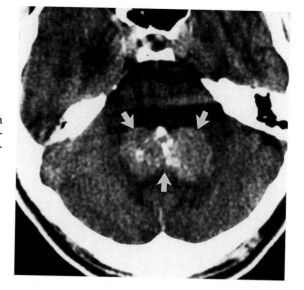

Fig. 12-57. Axial CECT scan in a 42-year-old patient with headaches shows a moderately enhancing, partially calcified fourth ventricular mass *(arrows)*. Choroid plexus papilloma was found at surgery.

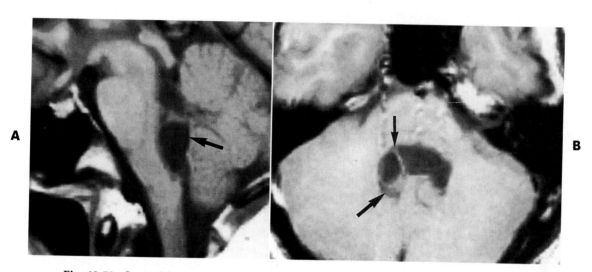

Fig. 12-58. Sagittal **(A)** and axial **(B)** T1-weighted MR scans show a cystic fourth ventricular mass *(arrows)*. Intraventricular cysticercosis cyst was found at surgery. (Courtesy C. Sutton.)

Cerebellopontine Angle Masses

Normal anatomy. The cerebellopontine angle (CPA) cistern lies between the anterolateral surface of the pons and cerebellum and the posterior surface of the petrous temporal bone (Fig. 12-59). Important structures within the CPA cistern include the fifth, seventh, and eighth cranial nerves, the superior and anterior inferior cerebellar arteries, and tributaries of the superior petrosal veins.[65]

The trigeminal nerve (CN V) arises from the middle of the pons at the cerebellopontine angle and courses anteriorly through the superolateral aspect of the cistern. The facial (CN VIII) and vestibulocochlear (CN VIII) nerves arise in the inferior part of the cistern and course laterally across the CPA cistern into the internal auditory canal. The flocculus, a lobe of the cerebellar hemisphere, projects into the CPA cistern behind the seventh and eighth cranial nerves.

The superior and anterior inferior cerebellar arteries arise from the basilar artery and course posterolaterally through the CPA cistern *(see* Chapter 6). Veins from the pons, middle cerebellar peduncle, and cerebellopontine fissure unite near the trigeminal nerve and form the superior petrosal veins.[65]

Lesions in the CPA cistern can arise from the brain, temporal bone, or subarachnoid space and its contents. The majority of CPA masses are located primarily in the cistern. Others arise within the internal auditory canal itself, and some originate in the adjacent brain or skull and extend into the CPA secondarily (Fig. 12-60).

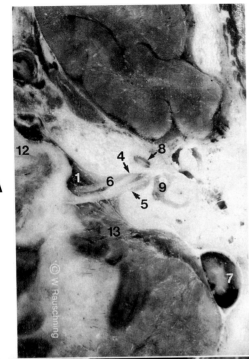

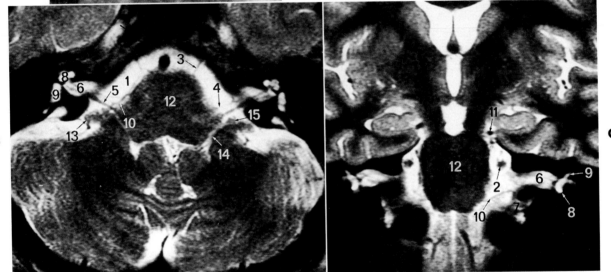

Fig. 12-59. Anatomy of the cerebellopontine angle is depicted. **A,** Axial cryomicrotome section through the cerebellopontine angle cistern and temporal bone. Axial **(B)** and coronal **(C)** T2-weighted MR scans are shown: *1,* Cerebellopontine angle cistern. *2,* CN V (trigeminal nerve). *3,* CN VI (abducens nerve). *4,* CN VII (facial nerve). *5,* CN VIII (vestibulocochlear nerve). *6,* Internal auditory canal. *7,* Jugular foramen. *8,* Cochlea. *9,* Vestibule, semicircular canals. *10,* Anterior inferior cerebellar artery. *11,* Petrosal veins. *12,* Pons. *13,* Flocculus of cerebellum. *14,* Lateral recess of fourth ventricle. *15,* Choroid plexus. (Courtesy W. Rauschning.)

Cerebellopontine Angle (CPA) Cistern Lesions
Imaging signs of extraaxial masses

Ipsilateral CPA cistern enlarged
CSF/vascular "cleft" between mass and cerebellum
Displaced gray-white matter interface around mass
Brainstem rotated
Fourth ventricle compressed (nonspecific)

Modified from Curnes JT: MR imaging of peripheral intracranial neoplasms: extraaxial versus intraaxial masses, *J Comp Asst Tomogr* 11:932-937, 1987.

Cerebellopontine angle (CPA) cistern masses. CPA masses are uncommon in children but very common in adults. The majority of CPA tumors in adults are extraaxial.[66] Imaging findings that distinguish extra- from intraaxial masses (*see* box) include the following:

1. Enlarged CPA cistern
2. A CSF "cleft" between the mass and adjacent brain
3. Brainstem rotation
4. Displaced cerebellar hemisphere cortex (Fig. 12-61).

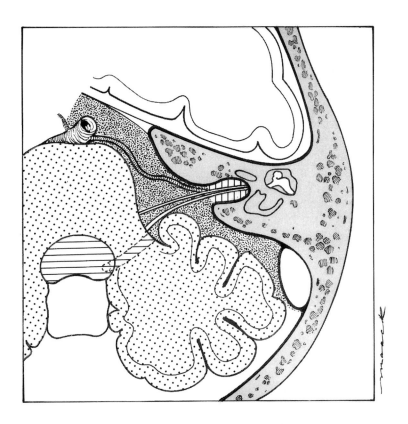

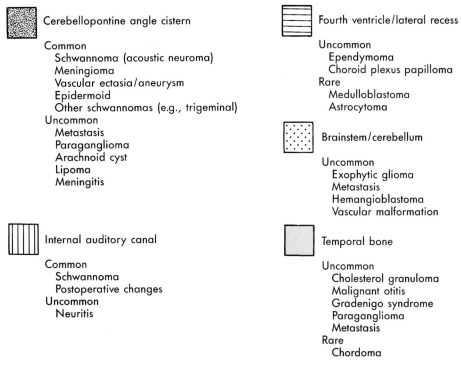

Cerebellopontine angle cistern

Common
  Schwannoma (acoustic neuroma)
  Meningioma
  Vascular ectasia/aneurysm
  Epidermoid
  Other schwannomas (e.g., trigeminal)
Uncommon
  Metastasis
  Paraganglioma
  Arachnoid cyst
  Lipoma
  Meningitis

Internal auditory canal

Common
  Schwannoma
  Postoperative changes
Uncommon
  Neuritis

Fourth ventricle/lateral recess

Uncommon
  Ependymoma
  Choroid plexus papilloma
Rare
  Medulloblastoma
  Astrocytoma

Brainstem/cerebellum

Uncommon
  Exophytic glioma
  Metastasis
  Hemangioblastoma
  Vascular malformation

Temporal bone

Uncommon
  Cholesterol granuloma
  Malignant otitis
  Gradenigo syndrome
  Paraganglioma
  Metastasis
Rare
  Chordoma

Fig. 12-60. Anatomic diagram depicts the cerebellopontine angle anatomy. Lesions that arise from each component are indicated.

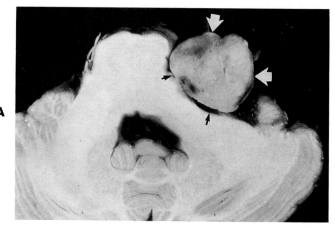

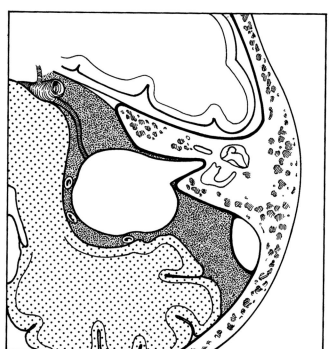

Fig. 12-61. Characteristic pathology and anatomy of the most common cerebellopontine angle (CPA) mass, vestibulocochlear schwannoma. **A,** Anatomic specimen shows a large CN VIII schwannoma *(large arrows)*. Note the "cleft" *(small arrows)* between the mass and the adjacent cerebellum. **B,** Anatomic diagram depicts the characteristic abnormalities seen with an extraaxial CPA mass: enlarged ipsilateral CSF cistern, CSF "cleft" between the mass and adjacent cerebellum, displaced or "buckled" cerebellar cortex, and brainstem rotation. (**A,** Courtesy E. Ross.)

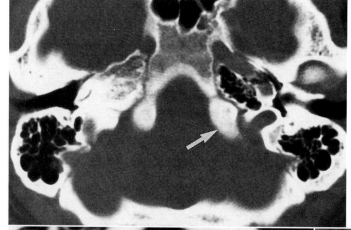

Fig. 12-62. "Pseudomasses" that can be mistaken for a CPA lesion. **A,** NECT scan with bone windows shows a prominent asymmetric jugular tubercle *(arrow)*. **B,** Normal choroid plexus on contrast-enhanced CT or MR *(arrows)*. **C,** Flocculus of the cerebellum. An incidental meningioma *(open arrows)* is seen on this T1-weighted MR scan. Floccular lobes *(curved arrows)*.

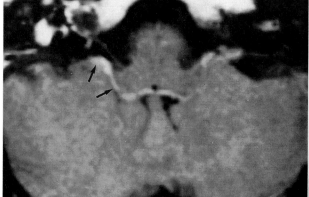

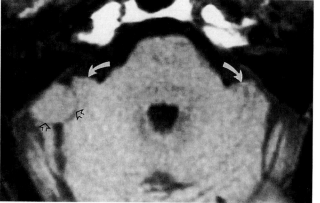

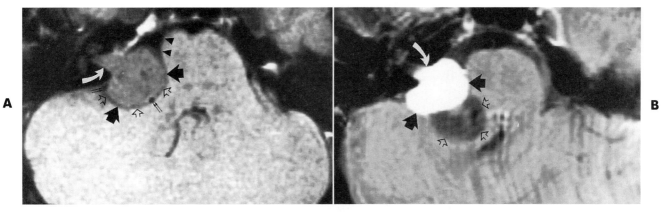

Fig. 12-63. Two patients with acoustic schwannomas. **A,** Axial unenhanced T1-weighted MR scan shows typical "ice cream cone" appearance of the schwannoma that consists of a larger CPA mass *(large black arrows)* and a smaller intracanalicular component *(curved white arrow)*. Note distinct CSF "cleft" *(open arrows)* between the extraaxial mass and the cerebellum. The ipsilateral CPA cistern is enlarged *(arrowheads)*. Note vessels *(double arrows)* displaced around the mass. **B,** Postcontrast axial T1WI in another patient shows the typical strongly enhancing CPA mass *(large black arrows)* with a small intracanalicular component *(curved white arrow)*. The mass has an associated cyst *(open arrows)*, either necrotic tumor or arachnoid with trapped CSF. Cystic acoustic neuroma was confirmed at surgery. (Courtesy H.R. Harnsberger. Reprinted from Swartz JD, Harnsberger HR: *Imaging of the Temporal Bone,* ed 2, New York, Thieme, 1992. With permission).

Table 12-1. Cerebellopontine angle cistern masses

Frequency of mass	Type of mass	Percent (%)
Common	Acoustic schwannoma	75
	Meningioma	8 to 10
	Epidermoid	5
	Other schwannomas	2 to 5
	Vascular (vertebrobasilar ectasia, aneurysm, vascular malformation)	2 to 5
	Metastases	1 to 2
	Paraganglioma	1 to 2
	Ependymoma, choroid plexus papilloma (primary in CPA or extension from fourth ventricle)	1
Uncommon		=/<1
	Arachnoid cyst	
	Lipoma	
	Dermoid	
	Exophytic cerebellar/brainstem astrocytoma	
	Chordoma	
	Osteocartilagenous tumors	

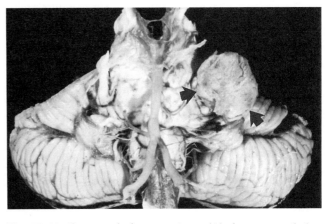

Fig. 12-64. Gross pathology specimen **(A)** shows a cerebellopontine angle meningioma *(arrows)*. (Courtesy E. Tessa Hedley-Whyte.) *Continued.*

Normal structures and anatomic variants that can be mistaken for a CPA mass include the cerebellar flocculus, prominent choroid plexus at the foramen of Luschka, a high jugular bulb, and prominent jugular tubercles (Fig. 12-62).

Vestibulocochlear (acoustic) schwannoma is by far the most common CPA mass, accounting for at least three quarters of all lesions in this location (Table 12-1; Figs. 12-61, *A,* and 12-63). In distant second, third, and fourth places are *meningioma* (Fig. 12-64), *epidermoid* tumor (Fig. 12-65), and *other cranial nerve schwannomas* (Fig. 12-66) (trigeminal schwannoma is the most common nonacoustic schwannoma).[66]

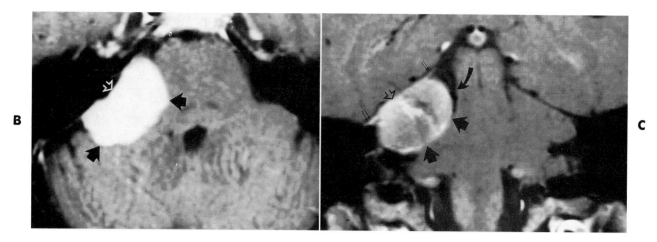

Fig. 12-64, cont'd. Axial **(B)** and coronal **(C)** contrast-enhanced MR scans in a 39-year-old man with right-side sensorineural hearing loss show a CPA meningioma *(large arrows)*. **C,** Note broad, flat base toward the dural surface *(open arrows)*. A subtle dural "tail" is present *(double arrows)*. The ipsilateral CPA cistern is widened *(curved arrow)*, indicating the mass is extraaxial.

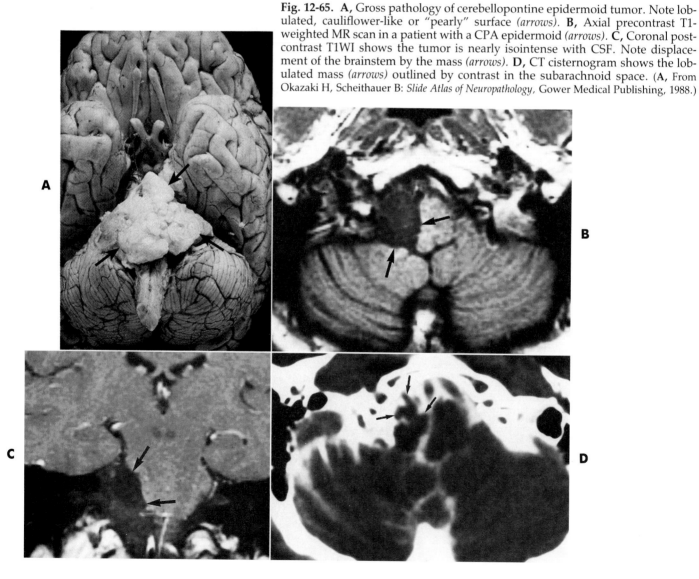

Fig. 12-65. A, Gross pathology of cerebellopontine epidermoid tumor. Note lobulated, cauliflower-like or "pearly" surface *(arrows)*. **B,** Axial precontrast T1-weighted MR scan in a patient with a CPA epidermoid *(arrows)*. **C,** Coronal post-contrast T1WI shows the tumor is nearly isointense with CSF. Note displacement of the brainstem by the mass *(arrows)*. **D,** CT cisternogram shows the lobulated mass *(arrows)* outlined by contrast in the subarachnoid space. (**A,** From Okazaki H, Scheithauer B: *Slide Atlas of Neuropathology,* Gower Medical Publishing, 1988.)

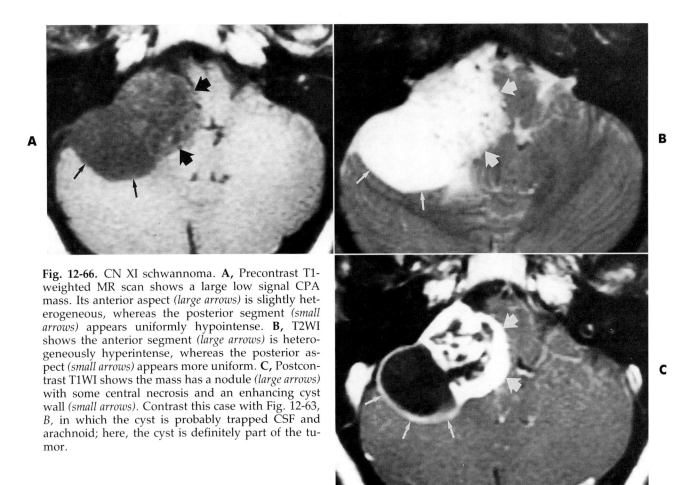

Fig. 12-66. CN XI schwannoma. **A,** Precontrast T1-weighted MR scan shows a large low signal CPA mass. Its anterior aspect *(large arrows)* is slightly heterogeneous, whereas the posterior segment *(small arrows)* appears uniformly hypointense. **B,** T2WI shows the anterior segment *(large arrows)* is heterogeneously hyperintense, whereas the posterior aspect *(small arrows)* appears more uniform. **C,** Postcontrast T1WI shows the mass has a nodule *(large arrows)* with some central necrosis and an enhancing cyst wall *(small arrows)*. Contrast this case with Fig. 12-63, *B,* in which the cyst is probably trapped CSF and arachnoid; here, the cyst is definitely part of the tumor.

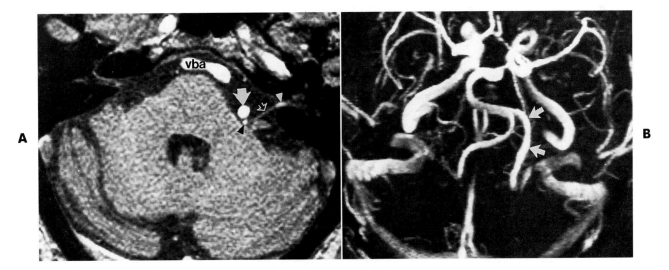

Fig. 12-67. A, Axial postcontrast T1-weighted MR scan shows a well-delineated, strongly enhancing mass *(large arrow)* adjacent to the left vestibulocochlear nerve *(open arrow)*. Smaller enhancing foci *(arrowheads)* are seen, probably representing anterior inferior cerebellar branches of this tortuous vertebrobasilar artery *(vba)*. **B,** Multiple overlapping thin-slab acquisition MR angiogram confirms the tortuous vertebrobasilar artery *(arrows)*.

Vascular lesions such as *vertebrobasilar dolichoectasia* (Fig. 12-67) and *aneurysm* (Fig. 12-68) account for 2% to 5% of CPA masses. *Metastases* account for 1% to 2% of CPA masses (Fig. 12-69). Metastases usually have multiple or bilateral cranial nerve and leptomeningeal lesions; coexisting parenchymal lesions are identified in 75% of these cases (Fig. 12-70).[67] The trigeminal nerve is a common site for perineural spread of head and neck malignancies such as adenoid cystic or squamous cell carcinoma. An enlarged nerve with irregular or nodular enhancement following contrast administration is seen in these cases (Fig. 12-71).[68,69]

Miscellaneous CPA masses include extension from fourth ventricular tumors such as *ependymoma* and *choroid plexus papilloma*, exophytic cerebellar and brainstem *gliomas* or *vascular malformations* (Fig. 12-72), and jugular foramen masses such as *paraganglioma*. Rarely, a choroid plexus papilloma originates within the CPA itself (Fig. 12-73).[70] *Arachnoid cyst, dermoid cyst, lipoma, hemangioma,* and *chordoma* are rare entities that occasionally cause a CPA mass (Fig. 12-74).

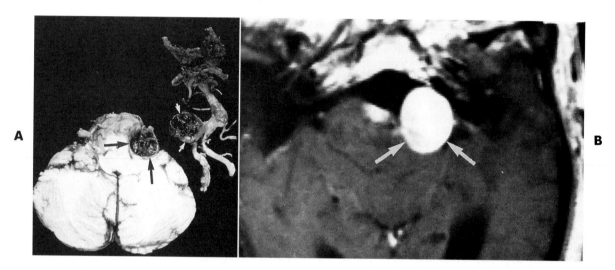

Fig. 12-68. A, Gross pathology specimen shows a CPA mass *(large arrows)* caused by a vertebral artery aneurysm *(small arrows)*. **B,** Axial postcontrast T1-weighted MR scan shows a left CPA mass from a patent aneurysm *(arrows)* with slow intravascular flow. (*A*, Courtesy E. Tessa Hedley-Whyte.)

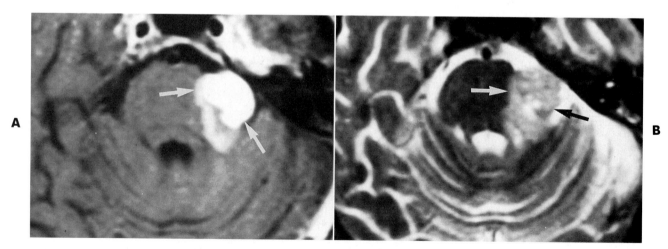

Fig. 12-69. Axial postcontrast T1- **(A)** and T2-weighted **(B)** MR scans in a 75-year-old patient with left-side sensorineural hearing loss. A nodular exophytic brainstem mass *(arrows)* is identified. The internal auditory canal is normal. Colon carcinoma metastasis. (Courtesy L. Tan.)

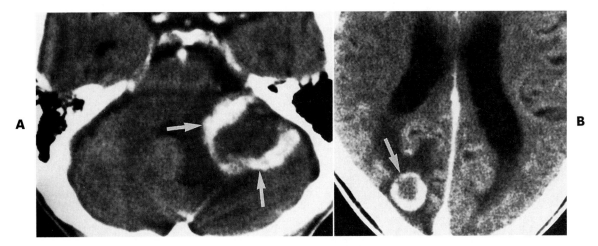

Fig. 12-70. A, Axial CECT scan shows a ring-enhancing left cerebellar hemisphere mass *(arrows)*. **B,** A second lesion *(arrow)* is present in the right occipital lobe. Metastatic carcinoma from unknown primary source was found at operation.

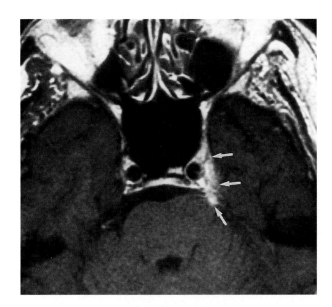

Fig. 12-71. Postcontrast T1-weighted MR scan in a patient with trigeminal neuralgia secondary to perineural tumor spread from malignant sinonasal carcinoma. Note nodular irregular enhancement along CN V *(arrows)* posteriorly into the root entry zone.

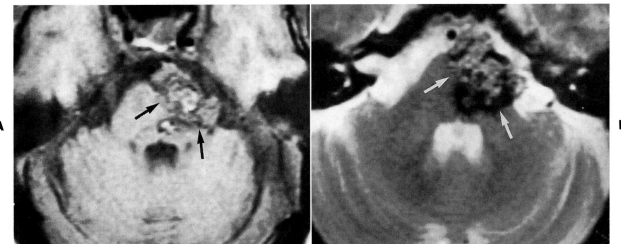

Fig. 12-72. A 51-year-old man has left facial and right extremity weakness. Axial T1- **(A)** and T2-weighted **(B)** MR scans show the mixed signal appearance of a typical cavernous angioma *(arrows)*. The mass is partially exophytic and extends anterolaterally into the CPA cistern.

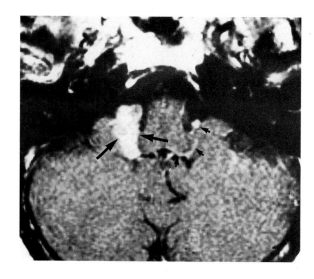

Fig. 12-73. A 37-year-old man has right CN IX to XI palsies. Postcontrast T1-weighted MR scan shows a strongly enhancing lobulated CPA mass *(large arrows)* located at the foramen of Luschka. Compare with normal choroid plexus *(small arrows).* Choroid plexus papilloma was found at surgery.

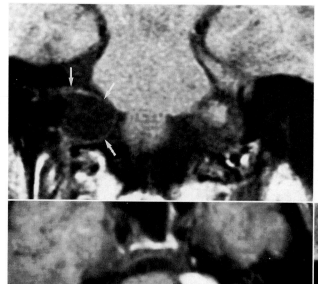

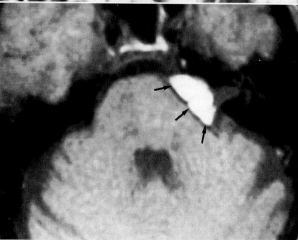

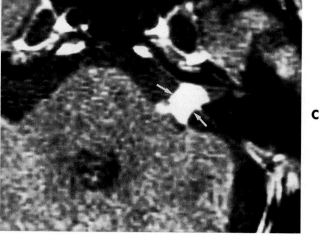

Fig. 12-74. Uncommon CPA masses illustrated by three cases. **A,** Coronal T1-weighted MR scan shows an arachnoid cyst *(arrows).* The cyst contents are similar to CSF; the wall is smooth. **B,** T1-weighted MR scan shows a high signal left CPA mass *(arrows).* The underlying internal auditory canal is normal. CNs VII and VIII course through the mass. Incidental lipoma. **C,** Axial postcontrast T1-weighted MR scan shows a lobulated, slightly irregular but strongly enhancing CPA mass *(arrows)* that partially extends into the internal auditory canal (IAC). Hemangioma.

Internal auditory canal and temporal bone masses

Internal auditory canal (IAC) masses (see box, p. 448, *top of page).* A small *acoustic schwannoma* is the most common intracanalicular mass (Fig. 12-75), followed by *postoperative reactive dural changes* (Fig. 12-76).[71] Facial schwannomas are rare. Occasionally, cerebellopontine angle *meningiomas* extend into the IAC. They can cause focal or diffuse enhancement within the IAC, possibly secondary to vascular stasis. In these cases, abnormal dural enhancement is always observed in other adjacent sites *(see* Fig. 14-28).[72] Rarely, a CP angle meningioma exhibits extensive calcification (Fig. 12-77).

Although facial nerve enhancement within the facial canal is normal, CN VII enhancement within the

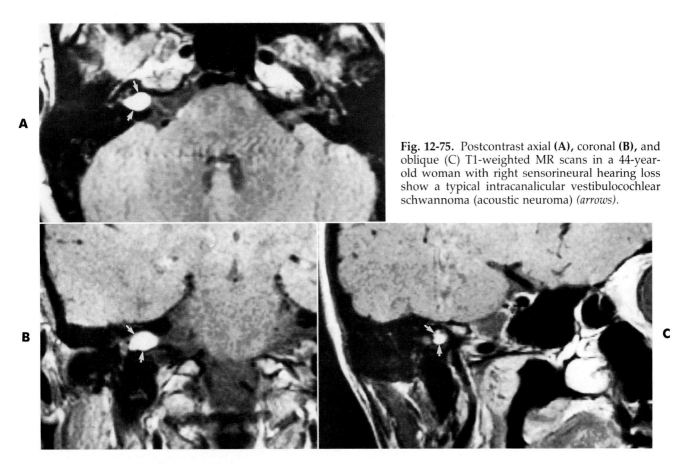

Fig. 12-75. Postcontrast axial **(A)**, coronal **(B)**, and oblique **(C)** T1-weighted MR scans in a 44-year-old woman with right sensorineural hearing loss show a typical intracanalicular vestibulocochlear schwannoma (acoustic neuroma) *(arrows).*

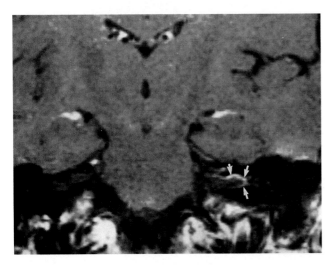

Fig. 12-76. Coronal postcontrast T1-weighted scan obtained 6 months after acoustic neuroma resection. Note enhancing dura in the internal auditory canal *(arrows).* This is a normal postoperative scan.

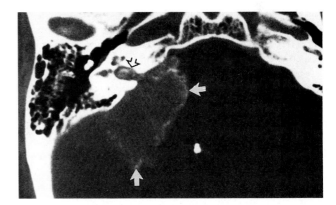

Fig. 12-77. Axial CT scan in a patient with a large, densely calcified right CPA meningioma *(white arrows)* shows the mass extends into the IAC *(open arrow).* (Courtesy HR Harnsberger. Reprinted from Swartz JD, Harnsberger HR: *Imaging of the Temporal Bone,* ed 2, New York, Thieme, 1992.)

Internal Auditory Canal Masses

Common

Intracanalicular acoustic schwannoma
Postoperative fibrosis

Uncommon

Neuritis (e.g., Bell's palsy, Ramsay Hunt syndrome)
Hemangioma
Lymphoma
Metastasis
Sarcoidosis
Meningioma

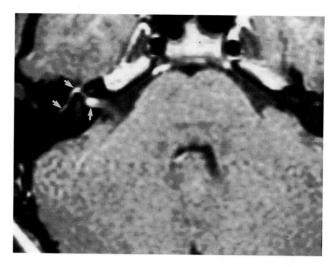

Fig. 12-78. A 10-year-old girl had a typical Bell's palsy. Contrast-enhanced T1-weighted MR scan shows enhancement along the intracanalicular, labyrinthine, and tympanic segments of the facial nerve *(arrows)*.

CPA cistern or IAC is not.[73] *Bell's palsy* (Fig. 12-78), *Ramsay Hunt syndrome* (herpes zoster otitis)[73a] (Fig. 12-79), and *viral infections* are benign conditions that can cause cranial nerve enlargement and enhancement.[74,75] *Lipoma, meningioma, hemangioma, lymphoma,* and nonneoplastic lesions such as *meningitis, postoperative fibrosis, sarcoidosis, hemorrhage, vascular loop, AVM,* or *aneurysm* can sometimes involve the IAC.[66,76,77] Some of these are among the many lesions other than acoustic neuroma that can cause sensorineural hearing loss.[78]

Temporal bone lesions. Primary temporal bone lesions that occasionally involve the CPA include Gradenigo's syndrome, malignant otitis, cholesterol granuloma, and paraganglioma (glomus tympanicum tumor) *(see box, right).*

Gradenigo's syndrome is osteomyelitis of the petrous apex with sixth nerve palsy, otorrhea, and retroorbital pain. NECT scans show a destructive lesion of the petrous apex with fluid in the adjacent middle ear and mastoid (Fig. 12-80).[79]

Malignant otitis externa is an uncommon but fulminant form of temporal bone osteomyelitis that is typically seen in insulin-dependent diabetics and immunocompromised patients. Extension into the parotid and masticator spaces, skull base, and occasionally the CPA cistern may occur (Fig. 12-81).[79]

Cholesterol granulomas, sometimes called giant cholesterol cysts, are expansile cystic lesions of the petrous apex that contain hemorrhage and cholesterol crystals. Cholesterol granulomas are hyperintense on both T1- and T2-weighted MR scans, unlike either cholesteatoma or epidermoid tumors (Fig. 12-82).[80] Other reported petrous apex masses include metastasis, petroclival meningioma, epidermoid tumors, off-axis chordomas, solitary plasmacytoma, paraganglioma, and mucocele.[81]

Paragangliomas are slowly growing hypervascular tumors that arise from neural crest cell derivates in many locations throughout the body.[82] Paraganglio-

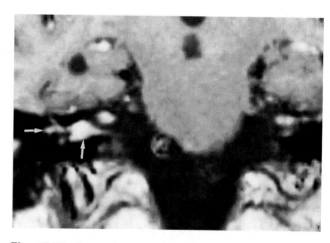

Fig. 12-79. Coronal contrast-enhanced T1-weighted MR scan in a patient with herpes zoster and Ramsay-Hunt syndrome shows a contrast-enhancing IAC and vestibular mass *(arrows).* (Courtesy of L. Hutchins.)

Temporal Bone Lesions that may Involve the Cerebellopontine Angle Cistern

Uncommon

Gradenigo's syndrome
Malignant external otitis
Cholesterol granuloma
Paraganglioma
Metastasis

Rare

Chordoma
Mucocele
Plasmacytoma

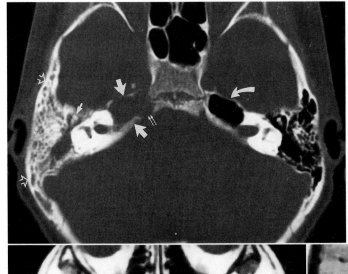

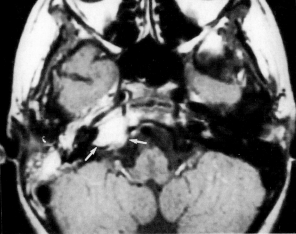

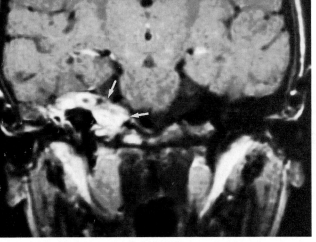

Fig. 12-80. A 6-year-old child with mastoiditis developed a right CN VI palsy. Axial NECT scan **(A)** shows complete opacification of the right mastoid *(open arrows)*. The middle ear cavity and mastoid antrum are also opacified, but the ossicles *(small single arrow)* are preserved. A destructive lesion of the right petrous apex is present *(large arrows)*, with involvement of the clivus and temporal bone perforation into the adjacent cerebellopontine angle cistern *(double arrows)*. Note the normal left temporal bone with large apex air cell *(curved arrow)*. Postcontrast axial **(B)** and coronal **(C)** T1-weighted MR scans show enhancing soft tissue in the mastoid, petrous apex, and cerebellopontine angle cistern *(arrows)*. Apical petrositis (Gradenigo's syndrome). (Courtesy H.R. Harnsberger. Reprinted from Swartz JD, Harnsberger HR: *Imaging of the Temporal Bone*, ed 2, New York, Thieme, 1992.)

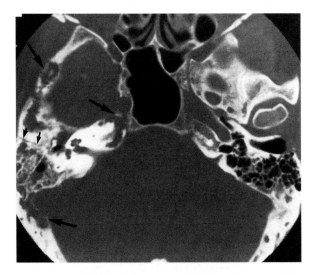

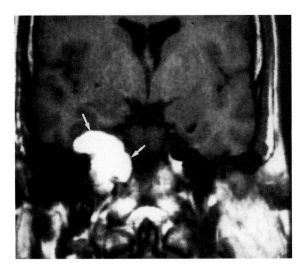

Fig. 12-81. Axial NECT scan. During long-term hospitalization this severely traumatized patient with multisystem injuries developed extensive skull base osteomyelitis *(large arrows)*, complicating a temporal bone fracture *(small arrows)*. Malignant external otitis was also present.

Fig. 12-82. Coronal T1-weighted MR scan shows a classic cholesterol cyst *(arrows)* of the petrous apex. The high signal mass extends into the adjacent cerebellopontine angle cistern. (Courtesy H.R. Harnsberger. Reprinted from Swartz JD, Harnsberger HR: *Imaging of the Temporal Bone*, ed 2, New York, Thieme, 1992.)

mas that are localized to the cochlear promontory in the middle ear cavity are termed *glomus tympanicum tumors*. Glomus jugulotympanicum tumors extend from the jugular foramen into the middle ear cavity. Large masses also extend into the CPA cistern (*see* Fig. 12-180). Paragangliomas are discussed in detail with posterior skull base masses (see subsequent discussion).

Intraaxial masses. *Metastasis* (Figs. 12-69 and 12-70), exophytic brainstem or cerebellar *astrocytoma*, and *hemangioblastoma* are intraaxial masses that may extend into or compress the CPA cistern. Fourth ventricular tumors such as *ependymoma* (Fig. 12-83) and *choroid plexus papilloma* often extend along the lateral recesses through the foramena of Luschka to involve the CPA cisterns (*see* box).

Differential diagnosis. Common CPA masses and their comparative imaging findings are summarized in Table 12-2.

Foramen Magnum Masses

Normal anatomy. The foramen magnum is a large aperture in the occipital bone through which the posterior fossa communicates with the cervical spinal canal. The foramen magnum transmits the medulla and its meninges, the spinal segment of CN XI (hypoglossal nerve), the two vertebral arteries, and the anterior and posterior spinal arteries and vertebral veins. The bony elements that contain these structures are collectively termed the *craniovertebral junction* (CVJ).

The CVJ is formed by the occiput and the C1 and C2 vertebrae (atlas and axis). Four joints are present between these three osseous components, as follows:
1. Atlantooccipital
2. Anterior median atlantoaxial
3. Posterior median atlantoaxial
4. Lateral atlantoaxial joints

Intraaxial Masses That May Involve the Cerebellopontine Angle Cistern

Common

Metastasis
Exophytic glioma

Uncommon

Hemangioblastoma
Extension from fourth ventricular neoplasm (ependymoma, choroid plexus papilloma)

Table 12-2. Comparative imaging findings of common CPA masses

| | MR (compared to brain) | | | | |
	T1	T2	Enhancement	Ca++	Other
Acoustic schwannoma	Hypo/iso	Hyper	Intense	Very rare	"Ice cream cone" appearance; bilateral in NF-2; large tumors may have cystic degeneration
Meningioma	Hypo/iso	Iso	Strong	Common	Broad dural base; dural "tail"; may cause hyperostosis; may extend into IAC and mimic schwannoma
Epidermoid	Iso to CSF	Iso/hyper to CSF	Rare	Rare	Insinuates along CSF cisterns
Other schwannoma	Hypo/iso	Hyper	Strong	Very rare	CNV most common
Vascular (VBD, aneurysm)	Varies	Varies	Varies	Frequent	May have "flow void"; phase artifact common; MRA helpful; IAC normal
Metastasis	Iso	Iso	Moderate	None	Coexisting brain metastasis in 75%; multiple cranial nerve/meningeal lesions common

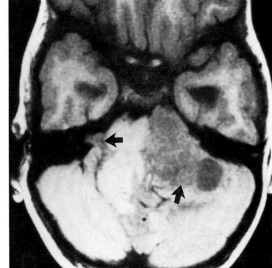

Fig. 12-83. Axial T1-weighted MR scan in a 5-year-old boy with a fourth ventricular ependymoma. The tumor has extended anterolaterally through the foramina of Luschka into both cerebellopontine angle cisterns *(arrows)*.

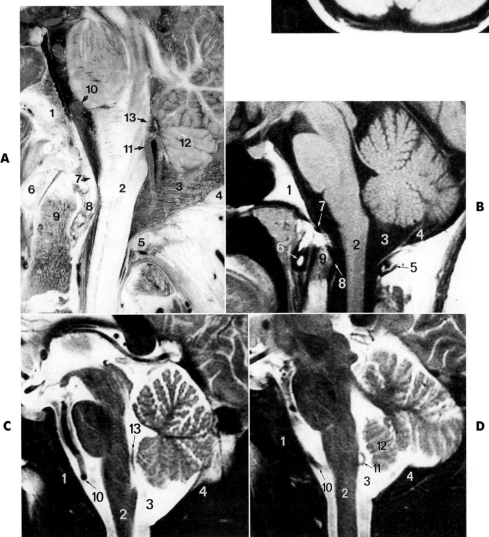

Fig. 12-84. Midline sagittal cryomicrotome section **(A)** demonstrates gross anatomy of the foramen magnum. Sagittal midline T1- **(B)**, T2- **(C)**, and paramedian **(D)** T2-weighted MR scans of the craniovertebral junction: *1,* Clivus. *2,* Cervicomedullary junction. *3,* Cisterna magna. *4,* Occiput. *5,* Posterior arch of C1. *6,* Anterior arch of C1. *7,* Tectorial membrane. *8,* Transverse ligament. *9,* Odontoid process of C2. *10,* Vertebrobasilar artery. *11,* Posterior inferior cerebellar artery. *12,* Tonsil. *13,* Choroid plexus of fourth ventricle. **(A,** Courtesy W. Rauschning.)

These four articulations are true synovial joints with hyaline articular cartilage and prominent lax capsules.[83] The CVJ and foramen magnum are illustrated in Fig. 12-84.

Pathology: overview. It is helpful to divide foramen magnum lesions into intraaxial (cervicomedullary) masses, extramedullary intradural masses, and extradural (i.e., osseous, CVJ) lesions (*see* box; Fig. 12-85).

Intraaxial (cervicomedullary) masses. Common intrinsic brainstem and spinal cord lesions that involve the cervicomedullary junction include benign

disorders such as syringohydromyelia and demyelinating disease and neoplasms.

Nonneoplastic intraaxial lesions. *Syringohydromyelia* is present in 25% of all patients with Chiari I malformation (*see* Fig. 2-2). Acquired syrinxes can also be seen with trauma and cystic neoplasms (*see*

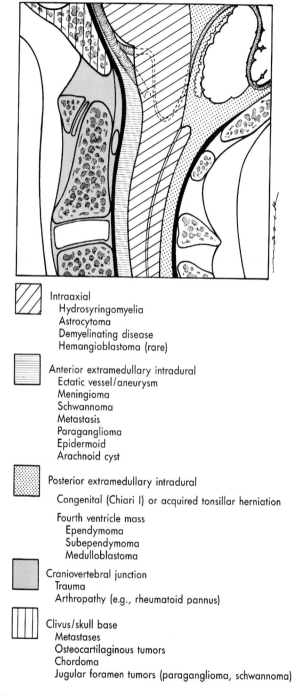

Fig. 12-85. Anatomic diagram depicts the foramen magnum and adjacent structures. Lesions and their locations are indicated.

Foramen Magnum Masses

Cervicomedullary masses

Common
Syringohydromyelia
Demyelinating diseases
Glioma
Fourth ventricle tumor (e.g., medulloblastoma)

Uncommon
Hemangioblastoma
Metastasis

Anterior extramedullary intradural masses

Common
Vertebrobasilar dolichoectasia
Meningioma
Aneurysm (vertebral artery, posterior inferior cerebellar artery)

Uncommon
Schwannoma
Epidermoid tumor
Paraganglioma
Metastases
Arachnoid cyst

Posterior extramedullary intradural masses

Common
Congenital/acquired tonsillar herniation
Ependymoma/subependymoma
Medulloblastoma

Extradural masses

Craniovertebral junction
Trauma
Arthropathies
Congenital anomalies

Clivus and skull base
Metastases
Chordoma
Osteocartilagenous tumors

Legend (from figure):

Intraaxial
Hydrosyringomyelia
Astrocytoma
Demyelinating disease
Hemangioblastoma (rare)

Anterior extramedullary intradural
Ectatic vessel/aneurysm
Meningioma
Schwannoma
Metastasis
Paraganglioma
Epidermoid
Arachnoid cyst

Posterior extramedullary intradural
Congenital (Chiari I) or acquired tonsillar herniation
Fourth ventricle mass
Ependymoma
Subependymoma
Medulloblastoma

Craniovertebral junction
Trauma
Arthropathy (e.g., rheumatoid pannus)

Clivus/skull base
Metastases
Osteocartilaginous tumors
Chordoma
Jugular foramen tumors (paraganglioma, schwannoma)

Chapters 20 and 21). A spectrum of *demyelinating disorders,* including multiple sclerosis, can be seen in the medulla and upper cervical spinal cord (*see* Chapter 19).

Neoplasms. Glial and nonglial neoplasms can involve the cervicomedullary junction. Half of *brainstem gliomas* occur here (*see* Chapter 13); cephalad extension of *cervical spinal cord tumors* into the distal medulla is also common (Figs. 12-86 and 12-87). Most primary cervicomedullary tumors are *low-grade astrocytomas* but ganglioglioma, anaplastic astrocytoma,

and ependymoma are also found in this location.[20] Inferior extension of *medulloblastoma* (PNET-MB) in children and *hemangioblastoma* in adults are common nonglial neoplasms of the cervicomedullary junction (Fig. 12-88). Intraaxial metastases in this location are rare.

Extramedullary   intradural   masses. Most extramedullary intradural foramen magnum masses arise anterior to the cervicomedullary junction. Posterior masses are much less common.

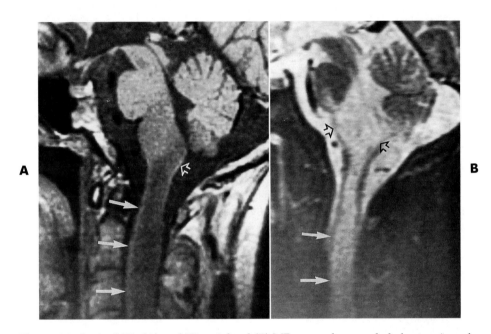

Fig. 12-86. Sagittal T1- **(A)** and T2-weighted **(B)** MR scans show cephalad extension of a cervical cord astrocytoma *(solid arrows)* through the foramen magnum into the lower medulla *(open arrows).*

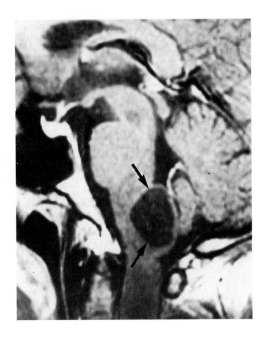

Fig. 12-87. Sagittal postcontrast T1-weighted MR scan in a patient with a cervical cord ependymoma shows an associated cystic component *(arrows)* in the medulla. (Courtesy J. Jones.)

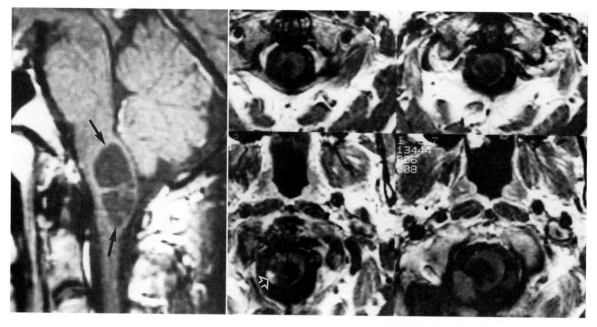

Fig. 12-88. Postcontrast sagittal **(A)** and axial **(B)** T1-weighted MR scans of an hemangioblastoma show a large cystic component at the cervicomedullary junction *(arrows)*. A very small enhancing mural nodule **(B,** *arrow)* is seen on one of the axial sections.

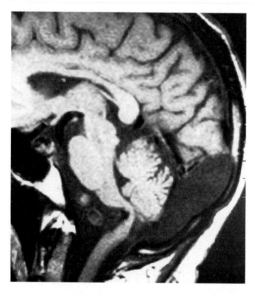

Fig. 12-89. Sagittal T1-weighted MR scan shows a tortuous, ectatic vertebral artery with severe cervicomedullary compression. (Courtesy J. Zahniser.)

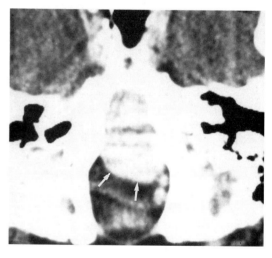

Fig. 12-90. Axial CECT scan shows a well-delineated, strongly enhancing mass *(arrows)* in the anterior foramen magnum. A large vertebral artery aneurysm was demonstrated at angiography (not shown).

Anterior foramen magnum masses. The most common intradural mass anterior to the medulla is a tortuous, *ectatic vertebral artery* (Fig. 12-89). Vascular grooves along the brainstem adjacent to ectatic arteries are seen in 8% to 10% of all MR examinations. There is no correlation between neurologic deficit and the presence of these grooves, regardless of their size.[84] Occasionally, vertebral or posterior inferior cerebellar artery *aneurysms* are seen at the anterior foramen magnum (Fig. 12-90).

Meningioma is the most common primary intradural extramedullary neoplasm in this location (Fig. 12-91). Nerve sheath tumors are the second most frequently encountered neoplasms. *Schwannomas* arising from CNs IX to XI (Fig. 12-92) and neurofibromas from exiting spinal nerve segments occur lateral to the cervicomedullary junction. *Epidermoid* tumors (Fig. 12-65) and *paragangliomas* (Fig. 12-93) as well as cisternal, perineural, and skull base *metastases* also occur here (Figs. 12-94 and 12-95).

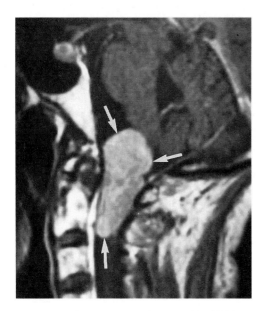

Fig. 12-91. Sagittal postcontrast T1-weighted MR scan in an elderly woman who suddenly became paraplegic. A strongly enhancing, lobulated anterior foramen magnum mass *(arrows)* is identified. Meningioma was found at surgery.

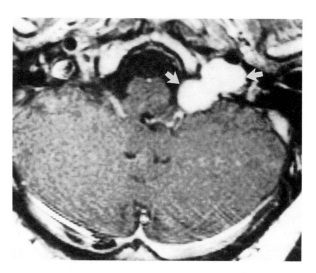

Fig. 12-92. Axial postcontrast T1-weighted MR scan shows a dumbbell-shaped jugular foramen schwannoma *(arrows)*.

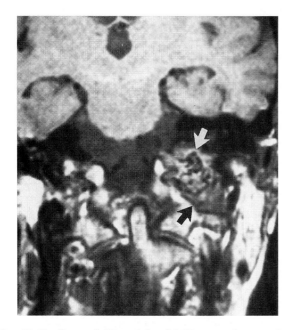

Fig. 12-93. Coronal T1-weighted MR scan shows a large mixed signal left jugular foramen mass *(arrows)*. The "salt and pepper" appearance is typical for paraganglioma.

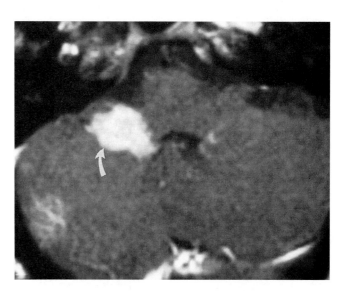

Fig. 12-94. Axial postcontrast T1-weighted MR scan shows a strongly enhancing mass *(arrow)* at the foramen of Luschka that extends into the lower cerebellopontine angle cistern. Metastatic lymphoma.

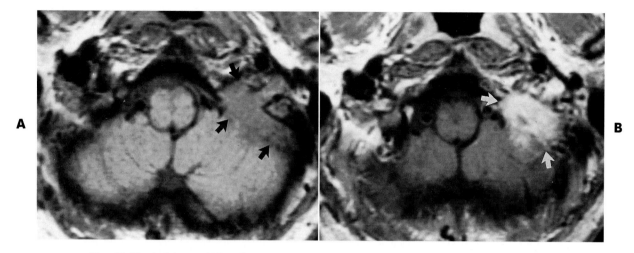

Fig. 12-95. Axial pre- **(A)** and postcontrast **(B)** T1-weighted MR scans in a patient with adenocarcinoma of the lung and left hypoglossal nerve palsy show a destructive mass at the left jugular foramen *(arrows)*. Presumed metastasis.

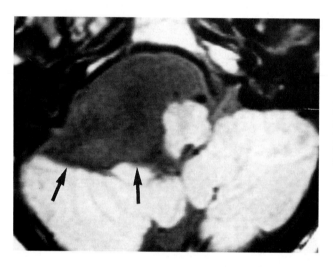

Fig. 12-96. A 25-year-old man with head trauma had a CT scan (not shown) that demonstrated a large low density posterior fossa extraaxial mass. Axial T1-weighted MR scan shows a CSF-intensity mass *(arrows)* that displaces the medulla. Arachnoid cyst.

Nonvascular, nonneoplastic anterior intradural extramedullary foramen magnum masses are uncommon. *Arachnoid, inflammatory* and *neurenteric cysts,* extraosseous intradural *chordomas* or notochordal rests (so-called *physaliphoras ecchordosis*),[85] and intradural *rheumatoid nodules* can occur in this location (Fig. 12-96).

Posterior foramen magnum masses. Congenital and acquired tonsillar herniations account for 5% to 10% of all foramen magnum masses. *Herniated tonsils* are the most frequent extramedullary intradural masses posterior to the cervicomedullary junction. Congenital tonsillar herniations occur with the Chiari malformations (Fig. 12-97) (*see* Chapter 2). Acquired herniations are usually caused by increased intracranial pressure or posterior fossa masses (Fig. 12-98). Tonsillar descent is common after lumboperitoneal shunting of the spinal subarachnoid space.[86] Caudal

tonsillar dislocation through the foramen magnum has also been reported with multiple traumatic lumbar punctures.[87] Imaging findings in these cases may be indistinguishable from those of congenital Chiari I tonsillar ectopia.

Ependymoma (Fig. 12-99), *subependymoma* (Fig. 12-100), and *medulloblastoma* are intraaxial neoplastic masses that sometimes extend posteroinferiorly behind the medulla.

Extradural masses. Most extradural masses at the foramen magnum are osseous lesions (Fig. 12-101). Common bony abnormalities in this location are trauma, arthropathies, congenital malformations, and tumors. High resolution MR best delineates the relationship between the osseous abnormalities, neural canal, and spinal cord in CVJ malformations.[88] Plain film tomography and CT with multiplanar or

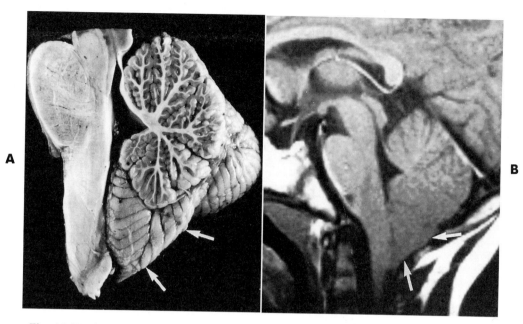

Fig. 12-97. A, Lateral view of gross pathology specimen with a Chiari I malformation. Inferiorly displaced tonsils *(arrows)* are a common cause of a mass behind the cervicomedullary junction. **B,** Sagittal T1-weighted MR scan in a patient with Chiari I malformation shows the classic appearance of inferiorly displaced, peglike cerebellar tonsils *(arrows)*. (**A,** From Okazaki H: Fundamentals of Neuropathology, ed 2, Igaku-Shoin Medical Publishers, New York, 1989.)

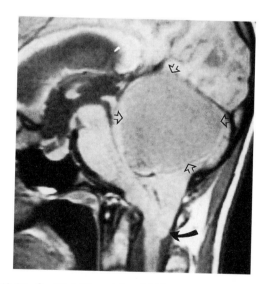

Fig. 12-98. Sagittal T1-weighted MR scan shows acquired descending tonsillar herniation *(curved arrow)* secondary to a large posterior fossa cystic astrocytoma *(open arrows)*.

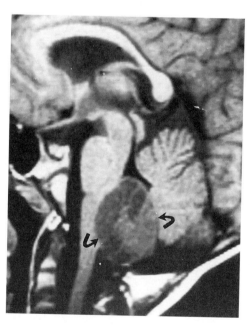

Fig. 12-99. Sagittal T1-weighted MR scan shows spread of a fourth ventricular ependymoma *(arrows)* posteroinferiorly through the foramen of Magendie into the cisterna magna, where it is seen behind the cervicomedullary junction.

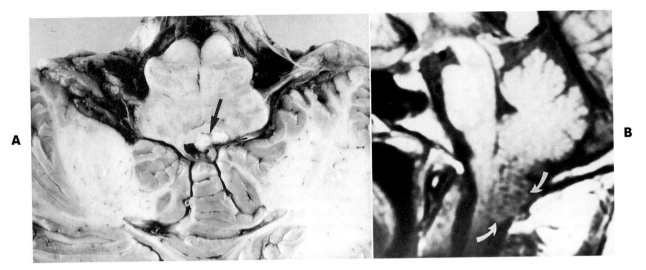

Fig. 12-100. A, Gross pathology of a fourth ventricular subependymoma *(arrow)* that was found incidentally at autopsy. **B,** A 62-year-old man had a CT scan (not shown) obtained after an auto accident. A partially calcified soft tissue mass at the foramen magnum was seen posterior to the cervicomedullary junction. An MR scan was then obtained. The sagittal T1-weighted scan shows a mottled isointense mass *(arrows)* behind the medulla. No enhancement was seen following contrast administration. Subependymoma was found at surgery. **(B,** From archives of the Armed Forces Institute of Pathology.)

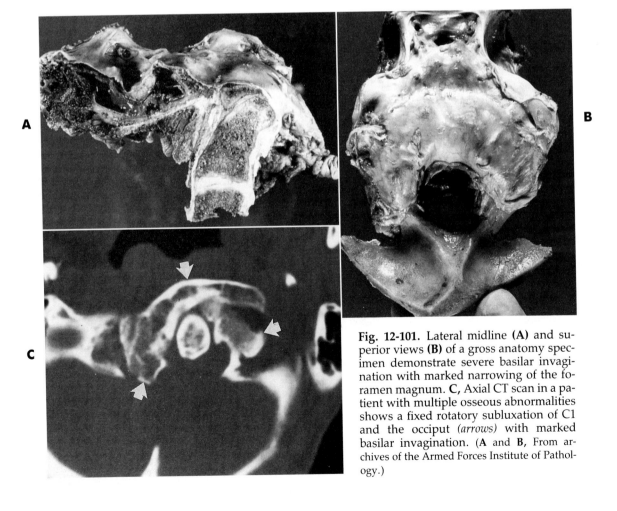

Fig. 12-101. Lateral midline **(A)** and superior views **(B)** of a gross anatomy specimen demonstrate severe basilar invagination with marked narrowing of the foramen magnum. **C,** Axial CT scan in a patient with multiple osseous abnormalities shows a fixed rotatory subluxation of C1 and the occiput *(arrows)* with marked basilar invagination. **(A** and **B,** From archives of the Armed Forces Institute of Pathology.)

three-dimensional reconstructions are helpful for detailing the complicated osseous abnormalities seen in these disorders (Fig. 12-101, C).[89]

Trauma. *Odontoid fractures* are relatively common, constituting nearly 20% of all cervical fractures. An estimated 25% to 40% of these injuries cause death at the accident scene. Most survivors do not experience immediate neurologic impairment. However, late-onset myelopathy secondary to nonunited dens fracture may occur.[90] Chronic instability can lead to spinal stenosis and irreversible cord damage. CT details the osseous abnormalities, and MR best delineates the relationship to the spinal subarachnoid space and cord itself.

Arthropathies. Because the osseous articulations that form the CVJ are true synovial joints the full spectrum of degenerative and inflammatory arthropathies may involve the foramen magnum region. *Rheumatoid arthritis* of the spine is second in incidence only to that of the hands and feet. The cervical spine is affected in up to 80% of these patients. Prominent *pannus* (Fig. 12-102) and *atlantoaxial subluxation* may cause severe CVJ narrowing with spinal cord compression. Sagittal MR scans in both flexion and extension delineate the dynamic relationship between osseous abnormalities and medulla particularly well (Fig. 12-103).

Occasionally, rheumatoid nodules may be present within the dura and perineurium. This is usually present only in advanced cases with widespread severe joint involvement.[91]

Less common CVJ lesions include *osteoarthritis,*

Paget disease, calcium pyrophosphate deposition disorders, and *osteomyelitis* with or without epidural abscess.

Congenital anomalies. *Congenital CVJ anomalies* are relatively uncommon. These include vertebralization of the occipital condyles, various arch hypoplasias and aplasias, os odontoideum or odontoid hypoplasia, assimilations, and ligamentous laxity (Fig. 12-104). These anomalies may occur in isolation or with

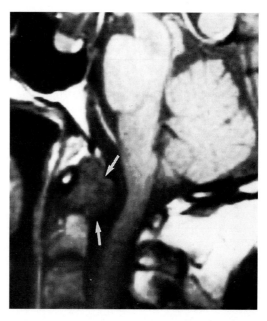

Fig. 12-102. Sagittal T1-weighted MR scan shows prominent rheumatoid pannus *(arrows)* with destruction of the odontoid process and mild foramen magnum narrowing.

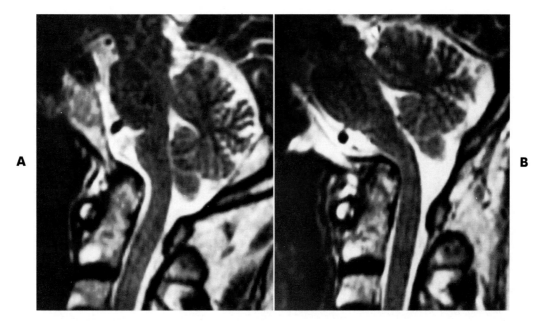

Fig. 12-103. Sagittal T2-weighted MR scans of a patient with rheumatoid arthritis show mild foramen magnum narrowing in neutral position **(A)** but marked narrowing with medullary compression in the flexed position **(B).**

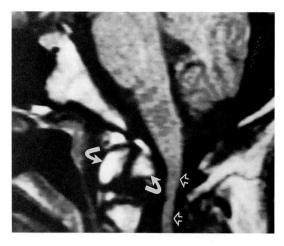

Fig. 12-104. Sagittal T1-weighted MR scan in a patient with os odontoideum. Segmented odontoid *(large arrows)*. The spinal cord is markedly atrophic *(open arrows)*.

basilar invagination (BI) (Fig. 12-105). In BI the vertebral column is abnormally high and indents the skull base (Fig. 12-101). CVJ anomalies may also be associated with other congenital abnormalities such as Down syndrome, Chiari I malformation, or syringohydromyelia.[92,93]

Neoplasms. Both primary and metastatic tumors occur at the CVJ. Most extradural tumors that affect the foramen magnum involve the clivus and are therefore anterior to the medulla. Primary neoplasms include *chordoma* and *osteocartilagenous tumors* such as chondroma and chondrosarcoma. *Metastases* can be either hematogenous or local extensions from nasopharyngeal or skull base tumors. Because they replace normal fatty marrow, most infiltrating skull base lesions exhibit low signal on T1-weighted MR scans and high signal on T2WI, regardless of etiology (Fig. 12-106).[94,95] The exception is chordoma. These tumors generally have very high but heterogeneous signal intensity on T2WI[96] (*see* Fig. 12-169).

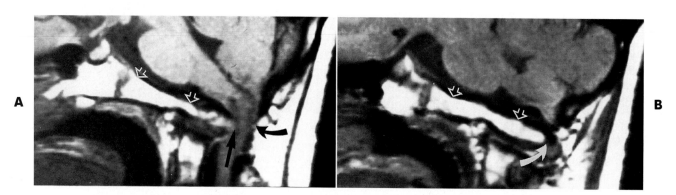

Fig. 12-105. A and **B,** Sagittal T1-weighted MR scans show platybasia with marked basilar invagination *(open arrows)*. Note severe medullary compression (**A,** *straight black arrow*) and foramen magnum narrowing *(curved arrows)*.

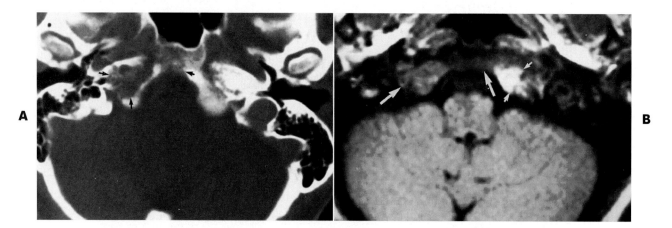

Fig. 12-106. A 40-year-old woman with known metastatic breast carcinoma had a right CN XII palsy. **A,** Axial CT scan shows a destructive clivus lesion *(arrows)*. **B,** Axial precontrast T1-weighted MR scan shows replacement of the normal high signal fatty marrow *(small arrows)* by soft tissue *(large arrows)* that is nearly isointense with brain.

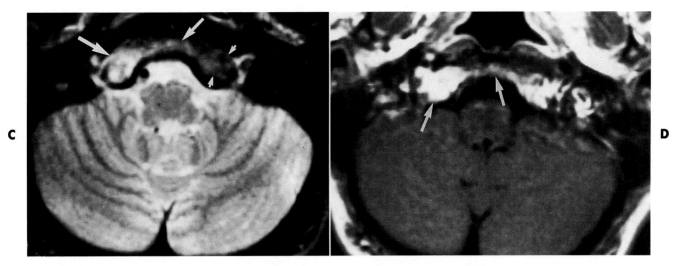

Fig. 12-106, cont'd. **C,** The lesion *(large arrows)* is high signal on the T2WI; compare with normal, low signal fatty marrow *(small arrows).* **D,** Postcontrast T1WI shows the lesion enhances *(arrows).* Presumed metastatic breast carcinoma.

Sellar/Suprasellar Masses

Normal anatomy and physiology. The sellar region is an anatomically complex area composed of the bony sella turcica, pituitary gland, and adjacent structures (Figs. 12-107 and 12-108).

Bony sella. The sella turcica is a cup-shaped depression in the central basisphenoid bone that contains the pituitary gland and inferior part of the infundibular stalk.

Pituitary gland. The pituitary gland is composed of two lobes that are physiologically and anatomically distinct.[97] Traditional embryology holds that the anterior lobe is derived from the primitive oral cavity and its embryonic ectoderm, the stomodeum. More recent studies indicate the anterior lobe actually may be of neuroectodermal, not stomodeal, origin.[98]

The anterior lobe or adenohypophysis is the largest part of the pituitary gland, comprising 75% of its total volume.[99] The adenohypophysis has the following three parts:

1. Pars tuberalis (part of the infundibular stalk and median eminence of the hypothalamus)
2. Pars intermedia
3. Pars distalis

The pars intermedia is very small in humans; the pars distalis forms most of the intrasellar adenohypophysis. It is composed of glandular epithelial cells plus blood vessels. The adenohypophysis does not have direct arterial supply. It receives its blood principally from the hypophyseal-portal system, which also serves as the pathway by which hypothalamic releasing hormones reach this structure.[98]

Hormones produced and secreted by the anterior lobe include growth hormone (GH), adre-

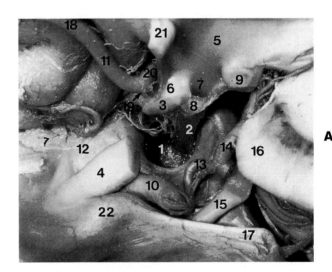

Fig. 12-107. **A,** Anatomic dissection shows anatomy of the sellar and suprasellar region. The optic chiasm has been sectioned to reveal the infundibular stalk, diaphragma sellae, and pituitary gland. The circle of Willis has also been partially removed. *1,* Pituitary gland. *2,* Infundibular stalk. *3,* Optic chiasm (cut across in anatomy section) and optic tracts. *4,* Optic nerve. *5,* Body of third ventricle. *6,* Optic recess of third ventricle. *7,* Infundibular recess of third ventricle. *8,* Hypothalamus with tuber cinereum. *9,* Mamillary body. *10,* Internal carotid artery. *11,* Anterior cerebral artery. *12,* Planum sphenoidale. *13,* Posterior communicating artery. *14,* Posterior cerebral artery. *15,* CN III. *16,* Cerebral peduncles/midbrain. *17,* Tentorial incisura. *18,* Anterior cerebral artery. *19,* Anterior communicating artery. *20,* Middle cerebral artery. *21,* Anterior commissure. *22,* Anterior clinoid process. *23,* Fornix. (From Bassett D: *A Stereoscopic Atlas of Human Anatomy: the central nervous system,* Section 1: Courtesy Bassett Collection, R. Chase (curator), Stanford University.)

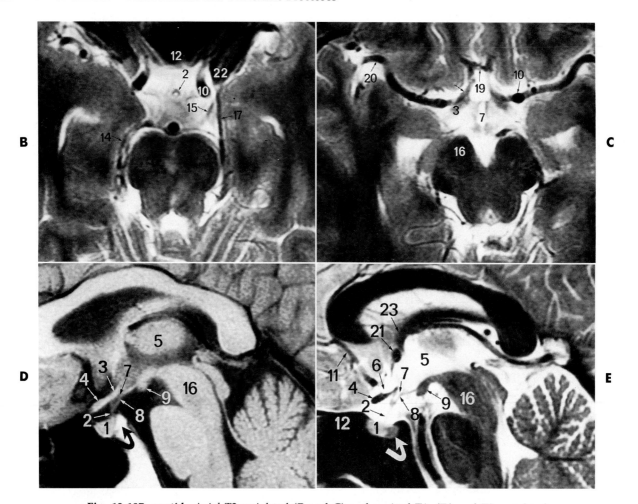

Fig. 12-107, cont'd. Axial T2-weighted (**B** and **C**) and sagittal T1- (**D**) and T2-weighted (**E**) MR scans show the suprasellar region (same key as **A**). The neurohypophysis is hyperintense on T1- and hypointense to brain on T2-weighted scans (**D** and **E**, *curved arrows*). *1*, Pituitary gland. *2*, Infundibular stalk. *3*, Optic chiasm (cut across in anatomy section) and optic tracts. *4*, Optic nerve. *5*, Body of third ventricle. *6*, Optic recess of third ventricle. *7*, Infundibular recess of third ventricle. *8*, Hypothalamus with tuber cinereum. *9*, Mamillary body. *10*, Internal carotid artery. *11*, Anterior cerebral artery. *12*, Planum sphenoidale. *13*, Posterior communicating artery. *14*, Posterior cerebral artery. *15*, CN III. *16*, Cerebral peduncles/midbrain. *17*, Tentorial incisura. *18*, Anterior cerebral artery. *19*, Anterior communicating artery. *20*, Middle cerebral artery. *21*, Anterior commissure. *22*, Anterior clinoid process. *23*, Fornix.

nocorticotropic hormone (ACTH), prolactin, thyroid-stimulating hormone (TSH), follicle-stimulating hormone (FSH), luteinizing hormone (LH), and melanophore-stimulating hormone.[100] Release of these hormones is mediated by the hypothalamus (Table 12-3). On T2- and unenhanced T1-weighted MR scans the adenohypophysis is isointense relative to gray matter (Fig. 12-107, *D* and *E*).[97]

The posterior pituitary lobe, infundibular stalk, and supraoptic and paraventricular hypothalamic nuclei form the neurohypophysis.[101] These structures are derived from diencephalic neuroectoderm. The posterior pituitary lobe is composed of axons and ter-

minal portions of the hypothalamohypophyseal tract, pituicytes (which are really astrocytic glial cells), and blood vessels.[102] The inferior hypophyseal arteries supply the pars nervosa, and the infundibular stalk is supplied by the superior hypophyseal ICA branches.[103]

Oxytocin and vasopressin are synthesized in the hypothalamus, coupled to carrier proteins known as neurophysins and enveloped by phospholipid membranes to form vesicles that are then transported to the posterior lobe along the hypothalamohypophyseal tract.[104]

The posterior pituitary lobe is normally hyperin-

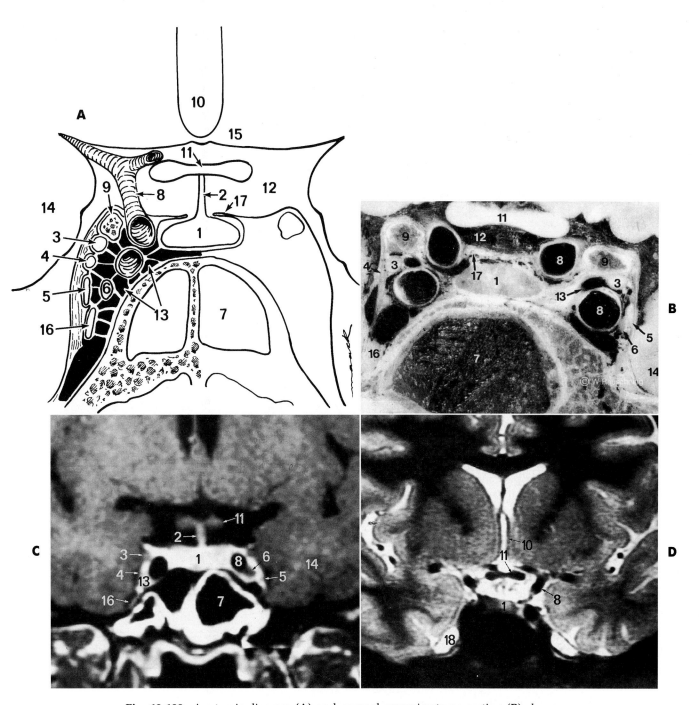

Fig. 12-108. Anatomic diagram **(A)** and coronal cryomicrotome section **(B)** show gross anatomy of the intrasellar region and cavernous sinus. Coronal postcontrast T1- **(C)** and T2-weighted **(D)** MR scans of the sella and cavernous sinus. *1,* Pituitary gland. *2,* Infundibular stalk. *3,* CN III. *4,* CN IV. *5,* CN V_1. *6,* CN VI. *7,* Sphenoid sinus. *8,* Internal carotid artery. *9,* Anterior clinoid process. *10,* Third ventricle. *11,* Optic chiasm. *12,* Suprasellar cistern. *13,* Venous spaces of cavernous sinus. *14,* Temporal lobe. *15,* Hypothalamus. *16,* CN V_2. *17,* Diaphragma sellae. *18,* Meckel's cave. (**A,** Diagram reproduced from Osborn A: *Handbook of Neuroradiology,* Yearbook Medical Publishers, 1990. **B,** Courtesy W. Rauschning.)

tense on T1WI (Fig. 12-107, *D*).[104] There may be more than one source of this high-intensity signal but in the majority of cases neurosecretory vesicles appear to be responsible.[105] Absent high signal is often—but not invariably—associated with central diabetes insipidus or compressive pituitary gland lesions.[106,107]

Adjacent structures. The sella is bordered superiorly by a dural reflection, the diaphragma sellae. The suprasellar subarachnoid space lies above the diaphragma sellae and is surrounded by the circle of Willis. The suprasellar cistern contains the optic nerves and chiasm and the upper part of the infundibular stalk. The hypothalamus and anterior third ventricular recesses lie just above the infundibular stalk.

Laterally the sella turcica is bordered by the thin medial dural reflection of the cavernous sinus. The cavernous sinus is a multiseptated venous channel that contains the cavernous internal carotid artery (ICA). The sixth cranial (abducens) nerve lies within the cavernous sinus adjacent to the ICA. CNs III, IV, and the ophthalmic (V1) and maxillary (V2) divisions of the trigeminal nerve lie in the lateral sinus wall (Fig. 12-108).

The sphenoid sinus lies directly below the sella. Anteriorly the sellar floor is continuous with the tuberculum sellae and limbus sphenoidale. The dorsum sellae demarcates the posterior sellar border.

Pathology: overview. Lesions in the anatomically complex sellar/juxtasellar region can arise from the pituitary gland or infundibular stalk, as well as adjacent brain, bone, dura, leptomeninges, vessels, cranial nerves, and extracranial structures such as the nasopharynx. At least 30 different pathologic entities have been described that affect the sella and juxtasellar region (*see* box).

Subdividing sellar/juxtasellar lesions into intra-, supra-, and juxtasellar masses facilitates diagnosis,

although some disease processes involve more than one area (Fig. 12-109). In this section we will discuss intra- and suprasellar masses. Juxtasellar masses, i.e., cavernous sinus, skull base, and nasopharyngeal lesions, are discussed later in this chapter.

Pathologic Entities
Sellar/Juxtasellar region

Abscess
Aneurysm
Arachnoid cyst
Cephalocele
Chloroma (granulocytic sarcoma)
Colloid/pars intermedia cysts
Craniopharyngioma
Dermoid
Ectopic neurohypophysis
"Empty" sella
Epidermoid tumor
Germinoma
Hamartoma (tuber cinereum/hypothalamus)
Histiocytosis
Hyperplasia
Hypophysitis
Lipoma
Lymphoma
Meningioma
Meningitis (bacterial, fungal, granulomatous)
Metastasis
Mucocele
Nasopharyngeal carcinoma
Opticochiasmatic-hypothalamic glioma
Osteocartilagenous tumors
Parasitic cyst
Pituitary adenoma
Rathke's cleft cyst
Sarcoid

Table 12-3. Principal Pituitary Hormones and Their Regulation

Pituitary lobe	Pituitary hormone	Releasing factor	Inhibitory factor	Target organ
Anterior	Corticotropin	Corticotropin-releasing hormone	Antidiuretic hormone	Adrenal gland
	Follicle-stimulating hormone, luteinizing hormone	Luteinizing hormone-releasing hormone	—	Gonads
	Growth hormone	Growth hormone-releasing hormone	Somatostatin	Liver, bone, adipocytes
	Prolactin	Vasoactive intestinal peptide	Dopamine	Breast
	Thyroid-stimulating hormone	Thyrotropin-releasing hormone	Somatostatin	Thyroid
Posterior	Antidiuretic hormone	—	—	Kidney
	Oxytocin	—	—	Breast, uterus

From Elster AD: Modern imaging of the pituitary, *Radiol* 187:1-14, 1993.

Intrasellar masses. Normal variations in pituitary gland size are common. Microadenomas and nonneoplastic cysts are the most common intrasellar masses. Although comparatively uncommon, other neoplastic, vascular, inflammatory, and congenital lesions can occasionally occur within the sella turcica itself (*see* box, p. 467).

Normal variants. The so-called *empty sella* is a very common anatomic variant in which the sella is partially filled with CSF. The infundibular stalk follows its normal course and inserts in the midline of the pituitary gland. The gland itself appears thinned and flattened against the bony floor (Fig. 12-110). Occasionally, intrasellar herniation of the optic nerve, chiasm, or tract and the anteroinferior third ventricle into a primary or secondary (i.e., postoperative) empty sella occurs (Fig. 12-111).[108] An acquired empty sella with anterior pituitary hormone deficiencies can occur secondary to pituitary gland necrosis following peripartum circulatory collapse (Sheehan syndrome).[109]

There are normal gender- and age-specific changes in pituitary size and shape.[110] The pituitary gland in neonates and young infants is rounder, brighter, and

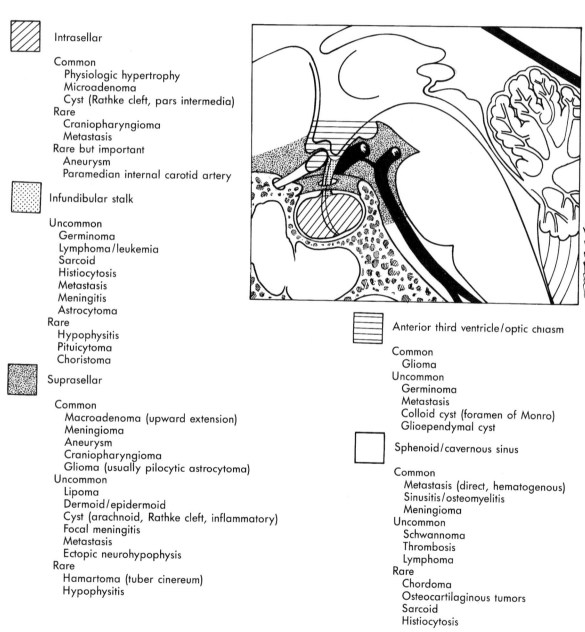

Intrasellar

Common
  Physiologic hypertrophy
  Microadenoma
  Cyst (Rathke cleft, pars intermedia)
Rare
  Craniopharyngioma
  Metastasis
Rare but important
  Aneurysm
  Paramedian internal carotid artery

Infundibular stalk

Uncommon
  Germinoma
  Lymphoma/leukemia
  Sarcoid
  Histiocytosis
  Metastasis
  Meningitis
  Astrocytoma
Rare
  Hypophysitis
  Pituicytoma
  Choristoma

Suprasellar

Common
  Macroadenoma (upward extension)
  Meningioma
  Aneurysm
  Craniopharyngioma
  Glioma (usually pilocytic astrocytoma)
Uncommon
  Lipoma
  Dermoid/epidermoid
  Cyst (arachnoid, Rathke cleft, inflammatory)
  Focal meningitis
  Metastasis
  Ectopic neurohypophysis
Rare
  Hamartoma (tuber cinereum)
  Hypophysitis

Anterior third ventricle/optic chiasm

Common
  Glioma
Uncommon
  Germinoma
  Metastasis
  Colloid cyst (foramen of Monro)
  Glioependymal cyst

Sphenoid/cavernous sinus

Common
  Metastasis (direct, hematogenous)
  Sinusitis/osteomyelitis
  Meningioma
Uncommon
  Schwannoma
  Thrombosis
  Lymphoma
Rare
  Chordoma
  Osteocartilaginous tumors
  Sarcoid
  Histiocytosis

Fig 12-109. Anatomic diagram depicts the sella turcica and suprasellar region as seen from the lateral view. Common lesions and their differential diagnosis by location are indicated.

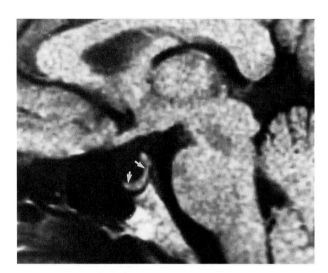

Fig. 12-110. Sagittal T1-weighted MR scan shows a partially empty sella turcica. The sella is mostly filled with CSF, and the pituitary gland *(arrows)* appears thinned and flattened against the bony floor and dorsum sellae.

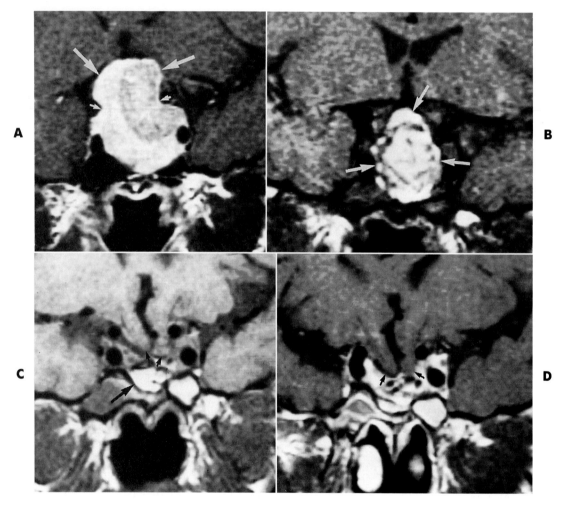

Fig. 12-111. Serial pre- and postoperative MR scans in a patient with a large pituitary adenoma. **A,** Preoperative coronal contrast-enhanced T1WI shows a large intra- and suprasellar enhancing mass *(large arrows).* Note "figure eight" appearance caused by slight constriction of the adenoma at the diaphragma sellae *(small arrows).* **B,** Coronal unenhanced T1WI 2 months after transsphenoidal hypophysectomy and fat graft packing *(arrows)* of the sphenoid sinus and tumor bed. Eighteen months later, pre- **(C)** and postcontrast **(D)** coronal T1WIs show nearly complete resorption of the fat graft. The gyri recti *(small arrows)* are herniated inferiorly into the sella. Some postoperative enhancing fibrosis is present within the sella.

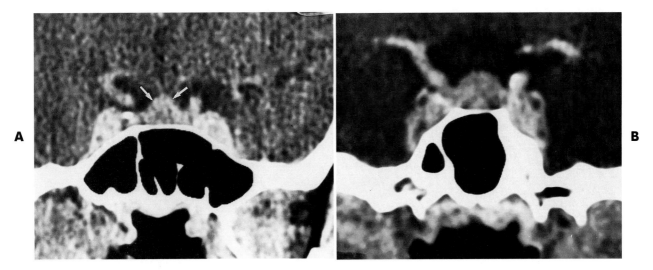

Fig. 12-112. A, Coronal CECT in a 31-year-old pregnant woman shows an upwardly convex pituitary gland that measures 10 mm in height *(arrows).* **B,** A 41-year-old woman with ovarian failure had this CECT scan. The upwardly convex pituitary gland measures 10 mm in height, abnormal at this age.

Intrasellar Masses

Common

Physiologic hyperplasia
Microadenoma
Nonneoplastic cyst (pars intermedia, colloid, Rathke's cleft)

Uncommon

Craniopharyngioma
Metastasis

Rare

Meningioma
Epidermoid or dermoid cyst

Rare but extremely important

Paramedian carotid arteries
Aneurysm

---

relatively larger during the first 2 months of life than in later childhood.[111]

The pituitary gland undergoes significant alterations during puberty, pregnancy, and the immediate postpartum period.[98,111,112] In adolescent girls and pregnant women the gland often appears spherical or upwardly convex and occasionally may reach 10 to 11 mm in height (Fig. 12-112).[112] The anterior lobe may also appear hyperintense in pregnant or postpartum women.[113] Pubertal males may have a slightly rounded, upwardly convex pituitary that measures 6 to 7 mm in height.[112,114] The pituitary

gland normally decreases in size with aging.[110,115]

Physiologic pituitary hypertrophy, pituitary hypertrophy secondary to *end-organ failure* (e.g., hypothyroidism), and some adenomas may appear virtually identical on imaging studies, all causing a diffusely enlarged pituitary gland (Fig. 12-112).[116] Central precocious puberty may also cause a large pituitary gland with a convex upper border.[117]

Pituitary cysts. Asymptomatic nonneoplastic pituitary cysts are found in approximately 20% of autopsy specimens.[118] Intrasellar cysts are derived either from arachnoid membrane or epithelial remnants along Rathke's pouch. Most are *pars intermedia, colloid,* or *Rathke cleft cysts;* other intrasellar cysts such as *epidermoid, dermoid,* and *cysticercosis cysts* are rare.[119] Signal intensity of these intrasellar cysts varies with cyst content, but on contrast-enhanced CT or MR scans, most appear as low density or low signal intensity foci within the intensely enhancing pituitary gland (Figs. 12-113 and 12-114).

Neoplasms. Microadenoma is by far the most common intrasellar neoplasm in adults. Pituitary adenomas are rare in children; less than 3% of adenomas occur in children under 18 years of age. Most pediatric pituitary tumors occur in adolescent girls and are ACTH- or prolactin-secreting adenomas.

Adenomas measuring 10 mm or less are defined as microadenomas. These tumors often fill the sella but do not have suprasellar extension.[100] Most microadenomas enhance less rapidly than surrounding normal pituitary tissue and are therefore seen as hypodense or hypointense areas on contrast-enhanced CT and MR studies (Fig. 12-115, *A*), particularly if dynamic sequences are acquired[120] (*see* Chapter 14). Ne-

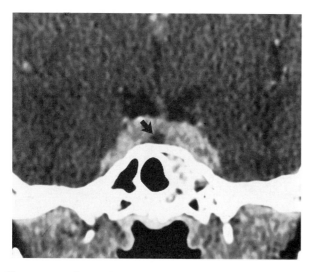

Fig. 12-113. Coronal CECT scan shows a low density lesion within the strongly enhancing normal pituitary gland. Presumed pituitary cyst in this endocrinologically normal patient.

crotic or hemorrhagic microadenomas are often hyperintense on T1-weighted sequences (Fig. 12-115, *B*).

Other than microadenoma, intrasellar neoplasms are uncommon. Only 5% to 10% of *craniopharyngiomas* are purely intrasellar.[121] Occasionally, an epidermoid or dermoid tumor occurs in this location. Truly intrasellar *meningiomas* are rare;[122] occasionally, a tuberculum or diaphragma sellae meningioma grows downward into the pituitary fossa. In some cases, direct visualization of a thickened, depressed diaphragma sellae below the enhancing mass may establish the diagnosis of intrasellar meningioma (Fig. 12-116).[123]

Metastases to the pituitary-hypothalamic axis account for 1% of sellar masses; most are suprasellar or combined intra- and suprasellar lesions (Fig. 12-117).[124] Purely intrasellar metastases are uncommon.[125]

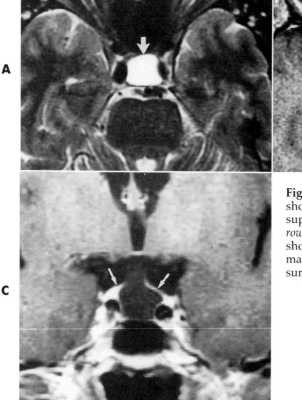

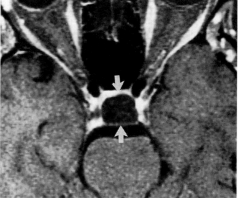

Fig. 12-114. A, Axial precontrast T2-weighted MR scan shows a high signal intrasellar mass *(arrow)*. **B,** Fat-suppressed postcontrast axial T1WI shows the mass *(arrows)* does not enhance. **C,** Coronal postcontrast study shows mass is surrounded by the intensely enhancing normal pituitary gland *(arrows)*. Rathke cleft cyst was found at surgery.

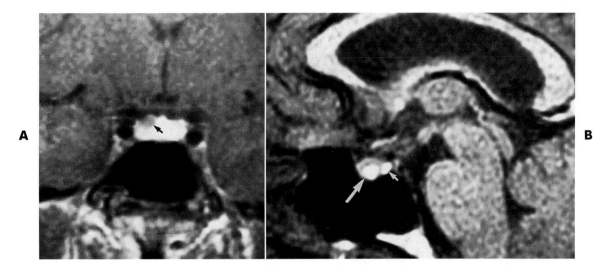

Fig. 12-115. A, Coronal postcontrast T1-weighted MR scan in a young woman with ga-lactorrhea shows a small focal mass *(arrow)* that enhances less intensely than the adja-cent normal pituitary gland. Microadenoma was found at surgery. **B,** Sagittal precon-trast T1-weighted MR scan in another patient with a small hemorrhagic microadenoma *(large arrow)*. Note normal high signal posterior pituitary lobe *(small arrow)* immediately behind the intrasellar adenoma.

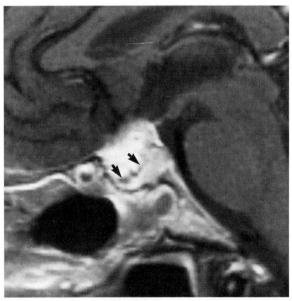

Fig. 12-116. Sagittal postcontrast T1-weighted MR scan of an intrasellar meningioma. Note inferior displacement of the diaphragma sellae *(arrows)*, indicating the mass is ex-trinsic to the pituitary gland. (Courtesy Ivan Ciric. Reprinted with permission from *Neurosurgery* 31:627, 1992.)

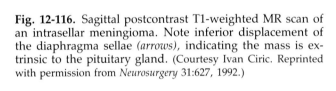

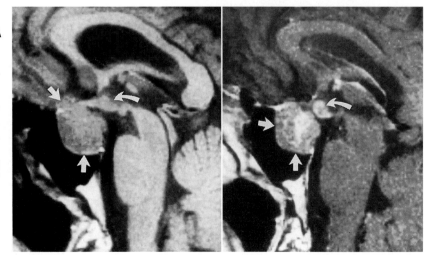

Fig. 12-117. Sagittal pre- **(A)** and postcontrast **(B)** T1-weighted MR scans in an elderly man with known lung carcinoma and bitemporal hemi-anopsia show an enlarged pituitary gland *(straight arrows)* that enhances mildly and inhomogeneously. A sec-ond, smaller mass is present in the hypothalamus *(curved arrows)*. Lung carcinoma metastatic to the pituitary gland. (Courtesy J. Creasey.)

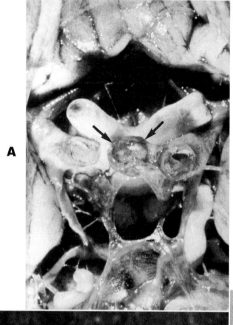

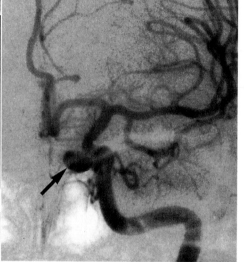

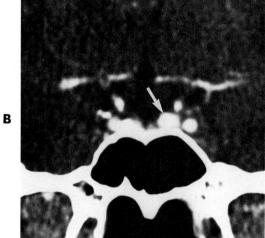

Fig. 12-118. **A,** Gross pathology specimen shows an incidental intrasellar carotid artery aneurysm *(arrows)* that was found at autopsy. **B,** Coronal CECT scan in another patient shows an intensely enhancing intrasellar mass *(arrow)*. This would be unusual for microadenoma, most of which appear hypodense compared to the adjacent pituitary gland. Cerebral angiography was performed for suspected aneurysm. **C,** Left internal carotid angiogram, arterial phase, AP view, shows an intrasellar aneurysm *(arrow)*. (**A,** Courtesy E. Tessa Hedley-Whyte.)

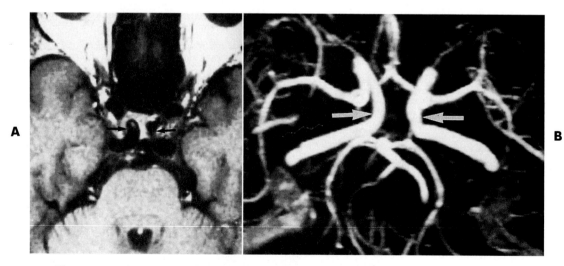

Fig. 12-119. Two cases of paramedian, or "kissing," internal carotid arteries (ICAs). **A,** Axial T1-weighted MR scan shows the two carotid arteries *(arrows)* nearly meet in the midline. **B,** In another case a multiple overlapping thin-slab acquisition MR angiogram, base view, shows paramedian course of the two ICAs *(arrows)*.

Vascular and inflammatory lesions. Important but uncommon intrasellar masses include intrasellar carotid artery *aneurysm* (Fig. 12-118) and *aberrant (kissing) carotid arteries* (Fig. 12-119). Inflammatory lesions such as *abscess* and *hypophysitis* are uncommon; when present they usually involve both the intra- and suprasellar regions (Fig. 12-120).

Congenital anomalies. True congenital anomalies of the pituitary gland are rare. The most common of these unusual abnormalities is a small or absent gland associated with primary panhypopituitarism. The infundibular stalk is usually small or absent. An *ectopic neurohypophysis* with hypothalamic "bright spot" is frequently observed in these cases (Fig. 12-121, *A*).[126] Occasionally, no suprasellar "hot spot" is identified

on T1-weighted MR scans. Instead, the sella may appear small, and the displaced neurohypophysis is isointense with brain but shows strong enhancement following contrast administration (Fig. 12-121, *B* and *C*).

High signal in the hypothalamus on T1WI is not specific for congenital ectopic neurohypophysis because any process (such as tumor or trauma) that disturbs transport of releasing hormones from the hypothalamus to the neural lobe can result in this finding (Fig. 12-122). The differential diagnosis of a suprasellar "hot spot" is noted in the box, p. 472.

Duplicated pituitary gland and stalk is a rare malformation that is probably a mild manifestation of median cleft face syndrome.[127]

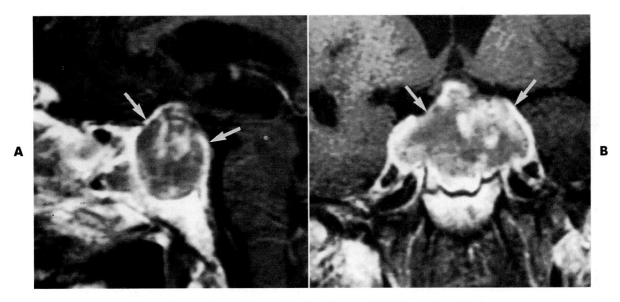

Fig. 12-120. Contrast-enhanced sagittal **(A)** and coronal **(B)** T1-weighted MR scans in an elderly patient with severe sphenoid sinusitis show a large intrasellar mass *(arrows)*. Infected, necrotic pituitary adenoma was found at surgery.

Fig. 12-121. A, Coronal T1-weighted MR scan in a 9-year-old child with growth hormone deficiency shows an absent infundibular stalk and ectopic posterior pituitary lobe, seen as a high signal focus or suprasellar "hot spot" *(arrow).* (Courtesy L. Tan.)

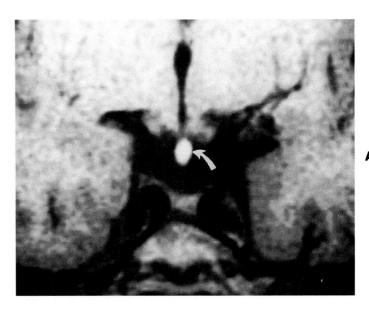

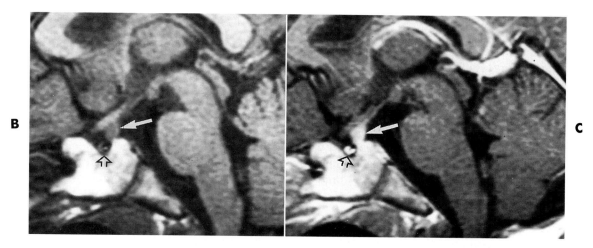

Fig. 12-121, cont'd. Sagittal pre- **(B)** and postcontrast **(C)** T1-weighted MR scans were obtained in a 7-year-old girl with small stature. All hormone levels were low. The precontrast study shows a very small pituitary fossa *(open arrows)* that appears devoid of glandular contents. A suprasellar mass in the hypothalamus is seen *(solid arrows)*. The mass is isointense with gray matter. **C,** The mass *(white arrow)* enhances strongly and uniformly after contrast administration. A small amount of enhancing intrasellar tissue is seen *(open arrow)*. Ectopic posterior pituitary lobe. (Courtesy L. Tan.)

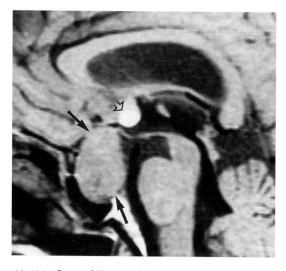

Fig. 12-122. Sagittal T1-weighted MR scan in a patient with a large pituitary adenoma *(large arrows)*. Note the high signal mass in the anterior third ventricular recesses *(open arrow)*, probably caused by displaced neurosecretory products. No intraventricular mass was identified at surgery.

Differential Diagnosis: Suprasellar "Hot Spot"
High signal focus on unenhanced T1-weighted MR scans

Common

Rathke's cleft cyst
Craniopharyngioma
Subacute hemorrhage
   Thrombosed aneurysm
   Hemorrhagic neoplasm (e.g., pituitary adenoma)
   Postoperative (hemorrhage, fat graft)

Uncommon

Lipoma
Dermoid
Congenital ectopic neurohypophysis
Disturbed transport of releasing hormones from
   hypothalamus to neural lobe
   Traumatic stalk transection
   Hypophysectomy
   Sarcoidosis, histiocytosis
   Pituitary or other tumor

Suprasellar masses. Four of the five most frequent suprasellar masses are tumors. The most common is suprasellar extension of pituitary adenoma. Meningioma, craniopharyngioma, hypothalamic/chiasmatic glioma, and aneurysm follow in varying order. These five entities account for more than three quarters of all sellar/juxtasellar masses.[97] Metastases, meningitis, and granulomatous disease account for another 10%. Typical MRI and CT appearance of common suprasellar lesions is described in Table 12-4.

Other suprasellar masses are uncommon; each is seen in less than 1% to 2% of all cases. Lesions that primarily or exclusively affect the infundibular stalk comprise a special diagnostic spectrum that is considered separately.

Neoplasms. In adults the two most common suprasellar neoplastic masses are suprasellar extension of pituitary adenoma and meningioma. In children, the most common lesions in this location are craniopharyngioma and hypothalamic-opticochiasmatic glioma.

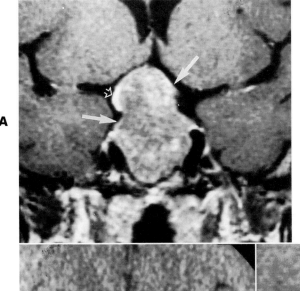

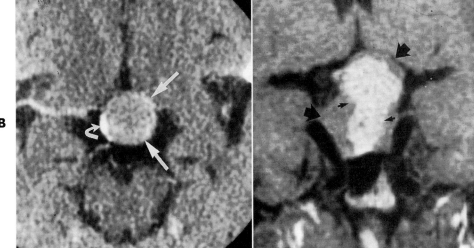

Fig. 12-123. Three different cases of pituitary adenoma. **A,** Coronal contrast-enhanced T1-weighted MR scan shows a large pituitary adenoma *(large arrows)*. Note the "figure eight" appearance. Higher signal at the periphery of the mass *(open arrow)* was subacute hemorrhage at surgery. **B,** Axial CECT scan shows a large enhancing suprasellar mass *(large arrows)* with rim calcification *(curved arrow)*. Pituitary adenoma was found at surgery. This appearance is more typical for aneurysm. **C,** Coronal T1-weighted MR scan of a macroadenoma *(large arrows)* with central necrosis and hemorrhage *(small arrows)*.

Upward extension of pituitary adenoma through the diaphragma sellae accounts for one third to one half of all suprasellar masses in adults. *Pituitary adenomas with suprasellar extension* typically have a "figure eight" appearance (Fig. 12-123, *A*). Most enhance strongly but somewhat inhomogeneously following contrast administration. Calcification is rare, occurring in 1% to 2% of cases (Fig. 12-123, *B*). Signal intensity on MR scans is variable but most often is similar to gray matter on all sequences. Hemorrhage, cyst formation, and postoperative changes may complicate the MR appearance of pituitary adenomas (Fig. 12-123, *C*)[108,128] (*see* Chapter 14).

Pituitary carcinoma is rare; malignancy can be diagnosed only if metastases are present.[129] Most malignant tumors in the pituitary gland are metastases from extracranial primary sources (see subsequent discussion).[130]

Meningiomas comprise 15% to 20% of all primary intracranial tumors and are the second most common suprasellar neoplasm in adults. Most parasellar meningiomas originate from the sphenoid ridge, diaphragma, or tuberculum sellae (Fig. 12-124). Contrast

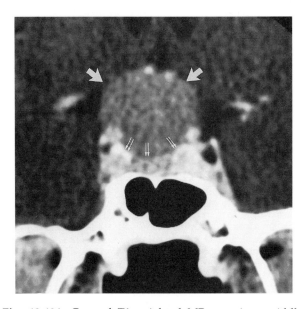

Fig. 12-124. Coronal T1-weighted MR scan in a middle-aged woman with bitemporal hemianopsia shows an enhancing suprasellar mass *(large arrows)*. Note that the mass does not enhance as intensely as, and can be distinguished from, the pituitary gland *(double arrows)*. Meningioma was found at subfrontal craniotomy.

Table 12-4. Typical MRI and CT appearance of common suprasellar lesions

Lesion	CT		MR signal compared to brain
	Unenhanced	Enhanced	T1W1
Pituitary macroadenoma	Isodense	Modest uniform enhancement	Isointense; enhances strongly, sometimes inhomogeneously
Pituitary macroadenoma (hemorrhagic)	Inhomogeneously hyperdense	Hyperdense	Often complex mixed signal; iso/hyperintense
Meningioma	Slightly hyperdense	Strong uniform enhancement	Isointense (may be inconspicuous); enhances strongly
Craniopharyngioma	Heterogeneous; cystic: hypodense; solid: iso- or slightly hyperdense	Variable; cystic: rim enhancement; solid: +/− enhancement	Variable; cystic: variable, often hyperintense; enhancement in rim or tumor nodule; solid: isointense
Glioma (optico-chiasmatic or hypothalamic)	Isodense or slightly hypodense	+/− enhancement	Isointense; variable enhancement
Aneurysm (patent)	Slightly hyperdense	Strong uniform enhancement	Flow void
Aneurysm (partially thrombosed)	Slightly hyperdense	Nonenhancing in area of thrombus; strongly enhancing patent lumen; may see rim enhancement	Thrombus: variable

T2W1	Comments
Isointense or slightly hyperintense	Calcification is rare; displacement rather than invasion of adjacent structures; often lobulated (figure eight); mass indistinguishable from pituitary
Complex mixed signal	Signal changes with age of clot
Variable: hypo- iso-, or slightly hyperintense	Smooth well-delineated lesion; calcification is common; look for dural "tail"; pituitary gland distinct from mass
Variable; cystic: hyperintense; solid: hyperintense	Focal calcification is common (rim, globular) location: 70% intra & suprasellar 20% suprasellar only 10% intrasellar only
Slightly hyperintense (may remain isointense)	May see chiasmal enlargement; calcification rare; retrochiasmatic extension is common (N.B.-occasionally compressive lesions such as craniopharyngioma or adenoma can cause hyperintensity in adjacent brain)
Flow void	Turbulent flow may give inhomogeneous signal; ICA or ACoA are most common locations; may see rim calcification
Variable	Thrombus may appear heterogeneous (laminated blood products in different stages)

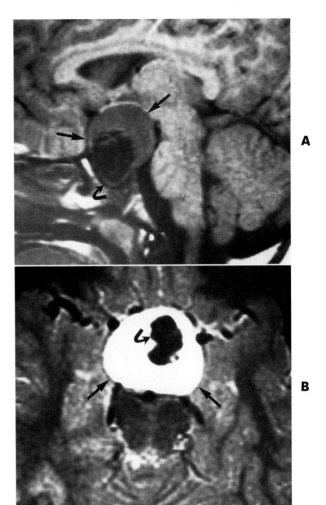

Fig. 12-125. A, Sagittal T1-weighted and, **B,** axial T2-weighted MR scans in an 8-year-old child show a large partially calcified intra- and suprasellar mass. The mass *(straight arrows)* is somewhat hypointense to brain on the T1WI but very hyperintense on the T2-weighted study. Calcification is seen as a central low signal focus *(curved arrows)* on both studies. Craniopharyngioma.

enhancement is strong and uniform but not as intense as the adjacent pituitary gland and cavernous sinus, allowing most meningiomas to be distinguished from adenoma.

Craniopharyngiomas account for half of all suprasellar tumors in children. A second peak occurs in adults between the fourth and sixth decades. At least 90% of all craniopharyngiomas exhibit calcification, enhance, and are at least partially cystic.[121] Signal intensity varies with cyst content, particularly on T1-weighted sequences, but the majority of craniopharyngiomas are hyperintense on T2WI (Fig. 12-125).[131] Most craniopharyngiomas are completely or at least partially suprasellar.[97]

Astrocytomas of the visual pathway, optic nerve, chiasm, and optic tracts account for 5% of childhood primary brain tumors and 25% to 30% of pediatric suprasellar neoplasms. Neurofibromatosis type 1 is present in 20% to 50% of these patients. Pathology is usually low-grade astrocytoma, often the juvenile pilocytic variety.[132] On CT these masses are iso- to hypodense and frequently enhance following contrast administration (Fig. 12-126). The lesions are hypointense on T1-weighted MR scans but hyperintense on T2WI. Post-chiasmatic enhancement or signal abnormality on T2WI is suggestive of—but not pathognomonic for—glioma because long-standing extraaxial compressive lesions such as adenoma or craniopharyngioma occasionally cause these findings.

Less common suprasellar tumors include germinoma, epidermoid and dermoid tumors, lymphoma and leukemia, and metastases.

Intracranial germinomas have a preference for midline sites. The pineal gland is the most common location, followed by the sellar/suprasellar region (Fig. 12-127). Synchronous pineal and suprasellar lesions account for 10% of intracranial germ cell tumors.[31]

Hypothalamoneurohypophyseal axis *germinomas* most often are both intra- and suprasellar; occasionally a germinoma involves only the infundibular stalk (see subsequent discussion).[133] Most patients are under 30 years of age and have endocrine dysfunction such as diabetes insipidus or panhypopituitarism.

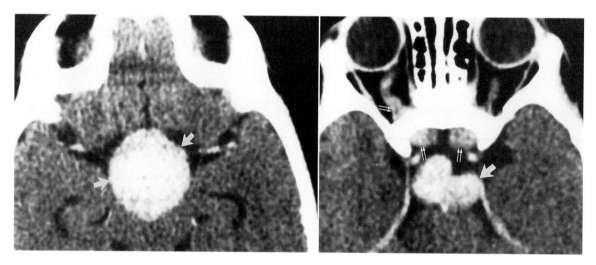

Fig. 12-126. CECT scans in a 3-year-old child with NF-1 show a strongly enhancing suprasellar mass *(large arrows)* that involves both optic nerves *(double arrows)*. Opticochiasmatic-hypothalamic glioma.

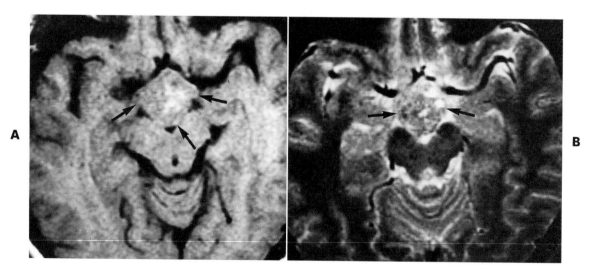

Fig. 12-127. Axial T1- **(A)** and T2-weighted **(B)** MR scans in a 22-year-old man with panhypopituitarism show a somewhat inhomogeneous suprasellar mass *(arrows)* that is predominately isointense with adjacent brain on both sequences.

MR scans typically demonstrate an infiltrating mass that is isointense to brain on T1WI, moderately hyperintense on T2-weighted studies, and enhances strongly and homogeneously after contrast administration.[97] CSF dissemination throughout the ventricular system and subarachnoid space is common.[121]

Epidermoid tumors occasionally occur in the suprasellar cistern (Fig. 12-128). These lesions are actually developmental epithelial inclusion cysts, not true neoplasms.[1] Epidermoids are most common between the fourth and sixth decades. Grossly, these tumors have a lobulated, irregular or frond-like surface. Squamous epithelium lines a central cystic area that

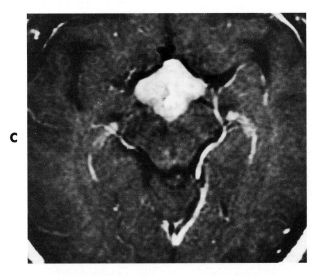

c

Fig. 12-127, cont'd. Postcontrast T1WI **(C)** shows the lesion enhances strongly. Germinoma.

is filled with desquamated cells and keratin debris. Most epidermoids appear similar to CSF on imaging studies.

Dermoid tumors are well-delineated, lobulated masses that typically occur in or near the midline. Most are found in the posterior fossa; suprasellar dermoids are uncommon. Similar to epidermoid cysts, dermoid tumors contain squamous epithelium and desquamated cellular debris. In addition, they contain dermal appendages (hair follicles plus sebaceous and sweat glands) and secretions. On imaging studies, dermoids usually appear similar to fat (Fig. 12-129). Calcification is relatively common. Ruptured dermoids may spill their contents throughout the CSF spaces and elicit severe chemical meningitis. Dermoids and lipomas (Fig. 12-130) are two uncommon causes of a suprasellar "bright spot" (*see* box, p. 472).

Lymphoproliferative disorders are uncommon causes of suprasellar masses. *Lymphoma* may involve the pituitary gland, hypothalamus, infundibular stalk, or a combination of these areas. A lesion with both an intra- and suprasellar component is typical. Most lymphomas occur in older adults. *Granulocytic sarcoma (chloroma)* is an unusual tumor composed of primitive myeloid cells. It occurs in younger patients with acute myelogenous leukemia. CNS involvement is rare. Dural and subarachnoid infiltration are common manifestations (see subsequent discussion). Orbit, sphenoid sinus, and hypothalamic-infundibular lesions occasionally occur (Fig. 12-131).[134]

Metastases to the hypothalamic-pituitary axis represent approximately 1% of sellar/parasellar masses.

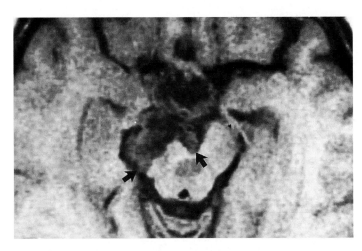

Fig. 12-128. Axial T1-weighted MR scan shows the typical cauliflower-like appearance of this suprasellar epidermoid tumor. The mass is mostly hypointense to brain, its core is very similar to CSF, and the lobulated surface is slightly higher in signal. Epidermoids insinuate themselves along CSF cisterns. Here, the tumor extends into the interpeduncular fossa and ambient cistern *(arrows)*.

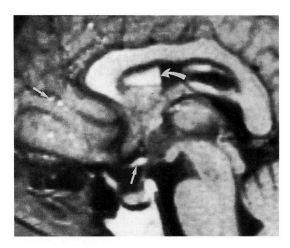

Fig. 12-129. Sagittal T1-weighted MR scan shows a ruptured dermoid cyst with high signal contents in the suprasellar cistern and interhemispheric fissure *(small arrows)*, as well as inside the lateral ventricle (where it forms a fat-fluid level, *[curved arrow]*).

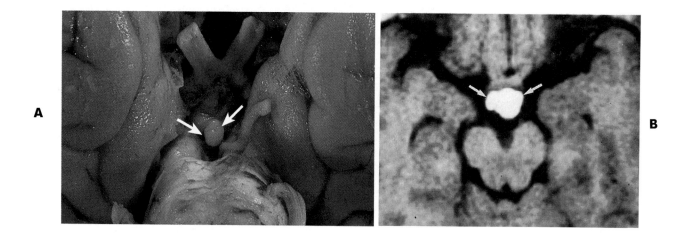

Fig. 12-130. A, Gross pathology specimen shows a suprasellar lipoma *(arrows)*. **B,** Axial T1-weighted MR scan shows a lobulated high signal suprasellar mass *(arrows)*. The lesion became profoundly hypointense on T2WI (not shown). Lipoma. (**A,** Courtesy B. Horten.)

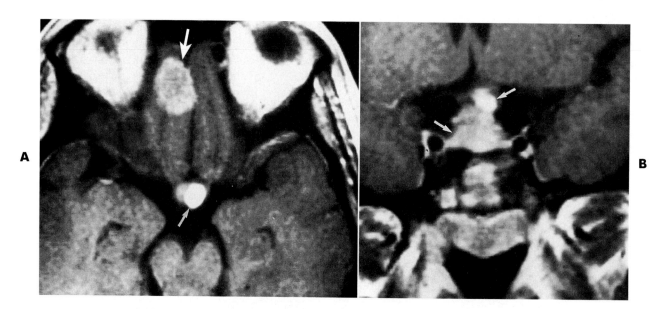

Fig. 12-131. Axial **(A)** and coronal **(B)** postcontrast T1-weighted MR scans in a 29-year-old woman with known leukemia show a combined intra- and suprasellar mass *(small arrows)*. A frontal lesion is also present (**A,** *large arrow*). Granulocytic sarcoma.

Overall, breast cancer is by far the most common, accounting for over half of all secondary pituitary neoplasms.[124] Primary sources of pituitary metastases in women in descending order of frequency are carcinomas of the breast, lung, stomach, and uterus. In men, common primary tumors are neoplasms of the lung, followed by prostate, bladder, stomach, and pancreas.

Pituitary metastases often cannot be distinguished clinically from pituitary adenomas.[124] Imaging studies disclose a suprasellar (Fig. 12-132) or combined intra- and suprasellar mass (Fig. 12-117). Metastases are typically isodense on T1-weighted MR scans and moderately hyperintense on T2WI. Moderate enhancement following contrast administration occurs.[125]

Vascular lesions. *Vascular ectasias* (Fig. 12-133) and *supraclinoid ICA aneurysms* (Fig. 12-134) are the most common nonneoplastic suprasellar masses in adults. Imaging appearance of aneurysms is variable, depending on the presence and age of thrombus and various flow parameters (*see* Chapter 9). Other than

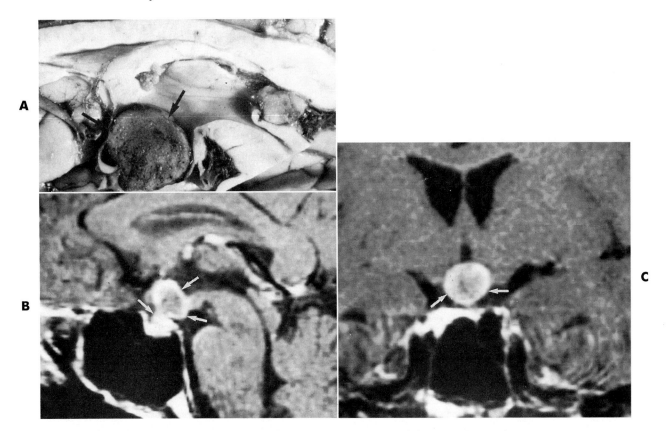

Fig. 12-132. **A,** Gross pathology specimen in a patient with lung carcinoma shows a metastasis that involves the hypothalamus and anterior third ventricle *(large arrows)*. A smaller metastasis is present in the pineal gland *(small arrow)*. Sagittal **(B)** and coronal **(C)** contrast-enhanced T1-weighted MR scans in another patient with lung carcinoma demonstrate a metastasis *(arrows)* that involves the hypothalamus and infundibular stalk. (**A,** Courtesy Rubinstein Collection, University of Virginia.)

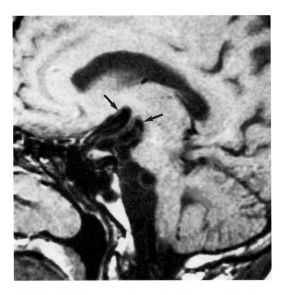

Fig. 12-133. Striking vascular ectasia *(arrows)* is shown on the sagittal T1-weighted MR scan in this elderly patient. The internal carotid and basilar arteries are elongated and tortuous, deeply indenting the third ventricle and thalamus *(arrows)*.

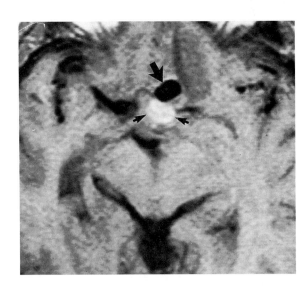

Fig. 12-134. Axial T1-weighted MR scan shows a partially thrombosed suprasellar ICA aneurysm. The patent lumen is seen as a well-delineated high-velocity signal loss *(large arrow)*, and the thrombosed segment is filled with hyperintense subacute clot *(small arrows)*.

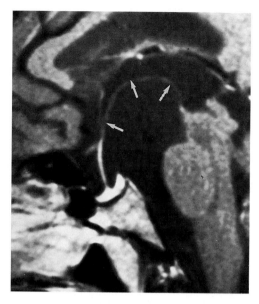

Fig. 12-135. Sagittal T1-weighted scan of a suprasellar arachnoid cyst (SSAC). The cyst elevates the third ventricle *(arrows)* and is slightly hyperintense compared to CSF.

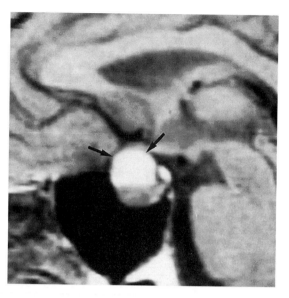

Fig. 12-136. Sagittal T1-weighted MR scan in a patient with headaches and no focal neurologic abnormalities on physical examination. A high signal suprasellar mass is present *(arrows)*. Surgery disclosed Rathke cleft cyst.

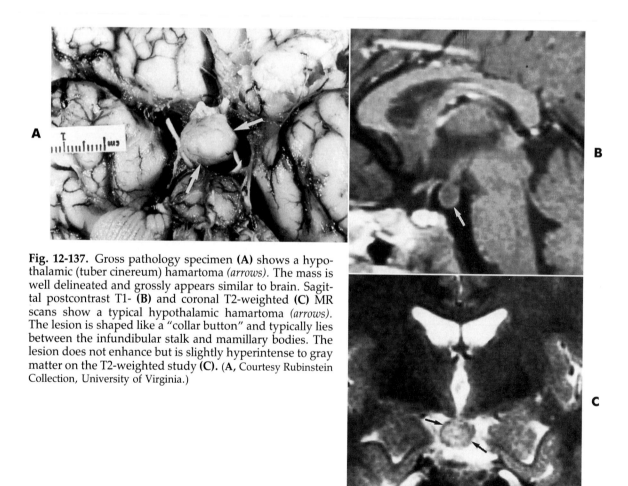

Fig. 12-137. Gross pathology specimen **(A)** shows a hypothalamic (tuber cinereum) hamartoma *(arrows)*. The mass is well delineated and grossly appears similar to brain. Sagittal postcontrast T1- **(B)** and coronal T2-weighted **(C)** MR scans show a typical hypothalamic hamartoma *(arrows)*. The lesion is shaped like a "collar button" and typically lies between the infundibular stalk and mamillary bodies. The lesion does not enhance but is slightly hyperintense to gray matter on the T2-weighted study **(C)**. (**A,** Courtesy Rubinstein Collection, University of Virginia.)

aneurysms and dolichoectatic vessels, suprasellar vascular masses are uncommon. Occasionally, cavernous angiomas occur in the hypothalamus.

Congenital. Important congenital lesions include suprasellar arachnoid cyst, Rathke's cleft cyst, and hypothalamic (tuber cinereum) hamartoma.

Arachnoid cysts account for about 1% of all intracranial space-occupying lesions.[135] Approximately 10% of arachnoid cysts occur in the suprasellar region. A suprasellar arachnoid cyst (SSAC) appears as a smoothly marginated mass that is similar to CSF in signal intensity. SSACs neither calcify nor enhance. A displaced, compressed third ventricle can usually be identified on MR studies (Fig. 12-135).

Rathke's cleft cyst (RCC) is a benign epithelium-lined cyst that probably arises from remnants of Rathke's pouch.[136] Intrasellar RCCs are usually asymptomatic and found incidentally at autopsy or MR imaging.[137] Symptomatic RCCs are usually combined intra- and suprasellar masses; purely suprasellar RCCs are rare.[138] RCCs have well-defined walls with intracystic material that ranges from serous to mucoid. CT density and MR signal vary with cyst content (Fig. 12-136). Calcification is absent, which helps distinguish RCCs from most craniopharyngiomas. The differential diagnosis includes arachnoid cyst, cystic pituitary adenoma, and the rare noncalcified cystic craniopharyngioma.[139]

Hypothalamic (tuber cinereum) hamartoma is a congenital nonneoplastic heterotopia.[140] Patients with hypothalamic hamartomas consist of two distinct clinical groups. The first group is characterized by isosexual precocious puberty.[141] Symptom onset is usually between birth and 3 years of age. In the second group, precocious puberty may be absent. Gelastic seizures of the partial complex type, intellectual impairment, and psychiatric disturbances may be present.[142]

Grossly, tuber cinereum hamartomas are pedunculated or sessile lesions that lie between the infundibular stalk anteriorly and the mamillary bodies posteriorly (Fig. 12-137, *A*). Microscopically, hamartomas closely resemble normal gray matter. Most are isointense to gray matter on T1-weighted and long TR/short TE scans but are often hyperintense on T2WI (Fig. 12-137, *B* and *C*). Hamartomas neither calcify nor exhibit enhancement following contrast administration. Occasionally, these lesions can be extensive and even form prominent cysts (Fig. 12-138). The differential diagnosis is hypothalamic glioma.

Inflammatory and infectious lesions. Exudative bacterial meningitis and tuberculous meningitis have a distinct predilection for the basilar subarachnoid spaces (*see* Chapter 16). Sarcoidosis can cause a thickened infundibular stalk, a focal hypothalamic mass or diffuse basilar leptomeningeal thickening (see subse-

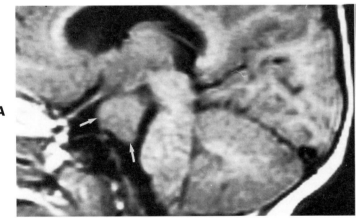

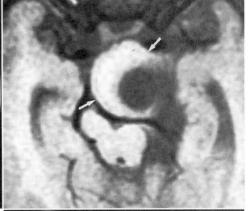

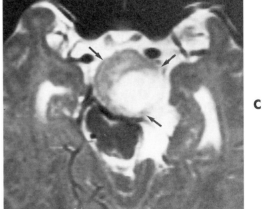

Fig. 12-138. Sagittal **(A)** and axial **(B)** T1- and axial T2-weighted **(C)** MR scans of an atypical tuber cinereum hamartoma. The lesion *(arrows)* is somewhat larger than usual and has a central cystic component. (Courtesy L. Tan and S. Lin.)

quent discussion). *Cysticercosis* may involve the suprasellar cistern. Parenchymal abscesses are rare in the hypothalamus.

Lymphocytic hypophysitis is a rare inflammatory process that affects the anterior pituitary lobe. It is characterized histologically by lymphocytic infiltration of the adenohypophysis. Clinically, the disorder is characterized by hypopituitarism and expanding suprasellar mass. Nearly all reported cases are in women. The disorder usually occurs during late pregnancy or the postpartum period.[143] Imaging studies in most patients disclose an enhancing intrasellar mass with suprasellar extension that resembles macroadenoma.

Giant-cell granulomatous hypophysitis is a chronic inflammatory disease of the pituitary gland. It presents with symptoms of hypopituitarism and an expanding sellar mass. In most cases, pituitary granulomas are caused by a specific lesion such as *syphilis, tuberculosis, sarcoidosis,* or Langerhans cell *histiocytosis* (formerly termed *histiocytosis X*). Idiopathic cases have been reported.[144] Imaging findings are nonspecific and resemble macroadenoma or lymphocytic hypophysitis.

Trauma. Traumatic lesions of the optic chiasm, intracranial optic nerves, hypothalamus, and pituitary gland produce various clinical signs and symptoms. Visual loss with or without bitemporal hemianopsia and endocrine dysfunction due to hypothalamic injury are the most common manifestations. MR imaging demonstrates a spectrum of abnormalities that ranges from *chiasm contusion* or *transection* and *traumatic tears* of the third ventricle to *avulsed third nerve* and *transected pituitary stalk*.[145] Interruption of the infundibular stalk can result in diabetes insipidus and hypothalamic high signal that appears similar to congenital ectopic neurohypophysis.

Infundibular stalk masses. The pituitary stalk tapers smoothly as it courses inferiorly from its hypothalamic origin to pituitary insertion. The normal stalk is 3 to 3.5 mm wide near the median eminence and 2 mm wide near its insertion on the pituitary gland.[146] Because it lacks a blood-brain barrier, the infundibulum normally enhances strongly and uniformly following contrast administration. Increase in stalk size or contour alteration from its normal symmetric tapering shape is abnormal. The differential diagnosis of an enlarged infundibulum is summarized in the box.

Infundibular masses in children. Pituitary stalk thickening in children occurs with *Langerhans cell histiocytosis* (LCH), formerly called histiocytosis X. The chronic, recurring, disseminated form of LCH (also known as Hand-Schuller-Christian disease) affects bone and extraskeletal sites in about 20% of LCH cases. Cranial involvement occurs in over 90% of

Infundibular Masses
Children
Common
Langerhans cell histiocytosis
Germinoma
Meningitis
Uncommon
Lymphoma
Glioma
Adults
Common
Sarcoidosis
Germinoma
Metastasis
Uncommon
Lymphoma
Glioma
Choristoma

these patients.[147] Many have overt diabetes insipidus, absent posterior pituitary "bright spot," and a thickened, enhancing infundibular stalk with or without associated hypothalamic mass (Fig. 12-139).[148,149] Dural and parenchymal masses can be present (*see* Fig. 12-194).[149a]

Infundibular stalk enlargement in children can also be caused by *germinoma* (Fig. 12-140) and *meningitis*. Isolated pituitary stalk glioma is a rare lesion. Sometimes termed infundibuloma, this lesion is usually a *pilocytic astrocytoma*. *Lymphoproliferative diseases* and inflammatory processes occasionally enlarge the infundibulum and hypothalamus in children but are more common in adults.

Infundibular masses in adults. Sarcoidosis, histiocytosis, and other inflammatory diseases may affect the hypophyseal region.[150] *Neurosarcoidosis* (NS) is relatively rare, affecting only 5% of all sarcoid cases. NS most commonly involves the meninges, cranial nerves, hypothalamus, infundibular stalk, and pituitary gland (Figs. 12-141).[151] Occasionally, NS causes a focal extraaxial or parenchymal mass and can mimic meningioma or glioma (*see* Fig. 12-195).[152]

An enlarged infundibular stalk can also occur with *lymphoma, germinoma,* and *metastases*. Primary tumors of the neurohypophysis and infundibulum are extremely rare. Two types are recognized: glioma (also known as infundibuloma or *pituicytoma*) and granular cell tumor (*choristoma,* myoblastoma, or granular cell myoblastoma).[153] Imaging findings of an enhancing suprasellar mass that is isointense to brain on MR and isodense on CT are characteristic but nonspecific (Fig. 12-142).

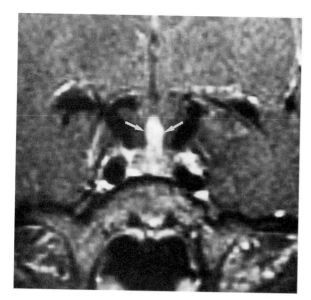

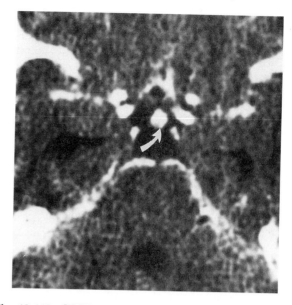

Fig. 12-139. Coronal contrast-enhanced T1-weighted MR scan in a 6-year-old child with diabetes insipidus and histiocytosis involving the infundibular stalk *(arrows)*.

Fig. 12-140. CECT scan in a 5-year-old child with diabetes insipidus shows a thickened, enhancing infundibular stalk *(arrow)* caused by germinoma.

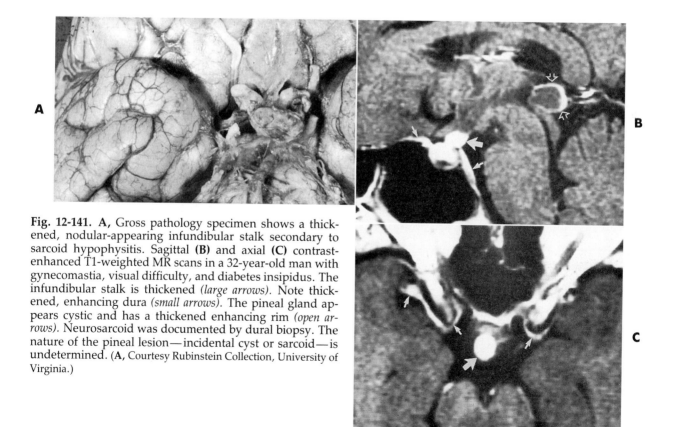

Fig. 12-141. A, Gross pathology specimen shows a thickened, nodular-appearing infundibular stalk secondary to sarcoid hypophysitis. Sagittal **(B)** and axial **(C)** contrast-enhanced T1-weighted MR scans in a 32-year-old man with gynecomastia, visual difficulty, and diabetes insipidus. The infundibular stalk is thickened *(large arrows)*. Note thickened, enhancing dura *(small arrows)*. The pineal gland appears cystic and has a thickened enhancing rim *(open arrows)*. Neurosarcoid was documented by dural biopsy. The nature of the pineal lesion—incidental cyst or sarcoid—is undetermined. **(A,** Courtesy Rubinstein Collection, University of Virginia.)

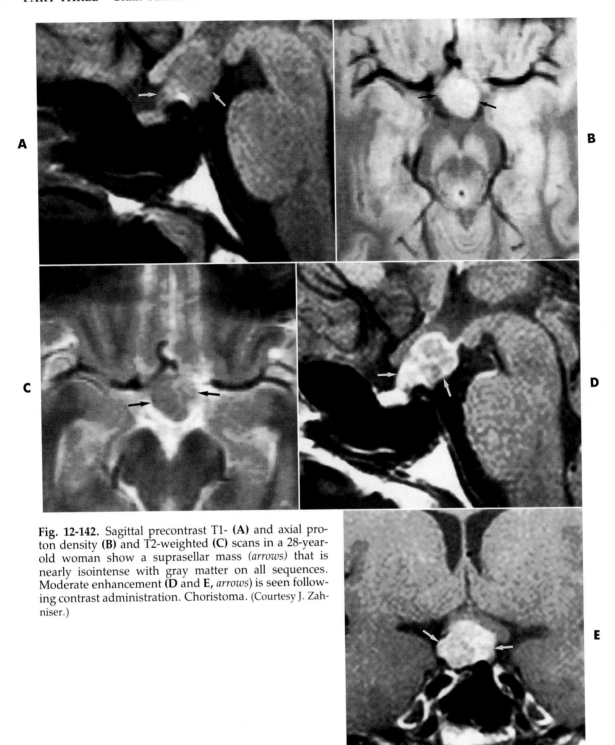

Fig. 12-142. Sagittal precontrast T1- **(A)** and axial proton density **(B)** and T2-weighted **(C)** scans in a 28-year-old woman show a suprasellar mass *(arrows)* that is nearly isointense with gray matter on all sequences. Moderate enhancement **(D** and **E,** *arrows)* is seen following contrast administration. Choristoma. (Courtesy J. Zahniser.)

Skull Base and Cavernous Sinus Masses

Normal anatomy. The skull base is composed of the ethmoid, sphenoid, and occipital bones and the paired frontal and temporal bones.[154,155] The principal foramina, fissures, and canals in the base of the skull (BOS) are illustrated in Fig. 12-143. These BOS "ins and outs" with their contents are summarized in Table 12-5.

Pathologic anatomy: overview. BOS lesions have been classified in several different ways. We will approach this complex anatomic region and its lesions by dividing the skull base into anterior, central, and posterior segments.

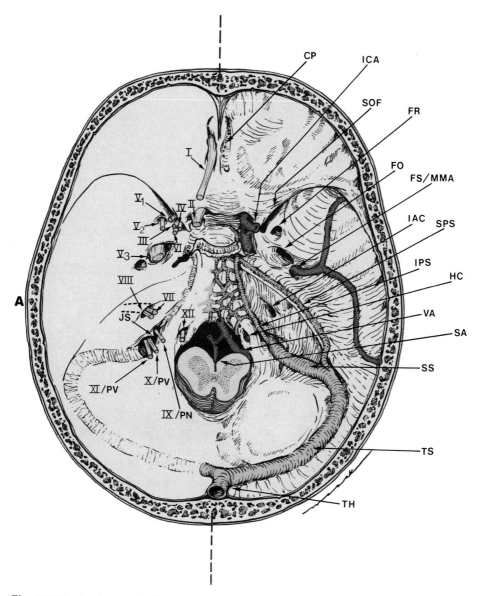

Fig. 12-143. A, Anatomic drawing depicts the endocranial aspect of the skull base. Foramina, fissures, and vascular anatomy *(arteries in red, dural sinuses in blue)* are shown on the right side of the drawing. Cranial nerves I to XII are shown on the left side and indicated by Roman numerals *(CNs and medulla are in yellow)*. *IAC,* Internal auditory canal. *SOF,* Superior orbital fissure. *VC,* Vidian canal. *CP,* Cribriform plate. *ICA,* Internal carotid artery. *SOF,* Superior orbital fissure. *FR,* Foramen rotundum. *FO,* Foramen ovale. *FS/MMA,* Foramen spinosum/middle meningeal artery. *IAC,* Internal auditory canal. *SPS,* Superior petrosal sinus. *IPS,* Inferior petrosal sinus. *HC,* Hypoglossal canal. *VA,* Vertebral artery. *SA,* Spinal artery. *SS,* Signmoid sinus. *TS,* Transverse sinus. *TH,* Torcular Herophili. *JS,* Jugular spine. *I,* Olfactory nerve (through cribriform plate). *II,* Optic nerve (through optic canal). *III,* Oculomotor nerve (through superior orbital fissure). *IV,* Trochlear nerve (through superior orbital fissure). V_1, Ophthalmic division, trigeminal nerve (through superior orbital fissure). V_2, Maxillary division, trigeminal nerve (through foramen rotundum). V_3, Mandibular division, trigeminal nerve (through foramen ovale). *VI,* Abducens nerve. *VII,* Facial nerve (through internal auditory canal; exits skull through stylomastoid foramen). *VIII,* Vestibulocochlear (auditory) nerve. *IX/PN,* Glossopharyngeal nerve/pars nervosa (through jugular foramen). *X/PV,* Vagus nerve/pars vascularis (through jugular foramen). *XI/PV,* Spinal accessory nerve/pars vascularis (through jugular foramen). *XII,* Hypoglossal nerve (through hypoglossal canal). (From Osborn AG et al: Sem US, CT, MR 7:91-106, 1986.)

Continued.

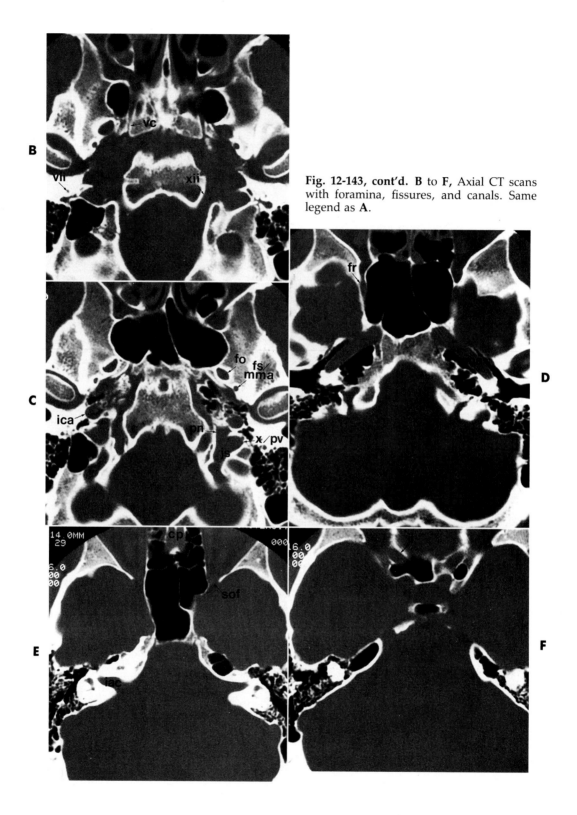

Fig. 12-143, cont'd. B to **F,** Axial CT scans with foramina, fissures, and canals. Same legend as **A.**

Table 12-5. Major Apertures of the Skull Base

Aperture	Location	Transmitted structure(s)	Connects
Cribriform plate	Medial floor of anterior cranial fossa	Olfactory nerve (CN* 1) Ethmoidal arteries (anterior and posterior)	Anterior fossa to superior nasal cavity
Optic canal	Lesser wing of sphenoid bone	Optic nerve (CN II) Ophthalmic artery Subarachnoid space, cerebrospinal fluid, and dura around optic nerve	Orbital apex to middle cranial fossa
Superior orbital fissure	Between lesser and greater sphenoid wings	CNs III, IV, V_1, VI Superior ophthalmic vein	Orbit to middle cranial fossa
Foramen rotundum	Middle cranial fossa floor inferior to superior orbital fissure	CN V_2 Emissary veins Artery of foramen rotundum	Meckel's cave to pterygopalatine fossa
Foramen ovale	Floor of middle cranial fossa lateral to sella	CN V_3 Emissary veins from cavernous sinus to pterygoid plexus Accessory meningeal branch of maxillary artery (when present)	Meckel's cave to nasopharyngeal masticator space (infratemporal fossa)
Foramen spinosum	Posterolateral to foramen ovale	Middle meningeal artery Recurrent (meningeal) branch of mandibular nerve	Middle cranial fossa to high masticator space (infratemporal fossa)
Foramen lacerum	Base of medial pterygoid plate at petrous apex	Meningeal branches of ascending pharyngeal artery (not internal carotid artery)	Not a true foramen; filled with fibrocartilage in life
Vidian canal	In sphenoid bone below and medial to foramen rotundum	Vidian artery	Foramen lacerum to pterygopalatine fossa
Carotid canal	Within petrous temporal bone	Internal carotid artery Sympathetic plexus	Carotid space to cavernous sinus
Jugular foramen	Posterolateral to carotid canal, between petrous temporal bone and occipital bone	Pars nervosa; inferior petrosal sinuses (CN IX and Jacobson's nerve) Pars vascularis: internal jugular vein, CNs X and XI, nerve of Arnold, small meningeal branches of ascending pharyngeal and occipital arteries	Posterior fossa to nasopharyngeal carotid space
Stylomastoid foramen	Behind styloid process	CN VII	Parotid space to middle ear
Hypoglossal canal	Base of occipital condyles	CN XII	Foramen magnum to nasopharyngeal carotid space
Foramen magnum	Floor of posterior fossa	Medulla and its meninges Spinal segment of CN XI Vertebral arteries and veins Anterior and posterior spinal arteries	Posterior fossa to cervical spinal canal

Modified from Osborn AG et al: *Sem US, CT, MR* 7:91-106, 1986.
*CN, Cranial Nerve.

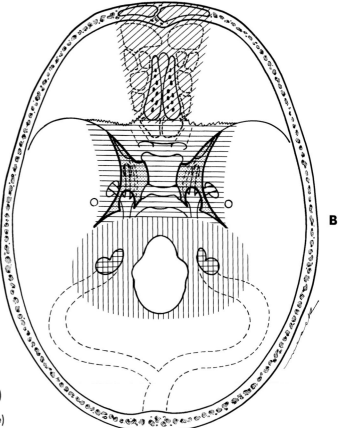

Anterior skull base

Common
  Sinonasal malignancy (e.g., squamous cell carcinoma)
  Meningioma (cribriform plate)
  Metastases (central skull base metastases more common)
Uncommon
  Benign sinonasal mass (e.g., osteoma, polyps, mucocele)
  Sinusitis/epidural abscess or empyema
  Some sinonasal malignant tumors (e.g., lymphoma, esthesioneuroblastoma)

Central skull base

Common
  Nasopharyngeal malignancy (e.g., squamous cell carcinoma)
  Extracranial metastases (e.g., breast carcinoma)
Uncommon
  Sinusitis (bacterial, fungal)
  Cocaine granuloma
  Meningioma
  Pituitary adenoma
Rare but important
  Sarcoidosis
  Histiocytosis
  Paget disease

Cavernous sinus

Unilateral
  Vascular lesion (aneurysm, C-C fistula)
  Meningioma
  Schwannoma
  Metastasis (hematogenous or perineural)
  Lymphoma
Bilateral
  Vascular lesion (some C-C fistulae)
  Pituitary adenoma
  Meningioma
  Metastases
  Lymphoma
  Thrombosis (septic, spontaneous)

Posterior skull base/clivus

Common
  Nasopharyngeal malignancy (e.g., squamous cell carcinoma)
  Metastasis
  Meningioma
Uncommon
  Chordoma
  Osteomyelitis (including Gradenigo syndrome)
  Myeloma/plasmacytoma
  Histiocytosis

Jugular foramen

Common
  Paraganglioma (glomus jugulare tumor)
  Metastases (e.g., breast)
  Asymmetric jugular bulb (can be very large)
  Thrombosed internal jugular vein
Uncommon
  Schwannoma of CNs IX to XI
  Osteomyelitis

Fig. 12-144. A, Axial cryomicrotome section depicts gross anatomy of the anterior and central skull base. *1,* Frontal, ethmoid sinuses. *2,* Crista galli. *3,* Cribriform plate. *4,* Gyrus rectus (frontal lobe). *5,* Planum sphenoidale. *6,* Spenoid sinus. *7,* Internal carotid artery. *8,* Superior orbital fissure. *9,* Pituitary gland. *10,* Cavernous sinus. **B,** Anatomic drawing of the skull base depicts locations of common lesions in this area. (**A,** Courtesy W. Rauschning.)

Anterior skull base lesions. The anterior BOS consists of the orbital plates of the frontal bones, the cribriform plate of the ethmoid bone and the planum sphenoidale (Fig. 12-144). Lesions in this area arise extracranially (from the nasal vault, frontal, and ethmoid sinuses), intrinsically (from the skull base itself), and intracranially (from the brain, meninges, and CSF spaces) (*see* box).

Extracranial lesions. Most extracranial anterior skull base masses originate from the nose and paranasal sinuses. Common benign lesions in this area are mucocele, polyposis, inverted papilloma, and osteoma. Malignant sinonasal tumors include squamous cell carcinoma, rhabdomyosarcoma, adenoid cystic carcinoma, and esthesioneuroblastoma.[156]

Mucoceles are caused by the accumulation of impacted mucus behind an occluded draining sinus ostium, most commonly from inflammatory obstruction. Posttraumatic or neoplastic obstruction can also cause a secondary mucocele. If a mucocele becomes infected it is termed *mucopyocele.* In descending order of frequency, mucoceles are found in the frontal, ethmoid, maxillary, and sphenoid sinuses.[156a]

Imaging studies typically show a well-delineated soft tissue mass with bone expansion and remodeling. Most mucoceles are low density on NECT scans, although inspissated secretions may appear hyperdense. MR signal is variable (Fig. 12-145).[157] Occasionally, mucoceles and *sinonasal polyposis* can simulate aggressive skull base erosion (Fig. 12-146). These changes are seen in 10% to 12% of cases.[158]

Inverted papilloma (IP) is a benign, slow-growing epithelial neoplasm that accounts for 1% to 4% of sinonasal neoplasms. IPs arise in the nasal vault near the junction of the ethmoid and maxillary sinuses. In these tumors, surface epithelium proliferates by in-verting into the underlying stroma rather than growing outward.[159]

The imaging appearance of inverted papilloma is distinctive but not pathognomonic. A unilateral, polypoid nasal fossa soft tissue mass widens the nasal vault, sometimes destroying bone and extending into the adjacent ethmoid and maxillary sinuses (Fig. 12-147). Focal erosion of the cribriform plate with cephalad extension occasionally occurs, mimicking sinonasal cavity malignancies.[158] There are no definitive MR findings that differentiate IPs from various malignant tumors.[160]

Anterior Skull Base Lesions

Common

Malignant sinonasal tumor (e.g., squamous cell carcinoma, rhabdomyosarcoma)
Meningioma
Metastases

Uncommon

Mucocele
Osteoma
Polyposis
Inverted papilloma
Esthesioneuroblastoma
Lymphoma
Complicated sinusitis (bacterial, fungal, granulomatous)

Rare

Cephalocele
Dermoid cyst

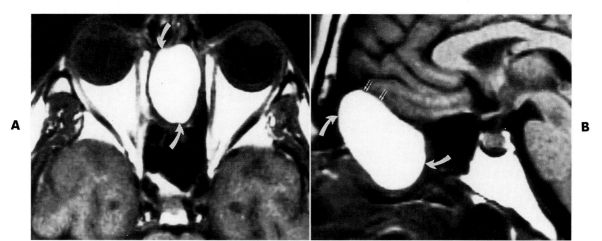

Fig. 12-145. Axial **(A)** and sagittal **(B)** TI- weighted MR scans show an ethmoid mucocele *(curved arrows).* The hyperintense mass expands and remodels bone. Anterior extension through the cribriform plate *(double arrows).*

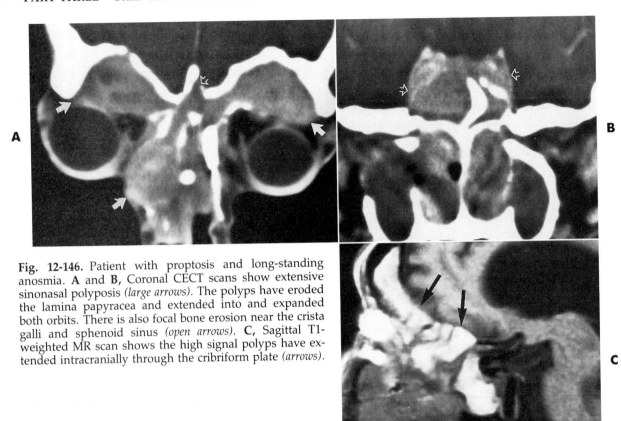

Fig. 12-146. Patient with proptosis and long-standing anosmia. **A** and **B**, Coronal CECT scans show extensive sinonasal polyposis *(large arrows)*. The polyps have eroded the lamina papyracea and extended into and expanded both orbits. There is also focal bone erosion near the crista galli and sphenoid sinus *(open arrows)*. **C**, Sagittal T1-weighted MR scan shows the high signal polyps have extended intracranially through the cribriform plate *(arrows)*.

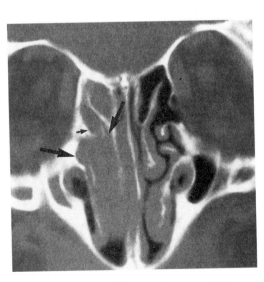

Fig. 12-147. Coronal NECT scan shows a soft tissue mass in the nasal vault *(large arrows)* that has eroded into the adjacent ethmoid sinuses (small arrow). Inverted papilloma was found at surgery.

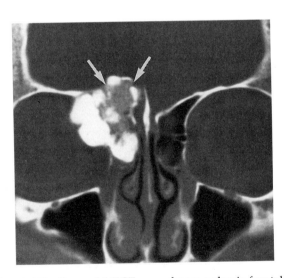

Fig. 12-148. Coronal NECT scan shows a classic frontal sinus osteoma. The osteoma has eroded through the sinus roof *(arrows)*.

Osteomas are benign bony tumors that have mature, well-delineated cortical bone as their primary component. The frontal sinus is the most common site in the head and neck. Osteomas can expand and then erode the posterior and superior frontal sinus walls (Fig. 12-148).

Intracranial extradural extension from *malignant sinonasal tumors* occurs in up to one third of cases. In children the most common extracranial malignancy that involves the skull base is rhabdomyosarcoma. *Rhabdomyosarcoma* is the most common soft tissue sarcoma in children, and the head and neck is the most common site of these malignant mesenchymal tumors. The orbit and nasopharynx are affected most often, followed by the paranasal sinuses and middle ear.[161,162]

Anterior skull base or cavernous sinus invasion occurs in approximately 35% of nasopharyngeal rhabdomyosarcomas.[163] Imaging studies show a bulky soft-tissue mass with areas of bone destruction. Signal intensity is similar to muscle on T1WI but becomes hyperintense on T2-weighted studies. Some contrast enhancement is usual.[162] Meningeal and perineural tumor spread are common (Fig. 12-149).

Ninety-eight percent of nasopharyngeal tumors in adults are carcinomas. *Squamous cell carcinoma* accounts for 80% of these tumors, and *adenocarcinoma* (most commonly from minor salivary glands) represents 18%. Nasopharyngeal carcinomas spread directly into the skull base (Fig. 12-150), as well as along muscles and their tendinous insertions. They extend intracranially along neural and vascular bundles via osseous foramina.[164]

A nasopharyngeal mass with obliterated soft tissue planes and adjacent bone destruction are the typical imaging findings with direct tumor invasion.[165] Serous otitis media can be seen because the eustachian tube is frequently obstructed.

Perineural tumor spread most commonly involves the second and third divisions of the trigeminal nerve (Fig. 12-71) and the facial nerve. Sometimes no dominant mass is present. Enhancement of the affected nerve or denervation atrophy of the muscles of mastication and face may be the only detectable abnormalities on imaging studies in some cases.[166]

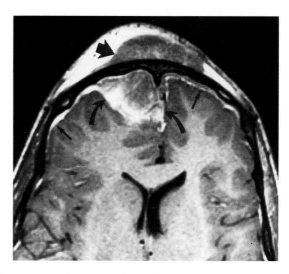

Fig. 12-149. Contrast-enhanced axial T1-weighted MR scan in an 8-year-old child with a forehead soft tissue mass. A large soft tissue mass is seen *(large arrow)* that has a significant intracranial extradural component *(curved arrows)*. Note meningeal extension *(small arrows)*. Rhabdomyosarcoma was found at surgery.

A, B   **C**

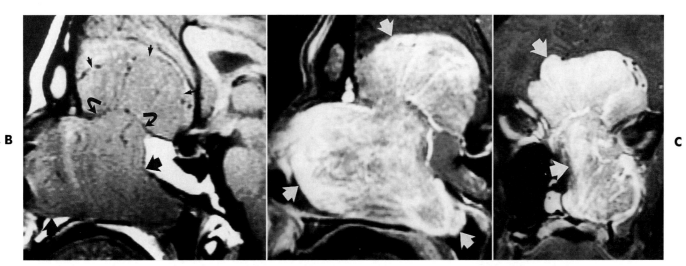

Fig. 12-150. Sagittal precontrast T1-weighted MR scan **(A)** shows a large sinonasal soft tissue mass *(large arrow)* that has extended through the cribriform plate *(curved arrows)*. A large intracranial extradural component is seen *(small arrows)*. Postcontrast sagittal **(B)** and coronal **(C)** T1WIs show the strongly but inhomogeneously enhancing mass *(arrows)*. Undifferentiated small cell carcinoma was found. (Courtesy L. Blas.)

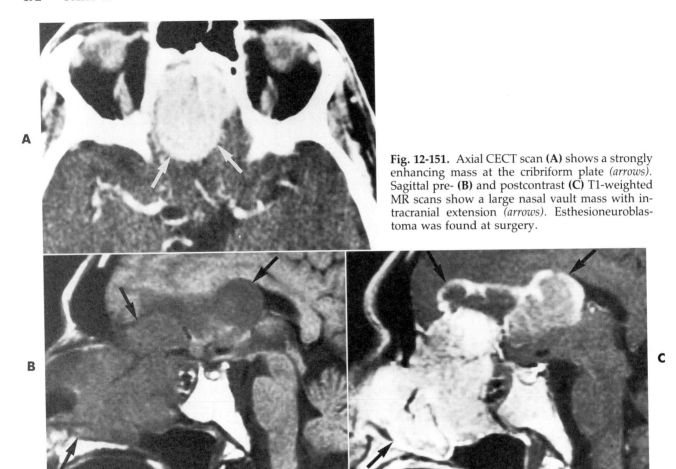

Fig. 12-151. Axial CECT scan **(A)** shows a strongly enhancing mass at the cribriform plate *(arrows)*. Sagittal pre- **(B)** and postcontrast **(C)** T1-weighted MR scans show a large nasal vault mass with intracranial extension *(arrows)*. Esthesioneuroblastoma was found at surgery.

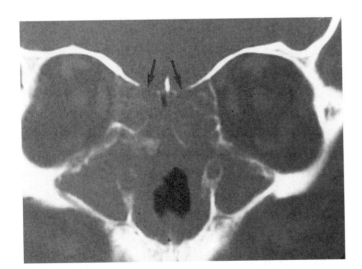

Fig. 12-152. Coronal NECT scan in a 46-year-old woman shows a midline sinonasal soft tissue mass with nasal septum and ethmoid bone erosion. The cribriform plate *(arrows)* is partially destroyed. Sarcoidosis was found at biopsy. The lesion is radiologically very similar to other aggressive sinonasal lesions such as Wegener granulomatosis, lymphoma, fungal sinusitis, or cocaine granuloma.

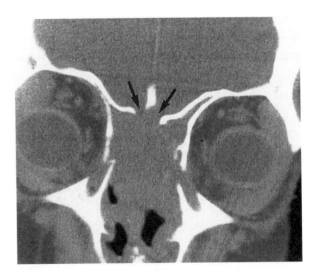

Fig. 12-153. Coronal NECT scan in a 43-year-old woman shows a midline sinonasal destructive soft tissue mass with ethmoid, nasal, and cribriform plate erosion *(arrows)*. The lacrimal glands and other orbital soft tissues are also involved. Lymphoma.

Esthesioneuroblastoma (ENB, or olfactory neuroblastoma) is an uncommon malignant tumor that arises from the bipolar sensory receptor cells in the olfactory mucosa. These cells originate in the neural crest and differentiate into the olfactory sensory elements. ENBs are histologically similar to adrenal or sympathetic ganglionic neuroblastomas and retinoblastomas.[167] In contrast to the typical childhood neuroblastoma, ENBs can occur at any age, although most reports show a bimodal distribution with a peak incidence in the second and fourth or fifth decades.[167,167a,b]

ENBs are often confined to the nasal cavity but may extend into the adjacent paranasal sinuses, orbit, or through the cribriform plate into the anterior cranial fossa. Imaging studies disclose a high nasal vault mass with focal bone destruction. These tumors have variable signal intensity on MR imaging. Moderate but inhomogeneous enhancement following contrast administration is typical (Fig. 12-151). CNS dissemination may occur as a late manifestation of ENB.[167]

Other radiologically aggressive processes that occasionally cause anterior skull base lesions include *bacterial* or *fungal sinusitis* (see subsequent discussion), *sarcoidosis* (Fig. 12-152), sinonasal *lymphoma* (Fig. 12-153), *cocaine granulomatosis* (Fig. 12-154), and *Wegener granulomatosis.*

Intrinsic lesions. Intrinsic anterior skull base lesions include entities such as *fibrous dysplasia* (Fig. 12-155), *Paget disease,* and osteopetrosis. These are discussed with scalp and skull abnormalities (see subsequent discussion).

Intracranial lesions. Intracranial lesions that involve the anterior skull base can arise from the meninges, CSF spaces, and the brain itself.

The most common meningeal lesion that involves the anterior BOS is *meningioma.* Planum sphenoidale and olfactory groove meningiomas account for 10% to 15% of all meningiomas. A broad-based, anterior basal subfrontal mass that enhances strongly and relatively uniformly after contrast administration is typical. Presence of a tumor-brain interface or cleft with

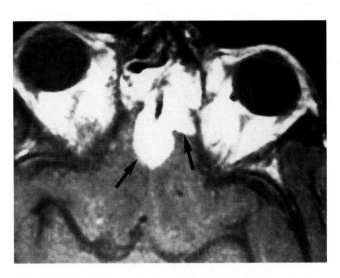

Fig. 12-154. Axial postcontrast T1-weighted MR scan in a 21-year-old man with seizures shows an enhancing mass *(arrows)* around the crista galli. Extensive sinonasal involvement was also present (not shown). Noncaseating granulomas were found at surgery. The patient later admitted long-standing cocaine use.

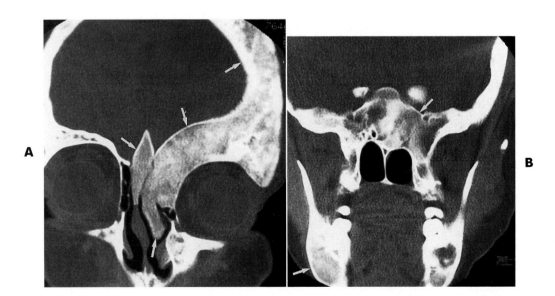

Fig. 12-155. Coronal CECT scans in a patient with polyostotic fibrous dysplasia. Note the expanded frontal bone, crista galli, and middle concha (**A,** *arrows*) by tissue that has the typical "ground glass" appearance of fibrous dysplasia. The sphenoid sinus and mandible are also affected (**B,** *arrows*).

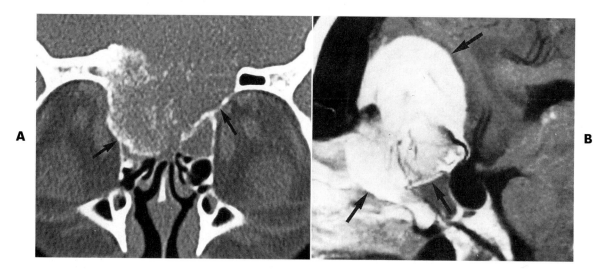

Fig. 12-156. A, Coronal NECT scan shows an extensive cribriform plate mass that has expanded and partially destroyed the planum sphenoidale. **B,** Sagittal T1-weighted MR scan shows a strongly enhancing mass that has both a large intracranial and extracranial *(arrows)* component. Meningioma. (Courtesy J. Fuentes.)

compressed cortex and white matter buckling indicate the extraaxial location *(see* Chapter 14).[168,169] Blistering and hyperostosis of the adjacent bone are common. Enlargement of the air-containing ethmoid sinus (pneumosinus dilatans) or even frank bone destruction is sometimes observed (Fig. 12-156).

The most common anterior skull base lesion that originates from the brain is a *nasoethmoidal cephalocele.* Fifteen percent of basal cephaloceles occur in the frontonasal area (Fig. 2-20).[163] Nasal *dermoid sinuses* and nasal *cerebral heterotopias* (nasal gliomas) are less common congenital lesions that occur in this location.[170]

Occasionally, slow-growing peripherally located *primary brain neoplasms* such as ganglioglioma cause pressure erosion of the adjacent skull. Frank dural invasion or calvarial destruction can occur with anaplastic astrocytoma and glioblastoma multiforme but is uncommon[171,172] *(see* Chapter 13).

Central skull base lesions. The central skull base includes the upper clivus, sella turcica, cavernous sinuses, and sphenoid alae.[162]

The cavernous sinuses are multiseptated, extradural venous spaces that lie on both sides of the sella turcica (Fig. 12-108). The cavernous sinuses communicate extensively with each other, the intracranial dural sinuses, and deep facial venous plexuses *(see* Figs. 6-57 and 6-58). The lateral cavernous sinus walls are composed of two layers: a thick outer dural layer and a thin inner membranous layer. The inner layer is formed by the perineurium of CNs III, IV, V$_1$, and sometimes V$_2$.[173] These nerves lie within the lateral wall, whereas the internal carotid artery and CN VI are inside the cavernous sinus proper. Medially, a

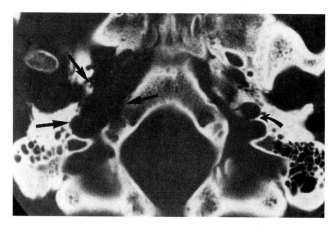

Fig. 12-157. Axial CT scan in a patient with diabetes mellitus and malignant external otitis. Note extensive right-side skull base destruction *(large arrows).* Compare with normal left side, where jugular foramen and jugular spine *(curved arrow)* are intact.

thin, poorly delineated medial dural wall separates the cavernous sinus from the sella turcica. Meckel's cave and its contents, the trigeminal ganglion, CSF, and investing arachnoid, invaginate into the cavernous sinus posteriorly *(see* Fig. 6-64).

Most lesions that affect the central skull base arise from the cavernous sinus, pituitary gland, nasopharynx, and basisphenoid bone. In this section we discuss the most important of these lesions: infections and neoplasms.

Infection and inflammatory disease. BOS *osteomyelitis* is a rare but potentially lethal complication of immunocompromised states, diabetes, chronic mastoiditis, paranasal sinus infection, trauma, or necrotizing otitis externa (Fig. 12-157).[174] Occasionally, skull base

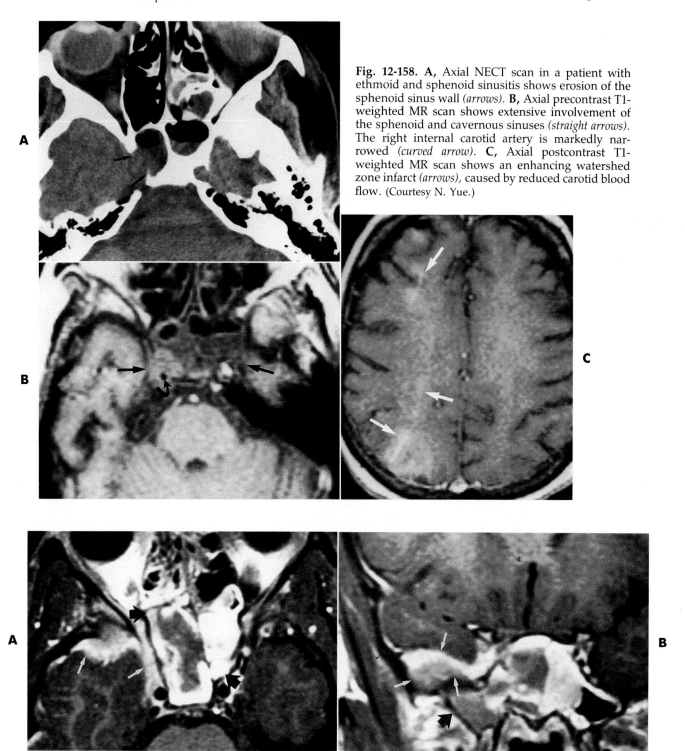

Fig. 12-158. A, Axial NECT scan in a patient with ethmoid and sphenoid sinusitis shows erosion of the sphenoid sinus wall *(arrows).* **B,** Axial precontrast T1-weighted MR scan shows extensive involvement of the sphenoid and cavernous sinuses *(straight arrows).* The right internal carotid artery is markedly narrowed *(curved arrow).* **C,** Axial postcontrast T1-weighted MR scan shows an enhancing watershed zone infarct *(arrows),* caused by reduced carotid blood flow. (Courtesy N. Yue.)

Fig. 12-159. Axial **(A)** and coronal **(B)** postcontrast T1-weighted MR scans in a patient with severe sphenoid sinusitis *(black arrows)* and secondary epidural abscess *(white arrows).*

infection occurs in the absence of these predisposing factors.

Osteomyelitis occasionally complicates *bacterial sinusitis.* Infection can extend directly from the frontal, ethmoid, or sphenoid sinuses or intracranially via skull emissary veins and the cavernous sinus. Cerebral infarct (Fig. 12-158), meningitis, subdural empyema (Fig. 12-159), and brain abscess may result (*see* Chapter 16).

Fungal sinusitis may also have serious complica-

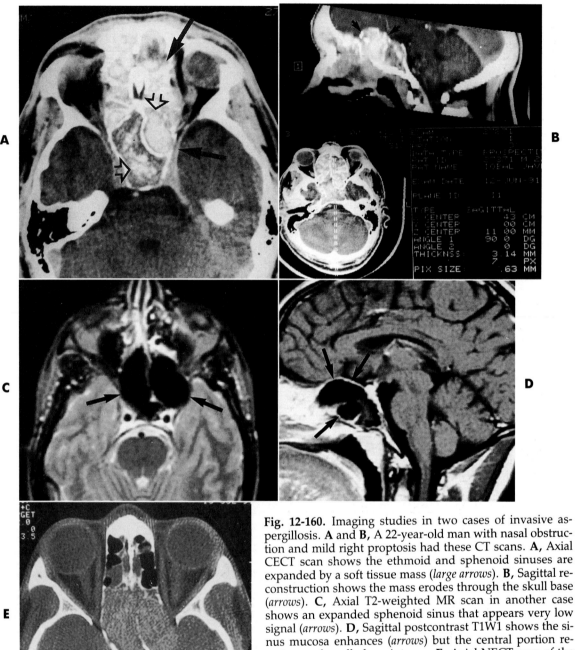

Fig. 12-160. Imaging studies in two cases of invasive aspergillosis. **A** and **B,** A 22-year-old man with nasal obstruction and mild right proptosis had these CT scans. **A,** Axial CECT scan shows the ethmoid and sphenoid sinuses are expanded by a soft tissue mass (*large arrows*). **B,** Sagittal reconstruction shows the mass erodes through the skull base (*arrows*). **C,** Axial T2-weighted MR scan in another case shows an expanded sphenoid sinus that appears very low signal (*arrows*). **D,** Sagittal postcontrast T1W1 shows the sinus mucosa enhances (*arrows*) but the central portion remains profoundly hypointense. **E,** Axial NECT scan of the same case shows central skull base destruction. (**A** and **B,** Courtesy A. Clifton, reprinted with permission from Breen DJ, Clifton AG et al: *Neurodiol* 35:216-217, 1992. **C** to **E,** Courtesy P.H. Demaeral. Reprinted with permission from *Br J Radiol* 66:260-263, 1993.)

tions. Paranasal sinus fungal infection has the following four predominant patterns (Fig. 12-160)[175]:

1. Extramucosal disease with cavitating mycetoma (fungus ball)
2. Allergic fungal sinusitis
3. Mucosal thickening from indolent, penetrating fungal sinusitis
4. Fulminant invasive mycosis

Manifestations of aggressive fungal infection include multiple cranial nerve palsies, septic cavernous sinus thrombosis, internal carotid occlusion, brain infarction, and brain abscess.[176,177] Various fungal granulomas, including candidiasis, aspergillosis, histoplasmosis, chromoblastomycosis, and rhinomucormycosis, have been implicated as causative organisms.[178]

Imaging studies in fungal sinusitis typically show multisinus nodular mucoperiosteal thickening. High attenuation foci within the soft tissue masses are seen on CT scans. Mycetomas may appear very hypointense on MR scans. A high signal rim that surrounds the very low signal fungus ball is often present. The differential diagnosis of low signal intensity lesions in the paranasal sinuses includes osteo- and chondrosarcomas, fibrous dysplasia, and acute hematoma.[179]

Aggressive mycosis may produce extensive skull base destruction. Cavernous sinus thrombosis, blood vessel invasion, and rapid intracranial dissemination may occur. Contrast-enhanced MR or CT demonstrates multiple filling defects within the cavernous sinus in these cases. Extensive skull base erosion with aggressive fungal infections can be indistinguishable from nasopharyngeal malignancy (*see* box).

Some nonfungal granulomas can also have extensive intracranial manifestations. *Wegener granulomatosis* (WG) has the potential for disseminated necrotizing granulomatous vasculitis in multiple organ systems, including the CNS. CNS manifestations of WG include BOS invasion by paranasal sinus granulomas, direct granuloma formation in the brain parenchyma or meninges, cranial arteritis, cranial neuropathies, and cerebral vascular thrombosis.[180]

Other granulomatous diseases, including *leishmaniasis, sarcoidosis, leprosy, rhinoscleroma, mycobacteria, treponemes,* and occasionally *cocaine* abuse, can cause extensive midfacial and central BOS lesions.[178] So-called lethal midline granuloma may cause similar imaging findings; these cases are immunopathologically very similar to *T-cell lymphomas.*[178]

Primary neoplasms. Common benign primary neoplasms that affect the central skull base include pituitary adenoma, meningioma, nerve sheath tumors, juvenile nasopharyngeal angiofibroma (JNA), chordomas, and osteocartilagenous tumors.

Pituitary adenomas are usually indolent, nonaggressive lesions that expand and slowly erode the bony sella turcica (*see* Chapter 14). Extension of these tu-

mors is typically superiorly through the diaphragma sellae and laterally into the cavernous sinus. Occasionally, some histologically benign pituitary adenomas behave more aggressively and may cause extensive destruction of the central skull base (Fig. 12-161).

Meningiomas of the central skull base are located along the sphenoid wing, diaphragma sellae (Fig. 12-

---

Destructive central skull base lesions
Differential Diagnosis

Common

Metastases
   Nasopharyngeal malignancy
   Hematogenous

Uncommon

Osteomyelitis
Fungal sinusitis
Nonfungal granulomas
   Wegener granulomatosis
   Cocaine abuse
   Midline granuloma (probably a lymphoma variant)
Aggressive pituitary adenoma
Lymphoma
Myeloma
Meningioma
Juvenile nasopharyngeal angiofibroma
Chordoma

Rare

Leprosy
Rhinoscleroma
Syphilis
Sarcoidosis

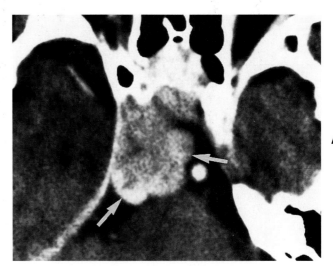

A

Fig. 12-161. A, Axial CECT scan shows a large lobulated enhancing pituitary adenoma *(arrows).*   *Continued.*

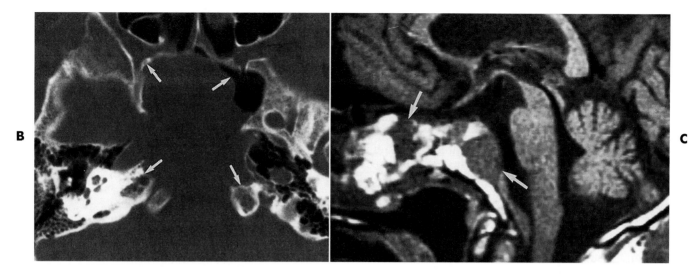

Fig. 12-161, cont'd. B, The lesion extends inferiorly, causing extensive central skull base destruction *(arrows).* **C,** Sagittal T1-weighted MR scan in another patient shows an extensive hemorrhagic pituitary adenoma that involves nearly the entire basisphenoid *(arrows).*

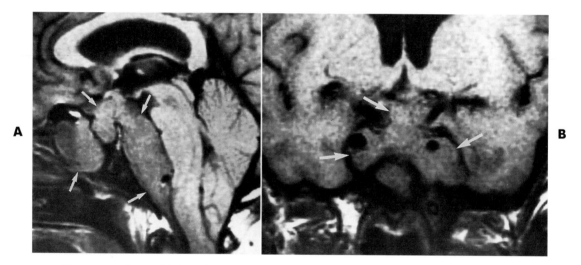

Fig. 12-162. Sagittal **(A)** and coronal **(B)** T1-weighted MR scans in a 52-year-old woman show a large meningioma *(arrows)* that extends along the clivus and diaphragma sellae into the sphenoid sinus and both cavernous sinuses.

124), clivus (Fig. 12-162), and cavernous sinus (Fig. 12-163). Meningiomas can appear as focal lobulated masses (globose meningioma) or flat, "en plaque" lesions. Occasionally, bony destruction or hyperostosis is striking. Cavernous sinus meningiomas may cause multiple cranial nerve palsies.

Nerve sheath tumors that involve the central BOS most often affect the cavernous sinus and Meckel's cave. *Plexiform neurofibromas* are unencapsulated, diffusely infiltrating masses that originate along peripheral nerves, usually the ophthalmic division of the trigeminal nerve, and involve the BOS by central extension. Extension along the mandibular and maxillary divisions of CNV is also common (Fig. 12-164).

Schwannomas (neurinomas, neurilemommas) cause

approximately one third of primary trigeminal nerve and Meckel's cave tumors[181]; neurinomas of the third, fourth, and sixth cranial nerves are rare.[182] Schwannomas are encapsulated, well-delineated tumors (Fig. 12-165). Most are quite vascular; hemorrhage or necrosis may occur.[183-185]

The most common schwannoma to involve the central skull base and cavernous sinus is a trigeminal schwannoma *(see* box, p. 501). Because these tumors may originate in any part of the nerve between the root and distal extracranial branches, their symptoms, signs, and imaging appearance vary with direction and extent of tumor growth.[186]

Schwannomas that arise from the trigeminal ganglion can remain localized within Meckel's cave or ex-

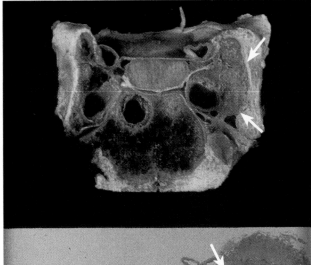

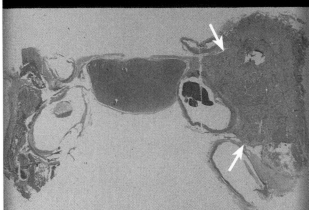

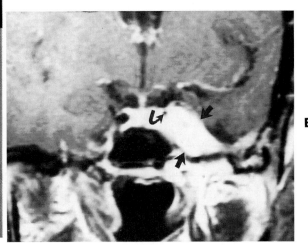

Fig. 12-163. A, Coronal gross pathology specimen shows a cavernous sinus meningioma *(arrows)*. **B,** Coronal postcontrast T1-weighted MR scan in a middle-aged woman with multiple left-side cranial nerve palsies shows an enhancing cavernous sinus lesion *(straight arrows)* that encases and severely narrows the internal carotid artery *(curved arrow)*. Meningioma. (**A,** From Okazaki H, Scheithauer B: *Slide Atlas of Neuropathology,* Gower Medical Publishing, 1989. With permission.)

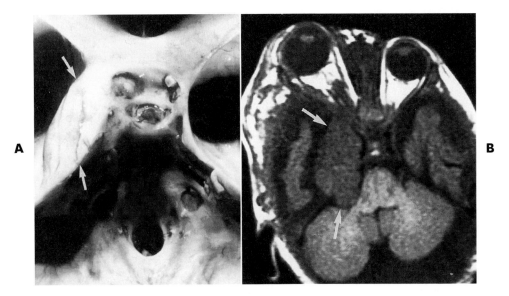

Fig. 12-164. An infant with neurofibromatosis type 1 had an extensive facial plexiform neurofibroma. Autopsy specimen **(A)** shows the enlarged cavernous sinus *(arrows)*. Axial precontrast T1-weighted **(B)** MR scan shows the large cavernous sinus mass *(arrows)*. (**A,** Courtesy M. Herrick. **B,** Courtesy R.S. Prieto, A. Kou, and J. Vaudagna.)   *Continued.*

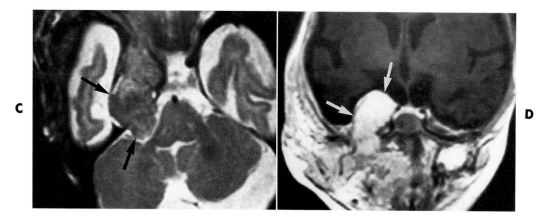

Fig. 12-164, cont'd. Axial precontrast T2-weighted **(C)** MR scan shows the large cavernous sinus mass *(arrows)*. Coronal postcontrast T1W1 **(D)** shows the plexiform neurofibroma *(arrows)* enhances intensely. (Courtesy R.S. Pretto, A. Kou, and J. Vaudagna.)

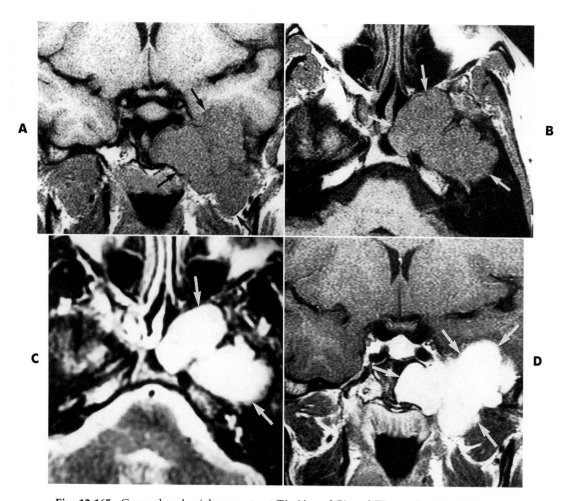

Fig. 12-165. Coronal and axial precontrast T1- **(A** and **B)** and T2-weighted MR **(C)** scans show a well-delineated lobulated cavernous sinus and skull base mass *(arrows)*. The lesion is isointense with gray matter on T1WI and hyperintense on T2WI. Postcontrast coronal T1WI **(D)** shows strong uniform enhancement *(arrows)*. Trigeminal schwannoma was found at surgery.

tend into the skull base. Tumors arising from the cisternal trigeminal nerve segment appear as a cerebellopontine angle mass. Schwannomas that involve both the gasserian ganglion and cisternal aspects of the trigeminal nerve have a "dumbbell" configuration

caused by the dural restriction of Meckel's cave (Fig. 12-166). Trigeminal schwannomas can also arise from, or extend along, the extracranial CN V branches.[186] Regardless of location most schwannomas are circumscribed rounded or lobulated soft tissue masses that enhance strongly but somewhat heterogeneously after contrast administration. Most are isodense with brain on CT and isointense on T1-weighted MR scans, but appear quite hyperintense on T2WI (Fig. 12-165).

Juvenile angiofibroma (JNA) is a highly vascular, locally invasive lesion that originates near the sphenopalatine foramen of adolescent males. JNA is the most common benign nasopharyngeal tumor.[163]

Cavernous Sinus Masses
Differential diagnosis

Unilateral

Common
Schwannoma
Meningioma
Metastasis
Aneurysm (cavernous internal carotid artery)
Carotid-cavernous fistula
Uncommon
Chordoma
Lymphoma
Rare
Lipoma
Epidermoid
Cavernous hemangioma
Osteocartilagenous tumors
Plexiform neurofibroma (NF-1)

Bilateral

Common
Invasive pituitary adenoma
Meningioma
Metastases
Uncommon
Lymphoma
Cavernous sinus thrombosis

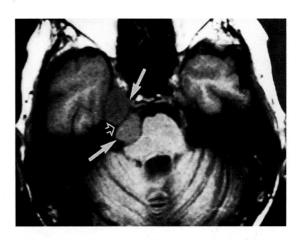

Fig. 12-166. Axial T1-weighted MR scan shows a "dumbbell" schwannoma that has both a cisternal and cavernous sinus (Meckel's cave) component *(solid arrows)*. Note the constriction caused by the dural orifice of Meckel's cave *(open arrow)*. (Courtesy W. Coit.)

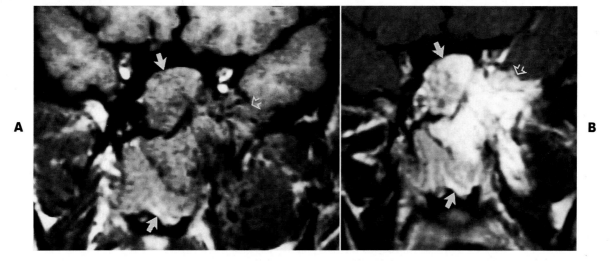

Fig. 12-167. Coronal pre- **(A)** and postcontrast **(B)** T1-weighted MR scans in a 17-year-old boy with epistaxis show a lobulated mass in the sphenoid sinus and nasopharynx *(solid arrows)*. Prominent "flow voids" are present, giving the lesion a salt-and-pepper appearance on the noncontrast study. The strongly enhancing tumor invades the left cavernous sinus *(open arrows)*.

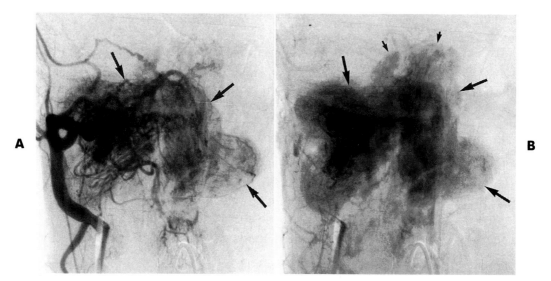

Fig. 12-168. An 18-year-old man had repeated epistaxis. Left external carotid angiogram, AP view, with early **(A)** and late **(B)** arterial phase studies shows a lobulated, highly vascular nasopharyngeal mass *(large arrows)*. Note extension into the sphenoid and cavernous sinuses, seen on the later phase film **(B,** *small arrows*). Juvenile nasopharyngeal angiofibroma.

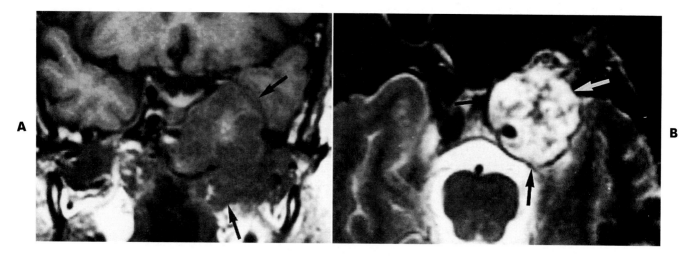

Fig. 12-169. Coronal T1- **(A)** and axial T2-weighted **(B)** MR scans of a chondroid chordoma *(arrows)*. The cavernous sinus and skull base mass is slightly hypointense to brain on T1WI but strikingly hyperintense on T2WI. (Courtesy T. Miller.)

JNAs typically spread along natural foramina and fissures into the pterygopalatine fossa, orbit, middle cranial fossa, sphenoid sinus, and cavernous sinus. Imaging findings are those of a strongly enhancing (Fig. 12-167), highly vascular (Fig. 12-168) nasopharyngeal soft tissue mass.

Chordomas are uncommon slow-growing, destructive tumors that are histologically benign but locally invasive. Approximately one third of all chordomas occur in the sphenooccipital region (*see* Chapter 21). Most occur in the midline and primarily involve the clivus. Off-midline locations within the petrous apex and Meckel's cave occasionally occur (Fig. 12-169).[187]

In contrast to the calvarium (which originates from the mesenchymal membranous neurocranium by intramembranous ossification), the clivus and skull base develop from the cartilaginous neurocranium by endochondral ossification.[188] Therefore a spectrum of benign and malignant osteocartilagenous neoplasms can arise within the central skull base.

Enchondroma is the most common benign osteocartilagenous tumor in this location. An expansile, lobulated soft tissue mass with scalloped endosteal bone resorption and curvilinear matrix mineralization are characteristic CT findings.[189] Most enchondromas are isointense with muscle on T1WI and hyperintense on

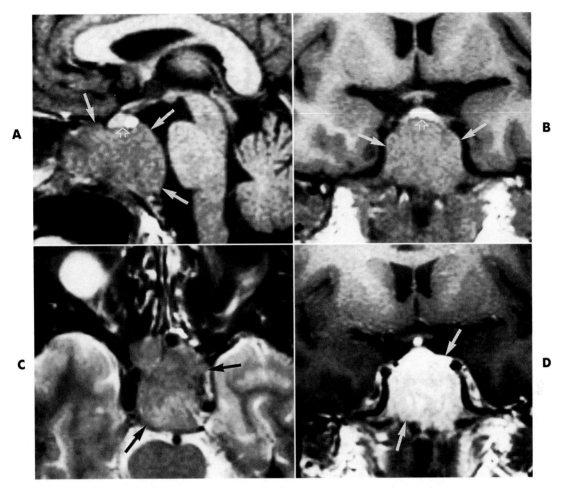

Fig. 12-170. A 45-year-old man with double vision had this MR examination. Precontrast sagittal **(A)** and coronal **(B)** T1-weighted scans show a destructive sphenoid mass *(large arrows)* that elevates and displaces the pituitary gland *(open arrows)*. Axial T2WI **(C)** shows the mass *(arrows)* is slightly hypointense relative to brain. Postcontrast coronal T1WI **(D)** shows strong, uniform enhancement *(arrows)*. Plasmacytoma. (Courtesy S. Sweriduk.)

T2-weighted studies. Postcontrast T1-weighted images show enhancement of the scalloped margins and curvilinear septae (ring-and-arc pattern).[189]

Miscellaneous benign tumors and tumorlike lesions that involve the cavernous sinus and Meckel's cave include *epidermoid* tumors, *lipomas,* and *cavernous hemangiomas.*[173,181]

Common primary malignant tumors that affect the central skull base are invasive *nasopharyngeal carcinomas* and *rhabdomyosarcoma* (see previous discussion). Other less common primary malignant tumors in this location are multiple myeloma and plasmacytoma, osteosarcoma, and chondrosarcoma.

Multiple myeloma (MM) can produce diffuse skull base and calvarial vault destruction. Solitary *plasmacytomas* in the absence of MM are uncommon. A focal destructive sphenoid sinus (Fig. 12-170) or calvar-

ial vault mass (*see* Fig. 12-189) is typical, although imaging findings are nonspecific.

Osteosarcoma is the second most common primary bone tumor (after multiple myeloma). Few osteosarcomas occur before age 5 or over age 50.[190] Craniofacial osteosarcomas are uncommon; when present, they often occur in older patients and commonly affect the maxilla or mandible. Skull base osteosarcomas are rare. They may occur spontaneously or in association with Paget disease or previous radiation therapy. A soft tissue mass with tumor matrix mineralization and aggressive bone destruction is characteristic in these cases. The differential diagnosis of a nonmineralized osteosarcoma is radiation osteitis, metastatic carcinoma, and myeloma.[190]

Chondrosarcomas of the skull base are rare, slow-growing, locally invasive tumors. A soft tissue mass

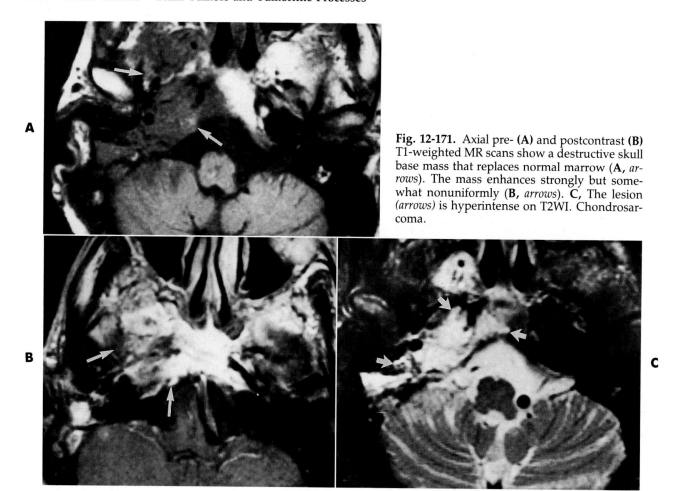

Fig. 12-171. Axial pre- **(A)** and postcontrast **(B)** T1-weighted MR scans show a destructive skull base mass that replaces normal marrow **(A,** *arrows*). The mass enhances strongly but somewhat nonuniformly **(B,** *arrows*). **C,** The lesion *(arrows)* is hyperintense on T2WI. Chondrosarcoma.

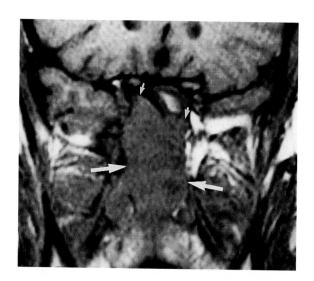

Fig. 12-172. Coronal T1-weighted MR scan in a patient with nasopharyngeal squamous cell carcinoma shows a destructive midline mass *(large arrows)* that obliterates normal soft tissue planes and extends cephalad into the sphenoid sinus *(small arrows).*

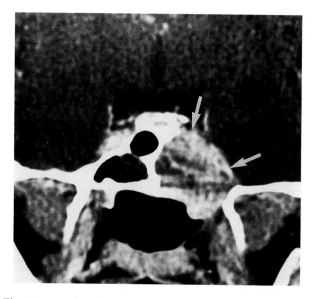

Fig. 12-173. Coronal CECT scan in a patient who had a mastectomy for breast carcinoma 4 years before developing a left sixth cranial nerve palsy. A large focal lytic enhancing cavernous sinus lesion *(arrows)* is present. No other metastases were identified.

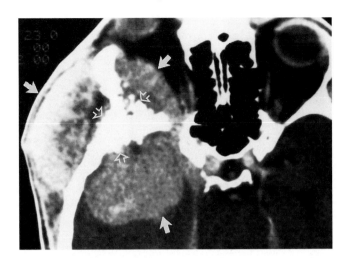

Fig. 12-174. CECT scan shows a large metastasis to the sphenoid wing and skull base *(solid arrows)*. Note mixed bony destruction and hyperostosis *(open arrows)*.

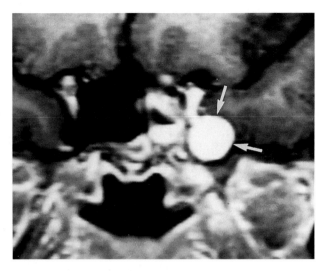

Fig. 12-175. Coronal contrast-enhanced T1-weighted MR scan in a patient with a facial sarcoma shows a well-delineated enhancing mass along the maxillary division of the trigeminal nerve *(arrows)*. This perineural metastasis appears very similar to a schwannoma.

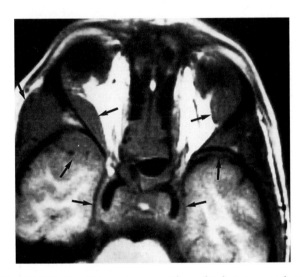

Fig. 12-176. B-cell lymphoma with multiple intra- and extracranial metastases is shown on this axial T1-weighted MR scan. Note right masticator space and lateral rectus, left lacrimal gland, bilateral cavernous sinus, and extradural masses *(arrows)*.

with focal bone destruction is typical. Matrix mineralization is seen in about half of all cases. These tumors are usually low to intermediate signal intensity on T1WI and hyperintense on T2-weighted scans. Strong but heterogeneous enhancement following contrast administration is usual (Fig. 12-171).[191]

Metastatic disease. Central skull base metastases are more common than primary bone neoplasms.[163] *Metastases* can arise via regional extension of head and neck malignancies (Fig. 12-172) or hematogenous spread from extracranial primary sites.

Prostate, lung, and breast carcinomas are the most common sources of hematogenous metastases. Lung and breast metastases can be focal (Fig. 12-173) or diffuse lytic destructive lesions. Prostate metastases often cause mixed hyperostosis and bone destruction with an associated soft-tissue mass that may resemble meningioma (Fig. 12-174).[163] The lateral orbital wall is a favorite site for prostate metastases. Perineural tumor spread can occur with regional head and neck, as well as remote, primary malignancies (Fig. 12-175).

CNS involvement by either primary or secondary *lymphoma* is uncommon but increasing in incidence. Leptomeningeal disease is the most common type of lymphomatous CNS metastasis, and cranial nerve palsies are the most common presenting signs (Fig. 12-176).[192] Focal masses (Fig. 12-177) or perineural tumor also occur.[166] MR scans show replacement of normal high signal marrow with infiltrating soft tissue that has decreased signal intensity. Enhanced scans with fat-suppression delineate tumor extent particularly well. Cavernous sinus lymphoma can be either uni- (Fig. 12-177) or bilateral (Fig. 12-176). The differential diagnosis of cavernous sinus masses is summarized in the box, p. 501.

Nonneoplastic processes that can mimic diffuse skull base metastases include *osteomyelitis, eosinophilic granuloma* (Fig. 12-178), and occasionally *sarcoidosis*.

Posterior skull base. The posterior skull base surrounds the foramen magnum and includes the clivus below the sphenooccipital synchondrosis, the petrous temporal bone, and the pars lateralis and squamae of the occipital bones.[193]

MR signal characteristics of the normal clivus and posterior skull base depend on the amount and na-

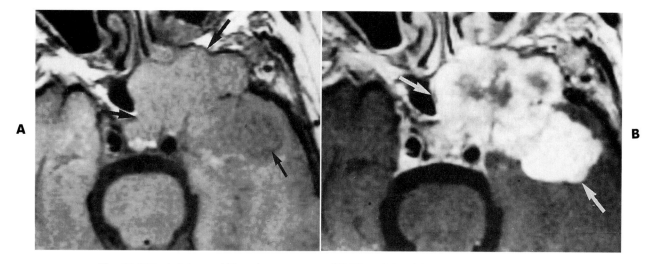

Fig. 12-177. Axial pre- **(A)** and postcontrast **(B)** T1-weighted MR scans show an extensive skull base soft tissue mass that invades the pterygopalatine fossa, sphenoid sinus, cavernous sinus, and middle cranial fossa **(A,** *arrows*). The mass enhances strongly but nonuniformly **(B,** *arrows*). Surgery disclosed lymphoma.

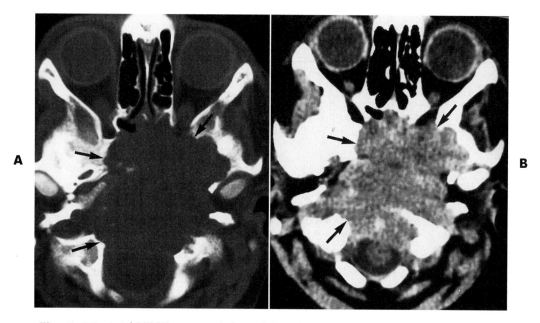

Fig. 12-178. Axial NECT scans with bone **(A)** and soft tissue **(B)** windows show a very extensive destructive central skull base lesion *(large arrows)* in this 4-year-old child. Some residual bone is seen within the mass. Eosinophilic granuloma.

ture of the marrow elements that comprise the cancellous bone. Red marrow (hematopoietic tissue) predominates up to approximately 3 years of age and results in low signal on T1WI.[194] In adults the normal clivus consists of low- and high-intensity portions mixed in various proportions on T1WI.[195] Enhancement of normal clival marrow sometimes occurs following contrast administration. This is mild and infrequent in adults, but is common and may even be quite striking in young children.[195] The skull base in

children normally has signal irregularity and patchy enhancement.[196]

Posterior skull base lesions in the temporal bone and foramen magnum lesions are discussed in preceding sections. Clival, paraclival, and jugular foramen masses are discussed next.

Clival and paraclival lesions. *Chordoma* and *metastasis* are the most common causes of a destructive clival mass.[188] The same *infectious* and *inflammatory processes* and *primary and metastatic tumors* that affect

Continued.

Jugular Foramen Masses
Differential diagnosis

Nonneoplastic masses

Common
Large jugular bulb (normal variant)
Jugular vein thrombosis
Uncommon
Osteomyelitis
Malignant external otitis

Neoplasms

Common
Paraganglioma
Metastasis
    Nasopharyngeal carcinoma
    Hematogenous
Uncommon
Schwannoma
Neurofibroma
Epidermoid tumor

---

the anterior and central skull base can also involve the clivus. Replacement of normal marrow that forms the cancellous clival bone by soft tissue masses is easily identified on MR studies in these cases. Compared to brain, most abnormalities exhibit low signal on T1WI and high signal on T2-weighted sequences.[194]

Jugular foramen masses (see box). A *prominent jugular bulb* occurs frequently as a normal variant and is the most common "pseudomass" in the jugular foramen (Fig. 12-179, *F* to *H*). The differential diagnosis of true jugular foramen masses includes paraganglioma, nerve sheath tumor, meningioma, and metastases.

Parasympathetic *paragangliomas* (chemodectomas, glomus tumors) arise from the paraganglia that exist in various locations throughout the body. The most common head and neck sites of these tumors are the carotid body, glomus jugulare, and glomus tympanicum. The glomus jugulare is situated in the jugular bulb adventitia immediately below the middle ear. Paragangliomas in this location expand the jugular foramen, eroding the jugular spine and surrounding

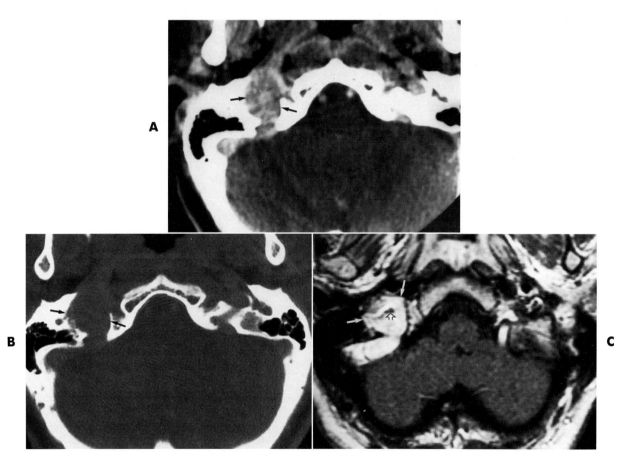

Fig. 12-179. Imaging studies of a typical jugular foramen paraganglioma are demonstrated. Axial CECT scans with soft tissue **(A)** and bone windows **(B)** show a strongly enhancing mass that has eroded the jugular foramen *(arrows)*. **(C)** Postcontrast axial T1-weighted MR scan shows the strongly enhancing jugular foramen mass *(arrows)*. Note central "flow voids" caused by high-velocity signal loss *(open arrow)*.   *Continued.*

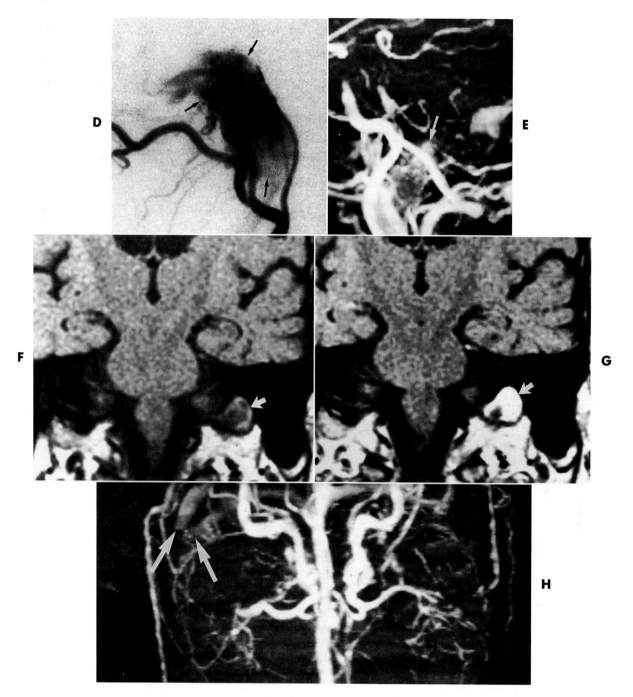

Fig. 12-179, cont'd.   (D) Distal external carotid angiogram, midarterial phase, lateral view, shows the extremely vascular mass *(arrows)*. Compare with the MR angiogram **(E).** For comparison, MR scans in a patient with a jugular foramen "pseudomass" are shown. Coronal precontrast T1-weighted study **(F)** shows an isointense mass in the left jugular foramen *(large arrow)*. Compare with normal "flow void" in the right jugular foramen. Postcontrast study **(G)** shows the "mass" *(large arrow)* enhances strongly. The patient was referred for surgery with the diagnosis of glomus jugulare. A multiple overlapping thin-slab MR angiogram **(H)** shows a prominent jugular bulb *(arrow)* as the cause of this jugular foramen "pseudomass." The isointense signal in this otherwise normal jugular bulb was caused by slow, turbulent flow. Diagnosis was confirmed at angiography (not shown).

cortex (Fig. 12-179, *A* to *E*). More extensive skull base involvement can be seen with large lesions. A lobulated, speckled-appearing mixed signal mass with internal foci of high-velocity signal loss is typical. These vascular tumors enhance strongly following contrast administration.[197]

Nerve sheath tumors. The jugular foramen is an uncommon location for nerve sheath tumors. *Schwannomas* of CNs IX to XI appear as smooth, well-delineated rounded or lobulated soft tissue masses that expand the jugular foramen. Pressure erosion is common, but in contrast to paragangliomas, frank bony invasion is rare. Regardless of location, most schwannomas are isointense with brain on T1WI, hyperintense on T2WI, and exhibit strong homogeneous contrast enhancement (Fig. 12-180).

Miscellaneous lesions. Less common lesions that involve the jugular foramen are listed in the box, p. 507.

Diffuse skull base masses. These are lesions that can occur in any or all BOS locations. They include metabolic and dysplastic lesions such as fibrous dysplasia and Paget disease, as well as histiocytosis, blood dyscrasias, myeloma, and metastases (*see* box, p. 511).

Fibrous dysplasia. *Fibrous dysplasia* (FD) is among the most common benign skeletal disorders. FD most often affects adolescents and young adults. FD can be monostotic or polyostotic; the monostotic form is seen in 70% of cases. The skull and facial bones are involved in 25% of patients with monostotic FD and 40% to 60% of patients with the polyostotic form (Fig. 12-155).[198] Clinical symptoms of FD vary from facial deformity to cranial nerve palsies. Albright syndrome is unilateral polyostotic fibrous dysplasia with precocious puberty.

FD expands and replaces the normal bony medullary spaces with vascular fibrocellular tissue.[198] Vary-

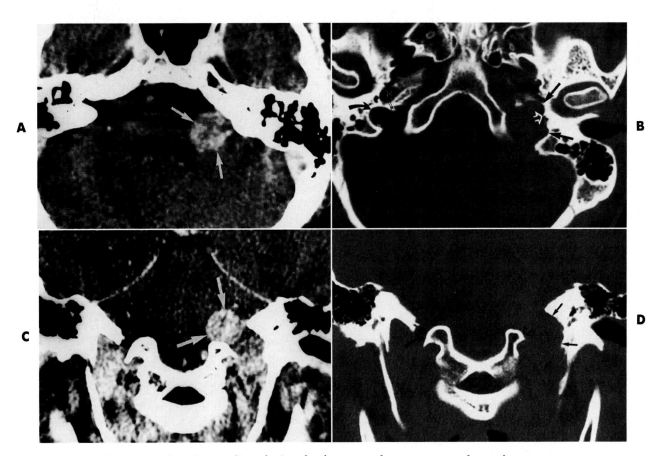

Fig. 12-180. Imaging studies of a jugular foramen schwannoma are shown for comparison to Fig. 12-179, the paraganglioma. Axial CECT scan (**A**) shows an enhancing cerebellopontine angle mass *(arrows)*. Axial bone windows through the skull base (**B**) show erosion of the left jugular foramen *(large arrows)* and jugular spine *(open arrow)*. Compare with the normal right jugular foramen *(curved arrow)* and spine *(double arrow)*. Coronal CECT scans with soft tissue (**C**) and bone windows (**D**) show the lobulated enhancing mass (**C**, *large arrows*) with erosion of the jugular foramen (**D**, *small arrows*) and jugular tubercle *(open arrow)*. Compare with normal right jugular tubercle *(curved arrow)*.

Continued.

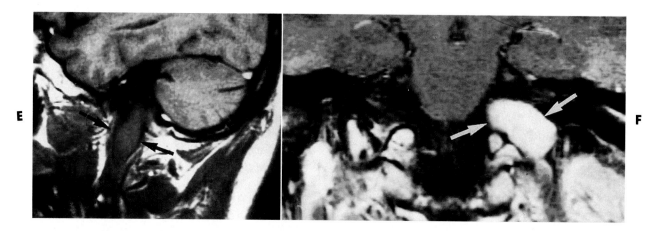

Fig. 12-180, cont'd. Sagittal T1-weighted MR scan **(E)** shows the mass *(arrows)* at the jugular foramen extending inferiorly within the carotid space. Coronal T1-weighted MR scan **(F)** shows the enhancing lesion is well-demarcated *(arrows)*. Glossopharyngeal schwannoma was found at surgery.

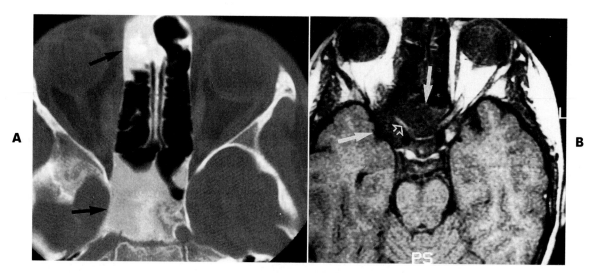

Fig. 12-181. A, Axial NECT scan in a patient with polyostotic fibrous dysplasia shows the typical "ground-glass" appearance in the sphenoid and frontal bones *(arrows)*. **B,** Axial T1-weighted MR scan shows the lesion *(large arrows)* is hypointense compared to brain. Note encasement of the optic nerve *(open arrow)*.

ing degrees of ossification may be seen. CT shows thickened, sclerotic bone with a "ground glass" appearance (Fig. 12-181, *A*). Cystic components may be present in the early active stage. The expanded, thickened bone is typically low to intermediate signal intensity on both T1- and T2-weighted MR scans, although scattered hyperintense regions may be present (Fig. 12-181, *B*). Variable enhancement following contrast administration occurs.[198]

Paget disease. *Paget disease* is an osseous lesion of unknown etiology that can be monostotic or polyostotic and focal or diffuse. Three phases are identified, as follows:

1. Early destructive phase (Fig. 12-182)

2. Intermediate phase with combined destruction and healing (*see* Fig. 12-187, *B* and *C*)
3. Late sclerotic phase

Imaging findings vary with stage. Bone expansion with variable destruction and sclerosis is typical. Paget disease may cause basilar invagination.

Langerhans cell histiocytosis. Solitary or monostotic eosinophilic granuloma (EG) is the most common presentation of *Langerhans cell histiocytosis* (LCH). EG is usually seen in children between 5 and 15 years of age and typically affects the skull vault. However, striking diffuse osteolytic skull base (Fig. 12-178) and calvarial lesions can occur. EG and diffuse LCH occasionally occur in young to middle-aged adults.[188,199]

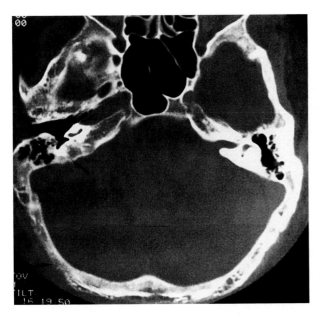

Fig. 12-182. Axial NECT scan shows diffuse skull base early Paget disease. The lesions are primarily destructive *(arrows)*.

Scalp, Cranial Vault, and Meningeal Masses

Scalp masses. Scalp masses are common, but rarely discussed in the imaging literature. Because scalp masses often present innocuously in otherwise healthy patients and may cause only cosmetic deformity, physicians tend to minimize their potential significance. Nontraumatic raised masses or "lumps" on the head may be benign local or diffuse scalp lesions. They may also represent the "tip of the iceberg" from large intracranial masses.[200]

The majority of nontraumatic scalp masses in children are caused by *dermoid* tumors. Other scalp masses include *cephalohematoma, eosinophilic granuloma, cephalocele, hamartomas* or *hemangiomas, lymphangioma, and plexiform neurofibroma* (Fig. 12-183).[200, 200a] In adults, common nontraumatic scalp masses include focal or diffuse *lipoma* (Fig. 12-184, *A*), *cutis gyrata* (redundant scalp tissue) (Fig. 12-184, *B*), *neurofibroma* (Fig. 12-184, *C*), *basal cell carcinoma* (Fig. 12-184, *D* and *E*), *lymphoma, angiomas,* and lesions that cover underlying calvarial masses such as *meningioma* or *metastasis*.[201] Miscellaneous scalp masses that can be found in both children and adults include *subgaleal hematoma,* scalp *edema, cellulitis,* and *fasciitis* (Figs. 12-185 and 12-186).

Cranial vault. Generalized or focal calvarial thickening and thinning are commonly observed on imaging studies. Some lesions are normal variants or abnormalities with minimal or no clinical significance. Others are indicators of significant underlying disease.

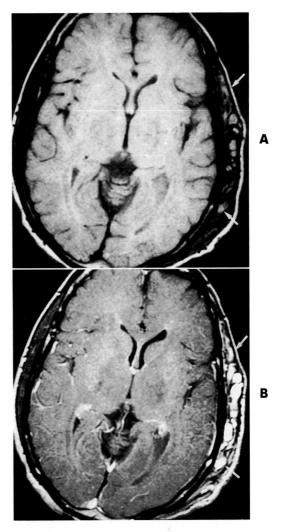

Fig. 12-183. Axial pre- **(A)** and postcontrast **(B)** T1-weighted MR scans in a 16-year-old boy with neurofibromatosis type 1 (NF-1) and a scalp mass. Extensive left-side subcutaneous unencapsulated soft tissue masses are present **(A,** *arrows*). The lesions enhance strongly following contrast administration **(B,** *arrows*). Plexiform neurofibroma.

Diffuse Skull Base Lesions
Nonneoplastic masses
Uncommon
Fibrous dysplasia
Paget's disease
Langerhans' cell histiocytosis
Neoplastic masses
Common
Metastases
Uncommon
Myeloma
Meningioma
Lymphoma
Rhabdomyosarcoma

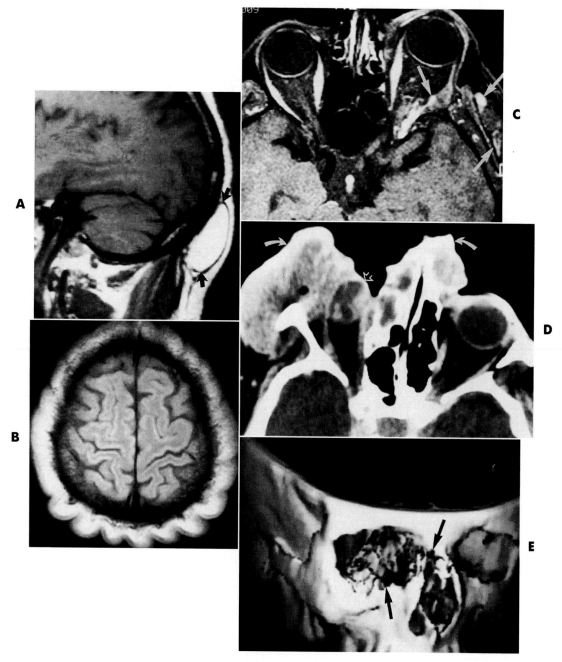

Fig. 12-184. Scalp masses are illustrated. **A,** Sagittal T1-weighted MR scan in a 68-year-old man with a suboccipital soft tissue mass. A well-delineated high signal lesion *(arrows)* that does not involve the underlying bone is identified. Lipoma. **B,** Axial T1-weighted MR scan in another patient shows redundant scalp with extensive subcutaneous fat. **C,** A 40-year-old man with NF-1 had a postcontrast T1-weighted axial MR scan with fat suppression. An extensive plexiform neurofibroma of the high deep masticator space and orbit is present *(arrows)*. **D,** Axial CECT scan in a patient with extensive basal cell carcinoma of the scalp, eyelid, and face *(solid arrows)*. Note phthsis bulbi *(open arrow)*. **E,** 3D CT of the face shows extensive destruction of the bony orbit and nose *(arrows)*.

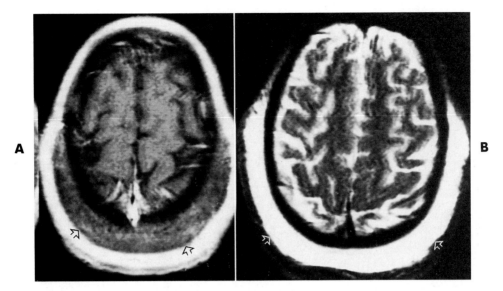

Fig. 12-185. Axial T1- **(A)** and T2-weighted **(B)** MR scans show extensive scalp edema *(arrows)*.

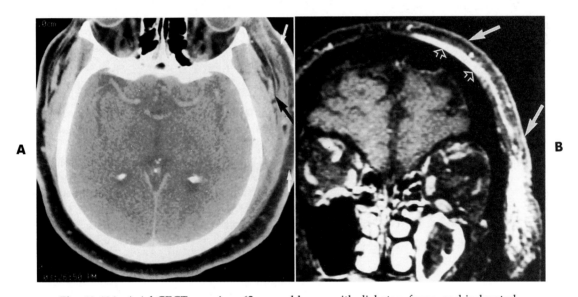

Fig. 12-186. Axial CECT scan in a 62-year-old man with diabetes, fever, and indurated, erythematous scalp. Subcutaneous cellulitis is present, seen as strandlike densities and "dirty fat" *(white arrows)* under the cutis. A focal low density fluid collection is present in the high deep masticator space, representing fasciitis *(black arrow)*. **B,** Coronal post-contrast T1-weighted fat-suppressed MR scan in a 74-year-old woman with herpes zoster shows extensive cellulitis *(large arrows)*. Some fasciitis is also present *(open arrows)*. (**A**, Courtesy T. Miller.)

Generalized calvarial thickening (see box, p. 515, *left).* The most common cause of a thick skull is a *normal variant.* Diffuse skull thickening also frequently occurs with *chronic phenytoin (Dilantin) therapy, shunted hydrocephalus, microcephaly, acromegaly, Paget disease,* and *fibrous dysplasia* (Fig. 12-187). *Blood dyscra-* sias such as sickle cell disease and iron deficiency anemia are uncommon hematologic disorders that cause diploic space enlargement. The parietal bones are most commonly affected, whereas the occipital squamae, which do not contain marrow, are spared.

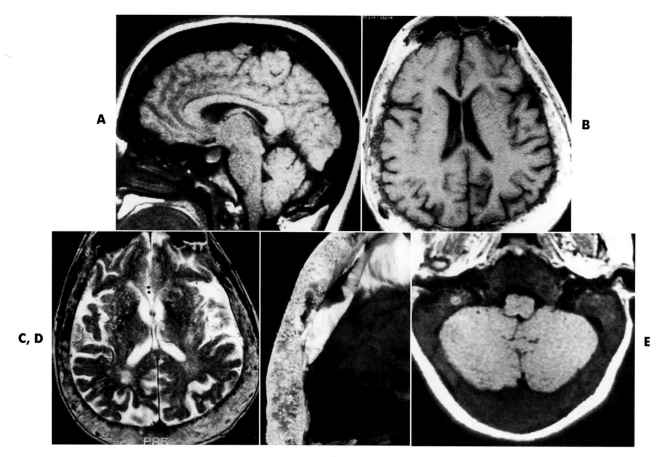

Fig. 12-187. Generalized calvarial thickening. Sagittal T1-weighted MR scan **(A)** in a patient with long-standing seizure disorder and chronic phenytoin therapy. The calvarium is markedly thickened, a side effect of the medication. Axial T1- **(B)** and T2-weighted **(C)** MR scans in an 80-year-old woman with severe generalized skull thickening secondary to Paget disease. Combined destruction and healing changes are seen. Gross pathology specimen **(D)** shows Paget disease (compare to **B** and **C**). Axial T1-weighted MR scan **(E)** in a 15-year-old girl with polyostotic fibrous dysplasia shows diffuse thickening of the skull and clivus. (**D,** Courtesy E. Tessa Hedley-Whyte.)

Regional and focal calvarial thickening (*see* box). The most common cause of regional skull thickening is *hyperostosis interna,* a benign process usually seen in the frontal bones of middle-aged and elderly women (Fig. 12-188, *A* to *C*). Hyperostosis frontalis interna spares the superior sagittal sinus and adjacent venous channels.

Other causes of focally thick skull include *Paget disease, fibrous dysplasia, osteoma, osteoblastic metastases* (Fig. 12-174) (prostate and breast carcinoma are the most common primary sites) and *neuroblastoma.* Neuroblastoma metastases often cause a striking "hairon-end" appearance (Fig. 12-188, *D*). *Hyperostotic meningioma,* another cause of focal calvarial thick-

ening, crosses the midline, sutures, and vascular channels. Hyperostosing en plaque meningioma causes a periosteal proliferating pattern, inward bulging of the calvarium and surface irregularities along the inner table (Fig. 12-188, *E*).[201] *Calcified cephalohematoma* or *calcified subdural hematoma,* are less frequent causes of focal skull thickening.[201a]

Generalized skull thinning (*see* box, p. 515, *right*). Prominent convolutional markings with gyriform thinning is a *normal variant. Severe untreated hydrocephalus* may cause striking generalized skull vault thinning. Congenital anomalies such as *osteogenesis imperfecta, Down syndrome,* and *lacunar skull* (with Chiari II malformation) also cause generalized skull

Common Causes of a Thick Skull
Diffuse
Common
Normal variant
Chronic phentoin (Dilantin) therapy
Microcephalic brain
Shunted hydrocephalus
Uncommon
Acromegaly
Hematologic disorders
Chronic calcified subdural hematomas
Regional/focal
Common
Hyperostosis frontalis interna
Paget disease
Fibrous dysplasia
Meningioma
Uncommon
Osteoma
Calcified cephalohematoma
Metastases (e.g., neuroblastoma, prostate)

Data from F. Guinto and R. Kumar.

Common Causes of a Thin Skull
Generalized
Common
Normal (prominent convolutional markings)
Long-standing hydrocephalus
Lacunar skull (with Chiari II malformation)
Uncommon
Osteogenesis imperfecta
Rickets
Cushing's disease
Regional/focal
Common
Parietal thinning
Temporal, occipital squamae
Pacchionian (arachnoid) granulations
Uncommon
Intracranial mass (arachnoid cyst, slow-growing neo-plasm)
Leptomeningeal cyst
Osteoporosis circumscripta

Data from F. Guinto and R. Kumar.

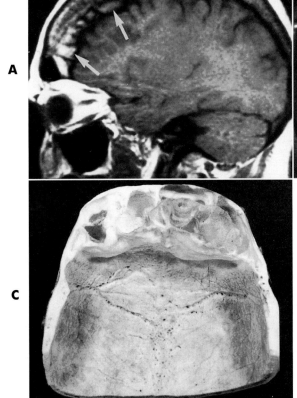

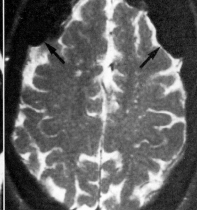

Fig. 12-188. Regional calvarial thickening is illustrated by these cases. Sagittal T1- **(A)** and axial T2-weighted **(B)** MR scans in an elderly woman show hyperostosis frontalis interna *(large arrows)*. Note that the calvarium is thickened to—but not beyond—the coronal suture *(open arrow)*. Gross pathology specimen **(C)** of hyperostosis frontalis interna with large frontal sinuses (compare to **A** and **B**).

Continued.

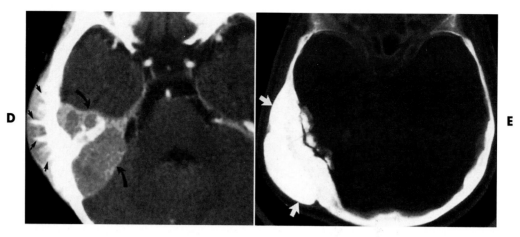

Fig. 12-188, cont'd. Axial CECT scan **(D)** in a child with neuroblastoma metastatic to the skull shows a large enhancing extradural soft tissue mass *(curved arrows)*. Note the "hair-on-end" appearance of the osseous metastases *(small arrows)*. Axial NECT scan **(E)** of a hyperostosing meningioma shows extensive but focal calvarial thickening *(arrows)*. (**C,** From the Royal College of Surgeons of England, *Slide Atlas of Pathology,* Gower Medical Publishing. By permission. **E,** Courtesy J. Jones.)

"Holes in the Skull"

Solitary

Common

Normal
  Fissure, foramen, canal
  Emissary venous channel
  Pacchionian (arachnoid) granulation
  Parietal thinning
Surgical/trauma (burr hole, shunt, surgical defect, fracture)
Dermoid
Eosinophilic granuloma
Metastasis (often multiple)

Uncommon

Osteoporosis circumscripta
Epidermoid
Hemangioma
Cephalocele
Intradiploic arachnoid cyst/meningioma
Leptomeningeal cyst (growing fracture)

Multiple

Common

Normal
  Fissures, foramina
  Diploic channels, venous lakes
  Pacchionian (arachnoid) granulations
Multiple burr holes/surgical defects
Metastases
Age-related osteoporosis

Uncommon

Hyperparathyroidism
Myeloma
Osteomyelitis

---

thinning (see Figs. 2-3 and 2-5). *Metabolic disorders* associated with calvarial thinning include rickets, hypophosphatasia, hyperparathyroidism, and Cushing disease.

Focal skull thinning can be *normal* (Pacchionian granulations, parietal foramina, venous lakes, temporal and occipital squamae). *Leptomeningeal cyst, arachnoid or porencephalic cysts,* and *slow-growing neoplasms* are intracranial processes that sometimes thin the adjacent skull (*see* box).

Focal "holes in the skull" can also be *normal* (fissures, foramina, vascular channels). Congenital anomalies that produce skull defects include *cephaloceles, dermoid cysts, cleidocranial dysostosis, intradiploic arachnoid cysts,* and *neurofibromatosis* type 1 (absent greater sphenoid wing, lambdoid sutural defects) (*see* Fig. 5-10).

Acquired solitary skull defects are *fractures, burr holes, bone flaps, craniotomies, shunts, infections,* and neoplasms, or tumorlike lesions such as hemangioma, epidermoid tumors, and eosinophilic granuloma.

Skull *hemangiomas* are usually solitary lytic diploic space lesions with well circumscribed margins and a "spoke-wheel" or reticulated pattern. Hemorrhagic changes can sometimes be seen on MR studies in these cases (Fig. 12-189, *A*). *Epidermoids* involve both the inner and outer tables and are well-defined lesions that lack central trabeculae and have a sclerotic rim. *Eosinophilic granulomas* are single or multiple well-circumscribed lytic lesions that have nonsclerotic "beveled" edges caused by asymmetric involvement of the inner and outer tables. The lytic phase of Paget disease can produce well-circumscribed sharply marginated defects (so-called *osteoporosis circumscripta*).

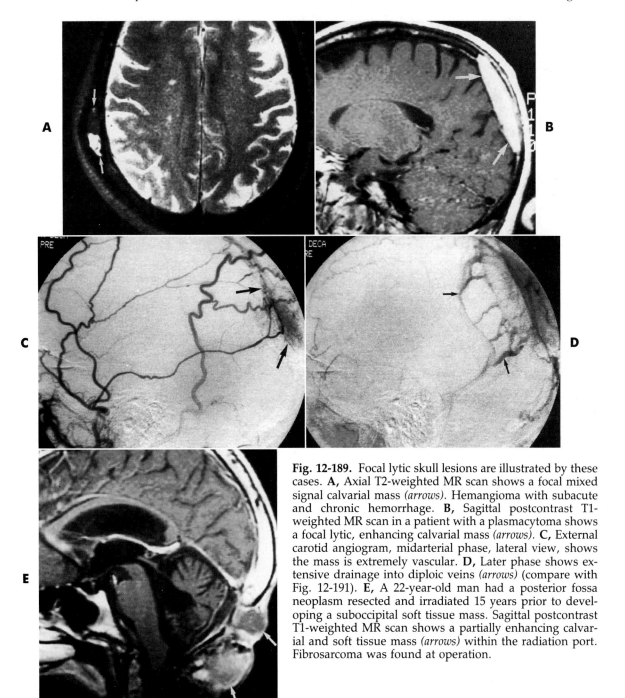

Fig. 12-189. Focal lytic skull lesions are illustrated by these cases. **A,** Axial T2-weighted MR scan shows a focal mixed signal calvarial mass *(arrows)*. Hemangioma with subacute and chronic hemorrhage. **B,** Sagittal postcontrast T1-weighted MR scan in a patient with a plasmacytoma shows a focal lytic, enhancing calvarial mass *(arrows)*. **C,** External carotid angiogram, midarterial phase, lateral view, shows the mass is extremely vascular. **D,** Later phase shows extensive drainage into diploic veins *(arrows)* (compare with Fig. 12-191). **E,** A 22-year-old man had a posterior fossa neoplasm resected and irradiated 15 years prior to developing a suboccipital soft tissue mass. Sagittal postcontrast T1-weighted MR scan shows a partially enhancing calvarial and soft tissue mass *(arrows)* within the radiation port. Fibrosarcoma was found at operation.

Less common causes of solitary lytic lesions include the rare primary calvarial neoplasms. *Plasmacytomas* (Fig. 12-189, *B* to *D*) and sarcomas (Fig. 12-189, *E*) are examples of such lesions.

Although *metastases* are sometimes solitary lytic lesions, they are more often multiple (Fig. 12-190). Reactive sclerosis is absent. *Multiple myeloma* and *hyperparathyroidism* are other causes of a stippled, or "salt and pepper," pattern caused by multiple small lytic defects.

Meninges

Anatomy. The cranial meninges consist of three layers: dura, arachnoid and pia mater (Fig. 12-191). The dura has two components: an outer (periosteal) and an inner (meningeal) layer. The outer dura consists of elongated fibroblasts and contains large extracellular spaces, as well as meningeal arteries and veins. The outer dura is tightly applied to the inner calvarial vault and is similar to periosteum. The inner dura is composed of epithelial cells and is con-

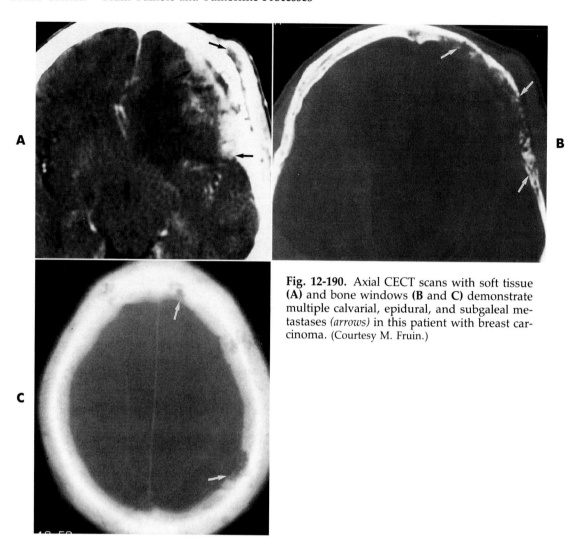

Fig. 12-190. Axial CECT scans with soft tissue **(A)** and bone windows **(B** and **C)** demonstrate multiple calvarial, epidural, and subgaleal metastases *(arrows)* in this patient with breast carcinoma. (Courtesy M. Fruin.)

Fig. 12-191. Anatomic diagram depicts the scalp, skull, and meninges. The potential epi- and subdural spaces are slightly exaggerated for illustrative purposes. These spaces, and lesions that occur within them, are coded on the diagram. Important anatomic structures are listed below: *1,* Scalp with subcutaneous fat. *2,* Scalp arteries and veins. *3,* Galea aponeurotica. *4,* Periosteum (the potential subgaleal space and periosteum are shown together here as a thin black line). *5,* Diploic veins in calvarium. *6,* Dura (outer and inner layers are shown). *7,* Arachnoid. *8,* Pacchionian granulations. Note projections from subarachnoid space into superior sagittal sinus (SSS). *9,* Cortical veins. These veins are shown as they course across the potential subdural space to enter the SSS. *10,* Pia mater. This, the innermost layer of the leptomeninges, is closely applied to the cerebral cortex. *11,* Pial arteries. *12,* Virchow-Robin spaces. These are pial-lined infoldings of CSF around penetrating cortical vessels. These spaces are exaggerated for illustrative purposes. *13,* Falx cerebri. Note potential subdural space adjacent to the falx.

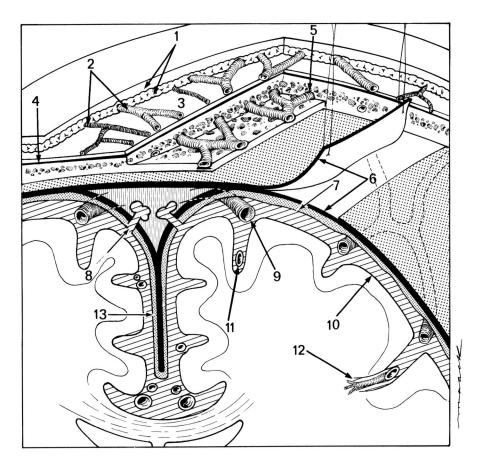

 Scalp, subcutaneous fat, galea aponeurotica

Common
  Dermoid, lipoma
  Contusion/laceration
  Subgaleal hematoma
  Underlying skull lesion (e.g., metastasis)
Uncommon
  Carcinoma/sarcoma (basal cell, lymphoma, Kaposi's)
  Plexiform neurofibroma
  Vascular malformation

 Calvarium

Common
  Hyperostosis frontalis interna
  Metastases
  Meningioma
  Paget disease
  Fibrous dysplasia
Uncommon
  Osteomyelitis
  Diploic tumor (e.g., epidermoid)
  Hematologic disorder

 Epidural space

Common
  Hematoma
  Metastasis (extension from skull lesion)
Uncommon
  Abscess

 Dura (periosteal, meningeal layers) and subdural space

Common
  Hematoma
  Meningioma enplaque
  Metastasis (e.g., breast, lymphoma)
  Effusion
  Postoperative change
Uncommon
  Empyema
  Leukemia
  Sarcoidosis
  Histiocytosis
  Pachymeningitis

 Dural venous sinus

Common
  Thrombosis
Uncommon
  Fibrosis (usually with long-standing thrombosis)
  Tumor (meningioma)

 Leptomeninges and subarachnoid space

Common
  Hemorrhage
  Meningitis ⎤ Penetrate parenchyma via
  Metastases ⎦ Virchow-Robin spaces
Uncommon
  Gliomatosis cerebri
  Histiocytosis
  Sarcoidosis

tinuous with the spinal dura, whereas the outer dura terminates at the foramen magnum.[202] The epidural space is the potential space between the outer dura and inner table of the skull.

The next layer is the arachnoid. The arachnoid is closely applied to the inner dura. The subdural space is the potential space between the inner dura and arachnoid layer of the cranial meninges. The subdural space is traversed by scattered trabeculae.[202] Cortical veins cross the subdural space as they course from the brain surface toward a dural sinus.

The innermost cranial meningeal layer is the pia. It is closely applied to the cortex and invaginates into the underlying sulci. The pia is composed of collagenous fibers externally and vermicular and elastic fibers internally.[202] Together the arachnoid and pia constitute the leptomeninges. The space in between these meningeal layers is the subarachnoid space. Virchow-Robin spaces are invaginations of pia and

CSF along cortical arteries that penetrate the brain parenchyma.

Dural microvessels lack tight junctions, unlike the arachnoid microvessels that are components of the blood-brain barrier.[203] Therefore some dural enhancement is normal following contrast administration. Normal meningeal enhancement is thin, smooth, discontinuous and symmetric. Enhancement is most prominent near the vertex and least striking around the anterior temporal lobes. Normally the meninges enhance less intensely than the dural venous sinuses (*see* box, *left*).

Pathology. The most common causes of abnormal meningeal enhancement are postsurgical changes, subarachnoid hemorrhage, infection, and neoplasm (*see* box, *below*). Eighty percent of patients demonstrate nonneoplastic meningeal enhancement following craniotomy.[204,205] *Postcraniotomy meningeal enhancement* can reflect focal inflammation or a diffuse chemical arachnoiditis caused by bleeding into the subarachnoid space during surgery. Postoperative meningeal enhancement is usually smooth and relatively thin (Fig. 12-192).

Meningeal fibrosis also occurs with aneurysmal subarachnoid hemorrhage (SAH) and long-term ventricular shunting.[206] *CSF leaks* and *intracranial hypotension*

Normal Meningeal Enhancement
Imaging characteristics

Thin
Smooth (not nodular, no focal masses)
Discontinuous
Most prominent near vertex
Less intense than cavernous sinus

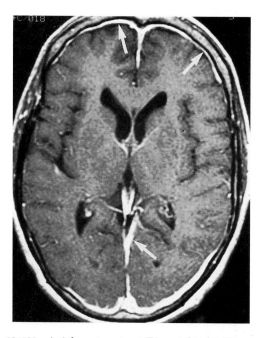

Fig. 12-192. Axial postcontrast T1-weighted MR scan in a patient 3 months postcraniotomy shows nonneoplastic meningeal enhancement (*arrows*). The meninges are mildly but diffusely thickened. Note smooth, linear enhancement without focal nodularity.

Abnormal Meningeal Enhancement
Differential diagnosis

Diffuse

Common
Postoperative
Infectious meningitis
Carcinomatous meningitis
Subarachnoid hemorrhage
Uncommon
Sarcoidosis
Histiocytosis
Idiopathic hypertrophic cranial pachymeningitis
Dural sinus thrombosis
Intracranial hypotension (e.g., with CSF leak)

Focal

Common
Meningioma
Postoperative (around craniotomy site)
Metastasis
Uncommon
Sarcoidosis
Histiocytosis
Rheumatoid nodules
Underlying cerebral infarction
Dural cavernous hemangioma, vascular malformation
Lymphoma/leukemia
Extramedullary hematopoiesis

can result in dural venous engorgement and striking enhancement.[203,203a] Dural venous sinus thrombosis can have similar findings.

Meningitis is a common cause of abnormally enhancing meninges. *Bacterial, viral, syphilitic,* and *granulomatous processes* can cause striking meningeal hypervascularity and enhancement (Fig. 12-193)[207,208] (*see* Chapter 16). Other less common nonneoplastic meningeal disorders include *histiocytosis* (Fig. 12-194), *sarcoidosis* (Fig. 12-195), *rheumatoid disease, extramedullary hematopoiesis* (Fig. 12-196), and *idiopathic hypertrophic cranial pachymeningitis* (Fig. 12-197). Diffuse and focal nodular meningeal lesions can be seen.[209-211] Focal meningeal sarcoid and pachymeningitis can be indistinguishable from meningioma.[212-214]

Meningioma and *carcinomatous meningitis* are the most common neoplasms that affect the dura. Men-

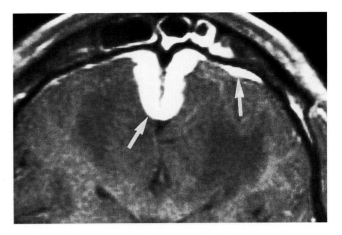

Fig. 12-193. Axial postcontrast T1-weighted MR scan in a patient with sinusitis and granulomatous meningitis *(arrows).* This particular case was related to cocaine abuse.

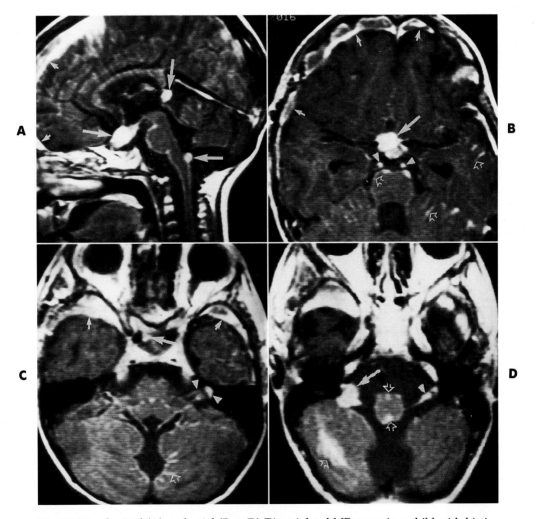

Fig. 12-194. Sagittal **(A)** and axial **(B to D)** T1-weighted MR scans in a child with histiocytosis. Note focal enhancing masses in the optic chiasm, optic nerves and hypothalamus, pineal gland, cerebellopontine angle, and fourth ventricle *(large arrows).* Extensive dural masses are seen in the anterior and middle cranial fossae *(small solid arrows).* Diffuse pial enhancement is present *(open arrows).* Numerous cranial nerves are affected, including III, VII, VIII, and IX to XI *(arrowheads).* (Courtesy W. Orrison.)

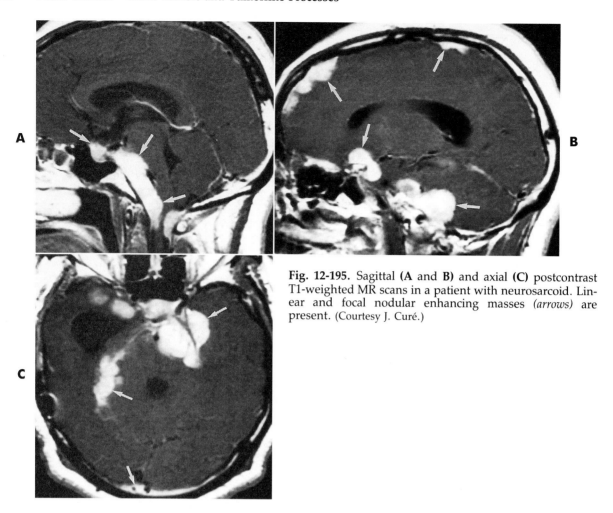

Fig. 12-195. Sagittal **(A** and **B)** and axial **(C)** postcontrast T1-weighted MR scans in a patient with neurosarcoid. Linear and focal nodular enhancing masses *(arrows)* are present. (Courtesy J. Curé.)

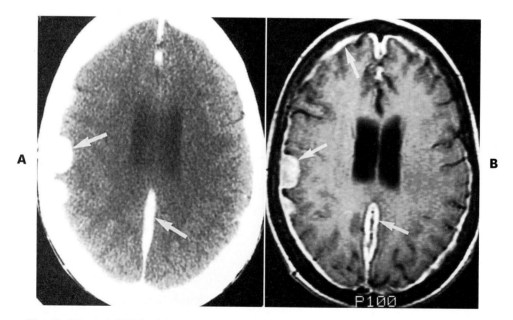

Fig. 12-196. Axial CECT **(A)** and postcontrast T1-weighted MR scans **(B)** in a patient with myelofibrosis and extramedullary hematopoiesis. Note diffuse and focal nodular enhancing dural masses *(arrows).* (Courtesy J. Curé.)

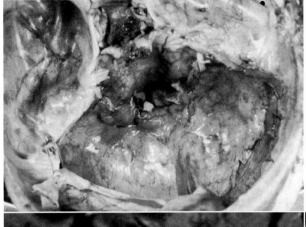

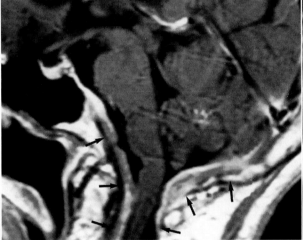

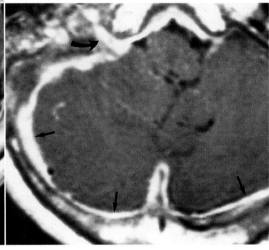

Fig. 12-197. Idiopathic cranial hypertrophic pachymeningitis. Gross pathology specimen (**A**) shows markedly thickened meninges. Sagittal (**B**) and axial (**C**) contrast-enhanced T1-weighted MR scans in a 65-year-old woman with neck pain, unsteady gait, and dysphagia show thickened, enhancing dura *(small arrows)* that extends into the jugular foramen (**C**, *curved arrow*). Hypertrophic pachymeningitis was found at surgery. (**A**, Courtesy Rubinstein Collection, Armed Forces Institute of Pathology. **B** and **C**, Courtesy D. Friedman, reprinted from *AJR* 160:900, 1993. With permission).

ingioma en plaque produces sessile dural thickening rather than a focal nodular mass (*see* Chapter 14). MR abnormalities can be demonstrated in one third to two thirds of patients with documented meningeal carcinomatosis.[202] Meningeal carcinomatosis can involve the dura, the leptomeninges, or both. Dural metastases are seen as curvilinear enhancing lesions under the skull that do not follow the gyral convolutions, whereas leptomeningeal tumor appears as thin, enhancing lines or small nodular deposits along the cortical surface (*see* Chapter 15).[202]

Extraskeletal mesenchymal osteocartilagenous tumors such as *osteochondroma* and *chondrosarcoma* can arise from the dura (*see* Chapter 14). These probably develop from pluripotential mesenchymal cells or embryonal cartilaginous rests in the falx and tentorium.[215]

Rare causes of leptomeningeal masses and abnormally enhancing dura include *amyloid, Gaucher disease* and other *mucopolysaccharidoses, glioneuronal heterotopias, meningioangiomatosis, gliomatosis cerebri, Wegener granulomatosis,* and *chordoma.*[202,215] Occasionally, primary brain parenchymal neoplasms such as *glioblastoma multiforme* extend directly into the adjacent meninges.[215]

REFERENCES

1. Okazaki H: Neoplastic and related conditions. In *Fundamentals of Neuropathology,* ed 2, pp 203-274, Igaku-Shoin, Tokyo, 1989.
2. Burger PC, Scheithauer BW, Vogel FS: Brain tumors. In *Surgical Pathology of the Nervous System and its Coverings,* Ed 3, pp 193-437, New York, Churchill Livingstone, 1991.
3. Rourke LB: Classification of basic tumors, *Categorical Course: Neoplasms of the Central Nervous System,* pp 3-4. American Society of Neuroradiology, 1990.
4. Russell DS, Rubinstein LJ: *Pathology of Tumors of the Nervous System,* ed 5, Baltimore, Williams and Wilkins, 1989.
5. Rourke LB, Gilles FH, Davis RL, Becker LE: Revision of the WHO classification of brain tumors for childhood brain tumors, *Cancer* 56:1869-1886, 1985.
6. Zulch KJ: *Brain Tumors. Their Biology and Pathology,* ed 3, Berlin, Springer, 1986.
6a. Kleihues P, Burger PC, Scheithauer BW: The new WHO classification of brain tumors, *Brain Pathol* 3:255-268, 1993.
7. Kyritsis AP, Yung WKA, Bruner J et al: The treatment of anaplastic oligodendrogliomas and mixed gliomas, *Neurosurg* 32:365-371, 1993.
8. Packer RJ: Clinical presentation of brain tumors/clinical areas of importance, *Categorical Course: Neoplasms of the Central Nervous System,* pp 23-27, American Society of Neuroradiology, 1990.
9. Harwood-Nash DC: Primary neoplasms of the central nervous system in children, *Cancer* 67:1223-1228, 1991.
10. Zimmerman RA: Posterior fossa pediatric tumors, *Categorical Course on Neoplasms of the Central Nervous System,* pp 33-35, American Society of Neuroradiology, 1990.

11. Buetow PC, Smirniotopoulos JG, Done S: Congenital brain tumors: a review of 45 cases, *AJNR* 11:793-799, 1990.

12. Haddad SF, Menezes AJ, Bell WE et al: Brain tumors occurring before 1 year of age: a retrospective review of 22 cases in an 11-year period, *Neurosurg* 29:8-13, 1991.

13. Hunt SJ, Johnsen PC, Coons SW, Pittman HW: Neonatal intracranial teratomas, *Surg Neurol* 34:336-342, 1990.

14. Kirk IR, Dominguez R, Castillo M: Congenital primary cerebral angiosarcoma: CT, US, and MR findings, *Pediatr Radiol* 22:134-135, 1992.

15. Hanna SL, Langston JW, Parham DM, Douglass EC: Primary malignant rhabdoid tumor of the brain: clinical, imaging, and pathologic findings, *AJNR* 14:107-115, 1993.

16. Zimmerman RA: Pediatric supratentorial tumors, *Sem Roentgenol* 25:225-248, 1990.

17. Gusnard DA: Cerebellar neoplasms in children, *Sem Roentgenol* 25:263-278, 1990.

18. Vandertop WP, Hoffman JH, Drake JM et al: Focal midbrain tumors in children, *Neurosurg* 31:186-194, 1992.

19. Stroink AR, Hoffman JH, Hendrick EB, Humphreys RP: Diagnosis and management of pediatric brainstem gliomas, *J Neurosurg* 65:745-750, 1986.

20. Epstein FJ, Farmer J-P: Brain stem glioma growth patterns, *J Neurosurg* 78:408-412, 1993.

21. Lizak PF, Woodruff WW: Posterior fossa neoplasms: multiplanar imaging, *Semin US, CT, MR* 13:182-206, 1992.

21a. Lavaroni A, Leonard M: Neuroradiological diagnostics of brain tumors in adults, *Riv di Neuroradiol* (suppl 2) :41-54, 1993.

22. Atlas SW: Adult supratentorial tumors, *Sem Roentgenol* 25:130-154, 1990.

23. Bilaniuk LT: Adult infratentorial tumors, *Sem Roentgenol* 25:155-173, 1990.

24. Naidich TP: Imaging evaluation of meningiomas, *Categorical Course on Neoplasms of the Central Nervous System*, pp 39-51. American Society of Neuroradiology, 1990.

25. Jelinek J, Smirniotopoulos JG, Parisi JE, Kanzer M: Lateral ventricular neoplasms of the brain: differential diagnosis based on clinical, CT, and MR findings, *AJNR* 11:567-574, 1990.

26. Zee C-S, Segall H, Apuzzo M et al: MR imaging of pineal region neoplasms, *J Comp Asst Tomogr* 15:56-63, 1991.

27. Smirniotopoulos JG, Rushing EJ, Mena H: Pineal region masses: differential diagnosis, *RadioGraphics* 12:577-596, 1992.

28. Edwards MSB, Hudgins RJ, Wilson CB et al: Pineal region tumors in children, *J Neurosurg* 68:689-697, 1988.

29. Ganti SR, Hilal SK, Stein BM et al: CT of pineal region tumors, *AJNR* 7:97-104, 1986.

30. Hoffman JH, Otsubo J, Hendrick EB et al: Intracranial germcell tumors in children, *J Neurosurg* 74:545-551, 1991.

31. Sugiyama K, Uozumi T, Kiya K et al: Intracranial germ-cell tumor with synchronous lesions in the pineal and suprasellar regions: report of six cases and review of the literature, *Surg Neurol* 38:114-120, 1993.

32. Chang T, Teng MMH, Guo W-Y, Sheng W-C: CT of pineal tumors and intracranial germ-cell tumors, *AJNR* 10:1039-1044, 1989.

33. Klein P, Rubinstein LJ: Benign symptomatic glial cysts of the pineal gland: a report of seven cases and review of the literature, *J Neurol Neurosurg Psychiatr* 52:991-995, 1989.

34. Todo T, Kondo T, Shinoura N, Yamada R: Large cysts of the pineal gland: report of two cases, *Neurosurg* 29:101-106, 1992.

35. Stern JD, Ross DA: Stereotactic management of benign pineal region cysts: report of two cases, *Neurosurg* 32:310-314, 1993.

36. Wisoff JH, Epstein F: Surgical management of symptomatic pineal cysts, *J Neurosurg* 77:896-900, 1992.

37. Constanzo A, Tedeschi G, DiSalle F et al: Pineal cysts: an incidental MRI finding? *J Neurol Neurosurg Psychiatr* 56:207-208, 1993.

38. Musolino A, Cambria S, Rizzo G, Cambria M: Symptomatic cysts of the pineal gland: stereotactic diagnosis and treatment of two cases and review of the literature, *Neurosurg* 32:315-321, 1993.

39. Martin N, Debroucker T, Mompoint D et al: Sarcoidosis of the pineal region: CT and MR studies, *J Comp Asst Tomogr* 132:110-112, 1989.

40. Hermann H-D, Winkler D, Westphal M: Treatment of tumors of the pineal region and posterior part of the third ventricle, *Acta Neurochirurgica* (Wien) 116:137-146, 1992.

41. Friedman DP: Extrapineal abnormalities of the tectal region: MR imaging findings, *AJR* 159:859-866, 1992.

42. Sherman JC, Citrin CM, Barkovich AJ, Bower BJ: MR imaging of the mesencephalic tectum: normal and pathologic variations, *AJNR* 8:59-64, 1987.

43. Sarwar M: *Computed Tomography of Congenital Brain Malformations*, St. Louis, Warren H. Green, 1985.

44. Dempsey PK, Kondziolka D, Lunsford LD: Stereotactic diagnosis and treatment of pineal region tumors and vascular malformations, *Acta Neurochir* (Wien) 116:14-22, 1992.

45. Truwit CL, Barkovich AJ: Pathogenesis of intracranial lipoma: an MR study in 42 patients, *AJNR* 11:665-674, 1990.

46. Choi SK, Starshak RJ, Meyer GA et al: Arachnoid cyst of the quadrigeminal plate cistern: report of two cases, *AJNR* 7:725-728, 1986.

47. Fitz CR: Disorders of ventricles and CSF spaces, *Sem US, CT, MR* 9:216-230, 1988.

48. DeMonte F, Zelby AS, Al-Mefty O: Hearing impairment resulting from a pineal region meningioma, *Neurosurg* 32:665-668, 1993.

49. Tien RD: Intraventricular mass lesions of the brain: CT and MR findings, *AJR* 157:1283-1290, 1991.

50. Pendl G, Ozturk E, Haselsberger K: Surgery of tumors of the lateral ventricle, *Acta Neurochir* (Wien) 116:128-136, 1992.

51. Degreef G, Lantos G, Bogerts B et al: Abnormalities of the septum pellucidum on MR scans in first-episode schizophrenics, *AJNR* 13:835-840, 1992.

52. Sarwar M: The septum pellucidum: normal and abnormal, *AJNR* 10:989-1005, 1989.

53. Yasargil MG, von Ammon K, von Deimling A et al: Central neurocytoma: histopathological variants and therapeutic approaches, *J Neurosurg* 76:32-37, 1992.

54. Coates TL, Hinshaw DB Jr, Peekman N et al: Pediatric choroid plexus neoplasms: MR and CT and pathologic correlation, *Radiol* 173:81-88, 1989.

55. Miyagi Y, Mannoji H, Akaboshi K et al: Intraventricular cavernous malformation associated with medullary venous malformation, *Neurosurg* 32:461-464, 1993.

56. Riebel T, Nasir R, Weber K: Choroid plexus cysts: a normal finding on ultrasound, *Pediatr Radiol* 22:410-412, 1992.

57. Nakase H, Morimoto T, Sakaki T et al: Bilateral choroid plexus cysts, *AJNR* 12:1204-1205, 1991.

58. Gaskill SJJ, Salvidar V, Rutman J, Morlin AE: Giant bilateral xanthogranulomas in a child: case report, *Neurosurg* 31:114-117, 1992.

59. Pappas CTE, Sonntag VKH, Spetzler RF: Surgical anatomy of the anterior aspect of the third ventricle, *BNI Quarterly* 6:2-10, 1990.

60. Maeder PP, Holtas SL, Basibuyuk LN et al: Colloid cysts of the third ventricle: correlation of MR and CT findings with histology and chemical analysis, *AJNR* 11:595-581, 1990.

61. Konovalov AN, Gorelyshev SK: Surgical treatment of anterior third ventricular tumors, *Acta Neurochir* (Wien) 118:33-39, 1992.

62. Lam AH, Villanueva AC: Symptomatic third ventricular choroid plexus cysts, *Pediatr Radiol* 22:413-416, 1992.

63. Barkovich AJ: Pediatric brain tumors, *Sem US, CT, MR* 13:412-448, 1992.

64. Nemoto Y, Inoue Y, Fukuda T et al: Displacement of the quadrigeminal plate in tumors of the fourth ventricle: MR appearance, *J Comp Asst Tomogr* 13:769-772, 1989.

65. Matsuno H, Rhoton AL Jr, Peace D: Microsurgical anatomy of the posterior fossa cisterns, *Neurosurg* 23:58-80, 1988.

66. Lo WWM: Cerebellopontine angle tumors, *Categorical Course on Neoplasms of the Central Nervous System*, pp 72-75, American Society of Neuroradiology, 1990.

67. Yuh WTC, Mayr-Yuh NA, Koci TM et al: Metastatic lesions involving the cerebellopontine angle, *AJNR* 14:99-106, 1993.

68. Laine FJ, Braun IF, Jensen ME et al: Perineural tumor extension through the foramen ovale: evaluation with MR imaging, *Radiol* 174:65-71, 1990.

69. Sevick RJ, Dillon WP, Engstrom J et al: Trigeminal neuropathy: Gd-DTPA enhanced MR imaging, *J Comp Asst Tomogr* 15:605-611, 1991.

70. Martin N, Pierot L, Sterkers O et al: Primary choroid plexus papilloma of the cerebellopontine angle: MR imaging, *Neuroradiol* 31:541-543, 1990.

71. Mueller DP, Gantz BJ, Dolan KD: Gadolinium-enhanced MR of the postoperative internal auditory canal following acoustic neuroma resection via the middle fossa approach, *AJNR* 13:197-200, 1992.

72. Aoki S, Sasaki Y, Machida T et al: Meningeal enhancement within the internal auditory canal caused by cerebellopontine angle meningiomas: 1.5T MRI with gadolinium-DTPA, *Neuroradiol* 33(suppl):309-310, 1991.

73. Gelbarski SS, Telian SA, Niparko JK: Enhancement along the normal facial nerve in the facial canal: MR imaging and anatomic correlation, *Radiol* 183:391-394, 1992.

73a. Carellas AR, Torres C, Isem EG et al: Ramsey-Hunt syndrome and high-resolution 3DFT MRI, *J Comp Asst Tomogr* 17:495-497, 1993.

74. Tien R, Dillon WP, Jackler RK: Contrast-enhanced MR imaging of the facial nerve in 11 patients with Bell's palsy, *AJNR* 11:735-741, 1990.

75. Han MH, Jabour BA, Andrews JC et al: Nonneoplastic enhancing lesions mimicking intracanalicular acoustic neuroma on gadolinium-enhanced MR images, *Radiol* 179:795-796, 1991.

76. Linskey ME, Jannetta PJ, Martinez AJ: A vascular malformation mimicking an intracanalicular acoustic neurilemoma, *J Neurosurg* 74:516-519, 1991.

77. Lhuillier FM, Doyon DL, Halimi PhM et al: Magnetic resonance imaging of acoustic neuromas: pitfalls and differential diagnosis, *Neuroradiol* 34:144-149, 1992.

78. Mark AS, Seltzer S, Harnsberger HR: Sensorineural hearing loss: more than meets the eye? *AJNR* 14:37-45, 1993.

79. Harnsberger HR: *Handbook of Head and Neck Imaging*, Year book Medical Publishers, Chicago, 1990.

80. Piazza P, Bassi P, Menozzi R: I tumori delle quaine nervose dei nervi cranici, *Riv di Neuroradiol* S(suppl 4):51-66, 1992.

81. (see above)

82. Olsen WL, Dillon WP, Kelly WM et al: MR imaging of paragangliomas, *AJNR* 7:1039-1042, 1986.

83. Schweitzer ME, Hodler J, Cervilla V, Resnick D: Craniovertebral junction: normal anatomy with MR correlation, *AJR* 158:1087-1090, 1992.

84. Reuther G, Masrur H, Müller S, Fahrendorf G: Assessment of vascular grooves at the brainstem, *Eur Radiol* 2:148-153, 1992.

85. Katayama Y, Tsubokawa T, Hirasawat et al: Intradural extraosseous chordoma in the foramen magnum region, *J Neurosurg* 75:976-979, 1991.

86. Chumas PD, Armstrong DC, Drake JM et al: Tonsillar herniation: the rule rather than the exception after shunting in the pediatric population, *J Neurosurg* 78:568-573, 1993.

87. Sathi S, Stieg PE: "Acquired" Chiari I malformation after multiple lumbar punctures: case report, *Neurosurg* 32:306-309, 1993.

88. Carella A, Resta M, Palma M: Malformazioni della cerniera cranio-cervicale: stato dell'arte, *Riv di Neuroradiol* 4:349-360, 1991.

89. Bassi P, Corona C, Contri P et al: Congenital basilar impression: correlated neurological syndromes, *Eur Neurol* 32:238-243, 1992.

90. Crockard HA, Heilman AE, Stevens JM: Progressive myelopathy secondary to odontoid fractures: clinical, radiological, and surgical features, *J Neurosurg* 78:579-586, 1993.

91. Kendall BE, Stevens JM, Crockard HA: The spine in rheumatoid arthritis, *Riv di Neuroradiol* (Suppl 2):23-28, 1992.

92. Smoker WRK, Keyes WD, Dunn VD, Menezes AH: MRI versus conventional radiologic examinations in the evaluation of the craniovertebral and cervicomedullary junction, *RadioGraphics* 6:953-994, 1986.

93. White KS, Ball WS, Prenger EC et al: Evaluation of the craniocervical junction in Down syndrome: correlation of measurements obtained with radiography and MR imaging, *Radiol* 186:377-382, 1993.

94. Kimura F, Kim KS, Friedman H et al: MR imaging of the normal and abnormal clivus, *AJNR* 11:1015-1021, 1990.

95. Chaljub G, Van Fleet R, Guinto FC Jr et al: MR imaging of clival and paraclival lesions, *AJR* 159:1069-1074, 1992.

96. Meyers SP, Hirsch WL Jr, Curtin HD et al: Chordomas of the skull base: MR features, *AJNR* 13:1627-1636, 1992.

97. Johnsen DE, Woodruff WW, Allen IS et al: MR imaging of the sellar and juxtasellar regions, *RadioGraphics* 11:727-758, 1991.

98. Elster AD: Modern imaging of the pituitary, *Radiol* 187:1-14, 1993.

99. Schwartzberg DG: Imaging of pituitary gland tumors, *Sem US, CT, MR* 13:207-223, 1992.

100. Schubiger O: Intrasellar tumors: neuroradiological diagnosis, *Riv di Neuroradiol* (Suppl 1)4:47-55, 1991.

101. Carlier R, Monmet O, Idir ABC et al: Insuffisance anté-et post-hypophysaire avec anomalies de la tige pituitaire, *J Radiol* 72:437-443, 1991.

102. Patel SC, Sanders WP: MRI of the pituitary gland: adenomas, *MRI Decisions*, pp 12-20, 1990.

103. Tien RD: Sequence of enhancement of various portions of the pituitary gland on gadolinium-enhanced MR images: correlation with regional blood supply, *AJR* 158:651-654, 1992.

104. Kucharczyk W, Lenkinski RE, Kucharczyk J, Henkelman RM: The effect of phospholipid vesicles on the NMR relaxation of water: an explanation for the MR appearance of the neurohypophysis? *AJNR* 11:693-700, 1990.

105. Mark LP, Haughton VM, Hendrix LE et al: High-intensity signals within the posterior pituitary fossa: a study with fat-suppression MR techniques, *AJNR* 12:929-932, 1991.

106. Colombo N, Berry I, Kucharczyk J et al: Posterior pituitary gland: appearance on MR imaging in normal and pathological states, *Radiol* 165:481-485, 1987.

107. Sato N, Ishizaka H, Yagi H et al: Posterior lobe of the pituitary in diabetes insipidus: dynamic MR imaging, *Radiol* 186:357-360, 1993.

108. Dina TS, Feaster SH, Laws ER Jr, Davis DO: Serial MR studies following transphenoidal resection, *AJNR* 14:763-768, 1993.

109. Dash RJ, Gupta V, Suri S: Sheehan's syndrome: clinical profile, pituitary hormone responses, and computed sellar tomography, *Aust NZ J Med* 23:26-31, 1993.

110. Doriswamy PM, Potts JM, Axelson DA et al: MR assessment of pituitary gland morphology in healthy volunteers: age- and gender-related differences, *AJNR* 13:1295-1299, 1992.

111. Cox TD, Elster AD: Normal pituitary gland: changes in shape,

size, and signal intensity during the 1st year of life at MR imaging, *Radiol* 179:721-724, 1991.

112. Elster AD, Chen MY, Williams DW, Key LL: Pituitary gland: MR imaging of physiologic hypertrophy in adolescence, *Radiol* 174:681-685, 1990.

113. Miki Y, Asato R, Okumura R et al: Anterior pituitary gland in pregnancy: hyperintensity at MR, *Radiol* 187:229-231, 1993.

114. Argyropoulou M, Perignon F, Brunelle F et al: Height of normal pituitary gland as a function of age evaluated by magnetic resonance imaging in children, *Pediatr Radiol* 21:247-249, 1991.

115. Lurie SN, Doraiswamy PM, Husain MM et al: In vivo assessment of pituitary gland volume with magnetic resonance imaging: the effect of age, *J Clin Endocrinol* 71:505-509, 1990.

116. Kuroiwa, Okabe Y, Hasuo K et al: MR imaging of pituitary hypertrophy due to juvenile primary hypothyroidism: a case report, *Clin Imaging* 15:202-205, 1991.

117. Kao SCS, Cook JS, Hansen JR, Simonson TM: MR imaging of the pituitary gland in central precocious puberty, *Pediat Radiol* 22:481-484, 1992.

118. Shanklin WM: Incidence and distribution of cilia in the human pituitary with description of micro-follicular cysts derived from Rathke's cleft, *Acta Anat* (Basel) 11:361-382, 1951.

119. Hua F, Asato R, Miki Y et al: Differentiation of suprasellar nonneoplastic cysts from cystic neoplasms by Gd-DTPA MRI, *J Comp Asst Tomogr* 16:747-749, 1992.

120. Sakamoto Y, Takahashi M, Korogi Y et al: Normal and abnormal pituitary glands: gallopentetate dimeglumine-enhanced MR imaging, *Radiol* 178:441-445, 1991.

121. Zimmerman RA: Imaging of intrasellar, suprasellar, and parasellar tumors, *Semin Roentgenol* 25:174-197, 1990.

122. Michael AS, Paige ML: MR imaging of intrasellar meningioma simulating pituitary adenomas, *J Comp Asst Tomogr* 12:949-946, 1988.

123. Taylor SL, Barakos JA, Harsh GR IV, Wilson CB: Magnetic resonance imaging of tuberculum sellae meningiomas: preventing preoperative misdiagnosis as pituitary adenoma, *Neurosurg* 31:621-627, 1992.

124. Wu JK, Hedges TR III, Anderson ML, Folkerth RD: Surgical reversal of a subacute complete unilateral visual loss from an ovarian metastasis to the pituitary gland, *Neurosurg* 31:349-352, 1992.

125. Schubiger O, Haller D: Metastases to the pituitary-hypothalamic axis, *Neuroradiol* 34:131-134, 1992.

126. Mucelli RSP, Frezza F, Magnaldi S, Proto G: Magnetic resonance imaging in patients with panhypopituitarism, *Eur Radiol* 2:42-46, 1992.

127. Ryals BD, Brown DC, Levin SW: Duplication of the pituitary gland as shown by MR, *AJNR* 14:137-139, 1993.

128. Steiner E, Knosp E, Herold CJ et al: Pituitary adenomas: findings of postoperative MR imaging, *Radiol* 185:521-527, 1992.

129. Popovic EA, Vattuone JR, Siu KH et al: Malignant prolactinomas, *Neurosurg* 29:127-130, 1991.

130. Juneau P, Schoene WC, Black P: Malignant tumors in the pituitary gland, *Arch Neurol* 49:555-558, 1992.

131. Ahmadi J, Destian S, Apuzzo MLJ et al: Cystic fluid in craniopharyngiomas: MR imaging and quantitative analysis, *Radiol* 182:783-785, 1992.

132. Loes DJ, Barloon TJ, Yuh WTC et al: MR anatomy and pathology of the hypothalamus, *AJR* 156:579-585, 1991.

133. Fujisawa I, Asato R, Okumura R et al: Magnetic resonance imaging of neurohypophyseal germinomas, *Cancer* 68:1009-1014, 1991.

134. Freedy RM, Miller KD Jr: Granulocytic sarcoma (chloroma): sphenoidal sinus and paraspinal involvement as evaluated by CT and MR, *AJNR* 12:259-262, 1991.

135. Armstrong EA, Harwood-Nash DC, Hoffman H et al: Benign suprasellar cysts: the CT approach, *AJR* 4:163-166, 1983.

136. Voelker JL, Campbell RL, Muller J: Clinical, radiographic, and pathologic features of symptomatic Rathke's cleft cysts, *J Neurosurg* 74:535-544, 1991.

137. Ross DA, Norman D, Wilson CB: Radiologic characteristics and results of surgical management of Rathke's cysts in 43 patients, *Neurosurg* 31:173-179, 1992.

138. Itoh J, Usui K: An entirely suprasellar symptomatic Rathke's cleft cyst: case report, *Neurosurg* 30:581-585, 1992.

139. Crenshaw WB, Chew FS: Rathke's cleft cyst, *AJR* 158:1312, 1992.

140. Boyko OB, Curnes JT, Oakes WJ, Burger PC: Hamartomas of the tuber cinereum: CT, MR, and pathologic findings, *AJNR* 12:309-314, 1991.

141. Albright AL, Lee PA: Neurosurgical treatment of hypothalamic hamartomas causing precocious puberty, *J Neurosurg* 78:77-82, 1993.

142. Cheng K, Sawamura Y, Yamauchi T, Abe H: Asymptomatic large hypothalamic hamartoma associated with polydactyly in an adult, *Neurosurg* 32:458-460, 1993.

143. Hashimoto M, Yanaki T, Nakahara N, Masuzawa T: Lymphocytic adenohypophysitis: an immunohistochemical study, *Surg Neurol* 36:137-144, 1991.

144. Higuchi M, Arita N, Mori S et al: Pituitary granuloma and chronic inflammation of hypophysis: clinical and immunohistochemical studies. *Acta Neurochir* 121:152-158, 1993.

145. Mark AS, Phister SH, Jackson DE Jr, Kolsky MP: Traumatic lesions of the suprasellar region: MR imaging, *Radiol* 182:49-52, 1992.

146. Simmons GE, Suchnicki JE, Rak KM, Damiano TR: MR imaging of the pituitary stalk: size, shape, and enhancement pattern, *AJR* 159:375-377, 1992.

147. Stull MA, Kransdorf MJ, Devaney KO: Langerhans cell histiocytosis of bone, *RadioGraphics* 12:801-823, 1992.

148. Tien RD, Newton TH, McDermott MW et al: Thickened pituitary stalk on MR images in patients with diabetes insipidus and Langerhans cell histiocytosis, *AJNR* 11:703-708, 1990.

149. Maghnie M, Arico M, Villa A et al: MR of the hypothalamic-pituitary axis in Langerhans cell histiocytosis, *AJNR* 13:1365-1371, 1992.

149a. Breidahl WH, Ives FJ, Khangure MS: Cerebral and brain stem Langerhans cell histiocysis, *Neuroradiol* 35:349-351, 1993.

150. Vogl TJ, Stemmler J, Scriba PC et al: Sarcoidosis of the hypothalamus and pituitary stalk, *Eur Radiol* 2:76-78, 1992.

151. Scott TF: Neurosarcoidosis: progress and clinical aspects, *Neurol* 43:8-12, 1993.

152. Seltzer S, Mark AS, Atlas SW: CNS sarcoidosis: evaluation with contrast-enhanced MR imaging, *AJNR* 12:1227-1233, 1991.

153. Cone L, Srinivasan M, Romanul FCA: Granular cell tumor (choristoma) of the neurohypophysis: two cases and a review of the literature, *AJNR* 11:403-406, 1990.

154. Laine FJ, Nadel L, Braun IF: CT and MR imaging of the central skull base. Part 1: Techniques, embryologic development, and anatomy, *Radiographics* 10:591-602, 1990.

155. Lang J: Anatomy of the skull base, *Riv di Neuroradiol* (Suppl 1):11-25, 1991.

156. Van Tassel P, Lee Y-Y: Gd-DTPA enhanced MR for detecting intracranial extension of sinonasal malignancies, *J Comp Asst Tomog* 15:387-394, 1991.

156a. Delfini R, Missori P, Iannetti G et al: Mucoceles of the paranasal sinuses with intracranial and intraorbital extension: report of 28 cases, *Neurosurg* 32:901-906, 1993.

157. Van Tassel P, Lee Y-Y, Jing B-S, DePena CA: Mucoceles of the paranasal sinuses: MR imaging with CT correlation, *AJNR* 10:607-612, 1989.

158. Som PM, Lawson W, Lidov MW: Simulated aggressive skull

base erosion: response to benign sinonasal disease, *Radiol* 180:799-759, 1991.

159. Brown JH, Chew FS: Inverted papilloma, *AJR* 159:278, 1992.

160. Yousem DM, Fellows DW, Kennedy DW et al: Inverted papilloma: evaluation with MR imaging, *Radiol* 185:501-505, 1992.

161. Castillo M, Pillsbury HC III: Rhabdomyosarcoma of the middle ear: imaging features in two children, *AJNR* 14:730-733, 1933.

162. Ginsberg LE: Neoplastic diseases affecting the central skull base: CT and MR imaging, *AJR* 159:581-589, 1992.

163. Laine FJ, Nadel L, Braun IF: CT and MR imaging of the central skull base, *Radiographics* 10:797-821, 1990.

164. Ruprecht A, Dolan KD: The nasopharynx in oral and maxillofacial radiology. II, Malignant lesions, *Oral Surg Oral Med Oral Pathol* 75:106-121, 1993.

165. Sham JST, Cheung YK, Choy D et al: Nasopharyngeal carcinoma: CT evaluation of patterns of tumor spread, *AJNR* 12:265-270, 1991.

166. Parker GD, Harnsberger HR: Clinical-radiologic issues in perineurial tumor spread of malignant diseases of the extracranial head and neck, *Radiographics* 11:383-399, 1991.

167. Mack EE, Prados MD, Wilson CB: Late manifestations of esthesineuroblastomas in the central nervous system: report of two cases, *Neurosurg* 30:93-97, 1992.

167a. Morita A, Ebersold MJ, Olsen KD et al: Esthesioneuroblastoma: prognosis and management, *Neurosurg* 32:706-715, 1993.

167b. Li C, Yousem DM, Hayden RE, Doty RL: Olfactory neuroblastoma: MR evaluation, *AJNR* 14:1167-1171, 1993.

168. Sheporaitis L, Osborn AG, Smirniotopoulos JG et al: Radiologic-pathologic correlation: intracranial meningioma, *AJNR* 13:29-37, 1992.

169. Zee CS, Chin T, Segall HD et al: Magnetic resonance imaging of meningiomas, *Sem US, CT, MR* 13:154-169, 1992.

170. Barkovich AJ, Vandermarck P, Edwards MSB, Cogen PH: Congenital nasal masses: CT and MR imaging features in 16 cases, *AJNR* 12:105-116, 1991.

171. Hasuo, Fukui M, Tamura S et al: Gliomas with dural invasion: computed tomography and angiography, *CT: J Comp Tomogr* 12:100-107, 1988.

172. Woodruff WW Jr, Djang WT, Voorhees D, Heinz ER: Calvarial destruction: an unusual manifestation of glioblastoma multiforme, *AJNR* 9:388-389, 1988.

173. El-Kalliny M, Van Loveren H, Keller JT, Tew JM Jr: Tumor of the lateral wall of the cavernous sinuses, *J Neurosurg* 77:508-514, 1992.

174. Malone DG, O'Boynick PL, Ziegler DK et al: Osteomyelitis of the skull base, *Neurosurg* 30:426-431, 1992.

175. Breen DJ, Clifton AG, Wilkins P et al: Invasive aspirgilloma of the skull base, *Neuroradiol* 35:216-217, 1993.

176. Ellie E, Houvang B, Lovail C et al: CT and high field MRI in septic thrombosis of the cavernous sinuses, *Neuroradiol* 34:22-24, 1992.

177. Anand V, Alemar G, Griswold JA Jr: Intracranial complications of mucormycosis: an experimental method and clinical review, *Laryngoscope* 102:656-662, 1992.

178. Marsot-Dupuch K, Cabane J, Raveau V et al: Lethal midline granuloma: impact of imaging studies on the investigation and management of destructive midfacial disease in 13 patients, *Neuroradiol* 34:155-161, 1992.

179. Demaerel P, Brown P, Kendall BE et al: Case report: allergic aspergillosis of the sphenoid sinus: pitfall on MRI, *Br J Radiol* 66:260-263, 1993.

180. Burlacoff SG, Wong FSH: Wegener's granulomatosis. The great masquerade: a clinical presentation and literature review, *J Otolaryngol* 22:94-105, 1993.

181. Yuh WTC, Wright DC, Barlan TJ et al: MR imaging of primary tumor of trigeminal nerve and Meckel's cave, *AJNR* 9:665-670, 1988.

182. Celli P, Ferrante L, Acqui M et al: Neuromas of the third, fourth, and sixth cranial nerves: a survey and report of a new fourth nerve case, *Surg Neurol* 38:216-224, 1992.

183. Abramowitz J, Dron JE, Jensen ME et al: Angiographic diagnosis and management of head and neck schwannomas, *AJNR* 12:977-984, 1991.

184. Al-Ghamadi S, Black MJ, Lafond G: Extracranial head and neck schwannomas, *J Otolaryngol* 21:186-188, 1992.

185. Mulkens TH, Parizel PM, Martin J-J et al: Acoustic schwannoma: MR findings in 84 tumors, *AJR* 160:395-398, 1993.

186. Pollack IF, Sekhar LN, Janetta PJ, Janecka IP: Neurilemmomas of the trigeminal nerve, *J Neurosurg* 70:737-745, 1989.

187. Meyers SP, Hirsch WL Jr, Curtin HD et al: Chordomas of the skull base: MR features, *AJNR* 13:1627-1636, 1992.

188. Sampson JH, Rossitch E Jr, Young JN et al: Solitary eosinophilic granuloma invading the clivus of an adult, *Neurosurg* 31:755-758, 1992.

189. Aoki J, Sone S, Fujioka F et al: MR of enchondroma and chondrosarcoma: rings and arcs of Gd-DTPA enhancement, *J Comp Asst Tomog* 15:1011-1016, 1991.

190. Lee Y-Y, Van Tassel P, Navert C et al: Craniofacial osteosarcomas: plain film, CT, and MR findings: 46 cases, *AJNR* 9:379-385, 1988.

191. Meyers SP, Hirsch WL Jr, Curtin HD et al: Chondrosarcomas of the skull base: MR imaging features, *Radiol* 184:103-108, 1992.

192. DePena CA, Lee Y-Y, Van Tassel P: Lymphomatous involvement of the trigeminal nerve and Meckel's cave: CT and MR appearance, *AJNR* 10:515-517, 1989.

193. Lang J: Anatomy of the posterior skull base, *Riv di Neuroradiol* 4(Suppl 1):125-134, 1991.

194. Chaljub G, Van Fleet R, Guinto FC Jr et al: MR imaging of clival and paraclival lesions, *AJR* 159:1069-1074, 1992.

195. Kimura F, Kim KS, Friedman H et al: MR imaging of the normal and abnormal clivus, *AJNR* 11:1015-1021, 1990.

196. Applegate GR, Hirsch WL, Applegate LJ, Curtin HD: Variability in the enhancement of the normal central skull base in children, *Neuroradiol* 34:217-221, 1992.

197. Vogl T, Bruning R, Schedel H et al: Paraganglioma of the jugular bulb and carotid body: MR imaging with short sequences and Gd-DTPA enhancement, *AJNR* 10:823-827, 1989.

198. Casselman JW, DeJonge I, Neyt L et al: MRI in craniofacial fibrous dysplasia, *Neuroradiol* 35:234-237, 1993.

198a. Yano M, Tajima S, Tanaka Y et al: Magnetic resonance imaging of craniofacial fibrous dysplasia, *Ann Plast Surg* 30:371-374, 1993.

199. Caresio JF, McMillan H, Batnitzky S: Coexistent intra- and extracranial mass lesions: an unusual manifestation of histiocytosis X, *AJNR* 12:80-81, 1991.

200. Ruge JR, Tomitashita T, Naidich TP et al: Scalp and calvarial masses of infants and children, *Neurosurg* 22:1037-1042, 1988.

200a. De Schepper AMA, Ramon F, Van Marck E: MR imaging of eosinophilic granuloma: report of 11 cases, *Skeletal Radiol* 22:163-166, 1993.

201. Kim KS, Rogus LF, Goldblatt D: CT features of hyperostosing meningioma en plaque, *AJNR* 8:853-859, 1987.

201a. Kaufman HH, Hochberg J, Anderson RP et al: Treatment of calcified cephalohematoma, *Neurosurg* 32:1037-1040, 1993.

202. Sze G: Diseases of the intracranial menengis: MR imaging features, *AJR* 160:727-733, 1993.

203. Fishman RA, Dillon WP: Dural enhancement and cerebral displacement secondary to intracranial hypotension, *Neuroradiol* 43:609-611, 1993.

203a. Pannullo SC, Reich JB, Krol G et al: MRI changes in intracranial hypotension, *Neurol* 43:919-926, 1993.

204. Burke JW, Podrasky AE, Bradley WG Jr: Meningitis: postoperative enhancement on MR images, *Radiol* 174:99-102, 1990.
205. Suzuki M, Takashima T, Kadoya M et al: Gadolinium-DTPA enhancement of dural structures on MRI after surgery, *Neurochir* 35:112-116, 1992.
206. Destian S, Heier LA, Zimmerman RD et al: Differentiation between meningeal fibrosis and chronic subdural hematoma after ventricular shunting: value of enhanced CT and MR scans, *AJNR* 10:1021-1026, 1989.
207. Mathews VP, Kuharia MP, Edwards NK et al: Gd-DTPA-enhanced MR imaging of experimental bacterial meningitis: evaluation and comparison with CT, *AJNR* 9:1045-1050, 1988.
208. Chang KH, Han MH, Roh JK: Gd-DTPA-enhanced MR imaging of the brain in patients with meningitis: comparison with CT, *AJNR* 11:69-76, 1990.
209. Mamelak AN, Kelly WM, Davis RL, Rosenblum ML: Idiopathic hypertrophic cranial pachymeningitis, *J Neurosurg* 79:270-276, 1993.
210. Song SK, Schwartz IS, Stauchen JA et al: Meningeal nodules with features of extranodal sinus histiocytosis with massive lymphadenopathy, *Am J Surg Pathol* 13:406-412, 1989.
211. Yuh WTC, Drew JM, Rizzo M et al: Evaluations of pachymeningitis by contrast-enhanced MR imaging: a patient with rheumatoid disease, *AJNR* 11:1247-1248, 1990.
212. Ranoux D, Devanx B, Laury C et al: Meningeal sarcoidosis, pseudomeningioma, and pachymeningitis of the convexity, *J Neurol Neurosurg Psychiatry* ss:300-303, 1992.
213. Mayer SA, Kim GK, Onesti ST et al: Biopsy-proven isolated sarcoid meningitis, *J Neurosurg* 78:994-996, 1993.
214. Friedman D, Flanders A, Tartaglino L: Contrast-enhanced MR imaging of idiopathic hypertrophic craniospinal pachymeningitis, *AJR* 160:900-901, 1993.
215. Salcman M, Scholtz H, Kristt D, Numaguchi Y: Extraskeletal myxoid chondrosarcoma of the face, *Neurosurg* 31:344-348, 1992.
216. Tishler S, Williamson T, Mirra SS et al: Wegener granulomatosis with meningeal involvement, *AJNR* 14:1248-1252, 1993.
217. Krol G, Simons B, Haines A: Meningeal and ependymal abnormalities associated with cranial neoplasms: MR findings, *Neuroradiol* 33(supp):31-32, 1991.

Astrocytomas and Other Glial Neoplasms

Astrocytomas
    Astrocytoma (Low-grade or "Benign" Astrocytoma)
    Anaplastic (Malignant) Astrocytoma
    Glioblastoma Multiforme
    Gliomatosis Cerebri
    Gliosarcoma
    Pilocytic Astrocytoma
    Pleomorphic Xanthoastrocytoma
    Subependymal Giant Cell Astrocytoma
Oligodendroglioma
    "Pure" Oligodendroglioma
    "Mixed" Oligodendroglioma
Ependymoma
    Cellular Ependymoma
    Subependymoma
Choroid Plexus Tumors
    Choroid Plexus Papilloma
    Choroid Plexus Carcinoma

Frequency of Gliomas

Two thirds of all brain tumors are primary neoplasms
Almost half of all primary brain tumors are gliomas
Three quarters of all gliomas are astrocytomas
More than three quarters of all astrocytomas are anaplastic astrocytomas and glioblastoma multiforme

---

Glial cells are the most common cellular component of the neuropil. They are five to ten times more frequent than the trillion brain neurons and compose half the CNS by volume.[1] Glial cells have an enormous potential for abnormal growth and are the chief source of CNS neoplasms (Fig. 12-1, *B*) (*see* box).

There are several different kinds of glial cells. Corresponding to the three histologic groups of glial cells are the following three major types of gliomas (*see* box, p. 530)[2]:

1. Astrocytoma
2. Oligodendroglioma
3. Ependymoma

Choroid plexus contains modified ependymal cells and therefore its neoplastic growths are generally considered with the other gliomas.

ASTROCYTOMAS

Approximately half of all primary brain tumors are glial cell neoplasms and more than three quarters of all gliomas are astrocytomas (Fig. 13-1). Astrocytomas are a histologically heterogeneous group of primary brain tumors that are both graded and classified.

Grading of astrocytomas. Tumor grading is important for prognosis and therapy. Grading of a ce-

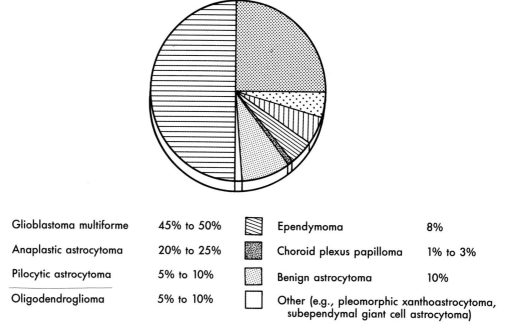

Glioblastoma multiforme	45% to 50%	Ependymoma	8%
Anaplastic astrocytoma	20% to 25%	Choroid plexus papilloma	1% to 3%
Pilocytic astrocytoma	5% to 10%	Benign astrocytoma	10%
Oligodendroglioma	5% to 10%	Other (e.g., pleomorphic xanthoastrocytoma, subependymal giant cell astrocytoma)	

Fig. 13-1. Frequency of glioma subtypes. Glioblastoma multiforme and anaplastic astrocytoma account for three quarters of all gliomas. So-called benign astrocytomas are uncommon.

rebral neoplasm ideally should be based on the most malignant cells present. Unfortunately, astrocytomas are often histologically heterogeneous, and focal biopsy specimens can be unrepresentative or misleading.

Several different grading and classification systems have been proposed. All are somewhat arbitrary and imprecise; none is universally accepted. Astrocytomas do not fall within discrete, easily definable categories but instead represent a biologic continuum that ranges from histologically well-differentiated tumors to poorly or undifferentiated neoplasms with nuclear and cellular pleomorphism, vascular endothelial proliferation, and necrosis.[2]

The traditional (Kernohan) astrocytoma grading scale uses a four point scale of ascending malignancy from 1 (benign) to 4 (glioblastoma multiforme). This has been modified by the National Brain Tumor Study Group and World Health Organization (WHO) into a three-tiered system for grading diffusely infiltrating astrocytomas:[4,5,5a]

WHO classification	Kernohan grade
Low grade or "benign" (grade II)	1 and 2
Anaplastic (grade III)	3
Glioblastoma multiforme (grade IV)	4

Regardless of the degree of histopathologic differentiation or anaplasia, all infiltrating gliomas are clinically malignant because without appropriate treatment they are usually fatal.[6,7]

Types of Gliomas

Astrocytomas
Oligodendrogliomas
Ependymomas
Choroid plexus papillomas/carcinomas

Classification. Astrocytomas can be subdivided and studied according to histologic type, patient age, and geographic location.

Histology. Astrocytomas are primary neoplasms that are composed of neoplastically transformed astrocytes. They are therefore appropriately described by the specific type of proliferating astrocyte (such as fibrillary or pilocytic) in addition to histologic grade. Cell types have great prognostic significance because some tumors (such as pilocytic astrocytomas) rarely become malignant, whereas others (such as fibrillary astrocytomas) are eventually fatal, even though they may initially have a low or "benign" numerical histologic grade.

Generally accepted astrocytoma subtypes are fibrillary, pilocytic, and subependymal giant cell astrocytomas and pleomorphic xanthoastrocytoma (*see* box, p. 531, *left*). Some astrocytomas contain prominent, plump cells with abundant eosinophilic cytoplasm (these are sometimes called "gemistocytic" astrocytomas, derived from the German word meaning

Astrocytoma Subtypes

Fibrillary (diffuse) astrocytoma
 	
Astrocytoma (low-grade or benign astrocytoma)
Anaplastic astrocytoma
    Protoplasmic astrocytoma
    Gemistocytic astrocytoma
Glioblastoma multiforme
    Gliomatosis cerebri
    Gliosarcoma
 	
Circumscribed astrocytomas
 	
Pilocytic astrocytoma
Pleomorphic xanthoastrocytoma
Subependymal giant cell astrocytoma

Low-Grade Astrocytoma
Pathology Either focal/well-delineated or diffusely infiltrating Kernohan grades 1 and 2, WHO grade II **Incidence** 10% to 15% of astrocytomas **Age** Children and young adults between 20 and 40 years **Location** Cerebral hemispheres +/− cortex **Natural history** 7 to 10 year survival **Imaging** Focal/diffuse mass Hypodense/intense on NECT/T1WI; hyperintense on   T2-weighted MR 15% to 20% calcify No necrosis; may have cystic degeneration Edema, hemorrhage rare Enhancement absent/mild, inhomogeneous

swollen) or stellate cells with delicate processes (protoplasmic astrocytomas).[2,3] Because these tumors may be considered subtypes of fibrillary astrocytomas we will consider all of the infiltrating or diffuse astrocytomas as a group.[8]

Age and location. Certain astrocytomas such as pilocytic astrocytomas are found primarily in children and young adults, whereas others such as glioblastoma multiforme typically are neoplasms of older patients. Some astrocytomas also have a strong predilection for specific anatomic sites. For example, most pilocytic astrocytomas are located around the third and fourth ventricles, whereas anaplastic astrocytomas and glioblastomas are primarily hemispheric neoplasms and rarely occur in the posterior fossa. Astrocytomas are illustrated according to age and location in Fig. 13-2, *A* and *B*.

In addition to their specific anatomic location, astrocytomas can be diffuse or focal. Most cerebral hemispheric astrocytomas are diffuse, unencapsulated tumors derived from fibrillary astrocytes that are located predominately—but not exclusively—in the white matter. Other astrocytic tumors are more focal neoplasms with histologic patterns and biologic behavior that differ significantly from diffuse fibrillary astrocytomas.

Focal astrocytomas are often found in specific areas such as the cerebellum, hypothalamus and optic chiasm, and at the foramen of Monro. Pilocytic astrocytomas and subependymal giant cell astrocytomas are examples of focal astrocytomas that occur in these areas. Pleomorphic xanthoastrocytoma is a focal hemispheric neoplasm.

Astrocytoma (Low-grade Astrocytoma)

In contrast to their more malignant counterparts, well-differentiated low-grade fibrillary astrocytomas of the cerebral hemispheres occur less frequently, affect a younger patient population, and have a more favorable prognosis[9] (*see* box, *above*).

Pathology. So-called low-grade astrocytoma is the most benign of the fibrillary astrocytomas. Often simply called "astrocytoma," such tumors are classified as grade 1 and 2 in the Kernohan system and grade II in the WHO system.[4,5a,10]

Gross appearance. Astrocytomas are unencapsulated tumors that may appear grossly circumscribed but usually infiltrate diffusely. Most low-grade astrocytomas are solid, slightly grayish masses that vary from soft to almost gelatinous in consistency.[10] Cystic degeneration may occur but necrosis is absent.

Histology. Microscopically, low-grade astrocytomas are characterized by proliferation of well-differentiated fibrillary astrocytes that demonstrate only mild nuclear pleomorphism. Mitoses are few and cell density is low to moderate. Vascular proliferation is absent and hemorrhage is rare. Most astrocytomas exhibit strong immunoreactivity with antibody to glial fibrillary acidic protein (GFAP).[7]

Incidence. Low-grade astrocytomas are uncommon tumors. Their true incidence is difficult to determine because sampling and grading vary substantially. So-called benign or low-grade astrocytomas are much less common than anaplastic astrocy-

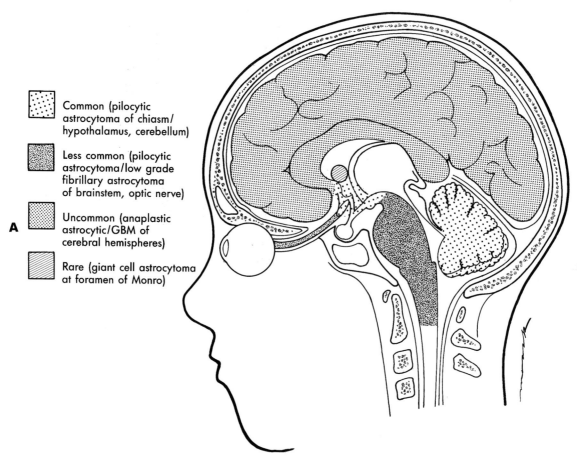

Common (pilocytic astrocytoma of chiasm/ hypothalamus, cerebellum)

Less common (pilocytic astrocytoma/low grade fibrillary astrocytoma of brainstem, optic nerve)

Uncommon (anaplastic astrocytic/GBM of cerebral hemispheres)

Rare (giant cell astrocytoma at foramen of Monro)

A

Fig. 13-2. Astrocytomas are illustrated according to age and location. **A,** Astrocytomas of childhood.

toma and glioblastoma multiforme. Low grade fibrillary astrocytomas probably represent 10% to 15% of gliomas.[11]

Age and clinical presentation. Low-grade fibrillary astrocytomas are neoplasms of children and adults from 20 to 40 years of age. These tumors are rare in older adults. Seizures are a common presenting symptom.

Location. Fibrillary astrocytomas are found throughout the hemispheres in proportion to the white matter present. Low-grade astrocytomas often involve the adjacent cortex as well.

Natural history. Astrocytomas are neither histologically nor biologically uniform tumors. The borderline between low-grade and anaplastic astrocytoma is at best indistinct.[6] Although many patients with low-grade astrocytomas survive for extended periods, 50% of surgically treated lesions evolve into anaplas-

tic astrocytomas or glioblastomas.[12] Degeneration into a higher-grade neoplasm is the most common cause of death in patients with low-grade astrocytoma (see Fig. 13-8); progressive low-grade disease occurs but is relatively rare.[13] Median survival is usually between 7 and 10 years.[7]

Imaging. Low-grade astrocytomas are most often diffusely infiltrating lesions, but focal, grossly circumscribed lesions can occur.

Angiography. Avascular mass effect without neovascularity or arteriovenous shunting is the usual pattern with focal astrocytomas. Diffusely infiltrating lesions may have minimal or no discernible angiographic abnormalities.

CT. Low-grade astrocytomas are iso- or hypodense compared to adjacent brain on NECT scans (Fig. 13-3). Despite their benign histology, the margins of many low-grade tumors are poorly delineated (Fig. 13-4).[14] Calcification is seen in 15% to 20% of cases. Although hemorrhage has been reported in gli-

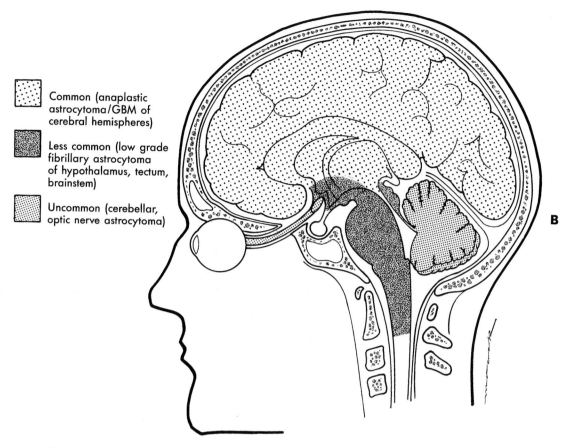

Common (anaplastic astrocytoma/GBM of cerebral hemispheres)

Less common (low grade fibrillary astrocytoma of hypothalamus, tectum, brainstem)

Uncommon (cerebellar, optic nerve astrocytoma)

B

Fig. 13-2, cont'd.   B, Adult astrocytomas have a distinctly different anatomic distribution and histology.

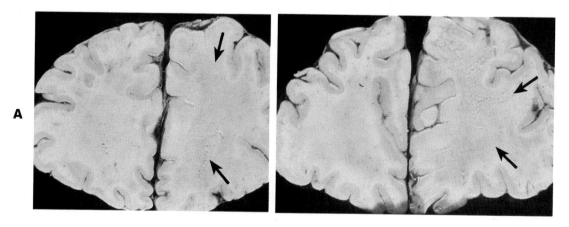

A

Fig. 13-3.   A, Coronal gross pathology section shows diffusely infiltrating low-grade astrocytoma. The cerebral white matter is slightly discolored, and both hemispheres appear mildly enlarged. (**A,** Courtesy Rubinstein Collection, Armed Forces Institute of Pathology.)

Continued.

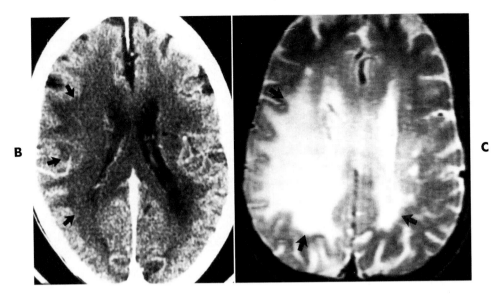

Fig. 13-3, cont'd. B, Axial CECT scan in a 60-year-old woman with dementia and progressive neurologic deterioration shows diffusely enlarged, low density right hemispheric white matter *(arrows).* **C,** Axial T2-weighted MR scan shows confluent white matter disease in both hemispheres and the corpus callosum. The patient expired, and autopsy disclosed diffusely infiltrating low-grade fibrillary astrocytoma. No anaplastic changes were seen. This case is unusual because most low-grade astrocytomas occur in younger patients. (**B** and **C,** Courtesy T. Burt.)

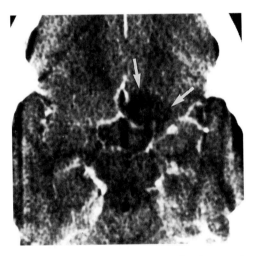

Fig. 13-4. Axial CECT scan shows a focal nonenhancing mass in the left posteromedial frontal lobe *(arrows).* The borders are indistinct and not clearly delineated from adjacent normal brain. Biopsy disclosed low-grade fibrillary astrocytoma.

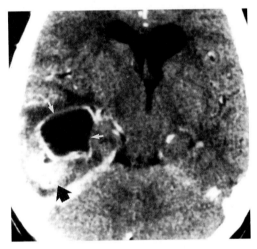

Fig. 13-5. Axial CECT scan in a 27-year-old patient with temporal lobe seizures. A ring-enhancing mass *(white arrows)* with surrounding edema, moderate mass effect, and a solid, enhancing component *(black arrow)* is present. Multiple biopsies of the tumor wall, nodule, and surrounding white matter disclosed grade I fibrillary astrocytoma.

omas of all grades, most low-grade astrocytomas are nonhemorrhagic.[15,16] Surrounding edema is typically minimal or absent.

Focal low-grade astrocytomas show mild-to-moderate inhomogeneous contrast enhancement in up to 40% of all cases (Fig. 13-5).[17] Occasionally, focal low-grade astrocytomas primarily involve the cor-

tex. Pressure erosion of the adjacent skull may occur with these slowly growing masses (Fig. 13-6). Occasionally, focal low-grade astrocytomas show prominent cystic changes (Figs. 13-5 and 13-7).

Diffusely infiltrating low-grade astrocytomas are poorly delineated hypodense lesions that typically show little or no enhancement and can be indistin-

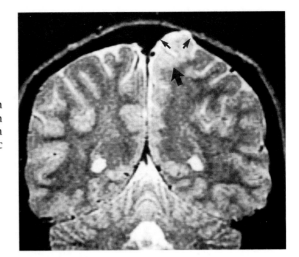

Fig. 13-6. A 15-year-old normotensive pregnant woman had a first-time seizure. Coronal T2-weighted MR scan shows a diffusely infiltrating cortical mass *(large arrow)* with focal bone erosion *(small arrows)*. Low-grade protoplasmic astrocytoma.

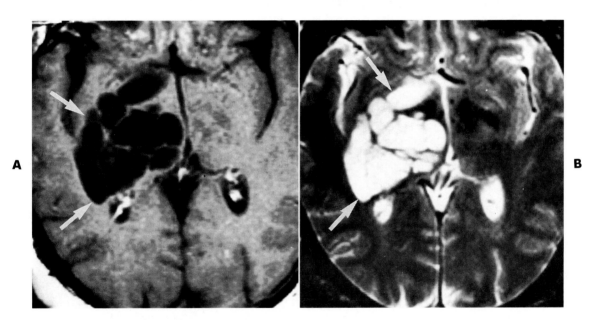

A

B

Fig. 13-7. Axial contrast-enhanced T1- **(A)** and T2-weighted **(B)** MR scans in a middle-aged man with low-grade astrocytoma diagnosed 13 years prior to this study show a well-delineated multicystic thalamic mass *(arrows)* without enhancing foci.

guishable from nonneoplastic white matter disease (Fig. 13-3).

MR. Low-grade astrocytomas are iso- to hypointense compared to adjacent brain on T1-weighted images and appear homogeneously hyperintense on T2WI (Fig. 13-3, *B*). Edema, hemorrhage, and contrast enhancement are relatively uncommon. Diffusely infiltrating lesions demonstrate confluent high signal areas in the cerebral white matter. Extension through compact white matter tracts with slight enlargement of the affected hemisphere can be seen in some cases and may be a form of gliomatosis cerebri (see subsequent discussion).

Most low-grade astrocytomas eventually undergo malignant degeneration. In these cases, contrast-enhancing foci within an otherwise benign-appearing mass may be the initial harbingers of more aggressive disease (Fig. 13-8).

Anaplastic (Malignant) Astrocytoma

Anaplastic astrocytomas are among the most common primary malignant brain tumors (*see* box, p. 537).

Pathology. Malignant or anaplastic astrocytomas (AAs) occupy an intermediate position between astrocytoma (benign or low-grade astrocytoma) and glioblastoma multiforme. A graded anaplasia also exists within the malignant astrocytoma group, with the upper extreme merging imperceptibly with glioblastoma.[5,10]

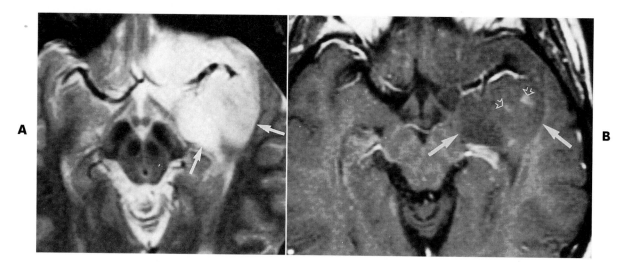

Fig. 13-8. This 29-year-old man with temporal lobe seizures had a biopsy performed 7 years ago that demonstrated "benign" astrocytoma. Increasing seizures prompted MR scan. **A,** Axial T2-weighted MR scan shows a relatively well-delineated hyperintense anterior temporal lobe mass *(arrows).* **B,** Axial postcontrast T1WI shows the mass *(large arrows)* is predominately hypointense to white matter. Two small enhancing foci *(open arrows)* are present. Stereotactic biopsy showed the enhancing areas are glioblastoma multiforme; the hyperintense but nonenhancing parts of the mass were still low grade astrocytoma.

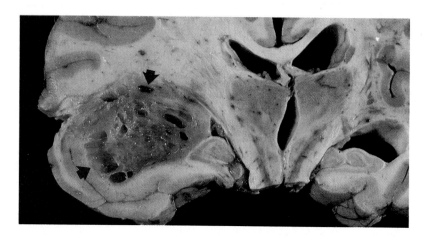

Fig. 13-9. Coronal cut brain section demonstrates gross pathology of anaplastic astrocytoma. A poorly delineated temporal lobe tumor with some hemorrhage and cystic degeneration is present *(arrows).* (Courtesy E. Tessa Hedley-Whyte.)

Gross appearance. AAs may appear grossly circumscribed, but most are diffusely infiltrating neoplasms with poorly delineated borders (Fig. 13-9). A heterogeneous mass with cystic areas is common. Hemorrhage can be present, but necrosis, the hallmark of glioblastoma multiforme, is absent.

Histology. Malignant fibrillary astrocytomas are less well differentiated and demonstrate greater hypercellularity and pleomorphism than their low-grade counterparts. Mitoses are frequent and vascular endothelial proliferation is common.

Ten to twenty percent of AAs have prominent plump, round-to-oval cells with abundant eosinophilic cytoplasm, one or more eccentric nuclei, and short glial fibers.[8] These tumors are sometimes called *"gemistocytic"* astrocytomas (from the German word gemastet, meaning bloating or swollen).[2] Because presence of at least 20% gemistocytes in a glial neoplasm is a poor prognostic sign, these tumors are classified with anaplastic astrocytomas and treated accordingly.[8]

Some astrocytomas have prominent stellate cells with delicate processes that form a fine, cobweblike matrix and are sometimes termed *protoplasmic* astrocytomas.[2] Protoplasmic astrocytes are normal components of gray matter, hence tumors of putative protoplasmic astrocytic origin are often located superficially in the cerebral cortex.[10] Because protoplasmic astrocytomas usually contain admixtures of proto-

plasmic and fibrillary cells, they are considered part of the anaplastic astrocytoma spectrum.

Incidence. AAs represent approximately one third of all fibrillary astocytomas and about one quarter of all gliomas (*see* Fig. 13-1).

Age and clinical presentation. Malignant astrocytomas can occur at any age but typically are found in older patients. Their peak incidence is in the fifth and sixth decades of life.[2] Seizures and focal neurologic deficits are common presenting symptoms.

Location. AAs occur throughout the cerebral hemispheres but are most common in the frontal and temporal lobes. Protoplasmic astrocytomas are often located peripherally in the cerebral cortex. Posterior fossa malignant astrocytomas of any type are rare.

Natural history. Malignant astrocytomas have a poor prognosis, with an average 2-year survival. Both anaplastic astrocytomas and glioblastomas spread through the extracellular space and along compact white matter tracts. Ependymal and CSF dissemination are common.[10]

Imaging
Angiography. Malignant astrocytomas typically demonstrate mass effect. Neovascularity, with tumor stain, arteriovenous shunting, and early draining veins, varies from none to striking.

Anaplastic Astrocytoma
Pathology
Diffusely infiltrating fibrillary astrocytoma
Kernohan grade 3, WHO grade III
May have gemistocytic/protoplasmic elements
Incidence
One third of astrocytomas
Age
Usually 40 to 60 years
Location
Cerebral white matter most common
Natural history
2 year survival
Imaging
Inhomogeneous mixed density/intensity mass
Calcification uncommon
Edema common; occasional hemorrhagic foci
Irregular rim enhancement common

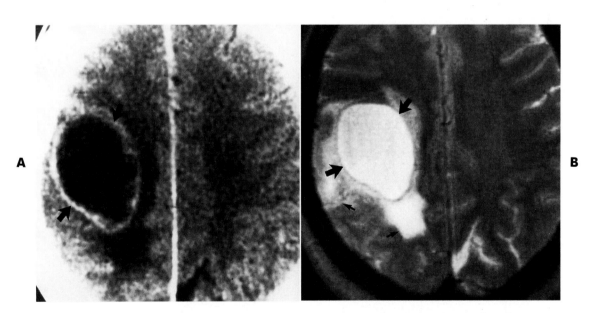

Fig. 13-10. **A,** Axial CECT scan in a 32-year-old woman with seizures shows a low density mass with irregular rim enhancement *(arrows)* and moderate surrounding edema. **B,** Axial T2-weighted MR scan shows the mass *(large arrows)* is uniformly hyperintense and has some peripheral edema *(small arrows)*. A grade 2 "gemistocytic" astrocytoma with anaplastic components was found at surgery.

CT. AAs are inhomogeneous, mixed density tumors on NECT. Calcification is uncommon unless malignant degeneration of a preexisting low-grade astrocytoma has occurred. AAs typically enhance strongly but nonuniformly following contrast administration. Irregular rim enhancement is common (Fig. 13-10).[13] Some AAs are diffusely infiltrating tumors that have little discernible mass effect (Fig. 13-11). Varying amounts of peripheral edema are usually present. Some intratumoral hemorrhage may occur (Fig. 13-12).

MR. AAs are poorly delineated lesions that have heterogeneous signal intensities on both T1- and T2WI. Mixed iso- to hypodense areas are seen on the T1-weighted sequences. Some hemorrhagic foci may be present (Figs. 13-13 and 13-14, *A*). A common appearance on T2WI is a central core of hyperintensity surrounded by an isointense rim with peripheral fingerlike high intensity projections secondary to vasogenic edema (Fig. 13-10, *B*).[18]

AAs usually have moderate mass effect.[15] Marked but irregular peripheral ringlike enhancement following contrast administration is usually evident.[18] AAs typically spread through white matter tracts. In most cases, biopsy will disclose tumor cells in the edematous areas that surround the enhancing mass and beyond the abnormal high signal areas demonstrated on T2WI.[18,19] AAs may also spread along the ependyma, leptomeninges, and CSF (Fig. 13-14).[20]

Uncommon imaging appearances of AA include a

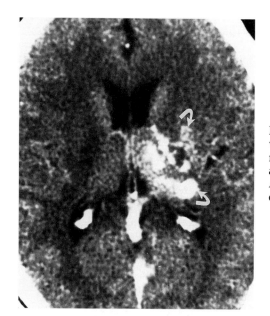

Fig. 13-11. Axial NECT scan (not shown) in this patient was normal. The contrast-enhanced study shows a poorly marginated enhancing thalamic mass *(arrows)*. The mass appears to infiltrate diffusely with virtually no mass effect. Anaplastic astrocytoma was diagnosed by stereotactic biopsy.

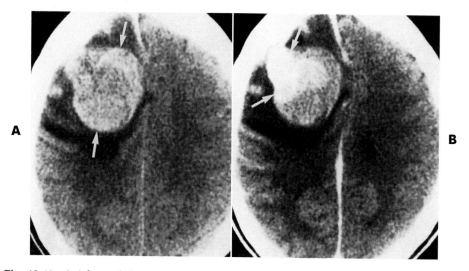

Fig. 13-12. Axial pre- **(A)** and postcontrast **(B)** CT scans in this 48-year-old woman show a hyperdense mass **(A,** *arrows)* that enhances slightly following contrast administration **(B,** *arrows)*. Hemorrhagic anaplastic astrocytoma was found at surgery.

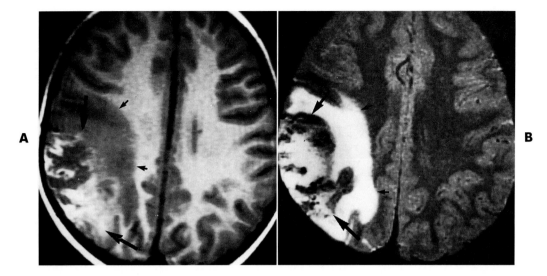

Fig. 13-13. A 15-year-old boy with seizures had this axial T1- **(A)** and T2-weighted **(B)** MR scan. A heterogeneous, mixed signal mass *(large arrows)* with moderate edema *(small arrows)* is present. Open biopsy showed anaplastic astrocytoma with subacute hemorrhage.

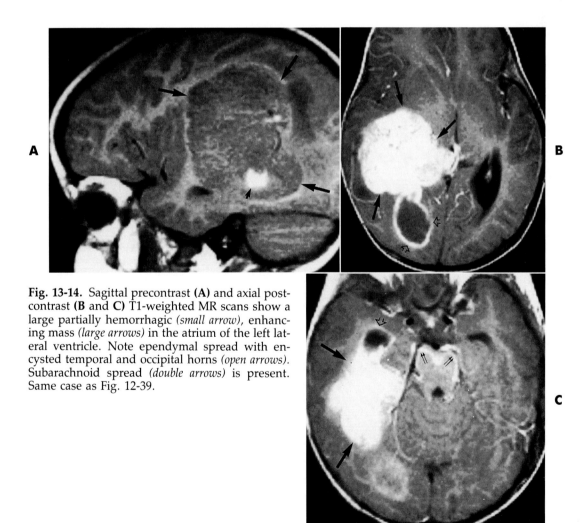

Fig. 13-14. Sagittal precontrast **(A)** and axial postcontrast **(B** and **C)** T1-weighted MR scans show a large partially hemorrhagic *(small arrow)*, enhancing mass *(large arrows)* in the atrium of the left lateral ventricle. Note ependymal spread with encysted temporal and occipital horns *(open arrows)*. Subarachnoid spread *(double arrows)* is present. Same case as Fig. 12-39.

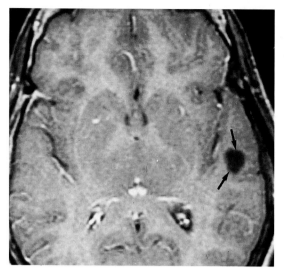

Fig. 13-15. A 29-year-old man with seizures since age 5 had this contrast-enhanced MR scan. The T1WI shows a focal, relatively well-delineated nonenhancing hypointense temporal lobe lesion *(arrows)*. Stereotaxic biopsy showed anaplastic astrocytoma.

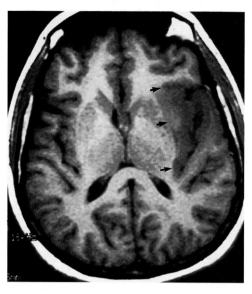

Fig. 13-16. Axial T1-weighted MR scan shows thickened left temporal lobe cortex *(arrows)*. Anaplastic astrocytoma was found at surgery.

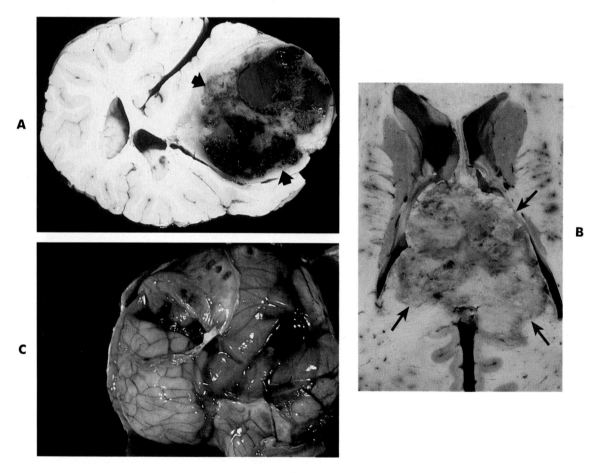

Fig. 13-17. Three autopsy cases demonstrate gross pathology of glioblastoma multiforme. **A,** Coronal section shows hemorrhagic, necrotic mass *(arrows)*. **B,** Axial section shows a corpus callosum GBM *(arrows)* with mixed necrotic and hemorrhagic areas. **C,** Gross pathology of a neonate with GBM. The tumor is huge, occupying most of the affected hemisphere. Note hemorrhagic and necrotic areas (**A** and **C,** Courtesy Rubinstein Collection, Armed Forces Institute of Pathology. **B,** Courtesy Rubinstein Collection, University of Virginia.)

focal, cystlike nonenhancing mass (Fig. 13-15) or cortical mass that resembles infarct or encephalitis (Fig. 13-16).

Glioblastoma Multiforme

Glioblastoma multiforme is the most common of all the primary intracranial CNS tumors. The highly variable gross and microscopic appearance of this malignant neoplasm gives rise to its "multiforme" appellation (*see* box).

Pathology. Glioblastoma multiforme (GBM) is the most malignant of all glial neoplasms and occupies the far end of the astrocytoma spectrum.

Gross pathology. Necrosis is the hallmark of GBMs.[10] Grossly, GBMs are usually large, heterogeneous masses with central necrosis, thick irregular "shaggy" walls, and increased vascularity. Intratumoral hemorrhage is common. Mass effect and edema are usually striking (Fig. 13-17).

Histology. As the name implies, the cellular composition of GBMs has multiple forms. Each GBM typically contains distinct subsets of neoplastic astrocytes that differ from each other in morphology, biologic activity, metastatic potential, and radiation sensitivity.[21]

Cellular composition is diverse and there is virtually no limit to the varied expression of GBMs. These highly cellular tumors have been described as ranging from monotonous small-cell neoplasms to "monstrocellular tumors with their Mardi Gras of grotesque forms."[22] Some tumor foci appear relatively well differentiated; others contain bizarre pleomorphic or undifferentiated cells. Mitoses are numerous and vascular proliferation is striking. As is the case with anaplastic astrocytoma, in GBMs, neoplastic cells are present well beyond the enhancing tumor margins and surrounding edema delineated on MR scans.[19]

Incidence. GBMs are the most common primary CNS neoplasm, representing 15% to 20% of these tumors. Approximately half of all astrocytomas are GBMs. GBM is the most common supratentorial neoplasm in adults.[23]

Age and clinical presentation. GBMs usually occur in patients over 50 and are rare in patients under 30. Like AAs, GBMs can occasionally be found at any age; AAs and GBMs are among the four most common primary brain tumors in infants and children under 2 years of age. Various symptoms occur with GBM, including seizure, focal neurologic deficit, and strokelike syndromes (*see* Chapter 11).

Location. The usual location for GBM is the deep cerebral white matter, particularly the frontal and temporal lobes. Basal ganglia involvement may be present. Multilobed and bihemispheric tumors that cross the corpus callosum are common. Posterior fossa GBMs are rare.

Natural history. Along with primary CNS lymphoma, GBMs have the worst prognosis of all primary brain tumors. GBMs disseminate early, rapidly, and widely (see subsequent discussion). CNS metastases are common, but distant metastases are rare. The median postoperative survival for patients with GBM is 8 months; the 5-year recurrence-free survival rate is essentially zero.[24]

Imaging. Imaging findings reflect the varied, "multiforme" pathology of this highly malignant tumor.

Angiography. A large mass with striking tumor blush, contrast stasis, and pooling in bizarre vascular channels is typical (Fig. 13-18, *A*). Arteriovenous shunting and early filling of draining cerebral veins are very common (Fig. 13-18, *B*). Occasionally an AA or GBM is so highly vascular that it resembles an arteriovenous malformation (Fig. 10-16). GBMs with a more diffuse gyriform blush can mimic cerebral infarcts with luxury perfusion.

CT. NECT scans typically demonstrate marked intratumoral heterogeneity. A central low density re-

---

Glioblastoma Multiforme

Pathology

Poorly delineated partially necrotic mass
"Mardi Gras" of cells
Kernohan grade IV

Incidence

Most common primary brain neoplasm
50% of astrocytomas are GBMS

Age

Older patients (>50); rare <30 years

Location

Cerebral hemispheric white matter

Natural history

Spreads rapidly, diffusely

Imaging

Thick irregular "rind" of tissue around necrotic core
Calcification rare
Highly vascular (may mimic AVM)
Hemorrhage, edema common
Strong inhomogeneous enhancement

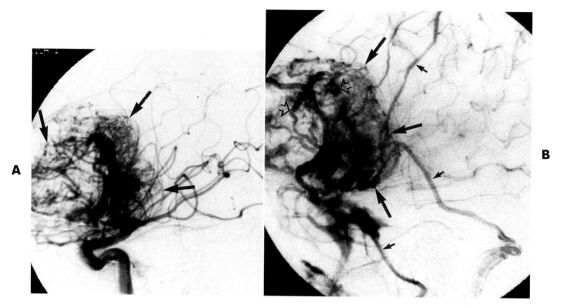

Fig. 13-18. Typical angiographic findings in GBM. **A,** Left internal carotid angiogram, early arterial phase, lateral view, shows an extremely vascular frontal lobe mass *(arrows)*. **B,** Late arterial phase study shows the mass *(large arrows)* with contrast pooling in irregular vascular spaces *(open arrows)*. Arteriovenous shunting with numerous early draining veins is present *(small arrows)*.

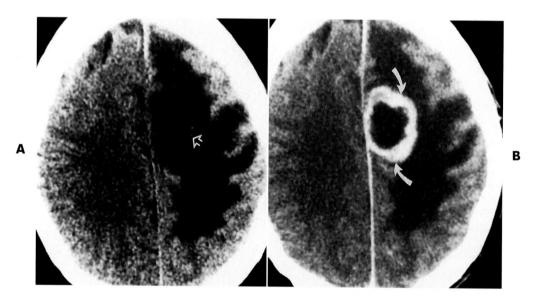

Fig. 13-19. Axial pre- **(A)** and postcontrast **(B)** CT scans in a patient with GBM show extensive edema that surrounds a thick, shaggy, irregular rim-enhancing mass *(curved arrows)*. Note that the underlying mass *(open arrow)* is virtually invisible on the unenhanced study.

gion that reflects necrosis or cyst formation is present in 95% of all GBMs (Fig. 13-19).[1] Calcification is rare unless the GBM developed from degeneration of a preexisting low-grade astrocytoma. Because cellularity varies from region to region within the neoplasm the mass has very inhomogeneous mixed density on NECT. Hemorrhages of differing ages are common.

Peripheral edema usually surrounds the tumor and extends along central white matter tracts.

Enhancement following contrast administration is strong but very inhomogeneous; thick, irregular rim enhancement is common (Fig. 13-19). Occasionally, GBMs do not have a dominant mass, infiltrate widely throughout the hemispheres, and have minimal or no

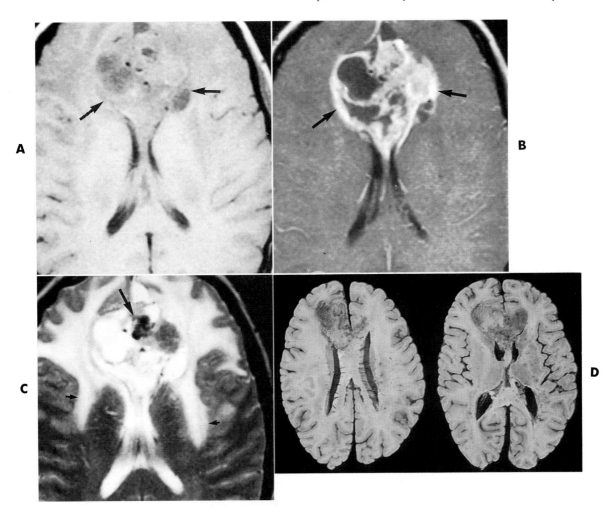

Fig. 13-20. Axial pre- **(A)** and postcontrast **(B)** T1-weighted MR scans show a mixed signal, partially enhancing mass in the corpus callosum genu that involves both frontal lobes *(arrows)*. The T2WI **(C)** shows blood degradation products *(large arrow)*. Note extensive edema tracking along the external capsule *(small arrows)* and subcortical "U" fibers with relative gray matter sparing. For comparison, the gross pathology **(D)** of a so-called "butterfly" glioma (i.e., a corpus callosum tumor with bihemispheric involvement) is shown. **(D,** Courtesy E. Tessa Hedley-Whyte.)

blood-brain barrier breakdown. Contrast enhancement is mild or absent in these cases. A diffusely infiltrating GBM may be a form of gliomatosis cerebri (see subsequent discussion).

MR. MR also reflects the pathologically heterogeneous nature of GBMs. T1-weighted scans show a poorly delineated mixed-signal mass with necrosis or cyst formation and a thick irregular wall (Fig. 13-20, A).[15] Marked but inhomogeneous contrast enhancement is present in the majority of GBMs (Fig. 13-20, B).[18] Because these tumors are often highly vascular, prominent flow voids and hemorrhages of different ages are often present.[16]

T2-weighted studies show a very heterogeneous mass with mixed signal cellular components, central necrosis, and hemorrhages of varying ages (Fig. 13-

20, C). Peripheral edema is typically striking. Tumor margins often blend imperceptibly with the surrounding edema and actually represent "tumor plus edema."[19,23] Neoplastic cells can be found far beyond demonstrable T2 signal abnormalities.[19]

Multiple GBMs, spread of GBMs, recurrence of GBMs

Multiple GBMs. Glioblastoma can present as multiple tumor foci. Multifocal or multicentric gliomas occur in 0.5% to 1.0% of cases.[25] Lesions with microscopic parenchymal connections or masses that occur as satellite lesions from CSF spread are termed *multifocal* (Fig. 13-21). Occasionally, isolated gliomas with no detectable microscopic connections are identified; these are termed *multicentric* gliomas (Fig. 13-22).

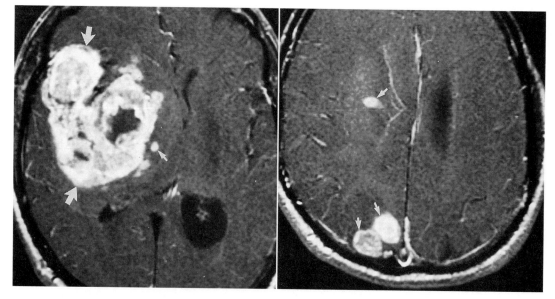

Fig. 13-21. Axial postcontrast T1-weighted MR scans in a patient with a large basal ganglia and temporal lobe GBM *(large arrows)*. Multiple satellite lesions are seen *(small arrows)*. The lesions appear grossly separated but were microscopically connected. Multifocal GBM.

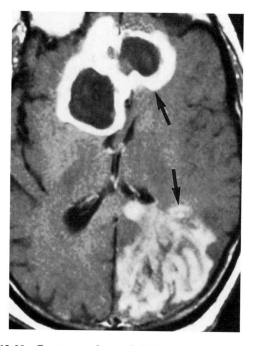

Fig. 13-22. Contrast-enhanced MR scan in this patient shows two widely separate enhancing masses *(arrows)*. Autopsy proven multicentric GBMs without demonstrable connection.

Multiple solid, enhancing masses that involve only one hemisphere are often seen in such cases.[26]

Spread of GBMs (*see* box) (Fig. 13-23). GBMs spread widely and rapidly. Extension along white matter tracts is the most frequent route. Bihemispheric spread across the corpus callosum, and

---

Spread of Glioblastoma/Anaplastic Astrocytoma

Common
Along compact white matter tracts
Around ventricular ependyma
Under pia
Into leptomeninges
CSF seeding of subarachnoid space

Uncommon
Dural invasion

Rare
Extracerebral metastases

---

anterior and posterior commissures is typical (Fig. 13-24), but extension along the internal and external capsules is also common. Spread down the cerebral peduncles and spinothalamic tracts into the posterior fossa can occur (Figs. 13-25, *A* to *C*, and 13-26).

Most patients with GBMs eventually develop satellite lesions that are grossly separate from, but microscopically connected to, the parent tumor (Fig. 13-21). Ependymal (Fig. 13-27), subpial (Fig. 13-28), and CSF dissemination throughout the cerebral and spinal subarachnoid spaces (Fig. 13-25, *D* to *F*) are frequent periterminal events.[20] Leptomeningeal invasion with subsequent CSF dissemination is common;

Fig. 13-23. Anatomic diagram illustrates common routes of spread of GBM. Tumor dissemination along white matter tracts, subpial space, and the subarachnoid space is indicated by the dots. Tumor also spreads along the ependyma and leptomeninges (*heavy black lines*). Note tumor spread along penetrating blood vessels and Virchow-Robin spaces, as shown in the right temporal lobe. Spread outside the CNS to sites such as bone and liver occurs but is rare. Dural (pachymeningeal) GBM spread is also uncommon.

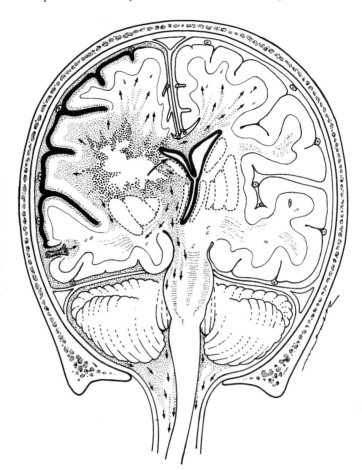

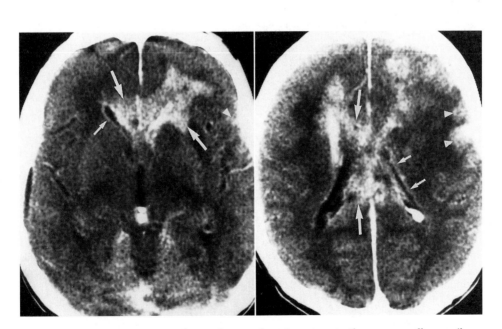

Fig. 13-24. Axial CECT scans show a large enhancing mass in the corpus callosum (*large arrows*). Subependymal (*small arrows*) and subarachnoid spread (*arrowheads*) is seen. Glioblastoma multiforme.

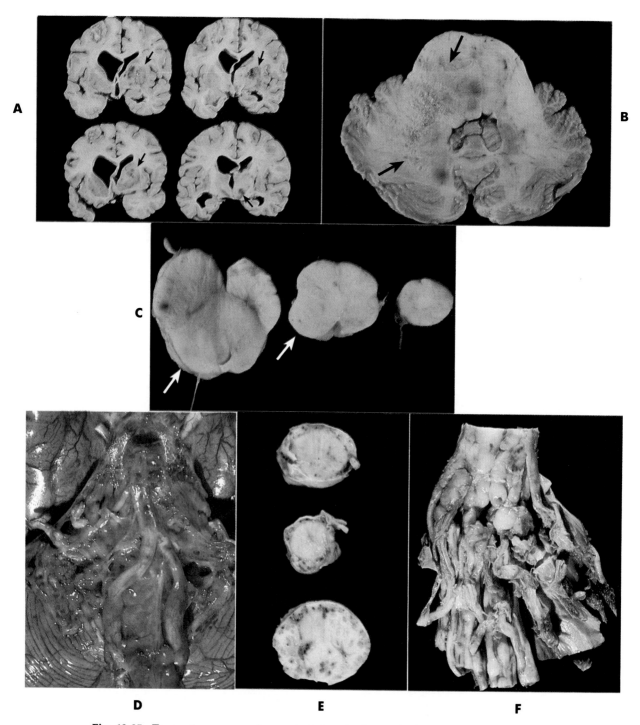

Fig. 13-25. Two autopsy cases demonstrate terminal spread of GBMs. **A,** Coronal gross autopsy specimen shows a thalamic GBM *(arrows).* **B** and **C,** Axial sections through the pons, midbrain, medulla, and upper cervical spinal cord show asymmetric enlargement secondary to infiltrating GBM *(arrows).* **D,** Diffuse leptomeningeal metastases from GBM coat the undersurface of the brain. **E,** Leptomeningeal metastases encase the spinal cord. **F,** Multiple nodular "drop" metastases are seen along the filum terminale (Courtesy E. Tessa Hedley-Whyte.)

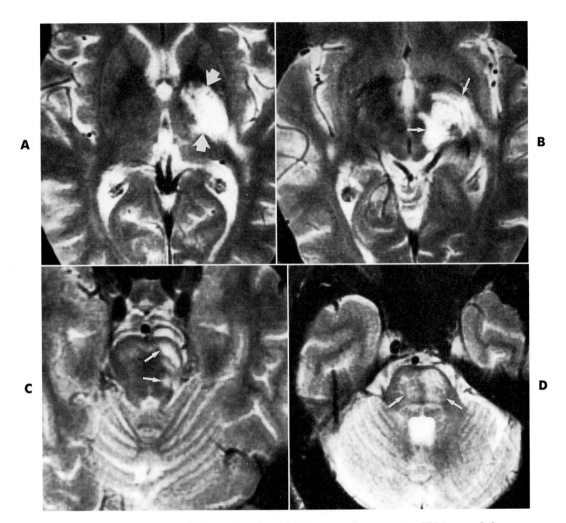

Fig. 13-26. **A** to **D,** Serial T2-weighted axial MR scans demonstrate GBM spread down white matter tracts. The primary tumor is located in the left thalamus (**A,** *arrows*), but abnormal signal is seen extending inferiorly into the ipsilateral internal capsule and cerebral peduncle (**B** and **C,** *arrows*). Bilateral pontine tumor is also present (**D,** *arrows*).

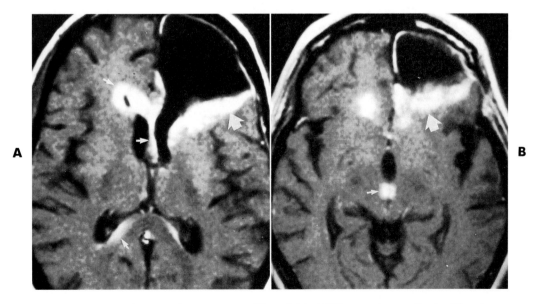

Fig. 13-27. **A** and **B,** Axial postcontrast T1-weighted MR scans in a patient with extensive subependymal spread after partial resection of a left frontal lobe GBM *(large arrows).* Tumor has spread along the ependyma of the lateral ventricles into the third ventricle.

Continued.

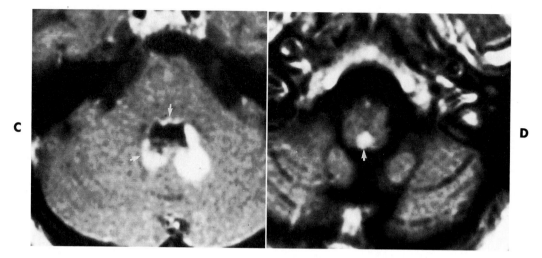

Fig. 13-27, cont'd. C and **D,** Axial postcontrast T1-weighted MR scans through the posterior fossa in the same patient show tumor has spread into the aqueduct, fourth ventricle, and obex *(small arrows).* (Courtesy K. Jaeckle.)

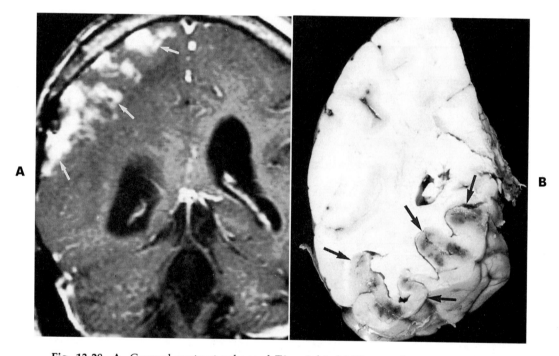

Fig. 13-28. A, Coronal contrast-enhanced T1-weighted MR scan shows extensive subpial spread of GBM *(arrows).* **B,** Coronal gross autopsy specimen shows diffuse subpial and cortical spread of an anaplastic astrocytoma *(arrows),* compare with **(A). (B,** Courtesy E. Tessa Hedley-Whyte.)

invasion of the pachymeninges is less common (Fig. 13-29). It is rare for high-grade gliomas to invade and destroy bone (Fig. 13-30).[27,28] Extracerebral metastases to lung, liver, bone, and other sites occur but are very uncommon (Fig. 13-31).

Recurrence of GBMs. The surgical resection of GBM is nearly always subtotal. Therefore it is important to evaluate accurately the presence and extent of

residual tumor for appropriate treatment strategies. Both contrast-enhanced CT and MR have been used to monitor the postoperative course of these patients, although the difficulty of distinguishing enhancement due to residual tumor from nonneoplastic postoperative change hampers evaluation.

In general, residual tumor is shown most reliably on contrast-enhanced MR scans obtained shortly af-

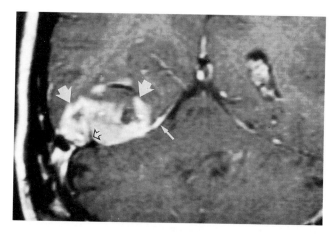

Fig. 13-29. Coronal postcontrast T1-weighted MR scan in a patient with a temporal lobe GBM *(large arrows)* shows abnormally enhancing dura *(small arrow)* and a vascular pedicle that arises from the dura *(open arrow)*. GBM with dural invasion was found at surgery.

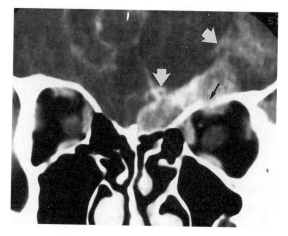

Fig. 13-30. Coronal CECT scan shows a large left frontal GBM *(white arrows)* that has invaded and partially destroyed the left orbital roof *(black arrow)*.

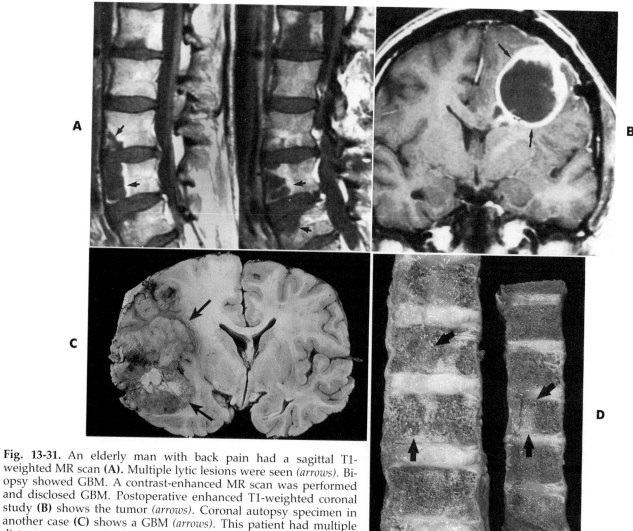

Fig. 13-31. An elderly man with back pain had a sagittal T1-weighted MR scan **(A)**. Multiple lytic lesions were seen *(arrows)*. Biopsy showed GBM. A contrast-enhanced MR scan was performed and disclosed GBM. Postoperative enhanced T1-weighted coronal study **(B)** shows the tumor *(arrows)*. Coronal autopsy specimen in another case **(C)** shows a GBM *(arrows)*. This patient had multiple distant metastases in the lung (not shown) and spine **(D,** *arrows)*. **(A** and **B,** Courtesy C. Truwit. **C** and **D,** Courtesy E. Tessa Hedley-Whyte.)

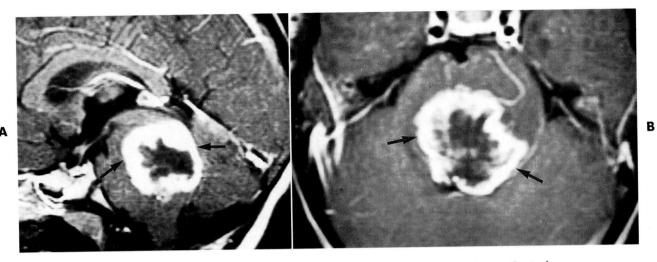

Fig. 13-32. Sagittal **(A)** and axial **(B)** postcontrast T1-weighted MR scans in a patient who received radiation therapy for a brain stem glioma. A thick, irregular rim-enhancing mass is seen *(arrows)* that expands and distorts the pons. Biopsy showed radiation necrosis with residual tumor.

ter surgery. After the fourth postoperative day and up to 3 months, surgically induced enhancement prevents recognition of residual tumor.[24] Blood degradation products can also mimic residual tumor if only contrast-enhanced MR scans are obtained.[29]

Radiation necrosis. Extensive radionecrosis and recurrent or persistent neoplasm produce a similar clinical and radiologic picture, i.e., an expanding contrast-enhancing mass.[10] Distinction between these two entities is often difficult because radiation-induced necrosis, reactive gliosis, and residual GBM often coexist and may appear identical on standard imaging studies (Fig. 13-32).[30] Positron emission tomography (PET) may be helpful for determining the extent of cerebral gliomas, as well as distinguishing radiation necrosis from residual neoplasm.[31]

Gliomatosis Cerebri

Pathology. Gliomatosis cerebri (GC) is characterized by diffuse overgrowth of the brain with neoplastic glial cells. GC probably represents an extreme form of diffusely infiltrating glioma.[32] Whether or how GC should be distinguished from highly infiltrative anaplastic astrocytoma or GBM is controversial.

Gross appearance. GC diffusely enlarges the cerebral hemispheres, cerebellum, or brain stem while preserving normal anatomic landmarks.[33] No grossly discernible focal masses form, although the neoplastic process may appear more concentrated in some areas than in others.[2]

Histology. Neoplastic glial cells in varying states of differentiation diffusely infiltrate the brain. There is relative preservation of the underlying cytoarchi-

tecture.[34] Although white matter is most commonly involved, gray matter can be affected as well. Tumor infiltration is typically perineuronal, perivascular, and subpial.[35]

Incidence, age at presentation, and natural history. GC is rare. It can occur at any age but is usually found in the third and fourth decades of life.[36] In older patients, clinical presentation can mimic normal pressure hydrocephalus (*see* Fig. 13-3, *B* and *C*).[33] A favorable response to radiation therapy has been reported, but long-term disease control has not.[37]

Location. Although any part of the brain or even spinal cord can be affected, the optic nerves and compact white matter pathways are the most common sites. The corpus callosum, fornices, and cerebellar peduncles are often involved.[10] Subpial extension with focal tumor aggregation is common. Primary leptomeningeal gliomatosis, a form of GC, can also occur.[38,39]

Imaging. The most common imaging appearance is a diffusely infiltrating, nonenhancing lesion that expands the cerebral white matter (Figs. 13-3, *B* and *C,* and 13-33). Some contrast-enhancing foci can develop late in the disease course. Leptomeningeal gliomatosis can mimic meningeal carcinomatosis or spreading CNS tumors (Fig. 13-34).[38,39]

Gliosarcoma

Pathology and etiology. Gliosarcoma is a rare primary brain tumor that is composed of neoplastic glial cells and a spindle-cell sarcomatous element. The gli-

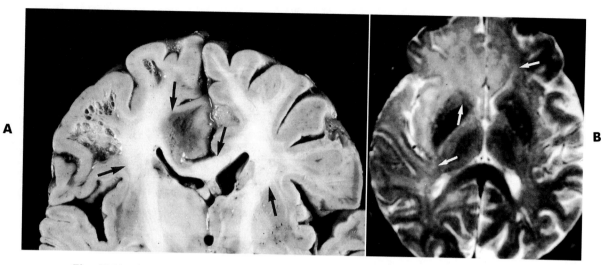

Fig. 13-33. A, Axial gross autopsy specimen in a patient with gliomatosis cerebri. Note expansion of the frontal white matter *(arrows).* **B,** Axial T2-weighted MR scan in a patient with gliomatosis cerebri. Note diffusely infiltrating mass throughout much of the white matter *(arrows).* Mild expansion of the right frontal lobe is present. (**A,** Courtesy Rubinstein Collection, University of Virginia. **B,** Courtesy T. Miller.)

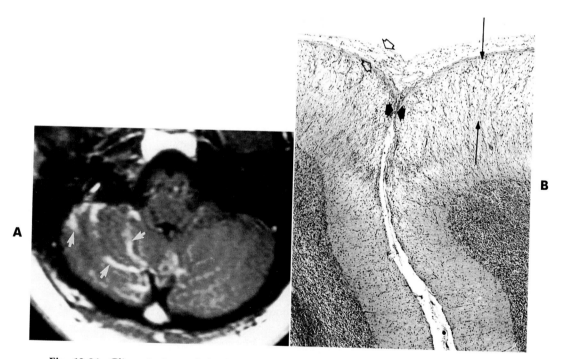

Fig. 13-34. Gliomatosis cerebri mimics leptomeningeal tumor dissemination. A 16-year-old boy had a right temporal lobe infiltrating glioma biopsied and radiated 1 year prior to this scan. **A,** Axial postcontrast T1-weighted image shows linear enhancing foci around the right cerebellum *(arrows).* Other scans (not shown) demonstrated other similar foci. **B,** Autopsy showed diffuse tumor infiltration along the cortex of the cerebellum and temporal lobe *(long arrows).* The intervening sulci are obliterated *(solid arrows).* The subarachnoid space *(open arrows)* is free of tumor. Gliomatosis cerebri. (Courtesy O. Boyko; **A,** reprinted from *AJNR* 11:801-802, 1990.)

oma is most often a GBM. The mesenchymal component theoretically could originate from endothelial, histiocytic, fibroblastic, or myoblastic elements.[40] In most cases the sarcomatous component probably arises from neoplastically transformed vascular elements within the GBM itself.

Gross pathology. Gliosarcomas are firm, lobulated tumors with central necrotic areas. The sarcomatous portion is sharply demarcated and often separable from the adjacent brain, whereas the astrocytic component is soft and poorly delineated from surrounding parenchyma.[41]

Histology. The pathologic diagnosis of gliosarcoma depends on identifying glial and mesenchymal tumor elements. The mesenchymal component is variable but most often resembles a typical fibrosarcoma or malignant fibrous histiocytoma. Cartilaginous and rhabdomyosarcomatous components have been described.[10] The infiltrating component of the gliosarcoma is almost always a GBM. Pleomorphic cells with vascular endothelial proliferation and necrosis are common.

Incidence, age at presentation, and natural history. Sarcomatous transformation occurs in less than 2% of GBMs.[10] Most patients with gliosarcomas are in the fifth to seventh decades. Survival is similar to that of GBM.[42] Extracranial metastases are common, occurring in 15% to 30% of all gliosarcomas. Disseminated hematogenous metastases to the viseral organs are common. Distant metastases do not significantly affect prognosis because the primary cause of death is the intracerebral neoplasm.[41]

Location. There is a pronounced tendency toward peripheral location and dural invasion.[41] The temporal lobes are a common site.[43] Most gliosarcomas contact the skull or falx cerebri.[42]

Imaging
Angiography. A prominent vascular stain with well-defined margins, irregular tumor vessels, and early cortical venous drainage is typical. Blood supply is pial or mixed pial-dural (Fig. 13-35, *A* and *B*).[41]

CT. Imaging findings are variable. Gliosarcomas can resemble meningioma or GBM. Gliosarcomas are usually less homogeneously hyperdense than meningiomas, do not have a broad dural attachment, and are virtually always associated with peritumoral edema. On NECT studies most gliosarcomas appear slightly but inhomogeneously hyperdense because of their high vascularity and cellularity.[42] Prominent homogeneous or irregular ringlike enhancement following contrast administration is typical.[41]

MR. Gliosarcomas also have a variable appearance on MR scans. Both T1- and T2WI show inhomogeneous signal intensity. Hemorrhage and necrosis are common; enhancement is strong but often somewhat heterogeneous (Fig. 13-35, *C* to *E*).

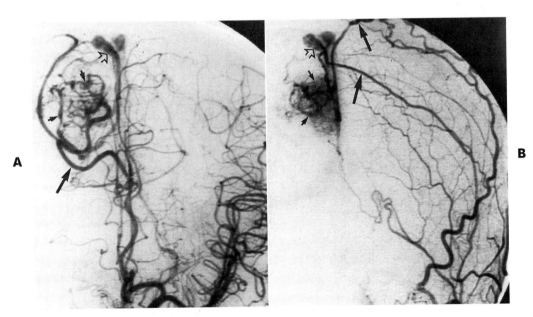

Fig. 13-35. Imaging studies in a patient with gliosarcoma. **A,** Left internal carotid angiogram, midarterial phase, AP view, shows a vascular mass supplied by enlarged anterior cerebral artery branches *(large arrow)*. Neovascularity *(small arrows)* and early draining veins *(open arrow)* are seen. **B,** Left external carotid angiogram, midarterial phase, AP view, shows dural supply via superficial temporal and middle meningeal artery branches *(large arrows)*. A highly vascular tumor stain *(small arrows)* with arteriovenous shunting and early draining veins *(open arrow)* is seen. (Courtesy H. K. Lu.)

Pilocytic Astrocytoma

Pilocytic astrocytoma (juvenile pilocytic astrocytoma, polar spongioblastoma) is a circumscribed, morphologically and biologically distinct astrocytoma subtype. The age at presentation, location, and prognosis of pilocytic astrocytoma (*see* box, p. 554) are all significantly different from diffusely infiltrating fibrillary astrocytomas (*see* boxes, pp. 531, 537, and 541). Pilocytic astrocytomas presumably arise from a class of astrocytes that is inconspicuous in normal brain but may become prominent in reactive gliosis and neoplasia.[10]

Pathology

Gross pathology. Pilocytic astrocytomas (PAs) have a gross appearance that varies with location. Cerebellar astrocytomas (sometimes termed *juvenile* or *cystic cerebellar* astrocytomas) are well-

circumscribed masses that typically have a large cyst with a small, reddish-tan mural nodule (Fig. 13-36). Opticochiasmatic-hypothalamic pilocytic astrocytomas are lobulated, grossly well-circumscribed but microscopically infiltrating tumors in the floor or walls of the third ventricle.[2] Brainstem pilocytic astrocytomas generally are uniform, nonfocal infiltrating neoplasms that diffusely expand the pons or medulla.

Histology. PAs have two histologic patterns: (1) densely compact regions of elongated cells with hairlike (pilocytic) processes and (2) more loosely organized spongiform foci with stellate astrocytes and microcystic changes.[10] PAs often have prominent Rosenthal fibers, small amorphous eosinophilic beadlike or corkscrew-shaped hyaline bodies that are surrounded by glial filaments.[10] Mitotic activity is low or absent. Although many PAs form cysts, tumor necrosis is absent.

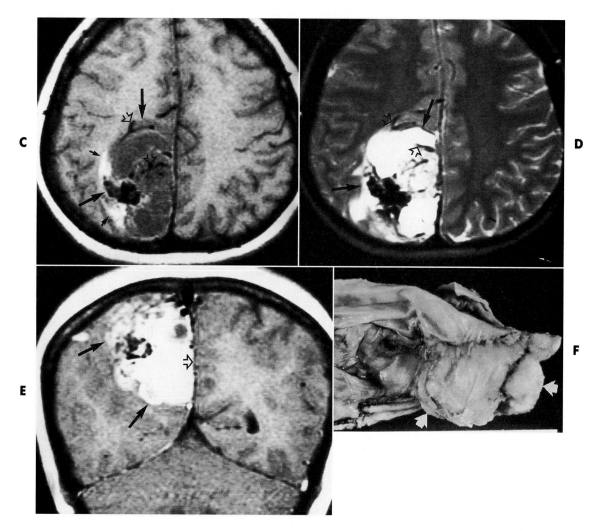

Fig 13-35, cont'd. Axial precontrast T1- **(C)** and T2-weighted **(D)** MR scans show the mixed signal lesion *(large arrows)* with prominent vessels *(open arrows)* and subacute hemorrhage *(small arrows)*. **E,** Coronal postcontrast T1WI shows the tumor *(large arrows)* enhances strongly but somewhat heterogeneously. Note tumor abuts the falx cerebri *(open arrow)*. **F,** Gross pathology specimen of a gliosarcoma. (**C** to **E,** Courtesy H. K. Lu. **F,** Courtesy Rubinstein Collection, University of Virginia.)

Pilocytic Astrocytoma

Pathology

Well-circumscribed but unencapsulated mass
"Hairlike" astrocytic processes; Rosenthal fibers
Cysts common; necrosis absent
WHO grade I

Incidence

5% to 10% of all gliomas
One third of pediatric gliomas
Second overall most common pediatric brain tumor

Age

Children, young adults

Location

Around third, fourth ventricles
Optic chiasm/hypothalamus most common
Cerebellar vermis/hemispheres next
Less common: cerebral hemispheres, ventricles

Natural history

85% to 100% 5-year survival rate

Imaging

Cystic/solid mass
10% calcify
Variable enhancement (mural nodule may enhance
intensely but inhomogeneously)

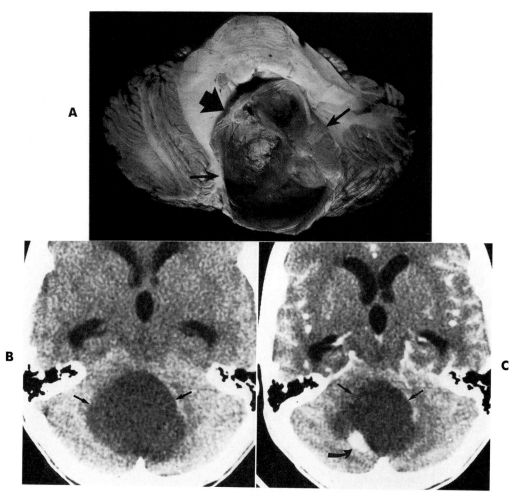

Fig. 13-36. A, Axial gross pathology specimen depicts a cerebellar pilocytic astrocytoma. A large, well-delineated cyst *(small arrows)* with a firm reddish-tan mural nodule *(large arrow)* is present. The cyst wall is nonneoplastic, composed of compressed brain. Axial pre- **(B)** and postcontrast **(C)** CT scans in this 6-year-old child with headaches and vomiting show a large midline posterior fossa cystic mass *(small arrows)*. A small, intensely enhancing mural nodule is seen **(C,** *curved arrow)*. Note obstructive hydrocephalus with enlarged third and lateral ventricles. Pilocytic astrocytoma. **(A,** From Okazaki H, Scheithauer B: *Slide Atlas of Neuropathology,* Gower Medical Publishing, 1988.)

Incidence. Pilocytic astrocytomas represent only 5% to 10% of all cerebral gliomas but account for nearly one third of pediatric glial neoplasms.[44] Opticochiasmatic-hypothalamic PAs are one of the most common supratentorial neoplasms in children, and cerebellar astrocytomas are the most common posterior fossa tumor in this age group (in some series medulloblastoma is the most common pediatric infratentorial tumor). Brainstem gliomas are the third most common pediatric infratentorial tumor.[45]

Age at presentation. PAs typically are tumors of children and young adults. Most tumors in the cerebellum become symptomatic during the first two decades of life and have a peak incidence at age 10. Cerebral hemispheric PAs occur a decade later with a peak age at 20 years.[46] Three quarters of optic pathway PAs occur in patients under 12 years of age.[47] Very rarely PAs occur in adults up to the fourth and fifth decades.[97a]

Natural history and clinical presentation. Pilocytic astrocytomas are indolent, slowly growing neoplasms. Natural history and presenting symptoms vary with location. The overall postoperative survival rate for PA is 86% to 100% at 5 years, 83% at 10 years, and 70% at 20 years.[48] Patients with gross total tumor resection have survival rates that approach 100%.[10] Even patients with unresectable hypothalamic-opticochiasmatic tumors can have long-term survival. The 5- and 10-year survivals in this group are 93% and 74% respectively.[47]

The natural history of brainstem gliomas is different. Brainstem gliomas are a biologically and histologically heterogeneous group of neoplasms. Intrinsic pontine tumors are infiltrative and all are considered malignant, regardless of histology at biopsy.[49] Symptoms are cranial nerve palsies, pyramidal tract signs, and ataxia. These tumors often reach an advanced state without developing increased intracranial pressure. Disease course is relentless and most patients die within 2 years.[49,50] At autopsy many of these tumors have anaplastic features.[50a]

Other brainstem gliomas arise in the fourth ventricular floor and have a dorsally exophytic growth pattern. Seventy-five percent of patients have hydrocephalus. In contrast to intrinsic pontine gliomas, cranial nerve deficits and long-tract signs are infrequent.[51] Prognosis is excellent. Patients with midbrain and medullary gliomas also have an excellent long-term prognosis; many of these neoplasms are nonpilocytic low-grade astrocytomas.[49-51]

Up to one third of pilocytic astrocytomas may be clinically aggressive.[52] However, frank malignant transformation is uncommon and leptomeningeal dissemination is very rare. Occasionally, histologically benign tumors disseminate without undergoing

either malignant degeneration or evidencing regrowth of the primary tumor. The growth rate of even distant PA metastases may remain very low.[53]

Location. Pilocytic astrocytomas are characteristically located around the third and fourth ventricles. Nearly half are found in the optic chiasm and hypothalamus, and about a third are located in the cerebellar vermis or hemispheres (*see* Fig. 13-1, *A*). Less common locations include the brainstem and basal ganglia.[54] Occasionally, cystic PAs occur in the cerebral hemispheres.[46] The frontal lobes are the most common location of hemispheric PAs[55]; intraventricular and subependymal PAs are the second most frequently encountered site.[54]

Imaging

Angiography. In most cases, cerebral angiograms demonstrate only an avascular mass effect with stretching and draping of otherwise normal vessels. Occasionally a mural nodule will show significant neovascularity.

CT. On NECT scans pilocytic astrocytomas typically are round or oval sharply demarcated and smoothly marginated hypo- or isodense masses. Calcification occurs in about 10% of all pilocytic astrocytomas.[54] Contrast enhancement is strong but variable. Some lesions enhance homogeneously and solidly; others have a small enhancing mural nodule in a large cyst (Fig. 13-36, *B* and *C*). Because the wall of most cystic astrocytomas consists of nonneoplastic compressed brain, it typically does not enhance, although occasionally some cases will show mural enhancement (Fig. 13-37). In others the cyst fluid en-

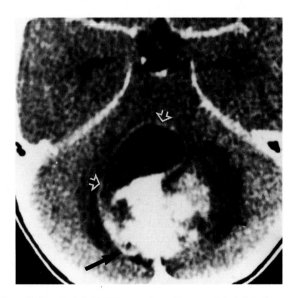

Fig. 13-37. Axial CECT scan in a 7-year-old child shows a mixed density midline cystic mass with a mural nodule that enhances strongly but heterogeneously *(black arrows)*. The cyst wall also enhances *(white arrows)*. Pilocytic astrocytoma.

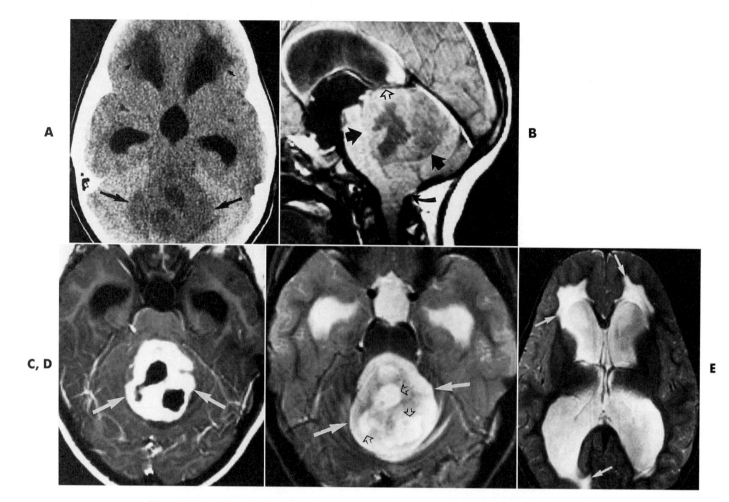

Fig. 13-38. A 4-year-old girl with headache, nausea, and vomiting. **A,** Axial NECT scan shows a hypodense mass in the midline posterior fossa *(large arrows).* Severe obstructive hydrocephalus is present, evidenced by markedly enlarged temporal and frontal horns of the lateral ventricles with transependymal CSF flow *(small arrows).* **B,** Sagittal precontrast T1-weighted MR scan shows the large mixed signal mass *(large black arrows)* is intraventricular. Note descending tonsillar *(curved arrow)* and ascending transtentorial *(open arrow)* herniations. **C,** Axial postcontrast scan shows the mass *(arrows)* enhances strongly but heterogeneously. **D,** Axial T2-weighted MR scan shows the lesion *(white arrows)* is inhomogeneously hyperintense. The intratumoral cysts *(open arrows)* are particularly high signal. **E,** Axial T2WI through the lateral ventricles shows severe obstructive hydrocephalus with transependymal CSF migration *(arrows).* Pilocytic astrocytoma of the fourth ventricle was found at surgery.

hances, with dependent layering that creates a contrast-fluid level, particularly if delayed scans are obtained.[55]

Obstructive hydrocephalus may occur relatively early and become moderately severe if a pilocytic astrocytoma is located in the vermis (Fig. 13-36) or fourth ventricle (Fig. 13-38, *A* to *E*). In contrast, brainstem tumors cause comparatively late-onset hydrocephalus that is usually mild to moderate (*see* Fig. 13-42).

MR. Most cerebellar pilocytic astrocytomas are cystic and therefore appear hypo- or isointense on T1-weighted images and hyperintense on T2-weighted scans. Mural nodules and solid tumors enhance strongly but somewhat inhomogeneously (Figs. 13-38 and 13-39).[54]

Brainstem gliomas are usually solid, infiltrating low-grade nonpilocytic tumors (Fig. 13-40), although cystic PAs may occur in this location. Pontine gliomas usually are diffusely infiltrating neoplasms that are inhomogeneously hypodense on T1WI and hyperdense on T2-weighted studies. Contrast enhancement is variable. These tumors may encase the basilar artery. Obstructive hydrocephalus is typically absent or mild even with advanced tumors. Medullary gliomas are low-grade fibrillary or pilocytic astrocytomas that infiltrate and expand the medulla (Fig. 13-41).

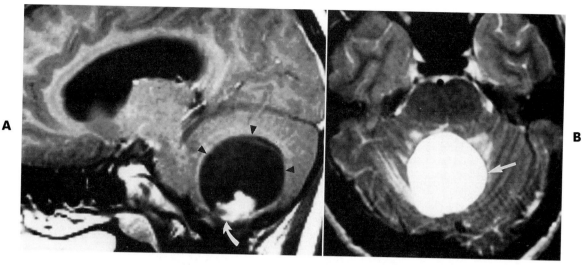

Fig. 13-39. A, Sagittal postcontrast T1-weighted image in a child with cerebellar pilo-cytic astrocytoma shows the typical findings of a cyst *(arrowheads)* with intensely enhanc-ing mural nodule *(white arrow).* **B,** Axial T2WI in another case shows the typical cystic astrocytoma is well delineated and hyperintense *(arrow).*

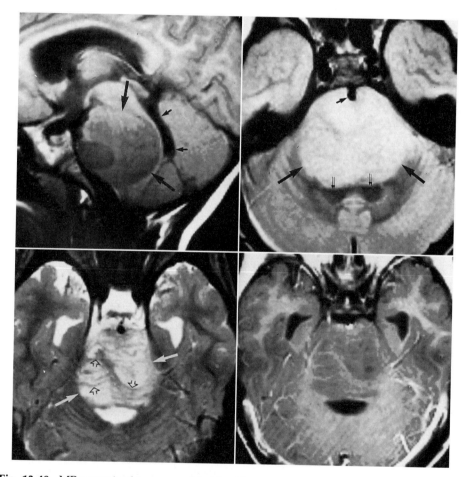

Fig. 13-40. MR scans in this 4-year-old girl with multiple cranial nerve palsies show typ-ical imaging findings of a large intrinsic pontine glioma. **A,** Sagittal precontrast T1WI shows the pons is markedly expanded by a mixed hypointense mass *(large arrows).* The fourth ventricle *(small arrows)* is distorted but not obliterated. **B,** Axial proton density-weighted mass shows the lesion *(large arrows)* is hyperintense relative to brain. The basi-lar artery *(small arrow)* is surrounded and nearly engulfed by tumor. The fourth ventricle is compressed *(double arrows)* but not obliterated. **C,** Axial T2WI shows the hyperintense mass *(large arrows)* infiltrates between white matter tracts that appear relatively preserved *(open arrows).* **D,** Axial postcontrast T1WI shows the mass does not enhance. Notice white matter tracts.

Continued.

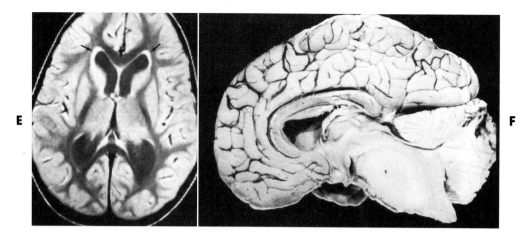

Fig. 13-40, cont'd. E, Axial proton density-weighted scan shows mildly enlarged lateral ventricles with smooth periventricular hyperintensity, indicating compensated hydrocephalus *(arrows).* **F,** Sagittal autopsy specimen of a large infiltrating pontine glioma is shown for comparison. The tumor was a grade I fibrillary astrocytoma. (**F,** Courtesy Royal College of Surgeons of England, *Slide Atlas of Pathology,* Gower Medical Publishing, 1988. With permission.)

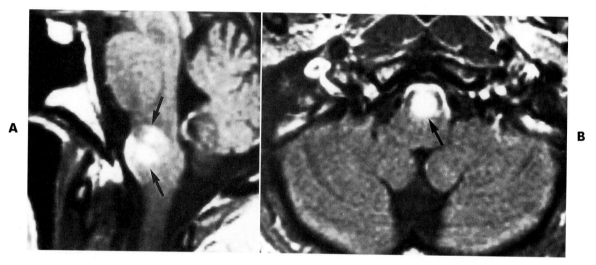

Fig. 13-41. Sagittal **(A)** and axial **(B)** postcontrast T1-weighted MR scans in an 18-year-old with a long-standing medullary pilocytic astrocytoma that has remained unchanged in size and configuration for several years. The tumor *(arrows)* enhances strongly but somewhat heterogeneously.

Typical opticochiasmatic-hypothalamic pilocytic astrocytomas are often solid. These tumors are hypo- to isodense with normal brain on T1WI and show mild to moderate enhancement following contrast administration (Fig. 13-42). Retrochiasmatic extension can sometimes be identified on T2-weighted scans or contrast-enhanced T1WI (Fig. 13-42). Occasionally, opticochiasmatic-hypothalamic PAs attain large size. Cyst formation and trapped pools of CSF may be prominent features in some cases (Fig. 13-43).

Hemispheric PAs are uncommon tumors. A cystic mass with enhancing mural nodule is typical (Fig. 13-44).[55]

Pleomorphic Xanthoastrocytoma

Pleomorphic xanthoastrocytoma is a rare neoplasm that represents a histologically and biologically distinct astrocytoma subtype (*see* box, p. 561).[5a,55a] Because of its indolent nature and generally benign clinical course, recognition of this uncommon but important entity is critical in avoiding overly aggressive treatment.

Pathology

Gross pathology. Pleomorphic xanthoastrocytomas (PXAs) are typically well-demarcated, partially cystic tumors with a discrete mural nodule. Lepto-

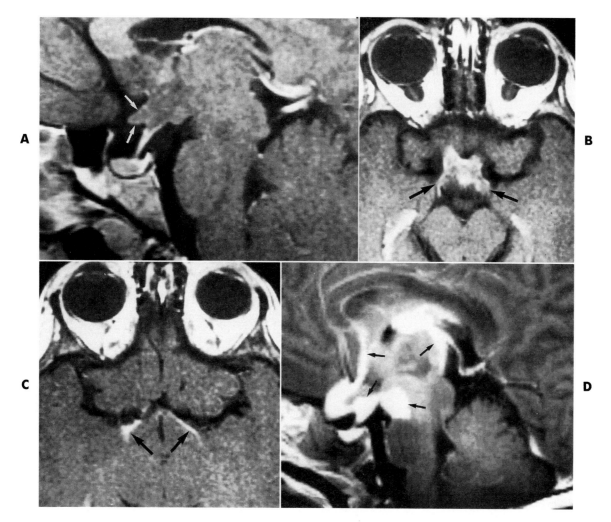

Fig. 13-42. Opticochiasmatic-hypothalamic pilocytic astrocytomas. **A,** Sagittal postcontrast T1WI in a 22-year-old with neurofibromatosis type 1 (NF-1) shows slight enlargement of the optic chiasm *(arrows)*. **B** and **C,** Axial postcontrast T1WIs in another case show the optic chiasm is enlarged and enhances strongly (**B,** *arrows*); there is subtle retrochiasmatic extension of the tumor (**C,** *arrows*). **D,** Sagittal postcontrast T1WI in another case shows an enhancing opticochiasmatic glioma with extensive involvement of the hypothalamus, fornix, thalami, and midbrain *(arrows)*.

Fig. 13-43. Three-year-old child with hypothalamic glioma. **A,** CECT scan shows a huge suprasellar mass that enhances strongly and uniformly *(large arrows)*. Note trapped CSF pooled around the mass *(small arrows)*.

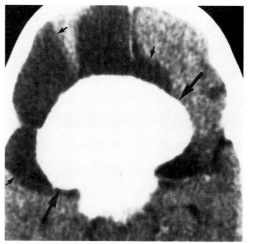

Continued.

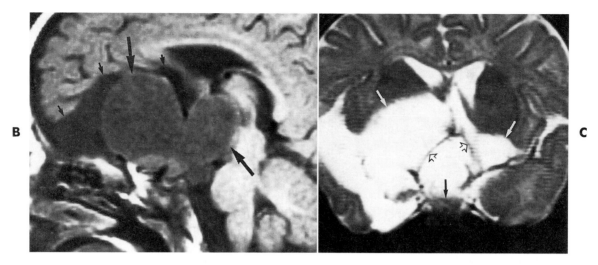

Fig. 13-43, cont'd.   B, Sagittal T1-weighted MR shows the extensive suprasellar mass *(large arrows)* is mostly hypointense to brain. Trapped CSF *(small arrows)*. C, Coronal T2WI shows the extremely hyperintense mass *(white arrows)* has elevated the A1 segments of both anterior cerebral arteries *(open arrows)*. Note the normal pituitary gland *(black arrow)* beneath the lesion.

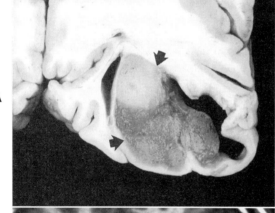

Fig. 13-44. Coronal gross pathology specimen **(A)** demonstrates a temporal lobe cystic pilocytic astrocytoma *(arrows)*. Coronal pre- **(B)** and postcontrast **(C)** MR scans in an 18-year-old man with temporal lobe seizures show a cystic mass *(small arrows)* with a mural nodule *(large arrows)* that enhances intensely after contrast administration. Pilocytic astrocytoma was found at surgery. (**A,** From Okazaki H, Scheithauer B: *Slide Atlas of Neuropathology,* Gower Medical Publishing, 1988.)

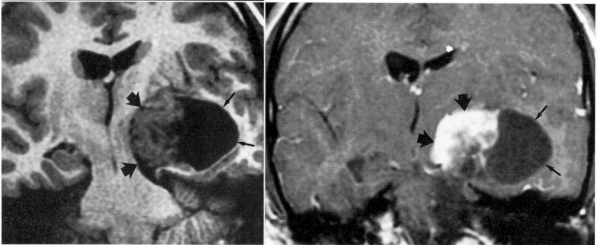

Pleomorphic Xanthoastrocytoma

Pathology

Partially cystic tumor with discrete mural nodule
Lipid-laden xanthomatous astrocytes

Incidence

Rare (<1% of astrocytomas)

Age

Children, young adults

Location

Superficial temporal lobe most common

Imaging

Superficial, partially cystic hemispheric mass with enhancing mural nodule is typical

---

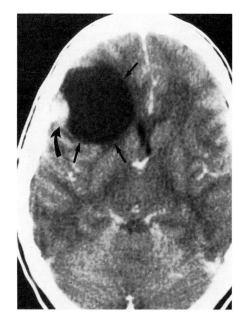

Fig. 13-45. CECT scan shows a well-demarcated cystic-appearing mass *(small arrows)* with a strongly enhancing peripheral mural nodule *(curved arrow).* The lesion was thought to be a pilocytic astrocytoma, but pathology review disclosed pleomorphic xanthoastrocytoma. (Courtesy J. Smirniotopoulos.)

meningeal adhesion or attachment is common, but most PXAs are easily separated from the adjacent normal brain. Occasionally PXAs appear more diffuse and have an infiltrating gyriform pattern or sulcal spread.[56,57]

Histology. Striking pleomorphic tumor cells with copious glassy cytoplasm and dark, multilobulated nuclei are seen.[10] A mixture of spindle-shaped cells, multinucleated giant cells, and foamy lipid-laden xanthomatous astrocytes is typical.[58] Focal cystic changes are common but endothelial proliferation is scanty or absent. Mitoses are few; necrosis is absent. An abundant reticulin network is usually present.[58]

Incidence, age, and clinical presentation. PXAs are rare. These are tumors of children and young adults. The average age in most reported series is in the second or third decade.[56] Some cases have been reported into the fifth decade.[59] Most patients have a long history of seizures.[56]

Location. A superficial cortical location is typical; the mural nodule usually abuts the leptomeninges. The temporal lobe is the most common site. Next in order are the parietal, occipital, and frontal lobes.[57]

Imaging

Angiography. Angiographic findings range from an avascular or hypovascular mass effect to intense neovascularity in the tumor nodule.[60]

CT. On NECT scans PXAs are typically hypodense cystic-appearing masses with distinct borders. Calcification is unusual.[60] A mural nodule that enhances strongly after contrast administration is common (Fig. 13-45).

MR. Most PXAs are well-delineated partially cystic masses that appear hypo- or isointense compared to normal brain on T1WI. A peripheral nodule is often present. Increased signal intensity of both the nodule and cystic component are seen on proton density- and T2WI. Marked contrast enhancement of the nodule can be seen following contrast administration.[60] Occasionally, PXAs are solid or infiltrating lesions.[56,57]

Subependymal Giant Cell Astrocytoma

Subependymal giant cell astrocytoma (SGCA) is a circumscribed tumor associated with tuberous sclerosis (TS) (*see* box, p. 562). Subependymal harmatomatous proliferations along the caudothalamic groove are common in TS. On occasion a nodule located at or near the foramen of Monro proliferates into a sizable mass that can cause ventricular obstruction and become symptomatic.[10] Whether or not SGCAs can occur in the absence of TS is debatable. So-called isolated or "spontaneous" cases may actually occur with a forme fruste of this neurocutaneous syndrome.

Pathology

Gross pathology. SGCAs are typically sharply defined lobulated masses that are often calcified. Cysts are common. SGCAs are often vascular tumors that may have a grossly angiomatous appearance.[3]

Histology. Large swollen astrocytes with abundant glassy eosinophic cytoplasm, prominent thick

---

Subependymal Giant Cell Astrocytomas

Pathology

Occurs with tuberous sclerosis (TS)
Large bi-, multinucleated astrocytes
Cysts common; necrosis, mitoses are rare
WHO grade I

Incidence

10% to 15% of patients with TS

Age

Usually <20 years

Location

Foramen of Monro

Natural history

Slow growing, indolent
Symptoms secondary to obstructive hydrocephalus
Long-term survival is usual

Imaging

Coexisting stigmata of TS
Focal partially calcified, partially cystic mass at foramen of Monro
Strong but heterogeneous enhancement

---

processes, and benign-appearing nuclei are present. Bi- and multinucleated forms occur. Mitoses are rare.[10] The prominent blood vessels that are often present in these tumors are thin-walled structures devoid of endothelial proliferation.[3] GFAP staining of SGCAs is variable.

Incidence, age, clinical presentation, and natural history. SGCAs occur in 10% to 15% of patients with tuberous sclerosis. Most patients become symptomatic before age 20. Symptoms are related to ventricular obstruction. SGCAs are characteristically slow growing, and long-term survival even after subtotal resection is typical.

Location. SGCAs occur at the foramen of Monro. They are virtually never found anywhere else in the brain.

Imaging. Most patients with SGCA also have imaging manifestations of tuberous sclerosis (*see* Chapter 5).
Angiography. SGCAs are variably vascular neoplasms. Venous phase films show elongated, stretched subependymal veins around the dilated lateral ventricles.
CT. A focal mass at the foramen of Monro with enlarged lateral ventricles is seen. Calcified subependymal nodules along the striothalamic groove can often

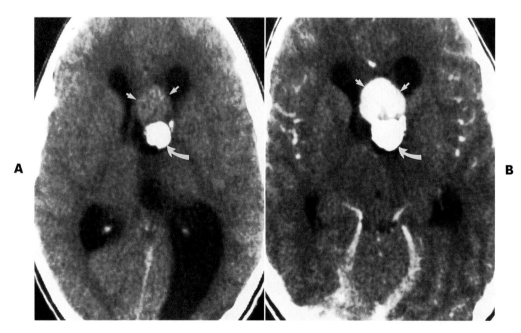

Fig. 13-46. Pre- **(A)** and postcontrast **(B)** axial CT scans in a patient with tuberous sclerosis (TS) show a mass *(small arrows)* at the foramen of Monro. The mass is partially calcified *(curved arrows)* and enhances strongly after contrast administration. (Courtesy R. Jahnke.)

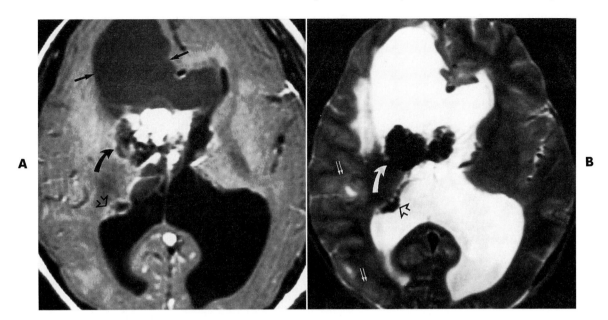

Fig. 13-47. A, Axial postcontrast T1-weighted MR scan in a patient with tuberous sclerosis shows a large partially cystic mass *(small arrows)* at the foramen of Monro. The solid portion of the mass *(curved arrow)* enhances strongly but nonuniformly. **B,** Axial T2WI shows the mass is partially calcified *(curved arrow)*. Other stigmata of TS are present, including a calcified subependymal nodule (**B,** *open arrow*) that enhances slightly (**A,** *open arrow*) and white matter lesions (**B,** *double arrows*). Note severe obstructive hydrocephalus, seen as markedly enlarged lateral ventricles. (Courtesy L. Tan.)

be identified. SGCAs are heterogeneous neoplasms with mixed hypo- and isodense regions. Calcification and cyst formation are common. Strong but inhomogeneous enhancement following contrast administration is typical (Fig. 13-46).

MR. The heterogeneous gross pathology of SGCAs is reflected by mixed signal intensities on both T1- and T2WI. Most SGCAs are hypo- and isointense on T1WI and iso- to hyperintense on T2-weighted sequences. Enhancement is strong but inhomogeneous (*see* Chapter 5). Other stigmata of TS are usually present in these cases (Fig. 13-47).

OLIGODENDROGLIOMA

Oligodendrogliomas are uncommon gliomas. Pure oligodendrogliomas are even more uncommon. Here, we consider so-called pure oligodendrogliomas, with the more common oligoastrocytoma or mixed glioma. Oligodendrogliomas arise from a specific type of glial cell, the oligodendrocyte, that makes and maintains the CNS myelin.

"Pure" Oligodendroglioma

Pathology

Gross appearance. Oligodendrogliomas are typically unencapsulated but well-circumscribed focal white matter tumors that may extend into the cortex and leptomeninges (*see* box, p. 564). Occasionally a poorly delineated, diffusely infiltrating lesion is seen.

Foci of cystic degeneration are relatively common, but hemorrhage and necrosis are less frequently seen.[2] Because oligodendrogliomas often calcify they may have a gritty texture.

Histology. Well-differentiated oligodendrogliomas are composed of uniform cells with regular spherical nucleoli that are surrounded by a clear halo (fried-egg appearance). Calcospherites are common but mitoses are few. As with most other gliomas, oligodendrogliomas also exhibit a spectrum of differentiation. Most are well-differentiated but others exhibit unequivocal anaplasia. Anaplastic or malignant oligodendrogliomas may show moderate pleomorphism and abundant mitotic figures.[10]

Incidence. Oligodendrogliomas comprise 2% to 5% of all primary intracranial tumors and 5% to 10% of all gliomas.[61,62] Pure oligodendrogliomas are uncommon.[63,64]

Age and clinical presentation. Oligodendrogliomas are tumors of adults. The ratio of adults to children with oligodendroglioma is 8:1. The peak incidence is between 35 and 45 years of age. Seizures are the most common presenting symptom.[62]

Natural history. Most oligodendrogliomas are slow-growing neoplasms; a minority are anaplastic.[65] Tumor grade is the single most important prognostic

Oligodendroglioma

Pathology

Arises from oligodendrocytes

Starts in hemispheric white matter, grows towards cortex

Foci of cystic degeneration common

Hemorrhage, necrosis uncommon

Cells have "fried egg" appearance

50% mixed histology (astrocytoma most common)

Incidence

2% to 5% of all primary brain tumors

5% to 10% of gliomas

Age

Adults>children (8:1); peak age 35 to 45 years

Location

Frontal lobes are most common; often involve cortex

Natural history

Slow-growing

75% 5-year survival for low-grade neoplasm

High-grade/mixed histology tumors have poorer prognosis

Imaging

Heterogeneous hemispheric mass that often involves cortex

Calcification in 70% to 90%

Overlying skull may show pressure erosion

Cysts common

Necrosis, gross hemorrhage rare

Mild/moderate inhomogeneous enhancement common

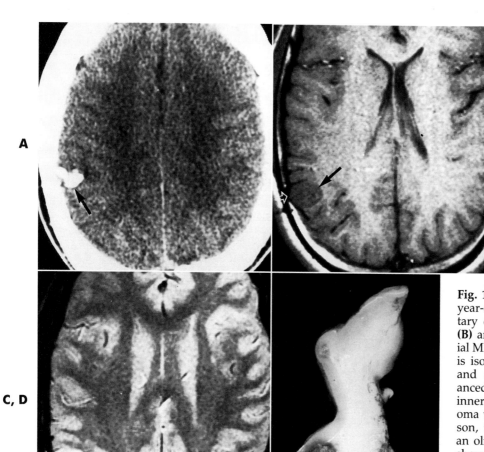

A

B

C, D

Fig. 13-48. Axial NECT scan **(A)** in a 32-year-old man with seizures shows a solitary calcified cortical lesion *(arrow)*. T1-**(B)** and proton density-weighted **(C)** axial MR scans show the mass *(large arrows)* is isointense with gray matter on T1WI and slightly hyperintense on the balanced study. Note pressure erosion of the inner table *(open arrows)*. Oligodendroglioma was found at surgery. For comparison, the gross resected specimen **(D)** of an oligodendroglioma in another case is shown. (D, From Okazaki H, Scheithauer B: *Slide Atlas of Neuropathology,* Gower Medical Publishing, 1988.)

variable. Patients with low-grade lesions have 5- and 10-year survival rates of 74% and 46% respectively; the rates are 41% and 20% for patients with grade 3 or 4 tumors.[63]

Location. Oligodendrogliomas are predominately lesions of the cerebral hemispheric white matter that grow toward the cortex. Eighty-five percent are supratentorial. The most common location is the frontal lobe.[61] Although they can be found anywhere, the posterior fossa is an uncommon site. Primary oligodendrogliomas can invade the ventricles, but a purely intraventricular tumor is rare.[66]

Imaging

Angiography. Low-grade "pure" oligodendrogliomas are typically avascular or faintly vascular masses that show focal stretching and draping of cortical vessels around the lesion. Malignant oligodendrogliomas may have significant neovascularity.

CT. Oligodendrogliomas are the most common in-tracranial tumor to calcify.[62] Nodular or clumped calcification is present in 70% to 90% of all cases. NECT scans typically show a partially calcified mixed density hemispheric mass that extends peripherally to the cortex. Scalloped erosion of the inner table of the skull is seen in some cases (Fig. 13-48). Cystic degeneration is common but gross hemorrhage and edema are relatively rare. Two thirds of oligodendrogliomas show mild to moderate enhancement following contrast administration (Fig. 13-49, *A* and *B*).[67] Intraventricular oligodendrogliomas are indistinguishable on imaging studies and light microscopy from central neurocytomas, neuronal neoplasms that arise in the midline or lateral ventricles (Fig. 13-49, *C*) (*see* Chapter 14).

MR. MR scans show mixed hypo- and isointense areas on T1WI and hyperintense foci on T2-weighted sequences (Fig. 13-50). Enhancement is typically patchy and moderate. MR is less sensitive than CT in detecting tumor calcification but is superior in delineating tumor extent.[67]

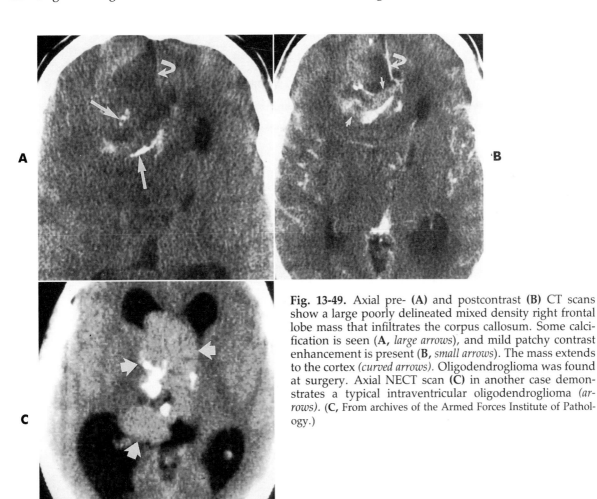

Fig. 13-49. Axial pre- **(A)** and postcontrast **(B)** CT scans show a large poorly delineated mixed density right frontal lobe mass that infiltrates the corpus callosum. Some calcification is seen (**A**, *large arrows*), and mild patchy contrast enhancement is present (**B**, *small arrows*). The mass extends to the cortex (*curved arrows*). Oligodendroglioma was found at surgery. Axial NECT scan **(C)** in another case demonstrates a typical intraventricular oligodendroglioma *(arrows)*. (**C**, From archives of the Armed Forces Institute of Pathology.)

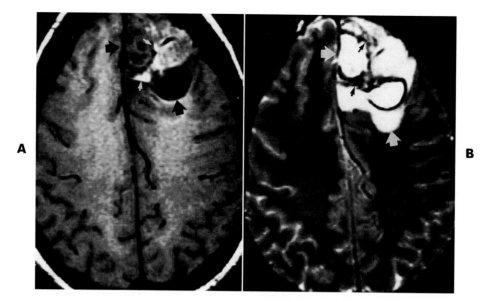

Fig. 13-50. Axial T1- **(A)** and T2-weighted **(B)** MR scans show a large mixed density left frontal lobe mass *(large arrows)*. Partially cystic oligodendroglioma with subacute and chronic hemorrhage *(small arrows)* was resected.

"Mixed" Oligodendroglioma (oligoastrocytoma)

Oligodendrogliomas often contain other glial elements. At least half the tumors generally classified as oligodendrogliomas consist of mixed-cell forms.[3,64] The most common mixture is with neoplastically transformed astrocytes. Transitional or ependymal elements are less common. Pathologic recognition of the mixed character of oligodendrogliomas is important when potential malignancy is assessed. However, these so-called mixed gliomas are indistinguishable on imaging studies from pure oligodendrogliomas.

EPENDYMOMA

The ependyma is a thin layer of ciliated cuboidal or columnar epithelium that lines the ventricular walls and central canal of the spinal cord.[1] Ependymal cells are embryologically related to other glial cell types, namely astrocytes and oligodendroglia. Neoplastically transformed ependymal cells often reflect this dual glial and epithelial heritage.[10]

There are several histologic variants of ependymoma (*see* box). The most common type, the so-called *cellular ependymoma*, has predominately glial features. "*Papillary*" ependymomas are uncommon. These tumors have single or multiple layers of neoplastic cells that cover glial papillae. A "*myxopapillary*" ependymoma is found exclusively in the conus medullaris or filum terminale of the spinal cord. An ependymoma variant, the so-called *subependymoma*, may represent a transitional form between ependymomas and astrocytomas.[67a]

Ependymal Tumors
Ependymoma (cellular, papillary)
Anaplastic (malignant) ependymoma
Myxopapillary ependymoma (conus medullaris/filum terminale)
Subependymoma

A rare, very immature form of ependymoma, the so-called *ependymoblastoma*, may represent a tumor that arises from a primitive neuroepithelial precursor cell and shows ependymal differentiation.[5a] This tumor is considered with other primitive neuroectodermal (PNET) tumors in Chapter 14.

In this chapter we discuss the two most common intracranial ependymomas: cellular ependymoma and subependymoma. Myxopapillary ependymomas are considered in Chapter 21 with other intramedullary spinal cord neoplasms.

Ependymoma

Pathology

Gross pathology. Ependymomas are slow-growing lobulated neoplasms that are often partly cystic. Calcification is common but gross hemorrhage is rare. When ependymomas occur in the fourth ventricle, the most common site, they arise from the floor or roof and protrude through the outlet foramina into the adjacent CSF cisterns. The term *plastic ependymoma* describes this tendency to ooze or extrude posteroinferiorly into the cisterna magna, anterolaterally

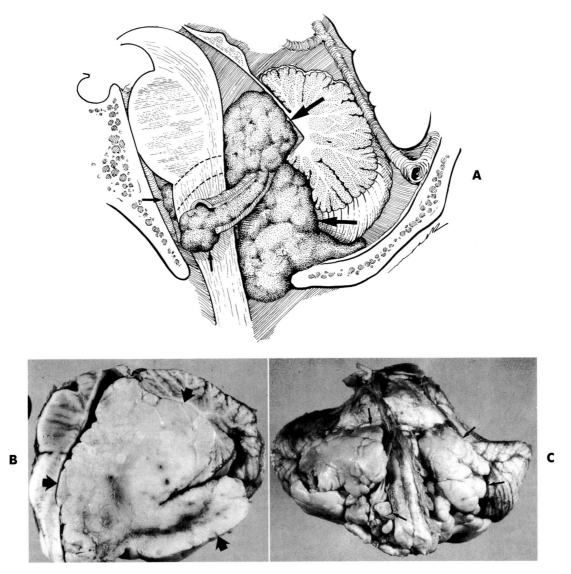

Fig. 13-51. Anatomic drawing **(A)** and gross pathology specimens **(B** and **C)** show a typical fourth ventricular ependymoma. The tumor *(large arrows)* expands the fourth ventricle and extends out the foramen of Magendie into the cisterna magna and through the foramina of Luschka into the cerebellopontine angle cisterns *(small arrows)*. The tendency of this tumor to squeeze out these foramina gives rise to the appellation "plastic" ependymoma. (**B** and **C,** Courtesy E.C. Alvord, Jr.)

into the cerebellopontine angle cisterns, and down through the foramen magnum into the upper cervical spine behind the cervicomedullary junction (Fig. 13-51) (*see* box, p. 568).[67b]

Histology. Ependymoma cellularity and architecture vary. Cellular ependymomas, the most frequent histologic subtype, are composed of fusiform cells arranged around small blood vessels. These so-called perivascular pseudorosettes are an important microscopic finding.[10] Occasionally, an ependymoma forms true ependymal rosettes, reproducing in miniature the lining of a normal ependymal cavity.[2]

Ependymomas demonstrate a spectrum of anaplasia that ranges from the typical well-differentiated neoplasm with infrequent mitoses, mild cellular pleomorphism, and minimal or no necrosis to lesions with high cell density, mitotic activity, cellular pleomorphism, vascular proliferation, and extensive necrosis.[10]

Incidence. Ependymomas represent from 2% to 8% of all primary intracranial brain tumors. They constitute 15% of posterior fossa neoplasms in childhood and are the third most common pediatric brain tumor.[68]

Ependymoma

Pathology

"Plastic" fourth ventricular tumor that extrudes through outlet foramina into adjacent CSF cisterns is most common

Variable cellularity, architecture, histologic differentiation

Incidence

2% to 8% of all primary brain tumors

15% of posterior fossa tumors in children

Third most common pediatric brain tumor

Age

Children 1 to 5 years of age

Location

60% infratentorial: >90% in fourth ventricle

40% supratentorial: extraventricular location more common than intraventricular sites

Natural history

45% 5-year survival rate

Imaging

Mixed density/intensity mass

50% calcify

Variable mild/moderate enhancement

Supratentorial extraventricular ependymomas resemble astrocytomas

---

Age and clinical presentation. Ependymomas are four to six times more common in children compared to adults. The peak age range is 1 to 5 years but there is a second, smaller peak in the mid-30s. Common presenting symptoms are disequilibrium, nausea and vomiting, and headache; the most frequent signs are ataxia and nystagmus.[69]

Natural history. The overall 5-year survival rate for infratentorial ependymomas in childhood is 45%. Tumor recurrence or progression at the primary site is by far the most common cause of death in these patients.[68,69] Spinal seeding is relatively uncommon.[69,70]

Location. Approximately 60% of intracranial ependymomas are located in the posterior fossa, and 40% are found above the tentorium. Ninety percent of infratentorial ependymomas occur in the fourth ventricle; the medulla and cerebellopontine angle cisterns account for the remaining posterior fossa sites.[67] Between two thirds and three quarters of supratentorial ependymomas are extraventricular.[70,71]

Imaging

Angiography. Angiographic findings vary from a hypovascular mass effect to extremely hypervascular lesions with intense vascular staining, contrast stasis, irregular tumor vessels, and arteriovenous shunting (Fig. 13-52).

CT. The CT findings of infratentorial ependymoma are variable. Most are isodense on NECT; approximately 50% exhibit calcification.[72,73] Mild to moderate inhomogeneous enhancement is seen in

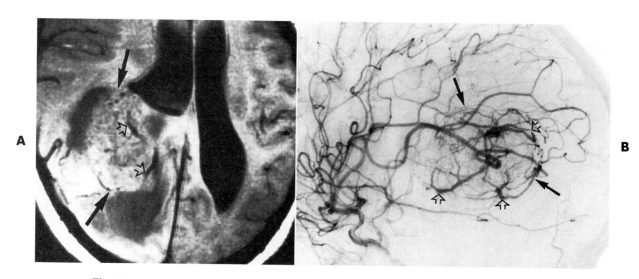

Fig. 13-52. A, Axial T1-weighted MR scan in a child with an ependymoma *(large arrows)* in the atrium of the right lateral ventricle (same case as Fig. 12-41). Prominent "flow voids" from high-velocity signal loss in tumor vessels *(open arrows)* are present. **B,** Common carotid angiogram, midarterial phase, lateral view, shows a hypervascular mass *(black arrows)* with irregular tumor vessels *(open arrows)*.

70% of cases (Fig. 13-53). Overt hemorrhage is uncommon.

MR. The MR differentiation of ependymomas from other gliomas is related to their location and morphology, not differences in signal intensity or enhancement patterns.[74] The classic appearance of a posterior fossa ependymoma is a somewhat lobulated soft tissue mass that appears to form a cast or mold of the fourth ventricle and extrudes through its outlet foramina into the adjacent subarachnoid cisterns (Figs. 13-53, *C,* and 13-54).

The solid components of ependymomas are typically hypo- or isointense compared to brain on T1WI and hyperintense on proton density- and T2-weighted scans (Fig. 13-54, *C*). The cystic portions of ependymomas are slightly hyperintense to CSF on T1WI and hyperintense to brain on T2WI. Intratumoral signal heterogeneity may represent necrosis, calcification, tumor vascularity, or blood degradation products. Moderate inhomogeneous enhancement following contrast administration is typical.

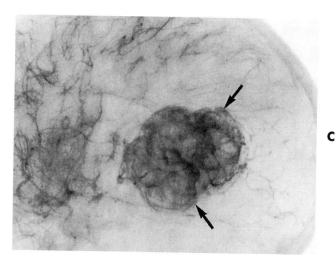

Fig. 13-52, cont'd.   C, Later phase film shows dense vascular stain *(arrows).*

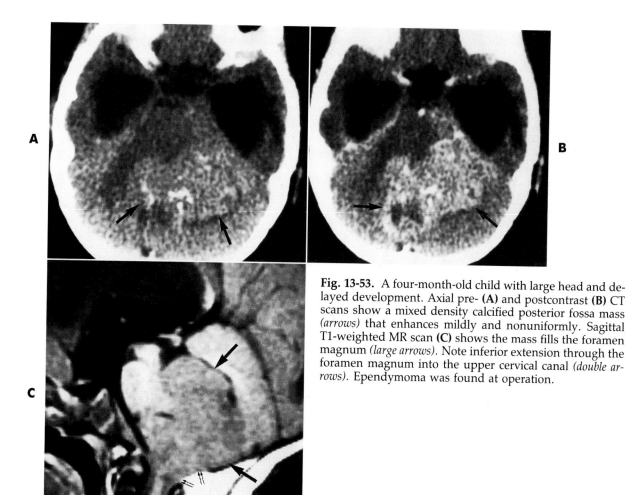

Fig. 13-53. A four-month-old child with large head and delayed development. Axial pre- **(A)** and postcontrast **(B)** CT scans show a mixed density calcified posterior fossa mass *(arrows)* that enhances mildly and nonuniformly. Sagittal T1-weighted MR scan **(C)** shows the mass fills the foramen magnum *(large arrows).* Note inferior extension through the foramen magnum into the upper cervical canal *(double arrows).* Ependymoma was found at operation.

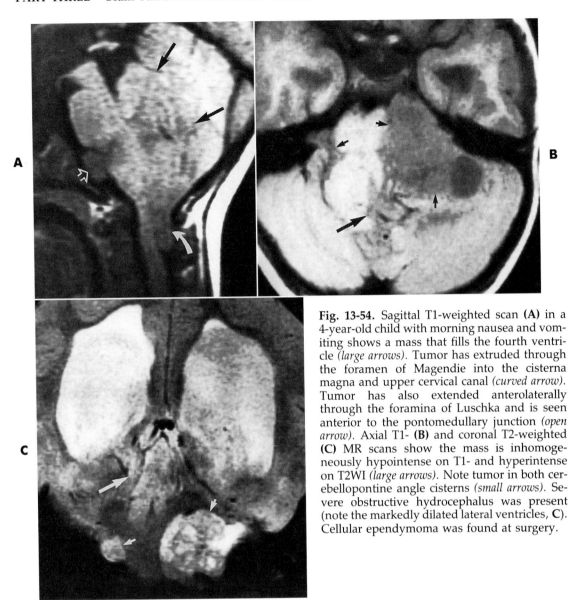

Fig. 13-54. Sagittal T1-weighted scan **(A)** in a 4-year-old child with morning nausea and vomiting shows a mass that fills the fourth ventricle *(large arrows)*. Tumor has extruded through the foramen of Magendie into the cisterna magna and upper cervical canal *(curved arrow)*. Tumor has also extended anterolaterally through the foramina of Luschka and is seen anterior to the pontomedullary junction *(open arrow)*. Axial T1- **(B)** and coronal T2-weighted **(C)** MR scans show the mass is inhomogeneously hypointense on T1- and hyperintense on T2WI *(large arrows)*. Note tumor in both cerebellopontine angle cisterns *(small arrows)*. Severe obstructive hydrocephalus was present (note the markedly dilated lateral ventricles, **C**). Cellular ependymoma was found at surgery.

Supratentorial ependymomas are often indistinguishable from other gliomas. Because they are primarily extraventricular lesions, supratentorial ependymomas can mimic astrocytoma. Homogeneous solid or ring-enhancing patterns are commonly seen (Fig. 13-55).[71]

Subependymoma

Subependymoma (SE) is a rare benign CNS tumor with distinctive histology, age at presentation, and clinical course (*see* box).[67a]

Pathology. On gross inspection, SEs are firm, well-delineated white to grayish avascular intraventricular masses that are attached to the septum pellucidum (*see* Fig. 12-38, *A*) or inferior fourth ventricle (*see* Fig. 12-100). Microscopic examination discloses a sparsely cellular neoplasm with a prominent fibrillary background. Microcystic changes are common but hypercellularity, ependymal rosette formation, neovascularity, mitoses and necrosis are absent.[2,75]

Age and clinical presentation. SEs occur in middle-aged and elderly adults; most are found incidentally at autopsy or on imaging studies performed for clinical indications that are unrelated to the neoplasm. The average age of SE patients depends on whether or not they are symptomatic. Symptomatic SEs occlude the CSF pathways and cause obstructive hydrocephalus. The average age of the symptomatic group is around 40 years of age. The average age of asymptomatic patients is nearly 60.[76]

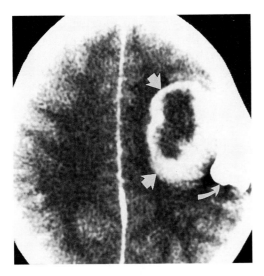

Fig. 13-55. Axial CECT scan in a child with seizures and right-side hemiparesis shows a large ring-enhancing mass *(large arrows)* with a prominent calcific focus *(curved arrow)*.

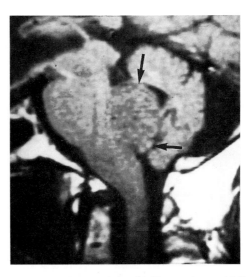

Fig. 13-56. Sagittal T1-weighted MR scan in a middle-aged patient shows a fourth ventricular mass *(arrows)*. Subependymoma was found at surgery. (Courtesy D. Tampieri.)

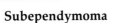

Subependymoma

Pathology, location

Firm, well-delineated mass
Inferior fourth ventricle, frontal horn of lateral ventricle most common sites

Incidence, age

Rare tumor in middle-aged/elderly

Imaging

Nonenhancing mass similar to brain

Location. SEs most often arise from the lower medulla and project into the caudal fourth ventricle. Another common location is in the frontal horn of the lateral ventricle where they attach to the septum pellucidum. A few SEs are found along the midbody of the lateral ventricle.[76]

Imaging

Angiography. Cerebral angiography may disclose arterial displacement around the mass and stretched subependymal veins, indicating ventricular dilatation. Neovascularity is absent.[77,78]

CT. NECT scans show a well-delineated mass that is hypo- or isodense to brain parenchyma. Calcification is sometimes identified. Minimal or no enhancement is seen on postcontrast studies.[74] Occasionally

these tumors are highly vascularized lesions with extensive hemorrhage.[79]

MR. Most subependymomas are homogeneously hypo- to isointense masses on T1WI (Fig. 13-56). Subependymomas may appear mildly hyperintense on T2-weighted scans.[74] There is some signal heterogeneity, reflecting multiple small intratumoral cysts.[76] Contrast enhancement is typically absent.[80] The differential diagnosis of a fourth ventricular SE is metastasis or cellular ependymoma; central neurocytoma and astrocytoma are the major differential diagnostic considerations for frontal horn SEs.

CHOROID PLEXUS TUMORS

Embryologically, choroid plexus epithelium arises from modified primitive ventricular neuroepithelial cells at certain sites along the developing neural tube. By virtue of its structure and its functions as both a secretory and absorptive organ, the choroid plexus resembles the surface epithelium that forms mucosal linings in other parts of the body. Like mucosa elsewhere, choroid plexus occasionally becomes the site of both benign and malignant neoplasms that respectively share the microscopic features of papilloma and carcinoma.[3]

The two primary choroid plexus tumors are choroid plexus papilloma and choroid plexus carcinoma. Other neoplasms that can involve the choroid plexus are meningioma (*see* Chapter 14) and metastases (*see* Chapter 15). Benign lesions that can arise in the choroid plexus include nonneoplastic cysts (*see* Chapter 15) and vascular malformations. In this section we consider choroid plexus papillomas and carcinomas.

Choroid Plexus Papilloma

Pathology

Choroid plexus papillomas>>carcinomas
Cauliflower-like mass
Multiple frondlike papillae with single epithelial layer around fibrovascular core
Histologically benign papillomas may show focal brain invasion, CSF spread

Incidence

<1% of all primary brain tumors
0.5% to 0.6% of adult primary brain tumors
2% to 5% of primary brain tumors in children
One of most common brain tumors in children under 2 years

Age

>85% in children ≧5 years of age

Location

Trigone of lateral ventricle in child
Fourth ventricle in adult
<10% other locations (third ventricle, cerebellopontine angle cistern)

Natural history

Long-term survival typical

Imaging

Mottled mass that is isodense/intense to brain
25% calcify
Enhance intensely
All ventricles usually enlarge with trigone CPPs

Choroid Plexus Papilloma

Pathology

Gross pathology. Choroid plexus papillomas (CPPs) are reddish-tan globular or cauliflower-like masses (Fig. 13-57) (*see* box). Although most CPPs are contained within the ventricle, some large masses may in part be buried in brain parenchyma, and limited focal invasion by otherwise benign-appearing papillomas can occasionally be seen.[2,3]

Histology. Microscopically these tumors are composed of numerous delicate frondlike papillae that closely resemble normal choroid plexus. A single layer of cuboidal or columnar epithelium surrounds a thin fibrovascular stromal core. These features differentiate CPPs from papillary ependymoma, which has papillae with a fibrillary neuroglial core that is covered with multilayered epithelium.[81] Cystic degeneration can occur but mitotic figures are rare.

Incidence and age. CPPs account for fewer than 1% of all primary brain tumors, representing 0.5% to 0.6% of intracranial neoplasms in adults and 2% to 5% in children.[3] Despite their relative overall rarity, CPPs are one of the most common brain tumors in children under 2 years of age. Eighty-six percent of CPPs in children occur in the first 5 years of life.[82]

Clinical presentation. Symptoms of a supratentorial CPP result from hydrocephalus. These tumors are typically characterized by asymmetric but striking ventricular enlargement. The precise etiology of the hydrocephalus is controversial. Enlargement of CSF spaces, ventricles, and cisterns not mechanically obstructed by the tumor is seen in 80% of CPPs, sug-

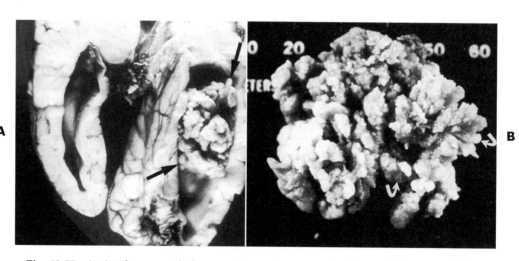

Fig. 13-57. **A,** Axial gross pathology specimen shows a typical choroid plexus papilloma (CPP) *(arrows)* in the atrium of the left lateral ventricle. **B,** Gross surgical specimen of a classic CPP shows the frondlike excrescences on the tumor surface *(arrows)*. (**A,** From Okazaki H, Scheithauer B: *Slide Atlas of Neuropathology,* Gower Medical Publishing, 1988. **B,** From archives of the Armed Forces Institute of Pathology.)

gesting overproduction of CSF or a resorption defect as the most likely etiology.[76] Hemorrhage with ependymitis could also contribute to the hydrocephalus that is almost invariably present with lateral ventricular CPPs.

CPPs that present below the tentorium usually occur in adults. Although fourth ventricular tumors often cause obstructive hydrocephalus with headaches and ataxia, CPPs that arise in the foramen of Luschka or cerebellopontine angle may cause cranial nerve palsies.[83]

Natural history. Although CPP is a benign, potentially curable neoplasm, and long-term survival is the rule, recurrences following resection are not uncommon.[10] Prognosis does not necessarily correlate with histologic grade of CPPs. Benign-appearing CPPs occasionally behave malignantly. Atypical CPPs with cytologic atypia, occasional mitoses, and microscopic tumor invasion often do not spread or recur.

Location. CPPs occur in proportion to the amount of choroid plexus that is normally present. Therefore the most common location is the lateral ventricle trigone (atrium), the site of nearly 50% of all CPPs. Forty percent occur in the fourth ventricle and 10% in other sites such as the third ventricle and cerebellopontine angle cistern. In children, CPPs are most common in the lateral ventricles; the fourth ventricle is the most common site in adults.[3] Bilateral tumors are very rare, accounting for only 3% to 4% of all CPPs.[84]

Extraventricular CPPs are rare. They are found in the following three situations[83,85]:

1. A primary intraventricular papilloma extends directly into an adjacent CSF cistern
2. The primary neoplasm sheds tumor and seeds the CSF pathways (drop metastases)
3. A primary tumor develops from the small choroid tuft that normally protrudes through the foramen of Luschka into the cerebellopontine angle cistern

Other extraventricular CPPs are extremely rare; they have been reported in the suprasellar cistern, pineal region, and even the brain parenchyma.[86]

Imaging

Angiography and ultrasound. CPPs are highly vascular neoplasms with a prominent, prolonged vascular stain (Fig. 13-58, *A* and *B*). Enlarged choroidal arteries are often present; occasionally early draining veins are observed. Transcranial ultrasound discloses a highly echogenic intraventricular mass with irregular borders and associated hydrocephalus (Fig. 13-58, *C*). Pulsatile vascular channels are sometimes identified.[87]

CT. Three quarters of CPPs are iso- or hyperdense compared to brain on NECT (Fig. 12-40); the remainder are hypodense or mixed density. Calcification is seen in about 25% (Fig. 13-59). Tumor margins are usually slightly irregular, reflecting the frondlike surface of these neoplasms (Fig. 13-60, *A*). Intense, slightly heterogeneous enhancement following con-

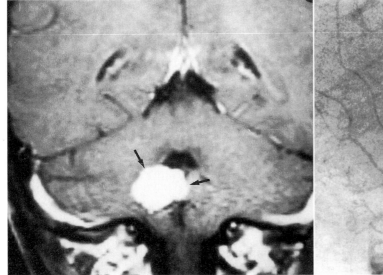
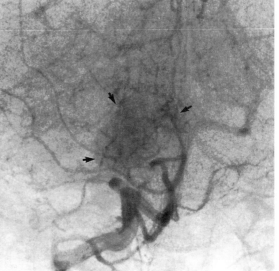

A **B**

Fig. 13-58. Imaging findings of choroid plexus papilloma are illustrated by this series of cases. **A,** Contrast-enhanced coronal T1-weighted MR scan in this 47-year-old woman with headaches shows an intensely enhancing fourth ventricular mass *(arrows)*. **B,** Right vertebral angiogram, midarterial phase, AP view, shows a hypervascular mass with prolonged contrast stain *(arrows).*   *Continued.*

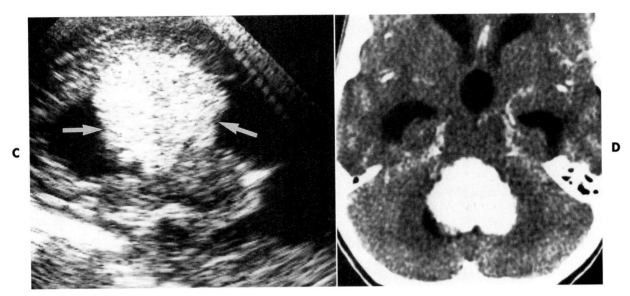

Fig. 13-58, cont'd.   C, Sagittal transcranial ultrasound study in a 7-month-old infant shows a strongly echogenic lateral ventricular mass with somewhat lobulated, irregular surface *(arrows)*. **D,** Axial CECT scan in another patient shows an intensely enhancing lobulated fourth ventricular mass *(arrows)*. Choroid plexus papilloma was found at surgery in all three cases. (**C,** From archives of the Armed Forces Institute of Pathology.)

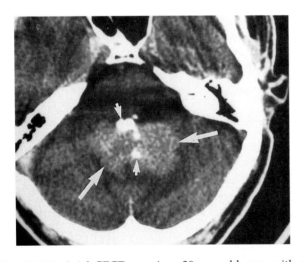

Fig. 13-59. Axial CECT scan in a 38-year-old man with a fourth ventricular choroid plexus papilloma *(large arrows)* shows prominent calcific foci *(small arrows)*.

trast administration is seen in virtually all CPPs (Fig. 13-60, *B*).[82]

MR. Regardless of location the typical MR appearance is that of a large, usually well-delineated lobulated mass that is predominately isointense to brain on T1WI. CSF trapped between the papillae gives most CPPs a somewhat mottled appearance (Fig. 13-60, *B*). CPPs are typically iso- to slightly hyperintense to brain on T2-weighted sequences (Fig. 13-60, *C*). Occasionally, signal voids from the vascular pedicle are observed. CPPs enhance intensely following con-

trast administration (Fig. 13-60, *D*). Hemorrhage occurs with some CPPs (Fig. 13-61).

Severe hydrocephalus that involves all components of the ventricular system is almost invariably present with large lateral ventricular masses (Fig. 13-60, *B*). Limited parenchymal invasion with edema is seen in some cases and does not indicate malignancy (Fig. 13-62). Occasionally, "drop metastases" are identified with histologically benign CPPs (Fig. 13-63).

The imaging differential diagnosis of CPP in a child includes choroid plexus carcinoma, papillary ependymoma, medulloblastoma, hemangioma, hematoma, and astrocytoma. In an adult, meningioma and metastasis can mimic CPP.[88]

Choroid Plexus Carcinoma

Pathology. Choroid plexus carcinomas (CPCs) almost always arise in the lateral ventricles. Grossly, these neoplasms infiltrate adjacent neural tissues. Microscopically, the regular papillary architecture of a CPP is lost and the cells themselves show conspicuous mitoses and histologic atypia.[3]

Incidence, age, clinical presentation, and natural history. Choroid plexus carcinomas (CPCs) are distinctly uncommon, representing only 10% to 20% of all choroid plexus neoplasms.[3] Almost all occur in infants and children 2 to 4 years of age; median age at diagnosis is 26 months.[89] Symptoms are due to hydrocephalus, less commonly to parenchymal inva-

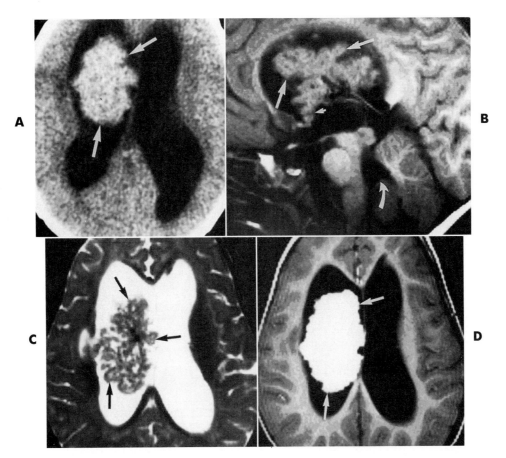

Fig. 13-60. A 10-month-old infant with large head and failure to thrive. **A,** NECT scan shows a hyperdense lobulated mass in the atrium and body of the left lateral ventricle *(arrows)*. **B,** Sagittal T1-weighted MR scan shows the lobulated, somewhat mottled-appearing mass *(large arrows)* has some tumor extension into the foramen of Monro *(small arrow)*. All ventricles, including the fourth *(curved arrow),* are enlarged. **C,** Axial T2WI shows the frondlike tumor surface *(arrows)* particularly well (compare with Fig. 13-57, *B*). The mass is mostly isointense to brain. **D,** Intense enhancement following contrast administration is seen on this axial T1WI. Choroid plexus papilloma was removed.

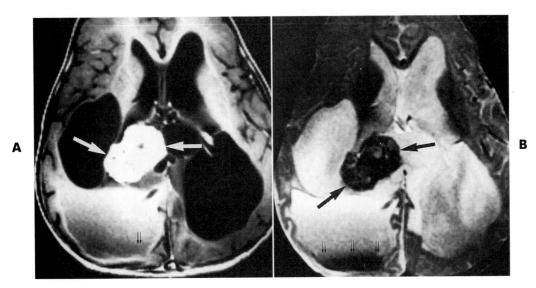

Fig. 13-61. Axial postcontrast T1- **(A)** and T2-weighted **(B)** scans in this 2-year-old child show a mass *(large arrows)* in the atrium of the right lateral ventricle. Note hemorrhage with intraventricular blood-fluid levels *(double arrows)*. The right occipital horn is also encysted and contains proteinaceous fluid that is hyperintense on both T1- and T2WI. Choroid plexus papilloma with intraventricular hemorrhage and xanthochromic fluid in the right occipital horn was found at surgery.

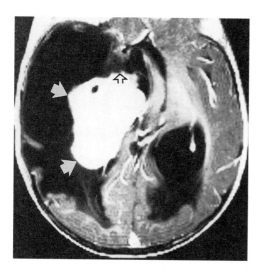

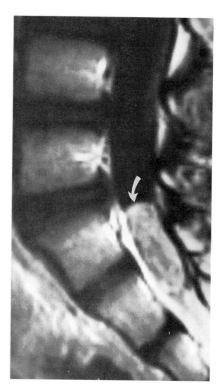

Fig. 13-62. Postcontrast T1-weighted MR scan in this 3-month-old infant with large head shows an intensely enhancing mass *(large arrows)* in the atrium of the right lateral ventricle. Some parenchymal invasion is seen *(open arrow)*. Note severe hydrocephalus. Choroid plexus papilloma was removed; focal thalamic invasion was seen at surgery but the tumor was histologically benign.

Fig. 13-63. Postcontrast sagittal T1-weighted MR scan of the lumbosacral scan was obtained in this 5-year-old child with a choroid plexus papilloma in the left lateral ventricle (not shown). An enhancing mass is seen at the distal thecal sac *(arrow)*. Choroid plexus papilloma was surgically removed; no microscopic evidence for malignancy was seen.

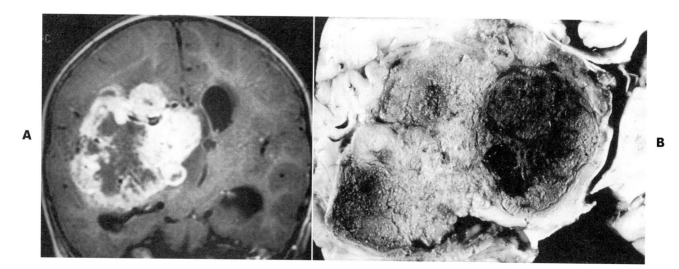

Fig. 13-64. A, Coronal contrast-enhanced MR scan in this 2-year-old child shows an inhomogeneously enhancing mass that invades the basal ganglia. **B,** Coronal gross pathology specimen shows the mass is hemorrhagic and partially necrotic. Choroid plexus carcinoma. (From archives of the Armed Forces Institute of Pathology.)

sion. Prognosis is favorable in patients with gross total surgical resection, although patients with partially resected lesions fare poorly with current treatment regimens.[89]

Imaging. Imaging findings are neither characteristic nor specific. Both benign (Fig. 13-62) and malignant choroid plexus neoplasms may show focal parenchymal invasion (Fig. 13-64). CSF dissemination can occur with either (Fig. 13-63). Signal characteristics and enhancement patterns do not distinguish benign from malignant tumors.

REFERENCES

1. Angevine JB Jr: The neuroglia, *BNI Quart* 4:21-34, 1988.
2. Okazaki H: Neoplasms and related lesions. In *Fundamentals of Neuropathology*, ed 2, pp 203-274, New York, Igaku-Shoin, 1989.
3. Russell DS, Rubinstein LS: *Pathology of Tumors of the Nervous System*, ed 5, Baltimore, Williams and Wilkins, 1989.
4. Zulch KJ: *Histological Typing of Tumors of the Central Nervous System*, International Histological Classification of Tumors, No. 21, World Health Organization, Gerrera, 1979.
5. Burger PC, Vogel FS, Green SB, Strike TA: Glioblastoma multiforme and anaplastic astrocytoma: pathologic criteria and prognostic implications, *Cancer* 56:1106-1111, 1985.
5a. Kleihues P. Burger PC, Scheithauer BW: The new WHO classification of brain tumors, *Brain Pathol* 3:255-268, 1993.
6. Hoshino T, Rodriguez LA, Cho KG et al: Prognostic implication of the proliferative potential of low-grade astrocytomas, *J Neurosurg* 69:839-842, 1988.
7. McCormack BM, Miller DC, Budzilovich GN et al: *Neurosurg* 31:636-642, 1992.
8. Krouwer HGJ, Davis RL, Silver P, Prados M: Gemistocytic astrocytomas: a reappraisal, *J Neurosurg* 74:399-406, 1991.
9. Vertosick FT Jr, Selker RG, Arena VC: Survival of patients with well-differentiated astrocytomas diagnosed in the era of computed tomography, *Neurosurg* 28:496-501, 1991.
10. Burger PC, Scheithauer BW, Vogel FS: *Surgical Pathology of the Nervous System and its Coverings*, ed 3, pp. 193-405, New York: Churchill Livingstone, 1991.
11. Fan KJ, Kovi J, Earle K: The ethnic distribution of primary central nervous system tumors: AFIP 1958 to 1970, *J Neuropathol Exp Neurol* 36:41-49, 1977.
12. Piepmeier JM: Observations in the current treatment of low-grade astrocytic tumors of the cerebral hemispheres, *J Neurosurg* 67:177-181, 1987.
13. Philippon JH, Clemenceau SH, Fauchon FH, Foncin JF: Supratentorial low-grade astrocytomas in adults, *Neurosurg* 32:554-559, 1993.
14. Castillo M, Scatliff JH, Bouldin TW, Sowki K: Radiologic-pathologic correlation: intracranial astrocytoma, *AJNR* 13:1609-1616, 1992.
15. Dean BL, Drayer BP, Bird CR et al: Gliomas: classification with MR imaging, *Radiol* 174:411-415, 1990.
16. Tervonen O, Forbes G, Scheithauer BW, Dietz MJ: Diffuse "fibrillary" astrocytomas: correlation of MRI features with histopathologic parameters and tumor grade, *Neuroradiol* 34:173-178, 1992.
17. Latchaw RE, Johnson DW, Kanal E: Primary intracranial tumors: neuroepithelial tumors, sarcomas, and lymphoma. In Latchaw R (editor), *MR and CT imaging of the Head, Neck, and Spine*, St Louis: Mosby, 1991.
18. Watanabe M, Tanaka R, Takeda N: Magnetic resonance imaging and histopathology of cerebral gliomas, *Neuroradiol* 35:463-469, 1992.
19. Earnest F IV, Kelly PJ, Scheithauer BW et al: Cerebral astrocytomas: histopathologic correlation of MR and CT contrast enhancement with sterotatic biopsy, *Radiol* 166:823-827, 1988.
20. Graff PA, Albright AL, Pang D: Dissemination of supratentorial malignant gliomas via the cerebrospinal fluid in children, *Neurosurg* 30:64-71, 1992.
21. Berkman RA, Clark WC, Saxena A et al: Clonal composition of glioblastoma multiforme, *J Neurosurg* 77:432-437, 1992.
22. Margetts JC, Kalyan-Raman VP: Giant-celled glioblastomas of brain: a clinical pathological and radiological study of ten cases (including immunohistochemistry and ultrastructure), *Cancer* 63:524-531, 1989.
23. Atlas SW: Adult supratentorial tumors, *Sem Roentgenol* 25:130-154, 1990.
24. Forsting M, Albert FK, Kunze S et al: Extirpation of glioblastomas: MR and CT follow-up of residual tumor and regrowth patterns, *AJNR* 14:77-87, 1993.
25. Barnard RO, Geddes JF: The incidence of multifocal gliomas: a histologic study of large hemisphere sections, *Cancer* 60:1519-1531, 1987.
26. Van Tassel P, Lee YY, Bruner JM: Synchronous and metachronous malignant gliomas: CT findings, *AJNR* 9:725-732, 1988.
27. Hasuo K, Fukui M, Tamura S et al: Gliomas with dural invasion: computed tomography and angiography, *CT: J Comp Tomogr* 12:100-107, 1988.
28. Woodruff WW Jr, Djang WT, Voorhees D, Heinz ER: Calvarial destruction: an unusual manifestation of glioblastoma multiforme, *AJNR* 9:388-389, 1988.
29. Meyding-Lamadé V, Forsting M, Albert F et al: Accelerated methaemoglobin formation: potential pitfall in early postoperative MRI, *Neuroradiol* 35:178-180, 1993.
30. Ashdown BC, Boyko OB, Uglietta JP et al: Postradiation cerebellar necrosis mimicking tumor: MR appearance, *J Comp Asst Tomogr* 17:124-126, 1993.
31. Ogawa T, Shishido F, Kanno I et al: Cerebral glioma: evaluation with methionine PET, *Radiol* 186:45-53, 1993.
32. Mineura K, Sasjima T, Kowada M et al: Innovative approach in the diagnosis of gliomatosis cerebri using carbon-11-L-methionine position emission tomography, *J Nuc Med* 32:726-728, 1991.
33. Dickson DW, Horoupian DS, Thal LJ, Lanto G: Gliomatosis cerebri presenting with hydrocephalus and dementia, *AJNR* 9:200-202, 1988.
34. Ross IB, Robitaille Y, Villemure J-G, Tampieri D: Diagnosis and management of gliomatosis cerebri: recent trends, *Surg Neurol* 36:431-440, 1991.
35. Spagnoli MV, Grossman RI, Packer RJ et al: Magnetic resonance determination of gliomatosis cerebri, *Neuroradiol* 29:15-18, 1987.
36. Koslow SA, Claassen D, Hirsch WL, Jungreis CA: Gliomatosis cerebri: a case report with autopsy correlation, *Neuroradiol* 34:331-333, 1992.
37. Yanaka K, Kamozaki T, Kobayashi E et al: MR imaging of diffuse glioma, *AJNR* 13:349-351, 1992.
38. Rippe DJ, Boyko OB, Fuller GN et al: Gadopentetate-dimiglumine-enhanced MR imaging of gliomatosis cerebri: appearance mimicking leptomeningeal tumor dissemination, *AJNR* 11:800-801, 1990.
39. Leproux F, Melanson D, Mercier C et al: Leptomeningeal gliomatosis: MR findings, *J Comp Asst Tomogr* 17:317-320, 1993.
40. Snipes GJ, Steinberg GK, Cane B, Horoupian DS: Gliofibroma, *J Neurosurg* 75:642-646, 1991.
41. Jack CR Jr., Bhansali DT, Chason JL et al: Angiographic features of gliosarcoma, *AJNR* 8:117-122, 1987.
42. Maiuri F, Stella L, Benvenuti D et al: Cerebral gliosarcomas: correlation of computed tomographic findings, surgical aspects, pathological features, and prognosis, *Neurosurg* 26:261-267, 1990.

43. Beute BJ, Fobben ES, Hubschmann O et al: Cerebellar gliosarcoma: report of a prolalle radiation-induced neoplasm, *AJNR* 12:554-556, 1991.

44. Zulch KJ: *Brain Tumors, Their Biology and Pathology,* pp 221-232, Springer-Verlag, 1986.

45. Zimmerman RA: Pediatric supratentorial tumors, *Sem Roentgenol* 25:225-248, 1990.

46. Palma L, Guidetti B: Cystic pilocytic astrocytomas of the cerebral hemispheres, *J Neurosurg* 62:811-815, 1985.

47. Rodriguez LA, Edwards MSB, Levin VA: Management of hypothalamic gliomas in children: an analysis of 33 cases, *Neurosurg* 26:242-247, 1990.

47a. Favre J, Deruaz J-P, de Tribolet N: Pilocytic cerebellar astrocytoma in adults: case report, *Surg Neurol* 39:360-364, 1993.

48. Obana WG, Cogen PH, Davis RL, Edwards MSB: Metastatic juvenile pilocytic astrocytoma, *J Neurosurg* 75:972-975, 1991.

49. Vandertop WP, Hoffman HJ, Drake JM et al: Focal midbrain tumors in children, *Neurosurg* 31:186-194, 1992.

50. Epstein FJ, Farmer J-P: Brain stem glioma growth patterns, *J Neurosurg* 78:408-412, 1993.

50a. Kane AG, Robles HA, Smirniotopoulos JG et al: Diffuse pontine astrocytoma, *AJNR* 14:941-945, 1993.

51. Stroink AR, Hoffman HJ, Hendrick EB, Humphreys RP: Diagnosis and management of pediatric brain-stem gliomas, *J Neurosurg* 65:745-750, 1986.

52. Strong JA, Hatten HP Jr, Brown MT et al: Pilocytic astrocytoma: correlation between the initial imaging features and clinical aggressiveness, *AJR* 161:369-372, 1993.

53. Mishima K, Nakamura M, Nakamura H et al: Leptomeningeal dissemination of cerebellar pilocytic astrocytoma, *J Neurosurg* 77:788-791, 1992.

54. Lee Y-Y, Van Tassel P, Bruner JM et al: Juvenile pilocytic astrocytomas: CT and MR characteristics, *AJNR* 10:363-370, 1989.

55. Smirniotopoulas JG, Parisi J, Murphy F: Cerebral hemispheric astrocytoma: radiologic-pathologic correlation. Presented at the 87th annual meeting of the American Roentgen Ray Society, Miami, Florida, April 26-May 1, 1987.

55a. Kepes JJ: Pleomorphic xanthoastrocytoma: The birth of a diagnosis and a concept, *Brain Pathol* 3:269-274, 1993.

56. Blom RJ: Pleiomorphic xanthoastrocytoma: CT appearance, *J Comp Asst Tomogr* 12:381-352, 1988.

57. Tien RD, Cardenas CA, Rajagopalan S: Pleomorphic xanthoastrocytoma of the brain: MR findings in six patients, *AJR* 159:1287-1290, 1992.

58. Hosokawa Y, Tsuchihashi Y, Okabe H et al: Pleomorphic xanthoastrocytoma, *Cancer* 68:853-859, 1991.

59. Kros JM, Vecht CJ, Stefanko SZ: The pleomorphic xanthoastrocytoma and its differential diagnosis, *Hum Pathol* 22:128-1135, 1991.

60. Yoshino MT, Lucio R: Pleomorphic xanthoastrocytoma, *AJNR* 13:1330-1332, 1992.

61. Shimizu KT, Tran LM, Mark RJ, Selch MT: Management of oligodendrogliomas, *Radiol* 186:569-972, 1993.

62. Dolinskas CA, Simeone FA: CT characteristics of intraventicular oligodendrogliomas, *AJNR* 8:1077-1082, 1987.

63. Shaw EG, Scheithauer BW, O'Fallon JR et al: Oligodendrogliomas: the Mayo clinic experience, *J Neurosurg* 76:428-434, 1992.

64. Kyritsis AP, Yung WKA, Bruner J et al: The treatment of anaplastic oligodendrogliomas and mixed gliomas, *Neurosurg* 32:365-371, 1993.

65. Cairncross JG, MacDonald DR, Ramsay DA: Aggressive oligodendroglioma: a chemosensitive tumor, *Neurosurg* 31:78-82, 1992.

66. Tekkok IH, Ayberk G, Saglam S, Onol B: Primary intraventricular oligodendroglioma, *Neurochir* 35:63-66, 1992.

67. Lee Y-Y, Van Tassel P: Intracranial oligodendrogliomas: imaging findings in 39 untreated cases, *AJNR* 10:119-127, 1989.

67a. Cheng TM, Coffey RJ, Gelber BR, Scheithauer BW: Simultaneous presentation of symptomatic subependymomas in siblings: case reports and review, *Neurosurg* 33:145-150, 1993.

67b. Ikezaki K, Matsushima T, Inoue T et al: Correlation of microanatomical localization with postoperative survival in posterior fossa ependymomas, *Neurosurg* 32:38-44, 1993.

68. Nazar GB, Hoffman HJ, Becker LE et al: Infratentorial ependymomas in childhood: prognostic factors and treatment, *J Neurosurg* 72:408-417, 1990.

69. Lyons MK, Kelly PJ: Posterior fossa ependymoma: Report of 30 cases and review of the literature, *Neurosurg* 28:659-672, 1991.

70. Palma L, Celli P, Cantore G: Supratentorial ependymomas of the first two decades of life: long-term follow-up of 20 cases (including two subependymoma), *Neurosurg* 32:169-175, 1993.

71. Armington WG, Osborn AG, Cubberley DA et al: Supratentorial ependymoma: CT appearance, *Radiol* 157:367-372, 1985.

72. Swartz GP, Zimmerman RA, Bilaniuk LT: Computed tomography of intracranial ependymoma, *Radiol* 143:97-101, 1982.

73. Lizak PF, Woodruff WW: Posterior fossa neoplasms: multiplanar imaging, *Sem US, CT, MR* 13:182-206, 1992.

74. Spoto GP, Press GA, Hesselink JR, Solomon M: Intracranial ependymoma and subependymoma: MR manifestations, *AJNR* 11:83-91, 1990.

75. Lobato RD, Sarabia M, Casto S et al: Symptomatic subependymoma: report of four new cases studied with computed tomography and review of the literature, *Neurosurg* 19:594-598, 1986.

76. Jelenik J, Smirniotopoulos JG, Parisi JE, Kanzer M: Lateral ventricular neoplasms of the brain: differential diagnosis based on clinical, CT, and MR findings, *AJNR* 11:567-574, 1990.

77. Artico M, Bardella L, Ciapetta P, Raco A: Surgical treatment of subependymomas of the central nervous system, *Acta Neurochir (Wien)* 98:25-31, 1989.

78. DiLorenzo N, Rizzo A, Ciapetta P: Subependymoma of the septum pellucidum presenting as subarachnoid hemorrhage, *Neurochir* 34:125-126, 1991.

79. Lindboe CF, Stolt-Nielsen A, Dale LG: Hemorrhage in a highly vascularized subependymoma of the septum pellucidum: case report, *Neurosurg* 31:741-745, 1992.

80. Kim DG, Han MH, Lee SH et al: MRI of intracranial subependymoma: report of a case, *Neuroradiol* 35:185-186, 1993.

81. Buchino JJ, Mason KG: Choroid plexus papilloma: report of a case with cytologic differential diagnosis, *Acta Cytol* 36:95-97, 1992.

82. Shoemaker EI, Romano AS, Gado M: Neuroradiology case of the day: choroid plexus papilloma, third ventricle, *AJR* 152:1333-1338, 1989.

83. Ken JG, Sobel DF, Copeland B et al: Choroid plexus papillomas of the foramen of Luschka: MR appearance, *AJNR* 12:1201-1202, 1991.

84. Cila A, Ozturk C, Senaati S: Bilateral choroid plexus carcinomas of the lateral ventricles, *Pediati Radiol* 22:136-137, 1992.

85. Domingues RC, Taveras JM, Reimer P, Rosen BR: Foramen magnum choroid plexus papilloma with drop metastases to the lumbar spine, *AJNR* 12:564-565, 1991.

86. Kimura M, Takayasu M, Suzuki Y et al: Primary choroid plexus papilloma located in the suprasellar region: case report, *Neurosurg* 31:563-566, 1992.

87. Schelhas KP, Siebert RC, Heithoff KB, Franciosi RA: Congenital choroid plexus papilloma of the third ventricle: diagnosis with real-time sonography and MR imaging, *AJNR* 9:797-798, 1988.

88. Coates TL, Hinshaw DBJ Jr, Peckman N et al: Pediatric choroid plexus neoplasms: MR, CT, and pathologic correlation, *Radiol* 173:81-88, 1989.

89. Packer RJ, Perilongo G, Johnson D et al: Choroid plexus carcinoma of childhood, *Cancer* 69:580-585, 1992.

14

Meningiomas and Other Nonglial Neoplasms

Approximately one half of all primary brain tumors are gliomas. The other half are derived from a spectrum of nonglial sources. We first turn our attention to an uncommon but fascinating group of primary neoplasms and neoplastic-like masses that represents a transition between glial and neuron-derived tumors. These are the ganglion cell tumors, dysplastic masses, and central neurocytoma.

We then consider the most common of all nonglial primary brain tumors: meningioma. Our discussion of primary brain tumors next turns to a spectrum of other nonglial neoplasms that ranges from pineal germinomas and pineal parenchymal tumors to embryonal, or "primitive," tumors such as primitive neuroectodermal tumor (PNET) and medulloblastoma (PNET-MB). We conclude this chapter by discussing the uncommon but increasingly more frequent primary CNS lymphoma.

MIXED GLIAL-NEURONAL AND NEURONAL TUMORS

This interesting group of unusual primary brain tumors includes the ganglion cell tumors, ganglioglioma and gangliocytoma, and central neurocytoma (*see* box p. 580). Neoplasms that contain mature neurons are designated ganglioglioma or gangliocytoma. Both are contingent on the microscopic identification of well-differentiated but neoplastic neurons within the tumor.[1]

Glial-neuronal tumors contain varying mixtures of differentiated but abnormal ganglion cells and glial

Ganglion Cell Tumors
Ganglioglioma (mixed glial, neuronal elements) and ganglioneuroma (pure ganglionic tumor) Gangliocytoma (probably dysplastic brain, not a true tumor) Lhermitte-Duclos disease (dysplastic cerebellar gangliocytoma; probably a malformation, not a true neoplasm) Dysembryoplastic neuroepithelial tumor (DNET)

Ganglioglioma
Pathology Cyst with mural nodule **Age, presentation** Children, young adults with seizures **Location** Typically temporal, frontal lobes **Imaging** Well-delineated cyst with partially calcified mural nodule most common; bone changes common if lesion is superficial

stroma.[2] Mixed tumors, designated ganglioglioma, are more common than pure ganglionic tumors (ganglioneuroma). Another type of ganglion cell tumor, gangliocytoma, is probably a dysplastic hamartoma similar to Lhermitte-Duclos disease. Gangliocytoma must also be distinguished from hamartomas and migrational abnormalities. Imaging studies can be critical in the preoperative diagnosis of these fascinating tumors.

Ganglioglioma and Ganglioneuroma

Courville first used the term *ganglioglioma* in 1930 to describe an unusual primary CNS tumor that contained both neuronal and glial elements. Ganglioglioma is thus conceptually a neoplasm that represents a transition between glial and nonglial tumors.

Pathology

Gross pathology. *Gangliogliomas* are usually small, firm, well-circumscribed masses. A cyst with a partially calcified mural nodule is common[3] (*see* box above *right*).

Microscopic appearance. Well-differentiated but neoplastic ganglion cells are mixed with glial stroma containing astrocytes or, occasionally, oligodendrocytes.[2] The abnormal neurons in these tumors must be distinguished from neoplastic glia that may resemble neurons and from normal neurons intermixed with infiltrative glioma.[1]

So-called *ganglioneuromas* are ganglion cell tumors in which mature neuronal components are the dominant component. Because they are histologically similar to and biologically indistinguishable from ganglioglioma, we will not consider them as a separate tumor.

Desmoplastic infantile ganglioglioma is an uncommon ganglioglioma subtype that occurs exclusively in infants. These neoplasms are typically large cystic frontal-lobe tumors. A meningeal-based nodule that has glial and ganglionic differentiation accompanied by an extreme desmoplastic reaction is usually present.[4,5]

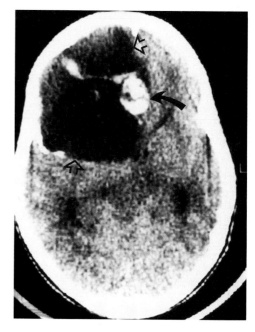

Fig. 14-1. Axial NECT scan in a 14-year-old with headache shows a large right frontal cystic mass *(open arrows)* with a calcified mural nodule *(curved arrow)*. No enhancement was seen following contrast administration. Ganglioglioma.

Age, clinical presentation, and natural history. Gangliogliomas occur in children and young adults. Between 60% to 80% of patients are under 30 years of age[3]; most become symptomatic during the second decade.[6] Seizures are the most common presenting symptom,[7,8,8a] followed by signs of increased intracranial pressure.[6]

Gangliogliomas are very slow-growing tumors. Symptoms have often been present for years, and long-term survival is the rule, even with incompletely resected lesions.[6] Very rare cases of leptomeningeal and subarachnoid dissemination of ganglioglioma have been reported.[9,10]

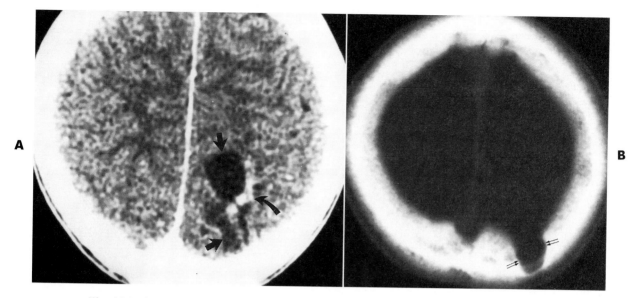

Fig. 14-2. A 9-year-old girl with long-standing seizures had a contrast-enhanced CT scan. **A,** Soft tissue windows show a cystic *(straight arrows)*, partially calcified *(curved arrow)* high left parietal mass. **B,** Slightly higher cut with bone window shows focal calvarial erosion *(arrows)*. Ganglioglioma was found at surgery.

Incidence. Reported incidence varies from 0.4% to 6%; the higher percentages reflect series with predominately pediatric patients.[11] The overall frequency is probably 0.5% to 1% of all primary CNS neoplasms.[8]

Location. Although gangliogliomas may occur in any location, the majority are supratentorial. The temporal lobe is the most common site, followed by the frontal and parietal lobes.[12,13] The cerebellum is also a reported site.[14,15]

Imaging

CT. The classic appearance is a cyst with an iso- or hypodense mural nodule that is often calcified (Fig. 14-1).[7,8] However, gangliomas have variable density and contrast enhancement patterns, and calcification may be inconspicuous.[6] Because these tumors are slow growing, peripherally located gangliogliomas may cause scalloped pressure erosion of the overlying calvarium (Fig. 14-2).

MR. MR findings are also nonspecific. The most common appearance is a well-delineated frontal or temporal lobe mass that is hypointense on T1- and hyperintense on T2-weighted sequences (Fig. 14-3 *A* and *B*).[16] Enhancement varies from none to striking.[15] Nodular, rim, and solid enhancement patterns all occur (Fig. 14-3 *C*).[8,15,16]

Gangliocytoma

The term *gangliocytoma* has been used to describe purely neuronal tumors that lack a glial component

and do not show neoplastic change.[17] Most, if not all, of the reported cases are probably dysplastic brain.[17,18] Histologic studies in patients with malformative disorders such as unilateral megalencephaly may show bizarre-appearing neurons associated with an increase in the number and size of astrocytes.[19] MR imaging in cases with the microscopic diagnosis of gangliocytoma often shows clear evidence for brain malformation and dysplasia rather than neoplasia (Fig. 14-4).

Lhermitte-Duclos Disease

Lhermitte-Duclos disease, also known as *dysplastic cerebellar gangliocytoma*, is characterized by progressive hypertrophy of the cerebellar folia. The etiology of this disorder is controversial, and satisfactory classification is difficult. Lhermitte-Duclos disease is probably a brain malformation and not a true neoplasm.

The normal cerebellar cortex consists of the following three layers:

1. Outer, or molecular, layer
2. Purkinje (middle) layer
3. Inner, or granular, layer

In Lhermitte-Duclos disease an abnormal population of large neurons is present in the granular layer and there is aberrant myelination in the molecular layer.[20] The cerebellar cortex appears grossly thickened and dysplastic. MR findings are those of an expanding mass with laminated, increased signal on T2WI (*see* Figs. 4-16 and 4-17).

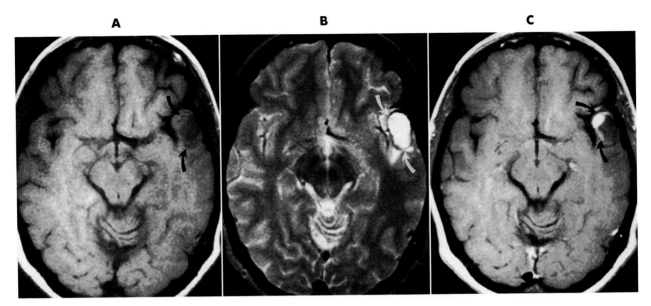

Fig. 14-3. Long-standing temporal lobe seizures in this 24-year-old patient prompted MR examination. **A,** Axial T1-weighted scan without contrast enhancement shows a well-delineated mass *(arrows)* that is slightly hypointense compared to surrounding brain. **B,** The mass *(arrows)* is hyperintense on T2WI. **C,** Postcontrast T1WI shows nodular rim enhancement *(arrows)*. Ganglioglioma was found at temporal lobe resection. (Reprinted from Osborn AG, Hendrick RE: Categorical course on MR imaging, Radiological Society of North America, 1990. With permission.)

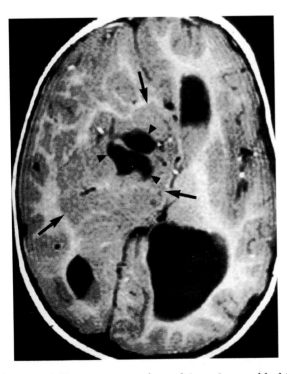

Fig. 14-4. MR scan was performed in a 6-year-old child with seizures. Axial T1WI shows a right hemisphere mass *(arrows)* that is isointense with gray matter. Low signal foci *(arrowheads)* are seen within the mass. Biopsy showed mature but disorganized neurons and ganglion cells and was called gangliocytoma. This is a dysplastic cerebral hemisphere with heterotopic gray matter. The low signal area is a partially formed ventricle. (Courtesy P. Davis.)

Dysembryoplastic Neuroepithelial Tumor (DNET)

Dysembryoplastic neuroepithelial tumor (DNET) is a newly described pathologic entity that is sometimes the underlying cause for partial complex seizures. Pathologically these tumors are benign lesions that are occasionally cystic and show at least one of the following three characteristics:[21,21a]

1. Specific glioneuronal element
2. Nodular component
3. Association with cortical dysplasia

MR scans show a focal cortical (usually temporal lobe) lesion that is hypointense on T1- and hyperintense on T2-weighted studies. Some cases resemble benign cysts with slightly increased signal on proton density-weighted sequences. Differentiation from low-grade astrocytoma and ganglioglioma on MR is not possible.[22]

Central Neurocytoma

Central neurocytoma is a recently recognized clinicopathologic entity that is histologically distinct from ganglion cell tumors, neuroblastomas, and primitive neuroectodermal tumors. Central neurocytomas have morphologic and immunohistochemical features of neuronal differentiation.[22a]

Pathology

Gross pathology. Central neurocytoma is a well-defined, sharply circumscribed, lobulated intraventricular mass that typically lies adjacent to the foramen of Monro or septum pellucidum[1] (*see* box). Necrosis and cyst formation are common.[3] Some neurocytomas are extensively vascularized[23]; frank intraventricular hemorrhage can occur but is uncommon.[24]

Microscopic appearance. Light microscopy shows features that are indistinguishable from oligodendroglioma. Electron microscopy demonstrates the neurosecretory granules, synapses, microtubules, and neuritic processes that confirm the neuronal origin of this tumor. Immunohistochemical studies show consistent and uniform expression of the neuronal marker proteins, neuron-specific enolase and synaptophysin.[23,25]

Age, clinical presentation, and natural history
Age. Neurocytomas are tumors of young adults. The average age of reported patients is 31 years, ranging from 17 to 53 years.[26] Duration of clinical symptoms is usually less than 6 months. Common presentation is headache with signs of increased intracranial pressure.[26]

A striking characteristic of central neurocytoma is its benign biologic activity. A recent review reported survival up to 19 years; no patients had died from tumor growth or recurrent neoplasm.[24]

Incidence. Central neurocytomas account for approximately 0.5% of primary brain tumors.[23,27]

Location. The lateral ventricle is the most common site; most central neurocytomas are located adjacent to the foramen of Monro. No tumor involved the occipital or temporal horns or atria of the lateral ventricles. All but one case were confined to the ventricles. A few cases that extended into the third ventricle were reported; to date, none is reported in the fourth ventricle.[26] Three cases of hemispheric (cerebral) neurocytomas have been reported.[28]

Imaging
Angiography. Angiographic findings are reported in only a few cases. Some tumors show moderate to marked vascularity, although most are avascular masses that produce moderate ventricular enlargement (Fig. 14-5, *A*).[23]

Central Neurocytoma

Pathology
Looks like oligodendroglioma on light microscopy
Electron microscopy shows neurosecretory granules, synapses
Immunohistochemistry shows neuronal marker proteins (e.g., synaptophysin)

Age
Young adults

Location
Lateral ventricles near foramen of Monro

Imaging
Inhomogeneous, partially calcified, mildly enhancing lateral ventricular mass

---

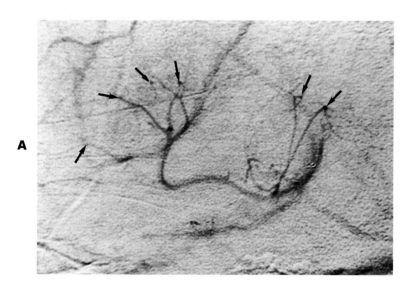

Fig. 14-5. Typical imaging findings of a central neurocytoma. Right internal carotid angiogram, venous phase, lateral view, **(A)** shows elongated, stretched subependymal veins *(arrows)*, indicating moderate hydrocephalus. No vascular stain was identified.

Continued.

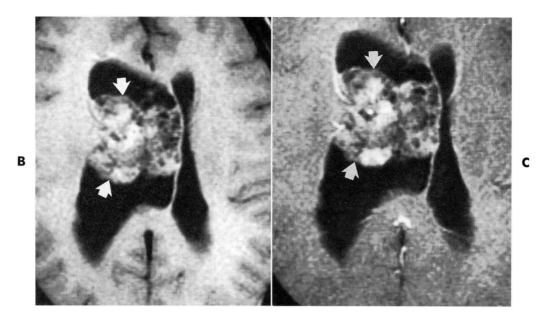

Fig. 14-5, cont'd. Pre- **(B)** and postcontrast **(C)** axial T1-weighted MR scans show a mixed hypo-/isointense right lateral ventricular mass *(arrows)* that enhances moderately but inhomogeneously following contrast administration. Central neurocytoma was found at surgery.

CT. NECT scans show an iso- or slightly hyperdense mass within the body of the lateral ventricle adjacent to the foramen of Monro. Most central neurocytomas contain multiple small cysts and exhibit a characteristic broad-based attachment to the superolateral ventricular wall.[29] Tumor calcification is seen in the majority of cases and is usually clumped, coarse, or globular.[26] Contrast enhancement is mild to moderate. Hydrocephalus is almost always present.[30]

MR. Most neurocytomas are inhomogeneously isointense on T1WI. Low or absent signal areas are seen with calcific foci and tumor vessels. Signal on T2-weighted sequences is variable; some neurocytomas remain relatively isointense with cortex, whereas others are moderately hyperintense. Contrast enhancement is inhomogeneous and varies from none to moderate (Fig. 14-5, *B* and *C*).[30]

The imaging differential diagnosis of central neurocytoma includes other intraventricular tumors that occur in young adults, i.e., oligodendroglioma, subependymal giant cell astrocytoma, low-grade or pilocytic astrocytoma, and ependymoma.[31]

MENINGEAL AND MESENCHYMAL TUMORS

The meninges have been called bland fibrous vestments of a magnificent organ. However, as the same neuropathologists who made that observation have noted, the cranial meninges have their own special spectrum of distinctive and important pathologic lesions.[1] In this section we consider meningeal neo-

---

Meningeal and Mesenchymal Tumors
Meningioma
Nonmeningotheliomatous mesenchymal tumors
Benign osteocartilagenous tumors (e.g., osteoma, enchondroma)
Malignant mesenchymal tumors (chondrosarcoma, fibrosarcoma, angiosarcoma)
Primary melanocytic lesions
Hemangiopericytoma
Hemangioblastoma

plasms, beginning with meningiomas, and then discuss nonmeningothelial mesenchymal neoplasms such as angiosarcoma and fibrosarcoma (*see* box). We conclude by discussing two related tumors: hemangiopericytoma and hemangioblastoma.

Meningioma

Although a broad spectrum of neoplasms can originate from the cranial meninges, meningioma is by far the most common.[32] Meningioma is the most common nonglial primary brain tumor.[3] We begin our discussion of these important neoplasms by delineating their etiology and pathology, then turn to the various imaging features of meningiomas.

Etiology. Histologic, chromosomal, biochemical, and receptor studies have significantly advanced the understanding of meningioma pathogenesis.[33,34]

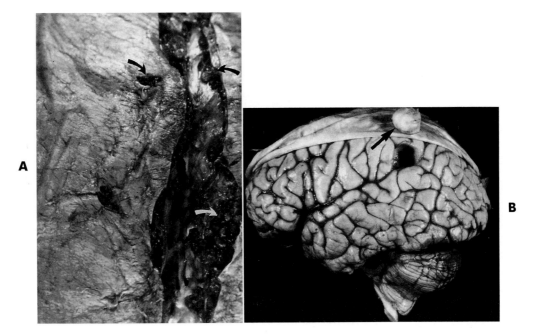

Fig. 14-6. A, The dura and superior sagittal sinus (SSS) from an autopsy case are seen from above. The SSS is opened to show the numerous arachnoid granulations *(arrows)* that project into its lumen. **B,** Autopsy specimen illustrates the location and appearance of a typical small convexity meningioma *(arrow).* Note invaginated adjacent brain. **(A,** Courtesy E. Ross. **B,** From Okazaki H, Scheithauer B: *Slide Atlas of Neuropathology,* Gower Medical Publishing. With permission.)

Histology. Any meningothelial cell, whether intracranial, intradiploic, spinal, or ectopic, can potentially give rise to a meningioma.[33] Most meningiomas originate from specialized meningothelial cells in arachnoid granulations, the so-called arachnoid cap cells (Fig. 14-6).[34] A few meningiomas probably arise from dural fibroblasts, whereas others arise from the arachnoid that is associated with cranial nerves and the choroid plexus.

Cytogenetics. Chromosome 22 is important in the pathogenesis of meningiomas.[34a] Monosomy occurs in 72% of cases and long-arm deletions are common.[34] Neurofibromatosis type 2 (NF-2) is the major genetic condition that predisposes to meningioma formation *(see* Chapter 5).

Receptor activity. Several clinical features suggest meningiomas may be related to sex hormones. Meningiomas are more common in women, are correlated positively with breast carcinoma, and sometimes increase in size during pregnancy. Progesterone and, possibly, estrogen or androgen receptors have been demonstrated in many meningiomas.[34]

Miscellaneous factors. Radiation therapy appears to be a predisposing factor in the development of some meningiomas.[34b]

Pathology

Gross pathology. Meningiomas assume two basic gross morphologic configurations: a spherical or lob-

ulated mass that is sometimes termed "globose" meningioma (Fig. 14-7, *A*) and a flatter, carpetlike "en plaque" lesion that infiltrates dura and also sometimes invades underlying bone (Fig. 14-7, *B*).[1] The dural attachment that underlies most meningiomas can be broad, giving rise to a sessile-appearing tumor, or narrow and stalklike with a pedunculated tumor mass.

Meningiomas are usually sharply circumscribed lesions with a well-delineated tumor-brain interface.[35] The surface of most meningiomas appears lobulated or bosselated. A distinct "cleft" of arachnoid with trapped CSF and prominent vessels that surround the extraaxial mass is often observed (Fig. 14-8).[36]

Consistency of meningiomas varies from soft to tough or even gritty, depending on the fibrous tissue or calcification present.[1] Necrotic and hemorrhagic foci are often present, although gross hemorrhage is uncommon. Cystic and xanthomatous changes are sometimes observed.[1] A "collar" of reactive thickened dura often surrounds the meningioma base (see subsequent discussion).

Classification and microscopic appearance. Recent advances in the pathologic delineation of meningiomas include the development of a simplified classification system, the use of markers to evaluate meningioma proliferative activity and potential aggressiveness, and the delineation of malignant phenotypes.

Several classification schemes for categorizing

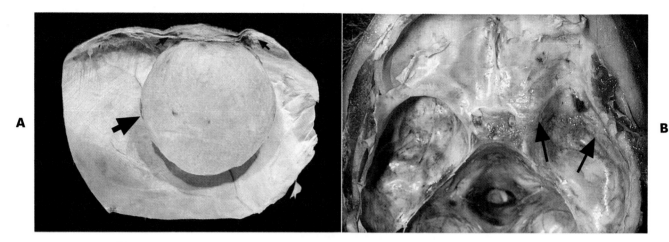

Fig. 14-7. A, Autopsy specimen illustrates a typical "globose" meningioma *(large arrow).* Note collar of thickened reactive dura *(small arrows)* that surrounds its attachment site. **B,** A sphenoid wing meningioma has a flatter, "en plaque" appearance *(arrows).* (**A,** From Royal College of Surgeons of England, *Slide Atlas of Pathology,* Gower Medical Publishing. By permission. **B,** From Okazaki H, Scheithauer B: *Slide Atlas of Neuropathology,* Gower Medical Publishing. With permission.)

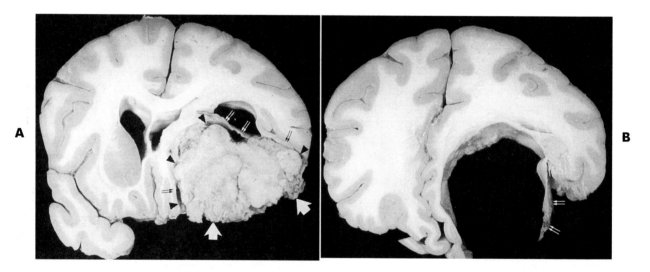

Fig. 14-8. Coronal autopsy specimens of a patient with a large sphenoid wing meningioma. **A,** The tumor is seen *in situ.* The mass *(large arrows)* has invaginated deeply into the brain. Note distinct cleft *(arrowheads)* that separates the tumor from adjacent brain. A fibrous pseudocapsule is indicated *(double white arrows).* Displaced cortex *(double black arrows)* indicates the extraaxial location of the mass. **B,** Specimen with the tumor removed shows the fibrous pseudocapsule *(arrows).* (Reprinted from Sheporaitis L, Osborn AG et al: Radiologic-pathologic correlation of intracranial meningioma, *AJNR,* 13:29-37, 1992.)

meningiomas have been promulgated *(see* box). Russell and Rubinstein's modification of Cushing's system divides these tumors into meningotheliomatous (syncytial), fibrous, transitional, and angioblastic types.[3] The World Health Organization (WHO) divides meningiomas into three basic categories: (1) meningioma (i.e., the common or typical "benign" meningioma), (2) atypical meningioma, and (3) anaplastic (malignant) meningioma.[36a]

Meningiomas are histologically heterogeneous neoplasms. Psammomatous calcifications and meningothelial cells that aggregate into whorls and lobules are present in many—but by no means all—meningiomas. These features characterize the so-called meningotheliomatous, or syncytial, meningioma. Other meningiomas have interlacing sheets and fascicles of markedly elongated spindle-shaped cells that sometimes exhibit a prominent storiform appearance. Abundant reticular and collagenous fibers are common in this type of meningioma, the so-called fibrous

<table>
<tr><td colspan="2">

Classification of Meningiomas

Classic description

Meningotheliomatous (syncytial) meningioma
Fibrous meningioma
Transitional meningioma
Angioblastic meningioma

World Health Organization (WHO)

Meningioma (typical "benign" meningioma)
Atypical meningioma
Anaplastic (malignant) meningioma

</td></tr>
</table>

<table>
<tr><td>

Meningioma: Etiology and Epidemiology

Etiology

Arise from specialized meningothelial cells called arachnoid "cap" cells
Chromosome 22 (association with NF-2)
Progesterone, estrogen receptors in meningiomas

Incidence

Most common nonglial primary CNS tumor
15% to 20% of primary brain tumors
Subtypes
  88% to 95% typical meningioma
  5% to 7% atypical meningioma
  1% to 2% anaplastic (malignant) meningioma
Multiple in 1% to 9%
Part of NF-2 syndrome

Age, gender

Peak incidence 40 to 60 years
Rare in children (often atypical location or histology)
Female:male = 2:1 to 4:1

Natural history

Most important factors are location, resectability
Local recurrence rate varies
Metastases rare, *but* both benign and malignant meningiomas can metastasize

</td></tr>
</table>

meningioma. Other meningiomas exhibit a mixture of these features and represent a "transitional" type.[1]

Some meningiomas are highly cellular and very vascular. These tumors, formerly called "angioblastic" meningiomas, are probably tumors that arise from blood vessels and are now classified as hemangiopericytomas (see subsequent discussion).

Little prognostic significance can be attached to the morphologic variations of meningiomas, described previously.[1] Many neuropathologists now use the simple WHO classification, which correlates with biologic behavior (see subsequent discussion) and is therefore the preferred system. In the WHO classification, 88% to 94% of meningiomas are benign or typical, 5% to 7% are atypical, and only 1% to 2% are anaplastic or malignant.[37,38]

Incidence. Meningiomas are the most common nonglial primary brain tumor and the most common intracranial extraaxial neoplasm[33] (*see* box, *right*). They account for 15% to 20% of all primary brain tumors. Meningiomas occur at a rate of 2 or 3 per 100,000 population.[34]

Age, gender, and clinical presentation

Age and gender. Meningiomas are basically adult tumors; the peak occurrence is between 40 and 60 years of age. Incidence in women outnumbers that in men—2:1 to 4:1.[33]

Only 1% to 2% of all meningiomas occur in children less than 16 years of age.[34] Meningiomas account for 1% to 3% of pediatric intracranial tumors.[39,40] When they occur in this age group they are often located in unusual sites such as the posterior fossa or lateral ventricles (Fig. 14-9).[34,34c]

Clinical presentation. Less than 10% of all meningiomas ever cause symptoms.[41] Many are discovered incidentally on imaging studies or at autopsy.

Clinical manifestations associated with symptomatic meningiomas vary significantly with location. Seizure and hemiparesis are common presentations

for convexity or parasagittal tumors. Basisphenoid lesions usually cause visual field defects, whereas cavernous sinus meningiomas are associated with multiple cranial nerve palsies. Frontal (cribriform plate) meningiomas often become very large before causing symptoms other than anosmia.

Location. (*see* box, p. 588). Most meningiomas are extraaxial dural-based lesions. Ninety percent are supratentorial.[42]

Meningiomas typically occur along intradural venous sinuses, at the confluences of multiple cranial sutures and at other sites where arachnoid granulations and arachnoid cell rests occur (Fig. 14-6).[42] The parasagittal region and cerebral convexities are common sites (Fig. 14-10; *see* box, p. 588), accounting for nearly half of all meningiomas. Convexity meningiomas arise from the dura that overlies the cerebral hemispheres. The coronal suture is a common site. Most parasagittal meningiomas arise along the middle third of the superior sagittal sinus (SSS); only 15% occur along the posterior SSS.[42] Parasagittal meningiomas often grow into and then occlude the SSS.

A third common site is the sphenoid ridge. Approximately one third of these tumors originate around the anterior clinoid process and often involve

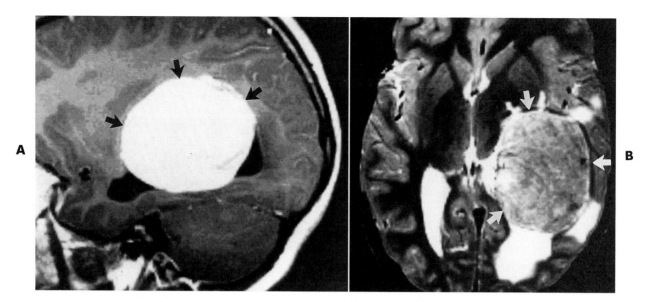

Fig. 14-9. **A,** Sagittal postcontrast T1-weighted MR scan in this 8-year-old girl without neurofibromatosis shows a large, intensely enhancing intraventricular mass *(arrows).* **B,** Axial T2WI shows the mass *(arrows)* is mostly isointense with cortex. Meningioma.

Meningioma
Location

General

Arachnoid granulations, along dural sinuses, at sutures

Specific

25% parasagittal
20% convexity
15% to 20% sphenoid ridge
5% to 10% olfactory groove
5% to 10% parasellar
10% posterior fossa (near porus acousticus, along clivus)
2% other (intraventricular, pineal region, optic nerve sheath)
1% extracranial (nose, sinuses, skull)

the optic canal. The remainder arise along the middle or lateral (pterional) aspects of the sphenoid wing.[42] Sphenoid wing meningiomas are often en plaque tumors.

Anterior basal or olfactory groove meningiomas account for 5% to 10% of meningiomas. These tumors often attain large size before causing symptoms other than anosmia. Another 5% to 10% of meningiomas arise in the sellar region. Juxta- and suprasellar meningiomas can originate from the cavernous sinus dura, tuberculum, dorsum, or diaphragma sellae and cause cranial nerve palsies or visual symptoms. Cav-

ernous sinus meningiomas can be either uni- or bilateral and often extend posteriorly to involve the tentorium.

Posterior fossa sites account for approximately 10% of meningiomas. The posterior surface of the petrous temporal bone and clivus are the most common infratentorial locations.

Approximately 2% of intracranial meningiomas have no dural attachment. These tumors arise from choroid plexus stromal cells or the tela choroidea and grow as intraventricular masses[43] (Fig. 14-9). They are usually confined to the ventricles but occasionally penetrate into adjacent brain (*see* Fig. 14-33).[42] Other uncommon meningioma sites include the optic nerve sheath and pineal region.

Approximately 1% of meningiomas arise outside the CNS dura. The most common extradural site is the paranasal sinuses. Other locations include the nasal cavity, parotid gland, and even the skin.[44-46] Primary calvarial meningiomas are rare. They have been reported in the diploic, calvarial, extra-calvarial, and subgaleal spaces.[47] Meningioma locations are depicted in Fig. 14-10.

Multiple meningiomas occur in 1% to 9% of imaged cases[48]; 16% are multiple at autopsy.[42] Most occur in women. Multiple meningiomas should be differentiated from meningiomatosis, a manifestation of neurofibromatosis type 2 (NF-2) (*see* Figs. 5-17 to 5-22).

Natural history. The most important factors in clinical outcome of meningioma are location and resectability.[49] Tumors with the same histologic pattern

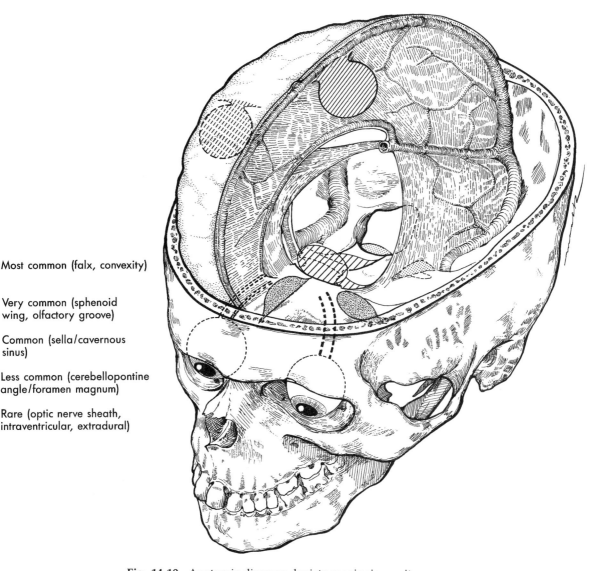

Most common (falx, convexity)

Very common (sphenoid wing, olfactory groove)

Common (sella/cavernous sinus)

Less common (cerebellopontine angle/foramen magnum)

Rare (optic nerve sheath, intraventricular, extradural)

Fig. 14-10. Anatomic diagram depicts meningioma sites.

and cytologic characteristics have significantly different outcomes that depend on location. For example, a convexity meningioma that is completely removed has a vastly better prognosis than an identical tumor that involves the cavernous sinus and skull base.[49]

Using the WHO criteria, there are also significant differences in recurrence rates for the different types of meningioma. For histologically typical (benign) meningiomas the 5-year recurrence rate is only 3% to 7%. For atypical tumors the recurrence rate is about one third, whereas it approaches 75% for anaplastic (malignant) meningiomas.[37,38]

Meningioma metastases are rare, occurring in 0.1% to 0.2% of these tumors. Location and even histopathology do not correlate with metastases; some metastatic tumors are histologically benign (Fig. 14-11), whereas some anaplastic meningiomas do not metastasize.[49]

Imaging (*see* box, p. 593)
Plain film radiography. Bone erosion, enlarged vascular channels, hyperostosis, tumoral calcification, and expanded paranasal sinus (pneumosinus dilatans, sometimes seen with anterior basal tumors) are plain film findings of meningioma (Fig. 14-12).[50,51]

Angiography. The majority of meningiomas are vascular tumors. Because most are dural-based (Fig. 14-13, *A*), they are initially supplied entirely by meningeal vessels such as the middle meningeal and anterior falcine arteries. Large tumors can also parasitize adjacent pial branches. In these cases there is a dual vascular supply (Fig. 14-13, *B*). The central portion is supplied by meningeal vessels, whereas the periphery is vascularized by the anterior, middle, or posterior cerebral arteries.[52]

The typical parasagittal or convexity meningioma

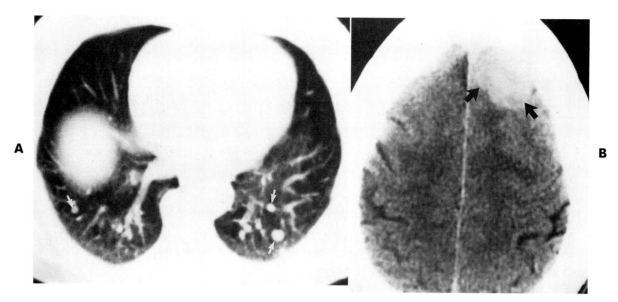

Fig. 14-11. A 62-year-old woman with unexplained weight loss had a chest radiograph (not shown) that demonstrated multiple pulmonary nodules. **A,** Axial CT scan shows the multiple nodules *(arrows).* The hilar areas were normal. An isotope bone scan was performed as part of the clinical evaluation and a skull lesion was identified. **B,** CECT scan showed an enhancing, dural-based left frontal mass *(arrows)* most consistent with meningioma. Biopsy of both the lung nodules and intracranial mass disclosed typical meningioma. The tumors in both sites were histologically benign. (Courtesy W. Coit.)

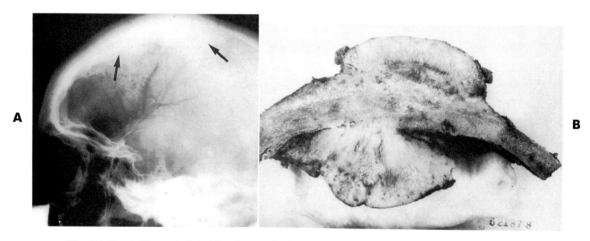

Fig. 14-12. A, Lateral plain film shows thickened, hyperostotic skull *(arrows).* **B,** Resected surgical specimen shows a meningioma that involves the skull and has large intracranial and subgaleal components. (From Archives of the Armed Forces Institute of Pathology.)

has an enlarged middle meningeal or anterior falcine artery that supplies the tumor nidus in a radial or "sunburst" pattern (Fig. 14-14, *A* to *C*). The periphery is supplied by numerous enlarged pial branches of the middle and anterior cerebral arteries (Fig. 14-14, *D* to *F*). Selective injection of the external and internal carotid arteries shows the dual supply of large meningiomas.

Late arterial and capillary phase films show a prominent, homogeneous prolonged vascular blush (Fig. 14-15) (an Armed Forces Institute of Pathology

colleague, Dr. James Smirniotopoulos, calls this the "mother-in-law sign": i.e., it "comes early and stays late!"). Occasionally, arteriovenous shunting with early opacification of draining veins occurs. Dural sinus occlusions can be identified on mid- and late venous phase films (Fig. 14-14, *F*).

CT. Plain and contrast-enhanced CT detect 85% and 95% of intracranial meninigiomas, respectively.[53]

NECT scans typically show a sharply circumscribed round or smoothly lobulated mass that abuts a dural surface, usually at an obtuse angle. Approx-

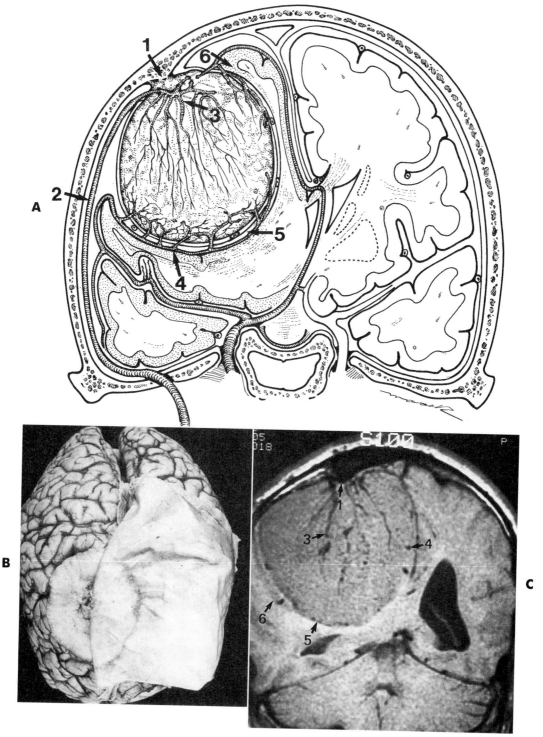

Fig. 14-13. A, Anatomic diagram, coronal plane, demonstrates the typical dual vascular supply of a large convexity meningioma. **B,** Gross autopsy specimen shows a large convexity meningioma and its dural attachment. Note "sunburst" of vessels that radiates outward from the central vascular pedicle. **C,** Coronal T1-weighted MR scan in a patient with a large convexity meningioma is shown for comparison: *1,* Enostotic "spur" with vascular pedicle. *2,* Enlarged middle meningeal artery. *3,* Dural-derived vessels supply center of the meningioma. *4,* Enlarged pial vessels supply the periphery. *5,* CSF/vascular cleft between the tumor and adjacent brain. *6,* Cortex displaced around the tumor confirms extraaxial location of the mass. (**B,** From archives of the Armed Forces Institute of Pathology.)

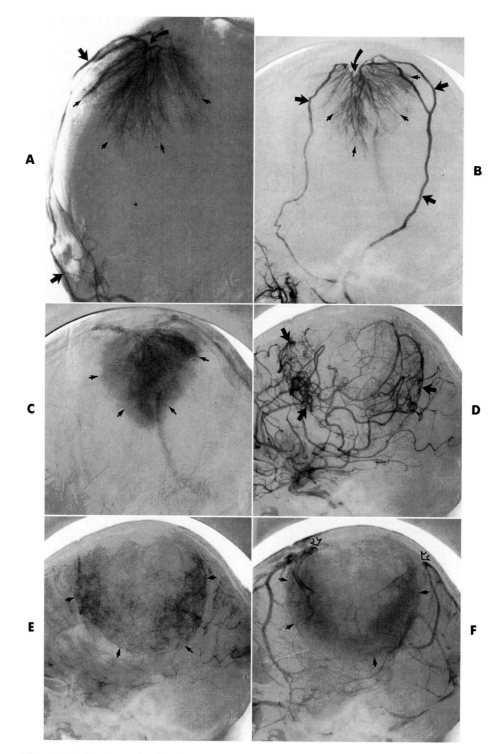

Fig. 14-14. Angiographic findings of a typical meningioma (compare with Fig. 14-13). **A** to **C**, Right external carotid angiogram, **(A)** AP and **(B)** lateral views, midarterial phase, shows an enlarged middle meningeal artery *(large straight arrows)* supplies the center of a large parasagittal meningioma. Note "sunburst" of dural vessels *(small arrows)* that radiates outward from the vascular pedicle *(curved arrows)*. **C,** Late arterial phase, lateral view, shows the dense prolonged vascular stain *(arrows)* that is characteristic of meningioma. **D** to **F,** Right internal carotid angiogram, lateral view, with midarterial **(D),** late arterial **(E),** and venous phase **(F)** studies shows enlarged pial branches of the middle and anterior cerebral arteries **(D,** *arrows)* supply the periphery of the tumor. Note prolonged vascular stain **(E** and **F,** *solid arrows).* The center of the mass is unopacified because it is supplied by the middle meningeal artery. Note occluded superior sagittal sinus **(F,** *open arrows).*

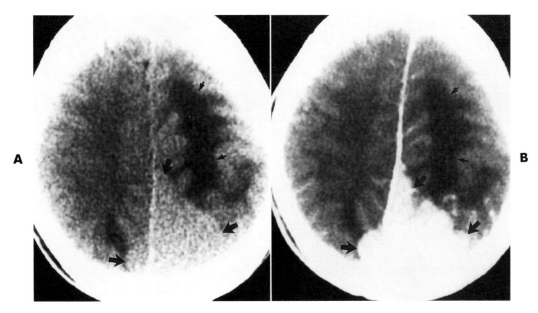

Fig. 14-15. Pre- **(A)** and postcontrast **(B)** axial CT scans show a typical parasagittal meningioma. The lobulated tumor is hyperdense on the NECT scan (**A**, *large arrows*). Strong uniform enhancement is seen (**B**, *large arrows*). Note white matter edema *(small arrows)*. (Courtesy M. Fruin.)

Meningioma
Imaging

Plain film radiography	CT
Hyperostosis	70% to 75% hyperdense
Erosion	20% to 25% calcified
Enlarged vascular channels	90% enhance strongly, uniformly
Tumor calcifications	10% to 15% cystic areas
Pneumosinus dilatans	60% peritumoral edema
	Hemorrhage rare
Angiography	
	MR
Dual vascular supply common (dural to center, pial to periphery)	Typically isointense with gray matter
"Sunburst" of enlarged dural feeders in tumor	>95% enhance strongly; heterogeneous enhancement common
Prolonged vascular stain	CSF/vascular "cleft"
	60% have dural "tail" (suggestive of, but not specific for, meningioma)

---

imately 70% to 75% of all meningiomas are homogeneously hyperdense relative to adjacent brain (Fig. 14-15); 25% appear isodense. Hypodense tumors are seen in 1% to 5% of cases (Fig. 14-16). Rarely, a lipoblastic or xanthomatous tumor has low negative attenuation numbers.[33]

Calcification is seen in 20% to 25% and can be diffuse or focal. Psammomatous (sandlike), sunburst, or globular and even rimlike patterns occur (Fig. 14-17, *A* and *B*). Occasionally, meningiomas appear densely calcified (Fig. 14-17, *C*). Hyperostosis can be striking

(*see* Fig. 12-188, *E*) or absent. Bone destruction sometimes occurs.

Gross hemorrhage is uncommon (*see* Fig. 7-49). Although true cystic meningiomas with large intratumoral fluid-filled cysts are uncommon (Fig. 14-18), small nonenhancing areas of cystic change or necrosis are seen in 8% to 23% of cases.[33] Degenerative brain parenchymal cysts and trapped arachnoid with pools of CSF between the meningioma and adjacent brain are common findings.[36] Peripheral edema is seen in 60% of cases and may be extensive, involv-

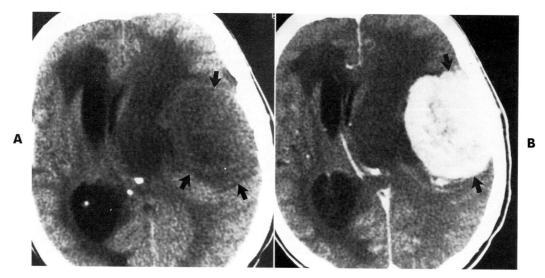

Fig. 14-16. Pre- **(A)** and postcontrast **(B)** axial CT scans show a convexity meningioma that is hypodense to brain on the NECT study **(A,** *arrows*). The tumor enhances strongly and uniformly following contrast administration **(B,** *arrows*).

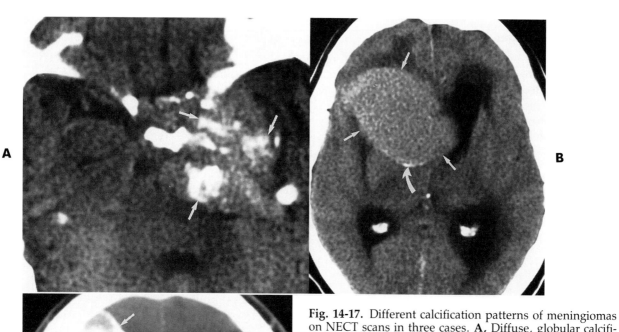

Fig. 14-17. Different calcification patterns of meningiomas on NECT scans in three cases. **A,** Diffuse, globular calcifications *(arrows)* are present in this cavernous sinus and tentorium meningioma. **(B)** Rimlike calcification *(curved arrow)* is seen around this hyperdense meningioma with fine diffuse psammomatous (sandlike) calcification *(small arrows).* **C,** Dense rocklike calcified meningioma *(arrows).*

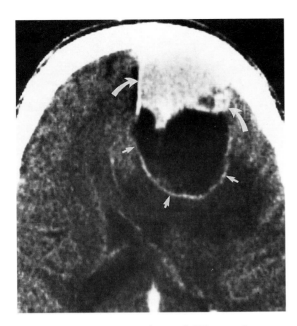

Fig. 14-18. Axial contrast-enhanced CT scan shows a partially cystic meningioma. A solid, dural-based mass *(curved arrows)* with a rim-enhancing cyst *(small arrows)* is identified.

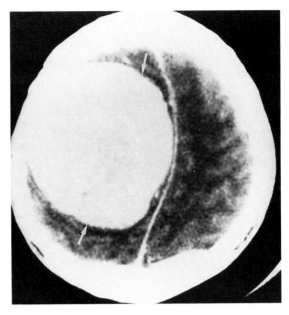

Fig. 14-19. Axial postcontrast CT scan in a patient with a large parasagittal meningioma shows the well-delineated, intensely enhancing mass *(arrows)*. Same case as Fig. 14-14.

ing the white matter tracts of an entire hemisphere.

CECT scans show intense, relatively uniform enhancement in 90% of all cases (Fig. 14-19; *see* Fig. 14-15, *B*). Ten to fifteen percent of meningiomas have an atypical pattern with rimlike tumor enhancement (Fig. 14-18) or imaging findings that suggest hemorrhage, prominent cyst formation, or metaplastic change.[54-58]

Some authors report that mushroomlike tumor projections, inhomogeneous contrast enhancement, and indistinct tumor-brain interface suggest an aggressive tumor.[59] "Mushrooming" is seen in approximately 10% of benign and 20% of malignant meningiomas[60]; benign meningiomas do not invariably have a sharply delineated brain-tumor interface.[36] Therefore malignant meningiomas cannot be distinguished from benign lesions solely on the basis of CT findings.[35,61]

MR. Meningiomas demonstrate imaging findings that are characteristic for all extraaxial masses (*see* box, p. 438), viz., gray-white interface "buckling" or displacement and a cleft or pseudocapsule of CSF and vessels that surrounds the mass, separating it from brain (Fig. 14-20; *see* Fig. 14-8).

The relationship between MR signal and meningioma histopathology is controversial. Some authors report that in the majority of cases, signal on T2WI correlates strongly with histopathologic features.[62,63] In their studies, up to 90% of fibroblastic/transitional tumors were hypointense relative to gray matter on balanced and T2WI (Fig. 14-21), whereas two thirds

of meningothelial/angioblastic tumors were hyperintense (Fig. 14-22).[63]

Other investigators conclude that although MR findings may be suggestive, the correlation is insufficient to permit an accurate histologic diagnosis based solely on imaging features.[64,65]

Regardless of histologic type, most meningiomas are iso- or slightly hypointense relative to cortex on T1-weighted studies, although signal on T2WI is variable (Figs. 14-23 and 14-24). The prominent radial or "sunburst" vascular pattern seen at cerebral angiography may be discernible in some cases (Fig. 14-24). In others the dural- and pial-supplied portions of the tumor vary slightly in signal intensity (Fig. 14-25).

A CSF cleft is often present around a meningioma, demarcating the brain-tumor interface and confirming its extraaxial location (Fig. 14-26). Enlarged, displaced pial vessels and draining veins may be striking. Moderate to severe peritumoral edema is present in two thirds of all cases (*see* Figs. 14-15 and 14-16) and is often associated with pial vascular supply.[66]

Nearly all meningiomas enhance rapidly and intensely following contrast administration.[67] There is no reliable correlation between the degree of contrast enhancement or surrounding edema with tumor size or histologic subtype.[68,68a] A tiny meningioma can incite tremendous edema (Fig. 14-27), and some very large meningiomas have comparatively little associated edema (*see* Fig. 14-19).

Enhanced MR scans are particularly useful in detecting small, inconspicuous meningiomas that are

Text continued on p. 600.

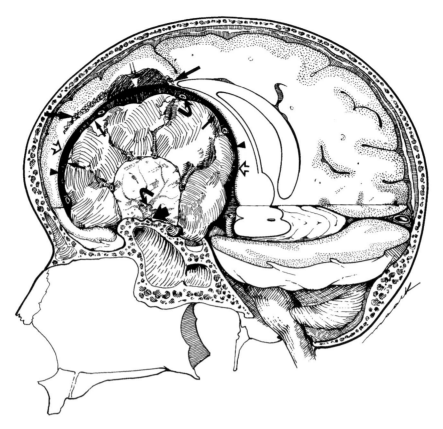

Fig. 14-20. Anatomic diagram depicts the gross pathology of meningioma. The large lobulated extraaxial mass is shown arising from the basisphenoid. Some bony hyperostosis is present, and the underlying sinus is enlarged (pneumosinus dilatans). Enostotic spur *(stubby large arrow)* and dural vascular pedicle *(curved arrow)*. Note CSF/vascular cleft *(small black arrows)* that surrounds the tumor, separating it from the adjacent brain, and pool of trapped CSF *(white arrowhead)*. The cortex *(open arrows)* is displaced around the mass. A thin fibrous pseudocapsule is indicated *(black arrowheads)*. Secondary changes in the adjacent brain include mass effect (note displaced corpus callosum and fornix), cystic encephalomalacia *(small double arrows)* and edema *(large black arrows)*. (Reprinted from Sheporaitis L, Osborn AG et al: Radiologic-pathologic correlation of intracranial meningioma, *AJNR*, 13:29-37, 1992. With permission.)

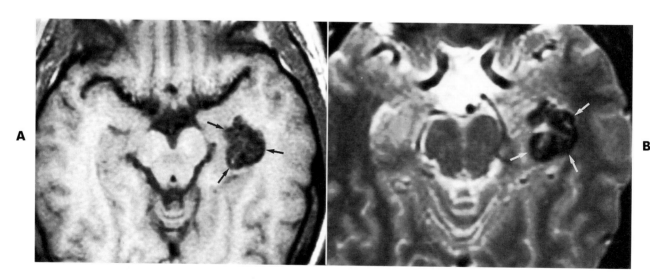

Fig. 14-21. For legend see p. 597.

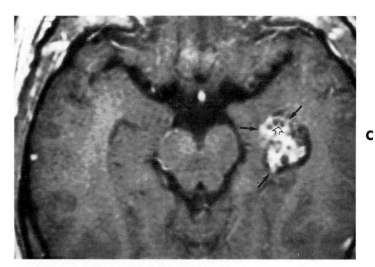

Fig. 14-21, cont'd. A, Axial precontrast T1-weighted MR scan shows a predominately hypointense mass *(arrows)* in the temporal horn of the left lateral ventricle. **B,** The mass remains hypointense on the T2WI. **C,** Following contrast administration the mass *(solid arrows)* enhances strongly but somewhat inhomogeneously. Fibroblastic, partially calcified meningioma with small foci of cystic degeneration *(open arrow)* was found at surgery. (Courtesy W. Gibby.)

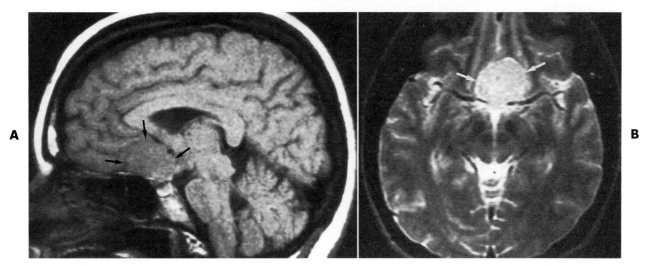

Fig. 14-22. Sagittal T1- **(A)** and axial T2-weighted **(B)** MR scans of a planum sphenoidal meningioma show the mass *(arrows)* is isointense with brain on the T1-weighted study but moderately hyperintense on the T2WI. Meningothelial meningioma.

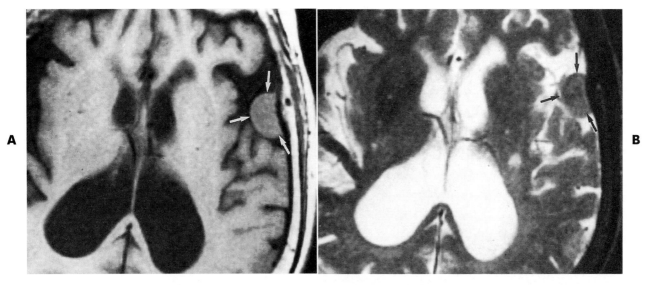

Fig. 14-23. A 69-year-old woman had a 1-month history of facial numbness. Axial T1- **(A)** and T2-weighted **(B)** MR scans show a small dural-based left middle cranial fossa mass *(arrows)* that is isointense with cortex on both sequences. The mass is apparent because the adjacent sylvian fissure is enlarged. Typical meningioma.

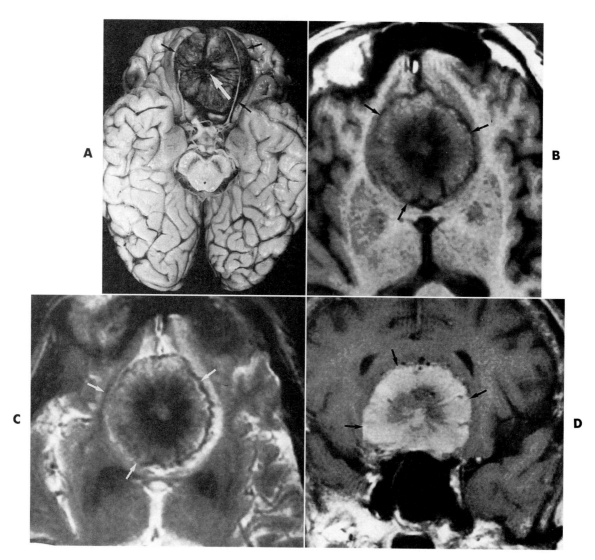

Fig. 14-24. Gross pathology specimen **(A)** shows a cribriform plate meningioma *(small arrows)*. Note "sunburst" pattern of vessels radiating outward from the central vascular pedicle *(large arrow)*. MR scans **(B to D)** in another patient with a cribriform plate meningioma demonstrate the imaging correlates of **(A)**. Axial T1- **(B)** and T2-weighted **(C)** scans show the mass *(small arrows)*. Coronal postcontrast T1WI **(D)** shows the mass *(small arrows)* enhances strongly. **(A,** From Okazaki H: Fundamentals of Neuropathology, ed 2, Igaku-Shoin Medical Publishers, New York, 1989. **B to D,** Courtesy J. Zahniser.)

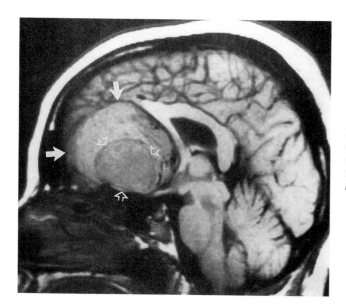

Fig. 14-25. Sagittal T1-weighted MR scan shows a large cribriform plate meningioma. The central portion *(open arrows)*, supplied by dural vessels, has slightly different signal from the outer (pial-supplied) part of the tumor *(large arrows)*.

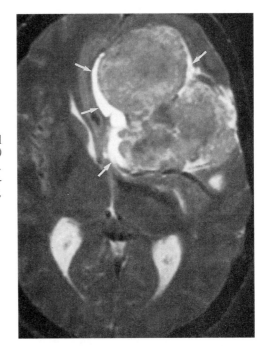

Fig. 14-26. T2-weighted axial MR scan of a large sphenoid wing meningioma shows a prominent CSF cleft *(arrows)* between the tumor and adjacent brain. Same case as Fig. 14-8. (Reprinted from Sheporaitis L, Osborn AG et al: Radiologic-pathologic correlation of intracranial meningioma, *AJNR,* 13:29-37, 1992.

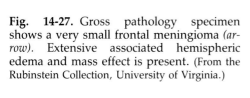

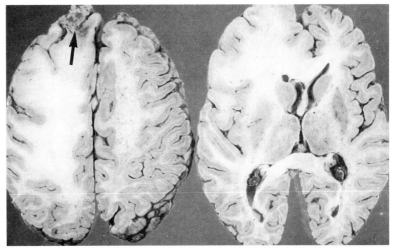

Fig. 14-27. Gross pathology specimen shows a very small frontal meningioma *(arrow).* Extensive associated hemispheric edema and mass effect is present. (From the Rubinstein Collection, University of Virginia.)

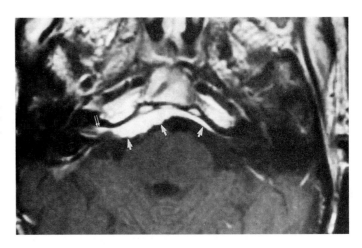

Fig. 14-28. Axial postcontrast T1-weighted MR scan shows an enhancing en plaque meningioma of the clivus *(single arrows).* Note extension into the right internal auditory canal *(double arrows).*

isointense with adjacent cortex on all pulse sequences. Postcontrast studies can also delineate the precise extent of en plaque lesions (Fig. 14-28).

Sixty percent of meningiomas have a collar of thickened, enhancing tissue that surrounds their dural attachment (Fig. 14-29).[69] The exact nature of this so-called dural tail is controversial. Some investigators report tumor cells infiltrating the thickened dura, suggesting that complete tumor removal requires resection of the dural "tail".[69-71]

Other investigators report that the abnormally enhancing dura surrounding most meningiomas represents reactive change and does not necessarily indicate neoplastic involvement.[72,73] What is clear is the following:

1. Sometimes meningiomas infiltrate adjacent dura
2. Meningiomas can induce nonneoplastic reactive dural changes
3. Other lesions such as schwannoma, glioblastoma multiforme, and metastases occasionally are associated with a dural tail[70,74,75]

4. The "dural tail sign" is highly suggestive but not specific for meningioma[76]

Predicting meningioma behavior on imaging studies and even histopathologic findings is difficult. The variable imaging features of meningiomas may not accurately reflect specific histologic subtypes, and the biologic behavior of meningiomas does not always correlate with histology.[33] From 20% to 30% of seemingly completely removed meningiomas recur.[41] Anaplastic meningiomas do not follow an invariably aggressive course, and histologically benign meningiomas can metastasize.[77]

Atypical meningiomas and meningioma "mimics" (*see* box). Although the imaging appearance of most meningiomas is characteristic, some meningiomas mimic benign tumors such as schwannoma, and others resemble malignant neoplasms such as anaplastic astrocytoma (Fig. 14-30).[78]

Several nonmeningotheliomatous lesions can resemble meningioma. Extramedullary hematopoiesis can appear as multiple contrast-enhancing dural-

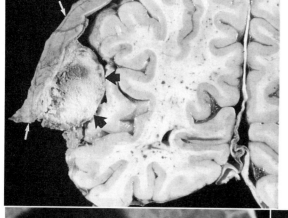

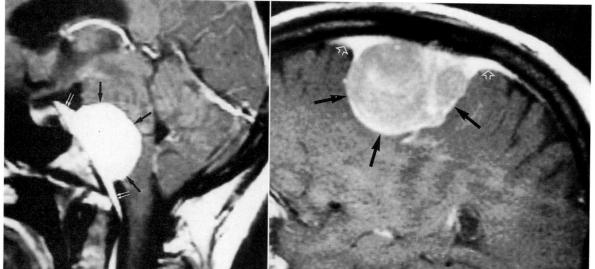

Fig. 14-29. A, Coronal section of gross autopsy specimen demonstrates a meningioma that has a collar of thickened dura *(small arrows)* surrounding the tumor *(large arrows),* the so-called dural tail. **B,** Sagittal postcontrast T1-weighted MR scan shows a clivus meningioma *(black arrows)* with prominent dural "tails" *(white arrows).* **C,** Sagittal postcontrast T1WI in another patient shows an enhancing parasagittal meningioma *(black arrows)* with a surrounding thickened dural collar *(white arrows)* that enhances even more intensely. (**A,** Courtesy E. Tessa Hedley-Whyte.)

based masses (*see* Fig. 12-196). Invasive skull base tumors with prominent dural vascular supply can mimic meningioma (*see* Fig. 12-150). Dural metastases from extracranial primary tumors such as breast or colon carcinoma can sometimes be indistinguishable from the typical benign meningioma on imaging studies (Fig. 14-31). Rarely, extracranial primary tumors metastasize *to* a meningioma. Cavernous angiomas and capillary hemangiomas occasionally occur in the dura or cavernous sinus and can mimic meningioma (Fig. 14-32).[78a]

Meningioma "Mimics"
Meningiomas can mimic:
Schwannomas
Gliomas
Metastases
Lesions that can mimic meningiomas
Dural vascular malformation or tumor (e.g., cavernous angioma, capillary hemangioma, hemangiopericytoma, metastasis)
Extramedullary hematopoiesis

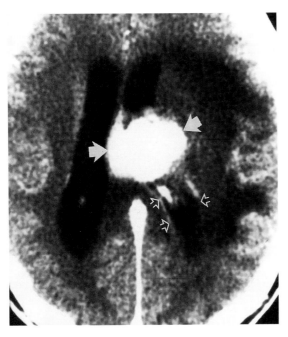

Fig. 14-30. Axial CECT scan shows an intensely enhancing mass (*large arrows*) adjacent to the left lateral ventricle. Note the ependymal enhancement (*open arrows*). Preoperative diagnosis was anaplastic astrocytoma. Intraventricular meningioma attached to the tela choroidea was found at surgery.

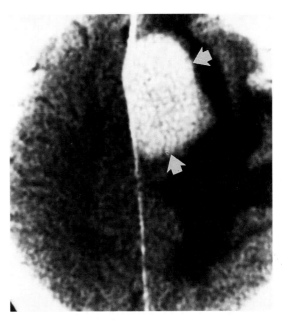

Fig. 14-31. Contrast-enhanced CT scan in a patient with colon carcinoma shows an enhancing falcine mass (*arrows*). Note associated white matter edema. Metastatic colon carcinoma was found at surgery. The imaging appearance is identical to meningioma.

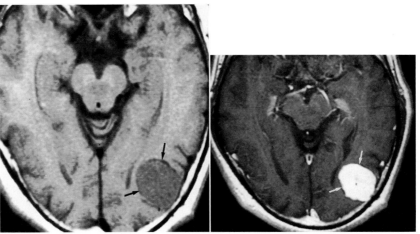

Fig. 14-32. Axial pre- (**A**) and postcontrast (**B**) T1-weighted MR scans show a dural-based extraaxial mass (*arrows*) that is isointense with cortex and enhances strongly following contrast administration.

Continued.

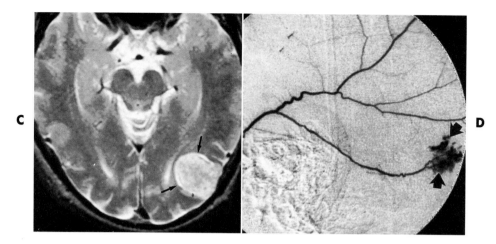

Fig. 14-32, cont'd. T2WI **(C)** shows the mass *(arrows)* is hyperintense. **(D)** External carotid angiogram *(arrows)* demonstrated an intensely vascular mass *(arrows)* that is supplied by the posterior division of the middle meningeal artery. Preoperative diagnosis was meningioma. Dural cavernous angioma was found at surgery.

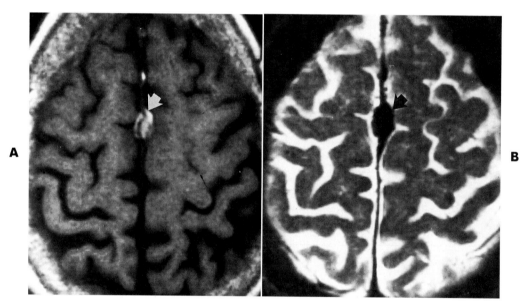

Fig. 14-33. Axial T1- **(A)** and T2-weighted **(B)** MR scans show an ossified falx with marrow *(arrows)*. The fatty marrow is hyperintense on T1WI and profoundly hypointense on the T2-weighted scan.

Nonmeningotheliomatous Mesenchymal Tumors

Primary mesenchymal tumors other than meningioma are uncommon. Benign neoplasms and neoplastic-like processes include ossified dura (Fig. 14-33) and osteocartilagenous tumors such as falx osteoma or enchondroma *(see* Chapter 12). Malignant mesenchymal neoplasms include the rare dural chondrosarcoma (Fig. 14-34), fibrosarcoma (Fig. 14-35), and angiosarcoma (Fig. 14-36).

Primary Melanocytic Lesions

Meningeal melanocytomas are rare CNS lesions. These tumors have a more benign course than the very rare primary malignant leptomeningeal melanoma. The usual sites of meningeal melanocytomas are the posterior fossa, cervical spinal canal, and Meckel's cave. The imaging appearance is that of an extraaxial mass that can resemble focal globose or en plaque meningioma. The few lesions with MR find-

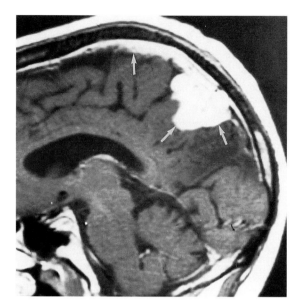

Fig. 14-34. Sagittal contrast-enhanced T1-weighted MR scan shows a lobulated mass with extension along the falx *(arrows)*. Dural chondrosarcoma was found at surgery.

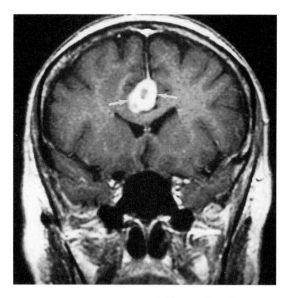

Fig. 14-35. Postcontrast coronal T1-weighted MR scan in this 67-year-old woman with seizures shows an enhancing mass *(arrows)* that arises from the inferior falx. Dural fibrosarcoma was found at surgery.

ings report isodense masses that enhance relatively homogeneously following contrast administration (Fig. 14-37).[79-81]

Primary malignant leptomeningeal melanoma is a highly malignant tumor that typically presents with hydrocephalus and diffuse meningeal enhancement on imaging studies.[82]

Hemangiopericytoma

Etiology. Hemangiopericytoma (HPC) is classified as a "tumor of uncertain origin" in the WHO system. Meningeal HPCs are considered by some to be a subtype of angioblastic meningioma. However, HPCs do not arise from the archetypal meningothelial arachnoid cap cell. They arise instead from contractile cells (pericytes) that surround capillaries.[83,84] Although some authors refer to these tumors as meningeal hemangiopericytomas or angioblastic meningioma (hemangiopericytic type),[85] others regard them as a distinctive mesenchymal neoplasm that is unrelated to meningioma.[1]

Pathology

Gross pathology. Macroscopically, many HPCs resemble meningioma.[1] Three quarters of all cases are firm, well-circumscribed, or encapsulated globular masses that can have either a narrow or broad-based dural attachment. HPCs are richly vascularized tumors with numerous penetrating blood vessels.[84]

Microscopic appearance. These highly cellular, vascular tumors have a dense, pervasive reticulin network. Lobules of neoplastic cells surround so-called staghorn vessels.[1]

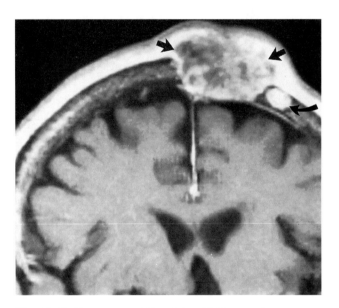

Fig. 14-36. Postcontrast T1-weighted MR scan shows an inhomogeneously enhancing calvarial, dural, and scalp mass *(straight arrows)*. A smaller diploic mass *(curved arrow)* is also present. Angiosarcoma was found at surgery.

Incidence. Hemangiopericytomas are rare tumors, accounting for less than 1% of all primary CNS neoplasms. Their overall frequency is 2.4% of meningiomas.[85]

Age and gender. Average age of onset is 42 years. In contrast to the female predominance in meningioma, there is a slight male preponderance with hemangiopericytoma.[85]

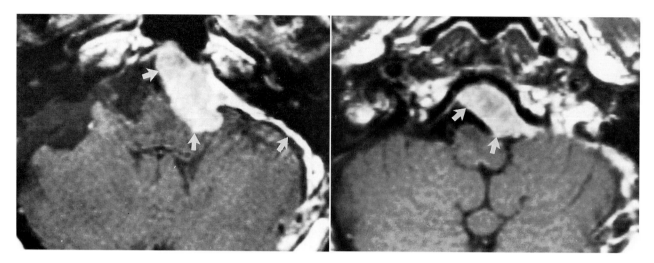

Fig. 14-37. Axial postcontrast T1-weighted MR scans show an extensive, strongly enhancing dural mass *(arrows)* that extends along the petrous temporal bone and clivus to the foramen magnum. Meningeal melanocytoma.

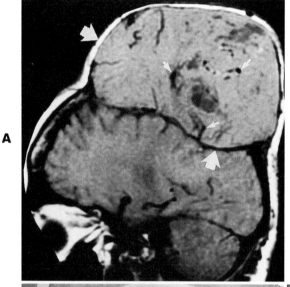

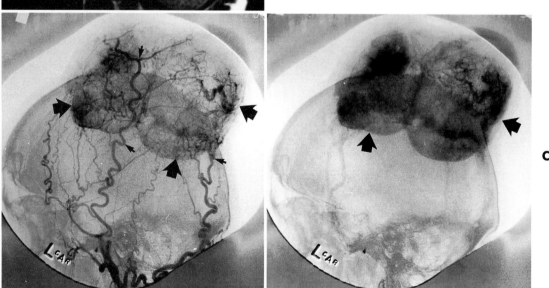

Fig. 14-38. Sagittal precontrast T1-weighted MR scan **(A)** shows a large extradural mass *(large arrows)* that has destroyed the calvarium. Numerous prominent vascular channels are seen within the mass *(small arrows)*. External carotid angiogram, lateral view, with midarterial **(B)** and capillary phase **(C)** shows an intensely vascular mass *(large arrows)* that is supplied primarily by branches of the superficial temporal and occipital arteries *(small arrows)*. Hemangiopericytoma. (Reprinted from Cosentino CM et al: Giant cranial hemangiopericytoma: MR and angiographic findings, *AJNR* 14:253-256, 1993. With permission.)

Natural history. The biologic behavior of hemangiopericytoma is considerably different from meningioma. There is a strong propensity for both local recurrence and extraneural metastasis, particularly to lung and bone. The survival rates at 5, 10, and 15 years following surgery are 67%, 40%, and 23% respectively.[85] A poor response to radiation therapy or chemotherapy is typical.[84]

Imaging

Angiography. Hemangiopericytomas are hypervascular lesions that typically have prolonged, dense, but heterogeneous tumor stain (Fig. 14-38, *B* and *C*). Arteriovenous shunting with early draining veins is uncommon. Mixed dural-pial vascular supply is typical.[85]

CT. Hemangiopericytomas are heterogeneous-appearing lesions on both pre- and postcontrast studies. Low density cystic or necrotic areas are common, and enhancement is typically strong but inhomogeneous.

MR. MR findings are also variable. Signs of an extradural mass are often, but not invariably, present. In the few reported cases, hemangiopericytomas are isointense with cortex on T1WI and slightly hyperintense on proton density-weighted sequences. Signal is typically heterogeneous on T2WI. Strong but inhomogeneous enhancement occurs following contrast administration. Prominent vascular channels are frequently identified (Fig. 14-38, *A*).[84]

Hemangioblastoma (Capillary Hemangioblastoma)

"The hemangioblastoma is a vascular neoplasm of unknown origin that appeals to the surgeon because of its curability, to the pathologist because of its distinctive morphology, to the geneticist because of its association with a phakomatosis, and to the internist because some of the tumors elaborate erythropoietin and stimulate erythropoiesis."[1] Hemangioblastomas also appeal to radiologists because of their striking imaging manifestations.

Etiology. The histogenetic origin of hemangioblastoma is discussed extensively but remains unknown. Whether these tumors arise from primitive vascular mesenchyme, hematopoietic stem cells, or another source remains to be determined.

Pathology (*see* box)

Gross pathology. Hemangioblastomas are typically well-circumscribed tumors. Sixty percent are cystic masses with a mural nodule that usually abuts a pial surface (Fig. 14-39, *A*); 40% are solid (Fig. 14-39, *B*).[86] Gross tumor necrosis and hemorrhage may occur but are uncommon.

Microscopic appearance. Hemangioblastomas are

histologically heterogeneous tumors that have varying mixtures of two principal cellular components: endothelial cells and pericytes, or interstitial "stromal" cells. The endothelial pericytic components usually predominate.[1] Thin-walled, tightly packed blood vessels that vary in size from capillary to cavernous are present. The cyst wall is composed of compressed brain parenchyma or reactive gliosis.[86]

Incidence. Hemangioblastomas are uncommon tumors, accounting for 1% to 2.5% of all primary CNS neoplasms and approximately 7% of primary posterior fossa tumors in adults.[87] Most hemangioblastomas occur sporadically; 10% to 20% occur as part of von Hippel-Lindau syndrome (VHL). Forty-four percent of all patients with VHL eventually develop a CNS hemangioblastoma[88] (*see* Chapter 5).

Age and clinical presentation. Hemangioblastomas are typically adult tumors and are very rare in children. Most become symptomatic during the third to fifth decades; the mean age at diagnosis in patients with VHL who develop a CNS hemangioblastoma is 39 years.[88]

Hemangioblastoma

Pathology

60% cystic with nodule, 40% solid
Gross hemorrhage, calcification, necrosis rare

Incidence

Uncommon (1% to 2.5% of primary CNS tumors)
10% to 20% occur with von Hippel-Lindau syndrome
Approximately 45% of patients with VHL develop hemangioblastoma

Age

Adults with peak during 40 to 60 years; rare in children

Location

80% to 85% cerebellum
3% to 13% spinal cord
2% to 3% medulla
Supratentorial lesions occur but are uncommon
60% of patients with VHL have retinal lesions

Imaging

Angiography: vascular nodule with intense, prolonged stain; +/− avascular cyst
CT: low density cyst with strongly enhancing mural nodule that abuts a pial surface
MR: cyst slightly hyperintense to CSF on T1WI; hyperintense to brain on T2WI; mural nodule variable but enhances strongly

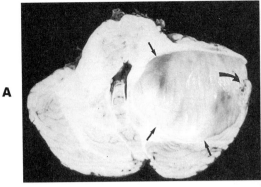

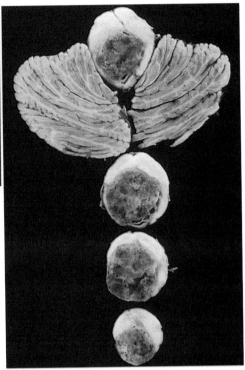

Fig. 14-39. A, Gross pathology of cystic cerebellar hemangioblastoma. A large cyst is present *(small arrows)* with a small mural nodule *(curved arrow)* that abuts a pial surface. **B,** Gross pathology of solid hemangioblastoma in the medulla and cervical spinal cord. (**A,** From Burger P, Scheithauer B: *Surgical Pathology of the Nervous System and its Coverings,* ed 3, New York, Churchill Livingstone, 1991. With permission. **B,** From Okazaki H: Fundamentals of Neuropathology, ed 2, Igaku-Shoin Medical Publishers, New York, 1989.)

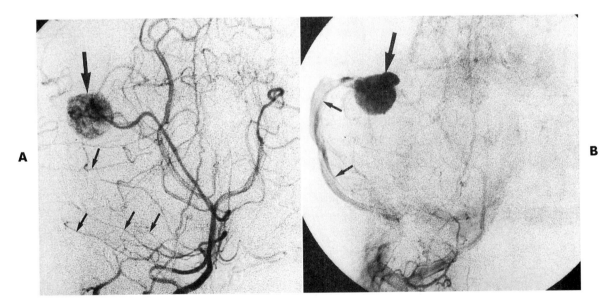

Fig. 14-40. Typical angiographic findings of a cystic cerebellar hemangioblastoma are illustrated by this case. **A,** Right vertebral angiogram, midarterial phase, AP view, shows a small but highly vascular tumor nodule *(large arrow)* is supplied by the superior cerebellar artery (SCA). Stretching and draping of posterior inferior cerebellar artery and SCA branches *(small arrows)* indicates a much larger avascular mass effect caused by an associated cyst. **B,** Capillary phase shows dense, prolonged tumor blush *(large arrow)* and arteriovenous shunting into the transverse sinus *(small arrows)*. The superficial location of the mural nodule is typical.

Common presenting symptoms of intracranial hemangioblastomas are headache, disequilibrium, nausea/vomiting, and dizziness/vertigo.[86]

Location. Between 80% to 85% of hemangioblastomas are found in the cerebellum. Other locations include the spinal cord (3% to 13%) and medulla (2% to 3%); supratentorial hemangioblastomas occur but are uncommon (1.5%).[86]

Multiple hemangioblastomas are seen only with VHL and occur in 42% of VHL-associated hemangioblastomas.[88] Approximately 60% of patients with VHL have retinal hemangioblastomas.

Natural history. Hemangioblastomas are potentially curable lesions, although they are the cause of death in 82% of patients with VHL.[88] Approximately one quarter of hemangioblastomas recur following surgical resection; most recurrences are associated with VHL. Death from disseminated disease is exceedingly rare.

Imaging

Angiography. The common angiographic pattern is a large avascular posterior fossa mass with a small highly vascular mural nodule (Fig. 14-40, *A*). An intense, prolonged vascular stain is typical. Arteriovenous shunting with early draining veins sometimes occurs (Fig. 14-40, *B*).

CT. The classic hemangioblastoma is seen as a large, low density, cystic-appearing cerebellar mass. A mural nodule may not be evident on NECT studies. Following contrast enhancement a mural nodule that enhances strongly and relatively uniformly can be identified adjacent to a pial surface in 70% to 75%

of cases.[89] Solid tumors enhance strongly and uniformly, although small cystic foci are sometimes identified (Fig. 14-41).

MR. The cystic component of a cerebellar hemangioblastoma is hypointense compared to brain on T1-weighted scans and hyperintense on T2WI (Fig. 14-42, *A* and *B*).[89] The mural nodule is more variable; most are inhomogeneously isointense on T1- and hyperintense on T2-weighted studies. A few nodules remain isointense with brain on T2WI. Enhancement following contrast administration is intense (Fig. 14-42, *C*). Prominent serpentine "flow voids" can often be identified (Fig. 14-42, *A*). Occasionally, hemangioblastomas demonstrate a solid or ringlike pattern of contrast enhancement (Fig. 14-43).

Pineal Region Tumors

A general overview of pineal region tumors can be found in Chapter 12. Here, we discuss in greater detail the two major categories of pineal gland tumors: germ cell and pineal cell neoplasms.

Germ Cell Tumors

Germ cell tumors include germinoma, teratoma, choriocarcinoma, endodermal sinus (yolk sac) tumor, embryonal carcinoma, and mixed germ cell tumors (*see* box, p. 608).

Germinoma. Germinoma, formerly called atypical teratoma, accounts for two thirds of germ cell tumors and about 40% of all pineal region neoplasms.[90] There is a strong male predominance. Most patients are between 10 and 30 years old; the peak age of presentation is the second decade.[90]

Germ cell tumors arise in or near the midline of

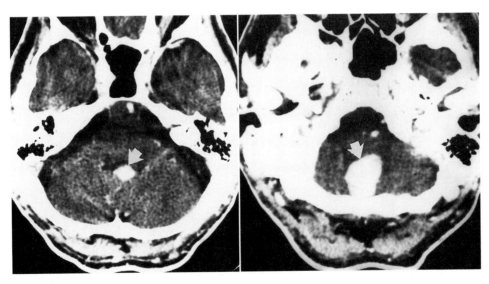

Fig. 14-41. Axial CECT scans in a 57-year-old man with a solid cerebellar hemangioblastoma show a uniformly enhancing mass *(arrows)* without associated cyst.

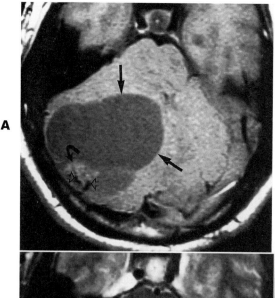

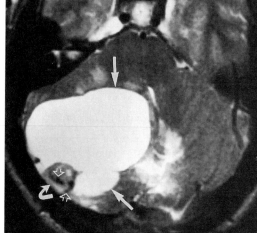

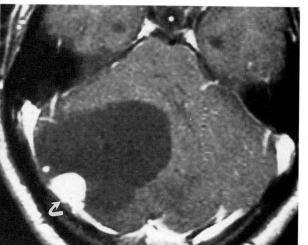

Fig. 14-42. Classic MR findings of cystic cerebellar hemangioblastoma are demonstrated by this case. **A,** Axial T1-weighted scan shows a large low signal cystic-appearing mass *(large arrows)* with a small isointense mural nodule *(curved arrow)* that abuts a pial surface (compare with Fig. 14-39, *A*). Note prominent "flow voids" *(open arrows)* from high-velocity signal loss in the vessels that supply the nidus. **B,** The cyst *(large arrows)* is very hyperintense on T2WI, but the mural nodule *(curved arrow)* remains mostly isointense with brain. **C,** The mural nodule *(arrow)* enhances strongly and uniformly following contrast administration. (Courtesy M. Fruin.)

Pineal Germ Cell Tumors

Germinoma

Most common germ cell tumor (67%); strong male predominance; patients between 10 and 30 years

Pineal gland most common location; second is anterior third ventricle; can occur in basal ganglia; ependymal spread common

Hyperdense on NECT; enhance strongly on CECT

MR signal usually like gray matter; contrast-enhanced studies best for ependymal, subarachnoid spread

Teratoma

Second most common germ cell tumor (15% of pineal masses); occurs in young children; strong male predominance

Two or more embryologic layers (ectoderm, mesoderm, endoderm)

Nonspecific imaging features; usually mixed density/intensity

Choriocarcinoma

Uncommon (<5% of pineal masses); occurs in first decade of life

Nonspecific imaging findings

Elevated serum HCG levels

Endodermal sinus (yolk sac) tumor

Rare; tumor of young children

Imaging features nonspecific

Embryonal cell carcinoma

Rare

Imaging findings nonspecific

Serum HCG, alpha-fetoprotein both elevated

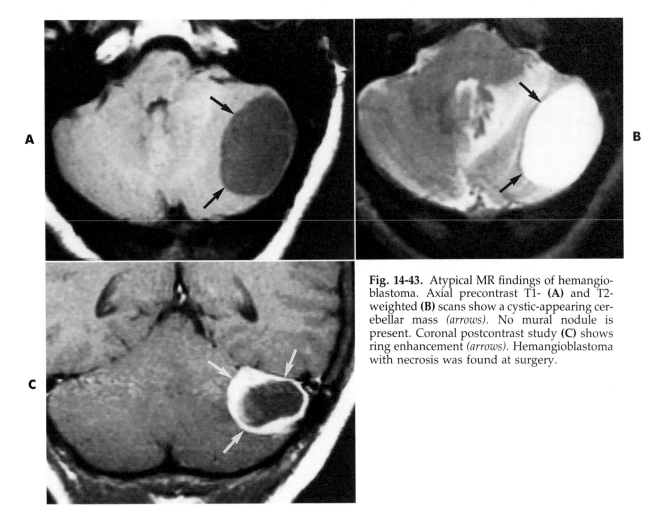

Fig. 14-43. Atypical MR findings of hemangioblastoma. Axial precontrast T1- **(A)** and T2-weighted **(B)** scans show a cystic-appearing cerebellar mass *(arrows)*. No mural nodule is present. Coronal postcontrast study **(C)** shows ring enhancement *(arrows)*. Hemangioblastoma with necrosis was found at surgery.

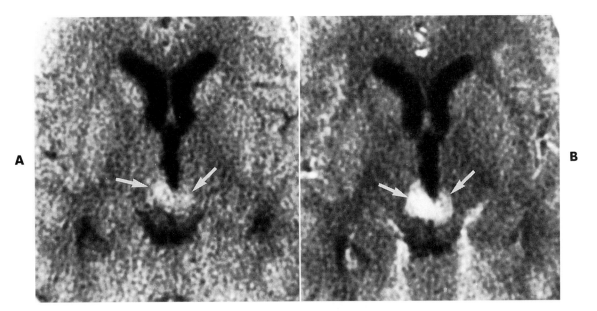

Fig. 14-44. A 24-year-old man with Parinaud's syndrome caused by pineal germinoma. **A,** NECT scan shows a slightly hyperdense posterior third ventricular mass *(arrows)*. **B,** Following contrast administration the mass *(arrows)* enhances intensely and uniformly. The tumor also involves the thalami.   *Continued.*

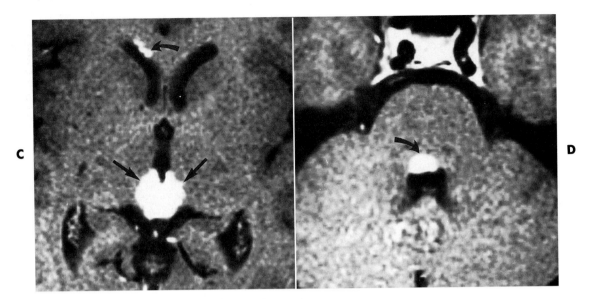

Fig. 14-44, cont'd. C and **D,** Axial contrast-enhanced T1-weighted MR scans show the tumor enhances strongly *(arrows).* Ependymal tumor spread to the frontal horns and fourth ventricle *(curved arrows)* is seen on the MR study but was not apparent on the CT examination.

the brain.[91] Although the pineal and suprasellar regions are preferred sites, 5% to 10% of intracranial germinomas arise in other locations such as the thalamus and basal ganglia.[92]

Precontrast CT scans typically show a slightly hyperdense mass that surrounds and engulfs a calcified pineal gland (Fig. 14-44, *A*). Enhancement is typically strong and uniform following contrast administration (Fig. 14-44, *B*).

Pineal germinomas often have secondary implants in the anterior third ventricular recesses *(see* Fig. 12-7). Because germinomas are unencapsulated, they can also invade the thalamus and adjacent structures (Fig. 14-44, *B*).[90] Diffuse ependymal and subarachnoid spread is also common (Fig. 14-45).

MR signal characteristics are nonspecific.[93] Germinomas are usually isointense with cortex on all pulse sequences (Fig. 14-46). Occasionally, they are hyperintense on T1- and hypointense on T2-weighted studies. Because germinomas are homogeneously hyperintense on contrast-enhanced T1WI, these studies are helpful in identifying tumor spread (Fig. 14-44, *C* and *D*).

Teratoma. Teratoma is the second most common pineal region tumor, accounting for 15% of pineal masses. Teratomas are tumors of multipotential cells that recapitulate normal organogenesis, producing tissues that represent a mixture of two or more embryologic layers of ectoderm, mesoderm, and endoderm.[90] As with germinomas, there is a male predominance that varies from 2:1 to 8:1.[90] Teratomas also are tumors of young children.[91] Teratomas

can be benign or malignant neoplasms and were formerly called teratocarcinoma.[94]

Imaging findings are variable. Teratomas are usually heterogeneous lesions with calcification and mixed CSF, lipid, and soft-tissue areas (Fig. 14-47).

Choriocarcinoma. Choriocarcinomas are uncommon, accounting for less than 5% of pineal masses. These tumors differentiate from pluripotential germ cells into extraembryonic placental-like tissues.[90] Serum and CSF beta human chorionic gonadotrophin levels are elevated.[91] Imaging findings are nonspecific; there are no known features that differentiate among choriocarcinoma, germinoma, teratoma, and teratocarcinoma.[94] Therefore some authors recommend resection of pineal and suprasellar germ-cell tumors to establish an accurate histologic diagnosis that can be used to guide adjuvant therapy.[91]

Endodermal sinus tumor. Also called "yolk sac" tumor, this germ cell neoplasm often has mixed histology. As with most other pineal tumors, no specific imaging features have been delineated.[90] Most patients with endodermal sinus tumors have elevated serum alpha-fetoprotein levels.[91]

Embryonal cell carcinoma. Embryonal cell carcinomas are composed of large, malignant, totipotential, undifferentiated embryonal-type epithelial cells.[90] Imaging findings in these tumors are also nonspecific. Both tumor markers, alpha-fetoprotein and human chorionic gonadotropin, are elevated with embryonal cell carcinomas.[94]

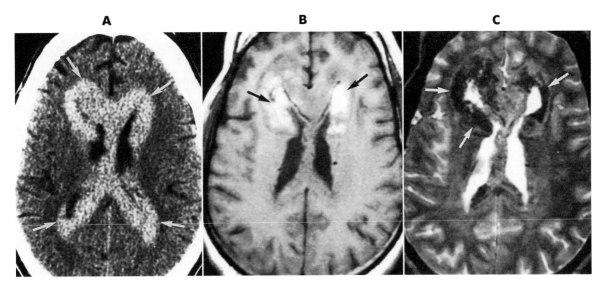

Fig. 14-45. Axial NECT scan **(A)** with diffuse ependymal spread of germinoma. A thick hyperdense rind of tumor *(arrows)* encases the lateral ventricles. MR scans show the tumor is hyperintense on T1WI **(B,** *arrows)* and quite hypointense on T2WI **(C,** *arrows).*

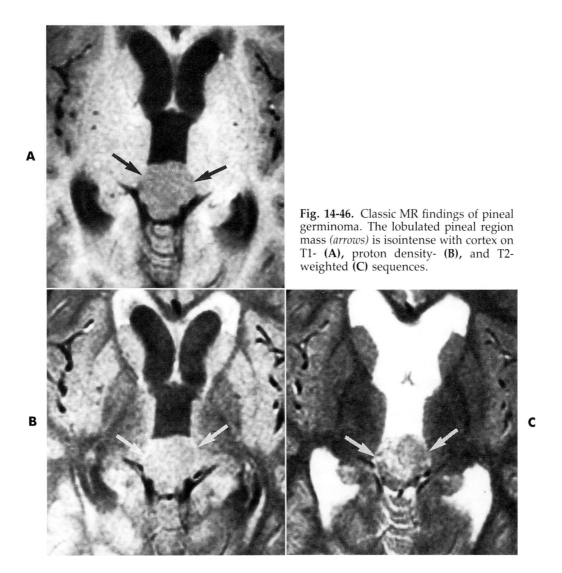

Fig. 14-46. Classic MR findings of pineal germinoma. The lobulated pineal region mass *(arrows)* is isointense with cortex on T1- **(A)**, proton density- **(B)**, and T2-weighted **(C)** sequences.

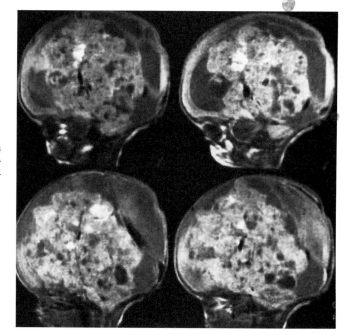

Fig. 14-47. Sagittal T1-weighted MR scans in a newborn infant with bulging fontanelles show a huge mixed signal mass that involves the third and both lateral ventricles. Teratoma was found at surgery.

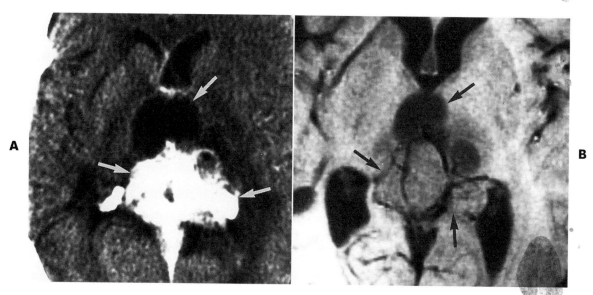

Fig. 14-48. A 32-year-old woman had a history of headache and Parinaud's syndrome at age 15. Pneumoencephalogram had demonstrated a "pinealoma." She was shunted and radiated. CT and MR scans were obtained 17 years later because of increasing headaches and recurrent Parinaud's syndrome. **A,** Axial CECT scan shows a mixed density enhancing pineal and thalamic mass *(arrows).* **B,** Axial T1-weighted MR scan shows a hypo- and isointense mass *(arrows).* Biopsy disclosed pineocytoma.

Pineal Cell Tumors

Pineal parenchymal neoplasms account for less than 15% of all pineal region tumors.[90] There are two basic types of pineal cell neoplasms: pineocytoma and pineoblastoma (*see* box).

Pineocytoma. Pineocytoma is a benign tumor that arises from pineal parenchymal cells. Pineocytomas are uncommon, accounting for only 0.4% to 1% of all primary brain tumors. Unlike other pineal neoplasms, there is no male preponderance. Pineocytomas also occur a decade or two later; the average age at diagnosis is 34 years.[95]

Pineocytomas grow slowly, closely resemble normal pineal gland parenchyma on histologic examination, and rarely disseminate in the CSF space.[96] No

Pineal Cell Tumors

Pineocytoma

Uncommon (<15% of pineal tumors; <1% of primary CNS tumors); average age is 34 years; no male predominance
Grows slowly, rarely disseminates
Sometimes discovered incidentally
Small tumors resemble benign pineal cysts on imaging studies

Pineoblastoma

Uncommon; a type of PNET; found in young children
Large, unencapsulated mass; imaging findings nonspecific

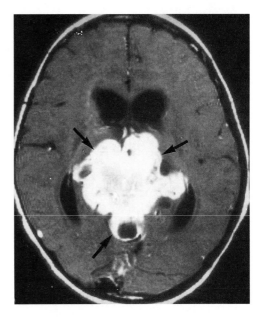

Fig. 14-49. Axial postcontrast T1-weighted MR scan in a 2-year-old child shows a large lobulated midline mass that involves the pineal region, third ventricle, and thalami *(arrows)*. Biopsy disclosed pineoblastoma. (From archives of the Armed Forces Institute of Pathology.)

characteristic imaging features have been described that differentiate pineocytoma from other pineal neooplasms.[95] Small pineocytomas are radiologically indistinguishable from benign pineal cysts *(see* Figs. 12-9 and 12-10); larger pineocytomas appear similar to other more aggressive pineal neoplasms (Fig. 14-48).

Pineoblastoma. Pineoblastomas are malignant neoplasms that are composed of undifferentiated, immature pineal cells. Pineoblastomas are a primitive neuroectodermal tumor similar to medulloblastoma and ependymoblastoma (see subsequent discussion)[90]; like these tumors, pineoblastomas occur in young patients.

Pineoblastomas are often large, unencapsulated masses that invade adjacent brain. Enhancement is strong but may be heterogeneous (Fig. 14-49).

PRIMITIVE NEUROECTODERMAL TUMORS

The embryonic neural tube contains multipotential neuroepithelial cells that give rise to all neuroectodermal elements of the CNS.[97] The concept of primitive neuroectodermal tumors (PNETs) was first introduced to describe largely undifferentiated tumors in children that could have focal areas of differentiation along neuronal or glial lines, as well as a mesenchymal component.

Subsequent authors expanded the PNET category to include other primitive tumors such as pineoblastoma and ependymoblastoma that have identical microscopic features and similar biologic behavior[98] *(see* box, *right)*. Other neuropathologists argue that well-established entities such as medulloblastoma, primary cerebral neuroblastoma, and pineoblastoma do not constitute a single pathologic entity and should

Primitive Neuroectodermal Tumors

Medulloepithelioma
Medulloblastoma (posterior fossa primitive neuroectodermal tumor or PNET-MB)
Primary cerebral neuroblastoma (supratentorial PNET)
Histologically similar tumors
Pineoblastoma
Ependymoblastoma

be treated separately. Because this issue has been—and still is—controversial, we will consider each primitive tumor separately.

Medulloepithelioma

Medulloepithelioma is the most undifferentiated of the primitive neuroectodermal tumors. It is an uncommon neoplasm that occurs in very young children and typically presents with increasing head size. Imaging studies show a large, bulky heterogeneous hemispheric mass. Hemorrhage, necrosis, and cyst formation are common (Fig. 14-50).

Medulloblastoma

Medulloblastoma is an infratentorial PNET and is sometimes termed *PNET-MB (see* box, p. 614).

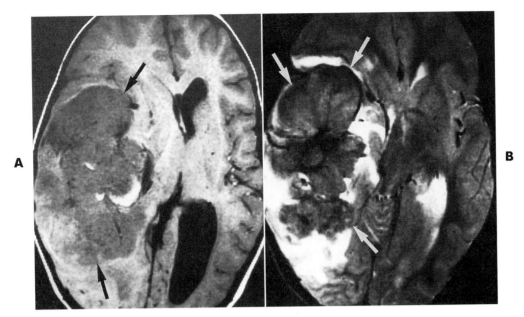

Fig. 14-50. Axial T1- **(A)** and T2-weighted **(B)** MR scans in a 3-year-old child with visual difficulties show a very large heterogeneous hemispheric mass *(arrows)*. Biopsy disclosed medulloepithelioma.

Medulloblastoma (PNET-MB)

Pathology

75% spherical midline posterior fossa mass
25% lateral cerebellum
Densely cellular (small round cells)

Incidence

15% to 25% of primary CNS tumors in children
One third of posterior fossa tumors in children
Rare in adults (<1% of primary CNS tumors)

Age

75% <15 years of age

Natural history

Early CSF dissemination (up to 50% at time of diagnosis)

Imaging

CT: hyperdense on NECT; enhance strongly; hemorrhage, calcification relatively rare
MR: hypointense on T1WI; variable on T2WI; cysts common; enhanced scans best for CSF dissemination (evaluate both brain and spine)

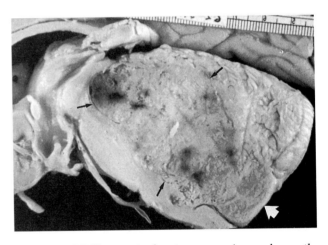

Fig. 14-51. Midline sagittal autopsy specimen shows the characteristic gross appearance of medulloblastoma. A large mass *(small arrows)* originates from the vermis and bulges anteriorly into the fourth ventricle. Note posteroinferior extension through the foramen of Magendie into the cisterna magna *(large arrow)*. (Courtesy E. Ross.)

Etiology. A so-called medulloblast has never been discovered. Medulloblastomas are thought to arise from bipotential embryologic cells located in the roof of the fourth ventricle. These cells normally migrate to form the external granular layer of the cerebellum.[97]

Pathology

Gross pathology. The classic medulloblastoma is an unencapsulated but relatively well-circumscribed spherical vermian mass that bulges anteriorly into the fourth ventricle (Fig. 14-51). Posterior extension into the cisterna magna is common. Unlike ependymomas, lateral extension into the cerebellopontine angles is rare.

Most medulloblastomas are friable, moderately homogeneous pale gray tumors. Gross calcification, cyst formation, and hemorrhage are uncommon.[2]

A

B

C

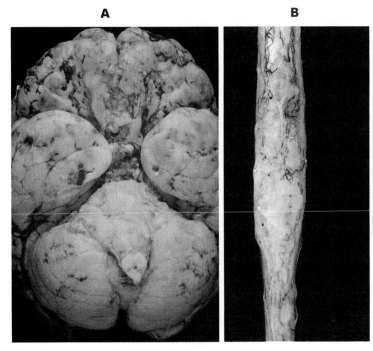

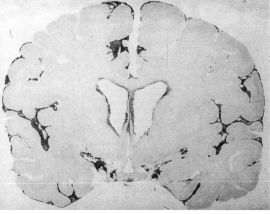

Fig. 14-52. A and **B.** Disseminated medulloblastoma coats the brain and spinal cord like icing on a cake. This has been termed *zuckerguss,* or sugar icing. **C,** Coronal section shows diffuse subarachnoid tumor spread (compare with Fig. 14-56). (From Okazaki H, Scheithauer B: *Slide Atlas of Neuropathology,* Gower Medical Publishing. With permission.)

Microscopic appearance. Medulloblastomas are densely cellular tumors composed of immature cells with hyperchromatic nuclei and relatively scanty cytoplasm. Some tumor cells are arranged radially around an eosinophilic center, forming pseudorosettes.[2]

Incidence. Medulloblastomas represent 15% to 25% of primary brain tumors in children and account for one third of all pediatric posterior fossa neoplasms.[99] Medulloblastomas account for 1% or less of CNS neoplasms in adults.[100]

Age and gender. Medulloblastomas are primarily, but not exclusively, childhood tumors. Nearly three quarters occur before age 15; 50% occur in the first decade.[2] There is a slight male predominance in children of 1.5 to 3:1.[2] A second, smaller peak of medulloblastomas occurs in adults 24 to 30 years of age.[101]

Clinical presentation. Symptoms are those of a posterior fossa mass and include headache, nausea, and vomiting. Visual and motor deficits are common.[90] Medulloblastoma may occur as part of the basal cell nevus (Gorlin) syndrome (*see* Chapter 5).

Location. Medulloblastomas occur in two posterior fossa locations. The most common site, seen in 75% of cases, is the vermis. These tumors are midline lesions that bulge anteriorly into the fourth ventricle and posteriorly into the cisterna magna.

A less common location is the lateral cerebellum. These tumors are more common in older children and adults.

Natural history. With surgery and radiation therapy, the overall 5-year survival rate exceeds 50%. Children with total tumor removal have 5 and 10 year survival rates of 75% and 25%, respectively.[101]

Medulloblastomas tend to metastasize early, widely, and massively throughout the CSF. Disseminated tumor is present in 20% to 50% of patients at initial operation.

Both diffuse and nodular metastases occur. Disseminated CSF metastases coat the brain like frosting on a cake, giving rise to the term "zuckerguss" (sugar icing) (Fig. 14-52). Brain parenchymal metastases occur by extension of tumor cells along the Virchow-Robin perivascular spaces.[2]

Imaging
Angiography. Most medulloblastomas are hypo- or avascular on cerebral angiograms. Signs of a posterior compartment mass are present, including an inferiorly displaced posterior inferior cerebellar artery and anteriorly displaced precentral cerebellar vein.

CT. The typical medulloblastoma is a pear- or heart-shaped midline vermian mass that displaces the fourth ventricle anteriorly. A thin crescent of CSF can sometimes be identified. Medulloblastomas are often homogeneously hyperdense on NECT scans (Fig. 14-53, *A*). Obstructive hydrocephalus is common. Calcification is reported in 15% of cases but may be as high as 50%.[97] Gross hemorrhage is rare. Moderately strong, relatively homogeneous enhancement is seen following contrast administration (Fig. 14-53, *B*).

The "typical" CT appearance of medulloblastoma is seen in only 30% of patients. So-called atypical changes are common. These include cystic changes

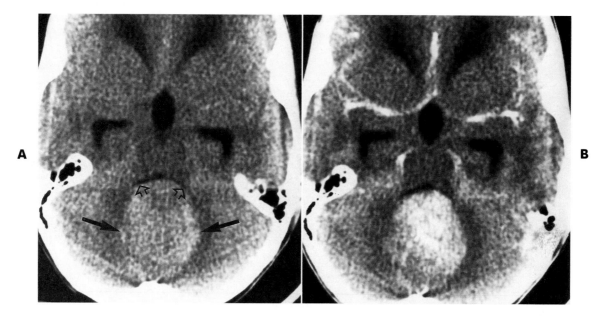

Fig. 14-53. A 7-year-old child had morning nausea and vomiting. Severe papilledema was seen on funduscopic examination. **A,** Axial NECT scan shows a round homogeneously hyperdense midline posterior fossa mass *(large arrows)*. Note anteriorly displaced crescent of CSF-filled fourth ventricle *(open arrows)*. **B,** CECT scan shows moderate enhancement. Note obstructive hydrocephalus with dilatation of the third ventricle and both lateral ventricles.

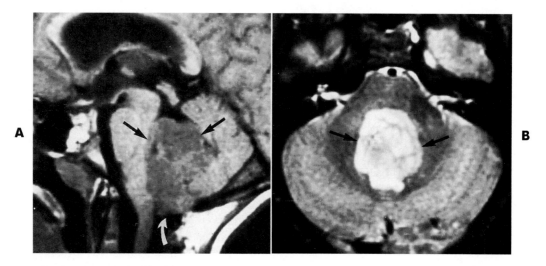

Fig. 14-54. MR findings in medulloblastoma. **A,** Sagittal precontrast T1WI shows a lobulated midline mass *(black arrows)* that bulges into the fourth ventricle and extends through the foramen of Magendie into the cisterna magna *(white arrow)*. The mass is inhomogeneously hypointense compared to cortex. **B,** The mass *(arrows)* is hyperintense on T2WI.

(65%), isodense attenuation on NECT (3%), and absent contrast enhancement (3%).[102] Between 15% and 20% of medulloblastomas in children are located off midline.[102]

MR. The "typical" medulloblastoma fills the fourth ventricle, often extending inferiorly through the foramen of Magendie into the cisterna magna (Fig. 14-54, *A*). Obstructive hydrocephalus is common (Fig. 14-54, *D*). Most medulloblastomas are heterogeneously hypointense to gray matter on T1WI. Cysts are seen in 75% to 80% of cases.[103] Signal on T2WI varies from hypo- to hyperintense (Fig. 14-54, *B*).

Contrast enhancement is quite variable. Moderately intense enhancement is typical (Fig. 14-54, *C*), but heterogeneous patterns are the rule. Many

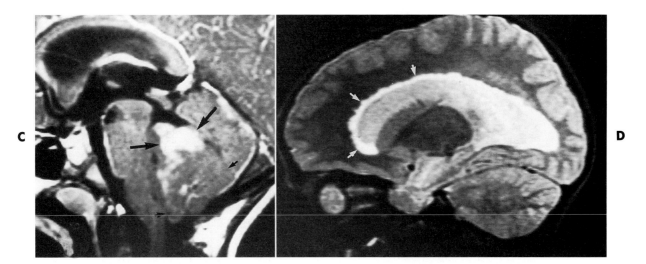

Fig. 14-54, cont'd. C, Following contrast administration, parts of the mass enhance moderately strongly *(large arrows),* and some components *(small arrows)* show little or no enhancement. **D,** Sagittal T2-weighted MR scan in another child with medulloblastoma shows the obstructive hydrocephalus with transependymal CSF flow *(arrows)* that is characteristic in these cases.

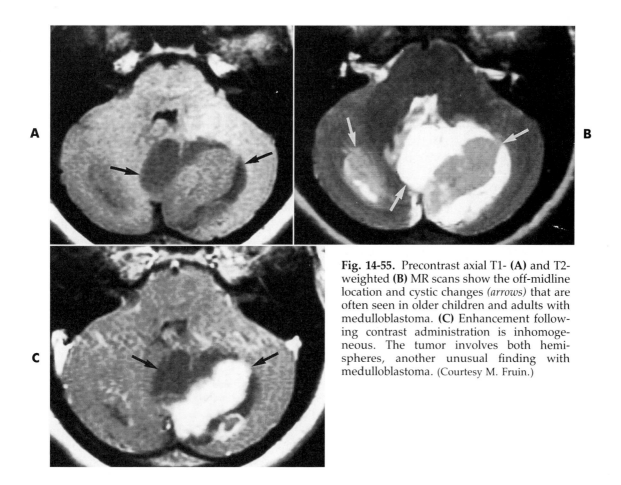

Fig. 14-55. Precontrast axial T1- **(A)** and T2-weighted **(B)** MR scans show the off-midline location and cystic changes *(arrows)* that are often seen in older children and adults with medulloblastoma. **(C)** Enhancement following contrast administration is inhomogeneous. The tumor involves both hemispheres, another unusual finding with medulloblastoma. (Courtesy M. Fruin.)

medulloblastomas show only partial enhancement following contrast administration (Figs. 14-54, C, and 14-55).[99]

Medulloblastomas in older children and adults have a more varied appearance (Fig. 14-55). Half the tumors are found in the cerebellar hemispheres, with the other half in the midline. Cystic changes are present in 80%, and tumor margins are often less well defined.[104] Some medulloblastomas may resemble meningioma.[100]

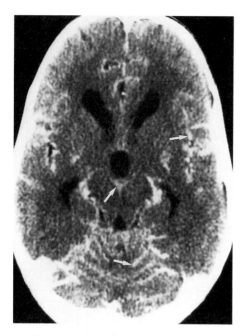

Fig. 14-56. CECT scan in this child with medulloblastoma was obtained 10 months after surgical resection. Disseminated leptomeningeal tumor (zuckerguss) is seen as diffuse sulcal-cisternal enhancement. Some of the many involved sites are indicated *(arrows).*

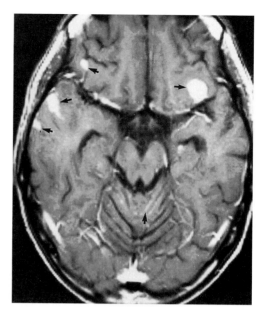

Fig. 14-57. Postcontrast axial T1-weighted MR scan in a patient with medulloblastoma shows diffuse linear and nodular enhancing lesions *(arrows)* that are characteristic of disseminated tumor.

Metastatic medulloblastoma. Disseminated medulloblastoma develops in 50% of cases. Two thirds of these metastatic lesions are to other CNS locations. The remaining one third disseminate to extracranial sites, primarily bone. Osseous metastases are typically lytic, but osteoblastic lesions also may occur.[105,106]

Leptomeningeal metastases can be identified on the initial imaging studies in 10% to 50% of patients. CECT scans in disseminated medulloblastoma show linear enhancing cisternal foci (Fig. 14-56).

Contrast-enhanced MR is superior to unenhanced MR, CT, myelography, and CT myelography for diagnosing subarachnoid dissemination and for monitoring disease response to therapy.[106] Postcontrast T1WI shows linear and nodular enhancing foci (Fig. 14-57). Both the brain and spine should be screened for metastases.

Primary Cerebral Neuroblastoma

Primary cerebral neuroblastoma is also known as PNET, cerebral medulloblastoma, undifferentiated small cell neoplasm, and PNET with neuronal differentiation (*see* box). Primary cerebral neuroblastoma is the prototypical supratentorial PNET, and we will refer to it as such.[97]

Pathology

Gross pathology. Supratentorial PNETs are typically large hemispheric masses that appear sharply circumscribed. Necrosis, hemorrhage, neovascularity, and cyst formation are common (Fig. 14-58).

Microscopic appearance. Supratentorial PNETs are composed of small undifferentiated cells with hyperchromatic nuclei, scanty cytoplasm, and numerous mitoses. These cells tend to cluster around a fibrinoid matrix, forming the so-called Homer-Wright rosettes.[97] A desmoplastic variant contains abundant connective tissue.

Incidence. Neuroblastoma is the third most common malignant neoplasm of childhood, after leukemia and brain tumors. Only 2% of all neuroblastomas arise in the brain.[107] Supratentorial PNET is a rare tumor, accounting for less than 1% of all primary CNS neoplasms. However, supratentorial PNET is one of the most common congenital brain tumors, accounting for 18% of neoplasms within the first 2 months of life (*see* Chapter 12).

Age, gender, and clinical presentation. Supratentorial PNETs are tumors of infants and young children; at least 80% occur in the first decade, usually before the age of 5 years. There is no gender predilection. Most children present with signs of increased intracranial pressure. Macrocrania is common in infants.

Location. Primary neuroblastomas can occur in any part of the CNS. Intraparenchymal, intraventric-

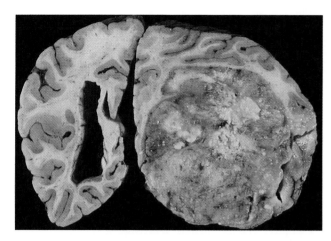

Fig. 14-58. Coronal autopsy specimen demonstrates gross pathologic findings with primary cerebral neuroblastoma (supratentorial PNET tumor). The large, bulky deep hemispheric mass appears grossly circumscribed. Necrosis, hemorrhage, and cyst formation are present in this very heterogeneous-appearing mass. (Courtesy Okazaki H, Scheithauer B: *Slide Atlas of Neuropathology,* Gower Medical Publishing.)

Primary Cerebral Neuroblastoma
Supratentorial PNET

Pathology

Large, bulky hemispheric mass with necrosis, cyst formation, hemorrhage, prominent vessels

Incidence

Rare (<1% of primary CNS tumors) except in neonates, infants

Age

80% in first decade, usually <5 years

Location

Anywhere; frontal, parietal lobes next to lateral ventricle are most common sites

Imaging

Heterogeneous density/intensity, variable enhancement

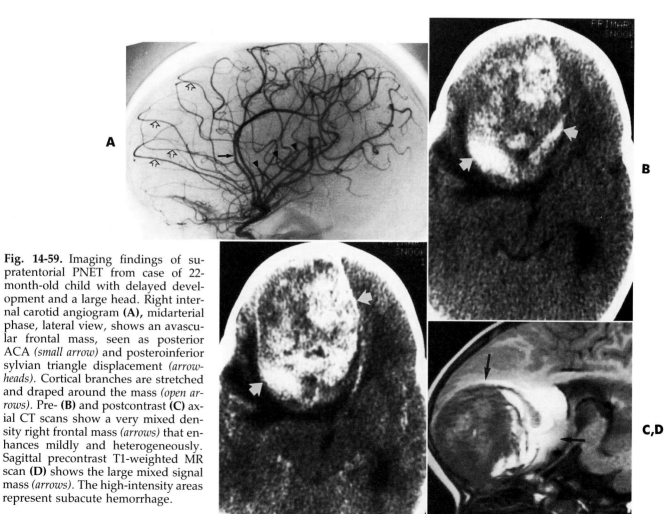

Fig. 14-59. Imaging findings of supratentorial PNET from case of 22-month-old child with delayed development and a large head. Right internal carotid angiogram **(A),** midarterial phase, lateral view, shows an avascular frontal mass, seen as posterior ACA *(small arrow)* and posteroinferior sylvian triangle displacement *(arrowheads).* Cortical branches are stretched and draped around the mass *(open arrows).* Pre- **(B)** and postcontrast **(C)** axial CT scans show a very mixed density right frontal mass *(arrows)* that enhances mildly and heterogeneously. Sagittal precontrast T1-weighted MR scan **(D)** shows the large mixed signal mass *(arrows).* The high-intensity areas represent subacute hemorrhage.

Continued.

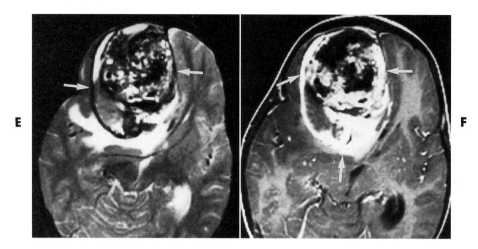

Fig. 14-59, cont'd. Axial T2WI **(E)** shows the mass *(arrows)* is extremely heterogeneous. Postcontrast T1WI **(F)** shows strong but very inhomogeneous enhancement.

ular, and even spinal cord lesions have been reported.[107] Most supratentorial PNETs are located in the frontal or parietal lobes, adjacent to the lateral ventricles.

Natural history. Prognosis is generally poor. Local recurrence following excision is the rule, and CSF dissemination is a recognized complication. The overall 5-year survival rate is 30%.[1]

Imaging
Angiography. Cerebral angiography has limited use in the evaluation of supratentorial PNETs.[97] A large hypo- or avascular mass effect is usually seen (Fig. 14-59, *A*), although occasional hypervascular masses are identified.

CT. NECT scans show a large, bulky heterogeneous hemispheric mass. Calcification, hemorrhage, necrosis, and cyst formation are common (Fig. 14-59, *B*). Enhancement is variable but typically heterogeneous (Fig. 14-59, *C*).

MR. MR also demonstrates a grossly heterogeneous hemispheric mass with variable signal on T1- and T2-weighted sequences (Fig. 14-59, *D* and *E*).[108] Contrast enhancement is mild to moderate (Fig. 14-59, *F*). Enhanced scans are helpful in detecting meningeal spread and subarachnoid seeding.[109] Both the brain and spine should be screened for disseminated disease.[97]

HEMOPOEITIC NEOPLASMS

CNS lymphomas and leukemias that are secondary manifestations of systemic disease will be discussed in Chapter 15 with other metastases. Parenchymal lymphomas that occur in the absence of recognized extracranial disease are considered in this

---

Primary CNS Lymphoma

Pathology
Non-Hodgkin lymphoma, usually B-cell

Incidence
1% to 2% of primary CNS tumors, but incidence in both AIDS and non-AIDS patients rapidly rising

Age
Any age, but most commonly 60s in immunocompetent individuals, 30s if immunocompromised

Location
Deep white matter, periventricular

Imaging
Hyperdense on NECT, enhance strongly and uniformly (unless AIDS, where ring-enhancement, hemorrhage common); like gray matter on MR. Can infiltrate diffusely, mimic white matter disease

---

chapter with other primary nonglial CNS neoplasms. Primary CNS leukemia is extraordinarily rare.

Primary CNS Lymphoma

Primary cerebral lymphoma (PCL) occurs in two different settings: immunologically normal patients and immunoincompetent patients.

Pathology
Gross pathology. PCLs are relatively well-circumscribed focal masses or poorly delineated, diffusely infiltrating lesions[1] (*see* box). Frank necrosis

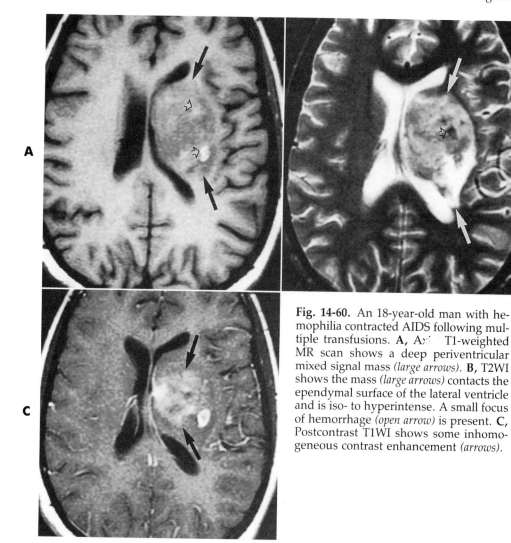

Fig. 14-60. An 18-year-old man with hemophilia contracted AIDS following multiple transfusions. **A,** A*xi* T1-weighted MR scan shows a deep periventricular mixed signal mass *(large arrows).* **B,** T2WI shows the mass *(large arrows)* contacts the ependymal surface of the lateral ventricle and is iso- to hyperintense. A small focus of hemorrhage *(open arrow)* is present. **C,** Postcontrast T1WI shows some inhomogeneous contrast enhancement *(arrows).*

and hemorrhage are uncommon in the absence of AIDS.

Microscopic appearance. Small neoplastic lymphocytes concentrated in a perivascular pattern are typical. Most are B-cell lymphomas, although a few primary CNS T-cell lymphomas occur.[110,111]

Incidence. PCL represents about 1% to 2% of all intracranial neoplasms and approximately 1% of primary non-Hodgkin lymphomas. Approximately 20% to 40% are multiple.[110,112]

Both AIDS-related and non-AIDS-related lymphomas are increasing in frequency. PCL occurs in about 2% of AIDS cases. Primary CNS lymphomas in immunologically normal patients have increased threefold in the last decade.[112]

Age. Primary CNS lymphomas are seen at all ages. The average age in immunologically normal pa-

tients is 60 years,[112] and in AIDS-related lymphoma it is 33 years.[113]

Location. Multiple centrally located lesions are frequent. The deep basal ganglia, periventricular region, and corpus callosum are common sites. Most PCLs abut the ependyma.[112]

Clinical presentation. Symptoms vary from seizure, headaches, and stupor to focal neurologic deficits such as hemiparesis.

Natural history. PCLs are highly radiosensitive tumors. Following radiotherapy, most cases regress almost completely. Unfortunately, this remission is short-lived. Recurrent or progressive disease typically appears within 1 year. Overall prognosis remains poor; the median survival after diagnosis is 13.5 months.[114]

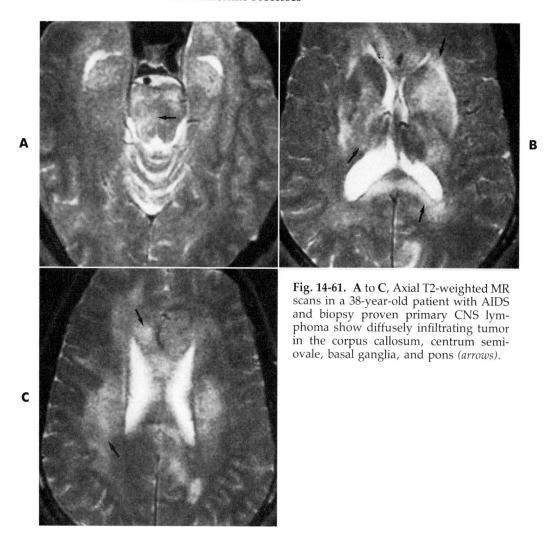

Fig. 14-61. A to **C,** Axial T2-weighted MR scans in a 38-year-old patient with AIDS and biopsy proven primary CNS lymphoma show diffusely infiltrating tumor in the corpus callosum, centrum semiovale, basal ganglia, and pons *(arrows).*

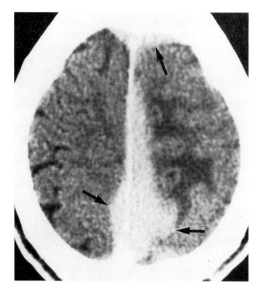

Fig. 14-62. Axial CECT scans in a patient with systemic leukemia show lobulated dural-based masses *(arrows)* along the falx and superior sagittal sinus. Chloroma was found at biopsy.

Imaging

CT. More than 90% of PCLs are iso- to moderately hyperdense on NECT and show strong, homogeneous enhancement following contrast administration. Nonenhancing tumors occur but are rare.[115] Ring enhancement is uncommon unless the patient is immunocompromised.

MR. Most focal PCLs are isointense to slightly hypointense compared to gray matter on T1WI and are iso- to slightly hyperintense on T2-weighted studies. Three quarters of all PCLs in immunologically normal patients enhance strongly and homogeneously.[112] AIDS-related PCLs may appear considerably more heterogeneous, with hemorrhage and necrotic foci (Fig. 14-60).

Primary CNS lymphoma can infiltrate the brain diffusely rather than form a dominant mass. Tumor involves both deep gray matter nuclei and white matter tracts. T2-weighted scans show extensive but poorly delineated hyperintensities in the pons, cerebellum, cerebral white matter, and basal ganglia. The imaging appearance of lymphomatosis cerebri is similar to gliomatosis cerebri (Fig. 14-61).

Leukemia

Primary CNS leukemia is extremely rare. Granulocytic sarcoma is a rare, solid tumor composed of immature granulocytes that is associated with systemic leukemia, usually acute myelogenous leukemia. Although granulocytic sarcoma can precede the development of leukemia by a few months, its occurrence without systemic leukemia is rare.[116] Imaging studies usually show an enhancing dural-based mass (Fig. 14-62).[117] Occasionally, the infundibular stalk and hypothalamus are affected (*see* Chapter 12).

REFERENCES

1. Burger PC, Scheithauer BW, Vogel FS: *Surgical Pathology of the Nervous System and its Coverings,* ed 3, pp 193-437, New York: Churchill Livingstone, 1991.
2. Okazaki H: *Fundamentals of Neuropathology,* ed 2, pp 204-275, Tokyo: Agaku-Shoin, 1989.
3. Russell DS, Rubinstein LJ: *Pathology of Tumors of the Nervous System,* ed 5, Baltimore: Williams and Wilkins, 1989.
4. VandenBerg SR, May EE, Rubinstein LJ et al: Desmoplastic supratentorial neuroepithelial tumors of infancy with divergent differentiation potential ("desmoplastic infantile gangliogliomas"), *J Neurosurg* 66:58-71, 1987.
5. Martin DS, Levy B, Awwad EE, Pitman T: Desmoplastic infantile ganglioglioma: CT and MR features, *AJNR* 12:1195-1197, 1991.
6. Diepholder HM, Schwechheimer K, Mohadjer M et al: A clinicopathologic and immunomorphologic study of 13 cases of ganglioglioma, *Cancer* 68:2192-2201, 1991.
7. Haddad SF, Moore SA, Menezes AH, VanGilder JC: Ganglioglioma: 13 years of experience, *Neurosurg* 31:171-178, 1992.
8. Otsubo H, Hoffman JH, Humphreys RP et al: Detection and management of gangliogliomas in children, *Surg Neurol* 38:371-378, 1992.
8a. Pilcher WH, Silbergeld DL, Berger MS, Ojemann GA: Intraoperative electrocorticography during tumor resection: impact on seizure outcome in patients with gangliogliomas, *J Neurosurg* 78:891-902, 1993.
9. Wacker MR, Cagan PH, Etzell JE et al: Diffuse leptomeningeal involvement by a ganglioglioma in a child, *J Neurosurg* 77:302-306, 1992.
10. Tien R, Tuori SL, Pulkingham, Burger PC: Ganglioglioma with leptomeningeal and subarachnoid spread: results of CT, MR, and PET imaging, *AJR* 159:391-393, 1992.
11. Silver JM, Rawlins CE III, Rossitch E Jr et al: Ganglioglioma: a clinical study with long-term follow-up, *Surg Neurol* 35:206-266, 1991.
12. Dorne HL, O'Gorman AM, Melanson D: Computed tomography of intracranial ganglioglioma, *AJNR* 7:281-285, 1986.
13. Tampieri D, Moumdjian R, Melanson D, Ethier R: Intracerebral gangliogliomas in patients with partial complex seizures, CT and MR findings, *AJNR* 12:749-755, 1991.
14. Castillo C, Davis PC, Takei Y, Hoffman JC Jr: Intracranial gangliogliomas: MR, CT, and clinical findings in 18 patients, *AJNR* 11:109-114, 1990.
15. Hashimoto M, Fujimoto K, Shinoda S, Masuzawa T: Magnetic resonance imaging of ganglion cell tumors, *Neuroradiol* 35:181-184, 1993.
16. Benitez WI, Glasier CM, Husain M et al: MR findings in childhood gangliogliomas, *J Comp Asst Tomogr* 14:712-716, 1990.
17. Altman NR: MR and CT characteristics of gangliocytoma: a rare cause of epilepsy in children, *AJNR* 9:917-921, 1988.
18. Duchowny MS, Resnick TJ, Alvarez L: Dysplastic gangliocytoma and intractable partial seizures in childhood, *Neurol* 39:602-604, 1989.
19. Townsend JJ, Nielsen SL, Malamud N: Unilateral megalencephaly: hamartoma or neoplasm? *Neurol* 25:448-453, 1975.
20. Vieco PT, del Cario-O'Donovan, Melanson D et al: Dysplastic ganglliocytoma (Lhermitte-Duclos disease): CT and MR imaging, *Pediatr Radiol* 22:366-369, 1992.
21. Daumas-Duport C, Scheithauer BW, Chidkiewicz J-P et al: Dysembryoplastic neuroepithelial tumor: a surgically curable tumor of young patients with intractable partial complex seizures, *Neurosurg* 23:545-556, 1988.
21a. Daumas-Duport C: Dysembryoplastic neuroepithelial tumors, *Brain Pathol* 3:283-295, 1993.
22. Koeller KK, Dillon WP: Dysembryoplastic neuroepithelial tumors: MR appearance, *AJNR* 13:1319-1325, 1992.
22a. Hassoun J, Söylemezoglu F. Gambarelli D et al: Central neurocytoma: a synopsis of clinical and histological features, *Brain Pathol* 3:297-306, 1993.
23. Yasargil MG, von Ammon K, von Deimling A et al: Central neurocytoma: histopathological variants and therapeutic approaches, *J Neurosurg* 76:32-37, 1992.
24. Smoker WRK, Townsend JJ, Reichman MV: Neurocytoma accompanied by intraventricular hemorrhage: case report and literature review, *AJNR* 12:765-770, 1991.
25. Kim DG, Chi JG, Park SH et al: Intraventricular neurocytoma: clinicopathological analysis of seven cases, *J Neurosurg* 76:759-765, 1992.
26. Goergen SK, Gonzales MF, McLean CA: Intraventricular neurocytoma: radiologic features and review of the literature, *Radiol* 182:787-792, 1992.
27. Nishio S, Tashima T, Takeshita I, Fukui M: Intraventricular neurocytoma: clinicopathological features of six cases, *J Neurosurg* 68:665-670, 1988.
28. Nishio S, Takeshita I, Kaneko Y, Fukui M: Cerebral neurocytoma: a new subset of benign neuronal tumors of the cerebrum, *Cancer* 70:529-537, 1992.
29. Wichmann W, Schubiger O, von Demling A et al: Neuroradiology of central neurocytoma, *Neuroradiol* 33:143-148, 1991.
30. Parker DR: Central neurocytoma, *AJR* 156:1311-1313, 1991.
31. Jelinek J, Smirniotopoulos JG, Parisi JE, Kanzer M: Lateral ventricular neoplasms of the brain: differential diagnosis based on clinical, CT, and MR findings, *AJR* 155:365-372, 1990.
32. Sze G: Diseases of the intracranial meninges: MR imaging features, *AJR* 160:727-733, 1993.
33. Buetow MP, Burton PC, Smirniotopoulos JG: Typical atypical, and misleading features in meningioma, *Radio Graphics* 11:1087-1100, 1991.
34. Black P McL: Meningiomas, *Neurosurg* 32:643-657, 1993.
34a. Vagner-Capodano AM, Grisoli F, Gambarelli D et al: Correlation between cytogenetic and histopathological findings in 75 human meningiomas, *Neurosurg* 32:892-900, 1993.
34b. Mack EE, Wilson CB: Meningiomas induced by high-dose cranial irradiation, *J Neurosurg* 79:28-31, 1993.
34c. Huang PP, Doyle WK, Abbott IR: Atypical meningioma of the third ventricle in a 6-year-old boy, *Neurosurg* 33:312-316, 1993.
35. Nakasu S, Hirano A, Llena J et al: Interface between the meningioma and the brain, *Surg Neurol* 32:206-212, 1989.
36. Sheporaitis L, Osborn AG, Smirniotopoulos JG, Clunie DA, Howieson J, D'Agostino AN: Radiologic-Pathologic correlation intracranial meningioma, *AJNR* 13:29-37, 1992.
36a. Kleihues P, Burger PC, Scheithauer BW: The new WHO classification of brain tumors, *Brain Pathol* 3:255-268, 1993.
37. Jaaskelainen J, Haltia M, Servo A: Atypical and anaplastic meningiomas: radiology, surgery, radiotherapy and outcome, *Surg Neurol* 25:233-242, 1986.

38. Maier H, Öffer D, Hittmair A et al: Classic, atypical and anaplastic meningioma: three histopathologic subtypes of clinical relevance, *J Neurosurg* 77:616-623, 1992.

39. Hope JKA, Armstrong DA, Babyn PS et al: Primary meningeal tumors in children: correlation of clinical and CT findings with histologic type and prognosis, *AJNR* 13:1353-1364, 1992.

40. Glasier CM, Husain MM, Chadduck W, Boop FA: Meningiomas in children: MR and histopathologic findings, *AJNR* 237-241, 1993.

41. Kallio M, Sankila R, Hakulinen T, Jaaskelainen J: Factors affecting operative and excess long-term mortality in 935 patients with intracranial meningiomas, *Neurosurg* 31:2-12, 1992.

42. Naidich TP: Imaging evaluation of meningiomas: categorical course on CNS neoplasms, American Society of Neuroradiology, 1990.

43. de la Sayette V, Rivaton F, Chapon F et al: Meningioma of the third ventricle, *Neuroradiol* 33:354-356, 1991.

44. Friedman CD, Constantino PD, Teitelbaum B et al: Primary extracranial meningiomas of the head and neck, *Laryngoscope* 100:41-48, 1990.

45. Halpin SFS, Britton J, Wilkins P, Uttley D: Intradiploic meningiomas, *Neuroradiol* 33:247-250, 1991.

46. Zee CS, Chin T, Segall HD et al: Magnetic resonance imaging of meningiomas, *Sem US, CT, MR* 13:154-169, 1992.

47. Nakao N, Kub K, Moriwaki H: Multiple growths of primary calvarial meningiomas, *Neurosurg* 29:452-455, 1991.

48. Roda JM, Bencosme JA, Perez-Higueias A, Fraile M: Simultaneous multiple intracranial and spinal meningiomas, *Neurochir* 35:92-94, 1992.

49. Kepes JJ: Presidential address: The histopathology of meningiomas: a reflection of origins and expected behavior, *J Neuropath Exp Neurol* 45:95-107, 1986.

50. Siegelman ES, Mishkin MM, Taveras JT: Past, present, and future of radiology of meningioma, *Radio Graphics* 11:899-910, 1991.

51. Dross PE, Lally JF, Bonier B: Pneumosinus dilatans and arachnoid cyst: a unique association, *AJNR* 13:209-211, 1992.

52. Osborn AG: The external carotid artery. In *Introduction to Cerebral Angiography*, pp 49-86, Hagerstown: Harper and Row, 1980.

53. New P, Aronow S, Hesselink J: National Cancer Institutes study: evaluation of computed tomography: the diagnosis of intracranial neoplasms IV meningiomas, *Radiol* 136:665-675, 1980.

54. Katayama Y, Tsubokawa T, Tanaka A et al: Magnetic resonance imaging of xanthomatous meningioma, *Neuroradiol* 35:187-189, 1993.

55. Martinez-Lage JF, Poza M, Martinez M et al: Meningiomas with hemorrhagic onset, *Acta Neurochir* (Wien) 110:129-132, 1991.

56. Zagzag D, Gomori JN, Rappaport ZH, Shalet MN: Cystic meningiomas presenting as a ring lesion, *AJNR* 7:911-912, 1986.

57. Kulali A, Ilcayto R, Fiskeci C: Cystic meningiomas, *Acta Neurochir* (Wien) 111:108-113, 1991.

58. Odake G: Cystic meningiomas report of three patients, *Neurosurg* 30:935-940, 1992.

59. Rohringer M, Sutherland GR, Louw DF, Sima AAF: Incidence and clinicopathologic features of meningioma, *J Neurosurg* 71:665-672, 1989.

60. Servo A, Porras M, Jaaskelainen J et al: Computed tomography and angiography do not reliably discriminate malignant meningiomas from benign ones, *Neuroradiol* 32:94-97, 1990.

61. Salcman M: Malignant meningiomas. In O. Al-Mefty (editor), *Meningiomas*, pp 75-85, New York: Raven Press, 1991.

62. Elster AD, Challa VR, Gilders TH et al: Meningiomas: MR and histopathologic features, *Radiol* 170:857-862, 1989.

63. Kaplan RD, Coon S, Drayer BP et al: MR characteristics of meningioma subtypes at 1.5 Tesla, *J Comp Asst Tomogr* 16:366-371, 1992.

64. Daemerel P, Wilms G, Lammeus M et al: Intracranial meningiomas: correlation between MR imaging and histology in fifty patients, *J Comp Asst Tomogr* 15:45-51, 1991.

65. Ray C Jr, Nijensohn E, Advana V, McDonald L: CT, MRI and angiographic findings of a highly aggressive malignant meningioma, *Clin Imaging* 17:59-63, 1993.

66. Inamura T, Nishio S, Takeshita I et al: Peritumoral brain edema in meningiomas: influence of vascular supply on its development, *Neurosurg* 31:179-185, 1992.

67. Fujii K, Fujita N, Hirabuki N et al: Neuromas and meningiomas: evaluation of early enhancement with dynamic MR imaging, *AJNR* 13:1215-1220, 1992.

68. Chen TC, Zee CS, Miller CA et al: Magnetic resonance imaging and pathological correlates of meningiomas, *Neurosurg* 31:1015-1022, 1992.

68a. Constantini S, Tamir J, Gomori MJ, Shohami E: Tumor prostaglandin levels correlate with edema around supratentorial meningiomas, *Neurosurg* 33:204-211, 1993.

69. Goldsher D, Litt AW, Pinto RS et al: Dural "tail" associated with meningiomas on Gd-DTPA-enhanced MR images: characteristics, differential diagnostic value, and possible implications of treatment, *Radiol* 176:447-450, 1990.

70. Wilms G, Lammeus M, Marchal G et al: Prominent dural enhancement adjacent to non-mengiomatous malignant lesions on contrast-enhanced MR images, *AJNR* 12:761-764, 1991.

71. Larson JJ, Tew JM Jr, Licot JG, de Courten-Myers GM: Association of meningiomas with dural "tails": surgical significance, *Acta Neurochir* (Wien) 114:59-63, 1992.

72. Tokumaru A, O'uchi T, Eguchi T et al: Prominent meningeal enhancement adjacent to meningioma on Gd-DTPA-enhanced MR images: histopathologic correlation, *Radiol* 175:431-433, 1990.

73. Aoki S, Sasaki Y, Machida T, Tanioka H: Contrast enhanced MR images in patients with meningiomas: importance of enhancement of the dura adjacent to the tumor, *AJNR* 11:935-938, 1990.

74. Lunardi P, Mastronardi L, Nardacci B et al: "Dural tail" adjacent to acoustic neuroma on MRI: a case report, *Neuroradiol* 35:270-271, 1993.

75. Toye R, Jeffree MA: Metastatic bronchial adenocarcinoma showing the "meningeal sign": case note, *Neuroradiol* 35:272-273, 1993.

76. Tien RD, Yang PJ, Chu PK: "Dural tail sign": a specific MR sign for meningioma? *J Comp Asst Tomogr* 15:64-66, 1991.

77. Celli P, Palina L, Domenicucci M, Scarpinati M: Histologically benign recurrent meningioma metastasizing to the parotid gland: case report and review of the literature, *Neurosurg* 31:1113-1116, 1992.Louw D, Sutherland G, Halliday W et al: Meningiomas mimicking cerebral schwannoma, *J Neurosurg* 73:715-719, 1990.

78. Louw D, Sutherland G, Halliday W et al: Meningiomas mimicking cerebral schwannoma, *J Neurosurg* 73:715-719, 1990.

78a. Williams SJ, Faye-Petersen O, Aronin P, Faith S: Capillary hemangioma of the meninges, *AJNR* 14:529-536, 1993.

79. Naul LG, Hise JH, Bauserman SC, Todd FD: CT and MR of meningeal melanocytoma, *AJNR* 12:315-316, 1991.

80. Litofsky NS, Zee C-S, Breeze RE, Chandrasoma PT: Meningeal melanocytoma: diagnostic criteria for a rare lesion, *Neurosurg* 31:945-948, 1992.

81. Uematsu Y, Yukawa S, Yokote H et al: Meningeal melanocytoma: magnetic resonance imaging characteristics and pathological features, *J Neurosurg* 76:705-709, 1992.

82. Hope JKA, Armstrong DA, Babyn PS et al: Primary malignant meningeal tumors in children: correlation of clinical and

CT findings with histologic type and prognosis, *AJNR* 13:1353-1364, 1992.

83. Parker DR, Rabinov JD: Recurrent meningeal hemaniopericy-toma, *AJR* 156:1307-1313, 1991.

84. Cosentino CM, Poulton TB, Esquerra JV, Sands SF: Giant cranial hemangiopericytoma: MR and angiographic findings, *AJNR* 14:253-256, 1993.

85. Guthrie BL, Ebersold MJ, Scheithauer BW, Shaw EG: Meningeal hemangiopericytoma: histopathologic features treatment and long-term follow-up of 44 cases, *Neurosurg* 25:514-522, 1989.

86. Ho VB, Smirniotopoulos JG, Murphy FM, Rushing EJ: Radiologic-pathologic correlation: hemangioblastoma, *AJNR* 13:1343-1352, 1992.

87. Lee SR, Sanches J, Mark AS et al: Posterior fossa hemangioblastomas: MR imaging, *Radiol* 171:463-468, 1989.

88. Neumann HPH, Eggert HR, Scheremet R et al: Central nervous system lesions in von Hippel-Lindau Syndrome, *J Neurol Neurosurg Psychiatr* 55:898-901, 1992.

89. Elster AD, Arthur DW: Intracranial hemangioblastomas: CT and MR findings, *J Comp Asst Tomogr* 12:736-739, 1988.

90. Smirniotopoulos JG, Rushing EJ, Mena H: Pineal region masses: differential diagnosis, *Radio Graphics* 12:577-596, 1992.

91. Hoffman HJ, Otsubo H, Hendrick EB et al: Intracranial germ-cell tumors in children, *J Neurosurg* 74:545-551, 1991.

92. Soijima T, Takeshita I, Yamamoto H et al: Computed tomography of germinomas is basal ganglia and thalamus, *Neuroradiol* 29:366-370, 1987.

93. Tien RD, Barkovich AJ, Edwards MSB: MR imaging of pineal tumors, *AJNR* 11:557-565, 1990.

94. Raaijmakers C, Wilms G, Demaerel P, Baert AL: Pineal teratocarcinoma with drop metastases: MR features, *Neuroradiol* 34:227-229, 1992.

95. Chang T, Teng MMH, Guo W-Y, Sheng W-C: CT of pineal tumors and intracranial germ-cell tumors, *AJNR* 10:1039-1044, 1989.

96. Nakagawa H, Iwasaki S, Kichikawa K et al: MR imaging of pineocytoma: report of two cases, *AJNR* 11:195-198, 1990.

97. Robles HA, Smirniotopoulos JG, Figueroa RE: Understanding the radiology of intracranial primitive neuroectodermal tumors from a pathological perspective: a review, *Sem US, CT, MR* 13:170-181, 1992.

98. Rorke LB, Gilles FH, Davis RL et al: Revision of the World Health Organization classification of brain tumors for childhood brain tumors, *Cancer* 56:1869-1886, 1985.

99. Meyers SP, Kemp SS, Tarr RW: MR imaging features of medulloblastomas, *AJR* 158:865-895, 1992.

100. Koci TM, Chiang F, Mehringer CM et al: Adult cerebellar medulloblastoma: imaging features with emphasis on MR, *AJNR* 14:929-939, 1993.

101. Maleci A, Cervoni L, Delfini R: Medulloblastoma in children and in adults: a comparative study, *Acta Neurochidr* (Wien) 19:62-67, 1992.

102. Nelson M, Diebler C, Forbes W StC: Pediatric medulloblastoma: atypical CT features at presentation in the SiOP II trial, *Neuroradiol* 33:140-142, 1991.

103. Mueller DP, Moore SA, Sato Y, Yuh WTC: MR spectrum of medulloblastoma, *Clin Imaging* 16:250-255, 1992.

104. Bourgouin PM, Tampieri D, Grahovac SZ et al: CT and MR imaging findings in adults with cerebellar medulloblastoma: comparison with findings in children, *AJR* 159:609-612, 1992.

105. Algra PR, Postma T, VanGroeningen CJ et al: MR imaging of skeletal metastases from medulloblastoma, *Skeletal Radiol* 21:425-430, 1992.

106. Kochi M, Mihara Y, Takada A et al: MRI of subarachnoid of dissemination of medulloblastoma, *Neuroradiol* 33:264-268, 1991.

107. David R, Lamki N, Fan S et al: The many faces of neuroblastoma, *Radio Graphics* 9:859-882, 1989.

108. Davis PC, Wichman Rd, Takei Y, Hoffman JC Jr: Primary cerebral neuroblastoma: CT and MR findings in 12 cases, *AJNR* 11:115-120, 1990.

109. Wiegel B, Harris TM, Edwards MK et al: MR of intracranial neuroblastoma with dural sinus invasion and distant metastases, *AJNR* 12:1198-1200, 1991.

110. Knorr JR, Ragland RL, Stone BB et al: Cerebellar T-cell lymphoma: an unusual primary intracranial neoplasm, *Neuroradiol* 35:79-81, 1992.

111. Dumas J-L, Visy J-M, Lhote F et al: MRI and neurological complications of adult T-cell leukemia/lymphoma, *J Comp Asst Tomogr* 16:820-823, 1992.

112. Róman-Goldstein SM, Goldman DL, Howieson J et al: MR in primary CNS lymphoma in immunologically normal patients, *AJNR* 13:1207-1213, 1992.

113. Cordoliani Y-S, Derosier C, Pharaboz C et al: Primary cerebral lymphoma in patients with AIDS: MR findings: 17 cases, *AJR* 159:841-847, 1992.

114. Watanabe M, Tanaka R, Takeda N et al: Correlation of computed tomography with the histopathology of primary malignant lymphoma of the brain, *Neuroradiol* 34:36-42, 1992.

115. DeAngelis LM: Cerebral lymphomas presenting as a nonenhancing lesion on computed tomographic/magnetic resonance scan, *Am Neurol* 33:308-311, 1993.

116. Wright DH, Hise JH, Bauserman SC, Naul LG: Intracranial granulocytic sarcoma: CT, MR, and angiography.

117. Williams MP, Ollift JFC, Rowley MR: CT and MR findings: parameningeal leukaemic masses, *J Comp Asst Tomogr* 14:736-742, 1990.

Miscellaneous Tumors, Cysts, and Metastases

TUMORS OF CRANIAL AND SPINAL NERVES

Schwannoma

Etiology and pathology

Etiology. Schwannomas are benign tumors that originate from schwann cells. The schwann cell is a neural crest derivative, and therefore schwannomas are classified as nonglial neuroectodermal tumors.[1]

Gross pathology. Schwannomas are round or lobulated well-delineated encapsulated tumors that arise eccentrically from their parent nerve.[2] Cystic or fatty degeneration and hemorrhagic necrosis are common (Fig. 15-1) (Table 15-1).

Microscopic appearance. Two histologic types have been identified: Antoni type A and Antoni type B. Antoni type A has compact interlacing bundles of fusiform neoplastic Schwann cells, reticulin, and collagen.[2] Well-developed cylindrical structures with palisading nuclei around a central core of cytoplasm, the classic "Verocay bodies," are seen.

Antoni type B consists of a loosely textured stroma with widely separated stellate cells and no distinctive pattern.[1]

Incidence. Schwannomas account for approximately 6% to 8% of all primary intracranial tumors.[3]

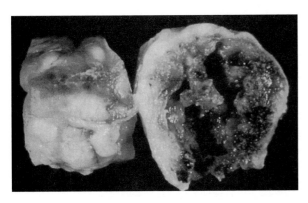

Fig. 15-1. Gross pathology of a schwannoma with central necrosis and hemorrhage. (Courtesy Rubinstein Collection, Armed Forces Institute of Pathology.)

Acoustic schwannoma is the most common cerebellopontine angle mass, accounting for 75% to 80% of all lesions in this location (*see* Chapter 12).

Schwannomas usually occur as isolated lesions. Multiple schwannomas are seen in approximately 5% of cases and are characteristic of neurofibromatosis type 2 (NF-2).[4] Approximately 18% of solitary schwannomas occur in the presence of neurofibromatosis.[5]

Age and gender

Age. Schwannomas are primarily adult tumors. They are most prevalent in older age groups (5th to 6th decades). When they occur with NF-2, schwannomas appear earlier, usually by the third decade.[6]

Schwannomas are rare in children, accounting for approximately 0.1% of pediatric intracranial tumors.[6] Schwannomas are especially rare in the absence of neurofibromatosis.

Gender. There is a slight female predominance (1.5-2:1).[7,8]

Clinical presentation. Symptoms depend on the specific cranial nerve affected.

Vestibulocochlear nerve. CN VIII is the most common location for intracranial schwannoma. Despite the fact that most acoustic schwannomas originate from the vestibular segment, the earliest symptoms are usually tinnitus and sensorineural hearing loss.[9] Vestibular symptoms are late manifestations. Other symptoms depend on tumor size and extent. These include symptoms of other cranial nerve involvement, brainstem compression, and obstructive hydrocephalus.[9]

Trigeminal nerve. Because the fifth cranial nerve has an extensive intracranial course and traverses several distinct anatomic regions, trigeminal schwannomas have various manifestations.[10] Eighty to ninety percent of gasserian ganglion schwannomas cause trigeminal dysfunction. Symptoms are pain,

Table 15-1. Comparison between schwannoma and neurofibroma

	Schwannoma	Neurofibroma (plexiform type)
Pathology	Schwann cells	Schwann cells + fibroblasts
	Encapsulated	Unencapsulated
	Focal	Infiltrating
	Round	Fusiform
	Cysts, necrosis, hemorrhage common	Cysts, necrosis, hemorrhage rare
	Don't undergo malignant degeneration	Malignant degeneration in 5% to 13%
	NF-2	NF-1
Incidence	Common (6% to 8% of primary brain tumors)	Uncommon (except in NF-1)
Age	40s to 60s	Any age
Location	Cranial nerves (especially CN VIII)	Cutaneous and spinal nerves (especially CN V_1 peripheral branches, exiting spinal nerves)
Imaging	Sharply delineated	Poorly delineated, infiltrating
	Heterogeneous (large lesions)	Homogeneous
	T1WI: 67% hypointense, 33% isointense	T1WI: mostly isointense with muscle
	T2WI: hyperintense	T2WI: hyperintense
	Enhance strongly	Enhance moderately/ intensely

paresthesias, and masticatory muscle weakness, in decreasing order of frequency.[11] Occult denervation atrophy can sometimes be identified on imaging studies in these patients (see subsequent discussion).

Ophthalmic division (V_1) involvement results in exophthalmos and diplopia. Posterior fossa trigeminal schwannomas cause ataxia and facial and auditory nerve dysfunction.[12] Atypical trigeminal neuralgia, lower cranial nerve palsies, pyramidal signs, and signs of increased intracranial pressure are found in 40% of patients.

Facial nerve. Regardless of location, facial nerve paresis is the most common presenting symptom. Schwannoma is nevertheless a rare cause of facial palsy, accounting for only 5% to 6% of cases; 80% are idiopathic (Bell palsy), with herpes zoster, otitis media, and trauma more common than schwannoma.[13,14]

Location

General. Excepting the first (olfactory) and second (optic) nerves, all cranial nerves have sheaths that are partially composed of Schwann cells and are therefore potential sites for intracranial schwannomas.[5] Cranial nerve sheaths have two anatomically distinct components. In one part the sheath surrounding the axons is formed by Schwann cells; in the other the sheath consists of oligodendroglial cells.[9] Most schwannomas arise at the point where the axonal sheath switches from glial (oligodendrocyte) to Schwann cell origin.[3] Schwannomas arise eccentrically from the outer nerve sheath layer and enlarge away from it, compressing rather than invading the nerve.[13]

Schwannomas have a distinct propensity to affect sensory nerves more than pure motor nerves. CN VIII is the most commonly affected, with the trigeminal nerve root or ganglion next in frequency of occurrence. Schwannomas arising from other cranial nerves are very rare.[5]

Vestibulocochlear nerve. Ninety to ninety-five percent of intracranial schwannomas arise from CN VIII. Most all "acoustic schwannomas" originate from the inferior or superior vestibular division; cochlear schwannomas are rare.[12]

Trigeminal nerve. Trigeminal schwannomas represent 0.07% to 0.28% of primary intracranial tumors and account for approximately 5% to 6% of all intracranial schwannomas.[7,10] The most common location is the middle cranial fossa, site of nearly half of all trigeminal schwannomas. CN V schwannomas that are totally or predominately within the posterior fossa account for another 15% to 20%. "Dumbbell"-shaped or "hourglass" tumors with significant components in both cranial fossae represent about one quarter of all trigeminal schwannomas.

Five percent of all schwannomas arise from distal intracranial CN V branches and extend extracranially (*see* Fig. 12-165). These rare tumors commonly originate from the ophthalmic division.[7,10,11] Completely extracranial head and neck schwannomas are uncommon. They usually arise from the sympathetic chain, cervical plexus, or vagus nerve.[1]

Facial nerve. The facial nerve is the third most common site of intracranial schwannomas. Most facial schwannomas are intratemporal; all segments of the intrapetrous facial nerve can be affected, although the geniculate ganglion is the most frequent site.[13,14] Involvement of multiple contiguous segments is also common.[13] Schwannomas involving the intracranial or intraparotid facial nerve segments are rare.

Other cranial nerves. Pure motor cranial nerves such as the oculomotor, trochlear, and abducens nerves are rarely involved by solitary schwannomas.[15] This is particularly true in the absence of NF-2.[4,5,16] Schwannomas of mixed cranial nerves (IX, X,

XI) are also uncommon.[17] These tumors occur as a purely cisternal mass, jugular foramen lesion, or a "dumbbell" lesion with both intra- and extracranial components.

Multiple schwannomas. Multiple cranial nerve schwannomas are common with NF-2[3]; bilateral acoustic nerve tumors are pathognomonic for NF-2 (*see* Chapter 5).

Intracerebral schwannoma. Schwannoma within the brain parenchyma is an exceedingly rare tumor; only 37 cases have been reported. These tumors may arise from perivascular nerve plexi in the tela choroidea.[18,18a]

Natural history. Schwannomas are very slow-growing benign neoplasms. Despite their potential for regrowth following incomplete excision, schwannomas rarely, if ever, undergo malignant degeneration.[2,19] Neurofibromas are much more likely than schwannomas to become malignant (see subsequent discussion).

Imaging

Plain film radiographs. Bone changes on plain film radiographs are comparatively late manifestations of intracranial schwannomas. Imaging findings vary with tumor location. Widening of the internal auditory canal can be seen with moderate-sized acoustic schwannomas; smooth, sharply marginated anteromedial petrous apex erosion is the most common plain film manifestation of trigeminal schwannoma.[7] The middle cranial fossa floor may also be affected with enlarged foramen ovale, foramen rotundum, or superior orbital fissure.[10] Hyperostosis and bone sclerosis are rare.

Angiography. Reported angiographic findings in schwannoma vary, and a typical pattern is not clearly established.[20] Many schwannomas are avascular or hypovascular lesions that are identified by focal displacement, stretching, and draping of adjacent vessels. One quarter of reported cases show hypervascularity, contrast pooling, and prominent capsular veins.[20] Diffuse vascular blush and arteriovenous shunting with early draining veins are uncommon. Benign and malignant nerve sheath tumors cannot be distinguished by their angiographic patterns alone.[21]

CT. Schwannomas are iso- or slightly hypodense to adjacent brain on NECT scans. Calcification and hemorrhage are uncommon.

Virtually all schwannomas enhance strongly following contrast administration. Small tumors usually show uniform enhancement, whereas larger lesions may have a heterogeneous pattern. This is due to cystic degeneration, xanthomatous change, or areas of relative hypocellularity adjacent to densely cellular or collagenous regions.[22] Peripheral arachnoid cysts or pools of trapped CSF are sometimes associated with schwannomas.[9] Trigeminal schwannomas with long-standing denervation cause atrophy and fatty infiltration of the masticatory muscles.

MR. Large acoustic schwannomas demonstrate the characteristic findings of an extraaxial mass (Fig. 15-2, *A*). There is a distinct CSF/vascular "cleft" between tumor and brain, the corticomedullary junction of the cerebellum is displaced, and the brainstem appears rotated (*see* Figs. 12-61, *B,* and 15-2, *B* and

C). Most acoustic schwannomas form an acute angle with the petrous temporal bone. The cisternal portion is typically larger than the intracanalicular segment, giving this particular tumor the appearance of ice cream on a cone (*see* Fig. 12-63).

Approximately two thirds of acoustic schwannomas are slightly hypointense to brain on T1WI (Fig. 15-3); one third are isointense. Most schwannomas have mild to markedly increased signal intensity on proton density- and T2-weighted sequences. Foci of

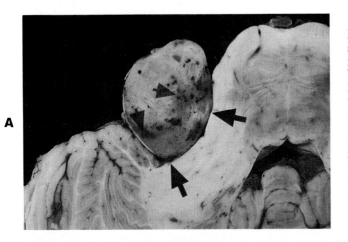

Fig. 15-2. Axial gross pathology **(A)** of a vestibulocochlear schwannoma with fatty degeneration and small hemorrhagic foci *(small arrows).* Note the distinct cleft *(large arrows)* between the extraaxial mass and the brain (compare with Figs. 12-61, *B* and 15-2, *B* and *C*). Axial postcontrast T1-weighted **(B)** and T2-weighted **(C)** MR scans in another patient show a typical large acoustic schwannoma. The tumor *(large arrows)* enhances strongly but heterogeneously. It is slightly hyperintense to brain on T2WI and has numerous intratumoral cysts *(open arrows).* Intracanalicular part of the tumor *(curved arrow).* Also note the compressed fourth ventricle *(arrowheads)* and rotated brainstem. (**A,** Courtesy B. Horten.)

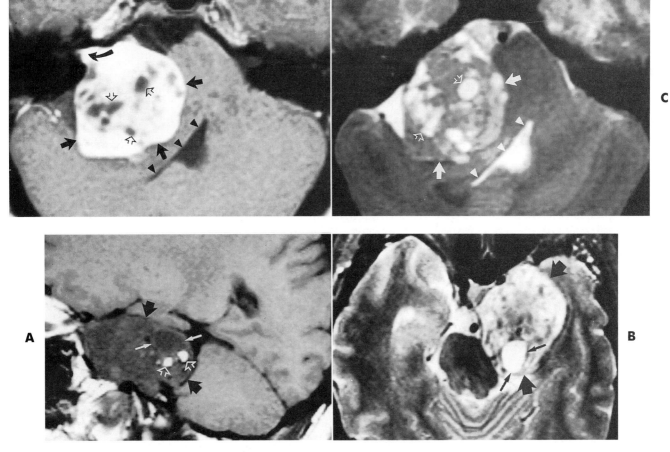

Fig. 15-3. Sagittal T1- **(A)** and axial T2-weighted **(B)** MR scans of a large trigeminal schwannoma *(large black arrows)* show intratumor cysts *(small arrows)* and hemorrhage *(open arrows).* (Courtesy Timothy J. Miller.)

cystic degeneration are common in larger lesions (Figs. 15-2, C and 15-3, C), but frank hemorrhage is rare (Fig. 15-3, A).[22a]

Nearly all schwannomas show intense enhancement following contrast administration (*see* Fig. 12-75). Enhancement patterns are homogeneous in 67% (*see* Fig. 12-63, B), mildly inhomogeneous in 10%, and heterogeneous with areas of intratumoral cystic degeneration in 22% (Fig. 15-2, B). Peritumoral edema is seen in 37%, and associated arachnoid cysts are present in 7% of cases (*see* Fig. 12-63, B).[23]

The major differential diagnosis of acoustic schwannoma is cerebellopontine angle meningioma. The latter is typically a broad-based lesion that forms an obtuse angle with the adjacent dura (*see* Fig. 12-64). A dural "tail" is highly suggestive of, but not diagnostic for, meningioma (*see* Chapter 14). Other lesions that can mimic acoustic schwannoma include metastasis, hemangioma (*see* Fig. 12-74, C), postoperative fibrosis (*see* Fig. 12-76), and inflammatory disease (*see* Fig. 12-79).[9,24]

Neurofibroma

Head and neck neurofibromas are usually plexiform tumors. Plexiform neurofibromas are a unique feature of neurofibromatosis type 1 (von Recklinghausen disease) and are considered pathognomonic of that neurocutaneous syndrome (*see* Chapter 5). Neurofibromas are not native to the intracranial cavity but occur in posterior ganglia as central extensions of peripheral tumors.[2]

Pathology

Gross pathology. Plexiform neurofibromas are unencapsulated tumors that diffusely infiltrate the affected subcutaneous tissue or nerve (Fig. 15-4). Fusiform enlargement of multiple nerve fascicles and branches is characteristic. In contrast to schwannomas, neurofibromas rarely undergo fatty degeneration, cystic necrosis, or hemorrhage[2] (*see* Table 15-1).

Microscopic appearance. Plexiform neurofibromas contain a mixture of Schwann cells, fibroblasts, reticulin, and collagen fibers, and a loose mucoid matrix interspersed between axons of the parent nerve.[2] In schwannomas, Schwann cells are the only proliferating cell type, mucopolysaccharide matrix is scanty or absent, and nerve fascicles are displaced rather than assimilated within the tumor.[19]

Incidence. Plexiform neurofibromas occur only with NF-1.

Age and gender. Plexiform neurofibromas can be found at any age. Both genders are equally affected.

Location. Neurofibromas can extend along cranial

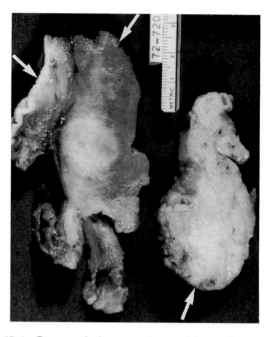

Fig. 15-4. Gross pathology specimen of the eyelid and adjacent scalp in a patient with an extensive plexiform neurofibroma. The unencapsulated tumor diffusely infiltrates the soft tissues *(arrows)*. (Courtesy Rubinstein Collection, Armed Forces Institute of Pathology.)

nerves from peripherally located tumors. The ophthalmic division of the trigeminal nerve is most commonly affected; the facial nerve is a less frequent site.

Natural history. Between 5% and 13% of plexiform neurofibromas undergo malignant degeneration.

Imaging. Plexiform neurofibromas are poorly delineated, diffusely infiltrating masses that can expand foramina and erode bone (Fig. 15-5, A). These lesions are typically isodense with muscle on NECT scans and show variable enhancement following contrast administration (Fig. 15-5, B). Most neurofibromas are isointense on T1-weighted MR scans, hyperintense on T2WI, and enhance moderately to intensely (*see* Figs. 12-164 and 12-183).

Malignant Peripheral Nerve Sheath Tumors

Malignant transformation of schwannomas is extremely rare. Between 5% and 13% of neurofibromas in von Recklinghausen disease become malignant. Malignant nerve sheath tumors can also arise *de novo* within an otherwise normal nerve. These so-called malignant peripheral nerve sheath tumors (MPNSTs) typically affect the retroperitoneum, mediastinum, and viscera, as well as large nerves of the neck and proximal extremities. Malignant tumors can arise from the eighth nerve, but the trigeminal nerve is the most commonly affected cranial nerve.[19]

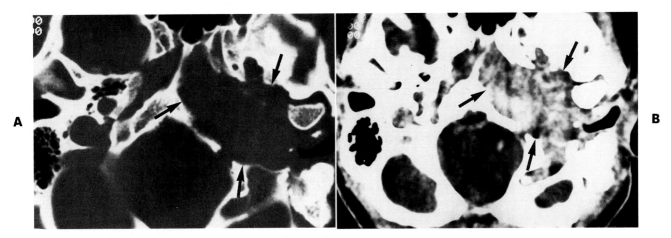

Fig. 15-5. Bone **(A)** and soft tissue windows **(B)** from an axial CECT scan in a patient with neurofibromatosis type 1 (NF-1) show an extensive plexiform neurofibroma *(arrows)* that erodes the skull base. The tumor enhances moderately.

NONNEOPLASTIC TUMORLIKE LESIONS
Epidermoid Tumor

Etiology. Both congenital and acquired epidermoid cysts occur. Congenital epidermoid "tumor" is actually a nonneoplastic inclusion cyst. Epidermoid cysts probably arise from inclusion of ectodermal epithelial elements at the time of neural tube closure or during formation of the secondary cerebral vesicles[24,25] (Table 15-2, p. 632).

Acquired epidermoid cysts develop as a result of trauma. Here, epidermis is implanted into deeper underlying tissues and forms a cyst that continues to desquamate keratin.[26] Intracranial implantation epidermoid cysts are uncommon; most epidermal inclusions cysts are found in the lumbosacral spine following nonstylet needle puncture (*see* Chapter 21).

Pathology
Gross pathology. Intracranial epidermoid tumors are well-delineated cystic lesions that insinuate along CSF cisterns. They have an irregular lobulated, or "cauliflower-like" outer surface that often has a shiny "mother of pearl" appearance (Fig. 15-6). The cyst interior is filled with soft, waxy, or flaky keratohyalin

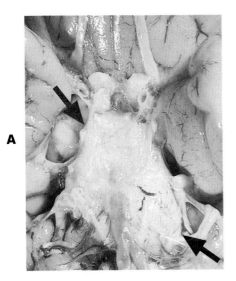

Fig. 15-6. Two gross pathology cases illustrate the typical appearance of epidermoid tumors. **A,** This suprasellar epidermoid tumor *(arrows)* is seen from below. Note the shiny "mother of pearl" appearance. The tumor insinuates throughout the suprasellar subarachnoid space, engulfing vessels and cranial nerves at the base of the brain. **B,** Close-up view of an epidermoid tumor that was removed from the cerebellopontine angle in another patient. Note the lobulated, "cauliflower-like" surface to the tumor. CSF is present between the tumor interstices. (**A,** Courtesy E. Tessa Hedley-Whyte. **B,** From Gao P-Y, Osborn AG et al: *AJNR* 13:863-872, 1992.)

Table 15-2. Comparison between epidermoid and dermoid tumors

	Epidermoid	Dermoid
Pathology	Ectodermal inclusion cyst	Ectodermal inclusion cyst (no mesoderm)
	Squamous epithelium	Squamous epithelium
	Keratinaceous debris	Keratinaceous debris
	Solid crystalline cholesterol	Liquid cholesterol
	No dermal appendages	Dermal appendages (hair, sebaceous glands)
	Grow by epithelial desquamation	Grow by epithelial desquamation + glandular secretion
	Rarely rupture	Commonly rupture
Incidence	0.2% to 1% of primary brain tumors	Uncommon (0.04 to 0.6% of primary brain tumors)
	4-9× more common than dermoid	
Age	20 to 60 years	30 to 50 years
	M = F	Slight male predominance
Location	Off-midline	Midline
	40% to 50% in cerebellopontine angle cistern; 10% to 15% parasellar, middle fossa space; 10% diploic space	Parasellar, frontobasal most common intracranial sites
	Insinuates along CSF spaces	Vermis, fourth ventricle most common infratentorial sites
		Subarachnoid spread from ruptured cyst
Imaging		
CT	NECT: low density (like CSF); calcification uncommon	NECT: very low density (like fat); calcification common; ± dermal sinus tract
	CECT: periphery occasionally enhances	CECT: no enhancement
MR	T1-, T2WI: often like CSF	Hyperintense on T1-, hypointense on T2WI

material that results from progressive desquamation of the cyst wall.[27] Epidermoid cysts encase vessels and engulf cranial nerves (Figs. 15-6, *A*, and 15-7). In some cases they invaginate deeply into adjacent brain.

Microscopic appearance. The cyst wall is composed of simple stratified cuboidal squamous epithelium, and the center is filled with keratinaceous debris and solid crystalline cholesterol. The keratin, produced in successive layers by desquamated epithelium from the cyst wall, has a laminated appearance. In contrast to dermoid cysts, epidermoid tumors do not contain hair follicles or sebaceous glands.[27]

Incidence. Epidermoid tumors represent 0.2% to 1% of all primary intracranial tumors.[3]

Age and gender. Epidermoid tumors typically occur between the ages of 20 and 60. The peak incidence is the fourth decade.[25] There is no gender predilection.

Location. Ninety percent of cranial epidermoid tumors are intradural. Intradural epidermoid tumors occur primarily in the basal subarachnoid spaces; off-midline sites are the common locations. Between 40% to 50% are found in the cerebellopontine angle cisterns, making epidermoid the third most common CPA mass (after acoustic schwannoma and meningioma). Supra- and parasellar (cavernous sinus or middle cranial fossa) regions account for 7% each (*see* Fig. 12-128).

Intraaxial epidermoid tumors are uncommon. The fourth ventricle is the most common site.[28] Rarely, these tumors occur in the cerebral hemispheres or brain stem.[27]

Ten percent of epidermoid cysts are extradural, mostly intradiploic. Primary intradiploic epidermoid cysts occur in the frontal, parietal, or occipital bones; the sphenoid bone is an uncommon site.[29] Cranial dermoids and epidermoid cysts are the most common scalp lesions in children[26] (*see* Chapter 12).

Natural history. The epithelium of epidermoid tumors proliferates at a rate comparable to normal epidermis, suggesting that these are not true neoplasms but benign cysts.[19] Although malignant degeneration does not take place, local recurrence following subtotal resection is common.

Imaging
Plain film radiographs. Diploic space epidermoid tumors can affect any part of the skull: the scalp, diploe (inner or outer table alone or both), and sometimes the epidural space as well.[30] Diploic epider-

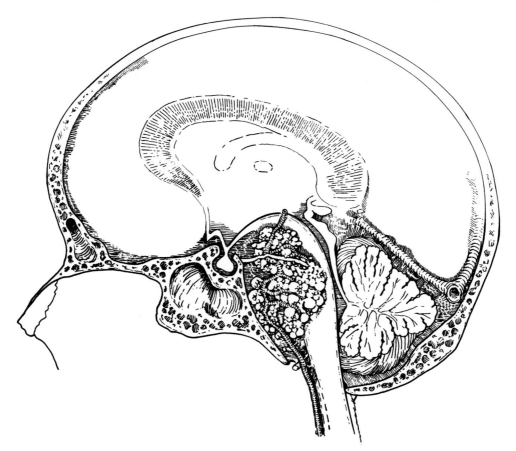

Fig. 15-7. Anatomic drawing of a typical posterior fossa epidermoid tumor. The lobulated tumor insinuates throughout the CSF cisterns, engulfing the basilar artery and its branches, as well as the trigeminal nerve. The tumor deeply invaginates the adjacent pons. (From Gao P-Y, Osborn AG et al: *AJNR* 13:863-872, 1992.)

moid cysts typically have round or lobulated, well-delineated focal bone erosions with sclerotic margins.

Angiography. Cerebral angiography is usually normal or discloses avascular mass effect.

CT. NECT scans show most epidermoid tumors are well-defined lucent-appearing lobulated masses with attenuation similar to CSF (Fig. 15-8). Calcification is present in 10% to 25% of cases.[27,31] Occasionally, epidermoid tumors appear hyperdense on NECT, possibly due to hemorrhage, high protein content, saponification of cyst debris to calcium soaps, or deposition of iron-containing pigment.[25,32,33]

Most epidermoids do not enhance following intravenous contrast administration, although enhancement at the tumor margin is sometimes observed.[27] Intrathecal contrast delineates the irregular, multilobulated tumor surface (*see* Fig. 12-65, *D*).

MR. Most intracranial epidermoid tumors are confined to, and insinuate along, the basilar CSF cisterns (Fig. 15-9; *see* Fig. 12-128). Epidermoid tumors typically have long T1 and T2 relaxation times, and signal characteristics that are similar to CSF (Figs. 15-8, *B* and *C*, and 15-9; and *see* Fig. 12-65, *B*

and *C*). Some epidermoid tumors have a lobulated rim that gives slightly higher signal than the hypointense central portion of the cyst (Fig. 15-10). A thin hyperintense rim that probably represents CSF trapped around the mass or within its frondlike interstices is sometimes seen on proton density-weighted sequences.[34]

Some epidermoid cysts appear iso- or even hyperintense to brain on T1WI. These so-called "white epidermoids" have high lipid content on magnetic resonance spectroscopy, whereas epidermoids with long T1 values (black epidermoids) have reduced lipid content on spectroscopy.[28,35] Rarely, epidermoids show mixed signal intensities on both CT and MR.[36]

Differential diagnosis. Although completely cystic schwannomas can sometimes mimic epidermoid tumor,[37] the major differential diagnostic consideration is arachnoid cyst (*see* Fig. 12-135).[31] Steady-state free-precession (SSFP) MR imaging is useful in differentiating tumors such as epidermoid from simple or complex benign cysts (see subsequent discussion).

Diffusion-weighted MR can also be useful in distinguishing between arachnoid cysts and epidermoid

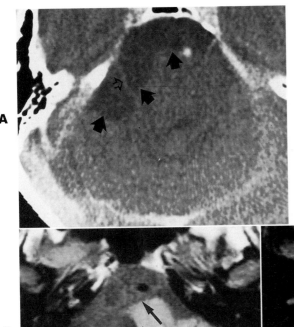

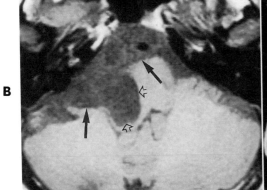

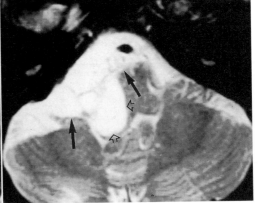

Fig. 15-8. Axial CECT scan **(A)** of a cerebellopontine angle epidermoid tumor shows the lesion *(large arrows)* is very low density and difficult to differentiate from CSF. The right trigeminal nerve *(open arrow)* is displaced and engulfed by the tumor. Axial T1- **(B)** and T2-weighted **(C)** MR scans in the same case show the tumor *(large arrows)* extends inferiorly along the cerebellopontine angle cistern, deeply invaginating into the adjacent medulla *(open arrows)*. (From Gao P-Y, Osborn AG et al: *AJNR* 13:863-872, 1992.)

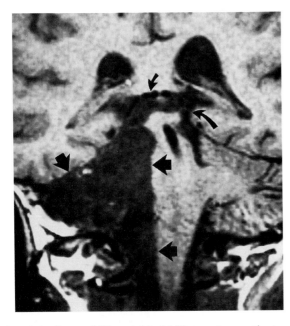

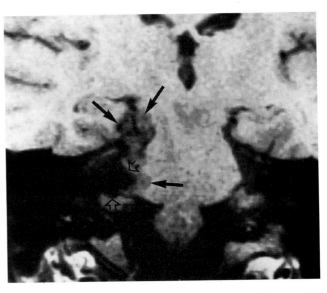

Fig. 15-9. Coronal T1-weighted MR scan in a patient with an epidermoid tumor shows the mass *(large arrows)* fills the cerebellopontine angle cistern and displaces the pons and medulla toward the opposite side. This case nicely demonstrates tumor insinuation into the adjacent ambient and quadrigeminal cisterns *(curved arrows)*. This epidermoid tumor is nearly isointense with CSF.

Fig. 15-10. Coronal T1-weighted MR scan in a 52-year-old woman with a right cerebellopontine angle epidermoid tumor shows the lobulated tumor rim *(large arrows)* is nearly isointense with gray matter, whereas the center *(open arrows)* is very low signal and is nearly isointense with CSF.

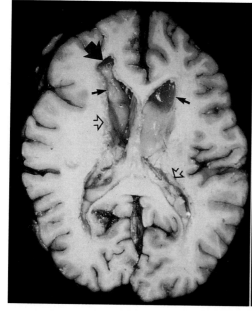

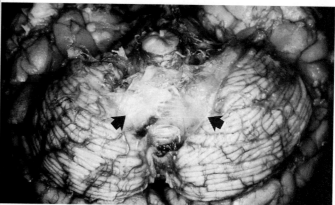

Fig. 15-11. Gross pathology of a dermoid cyst is demonstrated. **A,** The frontal mass *(large arrow)* ruptured into the lateral ventricles, filling both ventricles with an oily, cheesy fluid *(small arrows)*. Note ependymitis *(open arrows)*. **B,** Basal view of the cisterna magna shows opaque, thickened meninges *(arrows)*, caused by the intense chemical meningitis. (From archives of the Armed Forces Institute of Pathology.)

tumors. The apparent diffusion coefficient (ADC) of arachnoid cysts is similar to stationary water, whereas the ADC of epidermoid tumors is similar to brain parenchyma.[38] Cystic astrocytomas, hemangioblastomas, and other low density cisternal masses such as enteric cyst are rarely confused with epidermoid tumors.

Dermoid Tumors

Etiology. A common misconception about the origin and content of dermoid cysts is that they arise from inclusion of both ectodermal and mesodermal elements. This so-called myth of the mesoderm derives from the misconception that hair, sebaceous, and sweat glands are mesodermal in origin. They are not.[39] These elements lie within mesodermal connective tissue, but their origin is the embryonic ectoderm. Therefore *both* epidermoid and dermoid cysts are ectodermal inclusion cysts.[39]

Pathology

Gross pathology. Dermoid cysts are well-defined, lobulated cystic masses that contain a thick, viscous oily fluid with lipid metabolites and liquid cholesterol derived from decomposed epithelial cells.[40] A dermal sinus may be present with spinal and posterior fossa lesions.[2] If the cyst has ruptured, its fatty contents can spread into the ventricles and subarachnoid spaces, inciting intense meningeal inflammatory response (Fig. 15-11).[41]

Microscopic appearance. The outer cyst wall is composed of a dense fibrous capsule; the interior is lined with squamous epithelium, hair, and dermal appendages (see subsequent discussion). Desquamated debris containing cholesterol and keratin is common to both epidermoid and dermoid cysts. In

addition, dermoid cysts contain dermal appendages (hair follicles and sebaceous and sweat glands). Liquid secretions and breakdown products of these dermal appendages result in an oily mixture that contains lipid metabolites.[39] Calcifications are common, representing dystrophic changes or dental enamel, another ectodermal derivative.[40]

Incidence. Intracranial dermoids are rare, accounting for 0.04% to 0.6% of primary intracranial tumors. Intradural dermoid cysts are four to nine times less common than epidermoid cysts.[42]

Age and gender. Spinal dermoid tumors typically present during the first two to three decades of life (*see* Chapter 21); intracranial lesions become symptomatic during the third decade. There is a slight male predilection.[27]

Location. Dermoid tumors typically occur in or near the midline. The lumbosacral spinal canal is the most common site (*see* Chapter 21), followed by the parasellar, frontobasal, and posterior fossa regions.[41-43] The midline vermis or the fourth ventricle are the most frequent infratentorial locations. Following rupture, dermoid contents can disseminate widely throughout the subarachnoid space and ventricles.

Clinical presentation and natural history. Seizures and headaches are the most common symptoms of uncomplicated supratentorial dermoids.[42,44] Dermoids increase in size through both epithelial desquamation and glandular secretion.[45] Cyst rupture can result in chemical meningitis, seizure, vasospasm with infarction, and death.[40]

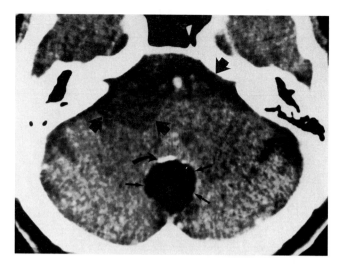

Fig. 15-12. Imaging findings that compare and contrast epidermoid with dermoid tumor are nicely demonstrated on the CECT scan of this patient who had both lesions present simultaneously. The epidermoid tumor *(large arrows)* is similar to CSF density, lobulated, and located off midline. The midline dermoid tumor *(small arrows)* is extremely hypodense and resembles fat. Note rim calcification *(curved arrow).* (Courtesy G. Wilms. From *AJNR* 11:1257-1258, 1990.)

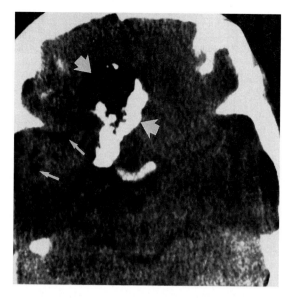

Fig. 15-13. Axial NECT scan of a typical frontobasal dermoid tumor shows the extremely low density, partially calcified paramedian mass *(large arrows).* The cyst has ruptured, spilling tiny fat droplets into the subarachnoid space *(small arrows).* (Courtesy D. Mendelsohn.)

Imaging

Angiography. Cerebral angiography is typically normal or demonstrates an avascular mass effect. Acutely ruptured dermoids can cause chemical meningitis, which, in turn, may induce vasospasm and cerebral ischemia. An association with intracranial aneurysm has been reported.[44]

CT. NECT scans typically show a rounded, well-delineated, uniformly hypodense (−20 to −40H) mass. Capsular calcification is common (Fig. 15-12). Ruptured dermoids may show low density fatty drops in the subarachnoid spaces or intraventricular fat-CSF levels (Fig. 15-13).[41] Hyperdense dermoid cysts have been reported but are uncommon.[46] Enhancement following contrast administration is uncommon.

MR. Increased signal intensity on T1WI is typical (Fig. 15-14, *A*).[40] Dermoids have variable signal on T2-weighted sequences that ranges from hypointense to inhomogeneously hyperintense (Fig. 15-14, *B*).[40,41] If the dermoid contains hair, fine curvilinear low signal components are sometimes present within the cyst.[41a] Ruptured dermoids typically have high signal fat droplets within the subarachnoid spaces and intraventricular fat-CSF levels.[41]

Lipoma

Intracranial lipomas are neither hamartomas nor true neoplasms.[47] Some pathologists classify lipomas as choristomas, i.e., they are a mass of tissue that would be histologically normal for an organ or body part other than the site at which it is located.[48] More than half of all intracranial lipomas are associated with specific brain malformations.[49] Lipomas probably represent a particular type of congenital brain malformation (see subsequent discussion).

Etiology and pathogenesis. Lipomas were once categorized as mesodermal-derived neoplasms. It is now apparent that lipoma formation results from abnormal persistence and maldifferentiation of the meninx primitiva, a mesenchymal neural crest derivative that normally forms the subarachnoid cisterns (*see box*).[49]

Pathology

Gross pathology. Lipomas are yellow fatty deposits that "contrast pleasurably with the functionally magnificent but tinctorially drab cerebrum" (*see* Fig. 12-19, *A*).[19] Lipomas can be separated into two groups with different gross morphologies and associated brain malformations. So-called *tubulonodular lipomas* are large, bulky, round or cylindrical masses that have a high incidence of associated corpus callosum dysgenesis, frontal lobe anomalies, and cephaloceles (*see* Fig. 2-28).[50]

Curvilinear lipomas are thin, posteriorly situated lesions that curve around the splenium (Fig. 15-15). The corpus callosum is normal or shows only mild dysgenetic changes (*see* Fig. 2-29).[50] Other lipomas appear as focal fatty deposits that are intimately adherent to, but do not invade, underlying brain parenchyma (Fig. 15-16; *see* Fig. 12-130).

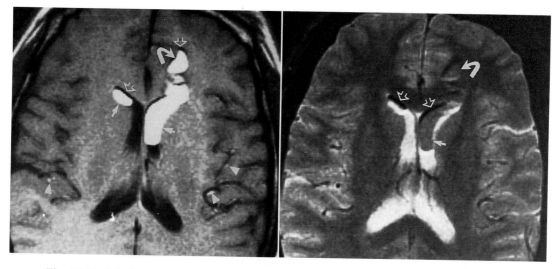

Fig. 15-14. MR findings of a typical ruptured dermoid. The left frontal lobe dermoid tumor *(curved arrows)* ruptured into the ventricles. Fat-CSF levels are present in both frontal horns. The fatty fluid cyst contents are hyperintense on T1- (**A,** *small arrows*) and hypointense on T2-weighted scans (**B,** *small arrows*). Note chemical shift artifact *(open arrows).* Tiny fat droplets are present in the sylvian cisterns *(arrowheads).*

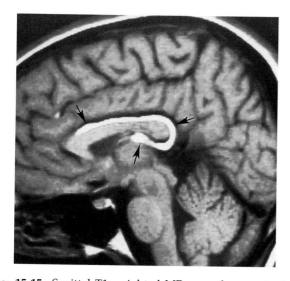

Fig. 15-15. Sagittal T1-weighted MR scan shows a typical curvilinear pericallosal lipoma *(arrows)* that was discovered incidentally in a patient being scanned for symptoms of vascular disease. Note the normally formed corpus callosum. (From Osborn AG, Hendrick RE: Basic MR physics, RSNA Categorical Course on MR Imaging, 1990.)

Calcification is common in lipomas; frank degenerative changes and hemorrhage are rare. Prominent vessels often course through tubulonodular lipomas. The seventh and eighth cranial nerves can become enveloped by cerebellopontine angle lipomas *(see* Fig. 12-74, *B).*

Intracranial Lipoma

Etiology

Persistence/maldifferentiation of meninx primitiva

Pathology

Gross: two types
  Tubulonodular (with callosal dysgenesis)
  Curvilinear (corpus callosum normal/nearly normal)
Microscopic: fat, calcification, vascular structures, sometimes glial ganglion cells

Incidence

Rare (0.1% to 0.5% of primary brain tumors)

Age and gender

Any age; M = F

Location

Midline 80% to 95%
50% dorsal pericallosal
Others: quadrigeminal/ambient, suprasellar, cerebellopontine angle cisterns

Imaging

Plain films: classic but rare = low density midline mass with "comma-shaped" Ca^{++}
CT: fat density mass +/− Ca^{++}
MR: like fat (hyperintense on T1-, hypointense on T2-weighted scans)

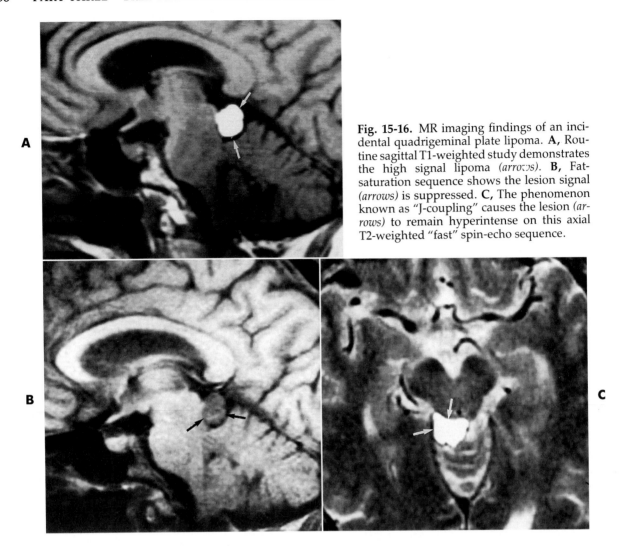

Fig. 15-16. MR imaging findings of an incidental quadrigeminal plate lipoma. **A,** Routine sagittal T1-weighted study demonstrates the high signal lipoma *(arrows).* **B,** Fat-saturation sequence shows the lesion signal *(arrows)* is suppressed. **C,** The phenomenon known as "J-coupling" causes the lesion *(arrows)* to remain hyperintense on this axial T2-weighted "fast" spin-echo sequence.

Microscopic appearance. Lipomas are composed of adipose tissue intermingled with a variable mixture of vascular elements, collagen and muscle fibers, glia and ganglion cells.[2] Calcification and ossification are common.

Incidence. Intracranial lipomas are rare, accounting for 0.1% to 0.5% of all primary brain tumors.[50a] They are found in 0.06% to 0.30% of all CT examinations and in 0.08% to 0.21% of autopsies.[51] Lipomas account for 5% of all corpus callosum tumors.[52]

Age and gender. The incidence of intracranial lipoma is neither age- nor gender-related.[53] Lipomas have been reported in neonates and ninety year olds.

Location. Between 80% and 95% of intracranial lipomas occur at or near the midline.[51] Eighty percent are supratentorial where the dorsal pericallosal area accounts for nearly 50% of these lesions. Occasionally, a pericallosal lipoma extends laterally through the choroidal fissure.[54] Isolated intraventricular lipo-

mas occur but are rare.[55] Lipomas of the cerebral cortex are extremely uncommon.[50a]

Other typical supratentorial sites include the quadrigeminal, ambient, interpeduncular, chiasmatic, and sylvian cisterns.[47] The cerebellopontine angle cistern is the most common posterior fossa site.[51]

Clinical presentation and natural history. Intracranial lipomas are often asymptomatic and discovered incidentally. Seizures, headache, and behavioral disturbances are common but usually are related to associated anomalies such as corpus callosum dysgenesis.

Encephalocraniocutaneous lipomatosis is a rare neurocutaneous syndrome that includes subcutaneous scalp and neck lipomas, intracranial and intraspinal lipomas, and leptomeningeal lipogranulomatosis. Cerebral abnormalities include microgyria, porencephaly, atrophy, parenchymal and leptomeningeal calcifications, and vascular malformations. Clinical manifestations include seizures and mental retardation.[56]

Cranial nerve palsies occasionally occur with infratentorial lipomas. Neurologic signs and symptoms are secondary to localized mass effect and compression of CNs VII and VIII, the nervus intermedius, and their accompanying vascular structures.[57]

Because vessels and nerves traverse many lipomas, attempts at total surgical extirpation historically have had poor neurologic outcomes.[57] When surgery is undertaken to relieve progressive neurologic abnormalities, decompression with minimal excision of the lipomatous mass has been recommended.[57]

Imaging

Plain film radiographs. Plain film findings of the typical bulky tubulonodular lipoma are distinctive but rare. They include a midline radiolucent lesion with symmetric, typically parenthesis-like, calcifications seen on anteroposterior projections (*see* Fig. 2-30).[53] Lipomas in other locations usually have normal plain film radiographs.

Ultrasound. Cranial sonography in infants with a corpus callosum lipoma shows an echodense lesion in the pericallosal area. Stigmata of callosal dysgenesis are often present.[58]

Angiography. Lipomas are typically avascular masses with neither tumor stain, contrast pooling, or vascular encasement.[53] Prominent vessels often course within lipomas, particularly the tubulonodular variety that is associated with callosal dysgenesis.

CT. NECT scans show a very low density mass that has attenuation characteristics similar to adipose tissue (-50 to -100H). Curvilinear or nodular calcification is occasionally seen. Lipomas do not enhance following contrast administration. Stigmata of associated congenital malformations such as callosal dysgenesis can be identified in many cases; in others, lipomas occur as an isolated anomaly.

MR. Lipomas appear similar to fat, i.e., they are hyperintense compared to brain on T1- and hypointense on standard T2-weighted spin echo sequences (*see* Figs. 2-31 and 15-16, *A*). They remain hyperintense on T2WI if "fast" spin-echo techniques are used (Fig. 15-16, *C*).[59] Typical chemical shift artifacts can be identified. Fat-suppression techniques can be used to confirm the diagnosis (Fig. 15-16, *B*). Low signal foci are often seen within lipomas and represent calcification or ossification, traversing arteries or engulfed nerves.[60]

NONNEOPLASTIC CYSTS

Various cysts are found in and around the central nervous system (*see* box). Cystic neoplasms are discussed in Chapters 13 and 14; congenital inclusion cysts such as epidermoid and dermoid cysts were discussed earlier in this chapter. Inflammatory cysts are described in Chapter 16. Nonneoplastic, noninflam-

---

Nonneoplastic Noninflammatory Intracranial Cysts
Arachnoid (leptomeningeal) cyst Colloid cyst Rathke cleft cyst Neuroepithelial cyst Enterogenous cyst Intraparenchymal cyst

---

matory intracranial cysts that will be discussed here include arachnoid, colloid, Rathke cleft, neuroepithelial, and enterogenous cysts.

Arachnoid Cysts

Arachnoid (leptomeningeal) cysts are benign, congenital, intra-arachnoidal space-occupying lesions that are filled with clear CSF-like fluid.[61] They have been increasingly well-recognized with the advent of noninvasive cross-sectional imaging.[62]

Etiology and pathology

Etiology. The precise etiology of arachnoid cysts is poorly understood and remains controversial.[62a] Mechanisms proposed for their origin and development have recently focused on meningeal maldevelopment. Minor aberrations of CSF flow through the loose primitive perimedullary mesenchyme may result in focal splitting of the developing meninges.[63] Formation of a pocket or diverticulum in the space thus created between the arachnoid and pia results in an arachnoid cyst.[64]

Gross pathology. True arachnoid cysts are fluid-filled cavities that lie entirely within the arachnoid membrane.[64] Grossly, these cysts consist of a thin but distinct transparent wall that is separated from the inner dural layer and the underlying pia-arachnoid (Fig. 15-17, *A*; *see* Fig. 4-11).[3] Arachnoid cysts range in size from small incidental cysts to large space-occupying lesions.[63] Compression of the underlying brain varies from none to severe. Temporal lobe dysgenesis is common with middle fossa arachnoid cysts[65] (Fig. 15-17, *B*) (*see* box, p. 640).

Arachnoid cysts are typically filled with clear, colorless liquid that resembles CSF. Occasionally, xanthochromic, proteinaceous, or hemorrhagic fluid is identified.[3] Arachnoid cysts can be loculated or communicate freely with the adjacent subarachnoid cisterns.

Microscopic appearance. The cyst wall consists of a vascular collagenous membrane lined by flattened arachnoid cells.[3] Arachnoid cysts do not have a glial limiting membrane or an epithelial lining.[64]

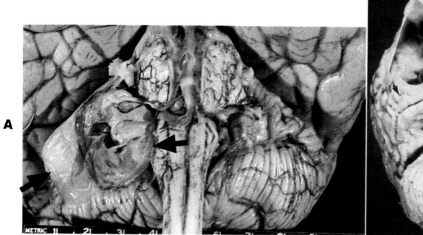
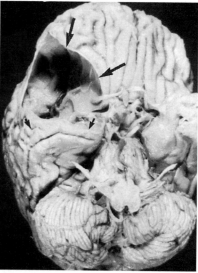

Fig. 15-17. Gross pathology of arachnoid cysts in two cases. **A,** Frontal view of the posterior fossa in a patient with a large cerebellopontine angle arachnoid cyst *(arrows).* The cyst is well delineated and has a thin, veil-like wall. **B,** Base view of a large middle fossa arachnoid cyst *(large arrows).* Note accompanying temporal lobe hypogenesis *(small arrows).* (**A,** Courtesy E. Tessa Hedley-Whyte. **B,** Courtesy J. Townsend.)

Arachnoid Cyst

Etiology

Meningeal maldevelopment

Pathology

Gross: thin-walled cyst filled with CSF (N.B. - temporal lobe hypogenesis common with middle fossa cyst)

Microscopic: lined by flattened arachnoid cells

Incidence

1% of nontraumatic intracranial masses

Age and gender

Any age, but 75% in children; M:F = 3:1

Location

Middle cranial fossa	50%-65%
Suprasellar cistern	5%-10%
Quadrigeminal cistern	5%-10%
Cerebral convexities	5%
Posterior fossa	5%-10%
Cerebellopontine angle	
Cisterna magna	

Imaging

CT, MR show extraaxial mass that resembles CSF

Differential diagnosis

Epidermoid tumor (others: cystic neoplasm, open-lip schizencephaly, infarct, loculated hygroma)

Incidence. Arachnoid cysts represent 1% of all nontraumatic intracranial masses.[65]

Age and gender. Arachnoid cysts occur in all age groups, although 75% occur in children.[66] There is a 3:1 male:female ratio.[67]

Location. Most arachnoid cysts are supratentorial. Between 50% and 65% occur in the middle cranial fossa, with another 10% each in the suprasellar and quadrigeminal regions. The frontal convexities account for another 5%.[65] Only 5% to 10% of arachnoid cysts occur in the posterior fossa; the cerebellopontine angles and cisterna magna are the most common infratentorial sites (*see* Fig. 4-12).

Clinical presentation and natural history. Between 60% and 80% of all arachnoid cysts are symptomatic. Common presenting symptoms include headaches, seizures, and focal neurologic signs.[65] The natural history of arachnoid cysts is unclear. Although most arachnoid cysts remain unchanged in size with advancing age, there is a subgroup of larger cysts that may expand with time.[63]

Controversy exists regarding the secretory capacity of cyst walls. Active intracystic fluid production by ectopic choroid plexus, glial, or ependymal cells has been proposed.[68] Most authors restrict this mechanism of expansion to choroidal-epithelial or ependymal cysts, postulating that when arachnoid cysts enlarge they do so by a ball-valve mechanism that en-

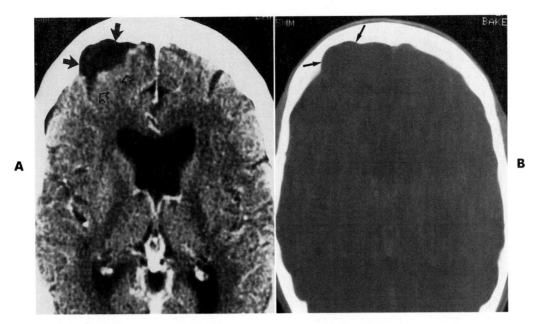

Fig. 15-18. Soft tissue **(A)** and bone windows **(B)** from the CECT scan in a patient scanned for headaches show a frontal convexity arachnoid cyst (**A,** *large arrows*). Note smooth, scalloped erosion of the overlying calvarium (**B,** *small arrows*) and the displaced cortex (**A,** *open arrows*).

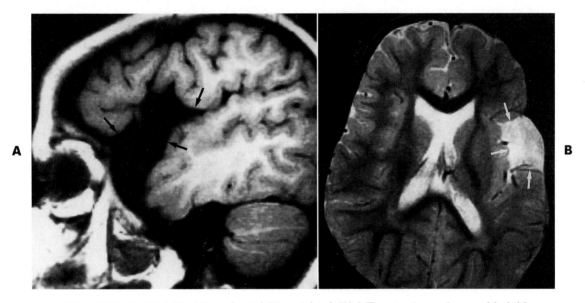

Fig. 15-19. Sagittal T1- **(A)** and axial T2-weighted **(B)** MR scans in an 8-year-old child with headaches show a typical middle fossa arachnoid cyst *(arrows).* The cyst is isointense with CSF on both sequences and has sharply marginated borders.

traps CSF.[63] An osmotic gradient between arachnoid space and cyst is an alternative possibility.[68]

Occasionally, arachnoid cysts are complicated by intracystic or subdural hemorrhage. Hemorrhage can be spontaneous or follow minor trauma with rupture of intracystic or bridging vessels.[62]

Imaging

CT. NECT scans show a smoothly demarcated noncalcified extraaxial mass that does not enhance following contrast administration (Fig. 15-18, *A*). Un-

less hemorrhage has occurred, most arachnoid cysts are similar to CSF in attenuation. Pressure erosion of the adjacent calvarium can occur (Fig. 15-18, *B*). Ipsilateral pneumosinus dilatans and asymmetric sinus aeration are sometimes present.[68a]

MR. Arachnoid cysts are sharply demarcated extraaxial masses that may displace or deform adjacent brain. They parallel CSF in signal intensity on all pulse sequences (Fig. 15-19).[69] The classic arachnoid cyst has no internal architecture and does not enhance (Fig. 15-20). Occasionally, hemorrhage or high

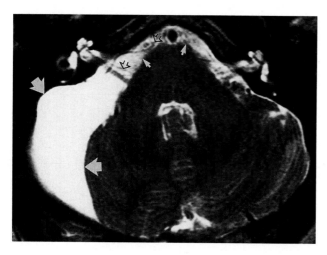

Fig. 15-20. Axial T2-weighted MR scan shows a moderately large cerebellopontine angle arachnoid cyst *(large arrows)*. Note featureless internal appearance of the cyst. Contrast the cyst with normal CSF in the prepontine angle cistern *(small arrows)*. Here, flow makes the CSF signal slightly heterogeneous. Vessels and nerves *(open arrows)* course through the normal cistern, in contrast to the cyst.

protein content may complicate the MR appearance of an arachnoid cyst.

Differential diagnosis. The most difficult lesion to distinguish from arachnoid cyst is an epidermoid tumor (see previous discussion). Epidermoid tumors can follow CSF signal intensity on all pulse sequences, although most are slightly hyperintense on proton density-weighted studies. Epidermoid tumors encase and engulf arteries and cranial nerves, whereas arachnoid cysts displace adjacent structures.[69] Diffusion or steady-state free-precession MR imaging can be helpful in some cases.[70,71]

Other lesions that occasionally resemble arachnoid cysts include cystic tumors, infarcts, open-lip schizencephaly, and loculated chronic subdural hygromas. Infarcts are lined by gliotic white matter, and schizencephalic clefts are bordered by heterotopic gray matter, whereas arachnoid cysts compress otherwise normal-appearing brain. Contrast-enhanced MR may be helpful in identifying enhancing tumor or subdural membranes.

Specific differentiation must be made between suprasellar arachnoid cyst and dilated third ventricle and between posterior fossa arachnoid cyst (PFAC) and Dandy-Walker malformation (DWM). In the former, MR scans usually delineate a displaced third ventricle (*see* Fig. 12-135). In the latter, a PFAC is separate from the vallecula and fourth ventricle that are normally formed but compressed, whereas in DWM the cyst appears as an extension of the fourth ventricle and the hypoplastic vermian remnant is everted anterosuperiorly over the large CSF space (*see* Chapter 4).

Colloid Cyst

Etiology
Endodermal-derived

Pathology
Gross: smooth, spherical gelatinous-filled cystic mass
Microscopic: collagenous/fibrous capsule lined by cuboidal/columnar epithelium

Incidence
0.5% to 1.0% of primary brain tumors; 15% to 20% of all intraventricular masses

Age and gender
Adults 20 to 40 years; rare in children; M = F

Location
Virtually always anterior third ventricle/foramen of Monro

Imaging
CT: ⅔ hyperdense, ⅓ isodense; noncalcified; occasionally rim enhances
MR: variable signal; most common = hyperintense to brain on T1WI, hypointense on T2WI

Colloid Cysts

Third ventricular colloid cyst is a well-established clinicopathologic entity with controversial etiology (*see* box). Because of their unique location at the foramen of Monro, symptoms of intermittent hydrocephalus are common, and death from sudden, acute obstruction has been reported.

Etiology and pathology

Etiology. The assumed neuroectodermal origin of colloid cysts is reflected in its other appellations: neuroepithelial or paraphyseal cyst.[3] Postulated precursors include choroid plexus, ventricular ependyma, the tela choroidea, and the paraphysis.[72] Recent immunohistochemical studies of colloid cyst epithelium demonstrate characteristics more consistent with endodermal than neuroepithelial tissue. Colloid cysts are therefore morphologically similar to bronchi and nasal cavity epithelium.[73]

Gross pathology. Colloid cysts are smooth, spherical, well-delineated cystic lesions that range in size from a few millimeters (*see* Fig. 12-47) to 3 to 4 cm in diameter. The cysts are filled with viscid gelatinous material or denser content that has the consistency of soft cartilage.[3] Other reported contents include blood degradation products, foamy cells, cholesterol crystals, and mucin.[74]

Microscopic appearance. Colloid cysts are lined by

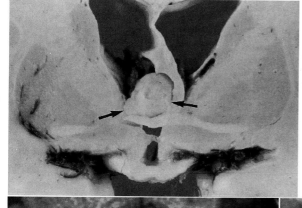

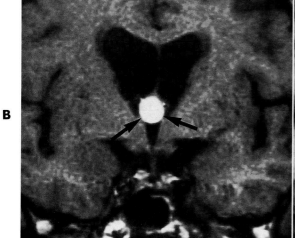

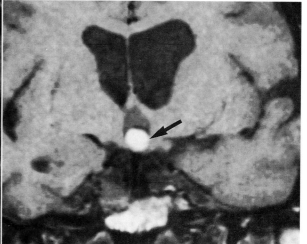

Fig. 15-21. A, Coronal gross pathology specimen demonstrates a classic colloid cyst *(arrows)*. The foramen of Monro location and attachment to the roof of the third ventricle are typical. **B,** Coronal T1-weighted MR scan demonstrates a typical colloid cyst *(arrows)*. **C,** Turbulent CSF flow *(arrow)* mimics a colloid cyst in this case. Note "pseudocyst" lies inferiorly in the third ventricle, whereas true colloid cysts are attached to the ventricular roof (contrast with **B**).

simple or pseudostratified, flattened cuboidal or columnar epithelial cells that rest on a thin capsule composed of collagen and fibroblasts.[73] Colloid cysts enlarge by accumulation of epithelial secretory and breakdown products.[19]

Incidence. Colloid cysts account for 0.5% to 1.0% of all intracranial tumors but represent approximately 15% to 20% of intraventricular masses.[75]

Age and gender. Colloid cysts are tumors of adults. Most become symptomatic between the third and fifth decades of life. Colloid cysts are remarkably rare in children; only 1% to 2% occur under 10 years of age. Men and women are equally affected.[3]

Location. Colloid cysts are located in the anterior third ventricle, typically positioned between the columns of the fornix (Fig. 15-21). They are attached to the third ventricular roof and choroid plexus.[19] Colloid cysts in other locations have been reported but are exceedingly rare.[76,77]

Clinical presentation and natural history. Colloid

cysts rarely become symptomatic before age 20. Symptoms of intermittent or prolonged increased intracranial pressure are frequent. The most common presenting symptom is headache, followed by vertigo, memory deficits, behavioral disturbances, and diplopia.[78] Sudden interruption of CSF circulation with coma and death have been reported. A few colloid cysts are asymptomatic and are discovered incidentally at autopsy or imaging (*see* Fig. 12-47, *A*).

Complete removal of a colloid cyst by open or stereotactic-guided microsurgery is curative; stereotactic aspiration of cyst contents fails to offer a radical or permanent treatment.[78] Malignant degeneration does not occur.

Imaging
CT. Approximately two thirds of colloid cysts are homogeneously hyperdense compared to brain on NECT scans, and one third are isodense. Hypodense colloid cysts are uncommon.[75] A well-delineated round or ovoid noncalcified anterior third ventricular mass at the foramen of Monro is characteristic.

Enhancement following contrast administration is

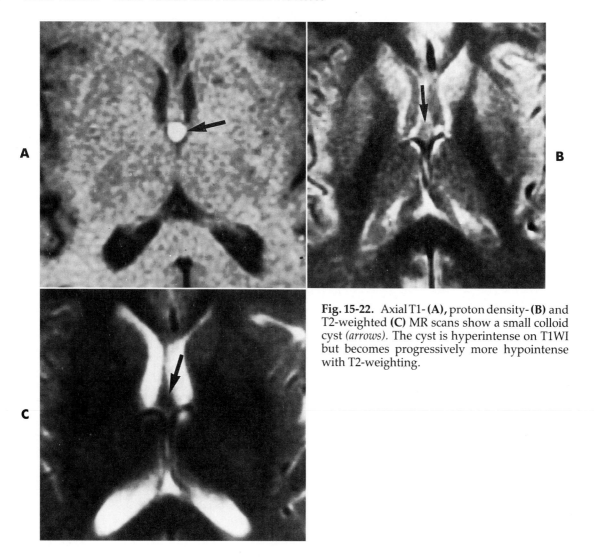

Fig. 15-22. Axial T1- (A), proton density- (B) and T2-weighted (C) MR scans show a small colloid cyst *(arrows)*. The cyst is hyperintense on T1WI but becomes progressively more hypointense with T2-weighting.

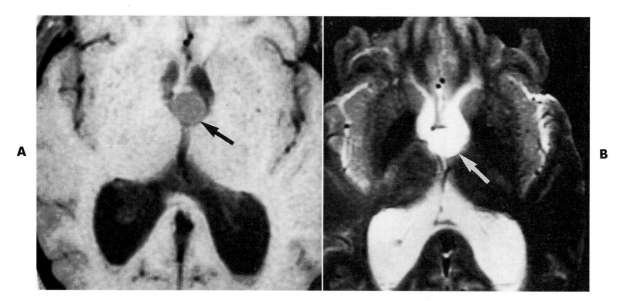

Fig. 15-23. The colloid cyst *(arrows)* in this case is hypointense to brain on T1WI (A) but very hyperintense on the T2-weighted study (B).

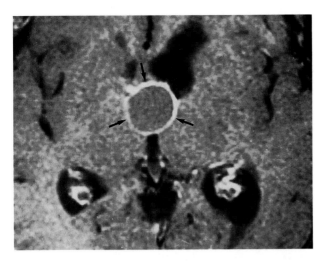

Fig. 15-24. Axial postcontrast T1-weighted MR scan shows rim enhancement *(arrows)* around this slightly hypointense colloid cyst.

usually absent. Occasionally, a thin rim of enhancing tissue around a colloid cyst is observed.

MR. The signal characteristics of colloid cysts vary widely. The most common appearance is a mass that is hyperintense on T1- and hypointense on T2-weighted studies (Fig. 15-22). However, colloid cysts can display virtually any signal intensity on any pulse sequence (Fig. 15-23). Some investigators report mixed-signal lesions with a hyperintense outer layer and profoundly hypointense center on T2WI.[79] Rim enhancement following contrast administration is observed in some cases (Fig. 15-24). CSF flow artifacts at the foramen of Monro can mimic colloid cyst (Fig. 15-21, C).

Rathke Cleft Cyst

Etiology and pathology
Etiology. Rathke's pouch develops as a rostral outpouching from the primitive stomodeum during the third or fourth gestational week. It is the embryologic precursor of the anterior lobe, pars intermedia, and pars tuberalis of the pituitary gland.[80] The cephalad elongation of Rathke's pouch forms the craniopharyngeal duct.[81] The proximal portion closes early during fetal development, but a remnant often persists into postnatal life as a cleft that lies between the pars distalis and pars nervosa.[3] Occasionally, this remnant gives rise to a macroscopic cyst, the Rathke cleft cyst (RCC) *(see* box).

Gross pathology. RCCs are smoothly marginated, well-delineated cysts that vary in size from a few millimeters to 1 to 2 centimeters. Cyst contents vary from serous to mucoid.[80]

Microscopic appearance. RCCs are lined by pseudostratified or single-layered columnar or cuboidal epithelium. Distinct cilia and scattered mucin-

---

Rathke Cleft Cyst

Etiology
Primitive stomodeal (Rathke's pouch) remnant

Pathology
Gross: cyst with variable contents (serous, mucoid)
Microscopic: columnar/cuboidal epithelium; goblet cells often present, squamous cells sometimes seen

Incidence
<1% of nontraumatic intracranial masses; small cysts common at autopsy

Age and gender
Any age, but mostly adults (4th to 6th decades); F:M = 2-3:1

Location
70% both intra/suprasellar; 20% to 25% intrasellar; <5% completely suprasellar

Imaging
CT: 75% hypodense to brain; noncalcified; 50% rim (capsular) enhancement
MR: most common = hyperintense to brain on T1WI, with variable signal on T2WI

Differential diagnosis
Arachnoid cyst, noncalcified craniopharyngioma, cystic pituitary adenoma, inflammatory cyst

---

secreting goblet cells are seen in most cases. Many RCCs have squamous differentiation, and cornified squamous pearls are occasionally identified.[73]

Incidence. Symptomatic RCCs are uncommon lesions, accounting for less than 1% of all primary intracranial tumorlike masses. Small asymptomatic cysts are found in the pars distalis or pars intermedia in 2% to 26% of routine autopsies.[82]

Age and gender. RCCs can be seen at any age, although most lesions are identified in adults. Mean age at presentation is 38 years. There is a 2-3:1 female predominance.[81,82]

Location. RCCs can be purely intrasellar or combined intra- and suprasellar masses. Approximately 70% are both intra- and suprasellar.[82] Completely suprasellar RCCs are rare.[83]

Clinical presentation and natural history. Intrasellar RCCs are usually asymptomatic and are found incidentally at autopsy or MR imaging. RCCs may also present with visual disturbances, symptoms of hypothalamic-pituitary dysfunction, and head-aches.[82,83a] Symptomatic masses may warrant surgical drainage or partial excision with cyst wall biopsy. The recurrence rate is low.[80,81]

Imaging

CT. CT density varies with cyst content. Three quarters of RCCs appear as discrete, low density lesions on NECT studies.[81] Mixed or high attenuation lesions occur but are uncommon. RCCs do not calcify. Capsular enhancement is seen in 50% of cases.[82]

MR. MR signal varies widely. Approximately two thirds are hyperintense to brain on T1WI (*see* Fig. 12-136); one third show low signal intensity similar to CSF.[81] Signal on T2WI is more unpredictable. Half are hyperintense, 25% are isointense, and 25% are hypointense.[81] RCCs typically do not enhance following contrast administration, although an intensely enhancing rim of displaced, compressed pituitary gland surrounding the cyst is sometimes present (*see* Fig. 12-114).[84]

Differential diagnosis. The differential diagnosis of RCC includes arachnoid cyst, cavitated pituitary adenoma, cystic craniopharyngioma, and inflammatory cyst.[80,83a] RCCs do not calcify, whereas calcified craniopharyngiomas are common. MR signal intensity does not distinguish nonneoplastic cysts from cystic tumors.[84] Dynamic contrast-enhanced studies are helpful in distinguishing wall enhancement from enhancing adjacent pituitary tissue.[84]

Neuroglial (neuroepithelial) Cysts

Intracranial neuroepithelial (NE) cysts comprise a heterogeneous group of lesions (*see* box). They are described using various names such as ependymal cyst, choroid plexus cyst, choroidal-epithelial cyst, and subarachnoid-ependymal cyst.[85,86] Colloid cysts were once included in this pathologic spectrum but are most likely of endodermal rather than neuroepithelial origin (see previous discussion).

Etiology and pathology

Etiology. The origin of NE cysts is controversial. These cysts have features of primitive ependyma or choroid plexus and probably arise from sequestration of the developing neuroectoderm or, in the case of choroid fissure cysts, infolded vascular pia mater.[87]

Gross pathology. NE cysts are well-delineated cystic lesions with specific appearances that vary slightly with particular location.

Microscopic appearance. These nonneoplastic cysts are lined by cells that morphologically resemble epithelium. Immunohistochemical studies are often strongly positive for glial fibrillary acidic protein (GFAP).[76]

Neuroepithelial Cysts
Ependymal (intraventricular) cyst
Trigone of lateral ventricle is most common site
Thin-walled, filled with CSF
Choroid plexus cyst
Often incidental
Frequently bilateral
Choroid fissure cyst
Medial temporal lobe between hippocampus, diencephalon
Ovoid/spindle-shaped CSF-like cyst

Incidence. The incidence of NE cysts varies with location. Small asymptomatic choroid plexus cysts are frequently seen on imaging studies and can be identified in more than 50% of autopsy cases (*see* Fig. 12-43).[86] Symptomatic NE cysts are rare. The majority are located in the lateral ventricles (Fig. 15-25).[85]

Age and gender. Although NE cysts can be seen at any age, most choroid plexus cysts are identified in older adults. The mean age at presentation of ependymal cysts is 33 years.[86] Moderate male predominance is reported in symptomatic ependymal cysts.[85,86]

Location. NE cysts can occur anywhere along the neuraxis. They are found in the choroid plexus, choroid fissure, cerebral ventricles, and, occasionally, within the brain parenchyma. The choroid plexus is the most common site (*see* Chapter 12). The choroidal fissure is a CSF space between the fimbria of the hippocampus and diencephalon that curves posterosuperiorly from the anterior temporal lobe to the atrium of the lateral ventricle. The choroidal fissure is also a common site for NE or arachnoid cysts (Fig. 15-26).[87]

Intraventricular and posterior fossa NE cysts are uncommon.[85,88] Most symptomatic NE cysts in the lateral ventricle are located in the trigone.[86]

Clinical presentation and natural history. Choroid plexus cysts are usually asymptomatic and discovered incidentally. Large lateral ventricular ependymal cysts occasionally cause obstructive hydrocephalus, although most have mild or no neurologic symptoms.[85] Headache and seizure have been reported.[86] The natural history of these cysts is unknown. Interval follow-up examinations disclose no clinical or imaging changes in asymptomatic lesions.[86]

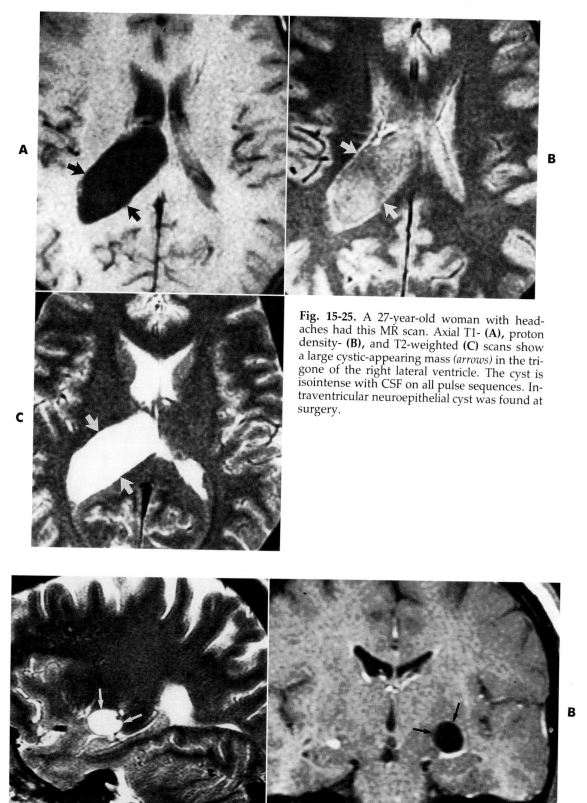

Fig. 15-25. A 27-year-old woman with headaches had this MR scan. Axial T1- **(A)**, proton density- **(B)**, and T2-weighted **(C)** scans show a large cystic-appearing mass *(arrows)* in the trigone of the right lateral ventricle. The cyst is isointense with CSF on all pulse sequences. Intraventricular neuroepithelial cyst was found at surgery.

Fig. 15-26. Sagittal T2- **(A)** and coronal postcontrast T1-weighted **(B)** MR scans show a classic choroid fissure cyst *(arrows)*. The shape and location between the medial temporal lobe near the choroid fissure and the diencephalon are typical. (Courtesy R. Dietz.)

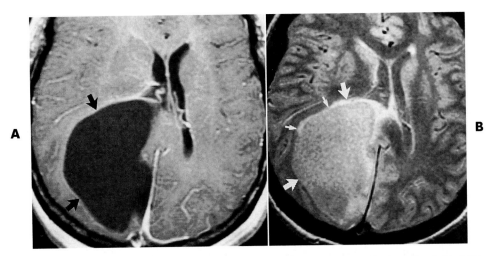

Fig. 15-27. A 54-year-old woman with headaches and bilateral papilledema had this MR scan. **A,** Axial postcontrast T1-weighted MR scan shows a large, nonenhancing low signal right occipital lobe mass *(arrows)*. The mass is slightly hyperintense to CSF and appears to displace the lateral ventricle. **B,** The proton density-weighted study shows the cyst *(large arrows)* is hyperintense compared to white matter and partially surrounded by a high signal rim that most likely represents gliotic brain *(small arrows)*. A nonepithelial, nonneoplastic intraparenchymal cyst was found at surgery.

Imaging

CT. NECT scans show a well-delineated homogeneous low density mass with attenuation characteristics similar to CSF. Calcification and contrast enhancement are absent.

MR. Signal characteristics generally approximate CSF on all sequences (Fig. 15-25), although some cysts appear slightly hyperintense, particularly on proton density-weighted sequences.[89] The cyst walls are thin but easily detected on MR studies. Contrast enhancement, surrounding edema, and gliosis are absent. Choroid fissure cysts have a characteristic spindle or ovoid shape on sagittal scans that, together with their location, indicates their probable origin and diagnosis (Fig. 15-26).[87]

Differential diagnosis. The differential diagnosis of NE cysts is comparatively limited. Inflammatory and parasitic cysts such as cysticercosis may resemble NE cysts but are usually smaller and often have mural nodules.[85] Intraaxial cystic tumors and infarcts are rarely confused with NE cysts.

Occasionally, benign, nonneoplastic intraparenchymal brain cysts occur. The cyst wall in these cases consists of neuroglial tissue with no arachnoidal layer, epithelial lining, tumor, or evidence of previous hemorrhage, infarction, or infection.[90] If such a brain cyst occurs near the ventricles, it can resemble a NE cyst. The fluid within these parenchymal cysts may have slightly different signal compared to CSF, and the adjacent brain may have minimal gliotic changes, seen as a mildly hyperintense rim on proton density-weighted sequences (Fig. 15-27).

Enterogenous Cysts

Enterogenous (neurenteric) cysts are rare intraspinal masses that are even less frequent intracranial lesions.[91]

Etiology and pathology

Etiology. The precise etiology of neurenteric cysts is unknown. Enterogenous cysts probably arise during notochordal development and transitory existence of the neurenteric canal. The notochord and foregut may fail to separate during formation of the definitive alimentary canal. Persistence of the temporary neurenteric canal could also interfere with notochordal development, resulting in enterogenous cyst formation.[92,93]

Gross pathology. Intracranial neurenteric cysts are well-delineated, comparatively thin-walled, fluid-containing masses. Cyst contents vary from colorless, transparent fluid resembling CSF to milky or mucinous-like secretions.[91,93]

Microscopic appearance. Neurenteric cysts contain only endodermal elements.[94] The cyst wall is composed of fibrous connective tissue with an underlying epithelium that resembles gastrointestinal or respiratory tract mucosa. A single layer of columnar or cuboidal ciliated and nonciliated epithelial cells with mucin-secreting goblet cells is typical.[92]

Incidence. Enterogenous cysts are rare CNS masses. More than 80% of enterogenous cysts are located in the spine *(see* Chapter 20), whereas only 10% to 15% are intracranial.[92]

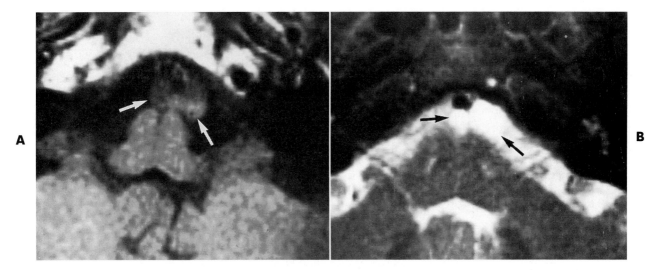

Fig. 15-28. Axial T1- **(A)** and T2-weighted **(B)** MR scans show a well-delineated mass *(arrows)* anterior to the medulla. The mass is isointense with brain on T1WI and very hyperintense on T2WI. The adjacent skull base appears normal. Enterogenous cyst was found at surgery. (**A,** From Harris CP et al: *Neurosurg* 29:893-897, 1991.)

Age and gender. Enterogenous cysts can occur at any age. A recent large series reports a patient age range from 2 to 70 years, with an average age of 21 years and a peak incidence in the first decade.[92] Slight male predominance was also noted.[92]

Location. Intracranial neurenteric cysts are typically intradural extramedullary posterior fossa masses. The cerebellopontine angles and craniocervical junction anterior to the brainstem are the most frequent sites of these uncommon lesions.[91,92] Intramedullary enterogenous cysts occur but are very rare.[94]

Clinical presentation and natural history. The clinical presentation of intracranial neurenteric cysts ranges from asymptomatic lesions that are discovered incidentally to gross ataxia, nystagmus, visual symptoms, and cranial nerve palsies. Prognosis is related to cyst size and location because these factors determine operability. Incompletely excised and intramedullary lesions have a poor prognosis.[94] Neoplastic transformation does not occur.

Imaging. NECT scans disclose a well-delineated, noncalcified, nonenhancing lobulated mass that is typically hypodense compared to adjacent brain parenchyma. MR signal varies with cyst content; most lesions are iso- or mildly hyperintense compared to CSF on T1WI and moderately hyperintense on proton density- and T2-weighted sequences (Fig. 15-28).[92,93]

The differential diagnosis of posterior fossa enterogenous cyst includes arachnoid and neuroepithe-lial cysts, epidermoid cyst, cystic schwannoma, and inflammatory cysts such as cysticercosis.

REGIONAL TUMORS THAT INVOLVE THE CNS BY LOCAL EXTENSION

Various head and neck neoplasms can involve the CNS by local geographic extension. Nasopharyngeal and skull base tumors were discussed previously (*see* Chapter 12). Here, we discuss in greater detail two diagnostically important lesions that occur between the skull and the brain: pituitary adenoma and craniopharyngioma.

Pituitary Adenoma

The normal gross anatomy of the sellar region and physiology of the hypothalamo-pituitary axis were discussed extensively in Chapter 12. Here, we concentrate specifically on the microscopic anatomy, pathology, and imaging spectrum of pituitary adenomas.

Microscopic anatomy

The various hormone-producing pituitary cells are not uniformly distributed in the adenohypophysis. PAS-positive ACTH- and TSH-producing cells are concentrated in the midline "mucoid wedge," whereas the generally chromophobic prolactin cells and the typically eosinophilic growth-hormone cells predominate in the "lateral wings." Gonadotrophs or follicle-stimulating hormone (FSH) and luteinizing hormone (LH) cells are diffusely distributed throughout the gland.[19] Antidiuretic hormone and oxytocin are found in the posterior lobe, i.e., the neurohypophysis.[95]

Pathology

Gross pathology. Microadenomas are defined as pituitary adenomas that are 10 mm or less in diameter; macroadenomas are larger than 10 mm. A useful guideline for determining the maximum normal height (in millimeters) of the pituitary gland is "Elster's rule of 6, 8, 10 and 12": 6 mm for infants and children, 8 mm in men and postmenapausal women, 10 mm in women of childbearing age, 12 mm for women in late pregnancy or postpartum women.[95a]

Pituitary adenomas have a variable gross appearance. Macroadenomas bulge superiorly, often extending through the diaphragma sellae into the suprasellar cistern. Combined intra- and suprasellar pituitary adenomas have a characteristic "figure eight" appearance on imaging studies. Lateral extension into one or both cavernous sinuses is common.[3] Necrosis, hemorrhage, and cyst formation are common in large adenomas.

Microscopic appearance. Pituitary adenomas show a remarkable range of histologic appearances. The "generic" adenoma has monotonous sheets of uniform cells, interrupted only by a delicate capillary network.[19] The traditional, so-called tinctorial classification of pituitary adenomas into acidophilic, basophilic, and chromophobe subtypes based on their tissue-staining characteristics has been abandoned in favor of a more sophisticated scheme that uses electron microscopic and immunohistochemical criteria (*see* box).[95]

Incidence. Pituitary adenomas are common lesions, accounting for approximately 10% of all primary intracranial neoplasms[3] and between one third and one half of all sellar/juxtasellar masses.[96]

Microadenomas. Pathologic studies indicate microadenomas are 400 times more common than macroadenomas.[97] Small incidental pituitary adenomas are identified at autopsy in 8% to 27% of all cases.[97] Fifteen percent of normal volunteers undergoing contrast-enhanced MR scans have focal intrapituitary areas of decreased signal intensity consistent with microadenoma or benign pituitary cysts.[98] Multiple microadenomas occur in 9% of autopsied or surgically documented cases.[97]

Macroadenomas. Imaging-based studies report macroadenomas are twice as frequent as microadenomas.[96] Pituitary macroadenoma is the single most common suprasellar mass, accounting for approximately one third to one half of all lesions in this area (*see* Chapter 12).

Malignant pituitary tumors. The most common malignant pituitary tumor is metastasis.[99,100] Pituitary carcinoma is very rare. So-called malignant adenomas represent less than 1% of all pituitary adenomas.[101]

Pituitary Adenoma

Pathology

Gross

  Macroadenoma >10 mm

  "Figure eight" appearance with suprasellar component

  Necrosis, cysts, hemorrhagic foci common

Microscopic: Classification based on staining characteristics (e.g., acidophilic, basophilic, chromophobe) no longer used

Incidence

10% of primary brain tumors

Most common sellar/juxtasellar mass (33% to 50%)

Microadenomas >>macroadenomas

Age and gender

Adult tumors (<10% in children)

F:M = 4-5:1 for prolactinomas; M:F = 2:1 for growth hormone-secreting tumors

Symptoms

75% endocrinologically active; symptoms vary with adenoma type (*see* Table 15-3)

Imaging

Microadenoma hypodense/hypointense compared to normal pituitary on dynamic contrast-enhanced CT/MR scans

Macroadenoma

  NECT: isodense; only 1% to 8% calcify

  CECT: enhance intensely

  MR: signal like cortex on T1-, T2WI is most common pattern; variable signal if hemorrhage, necrosis, cyst formation present

---

Age and gender. Age and gender incidence vary according to tumor type. In general, pituitary adenomas are tumors of adults; less than 10% occur in children.[3] Prolactinomas have a 4-5:1 female predominance and typically are seen in young adults. Corticotrophic adenomas also occur mostly in women; 22% of cases occur in children or adolescents.[97] Growth hormone-secreting tumors have a 2:1 male predominance and also often occur in children.[3]

Clinical presentation. Pituitary adenomas show a spectrum of hormonal activities.[102,102a] Endocrinologically active adenomas account for 75% of cases[97] (Table 15-3).

Prolactinoma. The most common pituitary adenoma is the prolactin-secreting adenoma, or prolactinoma.[3] Prolactinomas account for approximately 30% of all pituitary adenomas.[95] At least half of all prolactinomas are microadenomas. These tumors typically

Table 15-3. Modern classification of pituitary adenomas

Type of adenoma	Prevalence (%)	Characteristics
Prolactin-cell adenoma	27	Also called lactotroph adenoma or prolactinoma; produces amenorrhea and galactorrhea in women, decreased libido in men
Growth hormone-cell adenoma	13	Produces gigantism in children, acromegaly in adults; sparsely granulated variant is more infiltrative and aggressive
Mixed growth hormone-and prolactin-cell adenoma	8	Mammosomatotroph variant is slow growing, secretes predominantly growth hormone; acidophil stem cell variant is aggressive, secretes prolactin
Corticotroph adenoma	10	Typically small, secretes corticotropin, resulting in Cushing disease
"Silent" corticotroph adenoma	5	Corticotroph morphology; secretes propiomelanocortin and other clinically silent fragments instead of corticotropin; high propensity for dural invasion
Gonadotroph adenoma	9	Secretes follicle-stimulating hormone and fragments of luteinizing hormone, producing infertility or menstrual disturbances in women; clinically silent in men
Thyrotroph adenoma	1	Secretes thyroid-stimulating hormone and α-subunit of thyroid-stimulating hormone; generally causes hyperthyroidism, but clinical picture varies
Plurihormonal adenoma	1	Typically secretes thyroid-stimulating hormone, growth hormone, and prolactin; symptoms depend on dominant hormone produced
Null cell adenoma, including oncocytoma	26	Previously called "nonfunctioning" or "chromophobe" adenoma; now known to secrete many hormone subunits and fragments that are clinically silent; often are macroadenomas at diagnosis

From Elster AD: Modern imaging of the pituitary, *Radiol* 187:1-14, 1993.

cause amenorrhea and galactorrhea in young women. Serum prolactin levels are only moderately elevated; levels of 150 ng/mL are indicative of tumor.[97]

By contrast, prolactinomas in men occur in older patients, are often endocrinologically silent, may attain large size, and are associated with extremely high serum prolactin levels.[3]

Growth hormone adenoma. These tumors are the second most common endocrinologically active tumor type, representing approximately 15% of all pituitary adenomas.[95] Also known as somatotroph adenomas, these tumors cause gigantism in children and acromegaly in adults.[3,102b]

Eight different types of growth hormone-secreting adenomas are recognized; the sparsely and densely granulated tumors are the most common variants. Sparsely granulated somatotroph adenomas are more likely to be invasive or extend into the suprasellar cistern.[102c] Tumor size and preoperative basal growth-hormone levels are inversely correlated with surgical outcome.[102b]

Corticotrophic adenoma. These tumors represent 5% to 10% of pituitary adenomas. They can be endocrinologically silent. More often they secrete ACTH and are associated with Cushing disease or Nelson syndrome (pituitary adenoma in patient who previously had an adrenalectomy for Cushing disease). Be-

cause of their potent endocrinologic effects, very small ACTH-secreting adenomas may produce profound clinical symptoms.[97]

Gonadotrophic adenoma. Gonadotrophic adenomas account for 5% to 10% of pituitary adenomas. These tumors secrete follicle-stimulating hormone and luteinizing hormone fragments, producing menstrual disturbances or infertility in women. They are clinically silent in men.[95]

Other endocrinologically active adenomas. Thyrotrophic adenomas are rare, representing 1% to 4% of pituitary adenomas. They secrete thyroid-stimulating hormone and generally cause hyperthyroidism.[95] Mixed or multihormonal secretory tumors account for approximately 2.5% to 8% of cases[95,97]; the most common mixed adenoma secretes both prolactin and growth hormone. Tumors that secrete other combinations such as luteinizing and follicle-stimulating hormones are less common.[3]

Null-cell adenoma (including oncocytoma). Endocrinologically silent adenomas represent 25% of pituitary adenomas.[95] Formerly called "nonfunctioning" or "chromophobe" adenoma, they are now called null-cell adenoma or oncocytoma. Null cell adenomas are not truly nonsecretory tumors. They often secrete many hormone subunits and fragments that have little or no endocrine effect.[95,97] These tumors can attain large size and usually become symptomatic because of their mass effect. Hypopituitarism, visual abnormalities and cranial nerve palsies are common symptoms.[3]

Natural history. Pituitary adenomas are typically benign, slow-growing tumors. Many—if not most—microadenomas are clinically silent and are discovered only incidentally on imaging studies or at autopsy. Operated symptomatic adenomas have a reported recurrence rate as high as 16% at 8 years and 35% at 20 years.[103]

Imaging

CT. Microadenomas uncomplicated by hemorrhage or cyst formation are typically isodense with the adjacent normal pituitary gland and may be invisible on NECT scans. Enhancement following contrast administration occurs but is usually delayed compared to the immediate, intense enhancement of the normal pituitary gland. Two thirds of microadenomas therefore typically appear hypodense on dynamic, rapid-sequence CECT scans; one third show "early" enhancement.[103a]

Macroadenomas have a variable appearance. Most are isodense with cortex on NECT scans and show moderate enhancement following contrast administration. Calcification is rare, occurring in 1% to 8% of cases. Necrosis, cyst formation, and hemorrhage may result in mixed-density lesions.

MR. Microadenomas are sometimes difficult to detect unless dynamic techniques are used (*see* Chapter 12). Microadenomas enhance less rapidly than normal pituitary tissue and therefore appear relatively hypointense on rapid-sequence contrast-enhanced T1-weighted scans (Fig. 15-29).

Uncomplicated macroadenomas typically parallel gray matter signal on all imaging sequences (Figs. 15-30 and 15-31). Mixed intensity lesions are common, reflecting necrosis, cyst formation, or hemorrhage. Enhancement following contrast administration is typically intense but is often heterogeneous. Invasion of adjacent structures such as the cavernous sinus is reportedly more common with prolactin- or growth hormone-secreting adenomas than nonsecreting tumors.[102] Benign invasive adenoma cannot be distinguished from the rare pituitary carcinoma on imaging studies alone (Fig. 15-32).

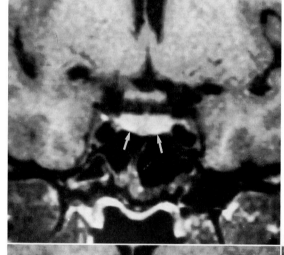

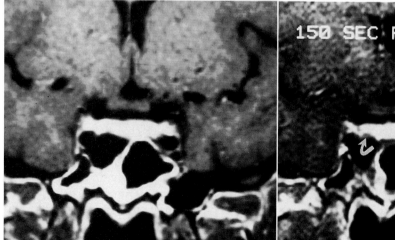

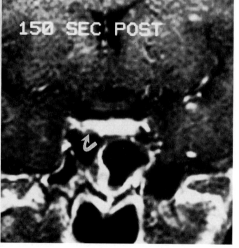

Fig. 15-29. This 21-year-old woman with amenorrhea and galactorrhea had elevated serum prolactin levels. A previous MR study was normal. **A,** Precontrast coronal T1-weighted MR scan shows a normal-appearing pituitary gland *(arrows).* **B,** Routine postcontrast T1WI appears normal. **C,** A "dynamic" sequence with multiple images obtained rapidly following bolus contrast injection was performed. At 150 seconds the normal gland enhances strongly and uniformly. A small comparatively hypointense focus is present *(curved arrow).* A 2 mm microadenoma was found at transsphenoidal hypophysectomy.

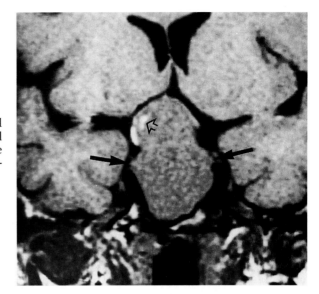

Fig. 15-30. Coronal T1-weighted MR scan shows a typical pituitary macroadenoma *(large arrows)*. Except for a small hyperintense focus caused by hemorrhage *(open arrow)*, the tumor is isointense with gray matter. The "figure eight" appearance on the coronal study is typical.

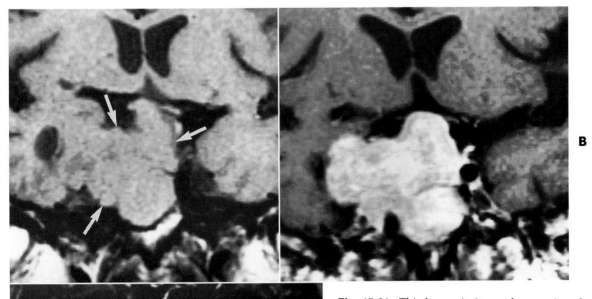

Fig. 15-31. This large pituitary adenoma invades the skull base and cavernous sinus. **A,** Precontrast coronal T1WI shows the lobulated mass *(arrows)* does not have a clear border between it and adjacent brain. **B,** Postcontrast study shows the mass enhances intensely but somewhat heterogeneously. **C,** Axial T2-weighted scan shows the mass *(large arrows)* is predominantly isointense with cortex. The right internal carotid artery *(curved arrow)* is encased but not narrowed.

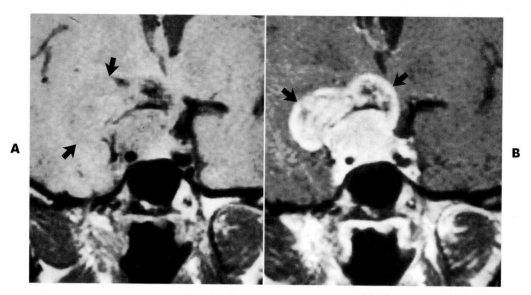

Fig. 15-32. Pre- **(A)** and postcontrast **(B)** coronal T1-weighted MR scan shows a large, somewhat heterogenous pituitary mass *(arrows)* that does not have a sharp tumor-brain interface (compare with Fig. 15-31). Pituitary carcinoma was found at surgery.

The MR imaging appearance of the postoperative sella was discussed in Chapter 12.[103a,103b] Serial MR scans can also be used to monitor long-term bromocriptine therapy, delineating changes in tumor size and detecting intrapituitary hemorrhage, cyst formation, and necrosis. Size reduction is often significant within 1 week of initiating therapy and may continue for several years.[104]

Craniopharyngioma

Etiology and pathology
Etiology. Craniopharyngiomas arise from squamous epithelial rests along the involuted hypophyseal-Rathke's duct.[105]

Gross pathology. The typical craniopharyngioma is a lobulated, well-delineated cystic mass with a mural nodule. Mixed cystic and solid tumors occur less frequently. Cyst contents range from straw-colored fluid to crankcase-like oily material rich in cholesterol. The mural nodule often contains gritty calcific foci.[2]

Microscopic appearance. Craniopharyngiomas are composed of an outside epithelial cell layer that rests on a collagenous basement membrane. Squamous epithelium with pearl-like keratin aggregations or loosely arranged stellate cells interspersed with stromal tissue line the cyst and form the nodule.[2] Fibrous tissue, necrotic debris, cholesterol clefts, and keratin pearls are commonly found within craniopharyngiomas.[19]

Incidence. Craniopharyngiomas account for 3% to 5% of all primary intracranial brain tumors. They are the most common nonglial brain tumor in children and account for half of all suprasellar masses in this age group.[106]

Age and gender. More than half of all craniopharyngiomas occur in children and young adults.[3] Forty percent of craniopharyngiomas in children occur between 8 and 12 years of age. A second, somewhat smaller, peak occurs in middle-aged adults. There is no gender predilection.[106]

Location. Craniopharyngiomas are essentially confined to the sellar region; only rarely do they occur in other intracranial locations.[19,106a] More than three quarters of all craniopharyngiomas are completely suprasellar or have a large suprasellar mass with a smaller intrasellar component; purely intrasellar craniopharyngiomas are rare.[105]

Clinical presentation and natural history. Headache is the most common symptom, followed by endocrine deficiencies and visual disturbances.[106]

Management of craniopharyngiomas is controversial. Despite the benign histology of craniopharyngiomas, in the past, many patients followed a progressively deteriorating course and eventually died of their disease. Prognosis has improved with earlier diagnosis and sophisticated microsurgical techniques.[106]

Imaging
CT. NECT scans typically show a cystic-appearing lobulated suprasellar mass with a solid mural nodule.

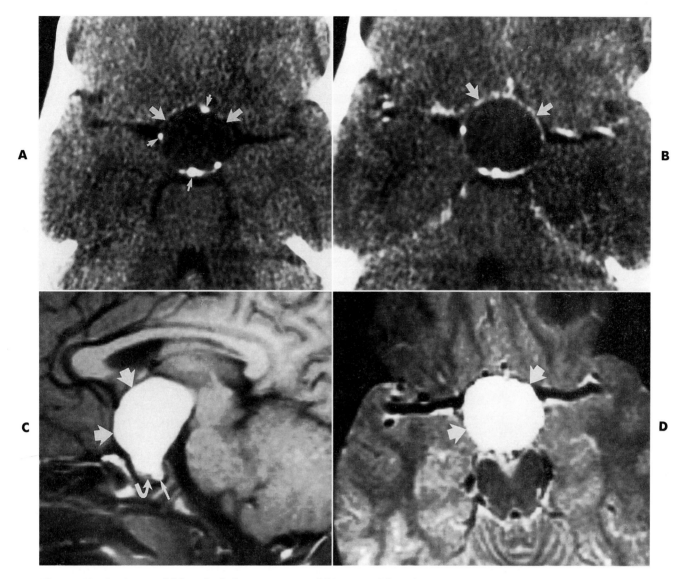

Fig. 15-33. An 8-year-old boy had short stature and bitemporal hemianopsia. **A,** Axial NECT scan shows a well-delineated low attenuation suprasellar mass *(large arrows)* that is slightly hyperdense compared to CSF. Rim calcification *(small arrows)* is present. **B,** The CECT study shows the rim enhances *(arrows)*. **C,** Sagittal T1-weighted MR scan shows a sharply demarcated mass that is hyperintense to adjacent brain. There is a large suprasellar component *(large arrows)* and a smaller intrasellar *(small arrow)* segment. Note the displaced pituitary gland *(curved arrow)* flattened against the sellar floor by the tumor. **D,** Axial T2WI shows the mass *(arrows)* remains strikingly hyperintense. Craniopharyngioma was found at surgery.

Craniopharyngioma

Etiology

Arise from squamous rests along Rathke's cleft

Pathology

Gross: well-delineated cyst with mural nodule most common

Microscopic: squamous epithelium with necrotic debris, cholesterol clefts, keratin pearls

Incidence

3% to 5% of primary brain tumors
50% of pediatric suprasellar tumors

Age

>50% in children, peak 8 to 12 years
Second peak in adults, 40 to 60 years

Location

70% combined suprasellar/intrasellar; completely intrasellar craniopharyngiomas are rare

Imaging

CT: 90% partially cystic, 90% Ca^{++}, 90% nodular/rim enhancement

MR: variable signal; most common is hypointense on T1-, hyperintense on T2WI

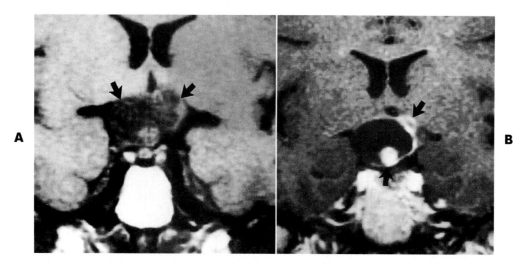

Fig. 15-34. This 54-year-old man complained of visual difficulties. Pre- **(A)** and postcontrast **(B)** coronal T1-weighted MR scans show a mixed signal suprasellar mass (**A,** *arrows*) that shows both nodular and rim enhancement (**B,** *arrows*) following contrast administration. Craniopharyngioma.

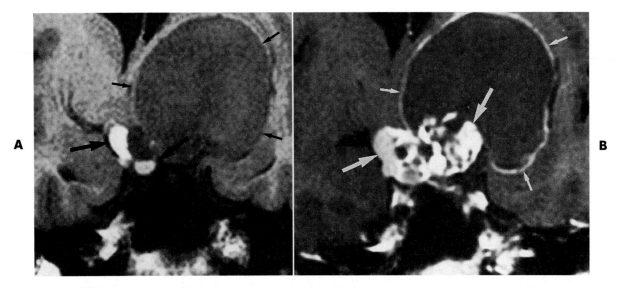

Fig. 15-35. Coronal pre- **(A)** and postcontrast **(B)** MR scans demonstrate the strikingly heterogeneous signal observed with some craniopharyngiomas. Both hyper- *(large arrows)* and hypointense areas *(small arrows)* are present on the precontrast study, **A.** Following contrast administration a thin enhancing rim is seen (**B,** *small arrows*). The solid tumor nodule enhances intensely but very heterogeneously (**B,** *large arrows.*) (Courtesy J. Zahniser.)

Intracranial Metastases	
Common	**Less common**
Skull	Dura
Leptomeninges (arachnoid/subarachnoid)	Pia/subpial
Parenchyma (gray-white junction most common)	
	Rare
	Carcinomatous encephalitis
	Limbic encephalitis (paraneoplastic disease)

Nodular or rim calcification is present in nearly all pediatric craniopharyngiomas (Fig. 15-33, *A*) and is identified in 50% of adult cases. Cyst contents are typically slightly higher in attenuation than CSF. Postcontrast studies demonstrate nodular or rim enhancement in more than 90% of all cases (Fig. 15-33, *B*).

MR. Of all sellar region masses, craniopharyngiomas have the most heterogeneous MR imaging spectrum.[96] Signal is highly variable (Fig. 15-33, *C* and *D*). The most common pattern is a cyst that is hypointense on T1- and hyperintense on T2-weighted sequences (*see* Fig. 12-125).[105] Studies analyzing the craniopharyngioma fluid content conclude that the increased signal intensity on T1WI seen in some tumors is caused by high protein concentration, blood degradation products in free solution, or both.[107]

Craniopharyngiomas enhance strongly but heterogeneously following contrast administration (Figs. 15-34 and 15-35) (*see* box, p. 655). The differential diagnosis of craniopharyngioma includes Rathke cleft cyst, necrotic pituitary adenoma, thrombosed aneurysm, and cystic hypothalamic opticochiasmatic glioma.[107a]

METASTATIC TUMORS

CNS metastatic disease from extracranial primary tumors has many manifestations (*see* box, *left*). Direct geographic extension from nasopharyngeal and skull base malignancy was delineated in Chapter 12. Here we discuss the numerous manifestations of hematogenous metastases to the skull and dura, leptomeninges, and brain parenchyma. We close our discussion of CNS metastatic disease by discussing an uncommon but important entity: limbic encephalitis.

Skull and Dural Metastases

Skull metastases. Calvarial metastases are common (*see* box). Breast and lung are the most frequent primary sites. [2] Lesions range from subtle intradiploic metastases to large masses with extensive areas of bone destruction. CT scans with bone algorithm reconstructions and wide window settings best delineate the osseous components. Contrast-enhanced MR studies are superior for detecting subtle intradiploic lesions, delineating lesion extent, and determining involvement of underlying dura or brain (Fig. 15-36).[108]

Dural metastases. Dural metastases are less common than skull lesions. Calvarial metastases commonly also involve the adjacent dura (Fig. 15-37).[2] Occasionally, focal dural metastases occur without associated calvarial lesions. In some cases a solitary focal dural metastasis can be indistinguishable on imaging studies from a typical benign meningioma (Fig. 15-38; *see* Fig. 14-31).[109]

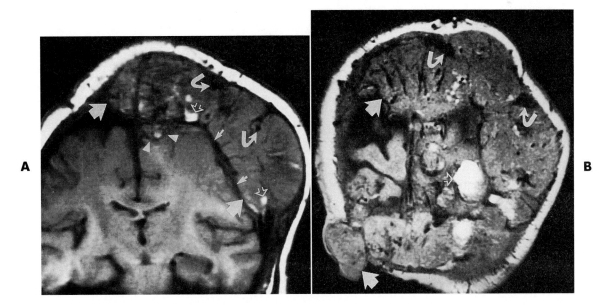

Fig. 15-36. This middle-aged woman with metastatic renal cell carcinoma has extensive diploic metastases. Coronal **(A)** and axial **(B)** T1-weighted scans show the large tumor mass *(large arrows)*. Note intratumoral hemorrhage *(open arrows)* and prominent foci of high-velocity signal loss *(curved arrows)*. The dura *(small arrows)* is largely intact and the mass remains mostly extradural. However, a small subdural tumor focus *(arrowheads)* is present near the vertex. The underlying cortex appears compressed and edematous.

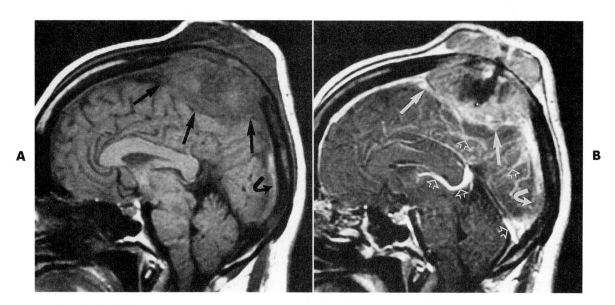

Fig. 15-37. This patient has lung carcinoma metastatic to the calvarium. Sagittal T1-weighted MR scans without **(A)** and with **(B)** contrast show an extensive enhancing mass *(large arrows)* that extends through the calvarial vault and under the galea. Some subacute thrombus is seen in the distal SSS *(curved arrow)*. The ISS, ICVs, vein of Galen, and torcular herophili show intense enhancement **(B,** *open arrows)*, indicating flow is present and possibly even increased as a result of collateral drainage.

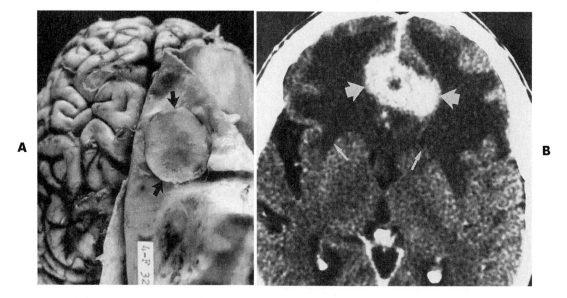

Fig. 15-38. A, Gross pathology specimen in a patient with metastatic breast carcinoma shows a focal dural mass *(arrow)* that resembles meningioma. **B,** Axial CECT scan in a 67-year-old woman with headaches and decreasing mental status shows an enhancing anterior falcine mass *(large arrows)* with extensive bifrontal edema *(small arrows)*. Because the patient had no known malignancy, the preoperative diagnosis was meningioma. Metastatic lung cancer was found at surgery. **(A,** Courtesy Rubinstein Collection, University of Virginia.)

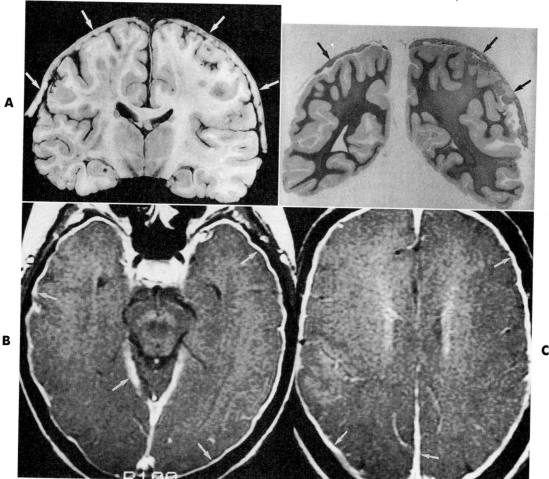

Fig. 15-39. Pathology and imaging manifestations of pachymeningeal (dural) carcinomatosis. **A,** Coronal gross specimen in this patient with disseminated breast carcinoma shows extensively thickened dura *(arrows)* with sparing of the brain and subarachnoid space. **B** and **C,** Axial postcontrast T1-weighted MR scans in another patient with breast carcinoma show diffusely thickened meninges *(arrows).* Biopsy disclosed pachymeningeal carcinomatosis. (**A,** From Okazaki H: Fundamentals of Neuropathology, ed 2, Igaku-Shoin Medical Publishers, New York, 1989.)

Isolated dural or pachymeningeal carcinomatosis is a rare form of intracranial metastatic disease. The meningeal fibrous layer of the dura is diffusely infiltrated by neoplastic cells, forming a thickened, somewhat nodular-appearing membrane that covers the brain and spares the underlying subarachnoid space (Fig. 15-39).[110]

Leptomeningeal Metastases

Leptomeningeal metastases are more common than pachymeningeal metastases. Although solitary leptomeningeal disease is rare, between 6% to 18% of CNS metastases also involve the arachnoid and subarachnoid space, pia, or both.[110]

Arachnoid/subarachnoid metastases. Diffuse or widespread multifocal tumor infiltrates and thickens the leptomeninges (Fig. 15-40). Focal tumor nodules are less common.[111,112] The subarachnoid space can be diffusely involved with metastatic tumor. The basal cisterns are the most common site.[2] Subtle leptomeningeal and subarachnoid metastatic disease is best delineated on contrast-enhanced MR scans (Fig. 15-41).[113]

Pial metastases. Pial metastases typically occur in combination with arachnoid and subarachnoid tumor. Isolated subpial tumor spread is more common with extension of anaplastic astrocytoma and glioblastoma multiforme than with extracranial primary tumors. A rare form of metastatic disease, carcinomatous encephalitis, occurs when there is diffuse tumor spread to the cortex and meninges without formation of macroscopic masses.[114] Diffuse tumor infiltration

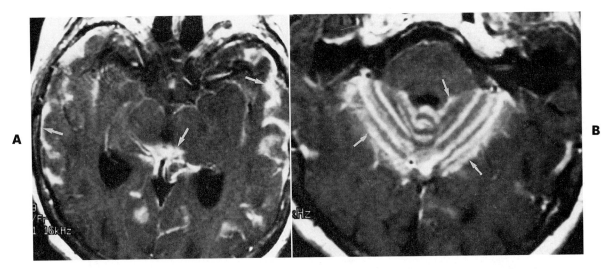

Fig. 15-40. Axial postcontrast T1-weighted MR scans show diffuse leptomeningeal and subarachnoid enhancing tumor *(arrows)* in this elderly woman with breast carcinoma.

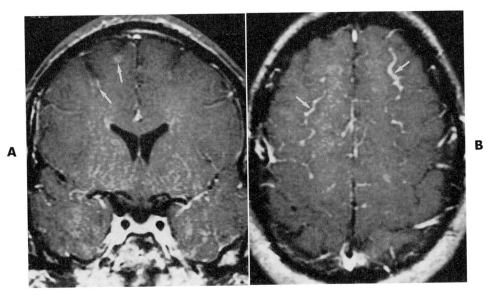

Fig. 15-41. Coronal **(A)** and axial **(B)** postcontrast T1-weighted MR scans in this 37-year-old man with end-stage acute myelogenous leukemia (AML) show subtle enhancing lesions in the cerebral sulci *(arrows)*. Lumbar puncture disclosed AML.

in a subpial perivascular distribution produces innumerable tiny tumor nodules with a miliary appearing pattern (Fig. 15-42).[115]

Parenchymal Metastases

Parenchymal metastases are by far the most common CNS manifestation of extracranial primary neoplasms *(see* box).

Etiology and pathology

Etiology. In descending order, the most common primary tumors to metastasize to brain are lung, breast, and malignant melanoma. Gastrointestinal and genitourinary primary tumors represent the fourth most common primary source.[116]

Pathology. Grossly, parenchymal metastases are typically well-defined circumscribed nodules of varying size that can be solid or partially cystic (filled with mucinous material, necrotic debris, or hemorrhagic fluid).[2] Extensive perifocal edema is common and frequently disproportionate to the size of the metastatic focus.[2] The microscopic appearance of metastases reflects the primary tumor source.

Age and incidence. Parenchymal metastases are uncommon in children. Intracerebral metastases in

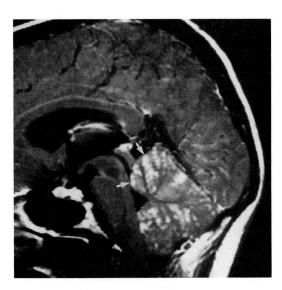

Fig. 15-42. Sagittal postcontrast T1-weighted MR scan in this patient with disseminated malignant melanoma shows innumerable tiny tumor nodules *(arrows)* in the vermis and occipital cortex. Carcinomatous encephalitis.

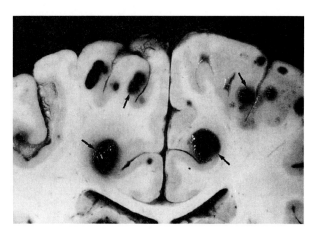

Fig. 15-43. Axial gross pathology specimen of metastatic melanoma shows numerous hemorrhagic tumor implants *(arrows)* at the corticomedullary junction, the most typical site for parenchymal metastases from extracranial primary tumors. (Courtesy B. Horten.)

adults are common, representing between one quarter and one third of all brain tumors.[116,117] Brain metastases are found in 10% to 25% of autopsied patients with extracranial malignant neoplasms.[116,118] Between 60% and 85% of metastases are multiple.[118a]

Location. All areas of the brain may be affected, but the corticomedullary junction is the most common site (Fig. 15-43).[2]

Clinical presentation and natural history. Clinical presentation varies from asymptomatic patients whose intracranial lesions are identified during evaluation for therapeutic protocols to nonambulatory patients with severe neurologic deficits. Despite treatment with standard whole-brain radiation therapy, median survival time is a dismal 3 to 6 months.[118] Aggressive treatments such as brachy- and neutron therapy, stereotactic gamma knife and linear accelerator radiosurgery, various radiation-chemotherapy combinations, and surgical resection for solitary metastases have had mixed results and remain controversial.

Imaging. Because detection of even a single brain metastasis in a cancer patient dramatically alters prognosis and may change therapy, the detection and characterization of cerebral metastases has received significant attention in the imaging literature.[119]

Parenchymal Metastases

Etiology

Lung > breast > melanoma > GI/GU tumors

Pathology

Rounded solid/partially cystic mass ±edema

Incidence

Most common site of CNS metastases from extracranial primary tumor
One quarter to one third of brain tumors
10% to 25% of autopsied cancer patients
>80% multiple

Age

Rare in children, most common in older adults (>40 years)

Location

Anywhere; gray-white junction most common site

Imaging

NECT: iso/hyperdense; Ca^{++} rare in untreated metastases
CECT: strong solid/ring enhancement
MR: most hypointense on T1-, hyperintense on T2WI; most enhance moderately intensely following contrast administration (dose of at least 0.1 mmol/kg recommended)

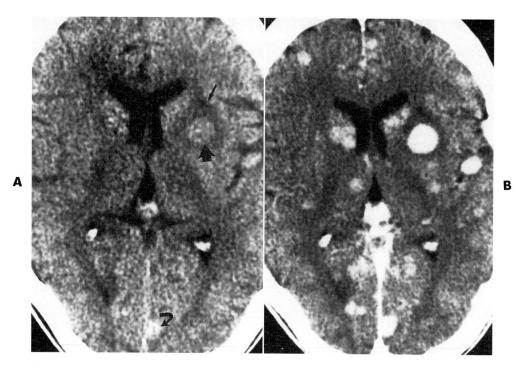

Fig. 15-44. A, Axial NECT scan in this patient with breast carcinoma appears nearly normal. A mass in the left basal ganglia *(large arrow)* is apparent only because the adjacent brain is edematous *(small arrow)*. A hyperdense left occipital lesion *(curved arrow)* is present. **B,** CECT scan shows numerous enhancing masses consistent with multifocal metastases.

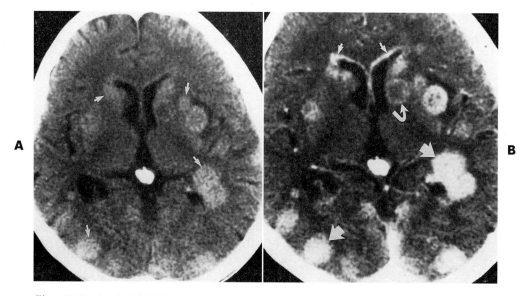

Fig. 15-45. A, Axial NECT scan in this middle-aged man with small cell lung cancer shows multifocal high density lesions *(arrows)*. **B,** CECT scan shows numerous enhancing masses. Note solid *(large arrows)*, ring *(curved arrow)* and ependymal *(small arrows)* enhancing patterns.

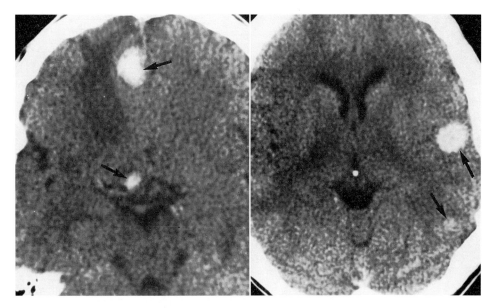

Fig. 15-46. Axial NECT scans in this patient with melanoma show multiple high density lesions *(arrows).* Autopsy disclosed hemorrhagic metastases (compare with Fig. 15-43).

CT. Attenuation of cerebral metastases on NECT scans varies. Most metastases are isodense with adjacent brain (Fig. 15-44). Hyperdense metastases are seen with small round cell tumors or other neoplasms with high nuclear to cytoplasmic ratios (Fig. 15-45). Hemorrhage can occur in virtually any metastatic tumor, but renal and breast carcinomas, melanoma, and choroicarcinoma are the most likely metastases to bleed (Fig. 15-46).

Cystic (Fig. 15-47) and calcified (Fig. 15-48) untreated metastases are rare, representing approximately 1% to 6.6% of reported cases.[120,120a] Lung and breast carcinoma are the most common primary sources.[120,121] Edema associated with metastases can be striking and in some cases is the only abnormality seen on NECT scans.

Most—but not all—parenchymal metastases enhance strongly following contrast administration. Both solid and ringlike patterns are seen (Fig. 15-45). Double-dose delayed CT scans significantly improve the sensitivity and specificity of cerebral metastatic disease detection.[117] False-negative studies occur in 11.5% of patients if scans are obtained immediately following administration of the standard contrast dose.[122]

MR. Signal intensity of brain metastases varies. Most nonhemorrhagic intracerebral metastases are slightly hypointense relative to brain on T1-weighted scans (Fig. 15-49, *A*).[116] Some nonhemorrhagic metastases, most noticeably malignant melanoma, are often hyperintense on T1WI (Fig. 15-50). T1 shortening in these cases correlates with melanin content, not hemorrhage or the presence of chelated metal ions.[123]

Most metastases demonstrate prolonged T2 relax-

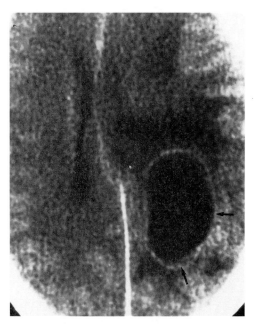

Fig. 15-47. Axial CECT scan in this patient with adenocarcinoma of the lung shows a solitary thin-walled left occipital lobe mass *(arrows).* No other lesions were present, and the patient had no known metastases elsewhere. Stereotactic biopsy disclosed metastatic tumor.

ation times and are therefore hyperintense on T2-weighted sequences (Fig. 15-49, *B*). Multifocal white matter and corticomedullary lesions on T2WI are common manifestations of metastatic disease (*see* Chapter 17). They therefore resemble the punctate high signal foci that are often observed on T2-weighted scans in normal elderly patients. If multifocal hyperintense foci do not enhance following con-

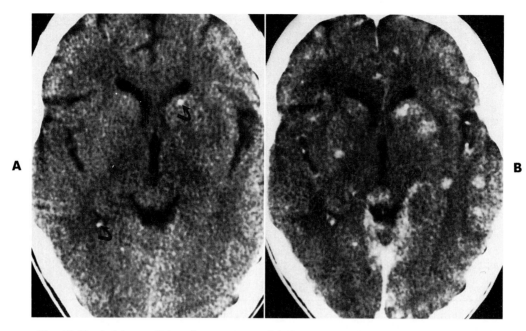

Fig. 15-48. Axial pre- **(A)** and postcontrast **(B)** CT scans in this patient with untreated metastatic breast carcinoma show some of the lesions *(arrows)* are calcified. Same case as Fig. 15-44.

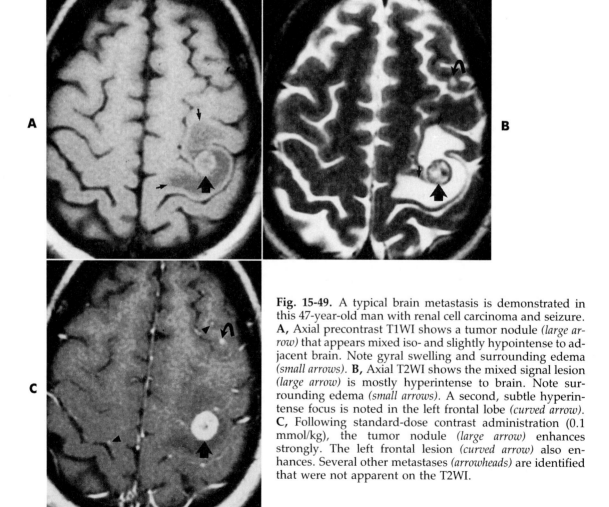

Fig. 15-49. A typical brain metastasis is demonstrated in this 47-year-old man with renal cell carcinoma and seizure. **A,** Axial precontrast T1WI shows a tumor nodule *(large arrow)* that appears mixed iso- and slightly hypointense to adjacent brain. Note gyral swelling and surrounding edema *(small arrows).* **B,** Axial T2WI shows the mixed signal lesion *(large arrow)* is mostly hyperintense to brain. Note surrounding edema *(small arrows).* A second, subtle hyperintense focus is noted in the left frontal lobe *(curved arrow).* **C,** Following standard-dose contrast administration (0.1 mmol/kg), the tumor nodule *(large arrow)* enhances strongly. The left frontal lesion *(curved arrow)* also enhances. Several other metastases *(arrowheads)* are identified that were not apparent on the T2WI.

trast administration, the probability that they represent metastases rather than small vessel disease or other benign entities is low.[119]

Some metastatic tumors are hypointense on T2WI. Examples are mucin-secreting neoplasms such as metastatic gastrointestinal adenocarcinoma[116] and densely cellular tumors with high nuclear to cytoplasmic ratios (Fig. 15-51). Hemorrhage can also complicate the appearance of metastases (Fig. 15-52; *see* Figs. 7-50 to 7-52).

Contrast-enhanced MR scans are the most sensitive imaging procedure for evaluating intracranial metastatic disease.[117] Most—but not all—metastases enhance strongly following contrast administration. Multifocal lesions located at the gray-white junction are typical (Fig. 15-49, *C*). Solid, rim, and mixed-

enhancement patterns occur (Fig. 15-53).

The optimum cost-effective contrast dosage has not been clearly established. The standard contrast dose (0.1 mmol/kg) is adequate in most cases; low-dose studies (0.05 mmol/kg) are suboptimal (Fig. 15-54). High-dose (0.2-0.3 mmol/kg) studies are even more sensitive than standard-dose (0.1 mmol/kg) examinations and may be helpful in detecting early, small, or additional metastatic lesions.[124,125] In contrast to CT, delayed postcontrast studies do not improve lesion-to-brain contrast.[125]

Limbic Encephalitis

Paraneoplastic syndromes are defined as clinical manifestations associated with cancer that are not due to tumor in the affected organ[126] (*see* box, p. 666).

Etiology and pathology
Etiology. The precise etiology of paraneoplastic syndromes is unknown, but autoimmune disorder and viral infection have been proposed as the most likely mechanisms.[126]

Small cell lung cancer (SCLC) is the extracranial malignancy most commonly associated with a range of neurologic paraneoplastic syndromes. These include Lambert-Eaton myasthenic syndrome, subacute sensory neuropathy, myelopathy, cerebellar degeneration, and encephalopathy.[127] Limbic encephalitis is a subacute encephalitis that predominately involves the limbic system and is frequently associated with malignant tumors, especially oat cell carcinoma.[128,129]

Other tumors associated with specific paraneoplastic syndromes include female genital tract tumors with cerebellar degeneration, neuroblastoma with opsoclonus, and Hodgkin's disease with demyelinating neuropathy.[127]

Pathology. Gross abnormalities are usually absent, and biopsy findings are nonspecific. Mononu-

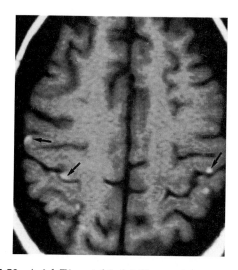

Fig. 15-50. Axial T1-weighted MR scan in a patient with metastatic melanoma shows multifocal corticomedullary junction lesions *(arrows)*. The lesions are hyperintense on this unenhanced study. The lesions were not seen on the T2WI (not shown). (Courtesy J. Stears.)

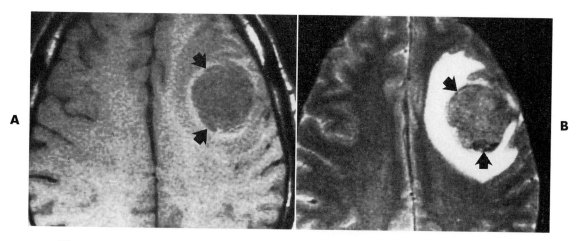

Fig. 15-51. Metastatic germ cell tumor is seen in this 38-year-old man. This densely cellular tumor *(arrows)* is hypointense on both T1- **(A)** and T2-weighted **(B)** scans.

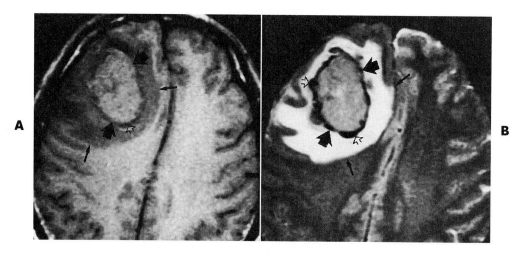

Fig. 15-52. This 50-year-old man with no known primary tumor had decreasing mental status. Axial T1- **(A)** and T2-weighted **(B)** MR scans show a right frontal lesion *(large arrows)* that is mostly isointense with cortex on both sequences. A hypointense rim *(open arrows)* surrounds the mass. Moderate peripheral edema *(small arrows)* is present. Surgery disclosed extensive acute hemorrhage. Underlying foci of metastatic hypernephroma were present on pathologic examination.

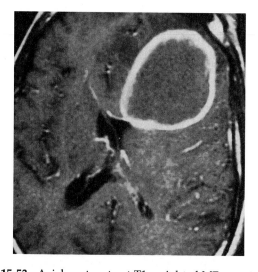

Fig. 15-53. Axial postcontrast T1-weighted MR scan in this patient with squamous cell lung cancer shows a left frontal rim-enhancing mass. This cystic metastasis resembles an abscess.

clear perivascular and parenchymal infiltrates with reactive gliosis, microglial proliferation, and neuronal loss have been reported.[128,129] No tumor cells or viral inclusion bodies are present.

Incidence. The exact incidence of paraneoplastic syndromes is unknown. Limbic encephalitis has been identified in 2% to 3% of patients with SCLC.[127]

Age and gender. The mean age of patients with SCLC is 64 years; nearly 80% of patients are men.[127]

Limbic Encephalitis

Paraneoplastic syndrome

Clinical manifestations associated with cancer but *not* due to tumor in affected organ

Etiology

Unknown (?autoimmune/viral)
Small cell lung cancer most commonly associated

Pathology

Gross: usually normal/mild nonspecific temporal lobe swelling
Microscopic: nonspecific inflammatory changes *without* viral inclusions/tumor

Incidence

(Rare, 2% to 3% of patients with small cell lung cancers)

Age and gender

Older men most commonly affected by paraneoplastic syndromes; M = F in limbic encephalitis

Location

Limbic system (temporal lobes, insula, cingulate gyri)

Imaging

Nonspecific (indistinguishable from viral encephalitis, especially herpes)

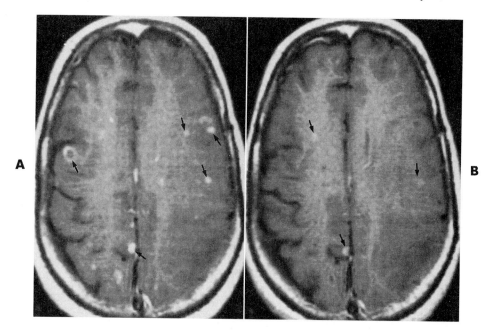

Fig. 15-54. Contrast-enhanced T1-weighted MR scans in this patient with parenchymal metastases were performed using standard (0.1 mmol/kg) and low dose (0.05 mmol/kg). Multile lesions are clearly identified on the standard dose study (**A**, *arrows*) but are barely seen on the low dose sequence (**B**, *arrows*). (Courtesy W.T.C. Yuh.)

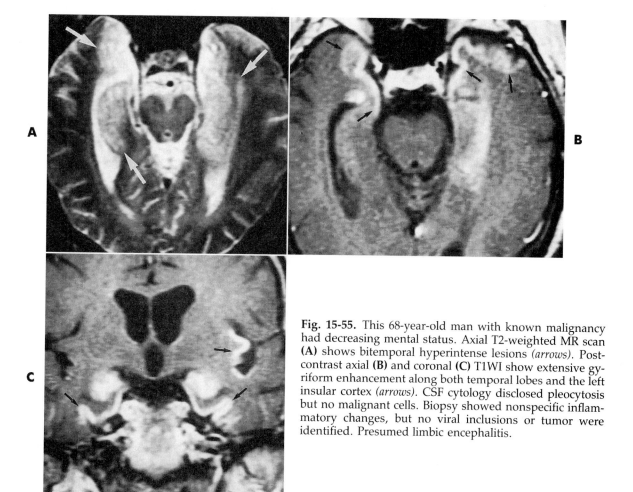

Fig. 15-55. This 68-year-old man with known malignancy had decreasing mental status. Axial T2-weighted MR scan (**A**) shows bitemporal hyperintense lesions *(arrows)*. Post-contrast axial (**B**) and coronal (**C**) T1WI show extensive gyriform enhancement along both temporal lobes and the left insular cortex *(arrows)*. CSF cytology disclosed pleocytosis but no malignant cells. Biopsy showed nonspecific inflammatory changes, but no viral inclusions or tumor were identified. Presumed limbic encephalitis.

Reported cases of limbic encephalitis are equally divided between both genders.[129]

Location. Hippocampal formations, amygdalae, and other medial temporal lobe structures are the most commonly involved sites in limbic encephalitis. Other paraneoplastic syndromes affect different anatomic areas such as the cerebellum or spinal cord.

Clinical presentation and natural history. The clinical hallmarks of limbic encephalitis are changing mental status with affective symptoms and memory impairment.[129] Treatment of the primary malignancy may reverse the course of this syndrome in some cases.

Imaging. Imaging findings are nonspecific. CT scans are usually normal.[128] High signal intensity in the medial temporal lobes can sometimes be identified on T2-weighted MR scans (Fig. 15-55, *A*).[129] Enhancement following contrast administration varies (Fig. 15-55, *B* and *C*). The major differential diagnosis of limbic encephalitis is viral encephalitis (e.g., herpes encephalitis).

REFERENCES

1. Al-Ghamadi S, Black MJ, Lafond G: Extracranial head and neck schawannomas, *J Otolaryngol* 21:186-188, 1992.
2. Okazaki H: *Fundamentals of Neuropathology*, ed 2, New York, Igaku-Shoin, 1989.
3. Russell DS, Rubinstein LJ: *Pathology of Tumors of the Nervous System*, ed 5, Baltimore, Williams and Wilkins, 1989.
4. Gentry LR, Mehta RC, Appen RE, Weinstein JM: MR imaging of primary trochlear nerve neoplasms, *AJNR* 12:707-713, 1991.
5. Tung H, Chen T, Weiss MH: Sixth nerve schwannomas, *J Neurosurg* 75:638-641, 1991.
6. Allcutt DA, Hoffman HJ, Isla A et al: Acoustic schwannomas in children, *Neurosurg* 29:14-18, 1991.
7. McCormick PC, Bello JA, Post KD: Trigeminal schwannoma, *J Neurosurg* 69:850-860, 1988.
8. Lizak PF, Woodruff WW: Posterior fossa neoplasms: multiplanar imaging, *Sem US, CT, MR* 13:182-206, 1992.
9. Bilaniuk LT: Adult infratentorial tumors, *Sem Roentgenol* 25:155-173, 1990.
10. Pollack IF, Sekhar LN, Jannetta PJ, Janecka IP: Neurilemmomas of the trigeminal nerve, *J Neurosurg* 70:737-745, 1989.
11. Beges C, Revel MP, Gaston A et al: Trigeminal neuromas: assessment of MRI and CT, *Neuroradiol* 34:179-183, 1992.
12. Brogan M, Chakeres DW: Gd-DTPA-enhanced MR imaging of cochlear schwannoma, *AJNR* 11:407-408, 1990.
13. Lidov M, Som PM, Stacy C, Catalano P: Eccentric cystic facial schwannoma: CT and MR features, *J Comp Asst Tomogr* 15:1065-1067, 1991.
14. Martin N, Sterkers O, Mompoint D, Nahum H: Facial nerve neuromas: MR imaging, *Neuroradiol* 34:62-67, 1992.
15. Celli P, Ferrante L, Acqui M et al: Neurinoma of the third, fourth and sixth cranial nerves: a survey and report of a new fourth nerve case, *Surg Neurol* 38:216-224, 1992.
16. Katsumata Y, Maehara T, Noda M, Shirouzu I: Neurinoma of the oculomotor nerve: CT and MR features, *J Comp Asst Tomogr* 14:662-664, 1990.
17. Sigal R, D'Anthouard F, David P et al: Cystic schwannoma mimicking a brain stem tumor: MR features, *J Comp Asst Tomogr* 14:662-664, 1990.
18. Casadei GP, Komori T, Scheithauer BW et al: Intracranial parenchymal schwannoma, *J Neurosurg* 79:217-222, 1993.
19. Burger PC, Scheithauer BW, Vogel FS: *Surgical Pathology of the Nervous System and its Coverings*, ed 3, New York, Churchill Livingstone, 1991.
20. Abramowitz J, Dion JE, Jensen ME et al: Angiographic diagnosis and management of head and neck schwannomas, *AJNR* 12:977-984, 1991.
21. Moscow NP, Newton TH: Angiographic features of hypervascular neurinomas of the head and neck, *Radiol* 114:635-640, 1975.
22. Cohen LM, Schwartz AM, Rockoff SD: Benign schwannomas: pathologic basis for CT inhomogeneities, *AJR* 147:141-143, 1986.
22a. Asari S, Katayama S, Itoh T et al: CT and MRI of haemorrhage into intracranial neuromas, *Neuroradiol* 35:247-250, 1993.
23. Mulkens TH, Parizel PM, Martin J-J et al: Acoustic schwannoma: MR findings in 84 tumors, *AJR* 160:395-398, 1993.
24. Vion-Dury J, Vincentelli F, Jiddane M et al: MR imaging of epidermoid cysts, *Neuroradiol* 29:333-338, 1987.
25. Braun IF, Naidich TP, Leeds NE et al. Dense intracranial epidermoid tumors, *Radiol* 122:717-719, 1977.
26. Ruge JR, Tomashitas T, Naidich TP et al. Scalp and calvarial masses of infants and children, *Neurosurg* 22:1037-1042, 1988.
27. Gao P-Y, Osborn AG, Smirniotopoulos JG, Harris CP: Epidermoid tumor of the cerebellopontine angle, *AJNR* 13:863-872, 1992.
28. Wagle WA, Jaufmann B, Mincy JE: Magnetic resonance imaging of fourth ventricular epidermoid tumors, *Arch Neurol* 48:438-440, 1991.
29. Bejarano PA, Burderick DF, Gado MH: Infected epidermoid cyst of the sphenoid bone, *AJNR* 14:772-773, 1993.
30. Pumar J, Otero E, Castñeira A et al: Intradiploic epidermoid tumor of the occipital bone: X-ray, CT, MR findings, *Eur Radiol* 3:183-185, 1993.
31. Tatler GLV, Kendall BE: The radiological diagnosis of epidermoid tumors, *Neuroradiol* 33(suppl):324-325, 1991.
32. Tekkok IH, Cataltepe O, Saglam S: Dense epidermoid cyst of the cerebellopontine angle, *Neuroradiol* 33:255-257, 1991.
33. Gualdi GF, Biasi C Di, Trasimeni G et al: Unusual MR and CT appearance of an epidermoid tumor, *AJNR* 12:771-772, 1991.
34. Tampieri D, Melanson D, Ethier R: MR imaging of epidermoid cysts, *AJNR* 10:351-356, 1989.
35. Horowitz BL, Chari MV, James R, Bryan RN: MR in intracranial epidermoid tumors: correlation of in vitro imaging with in vitro ^{13}C spectroscopy, *AJNR* 11:299-302, 1990.
36. Shen WC, Yang CF: Epidermoid cyst with variable contents shown on CT and MRI, *Neuroradiol* 33(suppl):317-318, 1991.
37. Kawamura Y, Sze G: Totally cystic schwannoma of the tenth cranial nerve mimicking an epidermoid, *AJNR* 134:1333-1334, 1992.
38. Tsuruda JW, Chew CM, Moseley ME, Norman D: Diffusion weighted MR imaging of the brain: value of differentiating between extraaxial cysts and epidermoid tumors, *AJNR* 11:925-931, 1990.
39. Smith AS: Myth of the mesoderm: ectodermal origin of dermoids, *AJNR* 10:449, 1989.
40. Smith AS, Benson JE, Blaser SI et al: Diagnosis of ruptured intracranial dermoid cyst: value of MR over CT, *AJNR* 12:175-180, 1991.
41. Wilms G, Casselman J, Demaerel Ph et al: CT and MRI of ruptured intracranial dermoids, *Neuroradiol* 33:149-151, 1991.
41a. Markus H, Kendall BE: MRI of a dermoid cyst containing hair, *Neuroradiol* 35:256-257, 1993.

42. Lunardi P, Missori P: Supratentorial dermoid cysts, *J Neurosurg* 75:262-266, 1991.

43. Searce TA, Shaw C-M, Bronstein AD, Swanson PD: Intraventricular fat from a ruptured sacral dermoid cyst: clinical, radiographic, and pathological correlation, *J Neurosurg* 78:666-668, 1993.

44. Ahmad I, Tominaga T, Ogawa A, Yoshimoto T: Ruptured suprasellar dermoid associated with middle cerebral artery aneurysm: case report, *Surg Neurol* 38:341-346, 1992.

45. Rubin G, Scienza R, Pasqualin A et al: Craniocerebral epidermoids and dermoids, *Acta Neurochir* (Wien) 97:1-16, 1989.

46. Drolshagen LF, Standefer M: Dense dermoid cyst of the posterior fossa, *AJNR* 12:317, 1991.

47. Uchino A, Hasuo K, Matsumoto S, Masuda K: Solitary choroid plexus lipomas: CT and MR appearance, *AJNR* 14:116-118, 1993.

48. Rorke LB: Demystifying malformations, *AJNR* 11:675, 1990.

49. Truwitt CL, Barkovich AJ: Pathogenesis of intracranial lipoma: an MR study in 42 patients, *AJNR* 11:665-674, 1990.

50. Tart RP, Quisling RG: Curvilinear and tubulonodular varieties of lipoma of the corpus callosum: an MR and CT study, *J Compt Asst Tomogr* 15:805-810, 1991.

50a. Britt PM, Bindal AK, Balko MG, Yeh H-SH: Lipoma of the cerebral cortex: case report, *Acta Neurochir* (Wieh) 121:88-92, 1993.

51. Donati F, Vassella F, Kaiser G, Blumberg A: Intracranial lipomas, *Neuropediatr* 23:32-38, 1992.

52. Rouhart F, Goas JY, Neriot P, Zagnoli F: Le lipome du corps calleux, *Sem Hôp Paris* 68:331-335, 1992.

53. Eghwrudjakpor PO, Kurisaka M, Fukuoka M, Mori K: Intracranial lipomas, *Acta Neurochir* (Wien) 110:124-128, 1991.

54. Melin GI, Keller MS: Pericallosal lipoma extending through the choroidal fissure: US/CT/MRI correlation, *Neuroradiol* 34:402-403, 1992.

55. Uchino A, Hasuo K, Matsumoto S, Masuda K: MRI of dorsal mesencephalic lipomas, *Clin Imaging* 17:12-16, 1993.

56. Wolpert SM, Barnes PD: Encephalocraniocutaneous lipomatosis. In *MRI in Pediatric Neuroradiology*, p. 329, St Louis: Mosby Year-Book, 1992.

57. Cohen TI, Powers SK, Williams DW III: MR appearance of intracanalicular eighth nerve lipoma, *AJNR* 13:1188-1190, 1992.

58. Beltinger C, Saule H: Imaging of lipoma of the corpus callosum and intracranial dermoids in the Goldenhar syndrome, *Pediatr Radiol* 18:72-73, 1988.

59. Dean B, Drayer BP, Berisini DC, Bird CR: MR imaging of pericallosal lipoma, *AJNR* 9:929-931, 1988.

60. Georgy BA, Hessilink JR, Jernigan TL: MR imaging of the corpus callosum, *AJR* 160:949-955, 1993.

61. van Burken, Sarioglu AC, O'Donnell HD: Supratentorial arachnoidal cyst with intracystic and subdural hematoma, *Neurochir* 35:199-203, 1992.

62. Eustace S, Toland J, Stack J: CT and MRI of arachnoid cyst with complicating intracystic and subdural hemorrhage, *J Comp Asst Tomogr* 16:995-997, 1992.

62a. Garcia Santos JM, Martinez-Lage J, Ubeda AG et al: Arachnoid cysts of the middle fossa: a consideration of their origins based on imaging, *Neuroradiol* 39:395-358, 1993.

63. Becker T, Wagner M, Hofmann E et al: Do arachnoid cysts grow? A retrospective CT volumetric study, *Neuroradiol* 33:341-345, 1991.

64. Flodmark O: Neuroradiology of selected disorders of the menengis, calvarium and venous sinuses, *AJNR* 13:483-491, 1992.

65. Robertson SJ, Wolpert SM, Runge VM: MR imaging of middle cranial fossa arachnoid cysts: temporal lobe agenesis syndrome revisited, *AJNR* 10:1007-1010, 1989.

66. Ciricillo SF, Cogen PH, Harsh GR, Edwards MSB: Intracranial arachnoid cysts in children: a comparison of the effects of fenestration and shunting, *J Neurosurg* 74:230-235, 1991.

67. Wester K: Gender distribution and sidedness of middle fossa arachnoid cysts: a review of cases diagnosed with computed imaging, *Neurosurg* 31:940-944, 1992.

68. Dhooge C, Govaert P, Martens F, Caemaert J. Transventricular endoscopic investigation and treatment of suprasellar arachnoid cysts, *Neuropediatrics* 23:245-247, 1992.

68a. García Santos JM, Martinez-Lage J, Gilabert Ubeda A et al: Arachnoid cysts of the middle cranial fossa: a consideration of their origins based on imaging, *Neuroradiol* 35:355-358, 1993.

69. Quint DJ: Retroclival arachnoid cysts, *AJNR* 13:1503-1504, 1992.

70. Tien RD, MacFall J, Heinz ER: Evaluation of complex cystic masses of the brain: value of steady-state free-precession MR imaging, *AJR* 159:1049-1055, 1992.

71. Maeda M, Kawamura Y, Tamagawa Y et al: Intravoxel incoherent motion (IVIM) MRI in intracranial, extraaxial tumors and cysts, *J Comp Asst Tomogr* 16:514-518, 1992.

72. Kondziolka D, Bilbao JM. An immunohistochemical study of neuroepithelial (colloid) cysts, *J Neurosurg* 71:91-97, 1989.

73. Lach B, Scheithauer BW, Gregor A, Wick MP: Colloid cyst of the third ventricle: a comparative immunohistochemical study of neuraxis cysts and choroid plexus epithelium, *J Neurosurg* 78:101-111, 1993.

74. Waggenspack GA, Guinto FC Jr: MR and CT of masses of the anterosuperior third ventricle, *AJNR* 10:105-110, 1989.

75. Hine AL, Chui MS: Hypodense colloid cyst of the third ventricle, *J Can Assoc Radiol* 38:288-291, 1987.

76. Shuangshoti S, Pitakdamrongwong N, Poneprasert B et al. Symptomatic neuroepithelial cysts in the posterior cranial fossa, *Surg Neurol* 30:298-304, 1988.

77. Sener RN, Jinkins JR: CT of intrasellar colloid cysts, *J Comp Asst Tomogr* 15:671-672, 1991.

78. Mathiesen T, Grane P, Lindquist C, von Holst H: High recurrence rate following aspiration of colloid cysts in the third ventricle, *J Neurosurg* 78:748-752, 1993.

79. Wilms G, Marchal G, Van Hecke P et al: Colloid cysts of the third ventricle: MR findings, *J Comp Asst Tomogr* 14:527-531, 1990.

80. Crenshaw WB, Chew FS: Rathke's cleft cyst, *AJR* 158:1312, 1993.

81. Ross DA, Norman D, Wilson CB: Radiologic characteristics and results of surgical management of Rathke's cysts in 43 patients, *Neurosurg* 30:173-179, 1992.

82. Voelker JL, Campbell RL, Muller J: Clinical radiographic and pathological features of Rathke's cleft cysts, *J Neurosurg* 74:535-544, 1991.

83. Itoh J, Usui K: An entirely suprasellar symptomatic Rathke's cleft cyst: case report, *Neurosurg* 30:581-585, 1992.

83a. Whyte AM, Sage MR, Brophy BP: Imaging of large Rathke's cleft cysts by CT and MRI: report of two cases, *Neuroradiol* 35:258-260, 1993.

84. Hua F, Asato R, Miki Y et al: Differentiation of suprasellar nonneoplastic cysts from cystic neoplasms by Gd-DTPA MRI, *J Comp Asst Tomogr* 16:744-749, 1992.

85. Numaguchi Y, Foster RW, Gum GK: Large symptomatic noncolloid neuroepithelial cysts in the lateral ventricle: CT and MR features, *Neuroradiol* 31:98-101, 1989.

86. Nakase H, Ishida Y, Tada T et al: Neuroepithelial cysts of the lateral ventricle, *Surg Neurol* 37:94-100, 1992.

87. Sherman JL, Camponovo E, Citrin CM: MR imaging of CSF-like choroidal fissure and parenchymal cysts of the brain, *AJNR* 11:939-945, 1990.

88. Ciricillo SF, Davis RL, Wilson CB: Neuroepithelial cysts of the posterior fossa, *J Neurosurg* 72:302-305, 1990.

89. Numaguchi Y, Kumra A, Schmidt RD, Martino C: Noncol-

loid neuroepithelial cysts in the lateral ventricles: magnetic resonance features, *CT: J Comp Tomogr* 12:174-181, 1988.

90. Wilkins RH, Burger PC: Benign intraparenchymal brain cysts without an epithelial lining, *J Neurosurg* 68:378-382, 1988.

91. Ito S, Fujiwara S, Mizoi K et al: Enterogenous cysts at the cerebellopontine angle: case report, *Surg Neurol* 37:366-370, 1992.

92. Gao P-Y, Osborn AG, Smirniotopoulos JG et al: Intraspinal and posterior fossa enterogenous cysts: imaging and pathologic spectrum, *AJNR*, in press.

93. Brooks BS, Durall ER, El Gammal T et al: Neuroimaging features of neurenteric cysts: analysis of nine cases and review of the literature, *AJNR* 14:735-746, 1993.

94. Malcolm GP, Symon L, Kendall B, Pires M: Intracranial neurenteric cysts, *J Neurosurg* 75:115-120, 1991.

95. Elster AD: Modern imaging of the pituitary, *Radiol* 187:1-14, 1993.

95a. Elster AD: Imaging of the sella: anatomy and pathology, *Sem US, CT, MR* 14:182-194, 1993.

96. Johnsen DE, Woodruff WW, Allen IS et al: MR imaging of the sellar and juxtasellar regions, *RadioGraphics* 11:727-758, 1991.

97. Schwartzberg DG: Imaging of pituitary tumors, *Sem US, CT, MR* 13:207-223, 1992.

98. Hall WA, Luciano MG, Doppman JL et al: A prospective double-blind study of high resolution pituitary MRI in normal human subjects: occult pituitary adenomas in the general population, *J Neurosurg* 72:342A, 1990.

99. Schubiger O, Haller D: Metastases to the pituitary-hypothalamic axis, *Neuroradiol* 34:131-134, 1992.

100. Juneau P, Schoene WC, Black P: Malignant tumors in the pituitary gland, *Arch Neurol* 49:555-558, 1992.

101. Popovic EA, Vattuone JR, Siu KH et al: Malignant prolactinomas, *Neurosurg* 29:127-130, 1992.

102. Lundin P, Nyman R, Burmas P et al: MRI of pituitary neuroadenomas with reference to hormonal activity, *Neuroradiol* 34:43-51, 1992.

102a. Bartuska DG, Kleinman DS, Kodroff KS, Piatok DJ: The sellar/paraseller endocrinopathies: a brief clinical overview, *Sem US, CT, MR* 14:178-181, 1993.

102b. Davis DH, Laws ER Jr, Ilstrup DM et al: Results of surgical treatment for growth hormone-secreting pituitary adenomas, *J Neurosurg* 79:70-75, 1993.

102c. Yamada S, Aita T, Sano T et al: Growth hormone-producing pituitary adenomas: correlations between clinical characteristics and morphology, *Neurosurg* 33:20-27, 1993.

103. Hsu DW, Hakim F, Biller BMK et al: Significance of proliferating cell nuclear antigen index in predicting pituitary adenoma recurrence, *J Neurosurg* 78:753-761, 1993.

103a. Bonneville J-F, Cattin F, Gorczyca W, Hardy J: Pituitary microadenomas: early enhancement with dynamic CT implications of arterial blood supply and potential importance, *Radiol* 187:857-861, 1993.

103b. Dina TS, Feaster SH, Laws ER Jr, Davis DO: MR of the pituitary gland postsurgery: serial MR studies following transsphenoidal resection, *AJNR* 14:763-769, 1993.

104. Lundin P, Bergstrom K, Nyman R et al: Macroprolatinomas: serial MR imaging in long-term bromocriptine therapy, *AJNR* 13:1279-1291, 1992.

105. Zimmerman RA: Imaging of intrasellar, suprasellar and parasellar tumors, *Sem Roentgenol* 25:174-197, 1990.

106. Hoffman HJ, de Silva M, Humphries RP et al: Aggressive surgical management of craniopharyngiomas in children, *J Neurosurg* 76:47-52, 1992.

106a. Demaerel P, Moseley IF, Scaravilli F: Recurrent craniopharyngioma invading the orbit, cavernous sinus, and skull base: a case report, *Neuroradiol* 35:261-263, 1993.

107. Ahmadi J, Destian S, Apuzzo MLJ et al: Cystic fluid in craniopharyngiomas: MR imaging and quantitative analysis, *Radiol* 182:783-785, 1992.

107a. Hershey BL: Suprasellar masses: diagnosis and differential diagnosis, *Sem US, CT, MR* 14:215-231, 1993.

108. West MS, Russell EJ, Breit R et al: Calvarial and skull base metastasis: comparison of nonenhanced and Gd-DTPA-enhanced MR images, *Radiol* 174:85-91, 1990.

109. Buff BL Jr, Schick RM, Norregaard T: Meningeal metastasis of leiomyosarcoma mimicking meningioma: CT and MR findings, *J Comp Asst Tomogr* 15:166-167, 1991.

110. Tyrrell RL, Bundschuh CV, Modic MT: Dural carcinomatosis: MR demonstration, *J Comp Asst Tomogr* 11:329-332, 1987.

111. Sze G, Soletsky S, Bronen R, Krol G: MR imaging of the cranial meninges with emphasis on contrast enhancement and meningeal carcinomatosis, *AJNR* 10:965-975, 1989.

112. Sze G: Diseases of the intracranial meninges: MR imaging features, *AJR* 160:727-733, 1993.

113. Rodesch G, Van Bogaert P, Mavroudakis N et al: Neuroradiologic findings in leptomeningeal carcinomatosis: the value interest of gadolinium-enhanced MRI, *Neuroradiol* 32:26-32, 1990.

114. Olsen WL, Winkler ML, Ross DA: Carcinomatous encephalitis: CT and MR findings, *AJNR* 8:553-554, 1987.

115. Nemzek W, Poirier V, Salamat MS, Yu T: Carcinomatous encephalitis (miliary metastases): lack of contrast enhancement, *AJNR* 14:540-542, 1993.

116. Egelhoff JC, Ross JS, Modic MT et al: MR imaging of metastatic GI adenocarcinoma in brain, *AJNR* 13:1221-1224, 1992.

117. Davis PC, Hudgins PA, Peterman SB, Hoffman JC Jr: Diagnosis of cerebral metastases: double-dose delayed CT vs contrast-enhanced MR imaging, *AJNR* 12:293-300, 1991.

118. Smalley SR, Laws ER Jr, O'Fallon JR et al: Resection for solitary brain metastasis, *J Neurosurg* 77:531-540, 1992.

118a. Bindal RK, Sawaya R, Leavens ME, Lu JJ: Surgical treatment of multiple brain metastases, *J Neurosurg* 79:210-216, 1993.

119. Elster AD, Chen MYM: Can nonenhancing white matter lesions in cancer patients be disregarded? *AJNR* 13:1309-1315, 1992.

120. Fukuda Y, Homma T, Kohga H et al: A lung cancer case with numerous calcified metastatic nodules of the brain, *Neuroradiol* 30:265-268, 1988.

120a. Hwang T-L, Valdivieso JG, Yang C-H, Wolin MJ: Calcified brain metastasis, *Neurosurg* 32:451-454, 1993.

121. Yamazaki T, Harigaya Y, Naguchi O et al: Calcified miliary brain metastases with mitochondrial inclusion nodules of the brain, *J Neurol Neurosurg Psychiatr* 56:110-111, 1993.

122. Shalen PR, Hayman LA, Wallace S et al: Protocol for delayed contrast enhancement in computed tomography of cerebral neoplasia, *Radiol* 139:397-401, 1981.

123. Atlas SW, Braffman BH, LoBuitto R et al: Human malignant melanomas with varying degrees of melanin in nude mice: MR imaging, histopathology, and electron paramagnetic resonance, *J Comp Asst Tomogr* 14:547-554, 1990.

124. Yuh WTC, Engelken JD, Muhonen MG et al: Experience with high-dose gadolinium MR imaging in the evaluation of brain metastases, *AJNR* 13:335-345, 1992.

125. Haustein J, Laniado M, Niendorf H-P et al: Triple-dose versus standard-dose gadopentetate dimeglumine: a randomized study in 199 patients, *Radiol* 186:855-860, 1993.

126. Hansen RA, Urich H: *Cancer and the Nervous System* pp 311-621, Oxford, Blackwell Scientific, 1982.

127. Elrington GM, Murray NMF, Spiro SG, Newsom-Davis J: Neurological paraneoplastic syndromes in patients with small cell lung cancer: a prospective survey of 150 patients, *J Neurol Neurosurg Psychiatr* 54:764-767, 1991.

128. Lacomis D, Koshbin S, Schick RM: MR imaging of paraneoplastic limbic encephalitis, *J Comp Asst Tomogr* 14:115-117, 1990.

129. Kodama T, Numagredri Y, Gella FE et al: Magnetic resonance imaging of limbic encephalitis, *Neuroradiol* 33:520-523, 1991.

PART FOUR

Infection, White Matter Abnormalities, and Degenerative Diseases

Infections of the Brain and Its Linings

CONGENITAL/NEONATAL INFECTIONS OF THE BRAIN

Congenital CNS infections are typically caused by the so-called *TORCH* agents: *TO*xoplasmosis, *Ru*bella, *C*ytomegalovirus, and *H*erpes simplex virus. Human immunodeficiency virus (HIV) and syphilis also are important causes of congenital CNS infections (*see* box, p. 674, *left*).

CNS infections are acquired in the following three ways[1,2]:

1. Through the maternal hematogenous-transplacental route (usual with toxoplasmosis and most viruses)
2. When the fetus travels through the birth canal (common with herpesviruses)
3. Via ascending infection from the cervix (common with bacteria)

Congenital infections often have devastating effects on the developing brain. Infectious sequelae reflect both the specific agent involved and the timing of the insult relative to fetal development. Intrauterine infections can result in developmental brain anomalies, encephaloclastic (destructive) lesions, or both.

Congenital CNS Infections

Agents

TORCH (TOxoplasmosis, Rubella, Cytomegalovirus, Herpes)

HIV

Routes

Hematogenous-transplacental (toxoplasmosis, most viruses)

Ascending cervical infection (bacteria)

At birth (herpesvirus)

Results (vary with timing of infection relative to fetal development)

Malformations (e.g., neuronal migrational abnormalities)

Brain destruction

Dystrophic calcifications

Cytomegalovirus

Ubiquitous DNA virus

Most common cause of congenital CNS infection

Predilection for germinal matrix

Periventricular calcifications

May cause abnormal neuronal migration

Cytomegalovirus

Etiology and pathology

Etiology. Human cytomegalovirus (CMV) is a ubiquitous DNA virus that belongs to the herpesvirus group. Humans are the only reservoir.[3] Congenital CMV results from transplacental virus transmission (*see* box, *above right*).

Gross pathology. Patchy spongiosis and encephalomalacia are common.[4] Hydranencephaly, porencephaly, and micrencephaly also occur.[1] CMV infection during the first or early second trimester can cause severe neuronal migration anomalies.

Microscopic appearance. Intranuclear and intracytoplasmic inclusions are present in glial cells and sometimes in neurons as well. Microglial nodules are common.[1]

Incidence.
In the United States, 50% to 85% of women of childbearing age are seropositive for CMV and 5% of pregnant women excrete CMV in the urine. Forty percent of the offspring from infected pregnant women become infected.[1]

CMV is the most frequent cause of congenital infections and is 2 to 3 times more frequent than toxoplasmosis, the next most common agent.[5] One percent of newborns excrete CMV in their urine; 10% of these have signs of CNS infection.[1]

Location.
Over 60% of infected fetuses have multiple organ systems involved.[6] Intracranial abnormalities are the most common manifestation, seen in nearly 70%. Cardiac anomalies and hepatosplenomegaly occur in one third of these cases.[6]

CMV has a particular affinity for the developing germinal matrix (Fig. 16-1, *A*). Widespread periventricular tissue necrosis with subsequent dystrophic calcification occurs. Other frequently affected sites are the cerebral white matter and cortex, cerebellum, brainstem, and spinal cord.

Clinical presentation. Infants infected with CMV are often born prematurely. Hepatosplenomegaly, jaundice, thrombocytopenia, and chorioretinitis are common manifestations during the newborn period.[5] Seizures, mental retardation, optic atrophy, sensorineural hearing loss, and hydrocephalus are later manifestations.[2]

CMV is diagnosed clinically by positive CMV cultures of body fluids, positive serum titers of CMV-specific immunoglobulin M, and demonstration of large intranuclear inclusions with small variable intracytoplasmic inclusions in CMV-infected visceral cells.[7]

Natural history. CMV may remain latent. Reactivation can occur, usually in patients who become immunocompromised.[2]

Imaging

Plain film radiography. The classic plain film finding of congenital CMV infection is microcephaly with eggshell-like periventricular calcifications.

Ultrasound. Bilateral periventricular calcifications, preceded by hypoechoic periventricular ringlike zones, may be specific for intrauterine CMV.[7] CMV may also result in widespread cerebral destruction with severe encephalomalacia.

CT. NECT scans show atrophy, ventricular enlargement, and parenchymal calcifications. CMV can cause widespread parenchymal calcifications in various locations but the periventricular region is the most common site (Fig. 16-1, *B*). Neuronal migration anomalies are also common (*see* Fig. 3-12).

MR. MR findings include migrational anomalies, encephalomalacia with nonspecific ventricular enlargement and prominent sulci, delayed myelination, and subependymal paraventricular cysts and calcification.[4,8]

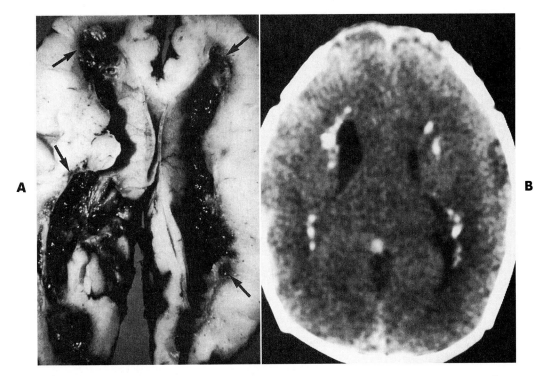

Fig. 16-1. A, Axial gross autopsy specimen in an infant born with severe cytomegalovirus (CMV) infection shows the striking periventricular lesions *(arrows)* caused by the predilection of this virus for the developing germinal matrix. **B,** Axial NECT scan in another case of a newborn infant demonstrates the typical periventricular calcifications seen with congenital CMV infection. (**A,** Courtesy archives of the Armed Forces Institute of Pathology.)

Toxoplasmosis

Etiology and pathology

Etiology. Toxoplasmosis is caused by *Toxoplasma gondii,* a ubiquitous protozoan that is an obligate intracellular parasite (*see* box). Oocysts in infected meat or cat feces are the usual sources of infection in humans. Hematogenous spread to the placenta and fetus occurs during maternal parasitemia. Over half of all infected fetuses develop CNS disease.[1]

Gross pathology. Toxoplasmosis infection is multifocal and scattered, without the prominent periventricular localization noted with CMV (Fig. 16-2, *A*). Toxoplasmosis causes necrosis but does not result in migrational anomalies.[1] Nonspecific findings include atrophy, microcephaly, and hydranencephaly.

Microscopic appearance. Toxoplasmosis induces a necrotizing granulomatous reaction with giant cells and eosinophilic infiltration with or without demonstrable intracellular organisms.[1]

Incidence. Toxoplasmosis is second only to CMV in causing congenital CNS infections. Toxoplasmosis affects between 1 in 1000 to 1 in 10,000 pregnancies in the United States.[5] Clinically significant abnormalities occur when the fetus is infected prior to 26 weeks gestional age.[3]

Toxoplasmosis
Intracellular parasite
Second most common cause of congenital CNS infection
Multifocal, scattered lesions (basal ganglia/periventricular, white matter, cortex)
Chorioretinitis
No migrational anomalies

Location. Basal ganglia, periventricular, and peripheral locations are all common (Fig. 16-2).[5]

Clinical presentation. The clinical presentation is diverse, ranging from mild cases that are initially undetected and present later as seizures to severely affected infants with microcephaly. Very early infections often result in spontaneous abortions.

Imaging. Hydrocephalus, bilateral chorioretinitis, and intracranial calcifications form the typical triad found in infants with congenital toxoplasmosis encephalitis.[3] Although the basal ganglia and cortex are common sites, calcifications can occur anywhere and

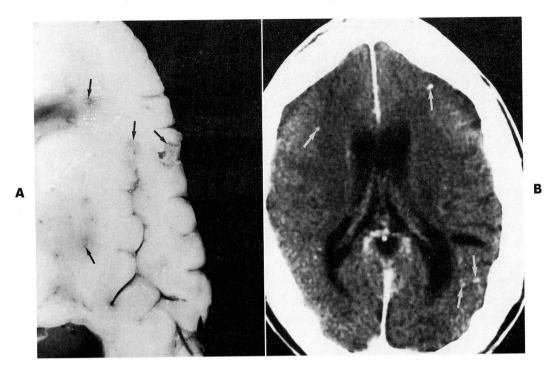

Fig. 16-2. A, Axial gross sutopsy specimen of congenital toxoplasmosis shows the scattered, nonfocal lesions characteristic of this infection. Note the subcortical, caudate and basal ganglia lesions (arrows) (courtesy Rubinstein Collection, University of Virginia). **B,** Axial CECT scan in a 27-year-old woman with severe mental retardation and seizures since birth. The brain is microcephalic and there are numerous scattered cortical and subcortical calcifications *(arrows)* consistent with residua of congenital toxoplasmosis.

are often more diffusely scattered than those associated with CMV encephalitis (Fig. 16-2, *B*). Hydrocephalus is due to ependymitis with periaqueductal necrosis that results in aqueductal stenosis.[1]

Rubella

Etiology and pathology
Etiology. Rubella is transmitted through the placenta to the fetus during maternal viremia. Rubella infection interferes with cellular multiplication, inhibiting proliferation of immature undifferentiated progenitor cells located in the germinal matrix.[1] The result is insufficient numbers of neurons and astroglia. Oligodendroglia may also be diminished, resulting in impaired myelination (*see* box).[9]

Gross pathology. The results of fetal infection are both teratogenic and destructive.[3] Rubella is characterized by meningoencephalitis, vasculopathy with ischemia and necrosis, micrencephaly, and delayed myelination.[1] Micrencephalia vera, a rare entity in which the brain is formed but is markedly diminished in size, has been reported.[9] It is probably related to inhibition of progenitor cell multiplication with insufficient generation of neurons and astroglia.[1]

Microscopic appearance. Inflammatory cells in the meninges and perivascular spaces are present. Lep-

Rubella
Rare
Too few neurons/glia result in small brain, impaired myelination
Prominent ocular abnormalities
Microcephalic brain with cortical, basal ganglia calcifications

tomeningeal and parenchymal vasculopathy is common. Small foci of perivascular necrosis are seen in the basal ganglia, periventricular region, and cerebral white matter.[1]

Incidence. Widespread rubella immunization has markedly diminished the incidence of this devastating neonatal infection. Nevertheless, congenital rubella syndrome remains a significant, albeit rare, cause of brain damage in newborn infants.[10]

Clinical presentation and natural history. Maternal rubella infection results in a spectrum of abnormalities ranging from mild manifestations to spontaneous abortion, stillbirths, and devastating abnormalities.[3] Gestational age at the time of infection is

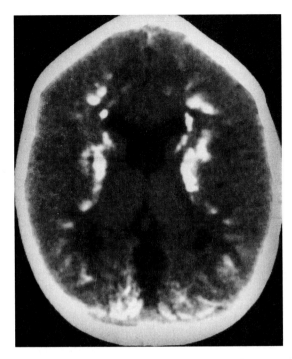

Fig. 16-3. Axial NECT scan in a deaf child with congenital rubella shows extensive calcifications in the basal ganglia, cerebral white matter, and cortex. (Courtesy H. Segall.)

Herpes Simplex
HSV-2 (genital herpes) causes 75% to 90% CNS manifestations 2 to 4 weeks after birth Brain diffusely affected (no temporal lobe localization) Cortex appears hyperdense, white matter hypodense; predilection of HSV for vascular endothelial cells may cause thrombosis/hemorrhagic infarction

the most important determinant of outcome.[2] Fetal infection before 8 to 12 weeks gestation causes more frequent infections with more severe consequences (see subsequent discussion), whereas infection during the last trimester is relatively mild with few or no significant lasting effects.[3]

Congenital rubella syndrome is usually caused by first trimester infections. A spectrum of abnormalities is seen. Cataracts, glaucoma, chorioretinitis, microphthalmia, cardiac malformations, and micrencephaly occur with early, severe infections; deafness is the most common late manifestation of congenital rubella.[2] Meningoencephalitis, thrombocytopenia, hepatosplenomegaly, and lymphadenopathy are transient abnormalities in neonates.[1]

Imaging. In general, imaging findings are similar to other congenital viral infections and are therefore nonspecific.

Ultrasound. Subependymal cysts in the caudate nucleus and striothalamic regions are seen but are not specific for rubella. Echogenic foci in the basal ganglia may represent mineralizing vasculitis with calcification.[10]

CT. Microcephaly and parenchymal calcifications are typically present. The cortex and basal ganglia are often affected (Fig. 16-3).[5]

MR. Deep and subcortical white matter lesions, possibly caused by vascular injury and ischemic ne-

crosis, have been reported.[10] Delayed myelination may occur, perhaps because there are insufficient numbers of oligodendroglia.

Herpes Simplex

Etiology and pathology

Etiology. Herpes simplex virus (HSV) is a DNA virus. There are two HSV serotypes: type 1 and type 2. Although either type can cause perinatal CNS infections, HSV type 2 (genital herpes) accounts for 75% to 90% of all neonatal herpesvirus infections (*see box, above*).[1,2]

Infection is rare during fetal development, possibly because the severe encephaloclastic effects of herpesvirus infection cause spontaneous abortions. Most neonatal infections are parturitional, acquired through direct contact between the infant's skin, eyes or oral cavity, and maternal herpetic lesions in the cervix or vagina.[1] Ascending infection can also occur after membranes rupture during delivery.

Postnatal infection is uncommon but can be transmitted from mothers with oral herpetic lesions, from other adults (such as hospital personnel), or from other infants. Defective macrophage function or impaired production of antiherpes antibody may contribute to the devastating effects of postnatal infections with HSV.[1]

Gross pathology. The neuropathology in HSV infection varies with timing and virus dose. Early gestational infection is rare and produces a spectrum of changes that ranges from minor focal calcifications to severe encephaloclastic lesions.[1] Microcephaly, hydrocephalus, microphthalmia, and chorioretinitis are seen.[11]

Microscopic appearance. All cellular CNS components may be infected. The particular predilection of HSV for endothelial cells results in vascular thrombosis and hemorrhagic infarction. Microglial nodules with intranuclear inclusions are present.[1] Secondary changes of infarction and multicystic encephalomalacia can be seen in surviving infants.

Incidence and age. Reported prevalence of neonatal HSV infection is between 1 in 200 and 1 in 5000

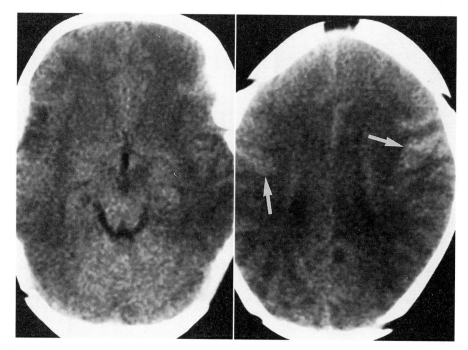

Fig. 16-4. A 20-day-old infant was born through herpes-infected vaginal canal. Initially healthy at birth, he then developed seizures. Axial NECT scans show diffuse, low density changes throughout the cerebral white matter. Note relatively dense-appearing cortex *(arrows)*. Presumed congenital herpes encephalitis. (Courtesy T. Miller.)

deliveries.[2] Neonates with disseminated HSV usually present between 9 and 11 days of age, whereas infants with isolated CNS herpesvirus infections become symptomatic approximatly 2 to 4 weeks after birth.[2,3]

Location. Acute neonatal HSV infections cause diffuse brain involvement. The limbic system localization (temporal lobes, cingulate gyrus) that is so characteristic in older children and adult infections does not occur.

Clinical presentation and natural history. Neonatal herpetic infections are divided into the following three clinical categories:
1. Skin, eye, and mouth lesions
2. Disseminated disease
3. CNS infections

Cutaneous infections are both the mildest and the most common manifestation, seen in 40% of cases. Untreated infection progresses to disseminated or CNS disease in 75% of infected infants.[2]

Disseminated disease causes signs and symptoms that suggest severe bacterial sepsis. CNS manifestations are present in approximately half of disseminated HSV cases. The overall mortality rate approaches 80% in untreated and 50% in treated infants.[2]

The CNS is affected in approximately 30% of infected infants. Clinical onset of isolated CNS herpes-virus infection occurs 2 to 4 weeks after birth. Fever, lethargy, and seizures are the most common manifestations; 20% of infected infants have no cutaneous lesions.[3]

Imaging

CT. Acute neonatal HSV encephalitis is seen on NECT scans as focal or diffuse white matter lucency (Fig. 16-4).[3] The relative hyperdensity of cortical gray matter appears accentuated. Hemorrhagic infarction may occur. Diffuse atrophy and multicystic encephalomalacia are long-term sequelae (Fig. 16-5).

MR. Because the neonatal brain is largely unmyelinated, diffuse white matter edema is difficult to detect. Hemorrhagic changes are occasionally identified. Parenchymal or meningeal enhancement following contrast administration is seen in some subacute cases.[3]

HIV Infection

Etiology and pathology

Etiology. Perinatal transmission is the most common route of human immunodeficiency virus (HIV) infection in children.[12] Nearly 80% of all childhood HIV infections are maternally transmitted, although only one third of HIV positive mothers pass on the infection.[5]

The HIV virus infects T_4 helper cells, allowing secondary infections such as *Pneumocystis carinii* and tumors (lymphoma, Kaposi's sarcoma) to develop. In

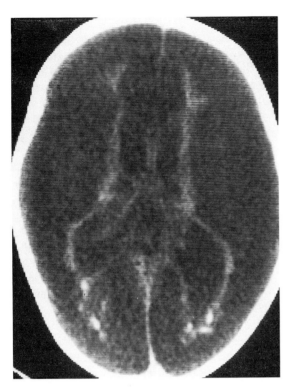

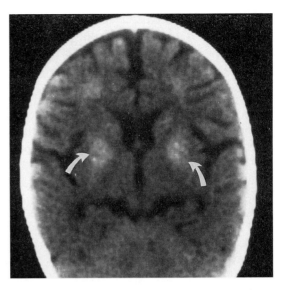

Fig. 16-6. Axial NECT scan in a 15-month-old infant with congenital HIV infection. Note generalized cerebral atrophy and bilateral basal ganglia calcifications *(curved arrows)*. (From C. Fitz, reprinted from *AJNR* 13:551-567, 1992.)

Fig. 16-5. Axial NECT scan shows residua of neonatal herpes encephalitis. Both hemispheres are severely encephalomalacic. Only a small amount of residual cerebral tissue is seen around the cerebral ventricles. (Courtesy H. Segall.)

Congenital HIV Infection
Maternally transmitted
CNS symptoms
Due to HIV encephalitis
Opportunistic infection, neoplasm rare
Most infected neonates die in first year
Atrophy, basal ganglia calcifications

children, opportunistic infections and tumors are less common manifestations of HIV infection. CNS signs and symptoms reflect the primary retroviral encephalitis (*see* box).[1]

Gross pathology. Atrophy with diminished brain weight is characteristic.

Microscopic appearance. Glial and microglial nodules are present in the basal ganglia, pons, and cerebral white matter. Multinucleated giant cells are seen. Perivascular calcifications are common, particularly in the putamen and globus pallidus. Demyelination and astrogliosis with relative cortical sparing is typical.[1]

Incidence. In the United States, approximately 2% of all patients with acquired immune deficiency syndrome (AIDS) are children. The reported worldwide incidence is between 5% and 25% of AIDS cases.[12] Transfusion-acquired HIV is waning.[12] Over 70% of seropositive cases in children are now linked to drug abuse in the child's mother or the mother's sexual partner.

Clinical presentation and natural history. Presenting signs of AIDS in children differ from those usually identified in adults. Weight loss, failure to thrive, chronic diarrhea, and chronic fever are seen. Minor signs include lymphadenopathy, oral thrush, repeated infections, and dermatitis.[12] Definitive diagnosis may require virologic tests because serologic tests are less reliable in newborn infants.

Thirty to fifty percent of HIV-infected infants and children develop a progressive encephalopathy that is characterized by loss of developmental milestones and bilateral pyramidal tract signs with progressive spastic quadriparesis.[13] Cognitive and psychomotor abnormalities are common manifestations in children; seizures are rare.[1] Infected infants may have cortical atrophy and microcephaly.

Most children with AIDS die in the first year of life. In the United States, AIDS is now the ninth highest-ranking cause of death in children between the ages of 1 and 4 years. More than 80% of children with AIDS diagnosed before 1 year of age have died.[12]

Imaging

CT. NECT scans show diffuse cerebral atrophy in nearly 90% of cases.[14] Basal ganglia calcifications are seen in one third of all cases (Fig. 16-6) but are virtually never identified before 1 year of age.[14] Hemorrhage can occur in children with thrombocytopenia. In contrast to adults, opportunistic infections and tumors are relatively rare, occurring in only 15% of cases.[13,15]

MR. Nonspecific cerebral atrophy is the most common finding. Foci of increased signal on T2WI are seen in the peripheral and deep white cerebral matter. Nonhemorrhagic cerebral infarcts have also been noted.[14]

Varicella

Varicella-zoster (VZ) infection during the first, second, or early third trimester causes a severe necrotizing encephalomyelitis. The anterior horn cells and the dorsal root ganglia are particularly affected.[1] Nonspecific changes include chorioretinitis, cataracts, microphthalmia, and optic atrophy.

VZ infection develops in approximately 25% of infants born to mothers with varicella during the last month of pregnancy.[1] Skin lesions of chicken pox and shingles are common clinical manifestations of these late in utero infections, whereas maternal herpes zoster has not been implicated as a cause of fetal infection or brain damage.[1]

Enteroviruses

Enteroviruses include *coxsackie A, coxsackie B, echovirus,* and *poliovirus.* These viruses, particularly the coxsackie B viruses, may produce acute neonatal infection with myocarditis and encephalitis.

Congenital intrauterine enterovirus infections have not been associated with CNS disease or malformations. Infection is typically seasonal and postnatal, and usually spread from infected parents to infants. A diffuse meningoencephalitis occurs with a high frequency of lesions in the inferior olivary nuclei and ventral horns of the spinal cord.[1]

Poliovirus is a picornavirus that affects adults and immunocompromised children. It has a single strand of RNA, replicates in the host cell cytoplasm, and is released by cell lysis. Most polio cases do not involve the CNS; only 0.1% to 1% progress to paralysis. Paralytic poliomyelitis is now uncommon in the United States with an average of 10 cases per year reported from 1980 to 1984, mostly vaccine-related.[16] Poliovirus involves the CNS by direct infection during viremia or by retrograde neural spread.

Paralytic poliomyelitis may present with spinal cord symptoms, bulbar (brainstem) symptoms, or both. Between 10% to 15% of paralytic polio cases are bulbar. The brainstem reticular formation and cranial nerves VII, IX, and X are most commonly involved.[16] MR imaging discloses high signal in the midbrain and medulla on T2WI; the findings are indistinguishable from other causes of brainstem encephalitis.[16]

MENINGITIS

Meningitis is the most common form of CNS infection.[17] Infectious meningitis is divided into the following three general categories[18,19]:

1. Acute pyogenic meningitis (mostly bacterial infections)
2. Lymphocytic meningitis (usually viral)
3. Chronic meningitis (classic examples are tuberculosis and coccidiodomycosis)

Acute Pyogenic Meningitis

Etiology and pathology

Etiology. Acute pyogenic meningitis is usually caused by bacteria. The specific agents involved vary among different age groups (*see* box). The most common cause of neonatal meningitis is group B streptococcus, followed by *Escherichia coli* and *Listeria monocytogenes.*[1,5] Factors involved in the pathogenesis of neonatal meningitis relate to delivery (e.g., maternal genitourinary tract infection or prolonged rupture of membranes), immaturity (deficiencies of cellular and humoral immunity), and environment (aerosols, catheters, inhalation therapy equipment).[1]

In children under 7 years of age, *Hemophilus influenzae* meningitis is common.[18] The older the child, the more adultlike is the infection.[5] *Neisseria meningitidis* is found in children and young adults, whereas *Streptococcus pneumoniae* is the most common infective agent in adults.

Meningitis

Agents

Neonates: group B streptococcus, *E. coli*
Children under 7: *H. influenzae*
Older children: *N. meningitidis*
Adults: *S. pneumoniae*

Pathology

Purulent exudate in basilar cisterns, sulci; perivascular inflammation, vasospasm common

Imaging

Early: may be normal/mild hydrocephalus
Effaced cisterns
Enhancing meninges, subarachnoid exudate

Complications

Hydrocephalus
Ventriculitis/ependymitis
Subdural effusion
Empyema
Cerebritis/abscess
Vasospasm/arterial infarcts
Dural sinus/cortical vein thrombosis, venous infarcts

Acute pyogenic meningitis begins in several ways. Hematogenous spread and local extension from contiguous extracerebral infection (e.g., otitis media, mastoiditis, or sinusitis) are the most common causes. Hematogenous infection probably occurs through the choroid plexus and CSF pathways.[18] Direct implantation of bacteria into the meninges is less frequent and is usually seen with penetrating head injury or comminuted skull fracture.

Gross pathology. The most striking feature of bacterial meningitis is a thick, creamy purulent exudate that is either confined to the basal cisterns or completely fills the subarachnoid space (Fig. 16-7, *A*). Complications of meningitis include perivascular inflammation and vasospasm with secondary venous or arterial infarction, subdural effusion or empyema, cerebritis, abscess, and ventriculitis (see subsequent discussion). Subarachnoid space compromise may cause extraventricular obstructive (communicating) hydrocephalus, whereas ventriculitis with cerebral aqueductal ependymitis causes intraventricular obstructive hydrocephalus.

Microscopic appearance. Bacterial and mycobacterial leptomeningeal inflammations are characterized by polymorphonuclear cell infiltration and extensive fibrinous exudation.[20] Vascular endothelial injury with altered blood-brain barrier permeability and vasogenic edema is common.[19] Inflammation often extends along the perivascular (Virchow-Robin) spaces into the underlying brain parenchyma.[20]

Age and incidence. Nonepidemic meningitis is most common in neonates, infants, and children. Neonatal sepsis occurs in 1.5 cases per 1000 births; meningitis is seen in 20% of these cases.[5] Epidemic meningitis can occur at any age.

New antibiotics have markedly diminished the incidence of bacterial meningitis and the once-high mortality rates associated with potentially devastating disease.[19]

Imaging. The diagnosis of meningitis is established by history, physical examination, and laboratory evaluation. Neuroimaging studies are typically

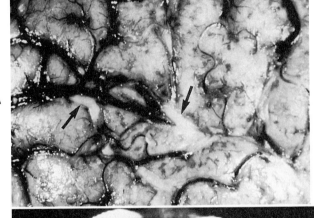

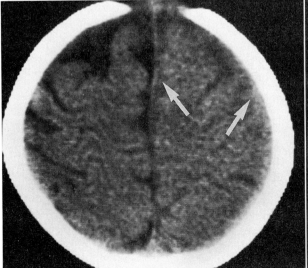

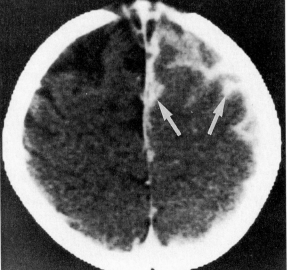

Fig. 16-7. A, Close-up view of gross pathology specimen in a patient who died with meningococcal meningitis. The typical thick, creamy fibrinopurulent exudate is seen filling the cerebral sulci *(arrows).* **B** and **C,** A 7-month-old infant had *H. influenzae* meningitis. **B,** Axial NECT scan shows subtle effacement of the subarachnoid cisterns over the left hemisphere *(arrows).* Compare with the normal CSF-filled cisterns on the right side. **C,** CECT study shows striking enhancement of the leptomeninges and subarachnoid inflammatory exudate *(arrows).*

used to monitor the complications of meningeal infection.[18]

CT. A normal scan is the most common finding in children with acute bacterial meningitis.[19] Mild ventricular dilatation and subarachnoid space enlargement are early abnormalities on NECT scans. Effacement of the basilar or convexity cisterns by inflammatory exudate can be seen in some cases (Fig. 16-7, *B*). Less than half of all children with clinically documented meningitis have abnormally enhancing meninges on CECT studies (Fig. 16-7, *C*).[5]

MR. MR imaging is superior to CT in the evaluation of patients with suspected meningitis.[21] Precontrast T1WI may show obliterated cisterns that enhance strongly following contrast administration. Extension of enhancing subarachnoid exudate deep into the sulci can be seen in severe cases (Fig. 16-8, *B* and *C*).

Complications of meningitis. CNS complications develop in 50% of adult patients with bacterial meningitis.[21a] These include hydrocephalus and ventriculitis, subdural effusion, subdural empyema, and parenchymal lesions such as cerebritis, abscess, edema with or without cerebral herniation, and cerebral infarction.[21a]

Hydrocephalus and ventriculitis. Extensive fibrinopurulent exudates can obstruct the subarachnoid space and result in extraventricular (communicating) hydrocephalus (Fig. 16-8, *A*). Aqueductal or outlet obstruction causes intraventricular (noncommunicating) hydrocephalus. Ventriculitis occurs in 30% of all patients and over 90% of neonates with meningitis.[17] The ependymal lining of the ventricles enhances intensely (*see* box). Choroid plexitis is sometimes present (Fig. 16-9).

Ependymal Enhancement
Differential diagnosis

Common

Ventriculitis/ependymitis (abscess rupture, meningitis, shunts, chemotherapy)
Primary brain tumor
    Anaplastic astrocytoma/GBM
    Lymphoma
    Pineal tumor (germinoma, pineoblastoma)
    PNET/medulloblastoma
    Ependymoma

Uncommon

Collateral venous drainage pathway (Sturge-Weber, dural sinus occlusion, vascular malformation)
Primary brain tumor (choroid plexus tumor)
Metastatic tumor (extracranial primary)

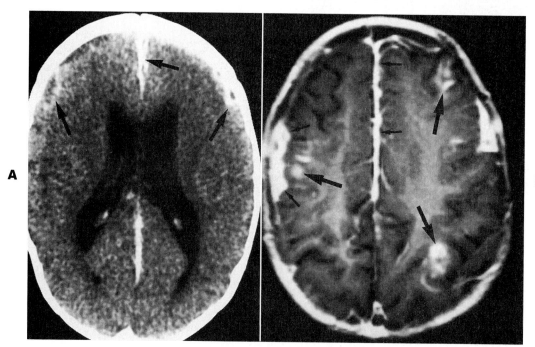

Fig. 16-8. A, Axial CECT scan in a child with *H. influenzae* meningitis shows mild nonspecific enlargement of the lateral ventricles. Subtle meningeal enhancement is present over the frontal lobes and within the anterior interhemispheric fissure *(arrows).* Axial **(B)** and coronal **(C)** contrast-enhanced T1-weighted MR scans show thickened, enhancing leptomeninges *(small arrows).* Note extension of inflammatory infiltrates deep into the sulci along the Virchow-Robin spaces with ill-defined contrast-enhancing areas that represent early cerebritis *(large arrows).*

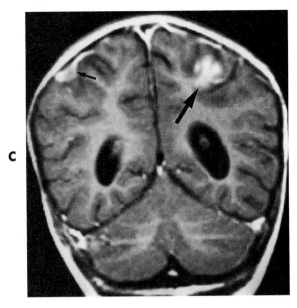

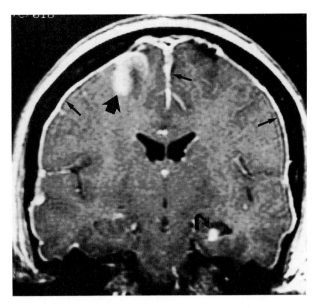

Fig. 16-8, cont'd. For legend see P. 682.

Fig. 16-9. Coronal postcontrast T1-weighted MR scan demonstrates meningitis *(small arrows)*, cerebritis *(large arrow)*, and choroid plexitis *(curved arrow)*.

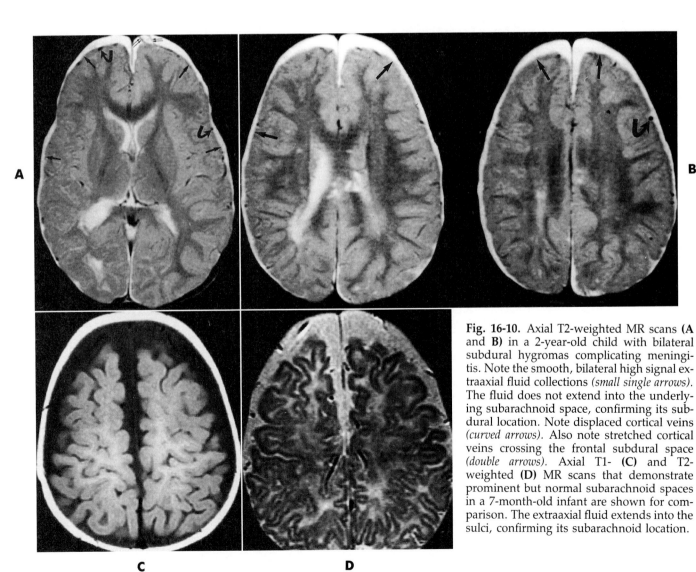

Fig. 16-10. Axial T2-weighted MR scans **(A** and **B)** in a 2-year-old child with bilateral subdural hygromas complicating meningitis. Note the smooth, bilateral high signal extraaxial fluid collections *(small single arrows)*. The fluid does not extend into the underlying subarachnoid space, confirming its subdural location. Note displaced cortical veins *(curved arrows)*. Also note stretched cortical veins crossing the frontal subdural space *(double arrows)*. Axial T1- **(C)** and T2-weighted **(D)** MR scans that demonstrate prominent but normal subarachnoid spaces in a 7-month-old infant are shown for comparison. The extraaxial fluid extends into the sulci, confirming its subarachnoid location.

Subdural effusion. Subdural effusion (SDE) is a common feature of some bacterial meningitides (Fig. 16-10, *A* and *B*). Twenty to fifty percent of meningitis cases in children less than 1 year old are complicated by sterile subdural effusions; 2% of these are infected secondarily and become subdural empyemas.[22] SDEs are probably caused by inflammation of subdural veins with fluid and albumin seepage into the subdural space.[18] SDEs should be distinguished from the prominent but normal subarachnoid spaces often seen in infants under 1 year of age (Fig. 16-10, *C* and *D*).[22a]

Imaging findings of SDE are crescentic extraaxial fluid collections that are similar to CSF on both CT and MR. Most SDEs resolve spontaneously and do not require treatment.[18] Cortical vein thrombosis and cerebritis are rare.[22]

Empyema. Sub- and epidural empyemas account for approximately 20% to 33% of all intracranial infections.[23] Nearly half of all cases are caused by sinusitis; the frontal sinus is the most common source.[22] Postcraniotomy infection accounts for another 30%. Between 10% to 15% of empyemas are complications of meningitis. Empyema carries an 8% to 12% mortality rate.[22]

Imaging studies in cerebral empyemas show crescentic or lentiform extraaxial fluid collections that are low density on CT (Fig. 16-11, *A*) and mildly hyperintense compared to CSF on T2-weighted MR studies. The cerebral convexities and interhemispheric fissure are common sites. A surrounding membrane that enhances intensely and uniformly following contrast administration is typically identified (Fig. 16-11, *B*, and 16-12).[24] Cortical vein thrombosis with venous

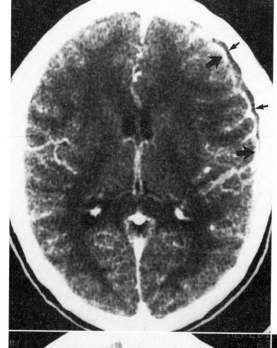

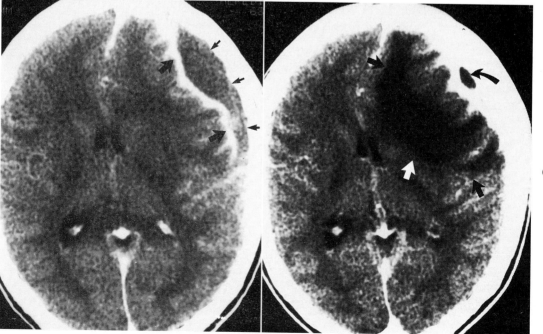

Fig. 16-11. A 29-year-old man with a history of otitis media presented with meningismus. **A,** Axial CECT scan shows a small left frontal subdural empyema (SDE) *(small arrows)* with meningitis, seen as an enhancing membrane *(large arrows)* underlying the small SDE. **B,** Follow-up CECT scan 9 days later shows the SDE *(small arrows)* has enlarged and the enhancing meninges *(large arrows)* appear thicker. Note increased mass effect with subfalcine herniation of the lateral ventricles. **C,** The SDE was drained but the patient deteriorated. This follow-up scan shows a small residual SDE *(curved arrow)*. Extensive left frontal lobe edema is seen *(large arrows)*, caused by venous infarction. The SDE caused cortical vein thrombosis.

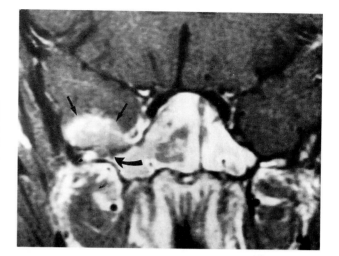

Fig. 16-12. Coronal postcontrast T1-weighted MR scan in this patient with sphenoid sinusitis shows osteomyelitis of the middle cranial fossa floor *(curved arrow)*. An intensely enhancing lentiform-shaped extraaxial mass is present *(straight arrows)*. Epidural empyema was found at surgery.

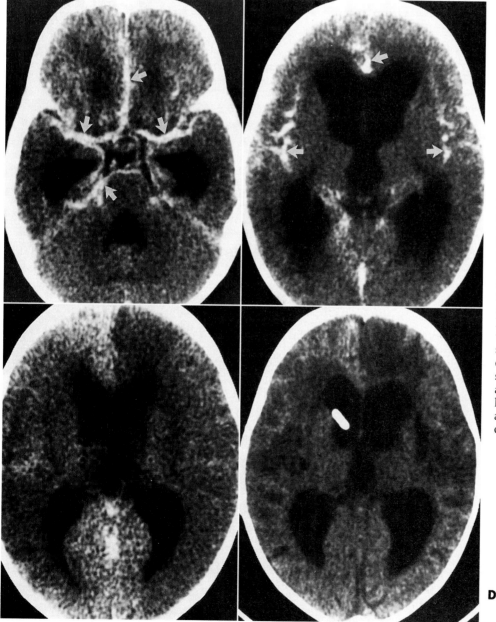

Fig. 16-13. A and **B,** Initial axial CECT scans in a child with acute tuberculous meningitis show extensive basilar and sylvian leptomeningeal enhancement *(arrows)*. Note severe extraventricular (communicating) hydrocephalus, seen as enlargement of the lateral, third, and fourth ventricles. **C,** Follow-up NECT scan 1 week later shows bilateral cerebral infarcts. **D,** NECT study 2 weeks after **(C)** shows a shunt in the right frontal horn. Note extensive encephalomalacic changes throughout both hemispheres.

infarction (Fig. 16-11, *C*) and cerebritis or abscess formation may ensue.

Cerebritis and abscess. Approximately 10% of patients with meningitis show parenchymal abnormalities on imaging studies (see Fig. 16-8). Cerebritis is seen in approximately 25% of these cases.[18] Cerebritis can evolve to frank abscess formation (see subsequent discussion).

Cerebrovascular complications. CNS infection is one of the most common causes of acquired cerebrovascular disease in children. Cerebral infarction develops in up to 27% of children with tubercular or complicated bacterial meningitis.[25] Cerebrovascular lesions are also the most frequent intracranial complication of bacterial meningitis in adults, accounting for 37% of all cases. Vessel wall irregularities, focal dilatations, arterial occlusion (Fig. 16-13), venous infarcts (Fig. 16-14), and dural sinus thrombosis occur.[26] The etiology is probably vasculitis, coagulopathy, vasospasm, or a combination of these factors.[25]

Acute Lymphocytic Meningitis

Acute lymphocytic meningitis is usually viral in origin. Most viral meningitides are benign and self-limited. Enteroviruses *(echoviruses, coxsackieviruses)* are thought to be responsible for 50% to 80% of viral meningitides. Other agents include *mumps virus, Epstein-Barr virus,* and *arbovirus.*[2] Signs and symptoms such as headache, fever, and meningismus are similar to those of bacterial meningitis but are often less severe.[18] Imaging findings are usually normal unless coexisting encephalitis occurs.

Chronic Meningitis

Etiology and pathology

Etiology. Chronic meningitis is a smoldering, indolent process that is typified by *Mycobacterium tuberculosis* (TB) infection. Hematogenous spread from pulmonary tuberculosis to the meninges is the putative mechanism in the development of TB meningitis.[27] Other organisms that are less commonly implicated in chronic meningitis include *Coccidiodomycosis imitans* and *Cryptococcus neoformans.*[28]

Gross pathology. Chronic meningitis is characterized by a thick, gray gelatinous exudate that predominately involves the basilar cisterns.[20]

Microscopic appearance. The exudate consists of polymorphonuclear cells, fibrin, and hemorrhage. In TB meningitis, pronounced caseous necrosis, chronic granulomas, endarteritis and perivascular parenchymal inflammatory changes occur.[20]

Age and incidence. After a decades-long decline, the incidence of TB is rising in the United States, particularly among immigrants, the homeless, IV drug abusers, HIV-infected persons, and residents of pris-

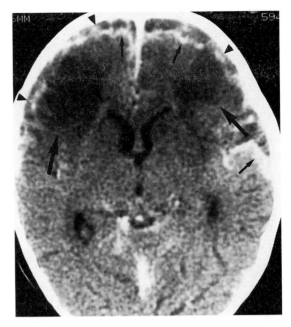

Fig. 16-14. Axial CECT scan in a 6-month-old child with *H. influenzae* meningitis *(small arrows)* demonstrates complications of bifrontal SDEs *(arrowheads)* and bilateral venous infarcts *(large arrows).*

ons and nursing homes.[29] TB remains a significant worldwide public health problem (see subsequent discussion).

Isolated TB meningitis is rare, representing less than 5% of childhood bacterial meningitis cases[27] and 17.5% of all intracranial TB cases.[30] Most children with tuberculous meningitis also have concomitant miliary brain infection,[27] and 11% of all patients have combined parenchymal/meningeal lesions.[30] Diffuse active and chronic meningitis both occur.

Location. TB and other chronic meningitides have a predilection for the basilar cisterns, although more generalized disease also occurs.[20]

Natural history. The overall mortality rate in TB meningitis is 25% to 30% with long-term morbidity ranging from 66% to 88% of survivors.[30] Sequelae of chronic meningitis, particularly tuberculosis, include pachymeningitis,[31] ischemia and infarction,[32] atrophy,[30] and calcifications. Three quarters of infarctions occur in the regions supplied by medial lenticulostriate and thalamoperforating arteries; one quarter involve the cerebral cortex. Bilateral infarctions occur in 70% of cases.[32]

Imaging

CT. NECT scans in chronic meningitis may disclose "en plaque" dural thickening. "Popcorn"-like dural calcifications can be seen in some cases, particularly around the basilar cisterns (Fig. 16-15, *A*).[33]

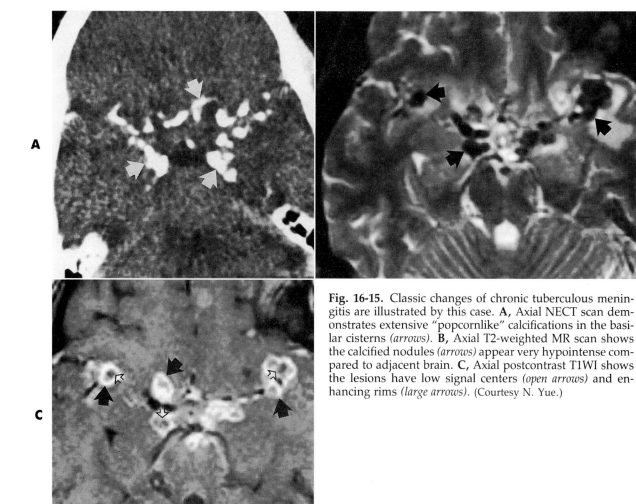

Fig. 16-15. Classic changes of chronic tuberculous meningitis are illustrated by this case. **A,** Axial NECT scan demonstrates extensive "popcornlike" calcifications in the basilar cisterns *(arrows)*. **B,** Axial T2-weighted MR scan shows the calcified nodules *(arrows)* appear very hypointense compared to adjacent brain. **C,** Axial postcontrast T1WI shows the lesions have low signal centers *(open arrows)* and enhancing rims *(large arrows)*. (Courtesy N. Yue.)

CECT may disclose abnormal meningeal enhancement years after the initial infection has been treated.[30] Sequelae of chronic meningitis, including atrophy and cerebral infarction, may be striking.

MR. Unenhanced MR images often do not detect active meningeal inflammation, whereas meningitis is conspicuous on postcontrast T1WI.[33,34] Contrast-enhanced T1-weighted MR scans in chronic meningitis show the characteristic basal meningeal inflammatory pattern seen on CECT studies (Fig. 16-16).[35]

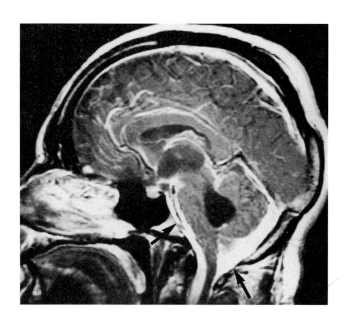

Fig. 16-16. MR findings of chronic meningitis are illustrated by this sagittal postcontrast T1-weighted scan in a patient with coccidiodomycosis granulomatous meningitis. Note the extensively thickened, intensely enhancing basilar meninges *(arrows)*.

Calcific meningeal nodules are markedly hypointense on all pulse sequences (Fig. 16-15, *B* and *C*). Peripheral enhancement often persists (Fig. 16-15, *C*).[34]

PYOGENIC PARENCHYMAL INFECTIONS
Cerebritis and Abscess

Cerebritis is the earliest stage of purulent brain infection.[17] Abscesses evolve from focal cerebritis in predictable stages (*see* box). The neuroimaging features of cerebral abscesses reflect the underlying pathophysiology of abscess formation.[36]

Etiology and pathology

Etiology. Infectious agents gain access to the CNS in several ways. The most common cause is hematogenous spread from an extracranial site. Mastoid and sinus infections spread directly to the CNS through retrograde thrombophlebitis and may be preceded by empyema, meningitis, or both (Fig. 16-17).[36] Congenital or acquired dural dehiscence and dermal sinuses are less common causes.

The specific organisms involved in cerebritis and abscess are quite variable; in one third of cases, more than one organism is found. Most abscesses are produced by pyogenic bacteria. Overall, the organisms most frequently isolated from cerebral abscesses are streptococci (both aerobic and anaerobic) and staphylococci, although gram-negative organisms are an increasing cause of cerebral abscess.[20] In neonates the most frequently implicated organisms are *Citrobacter, Proteus, Pseudomonas, Serratia,* and *Staphylococcus aureus.*[1] These abscesses are often large and have poorly formed capsules.[17]

Occasionally, organisms other than pyogenic bacteria cause cerebral abscesses. Examples include *Mycobacterium tuberculosis,* fungi such as *Actinomyces,* and parasites.

Pathology. The following four stages in abscess evolution have been described[37,38]:

1. Early cerebritis
2. Late cerebritis
3. Early capsule formation
4. Late capsule formation

Early cerebritis is the initial phase of abscess formation. During this stage, infection is focal but not yet localized.[1] An unencapsulated mass of congested vessels with perivascular polymorphonuclear cell in-

filtrates and edema is seen. Scattered necrotic foci and microscopic petechial hemorrhages without frank tissue destruction are present (Fig. 16-18, *A*).[20] The early cerebritis stage typically lasts from 3 to 5 days.

The *late cerebritis* stage then ensues. The infection becomes more focal as small necrotic zones coalesce. Vessels proliferate and a central necrotic core is formed that is surrounded by an ill-defined ring of inflammatory cells, macrophages, granulation tissue, and fibroblasts (Fig. 16-18, *B*). The late cerebritis stage lasts from 4 to 5 days to 10 to 14 days.

The *early capsule* stage begins around the end of the second week following the initial infection. Collagen and reticulin form a well-delineated capsule around a core consisting of liquefied necrotic and inflammatory debris. The abscess capsule is initially thin and incomplete but becomes thicker as more collagen is produced (Fig. 16-18, *C*). As the abscess matures, mass effect and surrounding edema begin to subside. Gliosis develops around the abscess periphery.

During the *late capsule* stage, the capsule is complete and consists of the following three layers[36]:

1. An inner inflammatory layer of granulation tissue and macrophages
2. A middle collagenous layer
3. An outer gliotic layer (Fig. 16-18, *D*)

The cavity gradually shrinks as the abscess heals. The late capsule stage lasts from several weeks to months.

Intracranial Abscess Development

Early cerebritis (3 to 5 days)
Late cerebritis (4 to 5 days to 10 to 14 days)
Early capsule (begins at about 2 weeks)
Late capsule (may last for weeks/months)

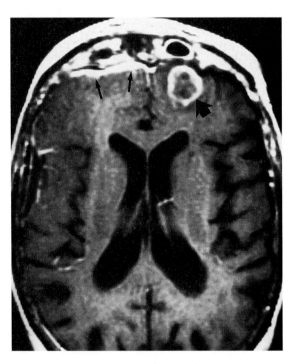

Fig. 16-17. Axial postcontrast T1-weighted MR scan in this patient with frontal sinusitis show complications of meningitis *(small arrows)* and abscess *(large arrow).*

Age and incidence. In developed countries, bacterial abscesses in children are rare, even in patients with congenital heart disease and immune problems.[5] Most abscesses in neonates and infants occur as a complication of bacterial meningitis.[1]

Location. The corticomedullary (gray-white matter) junction is the most common location, and the frontal and parietal lobes are the most frequent sites. Less than 15% of intracranial abscesses occur in the posterior fossa. Multiple abscesses are uncommon except in immunocompromised patients.[36]

Natural history. Improved diagnostic imaging techniques and new antibiotic treatments have dramatically improved the prognosis of cerebral abscess. Mortality has decreased from 40% to 50% to under 5%.[36]

Imaging

Nuclear medicine. Although CT or MR are the most common imaging modalities used to evaluate patients with possible abscess, it is occasionally difficult to distinguish between brain abscess and neoplasm or between postoperative changes and infec-

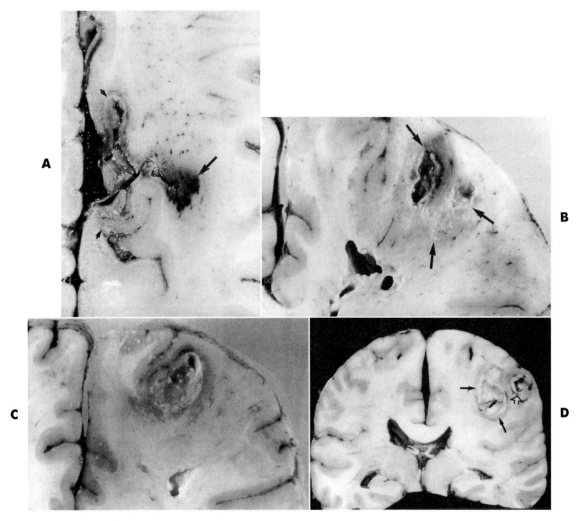

Fig. 16-18. Stages in abscess development are illustrated by these gross autopsy specimens. **A,** Meningitis *(small arrows)* is complicated by early cerebritis *(large arrow).* Vascular congestion with an unencapsulated mass that consists of edema, inflammatory infiltrate, and petechial hemorrhage is present. **B,** Late cerebritis stage is illustrated by this case. Several necrotic zones have coalesced and formed a central liquefied core. An ill-defined rim of inflammatory cells and granulation tissue is present *(arrows).* **C,** Late cerebritis/early capsule stage of abscess formation is shown. **D,** Late capsule stage has a well-delineated collagenous wall *(small arrows)* that surrounds the necrotic core. Note "daughter" or satellite lesion. *(open arrow)* (**D,** Courtesy Royal College of Surgeons of England, *Slide Atlas of Pathology,* Gower Medical Publishing.)

tion. [99m]Tc HMPAO, a new radionuclide imaging label for leukocytes, and radiolabeled polyclonal immunoglobulin (IgG) antibodies may be helpful in selected cases.[39,40]

CT. The neuroimaging features of brain abscesses vary with lesion stage. During the early cerebritis stage, NECT scans may be normal or show only a poorly marginated subcortical hypodense area.[36] In some cases CECT studies disclose an ill-defined contrast-enhancing area within the edematous region (Fig. 16-19, *A*).

As the lesion coalesces during the late cerebritis stage, a somewhat irregular enhancing rim that surrounds a central low density area is typical. Delayed scans may show contrast "fills in" the central low density region.[37,38] Peripheral edema is usually marked, and mass effect with sulcal obliteration is apparent.

The early capsule stage is characterized by formation of a distinct collagenous capsule (see previous discussion). A relatively thin, well-delineated capsule that enhances strongly, uniformly, and continuously

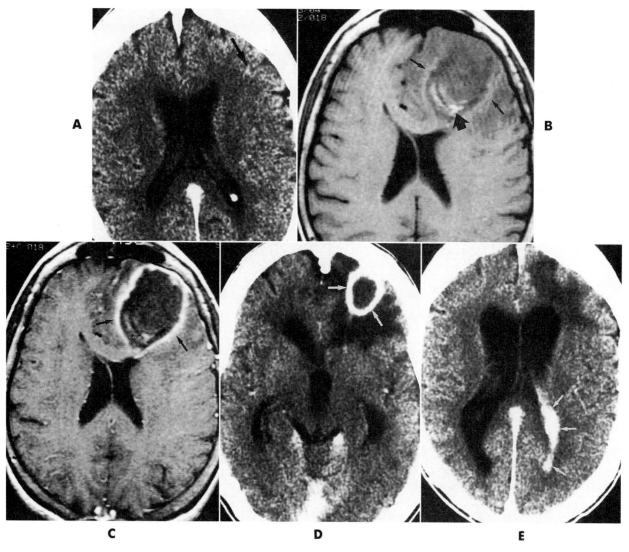

Fig. 16-19. This 57-year-old woman was found unresponsive. Axial CECT scan **(A)** was read as normal (in retrospect, a tiny ill-defined enhancing focus is present in the left frontal lobe *[arrow]*. This is very early cerebritis). Pre- **(B)** and postcontrast **(C)** axial T1-weighted MR scans performed 9 days later show a predominately low signal left frontal mass **(B,** *small arrows)* with focal hemorrhage *(large arrow)* and an irregularly enhancing rim **(C,** *arrows).* The rim is slightly hyperintense on the unenhanced T1WI **(B,** *small arrows).* This is the late cerebritis stage of abscess formation. Axial CECT scans **(D** and **E)** obtained 5 weeks after stereotactic drainage and antibiotic therapy show a small, ring-enhancing residual left frontal lobe mass **(D,** *arrows).* Some edema persists but is diminished. This is the late capsule stage of abscess formation. Note enlarged lateral ventricles and persistent choroid plexitis **(E,** *arrows).*

is typical (Fig. 16-20). Moderate vasogenic edema is present.[36] At this stage, the "ring-enhancing" mass is a nonspecific imaging finding that can be seen in various noninflammatory benign and neoplastic processes (*see* box). In contrast to other lesions such as tumor, an abscess rim typically is thickest near the cortex and thinnest near the ependyma.

Late capsule stage abscesses gradually shrink and the peripheral edema diminishes and then disappears (Fig. 16-19, *D*). Rim enhancement may persist for months, long after clinical resolution occurs.

MR. MR findings in brain abscess also vary with time. During the initial, early cerebritis stage an ill-defined subcortical hyperintense zone can be noted on T2WI. Postcontrast T1-weighted studies may disclose poorly delineated enhancing areas within the iso- to mildly hypointense edematous region (*see* Figs. 16-8, *B* and *C*, and 16-9).

During the late cerebritis stage, the central necrotic area is typically hyperintense to brain on proton-density and T2-weighted sequences. The thick, somewhat irregularly marginated rim appears iso- to mildly hyperintense on T1WI (Fig. 16-18, *B*) and iso- to relatively hypointense on proton density- and T2-weighted scans. Peripheral edema is nearly always present. The rim enhances intensely following contrast administration (Fig. 16-18, *C*). Satellite lesions are commonly present.[41]

During the early and late capsule stages, the collagenous abscess capsule is visible on unenhanced scans as a comparatively thin-walled, well-delineated iso- to slightly hyperintense ring that becomes hypointense on T2-weighted sequences (Fig. 16-21).

Abscesses in immunocompromised patients.

Impaired host response can alter the imaging appearance of cerebral abscesses. Steroid treatment reduces edema and mass effect; the capsule is thinner and enhances less intensely.[36] Patients with systemic diseases such as lymphoma or leukemia frequently develop multiple abscesses, often with unusual opportunistic organisms.[36] Abscess morphology also varies in these patients. Lesions may have thick and irregular walls, indistinguishable from primary or metastatic neoplasm (Fig. 16-22).

Patients with acquired immunodeficiency syndrome (AIDS) rarely develop pyogenic abscesses, although infections with opportunistic organisms are common (see subsequent discussion).

Complications of Cerebral Abscesses

Abscess complications include the following[20]:
1. Formation of satellite or "daughter abscesses"
2. Ventriculitis
3. Choroid plexitis
4. Purulent leptomeningitis

Satellite abscesses. "Daughter abscesses" are formed by rupture of poorly developed capsules and extension of the inflammatory process into the adjacent parenchyma.[20] Satellite abscesses can also be formed when adjacent areas of cerebritis coalesce.

Ventriculitis. Ventriculitis most often follows shunting procedures, intraventricular surgery, placement of indwelling prosthetic devices, intrathecal

---

Ring-Enhancing Lesions
Differential diagnosis

Common

Some primary brain tumors (e.g., anaplastic astrocytoma)
Metastatic brain tumor
Abscess
Granuloma
Resolving hematoma
Infarct

Less common

Thrombosed vascular malformation
Demyelinating disease (e.g., multiple sclerosis)

Uncommon

Thrombosed aneurysm
Other primary brain tumors (e.g., primary CNS lymphoma in AIDS)

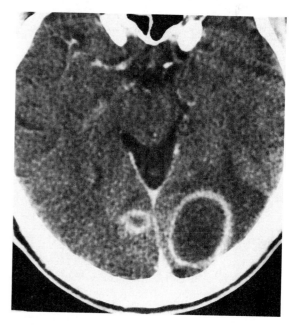

Fig. 16-20. Axial CECT scan in a patient with two occipital lobe abscesses. The well-delineated lesions with thin, ring-like enhancement patterns are typical of—but not pathognomonic for—abscess.

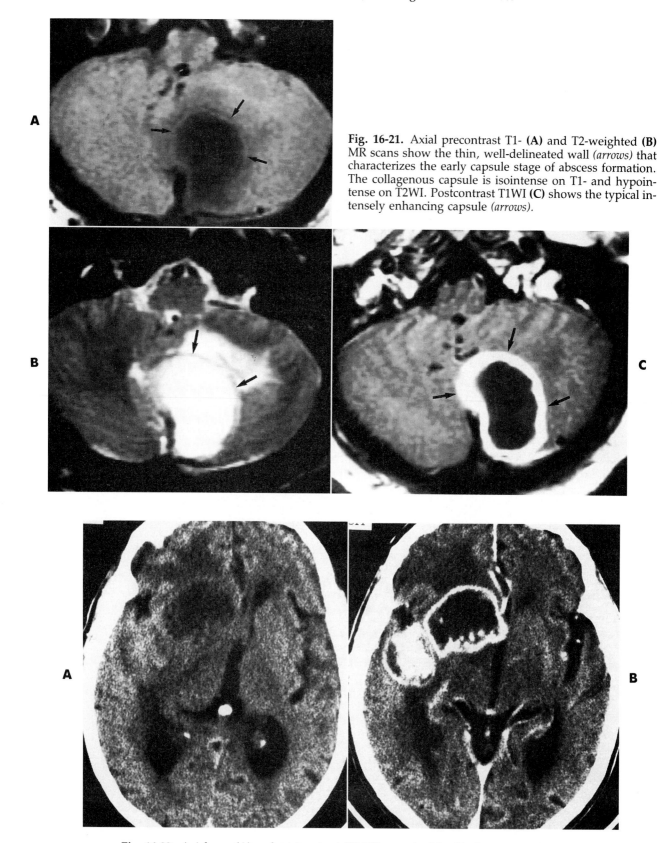

Fig. 16-21. Axial precontrast T1- **(A)** and T2-weighted **(B)** MR scans show the thin, well-delineated wall *(arrows)* that characterizes the early capsule stage of abscess formation. The collagenous capsule is isointense on T1- and hypointense on T2WI. Postcontrast T1WI **(C)** shows the typical intensely enhancing capsule *(arrows)*.

Fig. 16-22. Axial pre- **(A)** and postcontrast **(B)** CT scans in this elderly patient with poor nutritional status show an irregularly enhancing right frontal lobe mass with focal nodular thickening. Preoperative diagnosis was glioblastoma multiforme. Poorly loculated abscess was found at surgery.

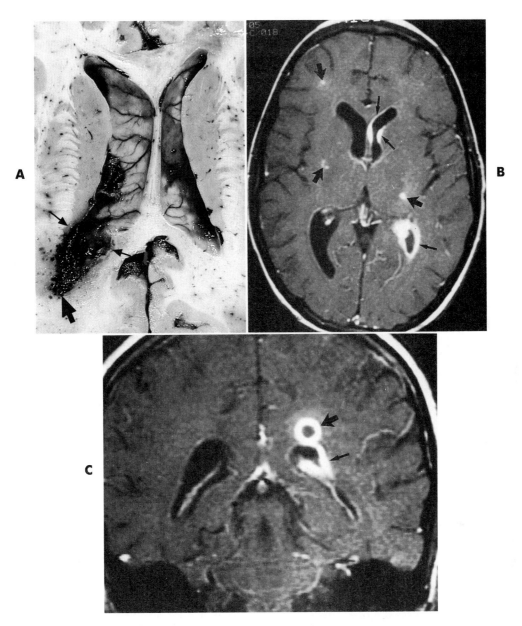

Fig. 16-23. Axial gross pathology specimen **(A)** shows an abscess *(large arrow)* that has ruptured into the atrium, causing ependymitis *(small arrows)*. Axial **(B)** and coronal **(C)** postcontrast T1-weighted MR scans in another case, a 12-year-old boy with acute leukemia, show multiple parenchymal brain abscesses *(large arrows)*. An abscess in the deep cerebral white matter ruptured into the left atrium, causing intense ventriculitis *(small arrows)*.

chemotherapy, or meningitis.[42] Purulent ependymitis is occasionally caused by intraventricular abscess rupture. The medial side of an abscess cavity is thinner than the well-vascularized cortical surface in 50% of cases. Abscesses expand centrally toward the white matter and may rupture through the adjacent ependyma, inciting a pyogenic ventriculitis. Diffusely thickened, intensely enhancing ependyma is seen on contrast-enhanced MR scans (Fig. 16-23).[42]

Choroid plexitis. The choroid plexus may serve as a primary portal through which infectious agents gain entry to the CNS. It can also be affected secondarily when there is associated meningitis (*see* Fig. 16-9), encephalitis, or abscess rupture with ependymitis (Fig. 16-19, *E*).[43] The choroid plexus appears enlarged and enhances prominently on postcontrast T1-weighted MR scans.

Meningitis. Occasionally, abscesses extend to the cortex and incite a focal meningitis that can become more generalized. This can occur with and without actual abscess rupture.[20]

ENCEPHALITIS

Encephalitis is a diffuse, nonfocal brain parenchymal inflammatory disease that can be caused by a broad spectrum of agents. The most common encephalitides are viral. Common nonepidemic causes of acute encephalitis in immunocompetent patients include herpes simplex virus (HSV) type 1 and HSV type 2. Sporadic epidemics of Eastern, Western, and Venezuelan equine encephalitis occur.[2,44]

Viral encephalitis in immunocompromised patients is usually caused by the human immunodeficiency virus (HIV), cytomegalovirus (CMV), and papovaviruses. Typical nonviral causes of encephalitis in these patients include *Toxoplasma gondii*, fungi (particularly *Aspergillosus fumigatus*), and *Listeria monocytogenes*.[45]

So-called slow virus encephalitides include Creutzfeldt-Jakob disease and subacute sclerosing panencephalitis (SSPE). Autoimmune or allergic encephalitides include acute disseminated encephalomyelitis (ADEM).

In this section we focus on the most common cause of viral meningoencephalitis in the United States and Europe: herpes simplex encephalitis. We also discuss the CNS manifestations of HIV infection and acquired immune deficiency syndrome (AIDS). We

then close this section by discussing briefly the slow virus infections and the allergic encephalitides.

Herpes Simplex Encephalitis

Etiology. Neonatal herpes simplex encephalitis (HSE) is usually caused by HSV 2 (genital herpesvirus), whereas HSE in older infants, children, and adults is caused by HSV 1 (oral herpesvirus).[5] During oral herpes infection, virus is transported along sensory nerve fibers to the olfactory nerve or gasserian ganglion. Encephalitis results from retrograde virus spread from the trigeminal ganglion and may occur with the primary infection, reinfection, or activation of latent infection (*see* box).[1]

Pathology
Gross pathology. HSV causes a fulminant hemorrhagic, necrotizing meningoencephalitis. Severe edema and massive tissue necrosis with petechial and some confluent hemorrhages are typical findings (Fig. 16-24).

Microscopic appearance. A focal necrotizing vasculitis with perivascular and meningeal lymphocytic infiltration, petechial hemorrhages, focal tissue necrosis, and eosinophilic intranuclear inclusions in glial cells and neurons is seen.[20]

Incidence and age. HSV 1 is the most common nonepidemic cause of viral meningoencephalitis in the United States and Europe.[2,46] Herpes encephalitis is common in both children and adults; approxi-

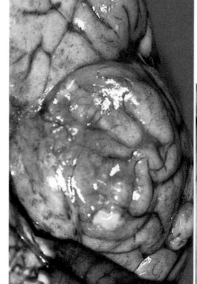
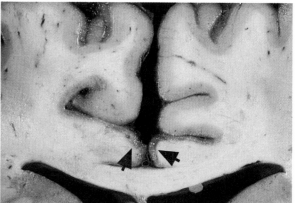

Fig. 16-24. A, Gross pathology specimen seen from below demonstrates the typical findings with acute herpes encephalitis. Note the markedly swollen, edematous temporal lobe has multifocal petechial hemorrhages. **B,** Coronal gross pathology specimen from a patient with herpes encephalitis graphically illustrates the limbic system involvement so typical with this infection. Note bilateral cingulate gyrus hemorrhagic necrosis *(arrows).*

mately one third of all patients are less than 20 years old.[2]

Location. Neonatal HSV type 2 encephalitis is a diffuse, nonfocal infection. In contrast, HSV 1 encephalitis has a particular predilection for the limbic system.[47] Infection is therefore often localized to the temporal lobes, insular cortex, subfrontal area, and the cingulate gyri (Fig. 16-24, *B*).[45,46] Involvement may initially appear unilateral but is typically followed by less severe contralateral disease. This "sequential bilaterality" is highly suggestive of HSE 1.[45]

Occasionally, HSE 1 affects the midbrain and pons, causing a mesenrhombencephalitis.[48] Infrequently, cranial nerve inflammation occurs. The trigeminal nerve is most commonly affected.

Herpes Simplex Encephalitis

HSV 2 in neonates, HSV 1 in children, adults (usually activation of latent infection in gasserian ganglion)

Most common viral encephalitis

Fulminant, necrotizing, hemorrhagic

Predilection for limbic system (temporal lobes, cingulate gyri, subfrontal region) in older children, adults (HSV 1)

Imaging
  CT: often normal early in disease
  MR: gyral edema; temporal lobe hyperintense on T2WI; +/−enhancement in early stage; hemorrhage uncommon early

---

Clinical presentation and natural history. Patients typically present with altered mental status. Seizures, fever, and headaches are also common. Early diagnosis and prompt therapy are essential as the disease progresses rapidly. The mortality rate with HSE is between 50% to 70%, with significant long-term morbidity in surviving patients. The diagnosis of HSE can be established by serology and CSF analysis but these can remain normal until the second week.[46] Identification of viral antigen on brain biopsy is definitive. Imaging findings can be highly suggestive of HSE in some cases.

Imaging

CT. Scans obtained early in the course of HSE type 1 may be normal or subtly abnormal (Fig. 16-25, *A*). Low-density lesions in the temporal lobes with mild mass effect are common initial abnormalities. Hemorrhage is highly suggestive of HSE but is a rare early finding and is usually seen on studies obtained later in the disease course (Fig. 16-25, *B*). CECT scans may demonstrate ill-defined patchy or gyriform enhancement.[45] Neonatal HSE 2 shows strikingly increased density of cortical gray matter and diffuse low attenuation in the white matter (*see* Fig. 16-4).[49]

MR. MR is more sensitive than CT in detecting early changes of HSE 1. Typical early findings include gyral edema on T1WI and high signal intensity in the temporal lobe or cingulate gyrus on T2-weighted scans (Fig. 16-26). The signal abnormalities often extend into the insular cortex and spare the putamen. Enhancement following contrast administration is

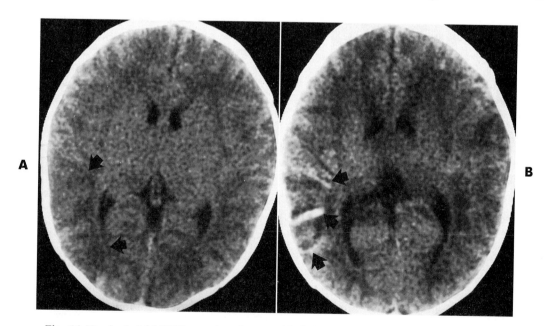

Fig. 16-25. **A,** Axial NECT scan in a 2-year-old child with seizure shows ill-defined low density changes in the right parietal lobe *(arrows)*. CECT scan (not shown) failed to demonstrate abnormal enhancement. **B,** Follow-up scan 10 days later shows gyriform hemorrhage *(arrows)*. Biopsy-proven herpes encephalitis.

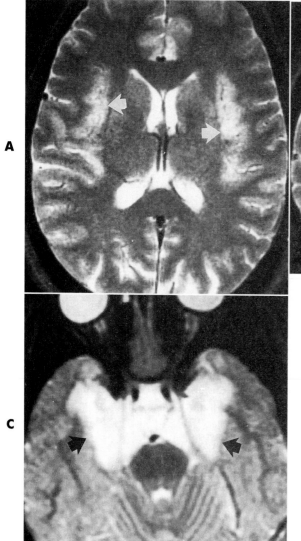

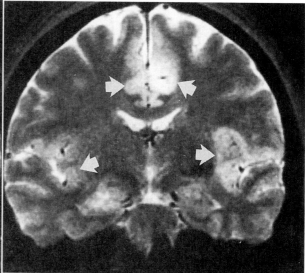

Fig. 16-26. Early MR findings of herpes encephalitis are illustrated by these two cases. Axial **(A)** and coronal **(B)** T2-weighted scans in this young woman with fever, confusion, and decreasing mental status show high signal edematous gray matter along the insular cortex and cingulate gyri *(arrows)*. The lesions are bilateral but asymmetric. Herpes encephalitis was found at biopsy. Axial T2-weighted MR scan **(C)** in this 3½-year-old child with new onset of seizures and abnormal EEG show striking increased signal in both medial temporal lobes. Herpes encephalitis. (C, Courtesy T. Miller.)

unusual in the early stages.[42] Petechial hemorrhages occur but are also uncommonly identified early in the disease process.

Follow-up scans obtained 1 to 2 weeks after disease onset demonstrate progressively more widespread abnormalities with involvement of the contralateral temporal lobe, insula, and cingulate gyri. Contrast enhancement and changes of subacute hemorrhage may become readily apparent (Fig. 16-27). Encephalomalacia, atrophy, and dystrophic calcifications are common late sequelae of HSE (Fig. 16-28).[45]

HIV Encephalitis and Other CNS Infections in AIDS

The retrovirus designated human immunodeficiency virus (HIV) causes acquired immunodeficiency syndrome (AIDS). Two HIV subtypes are recognized: HIV-1 and HIV-2. HIV-1 is the most widespread type and accounts for most AIDS cases in the United States and Europe. CNS involvement is both an early and a common feature of HIV infection.[50] Another retrovirus that can cause CNS infection is HTLV type 1. HTLV I is endemic in parts of Africa, South America, the Caribbean, and Japan. Although HTLV 1 is uncommon in North America, its incidence is rising.[50]

HIV is a neurotropic virus that can directly involve both the peripheral and central nervous systems. The HIV virus itself is the most common CNS pathogen in AIDS patients, followed by *Toxoplasma gondi* and *Cryptococcus neoformans*.[51] In this section we will discuss the pathology and imaging findings of HIV encephalopathy and AIDS encephalitis, toxoplasmosis and cryptococcosis, and other AIDS-related CNS infections (*see* box, p. 698).

HIV encephalopathy. HIV encephalopathy is a progressive subcortical dementia that is a form of subacute encephalitis.[52]

Etiology and pathology. HIV encephalopathy is caused by CNS infection with the HIV virus itself and is not an opportunistic infection.[53] Pathologic findings include atrophy and loss of axons, ill-defined areas of demyelination, gliosis, and infiltration with multinucleated giant cells.[52,54]

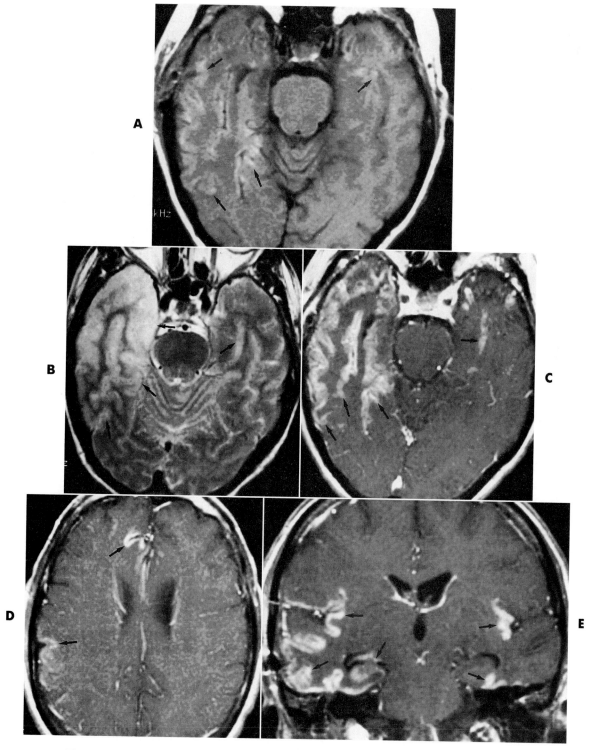

Fig. 16-27. A 65-year-old woman with high fever and coma had these MR scans 10 days after admission. Axial T1-weighted scan **(A)** shows subacute gyriform hemorrhage in the right temporal lobe *(arrows)*, with less striking changes in the left temporal lobe. Axial T2WI **(B)** shows gyriform edema *(arrows)* corresponds to the hemorrhagic areas seen in **(A)**. Axial **(C** and **D)** and coronal **(E)** postcontrast T1-weighted scans show the bilateral but asymmetric gyriform enhancement in the temporal lobes, insulae, and cingulate gyrus *(arrows)* that is characteristic for herpes encephalitis.

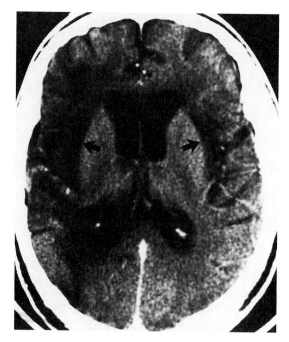

Fig. 16-28. Axial CECT scan in a patient who survived herpes encephalitis shows bilateral asymmetric encephalomalacic changes in the temporal lobes and insulae *(arrows)*.

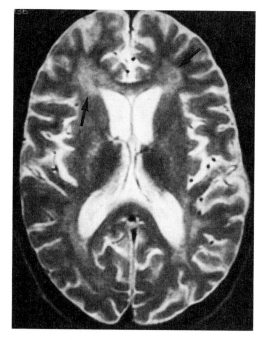

Fig. 16-29. Axial T2-weighted MR scan in this 24-year-old man with AIDS and HIV encephalopathy shows diffuse cerebral atrophy and multifocal white matter hyperintensities that are most prominent in the frontal lobes *(arrows)*.

CNS Infections in AIDS
HIV encephalitis most common (60%)
Toxoplasmosis most common opportunistic infection (20% to 40%)
Cryptococcosis (5%)
Progressive multifocal leukoencephalopathy (1% to 4%) (papovavirus)
Others
Tuberculosis (2% to 18%)
Neurosyphilis (1% to 3%)
Varicella zoster (<1%)
CMV encephalitis/ependymitis (rare)

Incidence. HIV encephalopathy eventually develops in up to 60% of AIDS cases. Approximately 10% of AIDS patients develop neurologic symptoms before other disease manifestations.[55]

Imaging. The most common finding on NECT scans in patients with HIV encephalopathy is atrophy.[56] Multifocal hypodense areas in the deep white matter are also common.[57]

T2-weighted MR scans show ill-defined diffuse or confluent patches of increased signal intensities in the deep white matter.[58] The frontal lobes are the most common sites (Fig. 16-29). White matter lesions in HIV encephalopathy are usually bilateral but are often asymmetric. Gray matter is typically spared, and mass effect is absent.[53] These lesions usually do not enhance following contrast administration. Histologic examination discloses demyelination with astrocytosis.[58a]

Toxoplasma gondii infections

Etiology and pathology. Toxoplasmosis is caused by the obligate intracellular parasite *Toxoplasma gondii.* Infection can result in focal lesions or a diffuse necrotizing encephalitis.[59]

Pathologically, toxoplasmosis lesions are characterized by three distinct zones and no capsule. The innermost zone consists of coagulative necrosis with few organisms. The intermediate zone is hypervascular and contains numerous inflammatory cells mixed with tachyzoites and encysted organisms. The peripheral zone is mostly composed of encysted organisms.[59] Vasogenic edema typically surrounds the mass.

Incidence and location. Toxoplasma is the most common opportunistic CNS infection in AIDS patients. The basal ganglia and cerebral hemispheres near the corticomedullary junction are the most common sites.[60]

Imaging. CECT scans show solitary or multiple ring-enhancing masses with peripheral edema. A "target" appearance is common (Fig. 16-30, *A*). Toxoplasmosis lesions are typically iso- to slightly hypointense on T1-weighted MR scans. Focal nodular or rim enhancement patterns are seen following contrast administration (Fig. 16-30, *B* and *C*); T2WI reportedly are more sensitive than enhanced T1-

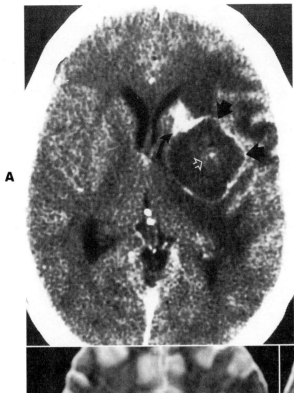

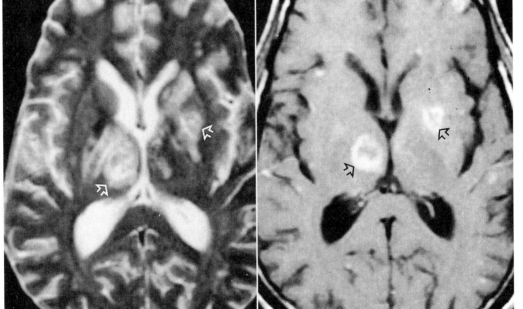

Fig. 16-30. AIDS-related *Toxoplasma gondii* infection is illustrated by these two cases. **A,** Axial CECT scan shows a solitary basal ganglia mass with a "target" appearance (*open arrow* points to the "bull's eye"). Note rim (*large arrows*) and nodular (*curved arrow*) enhancement. Biopsy-proven toxoplasmosis. Axial precontrast T2- **(B)** and postcontrast T1-weighted **(C)** MR scans in this HIV-positive patient show multiple "target"-appearing lesions *(open arrows)* that are most prominent in the basal ganglia. The lesions responded to toxoplasmosis therapy. (**B** and **C,** Courtesy T. Miller.)

weighted studies in identifying multifocal lesions.[61] Treated lesions often demonstrate calcification or hemorrhage on imaging studies.[60]

The major differential diagnostic consideration is primary CNS lymphoma.[62] The detection of more than one lesion increases the likelihood of toxoplasmosis rather than lymphoma[61]; periventricular location and subependymal spread favor lymphoma over toxoplasmosis.[62] CNS lymphomatoid granulomatosis, a rare lymphoproliferative disorder that primarily affects the lung, has been reported in AIDS. Leptomeningeal or parenchymal infiltrates and multifocal solid or ring-enhancing masses in the basal mul-

tifocal solid or ring-enhancing masses in the basal ganglia occur. The latter are indistinguishable from toxoplasmosis and CNS lymphoma.[62a]

Cryptococcosis
Etiology and pathology. Cryptococcus neoformans is a ubiquitous fungus that enters the body via the respiratory tract and then involves the CNS by hematogenous spread. Cryptococcosis causes meningitis, dilated perivascular spaces, and focal cryptococcomas. Meningitis is the most frequent manifestation of cryptococcus in immunocompetent patients, whereas disseminated infection is more common in AIDS patients.[51]

Fig. 16-31. Intracranial cryptococcosis in AIDS. **A,** Axial T2-weighted MR scan shows clusters of tiny hyperintense foci in both basal ganglia *(arrows)*. These represent multiple dilated Virchow-Robin spaces. **B,** Photomicrograph shows a dilated Virchow-Robin space. It is filled with numerous foamy macrophages that surround a pocket *(arrows)* containing small darkly stained circular organisms *(C. neoformans.* (**A,** Reprinted from Tien RD: *AJNR* 12:283-289, 1991.)

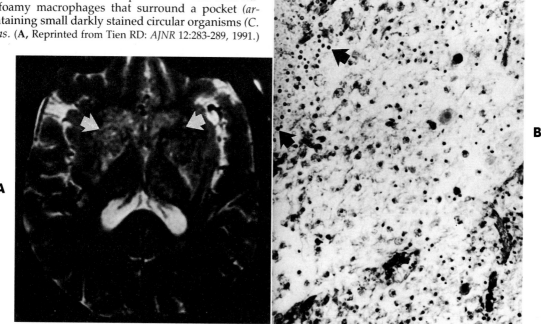

Typical lesions consist of organisms, inflammatory cells, and gelatinous mucoid material in or near prominent perivascular spaces.[51]

Incidence and location. *Cryptococcus neoformans* is the third most frequent CNS pathogen in AIDS patients, exceeded only by the HIV virus itself and *Toxoplasma gondii*. Approximately 5% of AIDS patients develop CNS cryptococcal infection.[59] The meninges, basal ganglia, and midbrain are the most commonly affected sites.[63]

Imaging. The most common finding is multifocal basal ganglia and midbrain hyperintensities on T2WI (Fig. 16-31). These represent both gelatinous pseudocysts (cryptococcomas) and dilated perivascular spaces.[63] Enhancement varies following contrast administration.[51,63a] Neither CT nor MR effectively identifies cryptococcal meningitis.[51]

Progressive multifocal leukoencephalopathy. Progressive multifocal leukoencephalopathy (PML) is a disease of immunocompromised patients.

Etiology and pathology. PML is caused by CNS infection with group B human papovaviruses (principally the JC virus). Papovaviruses infect and destroy oligodendroglia. Extensive demyelination occurs.[54] Multifocal areas of myelin and axon loss involving the deep and superficial white matter are typical, whereas the cortical gray matter is relatively spared.[64]

Incidence and age. Between 1% and 4% of adult AIDS patients develop PML. PML is extremely rare in children.[1]

Location. The subcortical areas are affected first. As spread to the deep white matter ensues, lesions become large and confluent.[64] PML is typically bilateral but asymmetric. The posterior centrum semiovale is the most common site.[59]

Imaging. MR scans are the most sensitive imaging modality for evaluating white matter disease. T2-weighted sequences initially show multifocal oval or round subcortical white matter hyperintensities in the parietooccipital area. Confluent white matter disease with cavitary change is a late manifestation of PML (Fig. 16-32).[59] Less common imaging manifestations of PML are unilateral white matter and thalamic or basal ganglia lesions.[64]

Other infections. Other agents that cause CNS infection in immunocompromised patients include CMV, herpes simplex (both HSV-1 and HSV-2), varicella-zoster, neurosyphilis, and tuberculosis. Pyogenic bacterial infection is uncommon.

CMV. CMV occasionally causes encephalitis in immunocompromised hosts and may represent reactivation of previously silent infection. CT and MR appearances often resemble CNS lymphoma. Findings are a thick, somewhat nodular confluent periventricular rim (Fig. 16-33). Subependymal enhancement is

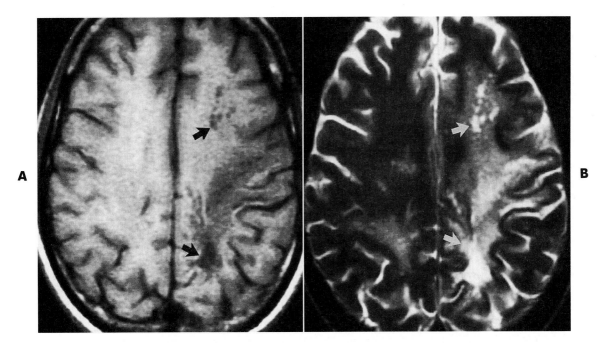

Fig. 16-32. Axial T1- **(A)** and T2-weighted **(B)** MR scans in this patient with AIDS demonstrate typical findings of late-stage progressive multifocal leukoencephalopathy (PML). Confluent white matter lesions with cavitary changes *(arrows)* are present in the left parietooccipital lobe. Note involvement of both deep and superficial white matter. (Courtesy M. Fruin.)

sometimes seen following contrast administration. The periventricular calcifications so typical of neonatal CMV are absent.[59]

Herpesvirus. Other than CMV, herpesvirus infection is relatively uncommon in immunocompromised patients. The perivascular inflammatory changes and temporal lobe encephalitis typically seen in immunocompetent patients are absent.[59]

Primary varicella zoster virus (VZV) infection causes varicella (chickenpox), whereas reactivation is known as herpes zoster. Less than 1% of immunocompetent patients develop neurologic complications from VZV infection.[64]

Deficiencies in cell-mediated immunity occur with lymphoproliferative malignancies, immunosuppressive therapy, radiation, AIDS, and advanced age.[65] CNS VZV infection in these patients causes multifocal plaquelike areas of myelin loss near the gray-white junction. These lesions progress in size and eventually coalesce. Necrosis and hemorrhage may occur. T2-weighted MR scans show multiple ovoid areas of high signal intensity in the deep and subcortical white matter. Subtle ring enhancement may occur following contrast administration.[65] Herpes zoster may also cause cranial neuritis; facial nerve involvement (Ramsay-Hunt syndrome) may be a striking manifestation.[66]

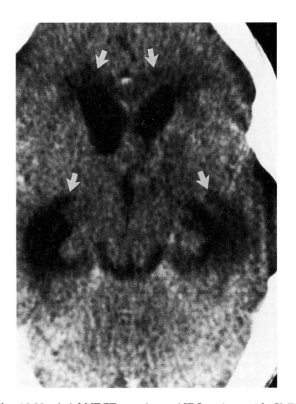

Fig. 16-33. Axial NECT scan in an AIDS patient with CMV encephalitis shows extensive periventricular low density changes *(arrows)*. (Courtesy N. Yue.)

Neurosyphilis. Syphilis is one of the most common sexually transmitted diseases. It is caused by the spirochete *Treponema pallidum.* Three well-characterized clinical phases have been described, but neurosyphilis can occur at any stage in the disease process and ensue weeks to decades after the initial infection.[67]

Neurosyphilis, strictly defined as presence of a reactive CSF VDRL test in association with positive serologic studies for syphilis in the blood, is present in approximately 1% to 3% of HIV-infected patients.[68] Neurosyphilis usually results from small-vessel endarteritis of the meninges, brain, and spinal cord. It may also develop after HIV-induced deficiencies in cell-mediated immunity adversely affect the course of primary syphilis.[67]

Imaging findings in neurosyphilis vary. Meningovascular neurosyphilis causes ischemic infarcts in the basal ganglia or middle cerebral artery territories, seen as patchy enhancing areas on postcontrast T1-weighted MR scans.[67] Syphilitic cerebral gummas are seen as isolated, peripherally located contrast-enhancing masses[68] (Fig. 16-34). Cranial nerve involvement also has been reported. The optic and vestibulocochlear nerves are most commonly affected.[67]

Tuberculosis. The reported incidence of intracranial tuberculosis (TB) in AIDS patients ranges from 2% to 18% and varies with TB prevalence in the general population.[69] In a recent series, over 90% of affected patients were intravenous drug abusers; TB was the first manifestation of AIDS in two thirds of these cases.[69]

The most frequent imaging findings in AIDS-related TB are hydrocephalus and meningeal enhancement, respectively seen in 50% and 40% of cases. Parenchymal involvement occurs in 37%. One quarter of affected patients have ischemic lesions, mostly in the basal ganglia.[69]

Miscellaneous Viral Encephalitides

In the United States and Europe, HSV is the most common sporadic nonepidemic viral encephalitis and is typically a reactivation of latent CNS infection. In contrast, the most common acute viral encephalitides are spread by arthropods (ticks and mosquitoes).[64] In North America, these viruses, sometimes epidemiologically called "arboviruses," include Eastern, Western, and Venezuelan equine encephalitis.

Other acute viral encephalitides include mumps encephalitis, varicella encephalitis, and measles encephalitis. All are rare.

Chronic viral infections that may involve the CNS include Epstein-Barr virus (EBV) and Rasmussen encephalitis. Infectious mononucleosis syndrome caused by EBV is generally an acute, monophasic illness. However, persistent or chronic EBV infection can cause prolonged or recurrent meningitis, cerebellitis, encephalitis, and relapsing acute disseminated encephalomyelitis (ADEM).[70] A more acute demyelinating disease complicating primary EBV infection

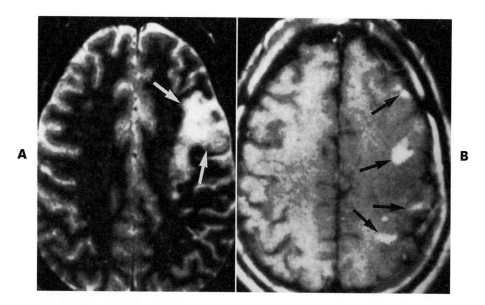

Fig. 16-34. Neurosyphilis in AIDS. This 32-year-old HIV-positive man had subacute right hemiplegia and expressive aphasia. **A,** Axial T2-weighted MR scan shows an area of increased signal in the left posterior frontal lobe *(arrows).* Both the cortex and subcortical white matter are involved. **B,** Axial T1-weighted study obtained after contrast administration shows multiple enhancing foci *(arrows).* Diagnosis of neurosyphilis was based on positive CSF VDRL test of 1=8; CSF VDRL decreased after penicillin treatment. Tests for other opportunistic organisms were negative. (Courtesy R. Tien.)

has also been described.[71] MR scans in neurologically complicated EBV infection usually show transient white matter lesions; the thalami are also often affected.[72]

Rasmussen's chronic encephalitis is a devastating childhood disease that causes progressive neurologic deficits and intractable seizures. Cytomegalovirus genome has been found in the resected cortical tissue of some patients.[73] Imaging findings in these patients show nonspecific atrophy and multifocal signal abnormalities isolated to one hemisphere (Fig. 16-35).[73,74] Positron emission tomography reveals a hypometabolism in the affected area.[73]

"Slow" virus infections probably account for Creutzfeldt-Jakob disease, a spongiform encephalopathy that behaves clinically like Alzheimer's disease and the primary degenerative dementias.[64] The pathological features of Creutzfeldt-Jakob disease resemble those of transmissible animal diseases such as scrapie of sheep and mink encephalopathy.[20]

Kuru is another disease of probable slow viral origin. It is a disease that is endemic in parts of New Guinea and is thought to be transmitted by ritualistic cannibalism (ingesting infected brain tissue). Histologic features resemble Creutzfeldt-Jakob disease, i.e., Kuru is a spongiform encephalopathy.[20]

Postinfection Encephalitis

Postinfection encephalitis is represented by two important entities: subacute sclerosing panencephalitis and acute disseminated encephalomyelitis.

Subacute sclerosing panencephalitis

Etiology. Subacute sclerosing panencephalitis (SSPE) is a progressive encephalitis that occurs several years after measles infection.[5] Elevated titers of neutralizing measles virus antibodies are present in the serum and CSF.[45] Measles virus genomic sequences have been isolated from tissue samples (*see* box).[5]

Pathology. Gross atrophy is typical (Fig. 16-36). Neuronal loss, gliosis, and perivascular lymphocytic infiltrates are seen in the gray matter; patchy demyelination and gliosis are present in the white matter. Eosinophilic intranuclear and intracytoplasmic inclusion bodies are found in oligodendrocytes and neurons.[20]

Incidence and age. SSPE is rare, with an estimated yearly incidence of 1 per million.[5] Children and young adults are affected.[75]

Clinical presentation and natural history. SSPE is

Subacute Sclerosing Panencephalitis
Measles virus implicated Occurs several years after initial infection Rare; affects children, young adults Gross atrophy, demyelination seen at pathology, imaging

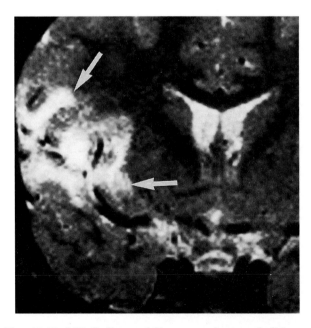

Fig. 16-35. MR findings of Rasmussen's encephalitis are demonstrated on the coronal T2-weighted MR scan in this 3½-year-old girl with chronic intractable and increasingly severe seizures. Note extensive right temporal lobe and insular signal abnormalities *(arrows)*. Hemispherectomy was performed with subsequent seizure resolution. (Courtesy T. Miller.)

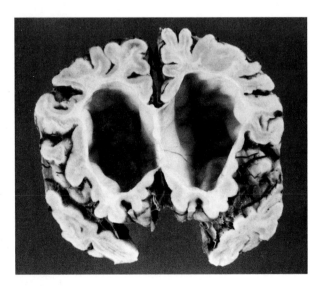

Fig. 16-36. Coronal gross pathology specimen in a patient with subacute sclerosing panencephalitis (SSPE). Severe atrophy of both gray and white matter is seen. (Courtesy Rubinstein Collection, University of Virginia.)

usually a slowly progressive disorder. The disease typically starts with mental or behavioral abnormalities and progresses to myoclonic jerks, tremors, and seizures.[76] Death occurs within 2 to 6 years. Occasionally, the disease course is fulminant and rapidly fatal.[75]

Imaging. NECT scans may be normal or show hypodense foci in the subcortical and periventricular white matter, as well as the basal ganglia.[45] Generalized atrophy is common. T2-weighted MR scans show multifocal hyperintense foci in the cerebral white matter and basal ganglia.[76]

Acute disseminated encephalomyelitis

Etiology. Acute disseminated encephalomyelitis (ADEM) is an immune-mediated response to a preceding viral infection or vaccination. ADEM occurs in several settings, as follows[77]:

1. Shortly after a specific viral illness, particularly exanthematous childhood diseases such as measles or chickenpox
2. Following a nonspecific, presumably viral, upper respiratory infection
3. Following vaccination against rabies, diphtheria, smallpox, tetanus, typhoid, or influenza
4. Spontaneously

The acute demyelination is believed to be an autoimmune phenomenon mediated by antibody-antigen complexes[78] (*see* box).

Pathology. Multiple perivascular (mostly perivenular) inflammatory (mostly mononuclear) infiltrates are seen. These are associated with a zone of demyelination that follows the course of affected venules.

Perivascular astrocytosis occurs as the disease resolves.[20]

Incidence and age. The true incidence of ADEM is unknown. ADEM occurs in all ages, although most reported cases are in children and young adults.

Clinical presentation and natural history. ADEM typically has an abrupt onset and a monophasic course.[77] Neurologic symptoms characteristically begin 1 to 3 weeks after infection. Initial symptoms may be mild; fever, headache, and drowsiness are common.[78] The clinical course is rapid, with development of multifocal symptoms that range from seizures and focal neurologic deficits to coma and death.[79] Some patients recover completely, but others have permanent neurologic impairment.[77,79a]

Imaging. MR is superior to CT in demonstrating ADEM. Multifocal subcortical hyperintense foci are present on T2-weighted studies (Fig. 16-37). The deep white matter, brainstem, and cerebellum can be affected.[80] Lesions are widely distributed and typically bilateral but asymmetric. Occasionally, confluent disease with basal ganglia involvement occurs (Fig. 16-38). Rarely, acute encephalopathy with bilateral stri-

---

Acute Disseminated Encephalomyelitis

Immune-mediated
Previous viral infection/vaccination
Pathology = perivenular demyelinating foci
Any age but mostly children, young adults
Subcortical hyperintense foci on T2WI

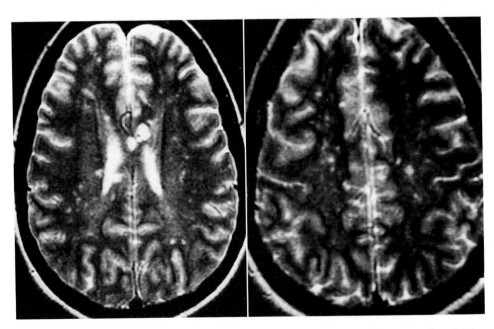

Fig. 16-37. Axial T2-weighted MR scans in a 20-year-old woman with onset of multiple neurologic abnormalities 2 weeks after a flulike illness show numerous hyperintense white matter lesions. Acute disseminated encephalomyelitis (ADEM).

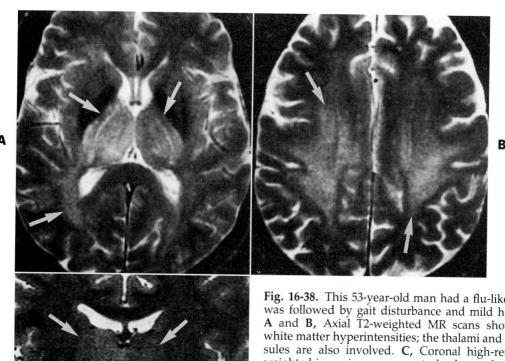

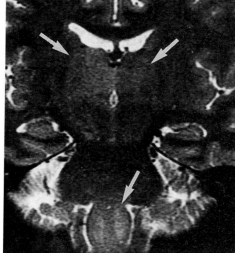

Fig. 16-38. This 53-year-old man had a flu-like illness that was followed by gait disturbance and mild hyperreflexia. **A** and **B,** Axial T2-weighted MR scans show confluent white matter hyperintensities; the thalami and internal capsules are also involved. **C,** Coronal high-resolution T2-weighted inversion recovery study shows abnormal signal in the medulla, as well as both thalami *(arrows)*. Biopsy disclosed ADEM.

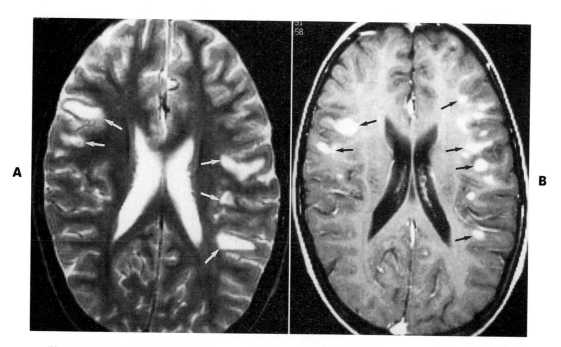

Fig. 16-39. Axial T2- **(A)** and postcontrast T1-weighted **(B)** MR scans in a 9-year-old boy show multifocal subcortical white matter lesions (**A,** *arrows*) that enhance following contrast administration (**B,** *arrows*). Biopsy disclosed subacute disseminated encephalomyelitis.

atal necrosis is seen as an infectious or parainfecitous complication.[79a]

Although petechial hemorrhages are sometimes identified on pathologic examination,[20] ADEM is usually nonhemorrhagic on MR.[78] Some—but not all—lesions enhance following contrast administration (Fig. 16-39).[78,79] Most abnormalities resolve.[20]

Lyme disease

Etiology and pathology. Lyme disease is a multisystem disorder caused by the tick-borne spirochete *Borrelia burgdorferi.* Although Lyme disease occurs worldwide, the geographic areas most commonly affected are the New England and Pacific states, Minnesota, and Wisconsin.[80a,80b]

The precise pathogenesis of Lyme disease is unknown. Both vasculitis and immune complex mechanisms have been proposed. Postviral demyelination similar to ADEM is the favored hypothesis.[80] Microscopic findings are similar to those of ADEM, i.e., perivascular inflammatory infiltrates with multiple demyelinating foci.

Incidence and clinical presentation. Between 10% and 15% of patients with Lyme disease develop neurologic complications. Cranial nerve palsies and peripheral neuropathies are common.[80a]

Imaging. Imaging findings vary from normal to extensive white matter lesions. Both superficial and deep, discrete and confluent lesions have been reported. Some lesions may enhance following contrast administration. The imaging appearance is indistinguishable from multiple sclerosis or other postviral encephalitides such as ADEM.[80a]

TUBERCULOSIS AND FUNGAL INFECTIONS
CNS Tuberculosis

Tuberculosis has been, and still remains, an important public health problem in both developing and industrialized nations. In emerging countries, poor socioeconomic conditions are responsible for persistant endemic disease, and high morbidity and mortality rates persist.[81] In developed countries such as the United States, substance abuse, immunocompromised states, homelessness, and crowded conditions in confined populations (i.e., prisons and nursing

homes) have contributed to a resurgence of TB. In many instances, the responsible mycobacterium is resistant to conventional therapies and is often lethal.

Several clinicopathologic forms of intracranial TB are recognized (*see* box). The most common acute presentation, tuberculous meningitis, has been discussed previously. In this section we discuss the pathology and imaging manifestations of the most common parenchymal TB infection: tuberculomas.

Etiology and pathology. Tuberculomas typically result from hematogenous dissemination and histologically are granulomas with central caseous necrosis.[20] The responsible organism is usually *Mycobacterium tuberculosis.* The *M. avium-intracellulare* complex rarely involves the CNS. *M. bovis,* a frequent pathogen in the past, is now rare.[81]

Incidence and age. Intracranial tuberculoma is uncommon in developed countries, although it is seen in immigrants from endemic areas and in immunocompromised patients.[82] It can be found at any age.

Location. The most common sites are the cerebral hemispheres and basal ganglia in adults and the cerebellum in children.[81] Cortical and subcortical locations are typical. The cerebral ventricles and brainstem are less common sites. Tuberculomas are usually solitary; multiple lesions occur in 10% to 35% of cases.[81] A "miliary" pattern with innumerable small parenchymal lesions is uncommon except in children with tuberculous meningitis.[83]

Imaging
CT. During the acute stage, NECT scans may show only a hypodense area caused by cerebritis. Immature tuberculomas are iso- or slightly hyperdense on NECT scans and show ring, nodular, or irregular enhancement following contrast administration (Fig. 16-40). Mature tuberculomas appear as welldelineated round or oval ring-enhancing masses.[81] Occasionally, a "target sign" is seen that consists of a ring-enhancing lesion with a central area of enhancement or calcification (Fig. 16-40).[81] Healed tuberculomas often calcify (Fig. 16-41).

MR. Tuberculomas are typically isointense to brain on T1-weighted images, have a central hyperintense region with hypointense rim on T2WI, and show marked enhancement following contrast administration.[84] Hypointense lesions on T2WI are associated with increased fibrosis, gliosis, and macrophage infiltration.[84a]

Differential diagnosis. Solitary tuberculomas may be indistinguishable from encapsulated abscess, malignant astrocytoma, or metastasis on imaging studies.[20] Tuberculomas are typically larger than cysticercus granulomas, another entity with which they can be confused.[85]

CNS Tuberculosis

Hematogenous dissemination of *M. tuberculosis,* usually from pulmonary infection

Most common: meningitis

Parenchymal lesions are caseating granulomas; up to 1/3 multiple

Cortical, subcortical, basal ganglia lesions

Ring/nodular enhancing pattern; old tuberculomas often calcify

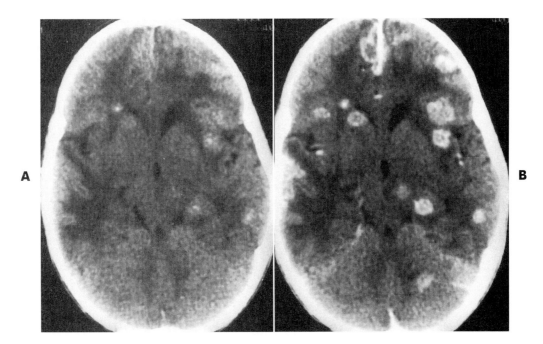

Fig. 16-40. Pre- **(A)** and postcontrast **(B)** axial CT scans in this patient with multiple tuberculomas show some of the lesions are hyperdense on the NECT study, whereas others are isodense with cortex. Following contrast enhancement, multiple "target"-enhancing lesions are seen. (Courtesy H. Segall.)

Fungal Infections

Fungi are ubiquitous single-celled organisms that are distinctly different from bacteria in size, structural complexity, chemical composition, and their pathologic effects on the central nervous system.[86] CNS manifestations of systemic mycoses are considered in this section.

Etiology. Common fungi that are considered "true" human pathogens and can infect immunocompetent individuals include *Histoplasma*, *Blastomyces*, and *Coccidioides*. Opportunistic infections occur in immunocompromised hosts. The majority of these infections are caused by *Aspergillus fumigatus*, *Candida albicans*, *Cryptococcus neoformans*, and *Rhizopus arrhizus* (*see* box, p. 708, *top left*).[86]

Pathology. In general, CNS fungal infection results in a granulomatous reaction.[64] An acute polymorphonuclear leukocytic reaction and abscess formation are also common.[20]

Some fungi are known for their ability to invade blood vessels and cause hemorrhagic infarcts. Aspergillosis is an example (*see* box, p. 708, *top right*) (Fig. 16-42).

Age and incidence. Fungal infections of the brain and meninges are relatively rare but are becoming more common with the general increase in immunocompromised patients.

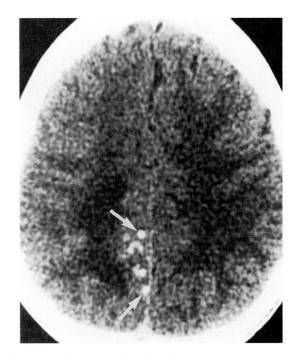

Fig. 16-41. Axial NECT scan in a child with seizures shows cortical and subcortical calcifications (*arrows*). Biopsy disclosed old tuberculomas.

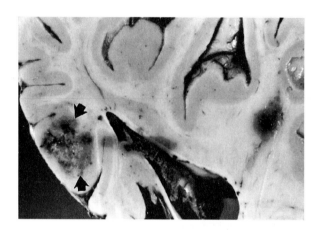

Fig. 16-42. Gross specimen of CNS aspergillosis shows hemorrhagic fungal abscesses *(arrows)* in the subcortical white matter. (Courtesy Rubinstein Collection, University of Virginia.)

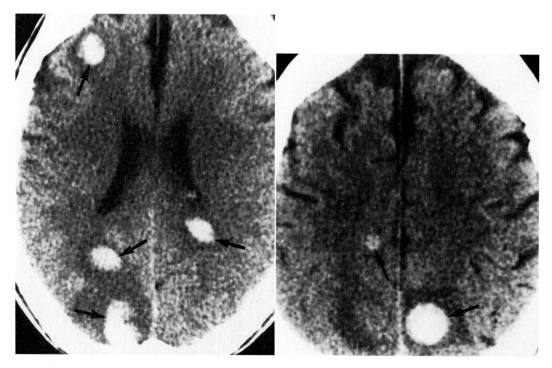

Fig. 16-43. Axial CT scans in a patient with necrotizing fungal vasculitis and multiple hemorrhagic foci *(arrows)*. Aspergillosis was seen at biopsy.

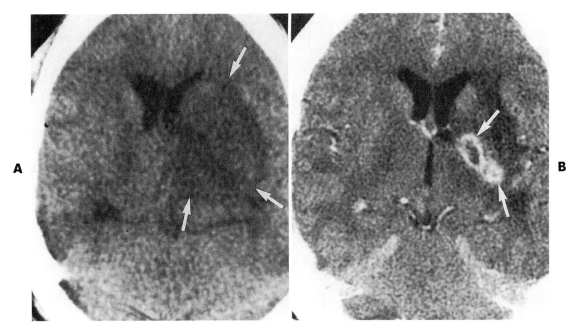

Fig. 16-44. Intracranial aspergillosis with basal ganglia infarct. **A,** Initial NECT scan shows low density changes in the left internal capsule, putamen, globus pallidus, and anterior thalamus *(arrows).* CECT scan (not shown) demonstrated slight patchy enhancement. **B,** Follow-up CECT scan 5 weeks later shows ring-enhancing lesions of subacute infarction. (Courtesy N. Yue.)

Location. Some fungal infections such as aspergillosis and mucormycosis involve the CNS by direct extension from nose and paranasal sites (*see* Chapter 12). Others, also including aspergillosis, reach the CNS via hematogenous spread from a pulmonary focus.

Imaging. Imaging findings vary somewhat according to the specific fungus involved. Cryptococcus produces gelatinous-appearing pseudocysts that extend along enlarged perivascular spaces, particularly in the basal ganglia (see previous discussion). Mucor tends to spread along perivascular and perineural channels through the cribriform plate into the frontal lobe or through the orbital apex into the cavernous sinus.[64] Intracranial mucor can also form a fungal abscess or invade blood vessels and cause cerebral infarction.[87,88]

Because aspergillosis is an angioinvasive fungus, its imaging findings are usually those of multifocal hemorrhagic mycetomas (Fig. 16-43) or penetrating or large vessel cerebral infarcts (Fig. 16-44).[89]

CNS coccidioidomycosis is usually seen as meningeal inflammation with infectious purulent and caseous granulomas. The basal meninges may appear strikingly thickened; communicating hydrocephalus is also common (*see* Fig. 16-16).[64]

PARASITIC INFECTIONS

Many parasites can cause CNS infections. Toxoplasmosis, cysticercosis, and schistosomiasis are

---

Parasitic CNS Infections

Immunocompetent individuals
Neurocysticercosis
Paragonimiasis
Sparganosis
Echinococcosis
Amebiasis
Malaria

Immunocompromised patients
Toxoplasmosis (exception: fetal infection)

---

common infections. Other parasitic infections with CNS manifestations include sparganosis, amebiasis, and echinococcosis (*see* box).

Toxoplasmosis has been discussed previously. In this section we emphasize the varied pathologic findings and imaging manifestations of neurocysticercosis, the most common parasitic CNS infection worldwide. We then briefly discuss less frequently encountered CNS parasitic infections.

Neurocysticercosis

Etiology. The larval form of the pork intestinal tapeworm *Taenia solium* is the agent responsible for neurocysticercosis (NCC). Humans are the definitive host for *T. solium* and usually harbor the adult tapeworm in the small intestine as an asymptomatic infestation. Fecal shedding of eggs by the definitive host, (i.e., man) leads to ingestion of eggs—usually in contaminated food or water—by the intermediate host, typically pig or man.[90]

Once inside the intestinal tract the eggs are released and produce oncospheres, the primary larvae. These larvae bore into the intestinal mucosa and enter the circulatory system. Hematogenous spread to neural, muscular, and ocular tissues occurs. Once inside the brain, the oncospheres develop into secondary larvae: the cysticerci.[64]

Because pathologic findings vary with lesion stage, these are discussed in concert with imaging manifestations of NCC (see subsequent discussion).

Incidence. NCC is the most common CNS parasitic infection worldwide[91] (*see* box). It is endemic in many areas such as Central and South America, eastern Europe, Africa, and parts of Asia. The general autopsy incidence of cysticercosis in such countries is approximately 4%.[92] Most cases in developed nations occur in immigrants from countries in which cysticercosis is endemic.

CNS involvement occurs in 60% to 90% of patients with cysticercosis.[93]

Location. The brain parenchyma is the most commonly affected site in NCC, seen in more than half of all cases.[94] The corticomedullary junction is the primary location. Intraventricular cysticercosis cysts are seen in 20% to 50% of cases (Fig. 16-45), with the fourth ventricle a common site.[95,96] Only 10% of NCC cases have isolated subarachnoid disease (Fig. 16-46). More than one anatomic compartment is often involved.[92]

Clinical presentation and natural history. Morbidity with NCC results from dead larvae that typically incite an intense host inflammatory response. NCC has a broad spectrum of clinical manifestations. Epilepsy is the most frequent symptom and is seen in 50% to 70% of cases.[91]

Pathology and imaging correlations. The pathologic manifestations of parenchymal cysticercosis have been classified into the following four stages: vesicular, vesicular colloidal, granular nodular, and

---

Neurocysticercosis

Most common CNS parasitic infection
Endemic in Central/South America, Africa, parts of Asia, Eastern Europe; immigrants from endemic areas
60% to 90% of patients with cysticercosis have CNS lesions
Brain parenchyma > ventricles > subarachnoid space
Dying larvae incite intense host inflammatory response
Imaging manifestations vary with stage (from nonenhancing cyst to ring-enhancing "target" lesion to calcified nodule)

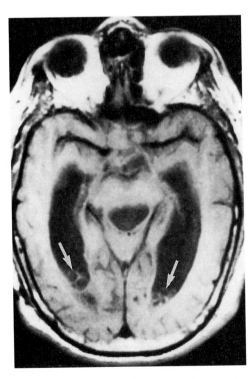

Fig. 16-45. Axial T1-weighted MR scan in a patient with cysticercosis shows multiple intraventricular cysts *(arrows)*. (Courtesy R. Jinkins.)

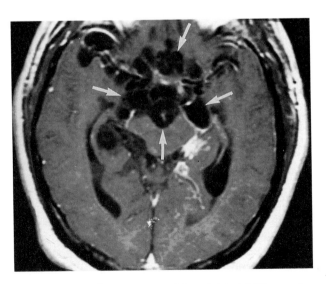

Fig. 16-46. Axial postcontrast T1-weighted MR scan in a patient with cystercosis shows multiple subarachnoid cysts *(arrows)*.

nodular calcified. Patients may have multiple lesions at different stages.[93]

Vesicular stage. During this first stage, a cysticercus consists of a thin capsule that surrounds a viable larva and its fluid-containing bladder. The fluid is clear, and little or no inflammatory reaction is present. On imaging studies obtained at this stage the larvum appears as a round CSF-like cyst with a mural nodule that represents its scolex (i.e., head). Edema and contrast enhancement are rare during this stage (Figs. 16-45, *A,* 16-47, *A*).[97]

Colloidal vesicular stage. When the larvum dies and begins to degenerate, the cystic fluid becomes turbid and the cyst shrinks as its capsule thickens. Degenerating larvae release metabolic products that disrupt the blood-brain barrier. Host inflammatory response ensues, resulting in edema and cyst wall enhancement on imaging studies (Figs. 16-45, *B* and *C;* 16-46, 16-47, *B;* and 16-48, *A*). Cyst fluid is hyperintense to CSF on MR scans performed during this stage (Fig. 16-48, *B*). Ringlike enhancement is seen in two thirds of cases[97] (Figs. 16-47, *C* and 16-48, *C*).

Granular nodular stage. The cyst retracts, its capsule thickens, and the scolex calcifies. NECT scans show an isodense cyst with a hyperdense calcified scolex. Surrounding edema is still present and en-

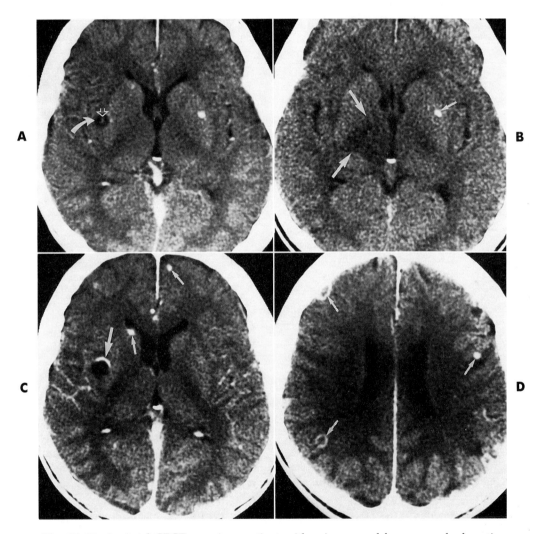

Fig. 16-47. A, Axial CECT scan in a patient with seizures and known cerebral cysticercosis shows a cystic lesion in the right external capsule *(curved arrow).* No edema is present and no cyst wall enhancement is seen. This represents the vesicular stage of infection. Note the scolex *(open arrow).* **B,** Axial NECT scan in the same patient obtained 10 weeks later shows edema in the right basal ganglia *(large arrows)* and a densely calcified mass in the left putamen *(small arrow).* The left-sided lesion represents the nodular calcified stage. The lesion on the right now represents the colloidal vesicular stage. **C,** CECT scan shows the cyst wall partially enhances *(large arrow).* Other lesions are seen that represent the granular nodular stage *(small arrows).* **D,** More cephalad CECT scan shows both micro-ring and nodular lesions *(small arrows).*

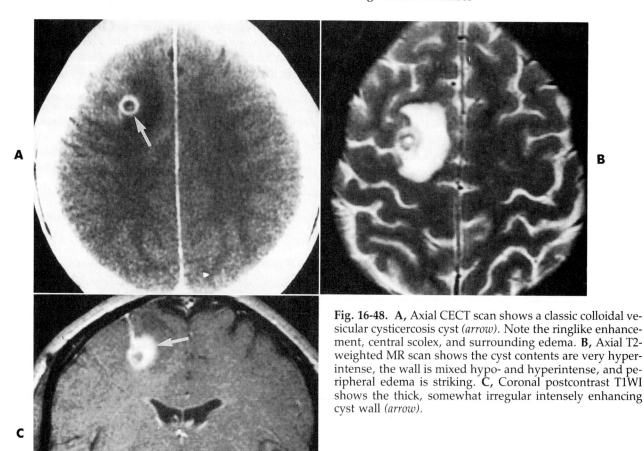

Fig. 16-48. A, Axial CECT scan shows a classic colloidal vesicular cysticercosis cyst *(arrow)*. Note the ringlike enhancement, central scolex, and surrounding edema. **B,** Axial T2-weighted MR scan shows the cyst contents are very hyperintense, the wall is mixed hypo- and hyperintense, and peripheral edema is striking. **C,** Coronal postcontrast T1WI shows the thick, somewhat irregular intensely enhancing cyst wall *(arrow)*.

hancement following contrast administration persists (Fig. 16-47, C). The residual cyst is typically isointense compared to brain on unenhanced T1WI and iso- to hypointense on T2-weighted sequences. Nodular or micro-ring enhancement is common at this stage, suggesting granuloma (Figs. 16-45, and 16-47, D).[97] Occasionally, a "target" or "bull's eye" appearance is seen with the calcified scolex in the center of the mass.

Nodular calcified stage. By this, the final stage, the granulomatous lesion has contracted to a fraction of its initial size and is completely mineralized (Fig. 16-45, B).[98] On NECT scans a small calcified nodule without mass effect or enhancement is typical.[97]

Miscellaneous Parasitic Infections

Paragonimiasis. Paragonimiasis is an infestation caused by a lung fluke of the genus *Paragonimus;* the most important human pathogen is *Paragonimus wes-*

termani. Paragonimiasis is endemic in East and Southeast Asia, parts of Africa, and Latin America.[93] Infection occurs when undercooked fish containing encysted larvae is ingested. Cerebral infection occurs in 1% of cases. Imaging findings vary with disease stage, although multiple conglomerate, ring-enhancing abscesslike lesions with striking peripheral edema are typical.[93]

Sparganosis. Sparganosis is an infection caused by sparganum, the migrating larva of *Spirometra mansoni.*[99] Sparganosis has been reported worldwide but is more common in East Asia.[100] Subcutaneous tissue or chest, abdominal wall, or limb muscles are the most commonly affected sites.

Cerebral sparganosis is rare.[99] An irregular mass that represents a granuloma encasing a sparganum is typical. Imaging findings are indistinguishable from other granulomas or neoplastic masses.[99]

Echinococcosis. Human echonococcosis, also known as hydatid disease, is caused by *Echinococcus granulosus*. The larval stage is known as the hydatid cyst.[101] Human echinococcosis is caused by ingestion of dog feces that contain tapeworm ova. Intermediate hosts infected by larval hydatid cysts are usually sheep and cattle.

Ingested ova hatch in the gastrointestinal tract. Liberated embryos can then spread to virtually every organ or tissue via the portal and systemic circulations. They subsequently develop into cystic larvae, classically termed an *echinococcal (hydatid) cyst*.[93]

Hydatid cysts occur most frequently in the liver (65%) and lung (20%). Skeletal involvement is less common; the skull and vertebrae are common sites.[93] Cerebral hydatid cysts are rare, seen in approximately 2% of cases. Hydatid cysts account for 1% to 5% of all intracranial masses in endemic areas.[101]

Imaging findings are striking. A single, thin-walled spherical CSF-density cyst in the parietal area is typical.[93] Multilocular or multiple lesions occur but are rare.

REFERENCES

1. Becker LE: Infections of the developing brain, *AJNR* 13:537-549, 1992.
2. Shaw DWW, Cohen WA: Viral infections of the CNS in children: imaging features, *AJR* 160:125-133, 1993.
3. Osborn RE, Byrd SE: Congenital infections of the brain, *Neuroimaging Clin N Amer* 1:105-118, 1991.
4. Sugita K, Ando M, Makino M et al: Magnetic resonance imaging of the brain in congenital rubella virus and cytomegalovirus infections, *Neuroradiol* 33:239-242, 1991.
5. Fitz CR: Inflammatory diseases of the brain in childhood, *AJNR* 13:551-567, 1992.
6. Drose JA, Dennis MA, Thickman D: Infection in utero: US findings in 19 cases, *Radiol* 178:369-374, 1991.
7. Tassin GB, Maklad NF, Stewart RR, Bell ME: Cytomegalic inclusion disease: intrauterine sonographic diagnosis using findings involving the brain, *AJNR* 12:117-122, 1991.
8. Boesch Ch, Issakainen J, Kewitz G et al: Magnetic resonance imaging of the brain in congenital cytomegalovirus infection, *Pediatr Radiol* 19:91-93, 1989.
9. Castillo M: Micrencephalia vera: CT findings, *AJR* 159:905-906, 1992.
10. Yamashita Y, Matsuishi T, Murakami Y et al: Neuroimaging findings (ultrasonography, CT, MRI) in 3 infants with congenital rubella syndrome, *Pediatr Radiol* 21:547-549, 1991.
11. Hutto C, Arvin A, Jacobs R et al: Intrauterine herpes simplex virus infections, *J Pediatr* 110:97-101, 1987.
12. Wood BP: Children with acquired immune deficiency syndrome, *Invest Radiol* 27:964-970, 1992.
13. Belman AL, Diamond G, Dickson D et al: Pediatric acquired immunodeficiency syndrome: neurologic syndromes, *Am J Dis Child* 152:29-35, 1988.
14. Kauffman WM, Sivit CJ, Fitz CR et al: CT and MR evaluation of intracranial involvement in pediatric HIV infection: a clinical-imaging correlation, *AJNR* 13:949-957, 1992.
15. Chamberlain MC, Nichols SL, Chase CH: Pediatric AIDS: comparative cranial MRI and CT scans, *Pediatr Neurol* 7:357-362, 1992.
16. Wasserstrom R, Mamourian AC, McGary CT, Miller G: Bulbar poliomyelitis: MR findings with pathologic correlation, *AJNR* 13:371-373, 1992.
17. Barkovich AJ: Infections of the nervous system. In AJ Barkovich: *Pediatric Neuroimaging*, pp 293-325, New York, Raven Press, 1990.
18. Harris TM, Edwards MK: Meningitis, *Neuroimaging Clin N Amer* 1:39-56, 1991.
19. Ashwal S, Tomasi L, Schneider S et al: Bacterial meningitis in children: pathophysiology and treatment, *Neurol* 42:739-748, 1992.
20. Okagaki H: *Fundamentals of Neuropathology*, ed 2, New York, Igaku-Shoin, 1989.
21. Chang KH, Han MH, Roh JK et al: Gd-DTPA-enhanced MR imaging of the brain in patients with meningitis: comparison with CT, *AJNR* 11:69-76, 1990.
21a. Pfister H-W, Feiden W, Einhäupl K-M: Spectrum of complications during bacterial meningitis in adults, *Arch Neurol* 50:575-581, 1993.
22. Chanalet S, Gense de Beaufort D, Gréselle JF et al: Clinical and radiological aspects of extracerebral empyemas: 39 cases, *Neuroradiol* 33(suppl):225-228, 1991.
22a. Wilms G, Venderschueren G, Demaerel PH et al: CT and MR in infants with pericerebral collections and macrocephaly: benign enlargement of the subarachnoid spaces versus subdural collections, *AJNR* 14:855-860, 1993.
23. Weingarten K, Simmerman RD, Becker RD et al: Subdural and epidural empyemas: MR imaging, *AJNR* 10:81-87, 1989.
24. Tsuchiya K, Makita K, Furui S et al: Contrast-enhanced magnetic resonance imaging of sub- and epidural empyemas, *Neuroradiol* 34:494-496, 1992.
25. Kerr L, Filloux FM: Cerebral infarction as a remote complication of childhood *Haemophilus influenzae* meningitis, *West J Med* 157:179-182, 1992.
26. Pfister H-W, Borasio GD, Dirnagl U et al: Cerebrovascular complications of bacterial meningitis in adults, *Neurol* 42:1497-1504, 1992.
27. Gee GT, Bazan C III, Jinks JR: Miliary tuberculosis involving the brain: MR findings, *AJR* 159:1075-1076, 1992.
28. Wrobel CJ, Meyer S, Johnson RH, Hesselink JR: MR findings in acute and chronic coccidioidomycosis meningitis, *AJNR* 13:1241-1245, 1992.
29. Buckner CB, Leithiser RE, Walker CW, Allison JW: The changing epidemiology of tuberculosis and other mycobacterial infections in the United States: implications for the radiologist, *AJR* 156:255-264, 1991.
30. Jinkins JR: Computed tomography of intracranial tuberculosis, *Neuroradiol* 33:126-135, 1991.
31. Callebaut J, Dormont D, Dubois B et al: Contrast-enhanced MR imaging of tuberculous pachymeningitis cranialis hypertrophic: case report, *AJNR* 11:821-822, 1990.
32. Hsieh F-Y, Chia L-G, Shen W-C: Locations of cerebral infarctions in tuberculous meningitis, *Neuroradiol* 34:197-199, 1992.
33. Chang K-H, Han M-H, Roh J-K et al: Gd-DTPA enhanced MR imaging in intracranial tuberculosis, *Neuroradiol* 238:340-344, 1991.
34. Mathews VP, Kuharik MA, Edwards MK et al: Gd-DTPA enhanced MR imaging of experimental bacterial meningitis: evaluation and comparison with CT, *AJNR* 9:1045-1050, 1988.
35. Offenbacher H, Fazekas F, Schmidt R et al: MRI in tuberculous meningoencephalitis: report of four cases and review of the neuroimaging literature, *J Neurol* 238:340-344, 1991.
36. Zimmerman RD, Weingarten K: Neuroimaging of cerebral abscesses, *Neuroimaging Clin N Amer* 1:1-16, 1991.
37. Enzmann DR, Britt RH, Yeager AS: Experimental brain abscess evaluation: computed tomographic and neuropathologic correlation, *Radiol* 133:113-122, 1979.

38. Enzmann DR, Britt RH, Placone R: Staging of human brain abscess by computed tomography, *Radiol* 146:703-708, 1983.

39. Grimstad IA, Hirschberg H, Rootwell K: ^{99m}Tc- hexamethyl-propyleneamine oxime leukocyte scintigraphy and C-reactive protein levels in the differential diagnosis of brain abscesses, *Neurosurg* 77:732-736, 1992.

40. Datz FL, Morton KA: New radiopharmaceuticals for detecting infection, *Invest Radiol* 28:356-366, 1993.

41. Haimes AB, Zimmerman RD, Morgello S et al: MR imaging of brain abscesses, *AJNR* 10:279-291, 1989.

42. Barloon TJ, Yuh WTC, Knepper LE et al: Cerebral ventriculitis: MR findings, *J Comp Asst Tomogr* 14:272-275, 1990.

43. Mathews VP, Smith RR: Choroid plexus infections: neuroimaging appearance of four cases, *AJNR* 13:374-378, 1992.

44. Morse RP, Bennish ML, Darras BT: Eastern equine encephalitis presenting with a focal brain lesion, *Pediatr Radiol* 8:473-475, 1992.

45. Jordan J, Enzmann DR: Encephalitis, *Neuroimaging Clin N Amer* 1:17-38, 1991.

46. Demaerel Ph, Wilms G, Robberecht W et al: MRI of herpes simplex encephalitis, *Neuroradiol* 34:490-493, 1992.

47. Mark LP, Daniels DL, Naidich TP, Borne JA: Limbic system anatomy: an overview, *AJNR* 14:349-352, 1993.

48. Soo MS, Tien RD, Gay L et al: Mesenchombencephalitis: MR findings in nine patients, *AJN* 160:1089-1093, 1993.

49. Enzmann D, Chang Y, Augustyn G: MR findings in neonatal herpes simplex encephalitis type II, *J Comp Asst Tomogr* 14:453-457, 1990.

50. Jarvik JG, Lenkinski RE, Grossman RI et al: Proton MR spectroscopy of HIV-infected patients: characterization of abnormalities with imaging and clinical correlation, *Radiol* 186:739-744, 1993.

50a. Whiteman MLH, Post MJD, Bowen BC, Bell MD: AIDS-related white matter diseases, *Neuroimaging Clin N Amer* 3:331-359, 1993.

51. Mathews VP, Alo PL, Glass JD et al: AIDS-related CNS cryptococcosis: radiologic-pathologic correlation, *AJNR* 13:1477-1486, 1992.

52. Meyerhoff DJ, MacKay S, Bachman L et al: Reduced brain N-acetylaspartate suggests neuronal loss in cognitively impaired human immunodeficiency virus-seropositive individuals, *Neurol* 43:509-515, 1993.

53. Balakrishnan J, Becker PS, Kumar AJ et al: Acquired immunodeficiency syndrome: correlation of radiologic and pathologic findings in the brain, *RadioGraphics* 10:201-215, 1990.

54. Hawkins CP, McLaughlin JE, Kendall BE, McDonald WI: Pathological findings correlated with MRI in HIV infection, *Neuroradiol* 35:264-268, 1993.

55. Flowers CH, Mafee MF, Crowell R et al: Encephalopathy in AIDS patients: evaluation with MR imaging, *AJNR* 11:1235-1245, 1990.

56. Chrysikopoulos HS, Press GA, Grafe MR et al: Encephalitis caused by human immunodeficiency virus: CT and MR imaging manifestations with clinical and pathologic correlation, *Radiol* 175:185-191, 1990.

57. Raininko R, Elovaara I, Virta A et al: Radiological study of the brain at various stages of human immunodeficiency virus infection: early development of brain atrophy, *Neuroradiol* 34:190-196, 1992.

58. Cohen WA, Maravilla KR, Gerlach R et al: Prospective cerebral MR study of HIV seropositive and seronegative men: correlation of MR findings with neurologic, neuropsychologic, and cerebrospinal fluid analysis, *AJNR* 13:1231-1240, 1992.

58a. Hawkins CP, McLaughlin JE, Kendall BE, McDonald WI: Pathological findings correlated with MRI in HIV infection, *Neuroradiol* 35:264-268, 1993.

59. Rovira MJ, Post MJD, Bowen BC: Central nervous system infections in HIV-infected persons, *Neuroimaging Clin N Amer* 1:179-200, 1991.

60. Revel M-P, Gray F, Brugieres P et al: Hyperdense CT foci in treated AIDS toxoplasmosis encephalitis: MR and pathologic correlation, *J Comp Asst Tomogr* 16:372-375, 1992.

61. Jensen MC, Brant-Zawadzki M: MR imaging of the brain in patients with AIDS: value of routine use of IV gadopentetate dimeglumine, *AJR* 160:153-157, 1993.

62. Dina TS: Primary central nervous system lymphoma versus toxoplasmosis in AIDS, *Radiol* 179:823-838, 1991.

62a. George JC, Caldemeyer KS, Smith RR, Czaja JT: CNS lymphomatoid granulomatous in AIDS: CT and MR appearances, *AJR* 161:381-383, 1993.

63. Tien RD, Chu PK, Hesselink JR et al: Intracranial crytocrocosis in immunocompromised patients: CT and MR findings in 29 cases, *AJNR* 12:283-289, 1991.

63a. Andreula CF, Luciani AR, Ladisa P, Carella A: L'aggressione subdola del criptocco al SNC, *Riv di Neuroradiol* 6:43-51, 1993.

64. Bowen BC, Post MJD: Intracranial infection. In SW Atlas, (editor), *Magnetic Resonance Imaging of the Brain and Spine,* pp 501-538, New York, Raven Press 1991.

65. Lentz D, Jordan JE, Pike GB, Enzmann DR: MRI in varicella-zoster virus leukoencephalitis in the immunocompromised host, *J Comp Asst Tomogr* 17:313-316, 1993.

66. Li J, Xiong L, Jinkins JR: Gadolinium-enhanced MRI in a patient with AIDS and the Ramsay-Hunt syndrome, *Neuroradiol* 35:269, 1993.

67. Tien RD, Gean-Marton AD, Mark AS: Neurosyphilis in HIV carriers: MR findings in six patients, *AJR* 158:1325-1328, 1992.

68. Berger JR, Washin H, Pall L et al: Syphilitic cerebral gumma with HIV infection, *Neurol* 42:1282-1287, 1992.

69. Villoria MF, de la Torre J, Fortes F et al: Intracranial tuberculosis in AIDS: CT and MRI findings, *Neuroradiol* 34:11-14, 1992.

70. Shoji H, Kusuhara T, Honda Y et al: Relapsing acute disseminated encephalomyelitis associated with chronic Epstein-Barr virus infection: MRI findings, *Neuroradiol* 34:350-342, 1992.

71. Bray PF, Culp KW, McFarlin DE et al: Demyelinating disease after neurologically complicated primary Epstein-Barr virus infection, *Neurol* 42:278-282, 1992.

72. Tolly TL, Wells RG, Sty JR: MR features of fleeting CNS lesions associated with Epstein-Barr virus infection, *J Comp Asst Tomogr* 13:665-668, 1989.

73. McLachlan RS, Girvin JP, Blume WT, Reichman H: Rasmussen's chronic encephalitis in adults, *Arch Neurol* 50:269-274, 1993.

74. Tien RD, Ashdown BC, Lewis DV Jr et al: Rasmussen's encephalitis: neuroimaging findings in four patients, *AJR* 158:1329-1332, 1992.

75. Sie TH, Weber W, Freling G et al: Rapidly fatal subacute sclerosing panencephlalitis, *Eur Neurol* 31:94-99, 1991.

76. Tsuchiya K, Yamauchi T, Furui S et al: MR imaging vs CT in subacute sclerosing panencephalitis, *AJNR* 9:943-946, 1988.

77. Atlas SW, Grossman RI, Goldberg HI et al: MR diagnosis of acute disseminated encephalomyelitis, *J Comp Asst Tomogr* 10:798-801, 1986.

78. Caldemeyer KS, Harris TM, Smith RR, Edwards MK: Gadolinium enhancement in acute disseminated encephalomyelitis, *J Comp Asst Tomogr* 15:673-675, 1991.

79. Broich K, Horwich D, Alavi A: HMPAO-SPECT and MRI in acute disseminated encephalomyelitis, *J Nucl Med* 32:1897-1900, 1991.

79a. Rosemberg S, Amaral LC, Kleimann SE, Arita FN: Acute encephalopathy with bilateral striatal necrosis: a distinctive clinicopathological condition, *Neuropediatr* 23:310-315, 1992.

80. Groen RJM, Begeer JH, Wilmink HT, le Coultre R: Acute cerebellar ataxia in a child with transient pontine lesions demonstrated by MRI, *Neuropediatr* 22:225-227, 1991.

80a. Caldemeyer KS, Edwards MK, Smith RR, Moran CC: Viral and postviral demyelination central nervous system infection, *Neuroimaging Clin N Amer* 3:305-317, 1993.

80b. Finkel MJ, Halperin JJ: Nervous system Lyme borreliosis: revisited, *Arch Neurol* 49:102-107, 1992.

81. de Castro CC, Hesselink JR: Tuberculosis, *Neuroimaging Clin N Amer* 1:119-139, 1991.

82. Bargallo N, Berenguer J, Tomas X et al: Intracranial tuberculosis: CT and MRI, *Eur Radiol* 3:123-128, 1993.

83. Gee DT, Bazan C III, Jinkins JR: Miliary tuberculosis involving the brain: MR findings, *AJR* 159:1075-1076, 1992.

84. Shen W-C, Cheng T-Y, Lee S-K et al: Disseminated tuberculomas in spinal cord and brain demonstrated by MRI with gadolinium-DTPA, *Neuroradiol* 35:213-215, 1993.

84a. Gupta RK, Pandey R, Khan EM et al: Intracranial tuberculomas: MRI signal intensity correlation with histopathology and localized proton spectroscopy, *Magnetic Resonance Imaging* 11:443-449, 1993.

85. Rajshekhar V, Haran RP, Prakash S, Chandy MJ: Differentiating solitary small cysticercus granulomas and tuberculomas in patients with epilepsy, *J Neurosurg* 78:402-406, 1993.

86. Bazan C III, Rinaldi MG, Rauch RR, Jinkins JR: Fungal infections of the brain, *Neuroimaging Clin N Amer* 1:57-88, 1991.

87. Yousem DM, Galetta SL, Gusnard DA, Goldberg HI: MR findings in rhinocerebral mucormycosis, *J Comp Asst Tomogr* 13:878-882, 1989.

88. Anand VK, Alemar G, Griswold JA Jr: Intracranial complications of mucormycosis: an experimental model and clinical review, *Laryngnscope* 102:656-662, 1992.

89. Cox J, Murtagh FR, Wilfong A, Brenner J: Cerebral aspergillosis: MR imaging and histopathologic correlation, *AJNR* 13:1489-1492, 1992.

90. Jackson A, Dobson MJ, Cooper PN: The Swiss cheese brain, *Br J Radiol* 65:1042-1044, 1992.

91. Del Brutto OH, Santibañez R, Noboa CA et al: Epilepsy due to neurocysticerosis: analysis of 203 patients, *Neurol* 42:389-392, 1992.

92. Couldwell WT, Zee C-S, Apuzzo MLJ: Definition of the role of contemporary surgical management in cisternal and parenchymatous cysticercosis cerebri, *Neurosurg* 28:231-237, 1991.

93. Chang KH, Cho SY, Hesselink JR, et al: Parasitic diseases of the central nervous system, *Neuroimaging Clin N Amer* 1:159-178, 1991.

94. Martinez HR, Rangel-Guerra R, Elizondo G et al: MR imaging in neurocysticerosis: a study of 56 cases, *AJNR* 10:1011-1019, 1989.

95. Teitelbaum GP, Otto RJ, Lin M et al: MR imaging of neurocysticercosis, *AJNR* 10:709-718, 1989.

96. Kramer J, Carrazana EJ, Cosgorve GR et al: Transaqueductal migration of a neurocysticercus cyst, *J Neurosurg* 77:956-958, 1992.

97. Chang KH, Lee JH, Han MH, Han MC: The role of contrast-enhanced MR imaging in the diagnosis of neurocysticercosis, *AJNR* 12:509-512, 1991.

98. Zee C-S, Segall HD, Boswell W et al: MR imaging of neurocysticercosis, *J Comp Asst Tomogr* 12:927-934, 1988.

99. Tsai M-D, Chang C-N, Ho Y-S et al: Cerebral sparganosis diagnosed and treated with stereotactic techniques, *J Neurosurg* 78:129-132, 1993.

100. Chang KH, Chi JG, Cho SY et al: Cerebral sparganosis: analysis of 34 cases with emphasis on CT features, *Neuroradiol* 34:1-8, 1992.

101. Diren HB, Ozcanli H, Bolok M, Kilic C: Unilocular orbital, cerebral and intraventricular cysts: CT diagnosis, *Neuroradiol* 35:149-150, 1993.

Inherited Metabolic, White Matter, and Degenerative Diseases of the Brain

"Things should be made as simple as possible. But no simpler."—Albert Einstein

The inherited metabolic and degenerative diseases are complex, heterogeneous brain disorders that defy easy categorization. Dividing white matter pathology into *dys*myelinating diseases (disorders with defective formation or maintenance of myelin) and *de*myelinating diseases (destruction of otherwise normally formed myelin) is a time-honored system. Recent classifications have focussed on the role of enzyme defects and organelle pathology in the pathogenesis of many metabolic disorders that affect the CNS. In this system the various neurodegenerative disorders are subdivided into lysosomal, peroxisomal, and mitochondrial diseases.[1]

Recognizing that simple is generally better and that no system yet devised is without flaws, we will discuss inherited metabolic brain disorders according to their pathologic-radiologic manifestations. We first briefly review normal myelination patterns in the developing brain, then turn our attention to the inherited metabolic disorders themselves. The first group of disorders mainly or exclusively involves the white matter, the so-called leukoencephalopathies. Other inherited diseases predominately affect gray matter. A few diseases affect both.

We close this chapter by considering neurodegenerative disorders in a special area, i.e., the basal ganglia.

Normal Myelination

Birth (full term)

Medulla
Dorsal midbrain
Inferior and superior cerebellar peduncles
Posterior limb of internal capsule
Ventrolateral thalamus

One month

Deep cerebellar white matter
Corticospinal tracts
Pre/postcentral gyri
Optic nerves, tracts

Three months

Brachium pontis, cerebellar folia
Ventral brainstem
Optic radiations
Anterior limb of internal capsule
Occipital subcortical U fibers
Corpus callosum splenium

Six months

Corpus callosum genu
Paracentral subcortical U fibers
Centrum semiovale (partial)

Eight months

Centrum semiovale (complete except for some fron-totemporal areas)
Subcortical U fibers (complete except for most rostral frontal areas)

Eighteen months

Essentially like adult

Table 17-1. MR Myelination/Developmental Markers

Structure	High signal (T1WI) first appears at:	Low signal (T2WI) first appears at:
Posterior fossa		
Dorsal medulla/midbrain	Birth	Birth
Inferior/superior cerebellar peduncles	Birth	Birth
Middle cerebellar peduncle	1 month	3 months
Cerebellar white matter (deep to peripheral)	1 to 3 months	8 to 18 months
Supratentorial		
Internal capsule		
Posterior limb	Birth	Birth
Anterior limb	3 months	3 to 6 months
Thalamus (ventro-lateral nuclei)	Birth	Birth
Pre/postcentral gyri	1 month	8 to 12 months
Corpus callosum		
Splenium	3 to 4 months	6 months
Genu	6 months	8 months
Centrum semiovale (deep)	Birth to 1 month	3 months
Optic radiations	3 months	3 months
Subcortical U fibers (posterior to anterior)	3 to 8 months (occipital first)	8 to 18 months (frontal last)

Modified from Byrd SE, Darling CR, Wilczynski NA: White matter of the brain: maturation and myelination on magnetic resonance in infants and children, *Neuroimaging Clin N Amer* 3:247-266, 1993; Bird CR, Hedberg M, Drayer BP et al: MR assessment of myelination in infants and children: usefulness of marker sites, *AJNR* 10:731-740, 1989; Barkovich AJ, *Pediatric Neuroimaging*, pp 13-24, New York, Raven Press, 1990; Barkovich AJ, Lyon G, Evrard P: Formation, maturation and disorders of white matter, *AJNR* 13:447-461, 1992; and Barkovich AJ: Brain development: normal and abnormal. In SW Atlas, editor, *Magnetic resonance imaging of the brain and spine*, p. 139, New York, Raven Press, 1991.

NORMAL MYELINATION

Normal brain myelination is a dynamic process that begins during the fifth fetal month and continues throughout life.[2] Myelination usually occurs in highly predictable, very orderly patterns. Delays in, or departures from, the expected patterns can be detected and exquisitely delineated with MR imaging.[2a]

In general, myelination progresses from caudad to cephalad, from dorsal to ventral, and from central to peripheral.[3] Sensory tracts also generally myelinate earlier than fiber systems that correlate sensory data into movement.[1] Myelination takes place rapidly during the first 2 years, by which time it is nearly completed. Some association tracts remain unmyelinated until age 20 to 30 years (*see* box.)

The MR imaging appearance of normal brain changes substantially as the pulse sequences are var-ied. Brain maturation occurs at different rates and times on T1- compared to T2-weighted images[4] (Table 17-1). We will therefore discuss the normal appearance of the developing brain on both T1- and T2-weighted sequences. Whereas the standard "T2-weighted" spin-echo sequences throughout this text used TRs between 2500 and 3000 msec and TEs of 70 to 90 msecs, to image the infant brain we typically use TRs of up to 3500 to 4000 msec and TEs between 80 and 120 msec.

Birth (Term Infant)

At birth, much of the brain is unmyelinated and there is relatively poor differentiation between gray and white matter, especially on T1- and proton density-weighted sequences.[5] The relative signal intensities of cortex and white matter are reversed compared to the pattern normally seen in older children and adults.[6]

T1-weighted scans. The following areas are myelinated at birth and therefore exhibit high signal intensity:

Medulla
Dorsal midbrain
Inferior and superior cerebellar peduncles
Posterior limb of the internal capsule

Small areas of myelinated white matter may extend a short distance from the posterior limb superiorly into the corona radiata. The ventrolateral thalamus of normal term infants also appears hyperintense on T1WI.[6,7]

T2-weighted scans. Unmyelinated white matter appears very hyperintense relative to the low signal cortex. Structures that are myelinated, and also therefore low signal on T2WI, include the dorsal midbrain, inferior and superior cerebellar peduncles, and parts of the posterior limb of the internal capsule (Fig. 17-1, A to C). The ventrolateral thalamus and perirolandic gyri are also low signal (Fig. 17-1, D).[7]

Three Postnatal Months

Myelination proceeds rapidly during the first few postnatal months.

T1-weighted scans. High signal can now be seen in the deep cerebellar white matter, folia, and middle cerebellar peduncles, the ventral brainstem, and corticospinal tracts, as well as the optic nerves, tracts, and optic radiations. The anterior limb of the internal capsule is now myelinated. The subcortical white matter in the occipital pole is also high signal.

T2-weighted scans. At 1 month there is little change from the appearance at birth. However, by 3 months low signal can be seen throughout the cerebellar white matter, anterior limb of the internal capsule, the optic radiations, and some parts of the centrum semiovale (Fig. 17-2).

Six Postnatal Months

T1-weighted scans. By 4 months, high signal is seen in the corpus callosum splenium; by 6 months, the genu also normally appears hyperintense. Myelination has proceeded further into the centrum semiovale and toward the more rostral subcortical white matter.

T2-weighted scans. There is little change at 4 months from the pattern seen at 3 months. However, by 6 months after birth the centrum semiovale begins to show decreased signal.

Eight Postnatal Months

By the eighth postnatal month the infant brain is largely myelinated and the appearance on MR imaging approaches the adult pattern.

T1-weighted scans. High signal is now present in virtually all white matter except in the most anterior frontal subcortical areas (Fig. 17-3).

T2-weighted scans. The centrum semiovale and all but the most rostral subcortical U fibers are hypointense relative to cortex.

Three Years of Age

T2-weighted scans. Very heavily myelinated, compact white matter fiber pathways such as the anterior commissure, internal capsule, corpus callosum, and uncinate fasciculus normally show very low signal intensity, whereas association fiber tracts around the ventricular trigones are still unmyelinated and therefore remain hyperintense (Fig. 17-3, C). These tracts often do not myelinate until age 30. Other areas that also normally appear hyperintense on T2WI are adjacent to the frontal horns. There are relatively fewer white matter fibers here, and therefore a "cap" of high signal intensity on T2WI is normal (Fig. 17-3, B).

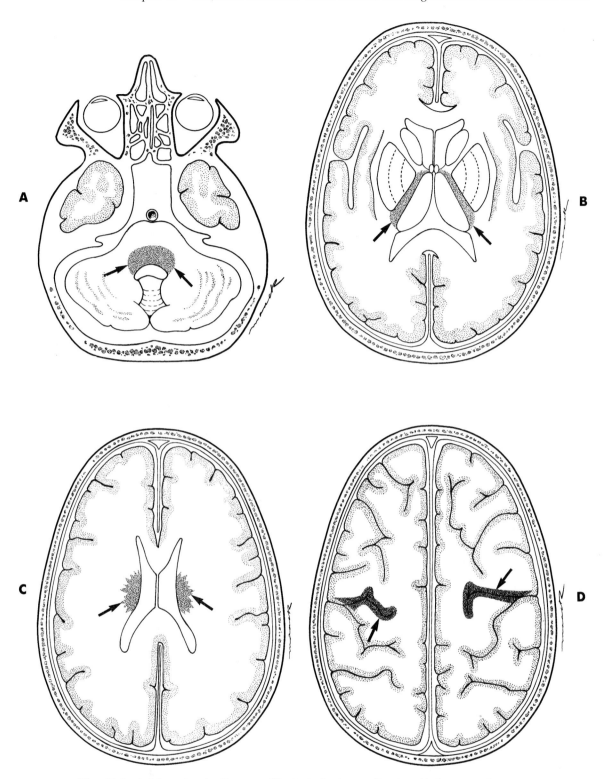

Fig. 17-1. Axial anatomic diagrams illustrate brain myelination *(dark patterned areas: arrows)* present at birth. **A,** Posterior fossa myelinated areas include the dorsal midbrain *(arrows),* as well as the medulla and inferior and superior cerebellar peduncles. **B,** The posterior limb of the internal capsule is myelinated; some myelination also extends superiorly into the deep centrum semiovale (**C,** *arrows*). **D,** No myelination is present in the subcortical U (arcuate) fibers but the pre- and postcentral gyri *(arrows)* often appear low signal on T2-weighted MR scans by the first postnatal month.

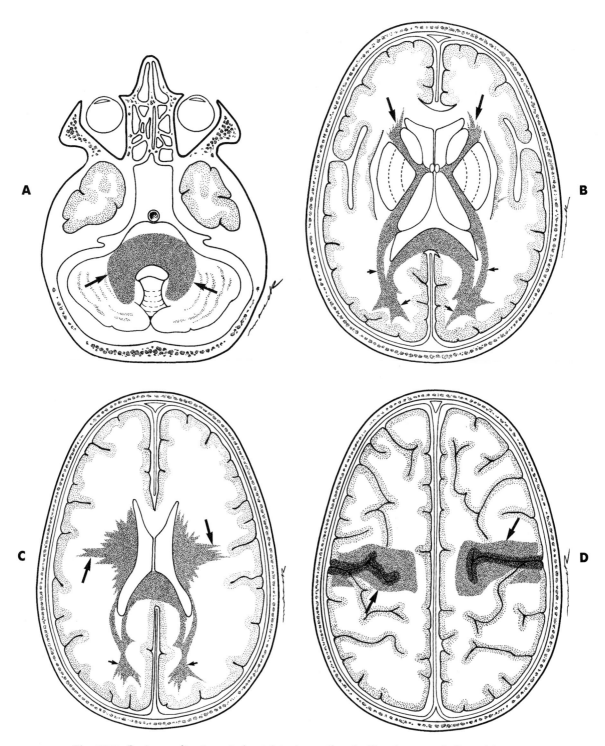

Fig. 17-2. Brain myelination at about 3 to 4 months. **A,** The deep cerebellar white matter and corticospinal tracts are myelinated. **B,** The anterior limb of the internal capsule *(large arrows)* and corpus callosum splenium are now at least partially myelinated. Occipital radiations and subcortical arcuate fibers are beginning to myelinate (**B** and **C,** *small arrows*). **C,** Myelination also extends further into the centrum semiovale *(large arrows).* **D,** Some arcuate fiber and centrum semiovale myelination around the pre- and postcentral gyri is present *(arrows).*

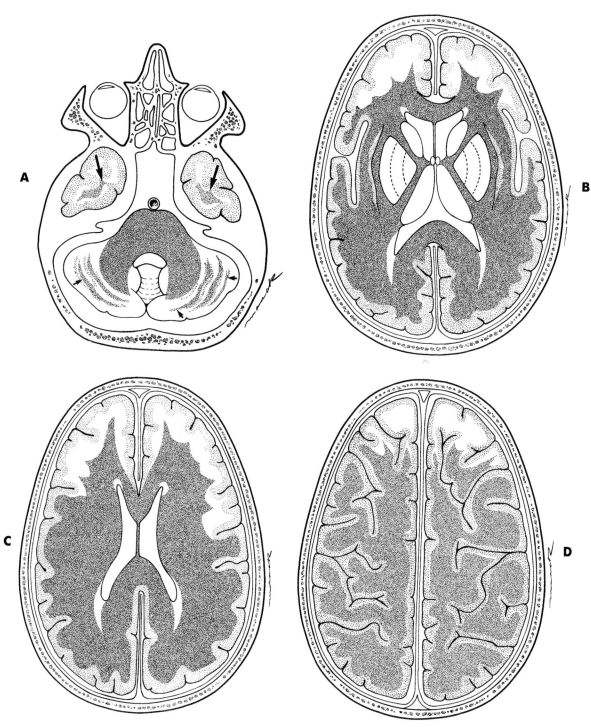

Fig. 17-3. Normal myelination between 6 and 8 months. **A,** Myelination of the cerebellar white matter is nearly completed and extends peripherally to the folia *(small arrows).* Temporal lobe myelination *(large arrows)* is present. **B,** The corpus callosum genu is also myelinated. **C** and **D,** Myelination extends through the centrum semiovale into the subcortical U fibers and is virtually complete except for some frontotemporal areas. The peritrigonal white matter may not myelinate completely until age 20 to 30 years.

DISORDERS THAT PRIMARILY AFFECT WHITE MATTER (LEUKODYSTROPHIES)

The leukodystrophies, also known as dysmyelinating diseases, are a heterogeneous group of disorders characterized by enzyme deficiencies that result in abnormal formation, destruction, or turnover of myelin.[8,9]

In some diseases such as metachromatic leukodystrophy the specific biochemical abnormalities have been identified; in others (e.g., Alexander disease), the enzyme defect has not been determined. Some leukodystrophies have distinctive imaging features (see box); many others have nonspecific findings.

There are many different leukodystrophies. In this chapter we focus on the more common and important of these disorders. The first two, metachromatic leukodystrophy and Krabbe disease, are lysosomal enzyme disorders (Table 17-2). The next, adrenoleukodystrophy, is caused by a single peroxisomal enzyme defect. Pelizaeus-Merzbacher disease is caused by defective biosynthesis of proteolipid protein,

whereas a cytosolic enzyme defect has been implicated in another striking leukodystrophy, Canavan disease. Leukodystrophies with unknown etiologies include Alexander disease, Cockayne disease, and sudanophilic leukodystrophy.[9] We close our discussion of inherited white matter diseases by considering the amino acid disorders.

Metachromatic Leukodystrophy

Etiology, inheritance, and pathology

Etiology and inheritance. Metachromatic leukodystrophy (MLD) is a lysosomal disorder caused by a deficiency of the catabolic enzyme arylsulfatase A. Inheritance is autosomal recessive.[10]

Pathology. Symmetric demyelination that spares the subcortical U fibers is characteristic (Fig. 17-4, *A* and *B*).[9] The cerebellum is often atrophic. Microscopic findings include axonal loss with astrogliosis.[9] A metchromatic lipid material, galactosylceramide sulfatide, accumulates in the peripheral and central nervous system white matter.[11]

Incidence and age. MLD is the most common hereditary leukodystrophy, with a prevalence of 1 in 100,000 newborns.[11] Three different types of MLD are recognized according to age at onset. These are

---

Leukodystrophies
Distinctive features

Complete/near complete lack of myelination
Canavan disease
Pelizaeus-Merzbacher disease

Frontal white matter most involved
Alexander disease

Occipital white matter most involved
Adrenoleukodystrophy (also callosal splenium)

Macrocephaly
Alexander disease
Canavan disease
Mucopolysaccharidosis type I (Hurler)
Mucopolysaccharidosrs type II (Hunter)

Thick meninges
Hurler syndrome

High density basal ganglia
Krabbe disease

Enhancement following contrast administration
Alexander disease
ALD

Strokes
Leigh syndrome
MELAS
MERRF
Homocystinuria

Table 17-2. Lysosomal Disorders

Disorder	Enzyme Deficiency
Sphingolipidoses	
Metachromatic leukodystrophy	Arylsulfatase A
Krabbe disease	Galactocerebroside beta-galactosidase
Niemann-Pick disease	Sphingomyelinase
Fabry disease	Alpha-galactosidase A
GM1 gangliosidosis (pseudo-Hurler)	Beta-galactosidase
GM2 gangliosidosis (Tay-Sachs, Sandhoff disease)	Beta-hexosaminidase A/B
Mucolipidoses (e.g., fucosidosis)	Varies (alpha-fucosidase with fucosidosis)
Canavan disease	Aspartoacylase
Mucopolysaccharidoses (e.g., Hurler, Hunter)	Varies (alpha-L-iduronidase with Hurler)
Ceroid lipofuscinoses (e.g., Batten disease)	Varies (ATP synthesase with Batten disease)

Data from Kendall BE: Disorders of lysosomes, peroxisomes, and mitochondria, *AJNR* 13:621-653, 1992.

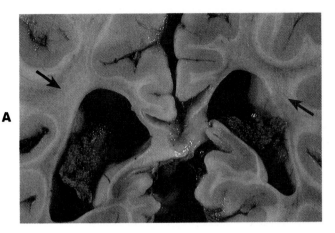

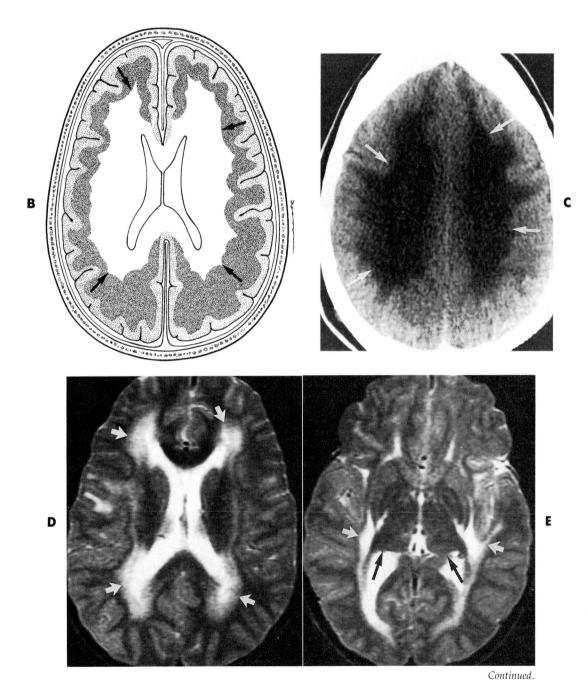

Fig. 17-4. A, Metachromatic leukodystrophy (MLD) is illustrated on this coronal autopsy specimen. Note extensive white matter demyelination *(arrows)* that spares the subcortical **U** fibers. Volume loss has caused moderate ventricular enlargement **B,** Axial anatomic diagram depicts MLD. Extensive, confluent periventricular demyelination is present *(arrows)*. Note sparing of the subcortical **U** fibers. **C,** Axial NECT scan in a 22-year-old man with MLD. Note bilateral symmetric low density areas in the centrum semiovale *(arrows)*. Involvement is more severe anteriorly and there is some arcuate fiber tract sparing, particularly in the occipital lobes. **D** and **E,** Axial T2-weighted MR scans in a 9-year-old boy with MLD. Note periventricular and deep white matter high signal areas *(white arrows)*. The thalami are abnormally hypointense (**E,** *black arrows*). (**A,** Courtesy E. Ross.)

Continued.

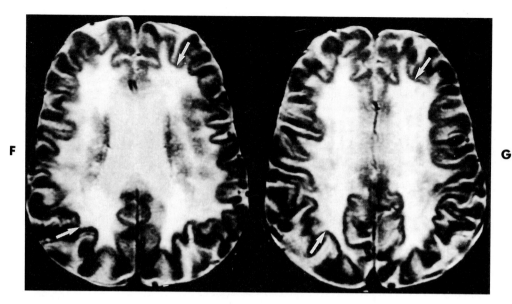

Fig. 17-4, cont'd. F and **G,** Axial T2-weighted scans in a 40-year-old man with adult-onset MLD. Note confluent white matter demyelination *(arrows)* and moderately severe cortical atrophy. Arcuate fiber involvement, present in this case, usually is not seen until late in the disease course.

the late infantile, juvenile, and adult forms. Approximately 80% of cases occur in childhood with onset typically between 1 and 2 years of age.[9,11]

Location. MLD involves the deep periventricular white matter and typically spares the arcuate fibers until late in the disease process (Fig. 17-4, *B*). The anterior white matter is more severely affected.[10]

Clinical presentation and natural history. In its most common form, late infantile MLD, motor signs of peripheral neuropathy are followed by deterioration in intellect, speech, and coordination. Within 2 years of onset, gait disorders, quadriplegia, blindness, and decerebrate posturing can be seen.[9] Disease progress is inexorable, and death occurs within 6 months to 4 years following symptom onset.[11]

Imaging
CT. NECT scans show moderate ventricular enlargement. Low density lesions are present, progressing anteriorly to posteriorly within the white matter (Fig. 17-4, *C*).[11] CT scans show no enhancement following contrast administration.[10]

MR. Diffuse confluent high signal is present in the periventricular white matter on T2WI (Fig. 17-4, *D*). Initially the arcuate fibers are spared. A striking feature in many cases is increased signal in the cerebellar white matter.[12] The thalami may appear mildly to extremely hypointense (Fig. 17-4, *E*). Corticosubcortical atrophy often occurs in later stages of the dis-

ease, particularly when myelin loss extends into the subcortical arcuate fibers (Fig. 17-4, *F* and *G*).[10]

Krabbe Disease
Krabbe disease is also known as globoid cell leukodystrophy (GLD).

Etiology, inheritance, and pathology
Etiology and inheritance. GLD is a lysosomal disorder that is caused by deficiency of the lysosomal hydrolase galactocerebroside beta-galactosidase.[13] Inheritance is autosomal recessive.

Pathology. The brain is small and atrophic. Extensive symmetric dysmyelination of the centrum semiovale and corona radiata with subcortical arcuate fiber sparing is seen. The cerebellar white matter is affected but to a lesser degree.[9] Microscopically, there is myelin loss with astrogliosis. Perivascular clusters of large multinucleated "globoid" and mononuclear epitheloid cells are present in the demyelinated zones.[11]

Incidence and age. There is a reported prevalence of 1:50,000 in Sweden but the incidence is much lower elsewhere.[11] Infantile, late infantile, and adult-onset Krabbe disease are recognized. The infantile form is the most common.[12,12a]

Location. The centrum semiovale and periventricular white matter are most severely affected; the subcortical U fibers are relatively spared (Fig. 17-5,

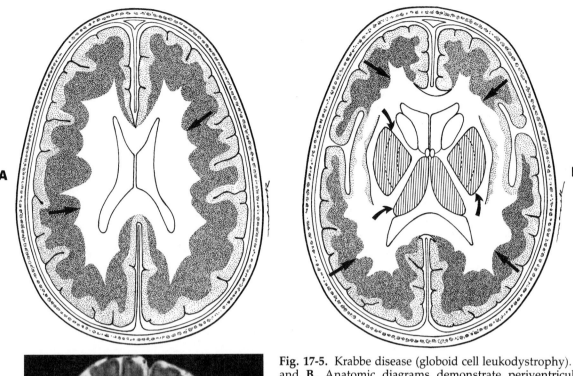

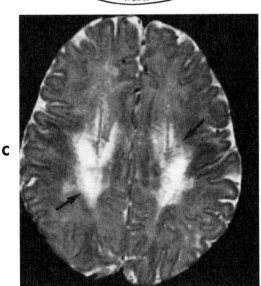

Fig. 17-5. Krabbe disease (globoid cell leukodystrophy). **A** and **B,** Anatomic diagrams demonstrate periventricular white matter demyelination *(white areas: large arrows)* and hyperdense basal ganglia and thalami *(vertical lines: curved arrows).* **C,** Axial T2-weighted MR scan in a 10-month-old child with Krabbe disease. The periventricular demyelination *(arrows)* is typical but not pathognomonic for Krabbe disease. Note early involvement of parietooccipital white matter.

A). The parietooccipital lobes may be selectively involved early in the disease course (Fig. 17-5, *C*).[12b]

Clinical presentation and natural history. Psychomotor deterioration, irritability, optic atrophy, and cortical blindness are seen. Seizures may occur in later stages. Krabbe disease typically is rapidly progressive and fatal.[11]

Imaging

CT. The thalami and basal ganglia often appear hyperdense on NECT scans (Fig. 17-5, *B*).[13] The corona radiata and cerebellum may show similar changes.[14] Diffuse low density is present in the periventricular white matter. No enhancement occurs following contrast administration.

MR. Nonspecific confluent, symmetric periventricular white matter hyperintensities are present on T2-weighted studies (Fig. 17-5, *C*). Late-onset disease may show changes limited to the posterior hemispheric white matter. Severe progressive atrophy occurs in the infantile form of GLD.[12,12a]

Adrenoleukodystrophy (X-linked)

Peroxisomes are small intracellular organelles that are involved in the oxidation of very long-chain and monounsaturated fatty acids.[15] Peroxisomal enzymes are also involved in gluconeogenesis, lysine metabolism, and glutaric acid catabolism.[1] Peroxisomal disorders are inborn errors of cellular metabolism caused by the deficiency of one or more of these enzymes. X-linked adrenoleukodystrophy is a leukodystrophy caused by a single peroxisomal enzyme deficiency, whereas Zellweger syndrome and neonatal adrenoleukodystrophy affect both the gray and white matter and are caused by multiple enzyme defects *(see box, p. 727) (see subsequent section).*[1]

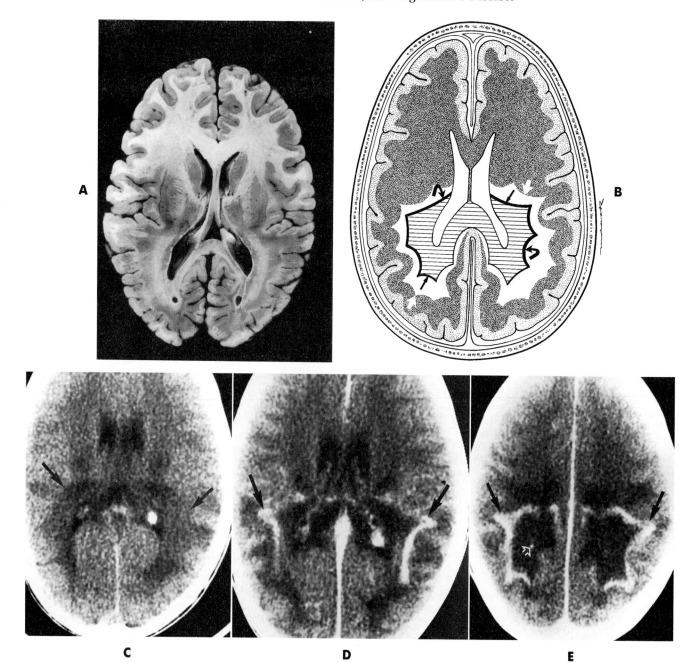

Fig. 17-6. X-linked adrenoleukodystrophy (ALD). **A,** Axial autopsy specimen demonstrates gross pathologic changes of ALD. Note striking bilateral demyelination in the peritrigonal areas and corpus callosum splenium **B,** Anatomic diagram illustrates the three zones typical of ALD. The central necrotic zone is indicated by the horizontal lines and small black arrows. The intermediate zone of active demyelination that enhances following contrast administration is indicated by the solid black line and curved arrows. The peripheral demyelinating area without inflammatory change is shown in white and indicated by the large white arrows. **C to E,** Pre- **(C)** and postcontrast **(D and E)** axial CT scans in a 6-year-old boy with 1-month history of progressive ataxia and dysarthria. The precontrast study shows bilaterally symmetric low density areas in both periatrial regions **(C,** *arrows*). The anterolateral margins enhance strongly following contrast administration **(D and E,** *arrows*). Note small focus of calcification **(E,** *open arrows*). Adrenoleukodystrophy. **F and G,** Axial postcontrast T1- **(F)** and T2-weighted **(G)** MR scans in another patient with ALD show striking bilateral periatrial enhancement **(F,** *arrows*) and active demyelination **(G,** *arrows*). **(A,** From Okazaki H, Scheithauer B, *Slide Atlas of Neuropathology,* Gower Medical Publishing. **F and G,** Courtesy C. Sutton.)

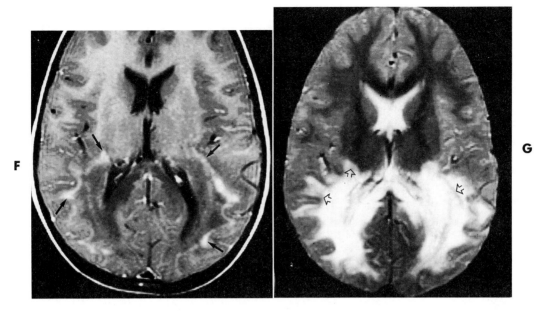

Fig. 17-6 cont'd.   For legend see p. 726.

Peroxisomal Disorders
Peroxisomes absent
Zellweger syndrome
Neonatal adrenoleukodystrophy
Infantile Refsum disease
Hyperpipecolic acidemia
Peroxisomes present with single enzyme deficiency
Adrenoleukodystrophy (X-linked)
Adrenomyeloneuropathy
Hyperoxaluria type 1
Acatalasia
Acyl-CoA oxidase deficiency
Pseudo-Zellweger syndrome
Peroxisomes present with multiple enzyme defects
Rhizomelic chondrodysplasia punctata

Data from Naidu SB, Moser H: Infantile Refsum disease, *AJNR* 12:1161-1163, 1991.

Etiology, inheritance, and pathology

Etiology and inheritance. Adrenoleukodystrophy-adrenomyeloneuropathy complex is a group of three closely related peroxisomal disorders, as follows:

1. Adrenoleukodystrophy (ALD)
2. Adrenomyeloneuropathy (AMN)
3. Adrenoleukomyeloneuropathy (ALMN)

Classic ALD is caused by deficiency of a single enzyme, acyl-CoA synthesase. This prevents breakdown of very long-chain fatty acids (VLFAs). VLFAs then accumulate in numerous tissues and plasma.[16] Inheritance is X-linked recessive.

A rare form of ALD, neonatal adrenoleukodystrophy, is an autosomal recessive disorder with multiple enzyme deficiencies.

Gross pathology. Autopsy specimens of ALD show enlarged ventricles and cerebral atrophy due to white matter volume loss. The cortex is normal. Demyelination classically first involves the occipital lobes and corpus callosum splenium in a bilaterally symmetric pattern (Fig. 17-6, *A*). Atypical ALD patterns include unilateral or predominately frontal disease (see subsequent discussion).

Microscopic appearance. The affected cerebral white matter typically has three zones,[1] as follows:

1. An innermost central and posterior zone with necrosis, gliosis, and, sometimes, calcification
2. An intermediate zone of active demyelination and inflammatory changes
3. A peripheral zone of demyelination without inflammatory reaction

Incidence, gender, and age. X-linked ALD is seen in males. Symptom onset typically occurs between 3 and 10 years of age. This childhood type of ALD represents 40% of all ALD-AMN cases.[17] AMN is the second most common form. Symptom onset is typical in young adulthood in members of families affected by childhood ALD.[18] AMN represents approximately 20% of ALD-AMN cases.[17]

Location. In the early stages of classical ALD, symmetric white matter demyelination occurs in the peritrigonal regions and extends across the corpus callosum splenium (Fig. 17-6, *A* and *B*).[1] Demyelination then spreads outward and forward as a confluent lesion until most of the cerebral white matter is affected. Auditory pathway involvement is common.[19] The subcortical white matter is relatively spared early but is often involved in later stages.[20,21]

Atypical cases with unilateral or predominately frontal lobe involvement occur.[16,22] Secondary degenerative changes in the posterior limb of the internal capsule, cerebral peduncles, pons, pyramid, and cerebellum are common.[9]

Adrenomyeloneuropathy typically involves the spinal cord and peripheral nerves.[12] The most common imaging manifestation is spinal cord atrophy, seen in approximately 30% of AMN patients. The thoracic cord is most commonly involved.[18]

Clinical presentation and natural history. The various ALD-AMN phenotypes involve the central and peripheral nervous systems and the endocrine systems differently.[18] In childhood ALD, neurologic abnormalities precede adrenal insufficiency in over 80% of cases.[17] Visual and behavioral disturbances are the most frequent initial symptoms.[9,19] Seizures, hearing loss, corticospinal tract involvement, and spastic quadraparesis occur. The interval between the first neurologic symptoms and vegetative state is approximately 2 years.[17]

Symptom onset in AMN is typically later, usually between the ages of 20 and 30 years.[18] Paraparesis is seen in virtually all cases, and adrenal dysfunction occurs in 87%. Cerebral involvement is seen in only 10% of cases.[17] Female heterozygotes are usually asymptomatic but approximately 12% have spastic paraparesis.[18]

Imaging. The definitive diagnosis of ALD is made by plasma, erythrocyte, or cultured skin fibroblast assay for the presence of increased VLFAs.[2] Imaging findings in most cases are characteristic.

CT. NECT scans typically show large, symmetric low density lesions in the parietooccipital (peritrigonal) regions (Fig. 17-6, *C*). Calcifications occasionally can be identified (Fig. 17-6, *E*). CECT scans show enhancement in the advancing rim, surrounded by a more peripheral nonenhancing edematous zone (Figs. 17-6, *D* and *E*).[17]

MR. The three histopathologic zones described in ALD can be delineated on MR (Fig. 17-6, *F* and *G*). The central necrotic zone is seen as a low signal region on T1WI and a homogeneously very hyperintense region on T2-weighted sequences. The intermediate zone of active demyelination and inflammation enhances following contrast administration. It is interposed between the central necrotic zone and the more peripheral, nonenhancing edematous area that is slightly hypointense on T1- and hyperintense on T2-weighted images.[20] Abnormal signal is usually present in the lateral geniculate bodies and auditory pathways, as well as the corpus callosum splenium and corticospinal tracts.[19]

Findings in AMN are symmetric hyperintensities in the posterior limb of the internal capsule on T2WI. The frontal, parietal, occipital, and temporal lobe white matter is spared.[21]

Pelizaeus-Merzbacher Disease

Etiology, inheritance, and pathology
Etiology and inheritance. Pelizaeus-Merzbacher disease (PMD) has been linked to a severe deficiency of myelin-specific lipids caused by a lack of proteolipid apoprotein (lipophilin).[9] The myelin-specific proteolipid protein is necessary for oligodendrocyte differentiation and survival.[11]

Two main forms of PMD are recognized: the classical form, type I, is X-linked recessive in inheritance. The connatal form, type II, is either X-linked or autosomal recessive.[23] A transitional form has also been described.[24]

Gross pathology. The brain and cerebellum are atrophic. The ventricles are large and there is patchy white matter demyelination. The cortex is normal (Fig. 17-7, *A*).[9]

Microscopic appearance. Patchy demyelination with characteristic sparing of perivascular white matter creates a "tigroid" or "leopard-skin" pattern. Lipid-laden macrophages are often present.[9]

Incidence, gender, and age. PMD is a rare neurodegenerative disorder that typically occurs in young boys, although rare cases in females have been reported. Symptom onset in type I PMD occurs during infancy or early childhood, whereas the connatal form, type II, is clinically more severe and symptoms begin in the neonatal period.[23]

Location. In the connatal type there is marked paucity to complete absence of myelin in all parts of the brain. Some residual myelin may be present in the diencephalon, brainstem, and cerebellum, as well as in the subcortical white matter.[24] Less pronounced changes are seen in the classical type I PMD. The internal capsule and subcortical U fibers are preserved and residual islands of perivascular white matter myelination are present (Fig. 17-7, *B*).

Clinical presentation and natural history. The classic PMD (type I) has its onset during infancy. Early symptoms are poor head control, nystagmus, and cerebellar ataxia.[21] The disease progresses slowly; death occurs in late adolescence or young adulthood.

The connatal type of PMD is a more severe variant. Abnormal eye movements are present in the neonatal period, and psychomotor development is severely

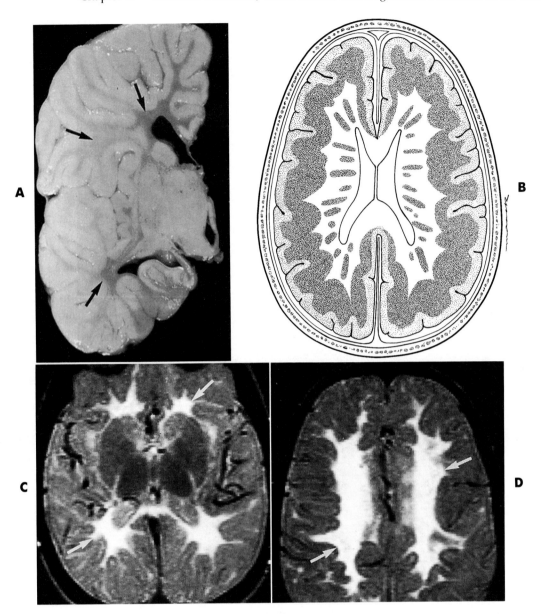

Fig. 17-7. Pelizaeus-Merzbacher disease (PMD). **A,** Coronal gross pathology specimen from an infant with connatal PMD shows marked white matter hypomyelination *(arrows).* **B,** Axial anatomic drawing of PMD shows extensive periventricular demyelination. Note islands of residual myelin around penetrating vessels, giving the "tigroid" appearance sometimes noted in PMD. **C** and **D,** Axial T2-weighted MR scans in an 8-year-old boy with PMD who was normal at birth. At age 3 years he developed progressive gait disturbance, limb ataxia, and nystagmus. Note extensive high signal throughout the white matter *(arrows).* Some residual myelination is present in the internal capsule and subcortical U fibers. (**A,** Courtesy Rubinstein Collection, University of Virginia. **C** and **D,** Courtesy D. Meyer.)   *Continued.*

retarded. Progression is comparatively rapid, and death typically occurs during the first decade.[21]

Imaging

CT. NECT scans show mild nonspecific cerebral and cerebellar atrophy. The white matter may appear normal, nearly normal, or show diffuse low density changes. The cortex is intact.[23,25]

MR. In contrast to CT, MR shows widespread white matter abnormality (Fig. 17-7, *C*). Severe cases show near-total lack of normal myelination with diffuse high signal on T2-weighted scans that extends peripherally to involve the arcuate fibers (Fig. 17-7, *D*).[26]

Some cases show heterogeneous high signal in the white matter with small scattered foci of more nor-

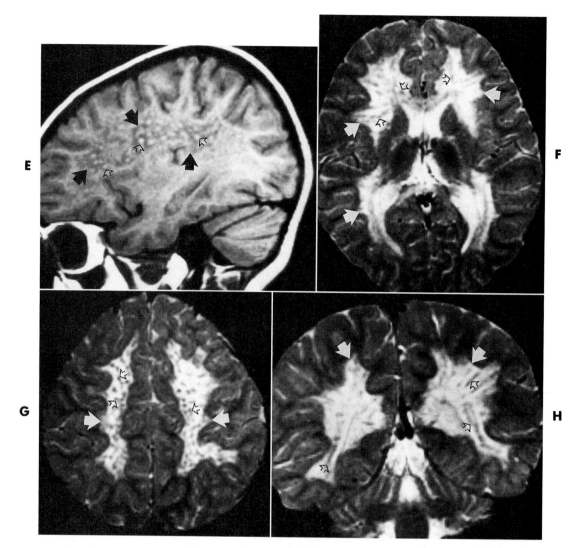

Fig. 17-7, cont'd. E to **H,** MR scans in another patient with probable PMD show a "tigroid" pattern of perivascular myelin preservation *(open arrows)* within the extensive confluent demyelinated area *(solid arrows).* The subcortical U fibers are spared. Note low signal in thalami **(F),** possibly reflecting abnormal iron deposition. Sagittal T1WI **(E),** axial **(F** and **G),** and coronal **(H)** T2WI are shown.

mal areas that may be the imaging manifestation of the "tigroid" pattern identified histopathologically (Fig. 17-7, *E* and *H*).[23,25] The brainstem, diencephalon, cerebellum, and subcortical white matter may demonstrate myelin preservation.[11] The basal ganglia and thalamus may appear unusually hypointense on T2WI, possibly representing abnormal iron deposition (Fig. 17-7, *F*).[26]

Alexander Disease

Etiology, inheritance, and pathology
Etiology and inheritance. Alexander disease (AD) is a sporadic leukoencephalopathy of unknown etiology. There is no definitive biochemical test for AD and the diagnosis is usually made by brain biopsy.[27]

Pathology. Grossly, the brain is *increased* in size and weight with massive deposition of Rosenthal fibers. These are dense eosinophilic rodlike cystoplasmic inclusions that are found in astrocytes.[27] Rosenthal fibers accumulate around blood vessels, in the subependymal region, and under the pia.[9] Extensive demyelination occurs in infantile-onset AD. The cortex is not involved.

Incidence, gender, and age. AD is a rare disorder that typically presents in infants, although juvenile and adult forms are recognized (see subsequent discussion). There is no gender predilection.

Location. AD has a predilection for the frontal lobe white matter early in its course (Fig. 17-8, *A*). Rosenthal fibers are also found in the basal ganglia, thalamus, and hypothalamus.

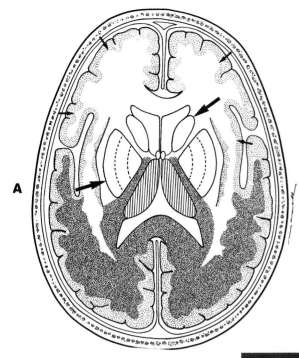

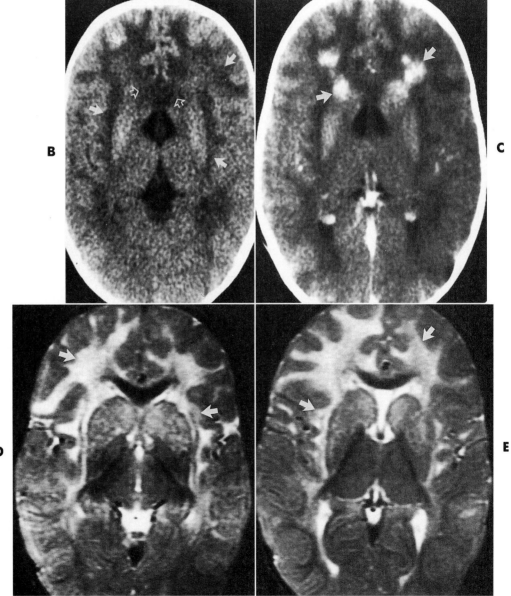

Fig. 17-8. Alexander disease (AD). **A,** Axial anatomic drawing shows the frontal lobe demyelination *(small arrows)* that is characteristic of early AD. The basal ganglia are also involved *(large arrows)*. **B,** Axial NECT scan in a 14-month-old boy who was healthy at birth but now has seizures and macrocephaly. The frontal white matter *(solid arrows),* caudate nuclei *(open arrows),* and external capsule show symmetric low density changes. **C,** Following contrast administration there is some enhancement in the deep frontal lobe white matter and caudate nuclei *(arrows).* **D** and **E,** Axial T2-weighted MR scans show the extensive demyelination in the frontal white matter and external capsules *(arrows).* Note sparing of the internal capsules, corpus callosum genu, and posterior white matter in this patient with AD.

Clinical presentation and natural history. Three clinical AD subgroups are recognized. The infantile group is characterized by early onset of megalencephaly, psychomotor retardation, spasticity, and seizures. Death occurs within 2 to 3 years.[28]

Juvenile AD is characterized by onset between 7 and 14 years. Progressive bulbar symptoms with spasticity are common. Disease duration in this group averages 8 years.[28]

In adult AD, symptom onset occurs between the second and seventh decades. The symptoms and disease course can be indistinguishable from classic multiple sclerosis.[28]

Imaging
CT. NECT scans show low attenuation in the deep frontal white matter (Fig. 17-8, *B*). The basal ganglia may also show low density changes. Enhancement following contrast administration occurs in the basal ganglia and periventricular regions (Fig. 17-8, *C*).

MR. The characteristic frontal lobe hyperintensities seen on T2-weighted scans in the early stages of AD distinguish it from other degenerative white matter disorders (Fig. 17-8, *D* and *E*).

Canavan Disease
Etiology, inheritance, and pathology
Etiology. Canavan disease (CD), also known as spongy degeneration of the brain or van Bogaert-Bertrand disease, is caused by a deficiency of *N*-acetylaspartylase that results in accumulation of *N*-acetylaspartic acid in the urine, plasma, and brain.[11,29] Inheritance is autosomal recessive.

Gross pathology. Striking megalencephaly is present with *increased* brain weight and volume. The white matter is demyelinated, gelatinous, and soft.

Microscopic appearance. There is widespread vacuolation that initially involves the subcortical white matter and then spreads to involve the deep white matter.[30] The white matter is demyelinated and replaced by a fine network of fluid-containing cystic spaces, described as having the "texture of a wet sponge."[9,11] Astrogliosis and Alzheimer-type II astrocytes are present.[9]

Incidence, gender, and age. CD is a rare disorder. There is no known gender predilection.[11]

Location. In contrast to other leukodystrophies, the demyelination seen in CD preferentially involves the subcortical U fibers. In severe cases the brain appears completely unmyelinated and only the internal capsule is relatively spared (Figs. 17-9, *A* and *B*). The occipital lobes are more involved than the frontal and parietal lobes.[9] In severe cases the basal ganglia and thalami can also be affected.[11]

Clinical presentation and natural history. Both infantile and juvenile forms are recognized. In the infantile form, symptoms appear between the second and fourth postnatal months. Hypotonia, loss of motor activity, and megalencephaly are typical. Death usually occurs before 5 years.[11]

Imaging
CT. NECT scans show diffuse low density throughout the cerebral white matter. The ventricles are usually normal in size.[29]

MR. T1-weighted scans in infantile CD demonstrate homogeneous, diffuse, symmetric low signal intensity throughout the white matter (Figs. 17-9, *C* and *D*).[30] T2-weighted images show near-total high signal in the supratentorial white matter (Fig. 17-9, *E*). The subcortical arcuate fibers are prominently involved. Relative sparing of the internal capsules is seen in some cases. The cortex may appear thin.[29]

Phenylketonuria and Amino Acid Disorders

Aminoacidopathies and aminoacidurias are autosomal recessive enzymatic defects that affect the amino acid (AA) metabolic pathways. Because amino acids are essential for formation of proteolipids (key components of myelin), defects in AA metabolism result in failure of myelin formation or failure to maintain otherwise normally formed myelin.[12]

AA disorders are due either to defective enzymes or failure to transport AAs to the appropriate site for metabolism. Deficiency of a specific enzyme (aminoacidopathy) causes accumulation of the affected AA (aminoacidemia) that is then excreted in the urine (aminoaciduria). In the aminoacidurias, a single amino acid is retained. Examples of enzymatic aminoacidopathies include phenylketonuria, maple syrup urine disease, glutaric acidemia type I, and methylmalonic acidemia (*see* box, p. 734).[12]

Occasionally, transport mechanisms are defective and result in failure to reabsorb AAs in the renal tubules (aminoaciduria without aminoacidemia). Transport defects involve multiple amino acids. Oculocerebral renal syndrome is an example of defective transport.[12]

Phenylketonuria. Phenylketonuria (PKU) is a relatively common autosomal recessive disorder that has an incidence of 1 in 14,000.[12] PKU is caused by defective hepatic phenylalanine hydroxylase, an enzyme that is required for the conversion of phenylalanine to tyrosine.[31] The block in phenylalanine degradation results in elevated levels of phenylalanine and its organic acid metabolites in blood and tissue.[32] Tissue damage occurs from continued exposure of the brain to high phenylalanine concentrations during critical periods of active organ growth.[11]

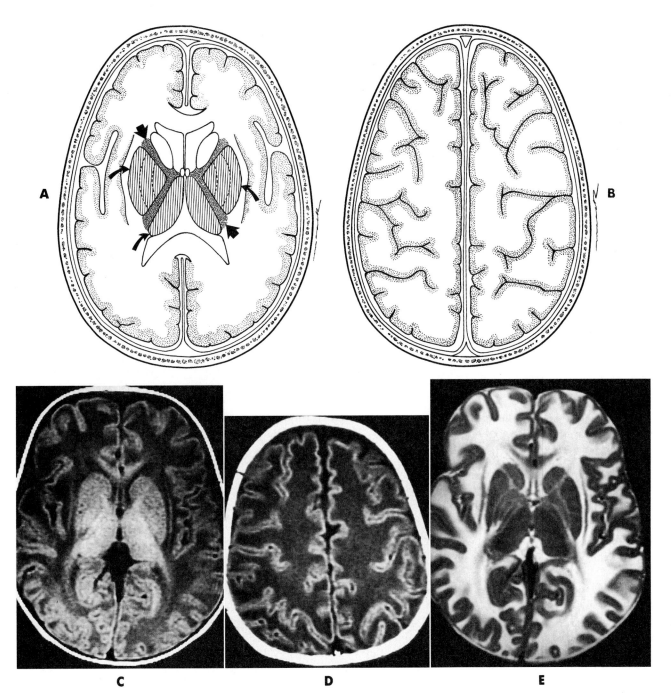

Fig. 17-9. Canavan disease (CD). **A** and **B,** Axial anatomic drawings depict CD. Note virtual complete lack of myelination except for the internal capsule (**A,** *dark pattern: large arrows*). The basal ganglia and thalami can appear very hypointense (**A,** *vertical pattern: curved arrows*). **B,** The near-total lack of myelination also involves the subcortical arcuate fibers. The appearance resembles that of a newborn infant (compare with Fig. 17-1, *D*). Axial T1- (**C** and **D**) and T2-weighted (**E**) MR scans in a 7-month-old with CD show nearly complete lack of myelination. Only parts of the internal capsule appear myelinated. The subcortical arcuate fibers are also involved. The appearance resembles that of a newborn infant. (**C** to **E,** Courtesy L. Tan and S. Lin.)

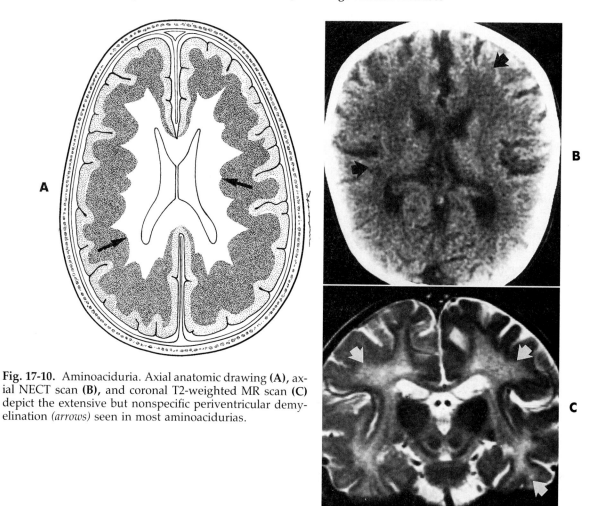

Fig. 17-10. Aminoaciduria. Axial anatomic drawing **(A)**, axial NECT scan **(B)**, and coronal T2-weighted MR scan **(C)** depict the extensive but nonspecific periventricular demyelination *(arrows)* seen in most aminoacidurias.

PKU patients are normal at birth but if untreated will develop mental retardation and other abnormalities such as autism, seizures, lack of coordination, hyperactive behavior, and hyperreflexia.[32] Recognition of this disorder is important because appropriately restricted diets should be instituted immediately. Cessation of dietary restrictions can cause neurologic deterioration within months.[31]

With some exceptions, imaging studies in most aminoacidurias, including PKU, are generally nonspecific. Varying degrees of demyelination occur, usually involving the periventricular white matter with relative sparing of the subcortical U fibers (Fig. 17-10, A). Periventricular hypodensity is seen on NECT scans (Fig. 17-10, B). Increased signal in the periventricular deep cerebral white matter can be identified on T2-weighted MR scans (Fig. 17-10, C).[33] The changes are most prominent posteriorly, particularly in the optic radiations.[32] Although MR imaging is not specifically diagnostic of PKU, it is a valuable tool in assessing the efficacy of dietary treatment and patient compliance.[34]

Amino Acid Disorders
Phenylketonuria
Maple syrup urine disease
Homocystinuria
Glutaric acidemia type I
Methylmalonic acidemia
Nonketotic hyperglycinemia
Oculocerebralrenal syndrome

Maple syrup urine disease. Maple syrup urine disease (MSUD) is caused by failure to catabolize branched-chain amino acids (leucine, isoleucine, and valine). The corresponding ketoacids accumulate and result in urinary excretion of a metabolite with a characteristic odor that resembles maple syrup.[35] Inheritance is autosomal recessive, and its estimated incidence is 1:224,000.[35]

MSUD typically presents within 4 to 7 days after birth with severe, rapidly progressive neurologic de-

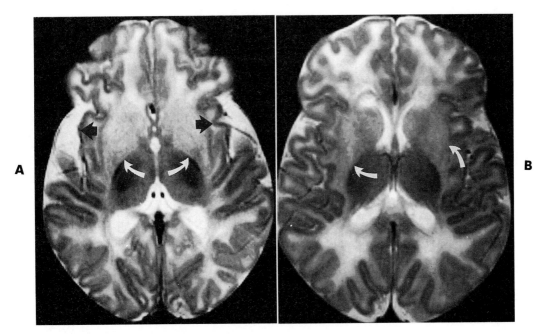

Fig. 17-11. Axial T1- **(A)** and T2-weighted **(B)** MR scans in a 3-month-old child with glutaric acidemia type I. Note the enlarged sylvian fissures with "bat wing" appearance (**A,** *large black arrows*). The caudate and lenticular nuclei have diffuse high signal (*curved arrows*).

fects. Without treatment, death occurs within 1 year.[12] Milder intermediate or even intermittent forms of MSUD have been described.[35]

Sequential imaging studies follow the natural disease course. CT scans typically are negative during the first few postnatal days. A marked, generalized diffuse edema appears and remains for 6 to 7 weeks in untreated infants. It then decreases and is transformed into better-demarcated periventricular white matter disease.[35]

A characteristic, more intense local edema (MSUD edema) involves the deep cerebellar white matter, dorsal brainstem, cerebral peduncles, and posterior limb of the internal capsule.[35] Low densities in the globus pallidus and thalami may also occur.[11] T2-weighted MR scans show high signal intensities in these areas.

Homocystinuria. Homocystinuria is an inborn error of methionine metabolism with autosomal recessive inheritance. Pathologically, homocytinuria is characterized by abnormalities in collagen and elastin formation. The intracranial vessels are often affected. Multiple small arterial thromboembolic infarcts, sagittal sinus thrombosis, and deep cerebral venous occlusion with infarction occur.[11]

Glutaric aciduria type I. Glutaric aciduria type I (GA-I) is an autosomal recessive metabolic disorder caused by a deficiency of glutaryl-CoA dehydroge-

nase, the coenzyme responsible for breakdown of lysine to tryptophan.[12,36] GA-I adversely affects mitochondrial activity and preferentially involves the basal ganglia.[12]

Clinically, GA-I is characterized by progressive dystonia and dyskinesia. Imaging studies show frontotemporal atrophy and "batwing" dilatation of the sylvian fissures (Figs. 17-11, A and B).[34,37] High signal changes in the basal ganglia and caudate nuclei are seen in some cases on T2-weighted MR scans (Fig. 17-11, C).

Methylmalonic acidemia. Methylmalonic acidemia (MMA) is an aminoacidopathy that also adversely affects mitochondrial activity. A block in the conversion of methylmalonyl-CoA to succinyl-CoA is present. Methylmalonate accumulates in the blood and urine, resulting in secondary hyperammonemia and severe ketoacidosis.[38] CT scans show bilateral low density lesions in the globus pallidi. T1-weighted MR studies show decreased signal in the corresponding areas with symmetric hyperintensities on T2WI (Fig. 17-12).[38]

Nonketotic hyperglycinemia. Nonketotic hyperglycinemia (NKH) is a disorder of glycine metabolism characterized by elevated glycine levels in the plasma, CSF, and urine.[39] Inheritance is autosomal recessive.

Two forms of NKH occur: a neonatal and a late-

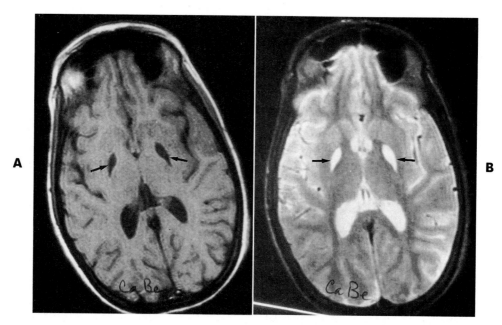

Fig. 17-12. Methylmalonic acidemia (MMA). Axial T1- **(A)** and T2-weighted **(B)** MR scans show the focal globus pallidus lesions *(arrows)* typically seen in MMA. (Courtesy M. Gado.)

onset type. In the more common neonatal type, disease onset occurs in early infancy. Clinical manifestations include seizures, hypotonia, severe developmental delay, lethargy, and coma.[39] Death usually occurs before 5 years of age.[40] Autopsy studies show severe white matter vacuolation. Imaging studies show decreased or absent myelination of the supratentorial white matter tracts.[40] The corpus callosum appears abnormally thin. Progressive supra- and infratentorial atrophy occur.

Oculocerebral renal syndrome. Oculocerebral renal syndrome (OCRS), also known as Lowe syndrome, is an example of defective amino acid transport.[12] OCRS is an X-linked recessive disorder that is characterized by congenital ocular abnormalities (cataracts), mental retardation, renal tubular disease (Fanconi syndrome), and metabolic bone disease (hypophosphatemic rickets).[41] Excessive excretion of multiple amino acids occurs.

MR studies in patients with OCRS show diffuse supratentorial white matter abnormalities. Two distinct lesions occur. Multiple small CSF-like spherical foci in the deep and subcortical white matter are identified. These discrete lesions are surrounded by confluent areas of diffuse white matter signal abnormality that appear slightly hypointense on T1- and hyperintense on T2-weighted sequences.[41]

DISORDERS THAT PRIMARILY AFFECT GRAY MATTER

The disorders that primarily affect gray matter are largely—but by no means exclusively—due to lyso-

somal enzyme defects (*see* Table 17-2). These enzymes are synthesized in the cytoplasm, then transported to the endoplasmic reticulum, where the Golgi apparatus packages them into primary lysosomes.[9] Microglia and phagocytic cells such as leukocytes and tissue macrophages have abundant lysosomes.[1] Lysosomes aid in the digestion of phagocytosed material. The eminent pediatric neuropathologist L.E. Becker has termed these organelles the *"Darth Vaders" of cells.*

When the activity of a specific lysosomal catabolic enzyme is deficient, undigested material accumulates within the affected cells. A lysosomal storage disorder is the result.[1] These disorders are often classified according to the abnormal material that accumulates, viz., lipid (lipidoses), mucopolysaccharide (mucopolysaccharidoses), or both (mucolipidoses). Enzyme deficiencies involved in carbohydrate (mainly glycogen) storage, synthesis, and degradation are termed *"glycogen storage diseases."*[9]

In this section we will consider some examples of each of the major lysosomal storage disorders that produce their most devastating effects on the cerebral gray matter.

Tay-Sachs Disease and Other Lipidoses

Lipid storage diseases are rare.[9] Two important lipidoses with gray matter manifestations include Tay-Sachs disease and neuronal ceroid-lipofuscinosis.

Tay-Sachs disease. Tay-Sachs disease (TSD) is classified as a GM2 gangliosidosis.[1] Sandhoff disease is a related but rarer related GM2 disorder. Although

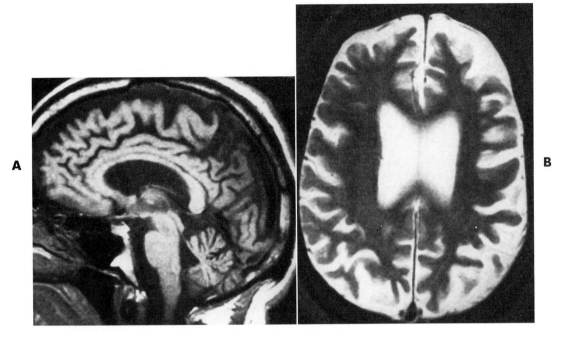

Fig. 17-13. Neuronal ceroid lipofuscinosis, Batten type. Sagittal T1- **(A)** and axial T2-weighted **(B)** MR scans in this young adult with long-standing neurodegenerative disease show strikingly enlarged sulci and ventricles. The T2WI shows the cortex is extremely atrophic but the underlying white matter is preserved.

genetically different, these two disorders are phenotypically indistinguishable.[42]

TSD is an inherited sphingomyelin lipidosis caused by deficiency of hexosaminidase A. As the abnormal GM2-ganglioside accumulates and interferes with intracellular function, neuronal deterioration and cell death ensue. Neuronal death also causes axonal deterioration and secondary demyelination. The latter can become prominent and be confused with diseases that produce primary demyelination, the leukodystrophies.[9]

TSD is diagnosed definitively by hexosaminidase leukocyte assay. Early in the disease process the caudate nuclei appear enlarged and protrude into the lateral ventricles.[43] CT scans typically show symmetrically, homogeneously hyperdense thalami.[42] MR scans in these patients show high signal intensity in the caudate nuclei, thalamus, and putamen on T2-weighted studies.[44] Progression is typically rapid, and severe cortical atrophy with widened sulci, shrunken gyri, and large ventricles is characteristically present later in the disease course.

Neuronal ceroid-lipofuscinosis. Neuronal ceroid-lipofuscinosis (NCL) is a clinically heterogeneous group of inherited neurodegenerative disorders that is subdivided into the following four groups, based on age at onset:[45]

1. Infantile
2. Late infantile
3. Juvenile (Batten disease)
4. Adult (Kufs disease)

The gene for infantile NCL is on chromosome 1, whereas juvenile NCL is located on chromosome 16.[44a] Because no specific enzyme defect has been identified in NCL,[9] diagnosis is currently established by electron microscopic examination of leukocytes or skin biopsies. NCL patients have characteristic curvilinear or "fingerprint" inclusions of an autofluorescent lipopigment (lipofuscin) within cytosomes.[9,45]

Imaging studies in these patients show mild to moderate cortical atrophy. Patients with infantile NCL may also have hyperintense white matter and low signal in the thalami and striatum on T2-weighted MR scans.[44a] No white matter changes are seen in Batten disease (Fig. 17-13).[9] Positron emission tomography (PET) studies of brain metabolism have shown decreased glucose utilization in all gray matter structures, most marked at the thalamus and posterior association cortex.[45]

Hurler Syndrome and the Mucopolysaccharidoses

The mucopolysaccharidoses (MPS) are lysosomal storage diseases that are marked by failure to degrade glycosaminoglycans (mucopolysaccharides).[46] Mucopolysaccharide accumulation due to specific catabolic enzyme defects produces 13 syndromes or variants; six are well recognized (Table 17-3, p. 739). Storage of undegraded mucopolysaccharides occurs in the cells of most organs, producing the typical gargoyle

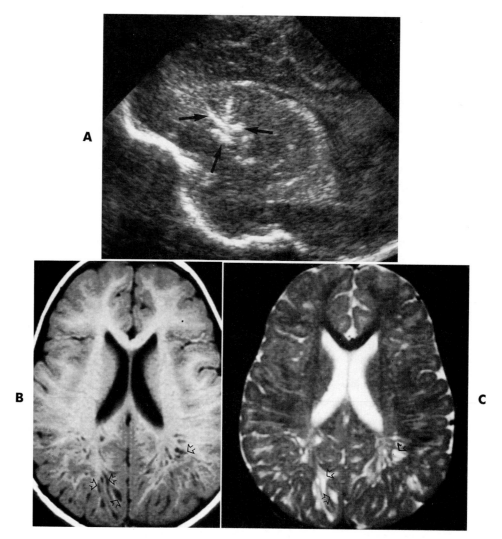

Fig. 17-14. **A,** Sagittal transcranial ultrasound in this 2-week-old infant with dysmorphic facies shows striking perivascular echogenicities in the basal ganglia *(arrows).* Probable mucopolysaccharidosis. The differential diagnosis includes toxoplasmosis, cytomegalovirus infection, trisomy 13, and lysosomal storage diseases. **B** to **C,** Axial T1- **(B)** and T2-weighted **(C)** MR scans in a 2-year-old child with mucopolysaccharidosis (MPS IH) show very prominent dilated Virchow-Robin spaces *(arrows)* in the peritrigonal areas. Margins of the enlarged perivascular spaces are obscured on the T2-weighted scan by surrounding demyelination or edema. **(A,** Courtesy K. Murray. **B** and **C,** Courtesy S. Blaser.)

features.[1] Hurler syndrome (MPS I) is the prototypical mucopolysaccharide storage disease.[9]

Hurler syndrome. Hurler syndrome, also known as MPS I, is an autosomal recessive mucopolysaccharidosis that results from deficiency of alpha-*L*-iduronidase.[46] Cortical and cerebellar neurons are ballooned from large intralysosomal accumulations of ganglioside, forming the so-called meganeurites. The perivascular spaces are grossly enlarged by accumulation of mucopolysaccharide-containing histiocytes (gargoyle cells) that surround the penetrating blood vessels.[9] Gross meningeal thickening is common. Death occurs between 5 and 10 years of age and is usually secondary to respiratory failure or cardiac involvement.[46]

Clinical features include gargoyle-like facies, dwarfism, progressive kyphosis, protuberant abdomen, hepatosplenomegaly, and severe psychomotor retardation.[9] Cerebral sonography in neonates with some lysosomal storage disorders shows stripelike perivascular echogenicities (Fig. 17-14, *A*).[46A] MR

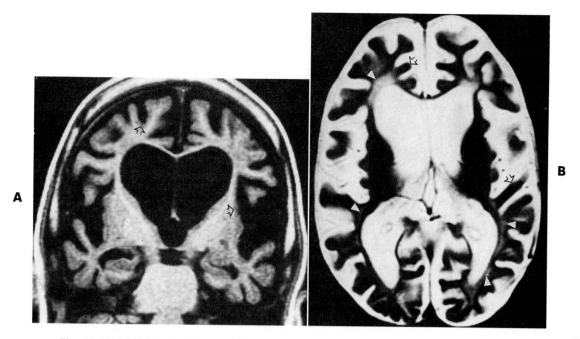

Fig. 17-15. MPS III (Sanfilipo syndrome). Coronal T1- **(A)** and axial T2-weighted **(B)** MR scans show large lateral ventricles and sulci with markedly thinned gray matter *(open arrows)*. Secondary white matter changes are also present **(B,** *arrowheads)*.

Table 17-3. Mucopolysaccharidoses

Number	Eponym	Distinctive imaging features
MPS IH	Hurler	Macrocrania, thick dura, perivascular "pits," concave or "hooked" thoraco-lumbar vertebrae with gibbus/kyphoscoliosis
MPS II	Hunter	Thick dura, perivascular "pits"
MPS III	Sanfilippo	Cortical atrophy
MPS IV	Morquio	Atlantoaxial subluxation, cord injury
MPS V	Not used	
MPS VI	Maroteaux-Lamy	Thick dura, ligamentous instability, subluxations, white matter lesions
MPS VII	Sly	Odontoid hypoplasia
MPS VIII	Not used	

studies typically disclose thickened dura, cortical atrophy, and perivascular "pits," seen as low and high signal cystic foci on T1- and T2WI, respectively (Fig. 17-14, *B* and *C*).[46] Communicating hydrocephalus is common.[46] Spinal cord compression secondary to the thickened dura may be present in some cases.[47]

Other mucopolysaccharidoses. Other MPS storage diseases that may have striking imaging findings include severe Hunter (MPS IIA) and Sanfilippo syndrome (MPS IIIB). T1-weighted MR scans show cortical atrophy; reduced gray-white matter contrast on T2WI is common (Fig. 17-15). Hyperintense white matter foci may also be present.

Mucolipidoses and Fucosidosis

The mucolipidoses are disorders associated with accumulation of mucopolysaccharide and lipids resulting from a single enzyme defect that affects both catabolic pathways. Examples of mucolipidoses include I-cell disease, fucosidosis, and mannosidosis.[9] Neuronal destruction with myelin loss, gliosis, and atrophy occur. Imaging studies show thin cortex with nonspecific white matter changes (Fig. 17-16).

Glycogen Storage Diseases

Glycogen storage diseases are a heterogeneous group of disorders resulting from deficiencies of enzymes involved in glycogen storage, synthesis, and degradation. Multisystem manifestations are common. Pompe disease is one disorder that has both CNS and peripheral lesions. Glycogen accumulates within neurons of the dorsal root ganglia, anterior horn cells, and motor nuclei of the brain stem.[9] Mild nonspecific cortical atrophy may be present.

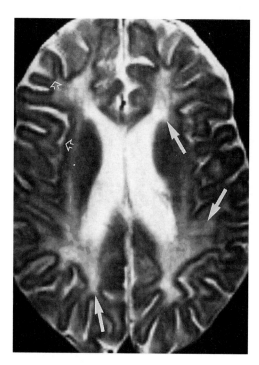

Fig. 17-16. Mucolipidosis (fucosidosis). Axial T2-weighted MR scan shows confluent periventricular demyelinated areas *(large arrows)*. The cortex *(open arrows)* is thinned secondary to myelin loss.

DISORDERS THAT AFFECT BOTH GRAY AND WHITE MATTER

A few inherited metabolic disorders affect gray and white matter to approximately the same extent. These are mostly diseases with mitochondrial or peroxisomal enzyme defects.[9]

Leigh Disease and Other Mitochondrial Encephalopathies

Mitochondria are threadlike cytoplasmic organelles that contain the DNA coding for production of numerous enzymes involved in the oxidative respiratory cycle. Krebs cycle enzymes and the cytochrome-electron transfer system required for adenosine triphosphate (ATP) formation are located in the mitochondria.[1,9]

Other than Leigh encephalopathy and focal cerebral ischemic lesions, the patterns of pathology associated with mitochondrial enzyme disorders have not been firmly established.[9] There is also considerable overlap with other entities. For example, certain aminoacidemias (e.g., glutaric acidemia type I and methylmalonic acidemia) are also involved with mitochondrial protein formation and result in basal ganglia abnormalities similar to those of primary mitochondrial defects.[12]

Despite these conceptual difficulties, three syn-

> **Mitochondrial Encephalopathies**
>
> Leigh disease (subacute necrotizing encephalomyelopathy)
> MELAS (mitochondrial encephalomyelopathy, lactic acidosis, and strokelike episodes)
> MERRF (myoclonic epilepsy with ragged red fibers)
> Kearns-Sayre syndrome
> Others (Alpers disease, Menkes disease)

dromes of mitochondrial dysfunction have emerged, as follows (*see* box):
1. Myoclonic epilepsy with ragged-red fibers (MERRF)
2. Mitochondrial encephalopathy, lactic acidosis, and strokelike syndromes (MELAS)
3. Kearns-Sayre syndrome (KSS)

A subacute necrotizing encephalomyelopathy, Leigh disease, represents end stage mitochondrial dysfunction and can occur from virtually any mitochondrial enzyme defect.[9] We will begin our discussion by considering Leigh disease, then turn our attention to MERRF, MELAS and KSS.

Leigh disease. Leigh disease, also known as subacute necrotizing encephalopathy, is a rare disorder that has been associated with several mitochondrial enzyme deficiencies: pyruvate dehydrogenase complex, pyruvate carboxylase, defects in the electron transport chain, and cytochrome c oxidase, among others.[11,48] Inheritance is autosomal recessive.

Leigh disease is characterized by spongiosis, demyelination, astrogliosis, and capillary proliferation.[9] Necrosis and capillary proliferation occur in the basal ganglia, spinal cord, and brainstem (Fig. 17-17, *A*). The periaqueductal, subependymal, and tegmental gray matter are commonly involved.[11]

Three clinical subtypes are recognized[49]:
1. An infantile form with symptom onset during the first 2 years of life
2. A juvenile form with disease manifestations in early childhood
3. An adult form with onset during the fifth or sixth decade

The infantile form of Leigh disease occurs with hypotonia, vomiting, seizures, and loss of head control. Slow progression with death from respiratory failure is typical.

NECT scans usually show low density areas in the putamina and caudate nuclei. The lesions typically do not enhance following contrast administration.[48] T2-weighted MR scans show striking symmetric hyper-

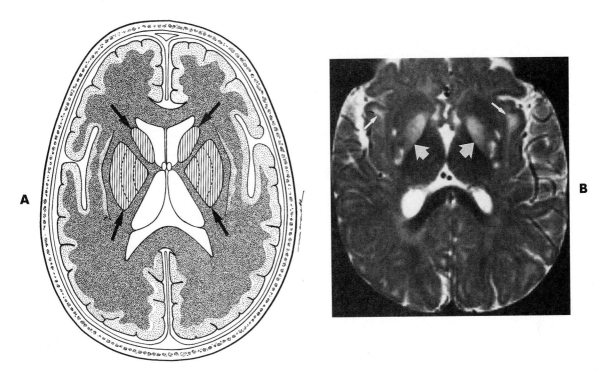

Fig. 17-17. Leigh disease is illustrated on the anatomic drawing **(A)** and axial T2-weighted MR scan **(B).** Note the bilaterally symmetric lesions in the caudate nuclei and basal ganglia *(large arrows).* Mild white matter disease is present *(small arrows).*

intense foci in the globus pallidus, putamen, and caudate (Fig. 17-17, *B*). The periventricular white matter and periaqueductal gray matter are often affected.[50]

MERRF syndrome. MERRF syndrome (for *my*oclonic *e*pilepsy with *r*agged *r*ed *f*ibers) is a mitochondrial encephalomyopathy that causes myoclonic epilepsy, muscle weakness, and progressive external ophthalmoplegia. Short stature, cardiac conduction defects, and endocrine deficiencies are common.[1] The definitive diagnosis is established by muscle biopsy that shows ragged red fibers with Gomori's modified trichrome stain.[54] Imaging findings are similar to those in MELAS syndrome, i.e., multiple infarcts in the cortex, subjacent white matter, and, sometimes, the basal ganglia.[12]

MELAS syndrome. MELAS syndrome (for *m*itochondrial *m*yopathy, *e*ncephalopathy, *l*actic *a*cidosis, and *s*trokelike episodes) is a familial disease that may have maternal inheritance.[51] A specific mutation in mitochondrial tRNA is associated with MELAS syndrome.[52] The patterns of brain damage with MELAS are related to cerebral infarcts. Although any part of the brain can be affected, the occipital lobes are the most common site.[1] Both large and multifocal small vessel occlusions occur (Fig. 17-18, *A*). Angiographic,

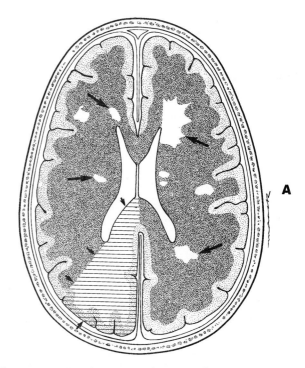

Fig. 17-18. A, Anatomic diagram depicts pathologic changes seen in MELAS syndrome. Multiple small vessel infarcts *(large arrows)* and major vessel occlusions *(vertical lines: small arrows)* occur. The occipital lobes are the most common site of large infarcts.   *Continued.*

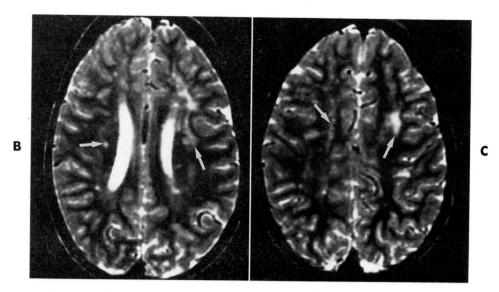

Fig. 17-18, cont'd. **B** and **C,** This 5-year-old boy with developmental delay and lactic acidosis has two siblings with known mitochondrial encephalopathy. Axial T2-weighted MR scans show ventriculomegaly and multifocal white matter lesions *(arrows).* (**B** and **C,** Courtesy P.D. Barnes.)

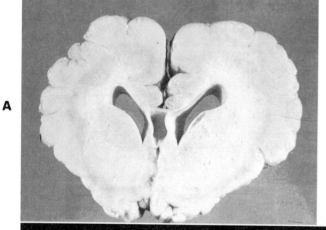

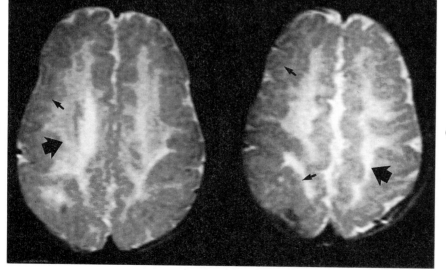

Fig. 17-19. A, Coronal gross autopsy specimen of Zellweger's syndrome shows hypomyelination with scanty white matter. The cortex is thickened and has foci of polymicrogyria. **B** and **C,** A 3-month-old girl with dysmorphic features, hypotonia, and seizures had these axial T2-weighted MR scans. Hypomyelination is seen as markedly diminished white matter volume *(large arrows).* Note polymicrogyria *(small arrows).* The diagnosis of Zellweger syndrome was confirmed at autopsy. (**A,** Courtesy Rubinstein Collection, Armed Forces Institute of Pathology. **B** and **C,** Courtesy P.D. Barnes.)

CT, and MR findings are those of nonspecific cerebral infarction (Fig. 17-18, *B*).[53]

Kearns-Sayre syndrome. Kearns-Sayre syndrome (KSS) is an autosomal dominant mitochondrial encephalopathy with elevated serum pyruvate. Pathologic and imaging findings are similar to Leigh disease (see previous discussion).[12]

Zellweger Syndrome and Other Peroxisomal Disorders

Peroxisomes are cell organelles responsible for metabolism of long-chain fatty acids. Their role in some inherited neurodegenerative disorders has been recently elucidated.

Two major groups of peroxisomal disorders are now recognized. The first group is caused by multiple enzyme defects with failure of peroxisomal development or maintenance. This category includes Zellweger syndrome, neonatal adrenoleukodystrophy, and infantile Refsum disease. The second group consists of disorders in which the peroxisomes appear structurally normal and only a single enzyme defect occurs. This class includes X-linked adrenoleukodystrophy.[55]

We have already discussed one of these important peroxisomal disorders that primarily affects white matter, i.e., X-linked adrenoleukodystrophy. In this section we discuss peroxisomal enzyme deficiencies that affect *both* gray and white matter approximately equally. The prototype disorder is Zellweger syndrome (*see* box, p. 727).

Zellweger Syndrome. Zellweger syndrome, also known as cerebrohepatorenal syndrome, is an autosomal recessive neurodegenerative disorder that is associated with deficiency of multiple peroxisomal enzymes.[1] Numerous organs are affected. In the brain, there is an unusual combination of abnormalities: neuronal migration disorders with heterotopic gray matter, pachygyria, and polymicrogyria occur, with a general decrease in white matter volume.[9,12] T2-weighted MR scans show pachygyria, periventricular heterotopias, cerebral white matter hypomyelination, and cortical neuronal loss (Fig. 17-19).[12,56]

BASAL GANGLIA DISORDERS

Numerous congenital and acquired metabolic disorders affect the basal ganglia. In this section we discuss inherited diseases whose primary or sole imaging manifestations are found in this location.

Huntington Disease

Huntington disease (HD) is a fully penetrant, autosomal dominant, inherited neurodegenerative disorder that is characterized clinically by movement, mentation, and behavioral disturbances.[57] Disease prevalence in North America is estimated at 10 cases per 100,000. Onset is typically in the fourth or fifth decade, although 5% of patients are under 14 years of age.[11,58] Disease duration averages between 15 and 30 years.

The most conspicuous neuropathologic finding is striking basal ganglia atrophy, although atrophy of other structures such as the cerebellum and brainstem are also common.[57] Imaging studies show both cortical and subcortical atrophy. Caudate nucleus volume loss causes focal enlargement of the frontal horns of the lateral ventricles (Fig. 17-20). Both increased and decreased putaminal signal intensity on T2-weighted scans have been reported in HD.[59]

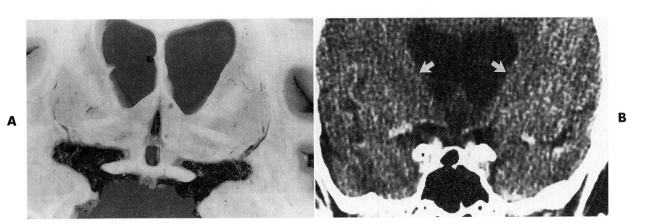

Fig. 17-20. A, Coronal gross pathology of Huntington disease shows striking caudate atrophy. **B,** Coronal CECT scan in a patient with known Huntington disease demonstrates caudate nucleus atrophy, shown by the laterally convex margin of the frontal horns *(arrows)*. **(A,** Courtesy J. Townsend.)

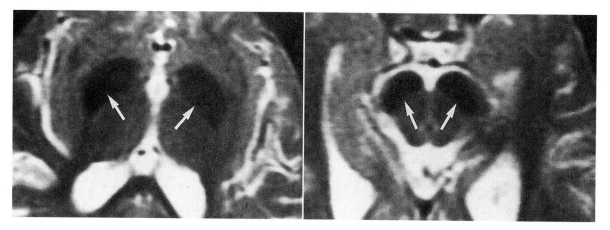

Fig. 17-21. Axial T2-weighted MR scans in this patient with Hallervorden-Spatz disease show characteristic low signal changes in the basal ganglia and substantia nigra *(arrows)*.

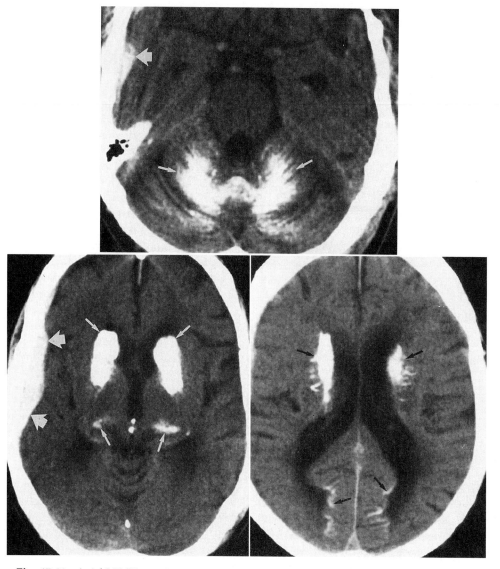

Fig. 17-22. Axial NECT scans in a patient with head trauma. A small right subdural hematoma is present *(large arrows)*. Incidentally noted are extensive calcifications in the caudate, lenticular and dentate nuclei, the thalamus, and the subcortical white matter *(small arrows)*. "Fahr's disease." (Courtesy M. Fruin.)

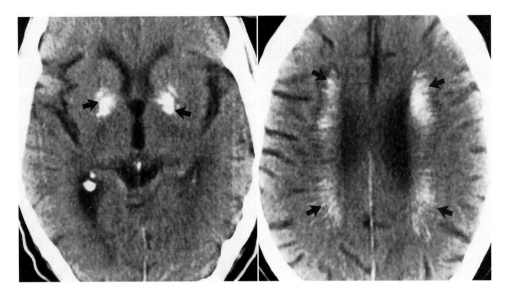

Fig. 17-23. Axial NECT scans show extensive idiopathic calcifications in the basal ganglia and centrum semiovale *(arrows)*. The deep white matter calcifications appear to follow the perivascular spaces. No metabolic abnormalities were present.

Bilateral Basal Ganglia Lucencies

Common

Normal (dilated perivascular spaces)
Arterial infarct (lacunar)
Hypoxic/ischemic encephalopathy (e.g., perinatal hypoxia, cardiac arrest, drowning)
Toxic encephalopathy (e.g., carbon monoxide, methanol, hydrogen sulfide, cyanide)

Uncommon

Metabolic (severe hypoglycemia, osmotic myelinolysis)
Infection (especially toxoplasmosis, cryptococcosis in AIDS; some encephalitides); postinfectious acute striatal necrosis
Inherited disorders (e.g., Leigh disease, Wilson disease, methylmalonic acidemia, juvenile Huntington disease; Alexander, Canavan and MLD)
Venous infarct (internal cerebral vein thrombosis)
Hemolytic-uremic syndrome

Bilateral Basal Ganglia Calcifications

Common

Idiopathic (no endocrine abnormality)
"Fahr disease" (familial cerebrovascular ferrocalcinosis)
Postinflammatory (TB, CID, toxoplasmosis, cysticercosis, congenital HIV)

Uncommon

Congenital (tuberous sclerosis, Down syndrome, MELAS/MERRF, Cockayne syndrome, neurofibromatosis, methemoglobinopathy)
Post-anoxic/toxic (e.g., carbon monoxide, chemotherapy and radiation therapy, lead intoxication)

Hallervorden-Spatz Disease

Hallervorden-Spatz disease (HSD) is a rare neurodegenerative disease with no known biologic marker to date. Both familial and sporadic cases have been reported.[60] Characteristic pathologic findings are iron deposits in the globus pallidus and substantia nigra. NECT scans show bilateral low densities in these areas. The differential diagnosis of congenital and acquired basal ganglia low densities is extensive, and summarized in the box, *above.*

Typical findings of HSD on T2-weighted MR scans include pallidonigral low signal intensity (Fig. 17-21).[61] Sometimes smaller anteromedial high signal intensities are also present (eye-of-the-tiger sign).[61,62]

Fahr Disease

So-called Fahr disease is not a single entity but a diverse group of disorders that have striking basal ganglia calcifications in common.[11] Some cases also have prominent calcifications in the dentate nuclei, centrum semiovale, and subcortical white matter (Figs. 17-22 and 17-23). The differential diagnosis of inherited and acquired basal ganglia calcifications is extensive, and summarized in the box, *above.*

Wilson Disease

Wilson disease (hepatolenticular degeneration) is an autosomal recessive inherited disorder of copper metabolism caused by a deficiency of ceruloplasmin, the serum transport protein for copper. Abnormal copper deposition occurs in various tissues, especially the liver, brain, cornea, bones, and kidneys.[63] Wilson disease (WD) is associated with cirrhosis of the liver and degenerative changes in the basal ganglia.

Although WD can occur at any age, most affected patients become symptomatic between the ages of 8 and 16 years.[58] Neurologic abnormalities result directly from copper deposition in the brain, indirectly as an encephalopathy complicating progressive liver disease, or a combination of both.[63,64]

Neuroimaging studies in some cases are normal or show only mild generalized atrophy.[63] Others show bilateral putaminal low density lesions on NECT scans and high signal in the thalami, putamen, dentate nuclei, and brainstem on T2-weighted MR scans.[58] Rarely, decreased signal intensity of the putamina and caudate nuclei occurs.[65,66]

REFERENCES

1. Kendall BE: Disorders of lysosomes, peroxisomes, and mitochondria, *AJNR* 13:621-653, 1992.
2. Barkovich AJ: *Pediatric Neuroimaging,* pp 13-24, New York, Raven Press, 1990.
2a. Staudt M, Schropp C, Staudt F et al: Myelination of the brain in MRI: a staging system, *Pediatr Radiol* 23:169-176, 1993.
3. Ballesteros MC, Hansen PE, Soila K: MR imaging of the developing human brain, *RadioGraphics* 13:611-622, 1993.
4. Barkovich AJ, Lyon G, Evrard P: Formation, maturation and disorders of white matter, *AJNR* 13:447-461, 1992.
5. Klycznik RL, Wolpert SM, Anderson ML: Congenital and developmental abnormalities of the brain. In Wolpert SM, Barnes PD, editors: *MRI in Pediatric Neuroradiology,* pp 83-91, St Louis, Mosby-Year Book, 1992.
6. Bird CR, Hedberg M, Drayer BP et al: MR assessment of myelination in infants and children: usefulness of marker sites, *AJNR* 10:731-740, 1989.
7. Byrd SE, Darling CR, Wilczynski NA: White matter of the brain: maturation and myelination on magnetic resonance in infants and children, *Neuroimaging Clin N Amer* 3:247-266, 1993.
8. Edwards MK, Bonnin JM: White matter diseases. In Atlas SW, editor: *Magnetic Resonance Imaging of the Brain and Spine,* pp 467-500, New York, Raven Press, 1991.
9. Becker LE: Lysosomes peroxisomes and mitochondria: function and disorder, *AJNR* 13:621-653, 1992.
10. Demaerel P, Faubert C, Wilms G et al: MR findings in leukodystrophy, *Neuroradiol* 33:368-371, 1991.
11. Wolpert SM, Anderson ML, Kaye EM: Metabolic and degenerative disorders. In Wolpert SM, Barnes PD, editors: *MRI in Pediatric Neuroradiology,* pp 121-150, St. Louis, CV Mosby, 1992.
12. Lee BCP: Magnetic resonance imaging of metabolic and primary white matter disorders in children, *Neuroimaging Clin N Amer* 3:267-289, 1993.
12a. Farley TJ, Ketonen LM, Bodensteiner JB, Wang DD: Serial MRI and CT findings in infantile Krabbe disease, *Pediatr Neurol* 8:455-458, 1992.
12b. Tada K, Taniike M, Ono J et al: Serial magnetic resonance imaging studies in a case of late onset globoid cell leukodystrophy, *Neuropediatr* 23:306-309, 1992.
13. Jardim LB, Giugliani R, Fensom AH: Thalamic and basal ganglia hyperdensities: a CT marker for globoid cell leukodystrophy? *Neuropediatr* 23:30-31, 1992.
14. Sasaki M, Sakuragawa N, Takashima S et al: MRI and CT findings in Krabbe disease, *Ped Neurol* 7:283-288, 1991.
15. van der Knaap MS, Valk J: The MR spectrum of peroxisomal disorders, *Neuroradiol* 33:30-37, 1991.
16. Uchiyama M, Hata Y, Tada S: MR imaging of adrenoleukodystrophy, *Neuroradiol* 33:25-29, 1991.
17. Kumar AH, Rosenbaum AE, Naidu S et al: Adrenoleukodystrophy: correlating MR imaging with CT, *Radiol* 165:497-504, 1987.
18. Snyder RD, King JN, Keck GM, Orrison WW: MR imaging of the spinal cord in 23 subjects with ALD-AMN complex, *AJNR* 12:1095-1098, 1991.
19. Jensen ME, Sawyer RW, Braun IF, Rizzo WB: MR imaging appearance in childhood adrenoleukodystrophy with auditory, visual, and motor pathway involvement, *RadiolGraphics* 10:53-66, 1990.
20. van der Knaap MS, Valk J: MR of adrenoleukodystrophy: histopathologic correlations, *AJNR* 10:512-514, 1989.
21. van der Knaap MS, Valk J, deNeeling N, Nauta JJP: Pattern recognition in magnetic resonance imaging of white matter disorders in children and young infants, *Neuroradiol* 33:478-493, 1991.
22. Hong-Magno ET, Muraki AS, Huttenlocher PR: Atypical CT scans in adrenoleukodystrophy, *J Comp Asst Tomogr* 11:333-336, 1987.
23. Scheffer IE, Baraitser M, Wilson J et al: Pelizaeus-Merzbacher disease: classical or connatal? *Neuropediatr* 22:71-78, 1991.
24. van der Knaap MS, Valk J: The reflection of histology in MR imaging of Pelizaeus-Merzbacher disease, *AJNR* 10:94-103, 1989.
25. Caro PA, Marks HG: Magnetic resonance imaging and computed tomography in Pelizaeus-Merzbacher disease, *Mag Res Imaging* 8:791-796, 1990.
26. Silverstein AM, Hirsh DK, Trobe JD, Gebarski SS: MR imaging of the brain in five members of a family with Pelizaeus-Merzbacher disease, *AJNR* 11:495-499, 1990.
27. Clifton AG, Kendall BE, Kingsley DPE et al: Computed tomography in Alexander's disease, *Neuroradiol* 33:438-440, 1991.
28. Shah M, Ross JS: Infantile Alexander disease: MR appearance of a biopsy-proved case, *AJNR* 11:1105-1106, 1990.
29. Brismar J, Brismar G, Gascon G, Oznan P: Caravan disease: CT and MR imaging of the brain, *AJNR* 11:805-810, 1990.
30. Marks HG, Caro PA, Wang Z et al: Use of computed tomography, magnetic resonance imaging, and localized 1H magnetic resonance spectroscopy in Canavan's disease: a case report, *Ann Neurol* 30:106-110, 1991.
31. McCombe PA, McLaughlin DB, Chalk JB et al: Spasticity and white matter abnormalities in adult phenylketonuria, *J Neuro Neurosurg Psychiatr* 55:359-361, 1992.
32. Pearsen KD, Gean-Marton AD, Levy HL, Davis KR: Phenylketonuria, MR imaging of the brain with clinical correlation, *Radiol* 177:437-440, 1990.
33. Shaw DWW, Maravilla KR, Weinberger E et al: MR imaging of phenylketonuria, *AJNR* 12:403-406, 1991.
34. Naidu SB, Moser HW: Value of neuroimaging on metabolic diseases in affecting the CNS, *AJNR* 12:413-416, 1991.
35. Brismar J, Aqeela A, Brismar G et al: Maple syrup urine disease: findings on CT and MR scans of the brain in 10 infants, *AJNR* 11:1219-1228, 1990.
36. Altman NR, Rovira MJ, Bauer M: Glutaric aciduria type 1: MR findings in two cases, *AJNR* 12:966-968, 1991.

37. Mandel H, Braun J, El-Peleg O et al: Glutaric aciduria type I, *Neuroradiol* 33:75-78, 1991.
38. Andreula CF, Blasi RD, Carella A: CT and MR studies of methylmalonic acidemia, *AJNR* 12:410-412, 1991.
39. Heidel W, Kugel H, Rah B: Noninvasive detection of increased glycine content by proton MR spectroscopy in the brains of two infants with nonketotic hyperglycinemia, *AJNR* 14:629-635, 1993.
40. Press GA, Barshop BA, Haas RH et al: Abnormalities of the brain in nonketotic hyperglycinemia: MR manifestations, *AJNR* 10:426-432, 2989.
41. Carroll WJ, Woodruff WW, Cadman TE: MR findings in culocerebrorenal syndrome, *AJNR* 14:449-451, 1993.
42. Brismar J, Brismar G, Crates R et al: Increased density of the thalamus on CT scans in patients with GM$_2$ gangliosidoses, *AJNR* 11:125-130, 1990.
43. Fukumizu M, Yoshikawa H, Takashima S et al: Tay-Sachs disease: progression of changes on neuroimaging in four cases, *Neuroradiol* 34:483-486, 1992.
44. Yoshikawa H, Yamada K, Sakuragawa N: MRI in the early stage of Tay-Sachs disease, *Neuroradiol* 34:394-395, 1992.
44a. Confort-Gouny S, Chabrol B, Vion-Dury J et al: MRI and localized proton MRS in early infantile form of neuronal ceroid-lipofuscinosis, *Pediatr Neurol* 9:57-60, 1993.
45. DeVolder AG, Cirelli S, de Barsy Th et al: Neuronal ceroid-lipofuscinosis: preferential alterations in the thalamus and posterior association cortex demonstrated by PET, *J Neurol Neurosurg Psychiatr* 53:1063-1067, 1990.
46. Murata R, Nakajima S, Tanaka A et al: MR imaging of the brain in patients with mucopolysaccharidosis, *AJNR* 10:1165-1170, 1989.
46a. Ries M, Deeg K-H, Wölfel D et al: Colour doppler imaging of intracranial vasculopathy in severe infantile sialidosis, *Pediatr Radiol* 22:179-181, 1992.
47. Gabrielli O, Salvolini U, Maricotti M et al: Cerebral MRI in two brothers with mucopolysaccharidosis type I and different clinical phenotypes, *Neuroradiol* 34:313-315, 1992.
48. Krageloh-Mann I, Grodd W, Niemann G et al: Assessment and therapy monitoring of Leigh disease by MRI and proton spectroscopy, *Ped Neuro* 8:60-64, 1992.
49. Geyer CA, Sartor KH, Prensky AJ et al: Leigh disease (subacute necrotizing encephalomyelopathy): CT and MR in five cases, *J Comp Asst Tomogr* 12:40-44, 1988.
50. Davis PC, Hoffman JC Jr, Braun IF et al: MR of Leigh's disease (subacute necrotizing encephalomyelopathy), *AJNR* 8:71-75, 1987.
51. Goto Y, Horai S, Matsuoka T et al: Mitochondrial myopathy, encephalopathy, lactic acidosis, and stroke-like episodes

(MELAS): a correlative study of the clinical features and mitochondrial DNA mutation, *Neurol* 42:545-550, 1992.
52. Moswich RK, Donat JR, DiMauro F et al: The syndrome of mitochondrial encephalyomyopathy, lactic acestosis, and stroke-like episodes presenting without stroke, *Arch Neurol* 50:275-278, 1993.
53. Ooiwa Y, Uematsu Y, Terada T et al: Cerebral blood flow in mitochondrial myopathy, encephalopathy, lactic acidosis, and stroke-like episodes, *Stroke* 24:304-309, 1993.
54. Sandhu FS, Dillon WP: MR demonstration of leukoencephalopathy associated with mitochondrial encephalopathy: case report, *AJNR* 12:385-379, 1991.
55. Naidu SB, Moser H: Infantile Refsum disease, *AJNR* 12:1161-1163, 1991.
56. Bruhn H, Kruse B, Korenke GC et al: Proton NMR spectroscopy of cerebral metabolic alterations in infantile peroxisomal disorders, *J Comp Asst Tomogr* 16:335-344, 1992.
57. Starkstein SE, Brandt J, Bylsma F et al: Neuropsychological correlates f brain atropy in Huntington's disease: a magnetic resonance imaging study, *Neuroradiol* 34:487-489, 1992.
58. Braffman BH, Trojanowski JQ, Atlas SW: The aging brain and neurodegenerative disorders. In Atlas SW: *Magnetic Resonance Imaging of the Brain and Spine*, pp 567-624, New York, Raven Press, 1991.
59. Chen JC, Hardy PA, Kucharczyk W et al: MR of human postmortem brain tissue: correlative study between T2 and assays of iron and ferritin in Parkinson and Huntington disease, *AJNR* 14:275-281, 1993.
60. Savoiardo M, Halliday WC, Nardocci N et al: Hallervoden-Spatz disease: MR and pathologic findings, *AJNR* 14:155-162, 1993.
61. Ambrosetto P, Nonni R, Bacci A, Gobbi G: Late onset familial Hallervorden-Spatz disease: MR findings in two sisters, *AJNR* 13:394-396, 1992.
62. Angelini L, Nardocci N, Rumi V et al: Hallervorden-Spatz disease: clinical and MRI study of 11 cases diagnosed in life, *J Neurol* 239:417-425, 1992.
63. Nazer H, Brismar J, Al-Kawi MZ et al: Magnetic resonance imaging of the brain in Wilson's disease, *Neuroradiol* 35:130-133, 1993.
64. Oder W, Prayer L, Grimm G et al: Wilson's disease, *Neurol* 43:120-124, 1993.
65. Brugieres P, Combes C, Ricolfi F et al: Atypical MR presentation of Wilson disease: a possible consequence of paramagnetic effect of copper? *Neuroradiol* 34:222-224, 1992.
66. Ho VB, Fitz CR, Chuang SH, Geyer CA: Bilateral basal ganglia lesions: pediatric differential considerations, *RadioGraphics* 13:269-292, 1993.

Acquired Metabolic, White Matter, and Degenerative Diseases of the Brain

N umerous inherited and acquired neurodegenerative disorders affect the central nervous system. Inherited metabolic, white matter, and degenerative diseases were delineated in Chapter 17. Here we briefly discuss the normal aging brain, then turn our attention to the broad spectrum of acquired neurodegenerative diseases.

NORMAL AGING BRAIN

Just as certain imaging findings reflect the dramatic changes in brain morphology that occur with fetal and postnatal development, others mirror normal alterations in the aging brain.[1] Specific age-related changes take place in the cerebral white and gray matter, the cerebrospinal fluid spaces, and the basal ganglia (see box, p. 750).

White Matter

Foci of increased signal intensity are often identified on T2-weighted MR scans in demented and healthy elderly patients. The clinical significance of these findings is uncertain, and their precise etiology remains unclear. These foci are found in several different locations: the subcortical, central, and periventricular white matter (Fig. 18-1).[2]

Subcortical lesions. Subcortical white matter hyperintensities (WMHs) are commonly identified on T2-weighted MR scans in healthy elderly patients.[3] WMHs have different etiologies, depending on location and configuration. Punctate lesions are characterized histologically by dilated perivascular spaces

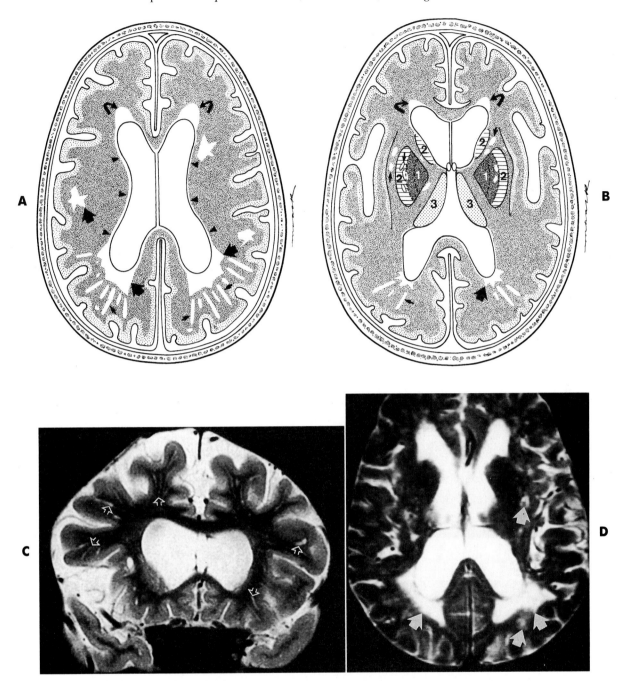

Fig. 18-1. A and **B,** Axial anatomic drawings depict basal ganglia iron deposition and white matter hyperintensities (WMHs) seen in the typical aging brain. Iron deposition is most noticeable in the globus pallidus (**B,** *1, black areas*), less prominent in the putamen and caudate nucleus, and even less prominent in the thalamus (**B,** *2, 3, dotted and cross-hatched areas*). Note triangular-shaped "caps" around the frontal horns *(curved arrows),* thin periventricular hyperintense halo (**A,** *arrowheads*), and dilated perivascular spaces, seen as punctate or linear hyperintensities *(small arrows)* in the subcortical white matter, centrum semiovale, and basal ganglia. Patchy periventricular and subcortical WMHs *(large arrows)* represent areas of myelin pallor and small vessel arteriosclerosis. **C,** Coronal T2-weighted MR scan in a normal 80-year-old woman shows WMHs in the subcortical white matter, centrum semiovale, and periventricular white matter. The linear WMHs represent dilated perivascular (Virchow-Robin) spaces *(arrows),* whereas more focal patchy lesions *(see* **D,** *arrows)* represent myelin pallor or atherosclerosis. Note prominent sulci and ventricles. **D,** Axial T2-weighted MR scan in a 76-year-old man with hypertension, confusion, and decreasing mental status shows numerous patchy subcortical and periventricular WMHs *(arrows).* The sulci and ventricles are enlarged but are not as prominent as seen in **C.**

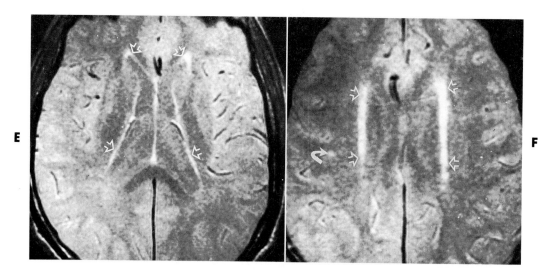

Fig. 18-1, cont'd. **E** and **F,** Axial proton density-weighted MR scans in a normal 72-year-old man show normal periventricular white matter hyperintensities. These consist of triangular, high signal "caps" around the frontal horns and a fine, thin hyperintense rim around the lateral ventricles *(open arrows).* Note WMHs *(curved arrow).*

Normal Aging Brain
Imaging findings

Scattered white matter hyperintensities on T2WI
Moderate enlargement of sulci, ventricles
Periventricular high signal rim on PD, T2WI
Iron deposition increases in globus pallidus, putamen

and perivascular gliosis, whereas more patchy lesions are associated with myelin pallor, dilated perivascular spaces, and arteriosclerosis (Fig. 18-1, *A* and *B*).[2]

Although early reports identified a history of ischemic stroke as predictive for the presence and severity of subcortical white matter lesions,[4] recent investigations indicate the major correlative factor is age.[5] Cognitive function is not related to presence or absence of WMHs.

Central lesions. WMHs in the corona radiata and centrum semiovale are typically found in a perivascular distribution.[5] Dilated perivascular spaces are round or linear lesions that are oriented perpendicularly to the ventricles and cortex (Fig. 18-1, *A* and *B*). Patchy, more confluent WMHs are probably related to small-vessel atherosclerosis and myelin pallor.[2,2a] They are most commonly located in the watershed zones between the middle and anterior or the middle and posterior cerebral arteries; they rarely occur in the temporal or occipital subcortical areas.[6]

The extent and frequency of central WMHs are closely related to age. Patients with hypertension (Fig. 18-1, *D*), diabetes, hyperlipidemia, and heart disease have more WMHs compared to patients without these risk factors but this becomes statistically significant only in the eighth decade.[6]

Periventricular lesions. Several different types of periventricular hyperintensities (Figs. 18-1 *A* and *B*) are seen on the T2-weighted MR scans in elderly patients, as follows:

1. Triangle-shaped "caps" around the frontal horns
2. Thin, smooth periventricular rims
3. Patchy periventricular hyperintensities

"Caps" adjacent to the frontal horns are a normal finding in patients of all ages (Figs. 18-1, *A, B,* and *E*). In this location, myelin is more loosely compacted and there is a relative increase in periependymal fluid.

Many healthy elderly patients also exhibit bilaterally symmetric thin rims of periventricular high signal intensity on T2-weighted scans (Figs. 18-1, *A, B, E,* and *F*). These are characterized histologically by subependymal gliosis and focal loss of the ependymal lining with increased periependymal CSF and are not indicative of normal pressure hydrocephalus.[2] This type of periventricular hyperintensity is also correlated with increasing age.[7]

Patchy periventricular hyperintensities represent deep white matter infarction and are more com-

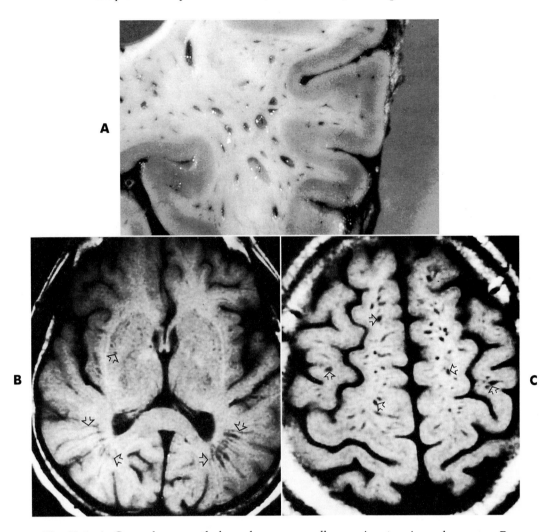

Fig. 18-2. A, Coronal gross pathology shows unusually prominent perivascular spaces. **B** and **C,** Axial T1-weighted MR scans in a normal 45-year-old man show numerous prominent Virchow-Robin spaces (VRSs) in the subcortical white matter (**B,** *arrows*) and centrum semiovale (**C,** *arrows*). Compare with **A.** Note that where the plane of the scan is parallel to the penetrating vessels, the VRSs appear linear (**B,** *arrows*), but if the scan plane is perpendicular to the VRSs, they appear more rounded (**C,** *arrows*). (**A,** Courtesy J. Townsend.)

mon in patients with hypertension or normal-pressure hydrocephalus (NPH) than age-matched controls, although there is significant overlap between these groups (Figs. 18-1, *A, B,* and *D*).[8,9] Some hypertension-related white matter lesions may resolve with blood pressure normalization.

Perivascular spaces. Perivascular spaces, also known as Virchow-Robin spaces (VRSs), are pial-lined extensions of the subarachnoid space that surround penetrating arteries as they enter either the basal ganglia or the cortical gray matter over the high convexities[10] (*see* Fig. 12-191). VRSs may extend deep into the basal ganglia and centrum semiovale (Figs. 18-1 to 18-3).

Small VRSs are found in patients of all ages and are a normal anatomic variant.[10] VRSs increase in size and frequency with advancing age.[10] Other factors such as hypertension, dementia, and incidental white-matter lesions are also associated with large VRSs but are considered part of the aging process and are not independent variables.[10]

High-resolution MR scans routinely demonstrate small rounded or linear perivascular foci that follow CSF on all pulse sequences (Fig. 18-2, *B* and *C*). VRSs surround the lenticulostriate arteries as they course through the anterior perforated substance into the basal ganglia (Fig. 18-3). VRSs are less frequently identified in the high-convexity gray matter and centrum semiovale. Prominent VRSs in the basal ganglia,

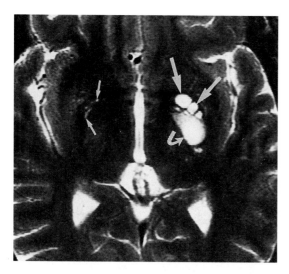

Fig. 18-3. Axial T2-weighted MR scan in a 67-year-old woman shows small perivascular spaces in the right basal ganglia *(small arrows)*, large Virchow-Robin spaces in the left basal ganglia *(large arrows)*, and a more focal, confluent hyperintense lesion *(curved arrow)* that probably represents a lacunar infarct.

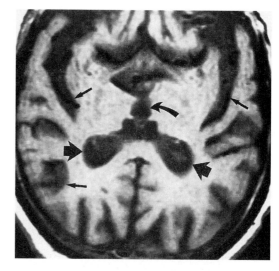

Fig. 18-4. Axial NECT scan in an intellectually normal 80-year-old man with head trauma shows prominent sulci and basilar cisterns *(small arrows)*. The third ventricle *(curved arrow)* and both lateral ventricles *(large arrows)* are also prominent.

Hydrocephalus
"Overproduction" hydrocephalus (questionable; may occur with choroid plexus tumors)
Hydrocephalus secondary to obstructed CSF flow (usually refers to intraventricular obstructive hydrocephalus, or IVOH; extraventricular obstructive hydrocephalus, or EVOH, is sometimes loosely termed *communicating hydrocephalus*)
Hydrocephalus secondary to decreased CSF absorption at the arachnoid villi
"Normal pressure" hydrocephalus

subcortical white matter, and centrum semiovale are a normal MR finding *(see* Figs. 18-1, *A* and *B,* and 18-2).

Sulci, Cisterns, and Ventricles

Sulci and cisterns. Sulcal and cisternal enlargement is part of the normal aging process (Figs. 18-1 and 18-4). Prominent CSF spaces are also common in children under 1 year of age; craniocortical widths up to 4 mm and interhemispheric widths up to 6 mm are normal (Fig. 18-5).[11] Large sulci in elderly patients have also been associated with diabetes, hypertension, chronic cerebrovascular disorders, and medications.[12] These factors often accompany the aging process and do not represent independent variables.[10] The degree and progression of additional atrophy in the senile dementias is uncertain. Overlap of all volumetric indices shows that imaging data alone can-

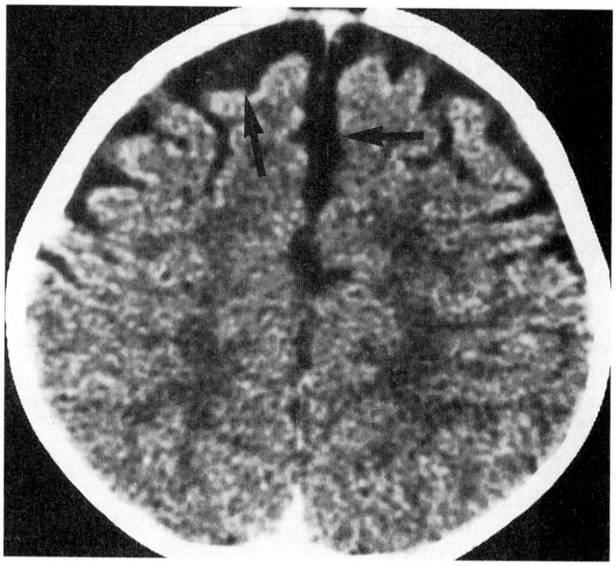

Fig. 18-5. Axial NECT scan in a normal 7-month-old baby shows prominent frontal and interhemispheric subarachnoid spaces *(arrows)*.

not be used to predict the presence or progression of dementia in individual cases (compare Figs. 18-1, *C* and *D*).[13]

Various inherited and acquired neurodegenerative disorders, toxic encephalopathies, trauma, and other such diseases also cause generalized atrophic changes, with concomitant enlargement of the intracranial CSF spaces (see subsequent discussion).

Ventricles and hydrocephalus. Under normal conditions the cerebral ventricular system has a volume of 20 to 25 ml.[14] Both hydrocephalus (Fig. 18-6,

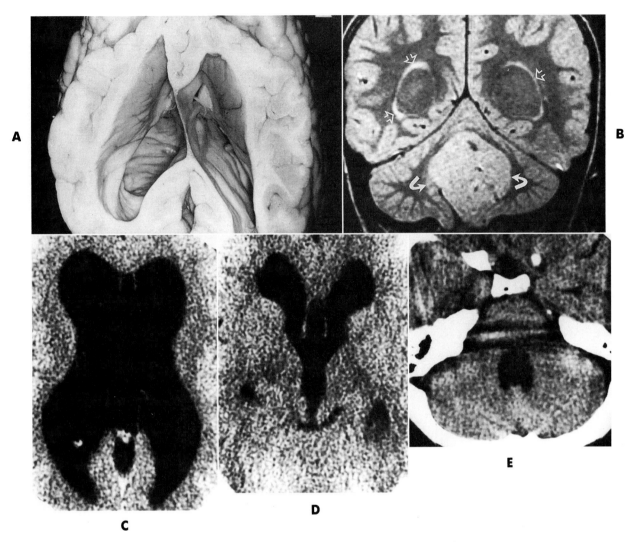

Fig. 18-6. A, Gross pathology of obstructive hydrocephalus secondary to a posterior fossa tumor (not shown). Note markedly enlarged lateral ventricles. The sulci are inapparent. **B** to **G,** Different types of hydrocephalus: **B,** Coronal proton density-weighted MR scan in a 4-year-old child with a fourth ventricular medulloblastoma *(curved arrows).* Note the enlarged lateral ventricles are surrounded by a thin hyperintense rim of transependymal CSF *(open arrows),* an abnormal finding in young patients but normal in elderly individuals (compare with Fig. 18-1, *E* and *F*). Obstructive hydrocephalus of the "noncommunicating" or intraventricular type (IVOH). **C** to **E,** Axial NECT scans in a 24-year-old man with a history of meningitis as a child show markedly enlarged lateral and third ventricles and a moderately enlarged fourth ventricle. The sulci are inapparent. Obstructive hydrocephalus of the "communicating" or extraventricular (EVOH) type. (**A,** From archives of the Armed Forces Institute of Pathology.)   *Continued.*

A) and atrophy *(see* Fig. 18-29, *A)* are characterized by ventricular dilatation.

Hydrocephalus. Three possible mechanisms account for the development of hydrocephalus *(see* box). With the exception of hydrocephalus caused by increased CSF production (choroid plexus tumors), hydrocephalus is caused by obstructed CSF flow, decreased CSF absorption, or a combination of both.[14] The term *hydrocephalus ex vacuo* is inappropriate and should be discontinued in favor of atrophy.

In so-called noncommunicating hydrocephalus (also sometimes termed *intraventricular obstructive hy-*

drocephalus, or IVOH), flow obstruction occurs inside the ventricular system down to and including the fourth ventricular outlet foramina (Fig. 18-6, *B*).

In "communicating" hydrocephalus (also sometimes termed *extraventricular obstructive hydrocephalus,* or EVOH), obstruction occurs within the subarachnoid spaces or cisterns (Fig. 18-6, *C* to *E*). This pattern of hydrocephalus can also occur with diminished CSF absorption at the arachnoid villi.

Imaging findings in obstructive hydrocephalus vary with the site and duration of the blockage. The ventricular system enlarges proximal to the obstruc-

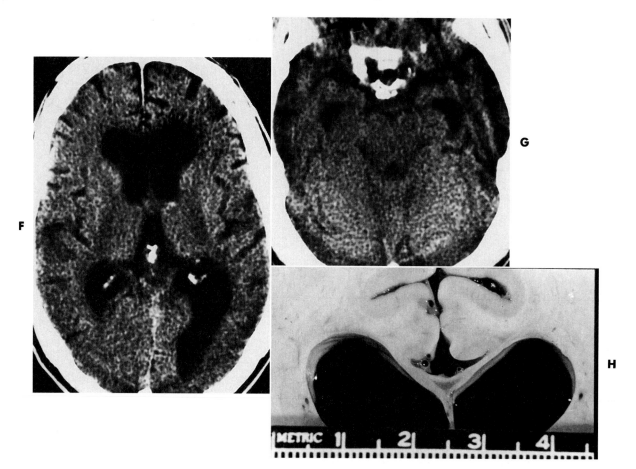

Fig. 18-6, cont'd. F and **G,** Axial NECT scans in a 66-year-old man with dementia, ataxia, and incontinence show disproportionately enlarged ventricles compared to the mildly prominent sulci. The patient improved after ventricular shunting. Normal pressure hydrocephalus. **H,** Coronal gross pathology of normal pressure hydrocephalus shows marked dilatation of the lateral ventricles with corpus callosum thinning. (**H,** Courtesy E. Tessa Hedley-Whyte.)

tion. With elevated intraventricular pressure, CSF extrudes across the ependyma into the adjacent white matter (Fig. 18-6, *B*). Periventricular high signal intensity rims or fingerlike CSF projections that extend outward from the ventricles can be delineated on proton density-weighted MR scans (*see* Figs. 13-38, *E,* and 18-6, *B*).

Normal pressure hydrocephalus (Fig. 18-6, *F* to *H*) is differentiated from generalized atrophy by ventricular dilatation out of proportion to sulcal enlargement on CT or MR scans (Fig. 18-6, *F* to *G*). Some investigators report CSF flow through the cerebral aqueduct is hyperdynamic, producing an accentuated "CSF flow void" on MR studies in patients with NPH.[8,15] Others disagree. Still others have recently suggested that symptoms seen in NPH (memory loss, gait disturbance, urinary incontinence) relate not to ventricular dilatation but rather to impingement of the corpus callosum by the falx cerebri.[16]

Atrophy. Aging causes enlargement of both the cerebral sulci and ventricles, indicating a process of mixed central and cortical volume loss.[13] Prominent sulci and ventricles are a normal finding on imaging studies, particularly in patients over 70 years of age (*see* Figs. 18-1, *C,* and 18-4).[14] Volumetric indexes in healthy aging patients remain fairly stable over time, whereas patients with Alzheimer-type senile dementias show progressive atrophy.[13] However, the overlap between groups is substantial and—as is also the case with the sulci and cisterns—ventricular size cannot be used to predict the presence or progression of dementia in individual cases.[13]

Brain Iron and the Striatonigral System

Iron is a trace element involved in brain function.[17] Iron is essential for cellular respiration, neurotransmitter synthesis, and brain development and maturation.[18] Iron deposition in certain parts of the brain occurs under normal and abnormal conditions and is easily detected on MR scans because magnetic susceptibility causes preferential T2 shortening.[19]

Nonheme iron deposition in the brain is indepen-

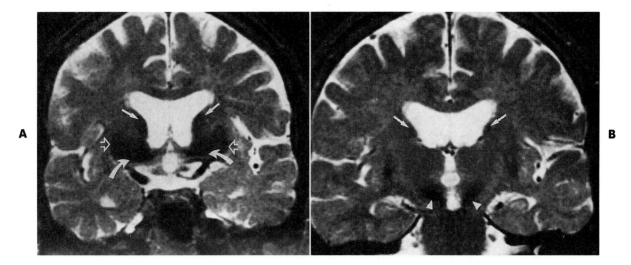

Fig. 18-7. A and **B,** Coronal T2-weighted MR scans in this 72-year-old patient show normal hypointensity in the putamen *(open arrow)*, globus pallidus *(curved arrows)*, caudate nuclei *(straight arrows)* and red nuclei *(arrowheads)*, caused by nonheme iron deposition. Same case as Fig. 18-1, *E* and *F.*

dent of hemoglobin metabolism and iron reserves in the rest of the body.[17] With aging the extrapyramidal gray matter nuclei normally become hypointense on T2-weighted MR scans (Fig. 18-7; *see* Fig. 18-1).[20] Small quantities of iron are first identified in the globus pallidus at 6 postnatal months, in the zona reticulata of the substantia nigra between 9 and 12 months, in the red nucleus at 18 to 24 months, and in the dentate nucleus at 3 to 7 years.[17]

Hypointense areas in the red nucleus, substantia nigra, and dentate nucleus seen on T2-weighted MR scans remain comparatively unchanged throughout all age groups, whereas hypointensity in the globus pallidus increases in middle-aged and elderly patients (Fig. 18-7).[21] Iron content in the putamen increases more slowly, reaching a maximum during the fifth decade.[19] The putamen normally appears hypointense only in the elderly (Fig. 18-7, *A*).[21] Although Perls' stain demonstrates some ferric iron deposition in the thalami and caudate nuclei of autopsied brains from elderly patients, hypointensity on T2WI is normally not seen in these areas.[21] Abnormal iron deposition in the caudate and other deep gray matter nuclei occurs with many neurodegenerative diseases and other pathological processes (see subsequent discussion).[20]

Cortical Gray Matter

Volume loss in the cortex with secondary enlargement of adjacent sulci and cisterns normally occurs with aging (*see* Fig. 18-4). Although patients with primary neurodegenerative disorders such as Pick disease or Alzheimer-type dementia have more marked sulcal enlargement (see subsequent discussion), substantial overlap between normal and abnormal elderly patients occurs (*see* Figs. 18-1, *C,* and 18-4).

Acquired White Matter Degenerative Disorders
Common
Multiple sclerosis
Arteriosclerosis
Trauma (diffuse axonal injury)
Uncommon
Viral/postviral demyelination
Toxic demyelination

WHITE MATTER NEURODEGENERATIVE DISORDERS

Some acquired neurodegenerative diseases primarily or exclusively involve the cerebral white matter (*see* box). These myelinoclastic diseases are sometimes termed *de*myelinating diseases to distinguish them from inherited or so-called *dys*myelinating disorders (*see* Chapter 17).

The most common and best-characterized of all the acquired demyelinating diseases is multiple sclerosis (MS).[22] In this section we first consider MS, then briefly review autoimmune-mediated demyelination disorders such as acute disseminated encephalomyelitis (considered in detail in Chapter 17). We then attend to toxic encephalopathies, concluding our discussion by delineating the effects of trauma and vascular disease on the cerebral white matter.

Multiple Sclerosis

Etiology and inheritance. The precise etiology of MS remains unknown, although most investigators favor autoimmune-mediated demyelination in genet-

Multiple Sclerosis
Possibly due to autoimmune-mediated demyelination
Most common demyelinating disease (after vascular and age-related demyelination)
Female preponderance, especially in children
Peak age between 20 and 40 years
Typical location   Calloseptal interface

Imaging
   Ovoid high signal foci on T2WI
   Perivenular extension (perpendicular to ventricles)
   Beveled or "target" (lesion within a lesion) appearance common on T1-, PD-weighted sequences
   Variable enhancement (solid, ring)
   Most lesions seen on MR are clinically silent
   Solitary lesions can mimic neoplasm, abscess

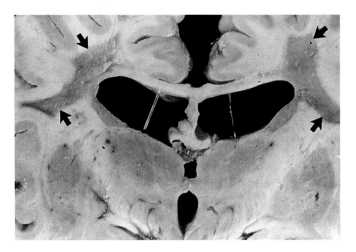

Fig. 18-8. Coronal gross autopsy specimen of multiple sclerosis shows confluent periventricular demyelinating plaques *(arrows)*. (Courtesy E. Tessa Hedley-Whyte.)

ically susceptible individuals (*see* box).[22-25a]

In experimental allergic encephalomyelitis (EAE), the animal model for MS, specific encephalitogenic peptides from myelin basic protein are presented on class II major histocompatibility complex molecules. These then induce T-cell receptor genes on CD4+ cells.[23] The exact role of such self-antigens in human MS is undetermined but epidemiologic and demographic studies suggest an exogenous infectious agent, possibly viral, as the most likely immunogen.[23]

The role of inheritance in MS is unknown but an increased incidence of subclinical demyelination has been demonstrated in asymptomatic first order relatives of MS patients.[24]

Pathology

Gross pathology. Both the gross and microscopic morphology of MS "plaques" are variable. The typical acute MS plaque is an edematous pink-gray white matter lesion.[22] Necrosis with atrophy and cystic changes are common in chronic lesions (Fig. 18-8). Hemorrhage and calcification are rare.[26]

Microscopic pathology. In MS, both myelin and the myelin-producing oligodendrocytes are destroyed. Lesions are defined as histologically active if moderate macrophage infiltration and at least mild perivascular inflammatory changes are present. Inactive lesions demonstrate minimal or no perivascular inflammation, mild or no macrophage infiltration, and well-established astrogliosis.[26]

Incidence. MS is by far the most common of all demyelinating diseases except for age-related vascular disease. Although MS preponderantly affects young adults of Northern European extraction and

occurs most often in temperate climates,[27] it has world-wide racial and geographic distribution.[28]

Age and gender. Symptom onset in MS is usually between 20 and 40 years of age. The female to male ratio in adults is 1.7-2:1. MS is less common in children and adolescents; when it occurs in these age groups, the female:male ratio is much higher, between 5 and 10:1.[29,30]

Location. More than 85% of MS patients have ovoid periventricular lesions that are oriented perpendicularly to the long axis of the brain and lateral ventricles.[31] This correlates well with the histologic localization of demyelination around subependymal and deep white matter medullary veins. The next most common site is the corpus callosum, involved in 50% to 90% of patients with clinically definite MS.[27,32] The callososeptal interface is a typical location; lesions here are optimally imaged in the sagittal plane (Fig. 18-9, *A*).[33]

In adults the brainstem and cerebellum are comparatively less common sites. Approximately 10% of MS plaques in adults are infratentorial, whereas the posterior fossa is a frequent site of MS plaques in children and adolescents (Fig. 18-9, *B*).[29] Occasionally, MS plaques are identified in the cortex (Fig. 18-9, *C*).

Multiple lesions are typical, although large, solitary plaques do occur and can be mistaken on imaging studies for neoplasm (see subsequent discussion).

Clinical presentation and natural history. The clinical spectrum and the natural history of MS are variable. The most typical course is prolonged relapsing-remitting disease.[34] Later, the disease often shifts into a chronic-progressive phase.[27] A rare ful-

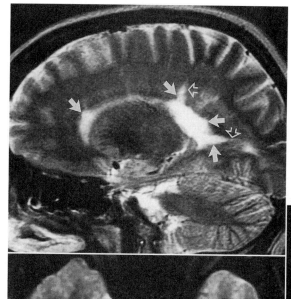

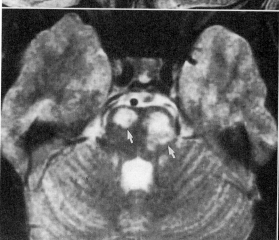

Fig. 18-9. A, Sagittal T2-weighted MR scan shows multiple ovoid areas of high signal intensity along the callososeptal interface *(large arrows)*. Note perivenular extension into the centrum semiovale *(open arrows)*, sometimes called "Dawson's fingers." Typical MS. **B,** Axial T2-weighted MR scan in a 16-year-old girl with facial numbness and MS shows multiple brainstem lesions *(arrows)*. **C,** Axial T2-weighted MR scan in this 23-year-old woman with MS and typical periventricular plaques *(straight arrows)* also shows a large right frontal plaque that involves the cortex *(curved arrow)*. (**B,** From Osborn AG et al: *AJNR* 11:489-494, 1990.)

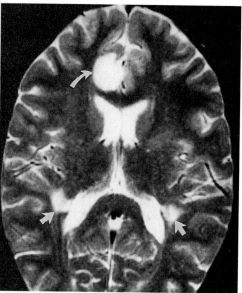

minant form, acute fulminant MS of the Marburg type, is associated with rapid clinical deterioration, substantial morbidity, and high mortality.[25]

Imaging. In a prospective 2-year study, the sensitivity of MR imaging in detecting MS was nearly 85% and exceeded all other tests, including oligoclonal bands, evoked potentials, and CT scans.[35] Imaging findings vary with disease activity, although clinical correlation with specific lesions is generally poor. Most foci identified on standard MR scans are clinically silent.[34,36]

CT. Scans are often normal early in the disease course. Lesions are typically iso- or hypodense with brain on NECT studies (Fig. 18-10, *A*). Enhancement following contrast administration is variable. Some lesions show no change, whereas others enhance intensely. Both solid (Fig. 18-10, *B* and *C*) and ringlike patterns are observed. Some lesions become apparent only after high-dose delayed scans are performed (Fig. 18-10, *C*).[28]

MR. Most MS plaques are iso- to hypointense on T1-weighted scans and hyperintense compared to

brain on T2-weighted scans. Because there are many causes of white matter hyperintensities on T2WI (see subsequent discussion), most authorities require the presence of three or more discrete lesions that are 5 mm or greater in size, as well as lesions that occur in a characteristic location and have a compatible clinical history, to establish the MR diagnosis of MS.[37,38, 38a] Oblong lesions at the callososeptal interface are typical (Fig. 18-11). Perivenular extension into the deep white matter, the so-called Dawson's finger, is characteristic (*see* Fig. 18-9, *A*).[38]

MS lesions are often seen as round or ovoid areas with a "beveled" (lesion within a lesion) appearance on T1- and proton density-weighted studies (Fig. 18-12, *A*). Confluent periventricular lesions are common in severe cases. Abnormal basal ganglia hypointensity is seen in about 10% of long-standing severe MS cases (Fig. 18-13).

Enhancement following contrast administration represents blood-brain barrier disruption. Enhancement is highly variable and typically transient, seen during the active demyelinating stage. Both solid (*see* Fig. 18-12, *C*) and ringlike (Fig. 18-14) enhance-

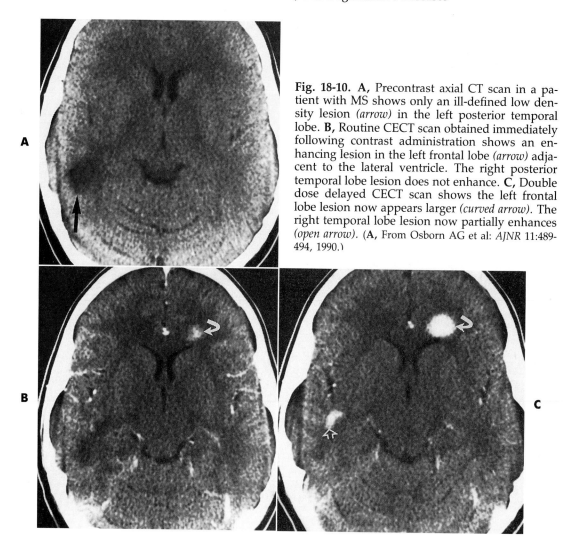

Fig. 18-10. A, Precontrast axial CT scan in a patient with MS shows only an ill-defined low density lesion *(arrow)* in the left posterior temporal lobe. **B,** Routine CECT scan obtained immediately following contrast administration shows an enhancing lesion in the left frontal lobe *(arrow)* adjacent to the lateral ventricle. The right posterior temporal lobe lesion does not enhance. **C,** Double dose delayed CECT scan shows the left frontal lobe lesion now appears larger *(curved arrow)*. The right temporal lobe lesion now partially enhances *(open arrow)*. (**A,** From Osborn AG et al: *AJNR* 11:489-494, 1990.)

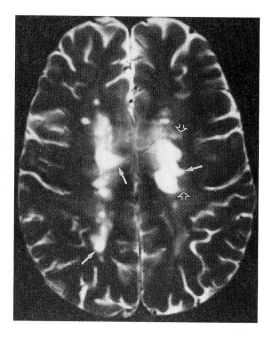

Fig. 18-11. Axial T2-weighted MR scan in this 42-year-old woman with long-standing MS shows multiple ovoid or oblong lesions in the deep periventricular white matter and corpus callosum *(solid arrows)*. Note extension into the centrum semiovale along the course of the deep medullary veins *(open arrows)*.

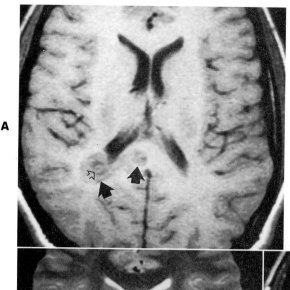

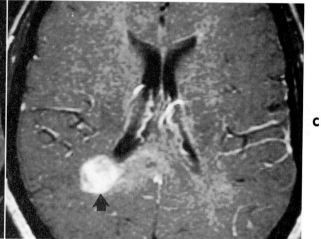

Fig. 18-12. Typical MS plaques are demonstrated on the MR scans obtained in this 23-year-old woman with clinically definite MS and CSF studies positive for oligoclonal bands. **A,** Axial precontrast T1-weighted scan shows a hypointense lesion in the corpus callosum splenium and deep periventricular white matter *(large arrows).* Note the beveled or "lesion within a lesion" appearance *(open arrow).* **B,** Axial T2WI shows the lesion *(arrows)* appears very hyperintense compared to normal white matter. **C,** Postcontrast T1WI shows the lesion *(arrow)* enhances strongly but somewhat inhomogeneously.

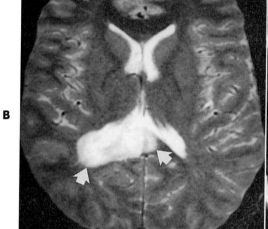

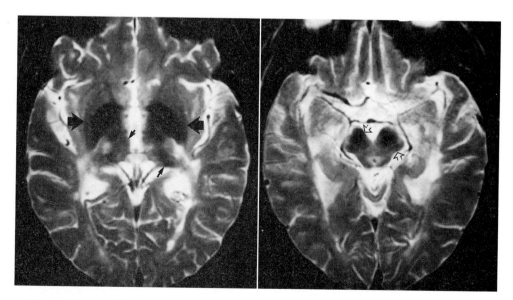

Fig. 18-13. Axial T2-weighted MR scans in this 42-year-old woman with long-standing, severe MS show abnormal nonheme iron deposition in the putamina *(large arrows),* thalami *(small arrows),* and midbrain *(open arrows).* Same case as Fig. 18-11.

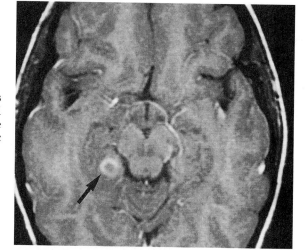

Fig. 18-14. Axial postcontrast T1-weighted MR scan in this 20-year-old woman with a temporal lobe seizure disclosed this solitary ring enhancing mass *(arrow)*. Because of the history, biopsy was performed. MS was found at histologic examination.

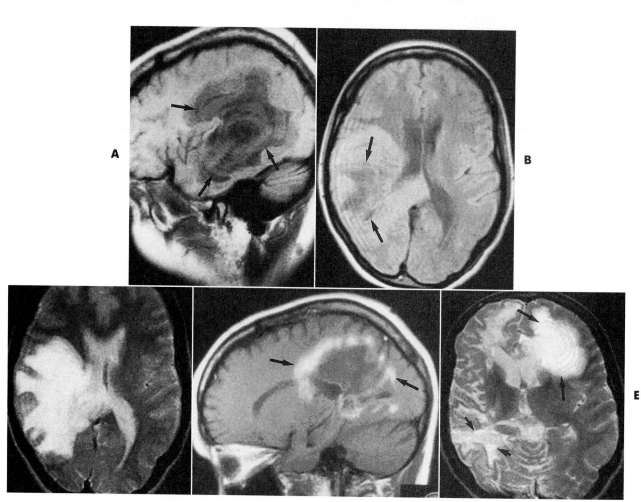

Fig. 18-15. This 32-year-old woman developed sudden onset of left extremity paresthesias. **A,** Sagittal T1-weighted MR scan shows a large, solitary parietotemporal mass with concentric ringlike hypointense areas *(arrows)*. Axial proton density- **(B)** and T2-weighted **(C)** studies show the mass is inhomogeneously hyperintense. The overlying cortical gray matter is spared. **D,** Sagittal postcontrast T1WI shows patchy ring enhancement *(arrows)*. **E,** Axial T2-weighted MR scan obtained 8 months later shows the right parietotemporal lesion *(short arrows)* has largely resolved. A new left frontal mass is now present *(long arrows)* that has concentric ringlike hyperintense areas. The patient expired; autopsy *(see* Fig. 18-15, **F)** showed multiple sclerosis. (**A** to **E,** From M. Tersegno; **A** and **C,** Reprinted from *AJR* 160:901, 1993.)

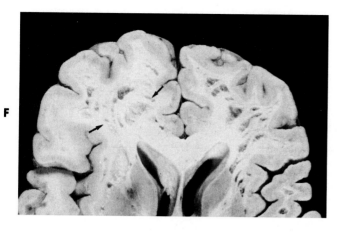

F

Fig. 18-15, cont'd. F, Axial brain specimen shows concentric laminae of spongiform demyelination *(arrows)* in the left frontal lobe (specimen seen from below). (**F,** From G.H. Collins.)

ment patterns are seen.[39] Enhanced T1-weighted scans can detect additional lesions that are not apparent on T2WI,[34] although most MS plaques do not enhance following contrast administration.[37] Some solitary or highly atypical MS lesions may be indistinguishable from abscess (Fig. 18-14) or neoplasm (Fig. 18-15).[40,40a]

Cranial neuropathies, particularly optic neuritis, are common in patients with MS. Lesions in the brainstem tracts and nuclei are seen on T2WI, whereas contrast-enhanced T1-weighted studies may delineate enhancement in the nerves themselves (Fig. 18-16). Fat-saturation and short inversion recovery scans are useful in separating optic nerve enhancement from high-signal orbital fat.[41]

Miscellaneous. Early evidence indicates that ^{1}H spectroscopy may be more sensitive than contrast-enhanced MR in delineating the true time course of demyelination in MS plaques.[42]

Viral and Postviral Diseases

Viral and postviral white matter diseases are discussed extensively in Chapter 16. Acute disseminated encephalomyelitis (ADEM) is characterized by immune-mediated disseminated demyelination. Multifocal high intensity lesions are seen on T2-weighted MR scans; both the supratentorial and posterior fossa white matter are typically affected (*see* Figs. 16-37 to 16-39). The basal ganglia are sometimes also involved.[43]

Toxic Demyelination

Toxic encephalopathy (TE) results from interaction of a chemical compound with the brain. A large number of chemicals are potential neurotoxins; some of the more common and important substances are listed in the box.

Toxins cause temporary or permanent disturbance of normal brain function in several ways,[44] including.

1. Depletion of oxidative energy
2. Nutritional deprivation

Toxic Demyelination
Common
Alcohol
Uncommon
Inherited leukodystrophies (e.g., storage diseases)
Osmotic demyelination
Hydrocarbons and other solvents
Cyclosporin toxicity
Methotrexate +/− radiation therapy
Rare
Lead
Mercury

3. Disturbances in neurotransmission
4. Altered ion balance

Toxins can be endogenous or exogenous to the CNS. Endogenous CNS toxins typically result from inborn errors of metabolism such as the amino acidopathies and globoid cell leukodystrophy (Krabbe disease). These inherited neurodegenerative disorders are detailed in Chapter 17.

Exogenous TE can be internal or external. Internal TEs are caused by systemic disorders that produce toxins, which then cross the BBB and damage the CNS. Examples are paraneoplastic syndromes (*see* Chapter 15) and ion balance disorders such as central pontine myelinolysis (CPM) and the hepatocerebral syndromes. External TEs include lead or mercury poisoning, solvent exposure, alcohol abuse, and chemotherapy.[44]

In this section we consider two of the more common exogenous TEs that primarily affect the white matter: osmotic myelinolysis and chronic alcoholism. Toxins that involve mostly the gray matter and basal ganglia are discussed in a later section of this chapter.

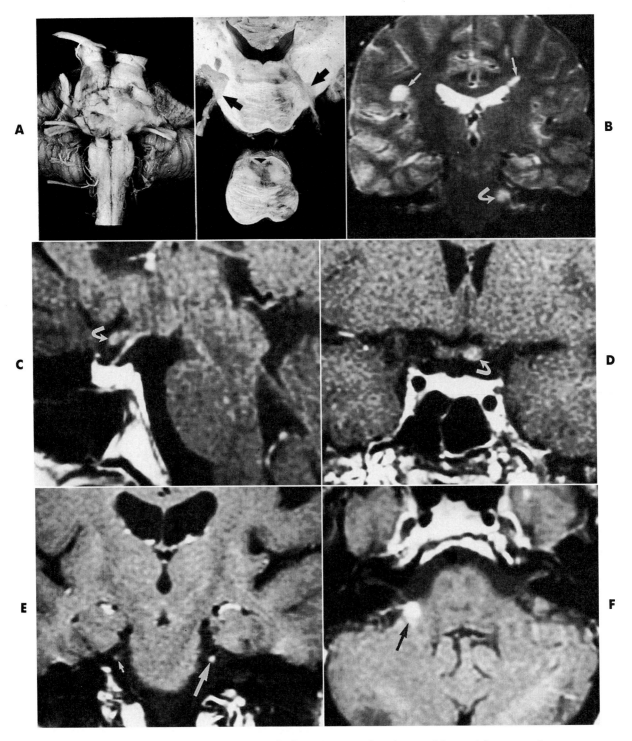

Fig. 18-16. Pathology and imaging findings in several patients with cranial nerve palsies caused by MS. **A,** Gross pathology specimen shows multiple plaques, including the root entry zones of the trigeminal nerves *(arrows)*. **B,** Coronal T2WI in this 15-year-old girl with left trigeminal neuralgia and MS show supratentorial white matter lesions *(straight arrows)* and a large plaque at the root entry zone of the left trigeminal nerve *(curved arrow)*. Compare with **A.** Sagittal **(C)** and coronal **(D)** postcontrast T1-weighted MR scans in this 44-year-old woman with optic neuritis show optic chiasm enhancement *(arrows)*. **E,** Coronal postcontrast T1WI in another patient who has left facial numbness shows left trigeminal nerve enhancement *(large arrow)*. Compare with the normal, unenhancing right CN V *(small arrow)*. **(F)** This 40-year-old woman with multiple neurologic symptoms and known MS developed right-sided sensorineural hearing loss. Postcontrast axial T1WI shows an enhancing plaque in the right restiform body and root entry zone of CN VIII *(arrow)*. (**A,** From Okazaki H, Scheithauer B: *Slide Atlas of Neuropathology,* Gower Medical Publishing.)

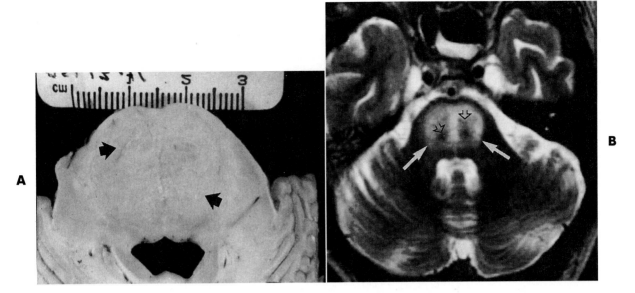

Fig. 18-17. A, Axial gross pathology shows central pontine myelinolysis *(arrows).* **B,** Axial T2-weighted MR scan in this 49-year-old man with rapid correction of severe hyponatremia shows the typical imaging findings of osmotic demyelination in the pons, also known as central pontine myelinolysis. The central pons appears hyperintense *(white arrows).* Note relative sparing of the descending corticospinal tracts *(black arrows).* (**A,** Courtesy E. Ross.)

Osmotic myelinolysis. Osmotic myelinolysis (OM) is a toxic demyelinating disease that classically occurs in alcoholic, malnourished, or chronically debilitated adults.[45] Over 75% of cases are associated with chronic alcoholism or rapid correction of hyponatremia, although other conditions such as hypernatremia have also been implicated.[46,47]

Pathologically, OM is characterized by myelin loss (myelinolysis) with relative neuron sparing. The central pons is the most common site *(central pontine myelinolysis,* or CPM), although OM also occurs in other locations (Fig. 18-17, *A*). So-called *extrapontine myelinolysis* (EPM) is identified pathologically in about half of all osmotic demyelination cases. Reported extrapontine sites include the putamina, caudate nuclei, midbrain, thalami, and subcortical white matter.[48]

Imaging manifestations of OM syndromes reflect increased water content in the affected areas. NECT scans are normal or disclose nonspecific hypodense areas. OM lesions are hypointense on T1- and hyperintense on T2-weighted MR scans (Fig. 18-17, *B*). Transverse pontine fibers are most severely affected, whereas the descending corticospinal tracts are often spared.[45] Enhancement following contrast administration varies; some lesions enhance but most do not.[49]

Pontine signal abnormalities have a broad differential diagnosis that includes infarct, metastasis, glioma, multiple sclerosis, encephalitis, and radiation or chemotherapy.[46] However, pontine plus concomitant basal ganglia involvement is fairly specific for OM.

In such cases the imaging differential diagnosis is much more narrow and includes hypoxia, Leigh disease, and Wilson disease. OM can usually be distinguished from these entities using a combination of imaging findings and clinical history.[45]

Chronic alcoholism. Various specific processes related to ethanol intoxication affect the CNS. These include Wernicke encephalopathy, Marchiafava-Bignami disease, and osmotic myelinolysis.[50] Ethanol adversely affects vascular, glial, and neural tissues and also causes myelin degeneration. Nonspecific deep white matter and periventricular demyelinating lesions are seen on the MR scans of patients with chronic alcoholism (Fig. 18-18).[50] Demyelination is the main pathological finding in Marchiafava-Bignami disease and is the earliest, most constant lesion in Wernicke disease.

Marchiafava-Bignami disease. Marchiafava-Bignami disease (MBD) is an uncommon disorder associated with chronic alcoholism.[51] This disorder was originally described in poorly nourished Italian men addicted to crude red wine consumption. MBD has now been reported in other population groups and with various alcoholic beverages.[52]

Pathologically, MBD is characterized by corpus callosum demyelination and necrosis, although the cerebral hemispheric white matter and other commissural fibers may also be affected.[52] Focal cystic necrosis occurs in the middle layers of the corpus callosum genu, body, or splenium. Sagittal MR scans show callosal atrophy and focal necrosis as linear or punctate

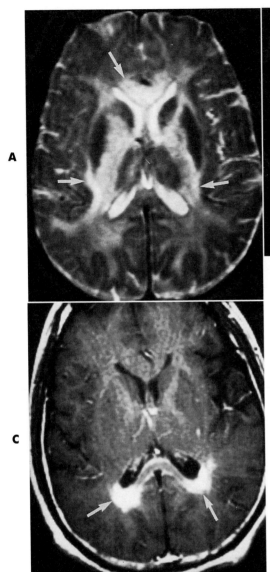

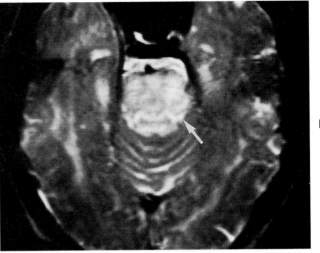

Fig. 18-18. A 47-year-old severe chronic alcoholic had these MR scans. **A** and **B,** Axial T2-weighted scans show diffuse deep white matter, periventricular, and pontine hyperintensities *(arrows).* **C,** Postcontrast T1WI shows some periventricular enhancement *(arrows).* Presumed alcohol-induced demyelination. (Courtesy L. Tan and S. Lin.)

hypointense regions on T1WI that become hyperintense on T2WI.[51,52]

Wernicke encephalopathy. Wernicke encephalopathy (WE) is caused by nutritional thiamine deficiency and occurs mainly—but not exclusively—in chronic alcoholics.[53,54] The classic clinical triad in WE consists of ophthalmoplegia, ataxia, and confusion, although these findings are not invariably present.[54,55]

WE shows a characteristic topographic distribution and involves both gray and white matter. The periventricular regions, the medial thalamic nuclei, massa intermedia, third ventricular floor, and mammillary bodies are most frequently affected (Fig. 18-19, *A*). The periaqueductal region, midbrain reticular formation, and tectal plate are also commonly involved.[56]

Imaging findings in acute WE seen on T2WI include hyperintense areas that surround the third ven-

tricle and aqueduct.[53] Postcontrast T1WI may show enhancement around the third ventricle, aqueduct, and in the mammillary bodies (Fig. 18-19, *B*).[55] Studies obtained after vitamin therapy sometimes show resolution of these abnormalities.[57] Third ventricular enlargement and mammillary body atrophy are seen in chronic WE.

Miscellaneous toxins. Myelin has a particularly high lipid content and very slow metabolic turnover. Therefore all myelinated tracts are especially vulnerable to lipid peroxidation and accumulation of toxic lipophilic substances.[44] Organic compounds such as solvents and toluene cause multifocal white matter lesions that are detectable on T2-weighted MR scans.[44]

Irradiation and chemotherapy. Neurotoxicity is a known complication of radiation therapy and some chemotherapeutic agents. Chemotherapeutic agents known specifically to cause leukoencephalopathy include cyclosporin A, methotrexate, cytarabine, and 5-fluorouracil (Fig. 18-20, *A*).[44,58,58a] Concomitant chemotherapy can also potentiate radiation-induced white matter damage. Intravenous or intrathecal methotrexate can cause leukoencephalopathy when used alone, although these effects are usually transient (Fig. 18-20, *B* and *C*).[59]

The pathophysiology of radiation- and chemother-

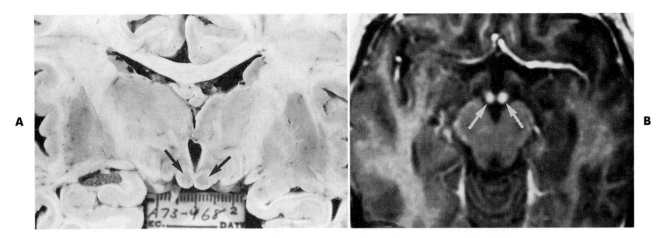

Fig. 18-19. A, Coronal gross pathology specimen of Wernicke encephalopathy shows necrotic changes in the mammillary bodies *(arrows)* **B,** Axial postcontrast T1-weighted MR scan in a patient with Wernicke encephalopathy shows enhancement of the mammillary bodies *(arrows).* (**A,** Courtesy E. Ross. **B,** Courtesy of M. Zagardo and M. Shagry.)

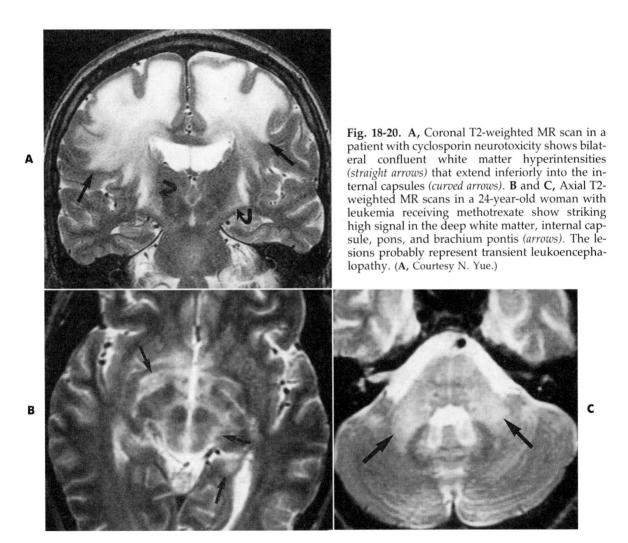

Fig. 18-20. A, Coronal T2-weighted MR scan in a patient with cyclosporin neurotoxicity shows bilateral confluent white matter hyperintensities *(straight arrows)* that extend inferiorly into the internal capsules *(curved arrows).* **B** and **C,** Axial T2-weighted MR scans in a 24-year-old woman with leukemia receiving methotrexate show striking high signal in the deep white matter, internal capsule, pons, and brachium pontis *(arrows).* The lesions probably represent transient leukoencephalopathy. (**A,** Courtesy N. Yue.)

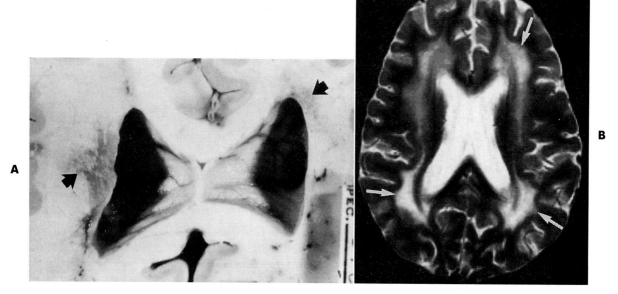

Fig. 18-21. A, Coronal gross pathology of disseminated necrotizing leukoencephalopathy *(arrows)* in a patient who had received intrathecal methotrexate and radiation therapy. **B,** Axial T2-weighted MR scan in a 12-year-old boy receiving radiation therapy and intravenous methotrexate shows diffuse, bilateral, confluent periventricular high signal intensity *(arrows)*. Note sparing of the subcortical arcuate fibers. Disseminated necrotizing leukoencephalopathy. (**A,** Courtesy Rubinstein Collection, University of Virginia.)

apy induced neurotoxicity is controversial. The most widely accepted explanation is that small and medium-sized vessel injury causes endothelial thickening, with ensuing obstruction, thrombosis, ischemia, infarction, and parenchymal necrosis.[60] Radiation- or chemotherapy induced neurotoxicity predominately involves the deep white matter with relative sparing of the cortex and underlying subcortical arcuate fibers.[60]

Imaging findings in the typical late "delayed" radiation injury range from a single focal mass to more diffuse white matter lesions. T1- and T2-relaxation times are both prolonged.[60] Confluent, diffuse white matter demyelination combined with rapid clinical deterioration is known as "necrotizing leukoencephalopathy" (Fig. 18-21).

Focal radiation necrosis also occurs and can be indistinguishable from recurrent or persistent neoplasm on routine contrast-enhanced CT or MR imaging (Fig. 18-22).[61] Dual-isotope single-photon emission computed tomography (SPECT) and positron emission tomography (PET) may be helpful in some cases.[62,63]

Widespread perivascular calcification, a condition known as mineralizing angiopathy (MA), typically occurs in children receiving both irradiation and chemotherapy for acute leukemia, although MA has been reported in other settings as well.[59] The basal ganglia and junction of the cortex with the subcorti-

cal white matter are the most common sites of MA (Fig. 18-23).[60]

Trauma

Trauma is one of the most common nonvascular causes of focal white matter lesions. Diffuse axonal injury (DAI) results from axonal shearing caused by sudden acceleration-deceleration or angular rotation forces on the brain. DAI typically occurs with severe trauma, not minor injury, has a characteristic clinical presentation (immediate loss of consciousness without an intervening "lucid interval"), and is seen on T2-weighted MR scans as multifocal hyperintensities in predictable locations (*see* Fig. 8-27). The gray-white matter interface, corpus callosum (*see* Fig. 8-29), internal capsule, and brainstem are common sites. Hemorrhagic shearing injuries may appear very low signal on T2WI (*see* Fig. 8-30).

Vascular Disease

Vascular disease can cause white matter lesions in children and in elderly patients (*see* box). Hypoxic-ischemic encephalopathy (HIE) and cerebral embolism occur in both groups, whereas small-vessel atherosclerosis is a disease of the elderly.

Hypoxic-ischemic encephalopathy. Imaging manifestations of HIE vary with length and severity of the insult, patient age, individual cerebral circulatory pat-

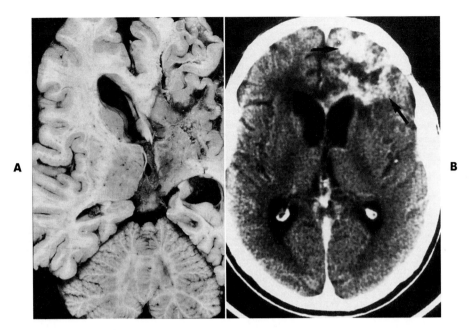

Fig. 18-22. **A,** Axial gross pathology specimen shows extensive frontal lobe radiation necrosis. **B,** Axial CECT scan in a patient with surgical resection of a left frontal anaplastic astrocytoma followed by radiation therapy. Note the extensive, irregularly enhancing mass *(arrows)*. Radiation necrosis without tumor recurrence was found at surgery. (**A,** Courtesy Rubinstein Collection, University of Virginia.)

Vascular Causes of White Matter Disease
Arteriosclerosis "Lacunar" infarcts Emboli Hypoxic-ischemic encephalopathy Vasculitis

terns, and the inherent vulnerability of certain anatomic regions and cell types to hypoxic-ischemic injury (*see* Chapter 11).

Premature infants. White matter of the developing brain is especially vulnerable to injury. The pathologic spectrum of lesions seen in HIE includes necrosis, gliosis, and disturbances in myelination.[64]

Periventricular leukomalacia (PVL) frequently occurs in premature infants and is probably caused by ischemic infarction of the periventricular white matter, the vascular watershed zone in the developing fetus (*see* Fig. 11-30). Isolated PVL typically reflects late second- or early third-trimester injury.[65] The most characteristic clinical presentation of PVL is spastic diplegia, a common form of cerebral palsy with nonprogressive but permanent impairment of movement and posture.[66]

Typical imaging findings in PVL include peritrigonal hyperintensities on T2-weighted MR scans, focal ventricular enlargement, and irregular ventricular

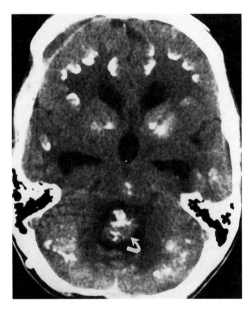

Fig. 18-23. Axial NECT scan in this 21-year-old man with radiation therapy 6 years earlier for a vermian astrocytoma *(arrow)*. Note widespread calcifications in the basal ganglia, dentate nuclei, and gray-white matter junction. Typical mineralizing angiopathy.

contours (Fig. 18-24). White matter volume is reduced, and the posterior corpus callosum often appears moderately atrophic. PVL is usually bilateral but is often asymmetric. PVL occasionally causes diffuse multifocal white matter lesions.[66]

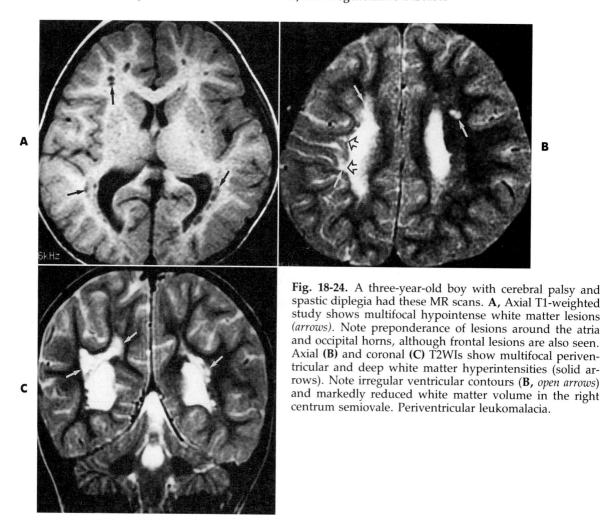

Fig. 18-24. A three-year-old boy with cerebral palsy and spastic diplegia had these MR scans. **A,** Axial T1-weighted study shows multifocal hypointense white matter lesions *(arrows)*. Note preponderance of lesions around the atria and occipital horns, although frontal lesions are also seen. Axial **(B)** and coronal **(C)** T2WIs show multifocal periventricular and deep white matter hyperintensities (solid arrows). Note irregular ventricular contours **(B,** *open arrows)* and markedly reduced white matter volume in the right centrum semiovale. Periventricular leukomalacia.

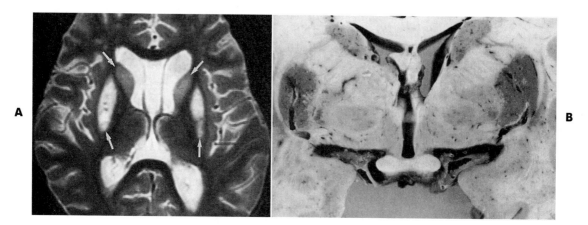

Fig. 18-25. A, Axial T2-weighted MR scan of a 5-year-old child who had respiratory arrest and profound hypotension following prolonged seizure activity. Note symmetric hyperintensity of the caudate nuclei and putamen *(arrows)*, caused by the hypoxic-ischemic event. **B,** For comparison, note bilateral putaminal necrosis in this autopsy specimen. Smoke inhalation and profound hypotension. **(A,** Courtesy L. Tan and S. Lin.)

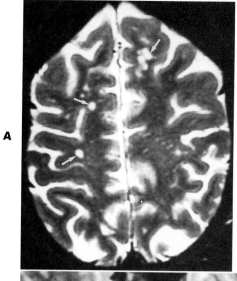

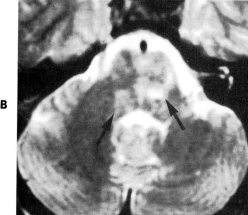

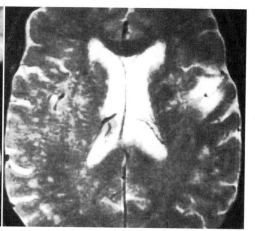

Fig. 18-26. Three cases of nonspecific white matter hyperintensities. **A,** Axial T2-weighted MR scan in this 42-year-old hypertensive but otherwise clinically normal woman without a history of trauma shows multifocal punctate subcortical white matter hyperintensities, or "unknown bright objects," *(arrows).* Diagnosis unknown. **B,** Axial T2WI in this 62-year-old man with gradual onset of multiple neurologic abnormalities shows multifocal pontine lesions *(arrows).* Primary CNS lymphoma. **C,** Axial T2WI in this elderly woman with known metastatic breast carcinoma shows multifocal white matter hyperintensities. Autopsy-proven metastases.

Term infants. Full-term infants with late third-trimester, perinatal, or postnatal injury have ischemic lesions located predominately in the cortex and subcortical white matter.[66] The deep gray nuclei are also commonly affected (*see* Fig. 11-35).[65]

Children and adults. HIE in these groups typically results in watershed infarction and bilateral selective neuronal necrosis within the globus pallidus, putamen, caudate nucleus, thalamus, parahippocampal gyrus, hippocampus, cerebellum, and brainstem nuclei (Fig. 18-25; *see* Figs. 11-32 and 11-33) (see subsequent discussion).[67]

Atherosclerosis. Focal white matter hyperintensities (WMHs) are frequently identified on T2-weighted MR scans (Fig. 18-26, *A*). These foci are variably referred to as leukoaraiosis, periventricular hyperintensities, white matter hyperintensities, and unidentified bright objects (UBOs). Their prevalence has been linked to numerous factors, including normal aging, carotid atherosclerosis, and hypertension.[68,68a]

The patchy hyperintense subcortical lesions observed on T2-weighted MR scans in both normal and demented elderly patients are often but not invariably associated with arteriosclerosis. Nonspecific myelin pallor accounts for some subcortical WMHs, whereas others are caused by dilated perivascular spaces (see previous discussion).[2]

Imaging findings of multifocal WMHs on T2-weighted MR scans are nonspecific, and the differential diagnosis of these lesions is very broad (*see* box, p. 771). The most common causes are age-related vascular changes, dilated perivascular spaces, and multiple sclerosis (MS). In contrast to MS, the T1-weighted images in patients with subcortical arteriosclerotic encephalopathy (SAE) are often normal.[69] Exceptions are focal hypointensities on T1WI caused by deep lacunar infarcts and widened Virchow-Robin spaces.[69]

Other causes of discrete multifocal WMHs include primary CNS lymphoma (Fig. 18-26, *B*), metastases (Fig. 18-26, *C*), and vasculitis (Fig. 18-27). Infiltrating astrocytoma (gliomatosis cerebri) can cause confluent white matter disease that is indistinguishable from benign leukoencephalopathies (Fig. 18-28).

Diabetes. Diabetes mellitus (DM) occurs in 1% to 2% of the population in the Western world. DM has

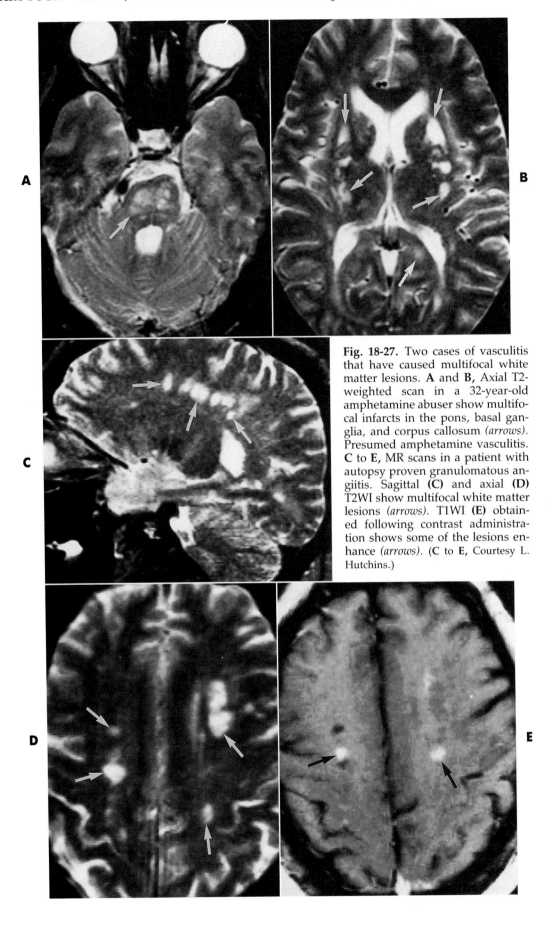

Fig. 18-27. Two cases of vasculitis that have caused multifocal white matter lesions. **A** and **B,** Axial T2-weighted scan in a 32-year-old amphetamine abuser show multifocal infarcts in the pons, basal ganglia, and corpus callosum *(arrows).* Presumed amphetamine vasculitis. **C** to **E,** MR scans in a patient with autopsy proven granulomatous angiitis. Sagittal **(C)** and axial **(D)** T2WI show multifocal white matter lesions *(arrows).* T1WI **(E)** obtained following contrast administration shows some of the lesions enhance *(arrows).* (**C** to **E,** Courtesy L. Hutchins.)

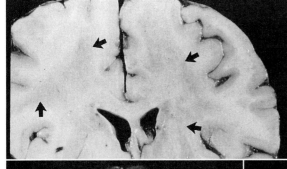

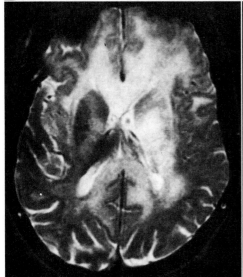

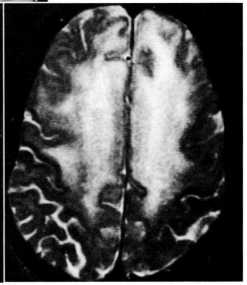

Fig. 18-28. A, Axial gross autopsy specimen shows diffuse white matter disease *(arrows).* Microscopic examination disclosed gliomatosis cerebri. **B** and **C,** Axial T2-weighted MR scans in a 68-year-old woman with a 3-month history of declining mental status show diffuse, confluent deep white matter hyperintensities. The left thalamus is also involved. Autopsy disclosed diffusely infiltrating anaplastic astrocytoma. (**A,** Courtesy E. Tessa Hedley Whyte. **B** and **C,** Courtesy M. Disbro.)

Multifocal White Matter Lesions
Differential diagnosis

Common	Uncommon
Perivascular (Virchow-Robin) spaces	Postviral demyelination
Aging/myelin pallor	Vasculitis
Arteriosclerosis	Primary CNS lymphoma
Multiple sclerosis	Multifocal glioma/gliomatosis cerebri
Multiple emboli	Inflammatory (e.g., multiple abscesses)
Metastases	Inherited leukoencephalopathy
Trauma (diffuse axonal or "shearing" injury)	Acquired leukoencephalopathy (e.g., toxic demyelination)
Inflammatory (e.g., cysticercosis)	Neurocutaneous syndromes (tuberous sclerosis, NF-1)

---

many manifestations. One of the most devastating complications is blindness, caused by proliferative retinopathy.[70] Imaging studies in these patients have not demonstrated an increased incidence of WMHs compared to age-matched nondiabetic volunteers. Therefore WMHs and ischemic changes in insulin-dependent diabetic patients under 40 years of age should not be attributed to diabetic vasculopathy. Other causes should be considered.[70]

Vasculitis. Systemic lupus erythematosus, Sjogren syndrome, Behcet disease, "moya moya" disease, polyarteritis nodosa, amyloid angiopathy, and other vasculitides are potential causes of WMHs on T2-weighted MR scans (Fig. 18-27).[71,72] Vasculitis and its imaging manifestations are discussed in detail in Chapter 11.

GRAY MATTER NEURODEGENERATIVE DISORDERS

Inherited neurodegenerative disorders that primarily or exclusively involve the gray matter and may present as dementia in adults include Kuf disease (adult-onset neuronal ceroid lipofuscinosis), GM_2 gangliosidosis (Tay-Sachs, Sandhoff disease) and mucopolysaccharidosis type III-B (Sanfilippo disease) (Fig. 17-15).[73] Other common "childhood" neurodegenerative diseases sometimes seen in adults include adult-onset adrenoleukodystrophy and metachromatic leukodystrophy, mitochondrial encephalopathies (e.g., MELAS and MERRF), and Wilson disease[73] (see box, below) (see Chapter 17).

Many acquired neurodegenerative disorders primarily, if not exclusively, involve the cortex or subcortical gray matter nuclei. Some disorders are temporary and potentially reversible. These include the brain volume loss that occurs with severe dehydration, steroid administration, anorexia, and starvation.[74]

Some Inherited Neurodegenerative Diseases That May Present in Adults as Dementing Disorders

Disorders that primarily affect gray matter

Lipidoses
  Neuronal ceroid lipofuscinosis (Batten, Kufs types)
  GM_2 gangliosidoses (Tay-Sachs, Sandhoff disease can become symptomatic in third decade)
Mucopolysaccharidoses (usually only MPS IIIB, Sanfilippo disease, presents in adults)
Fucosidosis (rare)
Glycogen storage disorders

Disorders that affect both gray and white matter

Mitochondrial encephalopathies
  MELAS
  MERRF

Disorders that affect white matter primarily or exclusively

Adult onset MLD
AMN, carrier state for ALD

Basal ganglia disorders

Wilson disease

Miscellaneous disorders

Gaucher type 1
Niemann-Pick II-C
Fabry disease
Lafora disease
Cerebrotendinous xanthomatosis

Data from Coker SB: *Neurology*: 41:794-798, 1991.

In this section we focus on the dementias, temporal lobe (hippocampal) atrophy, acquired extrapyramidal degenerative disorders, and striatonigral syndromes.

Alzheimer Disease and Other Cortical Dementias

The exact prevalence of dementia is unknown, but some estimate at least 5% of people over 65 years and 15% over 85 years of age are severely demented (see box, below).[20] Alzheimer and Pick disease are examples of cortical dementias. Multi-infarct dementia is an example of combined cortical and subcortical dementia.[74a]

Alzheimer disease. Alzheimer disease (AD) is the most common acquired brain degenerative disease.[20] AD is also the most common form of dementia in western industrialized countries, representing between 60% and 70% of all cases.[75] In the United States, AD affects 7% of the population over 65 years of age.

Grossly, the brains of patients with AD show diffuse cerebral atrophy with widened sulci and enlarged lateral ventricles (Fig. 18-29, *A*). Disproportionate atrophy of the temporal lobes, particularly the hippocampal formations, is a gross pathologic hallmark of AD.[76] The cortical gray matter is reduced, particularly in the temporal lobes.[77] Microscopically, AD is characterized by neuronal loss, gliosis, neurofibrillary tangles, senile (neuritic) plaques, Hirano bodies, granulovacuolar degeneration of neurons, and amyloid angiopathy.[20]

Although many imaging-based morphologic measurements have been proposed to differentiate AD from normal aging, a simple and reliable linear measurement that can be made on routine MR studies remains elusive.[78,78a,b] In general, imaging studies in AD patients show diffusely enlarged ventricles and prominent sulci. Annual increases in ventricular volume are significantly greater than in age-matched controls.[79]

AD patients have generalized cortical atrophy and

Alzheimer Disease

Most common acquired brain degenerative disease
Disproportionate temporal lobe atrophy on gross; neurofibrillary tangles and senile plaques on microscopic
Imaging studies show generalized atrophy, most severe in temporal lobes; white matter hyperintensities not a prominent feature
Differential diagnosis: normal aging

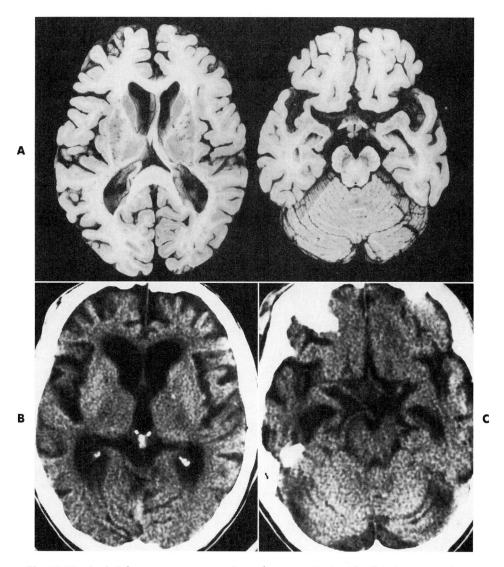

Fig. 18-29. A, Axial gross autopsy specimen from a patient with Alzheimer-type dementia shows diffuse ventricular and sulcal enlargement. The sylvian fissures are especially prominent. **B** and **C,** Axial NECT scans in a 69-year-old woman with a 10-year history of Alzheimer-type dementia show markedly enlarged ventricles and sulci. The sylvian fissures and temporal horns of the lateral ventricles are the most severely affected. (**A,** From Okazaki H, Scheithauer B; *Slide Atlas of Neuropathology,* Gower Medical Publishing.)

gray matter reduction with disproportionate volume loss in the anterior temporal lobes and hippocampi (Fig. 18-29, *B* and *C*).[76] The temporal horns, as well as the choroid and hippocampal fissures, appear particularly prominent.[80,81] Enlarged sylvian fissures are sensitive but less specific indicators of AD.[80]

White matter hyperintensities are not a particularly prominent feature of AD. Some WMHs do occur but there is significant overlap with normal age-matched controls and no definite correlation with dementia severity (see previous discussion). Severe subcortical and periventricular white matter disease is more typical of multi-infarct dementia than AD (see subsequent discussion).[20] Other diseases besides

multi-infarct dementia that can mimic AD clinically include subdural hematoma and primary brain tumor.[82] A variant of AD, *Lewy-body disease,* has eosinophilic cytoplasmic inclusions, prominent Parkinsonian features, and accentuated frontal lobe atrophy.[83]

Pick disease. Pick disease (PD) is a cortical dementia that is much less frequent than AD. Presenile onset (before age 65) is common.[84] The neuropathologic markers for PD are Pick bodies, distinctive round cytoplasmic inclusions.

Grossly, Pick disease is characterized by strikingly circumscribed lobar atrophy that may be very asymmetric. The frontal and temporal lobes are most com-

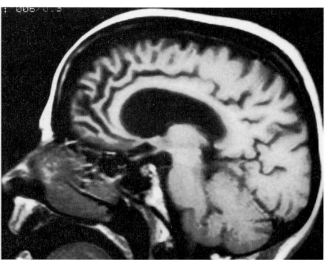

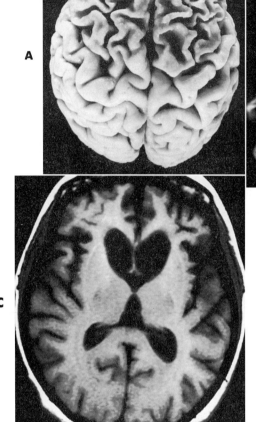

Fig. 18-30. A, Autopsy specimen of a patient with Pick disease, seen from above, shows gross frontal atrophy. The markedly shrunken gyri have a knifelike appearance. Sagittal **(B)** and axial **(C)** T1-weighted MR scans in a patient with Pick disease show striking frontotemporal lobe atrophy with sparing of the parietal and occipital lobes. (**A,** Courtesy B. Horten. **B** and **C,** Courtesy M. Fruin.)

monly and disproportionately affected, whereas the parietal and occipital lobes are relatively spared (Fig. 18-30).[20]

Vascular dementia. After AD, stroke is the second leading cause of progressive and irreversible dementia, accounting for 10% to 30% of all dementias.[85] Depending on their size, number, and location, multiple small or large single vessel infarcts can result in dementia.[20]

So-called *multi-infarct dementia* (MID) is defined clinically by several features, one of which is a history of multiple cerebral infarcts.[85] NECT scans in patients with clinical MID show more cortical and subcortical infarcts, larger ventricles and cortical sulci, and a higher prevalence of white matter lucencies than age-matched controls.[85]

Subcortical arteriosclerotic encephalopathy (SAE), also known as *Binswanger disease,* is probably a form of MID. Hypertension-induced arteriosclerotic change in long penetrating medullary arteries may induce hypoperfusion and secondary ischemic damage in the periventricular white matter.[86]

Temporal lobe (hippocampal) atrophic disorders. Disproportionate mesial temporal lobe atrophy, particularly the hippocampus, has been described in AD patients.[78b] Focal temporal lobe atrophy has also been implicated in intractable seizure disorders.[87] Hippocampal sclerosis is identified in the surgical specimens of approximately 65% of patients undergoing temporal lobectomy.[88,88a] In the remaining patients, various other lesions are found, including gliomas, hamartomas, heterotopias, cavernous angiomas, and arteriovenous malformations.[88a] Atrophy of mesial temporal lobe structures and increased signal on T2WI are also correlated with mesial temporal sclerosis (Fig. 18-31).[88b] The dentate gyrus and Ammon's horn are typically affected.[89,90]

Extrapyramidal Disorders and Subcortical Dementias

Movement is mediated by the pyramidal, extrapyramidal, and cerebellar systems. The major extrapyramidal motor circuit is a loop of projections from the cortex to the caudate nuclei and putamen, globus pallidus, subthalamic nuclei, and back to the cortex. Damage to this circuit may result in abnormal movements and subcortical dementia.[74a,91]

Extrapyramidal neurodegenerative disorders primarily or exclusively affect the extrapyramidal nuclei. With the exception of acquired hepatocerebral syndromes, most extrapyramidal degenerations are inherited disorders, discussed extensively in Chapter 17. In this section we focus on the pathology and im-

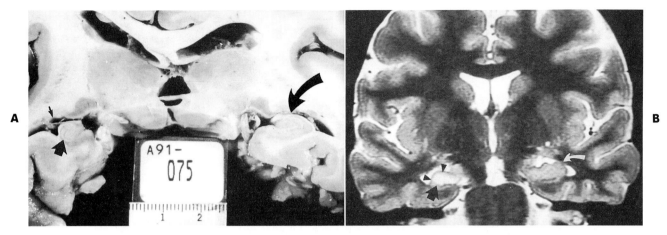

Fig. 18-31. A, Coronal autopsy specimen from a patient with hippocampal sclerosis shows marked atrophy of the right hippocampus *(large arrow)* with enlarged right temporal horn *(small arrow)*. Compare with the normal left hippocampus *(curved arrow)*. **B,** Coronal T2-weighted MR scan in this patient with long-standing right temporal lobe seizures shows striking atrophy of the right hippocampus *(arrowheads)*. Compare with the normal left hippocampus *(curved arrow)*. The right hippocampal gyrus also has abnormally high signal intensity *(large arrow)*. Surgically-proven hippocampal sclerosis. (**A,** Courtesy C. Petito.)

aging of acquired hepatocerebral degeneration, then turn to other causes of basal ganglia dysfunction. Parkinson disease and related nigrostriatal tract abnormalities are discussed separatelv in the next section.

Acquired hepatocerebral degeneration. Acquired hepatocerebral degeneration (AHCD) is an irreversible neurodegenerative syndrome that occurs with many types of chronic liver disease. It is most frequently associated with alcoholic cirrhosis, subacute or chronic hepatitis, and portal-systemic shunts.[92,93]

Pathologically the brain shows laminar or pseudolaminar necrosis with microcavitary changes at the gray-white matter junction, in the corpus striatum, and in the cerebellar white matter.[92] Imaging changes are strongly correlated with plasma ammonia levels.[94] The typical finding is bilateral basal ganglia hyperintensities on T1-weighted MR scans, seen in 50% to 75% of patients with advanced chronic liver disease (Fig. 18-32).[95] Other areas that may demonstrate signal intensity alterations are the pituitary gland, caudate nucleus, subthalamic region, and mesencephalon around the red nuclei.[96] Pallidal hyperintensities may resolve following liver transplantation.[95]

Another reported cause of increased signal intensity in the basal ganglia on T1WI is long-term total parenteral nutrition, probably caused by manganese toxicity (see subsequent discussion).[97]

Miscellaneous acquired basal ganglia disorders. There are numerous causes of focal, symmetric, bi-

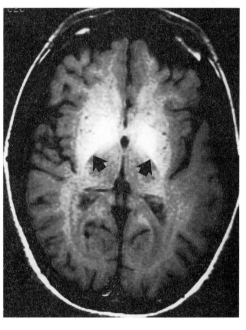

Fig. 18-32. Axial T1-weighted MR scan in a patient with acquired hepatocerebral degeneration shows bilateral high signal intensity in the basal ganglia *(arrows)*.

lateral basal ganglia lesions on MR scans (*see* box, p. 777). Some are vascular. These include hypoxic injury, severe osmotic imbalance, and deep cerebral venous infarction. Selective necrosis of the putamen or globus pallidus can also be caused by certain toxins. These include methanol intoxication, carbon monoxide inhalation, and manganese administrations.[98,99]

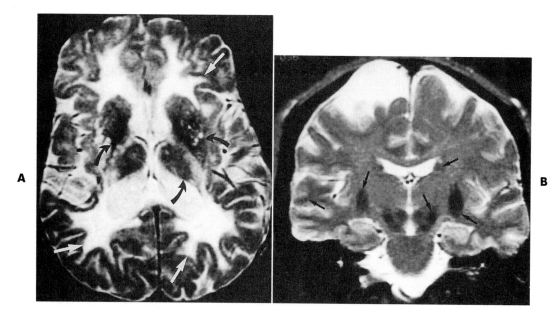

Fig. 18-33. A, Axial T2WI in a patient with adult-onset metachromatic leukodystrophy *(white arrows)* shows strikingly hypointense basal ganglia and thalami *(black arrows).* **B,** Coronal T2-weighted MR scan in a 60-year-old woman with ataxia shows striking iron deposition in the putamina, caudate nuclei, midbrain, and even the subcortical arcuate fibers *(arrows).* Neurodegenerative syndrome of unknown etiology. Note overlap with the iron deposition that occurs in the normal elderly (Fig. 18-7).

Increasing basal ganglia iron deposition occurs with normal aging. It is also seen as a secondary phenomenon associated with inherited neurodegenerative disorders (Fig. 18-33, *A*), acquired diseases such as long-standing severe multiple sclerosis (Fig. 18-13), Parkinson and Huntington diseases, and striatonigral degenerations (Fig. 18-33, *B*).[100,101] Abnormal basal ganglia iron accumulation also is seen following severe hypoxic-ischemic insults in children.[102]

Parkinson Disease and Related Striatonigral Degenerations

Age-related degenerative changes in the midbrain, particularly the striatonigral system, may play a role in the pathogenesis of several disorders, including Parkinson disease, striatonigral degeneration, Shy-Drager syndrome, and progressive supranuclear palsy.[103]

Parkinson disease. Parkinson disease (PD) is a common disorder. In the United States it affects approximately 1% of the population over the age of 50 years. Symptom onset is typically between 40 and 70 years of age.[20]

The neuropathologic hallmark of PD is loss of neuromelanin-containing neurons in the substantia nigra (particularly the pars compacta), the locus ceruleus, and the dorsal vagal nucleus (Fig. 18-34, *A*).[20] Imaging studies show decreased width of the pars compacta (Fig. 18-34, *B*).[104] Although tissue iron and ferritin concentrations are elevated in PD, in most

cases they do not cause detectable T2 shortening.[100,105]

Parkinson plus syndromes. Approximately 25% of patients with parkinsonian symptoms have more severe clinical manifestations and respond poorly to dopamine replacement therapy. These are sometimes grouped together and termed *Parkinson plus syndromes,* or *multisystem atrophy.*[17] This group of movement disorders includes striatonigral degeneration, Shy-Drager syndrome, progressive supranuclear palsy, and olivopontocerebellar degeneration. All the parkinsonian disorders have in common generalized atrophy with large supratentorial sulci and prominent posterior fossa subarachnoid cisterns.[17]

Striatonigral degeneration. Striatonigral degeneration (SD) is a parkinsonian-like syndrome with putaminal atrophy and abnormally hypointense signal on T2-weighted MR scans.[20] The pars compacta of the substantia nigra is also diminished in width.

Shy-Drager syndrome. Shy-Drager syndrome (SDS) is characterized clinically by autonomic nervous system failure. Orthostatic hypotension, urinary incontinence, inability to sweat, and extrapyramidal and cerebellar disturbances are typical symptoms. In SDS the putaminal hypointensity on T2-weighted MR scans equals or exceeds that of the globus pallidus.[106]

Progressive supranuclear palsy. Progressive supranuclear palsy (PSP) is characterized by axial rigidity without tremor, supranuclear gaze palsy, and

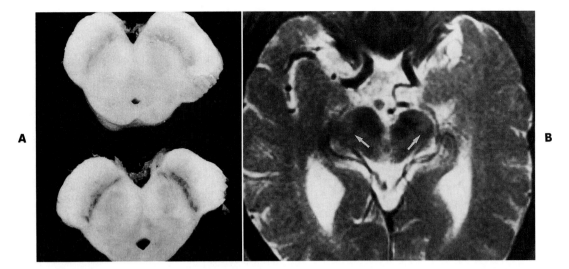

Fig. 18-34. A, Axial gross pathology of Parkinson disease *(upper specimen)* shows reduced iron deposition in the substantia nigra with a thinned pars compacta. The midbrain from a normal case *(lower specimen)* is shown for comparison. **B,** Axial T2WI in a patient with Parkinson syndrome shows reduced iron deposition in the substantia nigra and a thin pars compacta *(arrows)*. (**A,** From Okazaki H, Scheithauer B: *Slide Atlas of Neurpathology,* Gower Medical Publishing.)

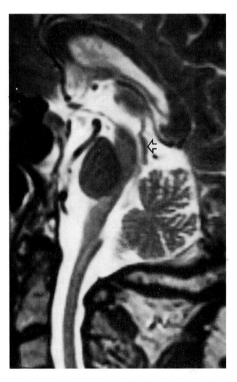

Bilateral Basal Ganglia Lesions on MR

High signal on T1WI

Hepatocellular degeneration
Calcification
Neurofibromatosis
Parenteral nutrition (manganese toxicity)

Low signal on T1WI

Leigh disease
Venous infarction
Hypoxic-ischemic encephalopathy
Toxic encephalopathy

Low signal on T2WI

Normal aging
Degenerative diseases (e.g., long-standing MS, hypoxic insults in children, parkinsonian syndromes)

High signal on T2WI

Venous infarcts
Hypoxic-ischemic encephalopathy
Toxic encephalopathy
Mitochondrial cytopathy

Fig. 18-35. Sagittal T2-weighted MR scan in this 55-year-old woman with progressive neurologic deterioration and supranuclear gaze palsy shows a strikingly atrophic tectum *(arrow)*. Probable progressive supranuclear palsy.

---

pseudobulbar signs. Imaging studies in PSP show marked midbrain and tectal atrophy (Fig. 18-35).[107]

Olivopontocerebellar degeneration. Olivopontocerebellar degeneration (OPCD) is a degenerative disease characterized by atrophy of the pons, middle cerebellar peduncles, and cerebellar hemispheres.[107] Imaging studies show small inferior olives and medulla, a small flattened pons, and atrophic cerebellar

hemispheres and vermis (Fig. 18-36).[17,107a] High signal intensity on T2-weighted MR scans is often seen in the transverse pontine fibers and brachium pontis.[107] The putamen, globus pallidus, and substantia nigra frequently show abnormally low signal intensity.[17]

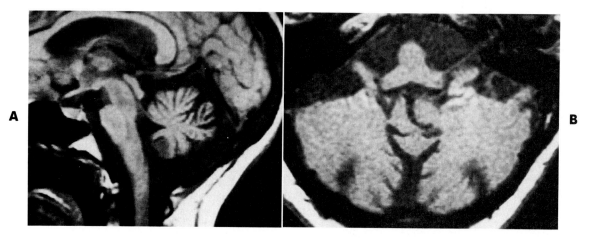

Fig. 18-36. Sagittal **(A)** and axial **(B)** T1-weighted MR scan in this 58-year-old woman with olivopontocerebellar degeneration shows marked atrophy of the pons, vermis, and medulla.

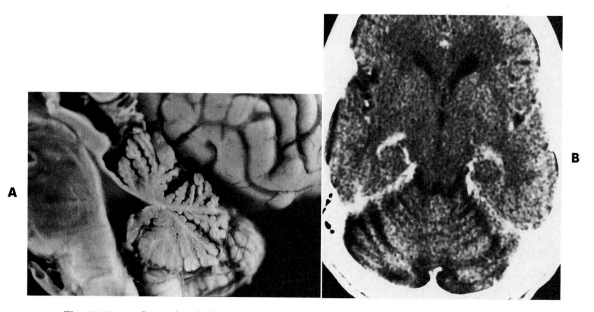

Fig. 18-37. A, Sagittal pathology shows the effect of severe ethanol abuse. Note prominent vermian atrophy. **B,** Axial CECT scan in another 41-year-old ethanol abuser shows marked cerebellar atrophy, seen as shrunken folia and widened posterior fossa subarachnoid spaces.

Miscellaneous Cerebellar and Motor Degenerations

Cerebellar degeneration. Age-related cerebellar degeneration is normal. The most dorsomedial vermian lobules (declive, folium, tuber) are commonly affected.[108] Acquired cerebellar degeneration syndromes occur with ethanol abuse, paraneoplastic syndromes, and some medications (e.g., dilantin) (Fig. 18-37). Uncommon developmental disorders that cause cerebellar atrophy include infantile autism, fragile X syndrome, Rett syndrome, and Down syndrome.[109] Freidreich's ataxia is a progressive familial cerebellar degenerative disease that also causes cervical spinal cord atrophy.[110]

Motor degenerations. Primary and secondary corticospinal (pyramidal tract) degenerations occur. The best-known and most common primary motor neuron disease is amyotrophic lateral sclerosis. Secondary pyramidal tract degeneration is termed Wallerian degeneration.

Amyotrophic lateral sclerosis. Amyotrophic lateral sclerosis (ALS) is characterized by progressive muscle weakness, limb and truncal atrophy, and bulbar signs and symptoms.[111] Mean age at diagnosis is 57 years.[111] Disease progression is relentless; half the patients are dead within 3 years and 90% have died by 6 years following symptom onset.[20]

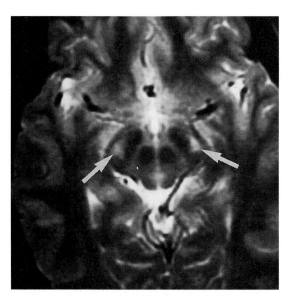

Fig. 18-38. Axial T2-weighted MR scan shows the bilateral high signal intensity foci in the cerebral peduncles *(arrows)* seen with amyotrophic lateral sclerosis.

T2-weighted MR scans disclose high signal areas along the large myelinated pyramidal tract fibers in the posterior limb of the internal capsule and cerebral peduncles in about 25% of cases (Fig. 18-38). Motor cortex lesions can be demonstrated on SPECT images.[111]

Wallerian degeneration. Wallerian degeneration refers to anterograde degeneration of axons and their myelin sheaths secondary to proximal axonal injury or death of the cell body.[20] Within 5 to 12 weeks after disease onset (e.g., cerebral infarct), Wallerian degeneration of the pyramidal tract can be detected as a high signal intensity area on T2-weighted MR scans.[112,113] Ipsilateral brainstem atrophy appears within 8 to 12 months after the ictus (*see* Chapter 11).[113]

REFERENCES

1. Coffey CE, Wilkinson WE, Parashos IA et al: Quantitative cerebral anatomy of the aging human brain: a cross-sectional study using magnetic resonance imaging, *Neurol* 42:527-536, 1992.
2. Chimowitz MI, Estes ML, Furlan AJ, Awad IA: Further observations on the pathology of subcortical lesions identified on magnetic resonance imaging, *Arch Neurol* 49:747-752, 1992.
2a. Munoz DG, Hastak SM, Harper B et al: Pathologic correlates of increased signals of the centrum ovale on magnetic resonance imaging, *Arch Neurol* 50:492-497, 1993.
3. Hendrie HC, Farlow MR, Austrom MG et al: Foci of increased T2 signal intensity on brain MR scans in healthy elderly subjects, *AJNR* 10:703-707, 1989.
4. Award IA, Spetzler RE, Hodak JA et al: Incidental subcortical lesions identified on magnetic resonance imaging in the elderly, I: correlation with age and cerebral vascular risk factors, *Stroke* 17:1084-1089, 1986.
5. Schmidt R, Fazekas F, Kleinert G et al: Magnetic resonance imaging spinal hyperintensities in the deep and subcortical white matter, *Arch Neurol* 49:825-827, 1992.
6. Horikoshi T, Yagi S, Fukamachi A: Incidental high-intensity foci in white matter on T2-weighted magnetic resonance imaging, *Neuroradiol* 35:151-155, 1993.
7. Meguro K, Yamaguchi T, Hishinuma T et al: Periventricular hyperintensity on magnetic resonance imaging correlated with brain aging and atrophy, *Neuroradiol* 35:125-129, 1993.
8. Bradley WG Jr, Whittemore AR, Watanabe AS et al: Association of deep white matter infarction with chronic communicating hydrocephalus: implications regarding the possible origin of normal-pressure hydrocephalus, *AJNR* 12:31-39, 1991.
9. Kimura M, Tanaka A, Yoshinaga S: Significance of periventricular hemodynamics in normal pressure hydrocephalus, *Neurosurg* 30:701-705, 1992.
10. Heier LA, Bauer CJ, Schwarts L et al: Large Virchow-Robin spaces: MR-clinical correlation, *AJNR* 10:929-936, 1989.
11. Libicher M, Tröger J: US measurement of the subarachnoid space in infants: normal values, *Radiol* 184:749-751, 1992.
12. Pirtilla T, Jarvenpaa R, Laippala P, Frey H: Brain atrophy on computed axial tomography scans: interaction of age, diabetes, and general morbidity, *Gerontology* 38:285-291, 1992.
13. Wippold FJ, Gado MH, Morris JC et al: Senile dementia and healthy aging: a longitudinal CT study, *Radiol* 179:215-219, 1991.
14. Cronqvist S: Hydrocephalus and atrophy, *Riv di Neuroradiol* 3(suppl 2):25-28, 1990.
15. Scroth G, Klose U: Cerebrospinal fluid flow, III: pathological cerebrospinal fluid pulsations, *Neuroradiol* 35:16-24, 1992.
16. Xiong G, Rauch RA, Hagino N, Jinkins JR: An animal model of corpus callosum impingement as seen in patients with normal pressure hydrocephalus, *Invest Radiol* 28:46-50, 1993.
17. Drayer BP: Magnetic resonance imaging and brain iron: implications in the diagnosis and pathochemistry of movement disorders and dementia, *BNI Quarterly* 3:15-30, 1987.
18. Pujol J, Junqué C, Vendrell P et al: Biological significance of iron-related magnetic resonance imaging changes in the brain, *Arch Neurol* 49:711-717, 1992.
19. Aoki S, Okada Y, Nishimura K et al: Normal deposition of brain iron in childhood and adolescence: MR imaging at I ST, *Radiol* 172:381-385, 1989.
20. Braffman BH, Trojanowski JQ, Atlas SW: The aging brain and neurodegenerative disorders. In Atlas SW, editor, *Magnetic resonance imaging of the brain and spine*, pp 567-624, New York, Raven Press, 1991.
21. Milton WJ, Atlas SW, Lexa FJ et al: Deep gray matter hypointensity patterns with aging in healthy adults: MR imaging at I.5T, *Radiol* 181:715-719, 1991.
22. Edwards MK, Bonnin JM: White matter diseases. In Atlas SW, editor, *Magnetic resonance imaging of the brain and spine*, pp 467-500, New York, Raven press, 1991.
23. Merrill JE, Graves MC, Mulder DG: Autoimmune disease and the nervous system: biochemical, molecular, and clinical update, *West J Med* 156:639-646, 1992.
24. Tienari PJ, Salonen O, Wikstrom J et al: Familial multiple sclerosis: MRI findings in clinically affected and unaffected siblings, *J Neurol Neurosurg Psychiatr* 55:883-886, 1992.
25. Niebler G, Harris T, Davis T, Raos K: Fulminant multiple sclerosis, *AJNR* 13:1547-1551, 1992.
25a. Kepes JJ: Large focal tumor-like demyelinating lesions of the brain: intermediate entity between multiple sclerosis and acute disseminated encephalomyelitis. A study of 31 patients, *Ann Neurol* 33:18-27, 1993.
26. Nesbit GM, Forbes GS, Scheithauer BW et al: Multiple sclerosis: histopathologic and MR and/or CT correlation in 37 cases at biopsy and three cases at autopsy, *Radiol* 180:467-474, 1991.

27. Wallace CJ, Seland TP, Fong TC: Multiple sclerosis: the impact of MR imaging, *AJR* 158:849-857, 1992.

28. Tan CT, Abdullah D, Zakariya AH: CT scan changes in multiple sclerosis among Malaysian patients, *Neuroradiol* 33:494-498, 1991.

29. Osborn AG, Harnsberger HR, Smoker WRK et al: Multiple sclerosis in adolescents: CT and MR findings, *AJNR* 11:489-494, 1990.

30. Ebner F, Millner MM, Justich E: Multiple sclerosis in children: value of serial MR studies to monitor patients, *AJNR* 11:1023-1027, 1990.

31. Horowitz AL, Kaplan RD, Grewe G et al: The ovoid lesions: a new MR observation in patients with multiple sclerosis, *AJNR* 10:303-305, 1989.

32. Gean-Marton AD, Vezina LG, Martin KI et al: Abnormal corpus callosum: a sensitive and specific indicator of multiple sclerosis, *Radiol* 180:215-221, 1991.

33. Wilms G, Marchal G, Kersschot E et al: Axial vs sagittal T2-weighted brain MR images in the evaluation of multiple sclerosis, *J Comp Asst Tomogr* 15:359-364, 1991.

34. Barkhof F, Scheltens P, Frequin STFM et al: Relapsing-remitting multiple sclerosis: sequential enhanced MR imaging vs clinical findings in determining disease activity, *AJR* 159:1041-1047, 1992.

35. Lee KH, Hashimoto SA, Hooge JP et al: Magnetic resonance imaging of the head in the diagnosis of multiple sclerosis: a prospective 2-year follow-up with comparison of clinical evaluation, evoked potentials, oligoclonal banding, and CT, *Neurol* 41:657-660, 1991.

36. Capra R, Marciano N, Vignolo LA et al: Gadolinium-pentetic acid magnetic resonance imaging in patients with relapsing remitting multiple sclerosis, *Arch Neurol* 49:687-689, 1992.

37. Runge VM: MRI of multiple sclerosis in the brain, *MRI Decisions*, pp 2-10, Nov/Dec 1992.

38. Yetkin FZ, Haughton VM: Common and uncommon manifestations of MS on MRI, *MRI Decisions*, pp 13-18, Nov/Dec 1992.

38a. Offenbacher H, Fazekas F, Schmidt R et al: Assessment of MRI criteria for a diagnosis of MS, *Neurol* 43:905-909, 1993.

39. Powell T, Sussman JG, Davies-Jones GAB: MR imaging in acute multiple sclerosis: ring-like appearance in plaques suggesting the presence of paramagnetic free radicals, *AJNR* 13:1544-1546, 1992.

40. Giang DW, Poduri KR, Eskin TA et al: Multiple sclerosis masquerading as a mass lesion, *Neuroradiol* 34:150-154, 1992.

40a. Zagzag D, Miller DC, Kleinman GM et al: Demyelinating disease versus tumor in surgical neuropathology, *Am J Surg Path* 17:537-545, 1993.

41. Miller DH, MacManus DG, Bartlett PA et al: Detection of optic nerve lesions in optic neuritis using frequency-selective fat-saturation sequences, *Neuroradiol* 35:156-158, 1993.

42. Grossman RI, Lenkinski RE, Ramer KN et al: MR proton spectroscopy in multiple sclerosis, *AJNR* 13:1535-1543, 1992.

43. Kimura S, Unayama T, Mori T: The natural history of acute disseminated leukoencephalitis: a serial magnetic resonance imaging study, *Neuropediatr* 23:192-195, 1992.

44. Valk J, van der Knaap MS: Toxic encephalopathy, *AJNR* 13:747-760, 1992.

45. Ho VB, Fitz CR, Yoder CC, Geyer CA: Resolving MR features in osmotic myelinolysis (central pontine and extrapontine myelinolysis), *AJNR* 14:163-167, 1993.

46. Miller GM, Baker HL Jr, Okozaki H, Whisnant JP: Central pontine myelinolysis and its imitators: MR findings, *Radiol* 168:795-802, 1988.

47. Clark WR: Diffuse demyelinating lesions of the brain after the rapid development of hypernatremia, *West J Med* 157:571-573, 1992.

48. Koci TM, Chiang F, Chow P et al: Thalamic extrapontine lesions in central pontine myelinolysis, *AJNR* 11:1229-1233, 1990.

49. Koragi Y, Takahashi M, Shinzato J et al: MR findings in two presumed cases of mild central pontine myelinolysis, *AJNR* 14:651-654, 1993.

50. Gallucci M, Amicarelli I, Rossi A et al: MR imaging of white matter lesions in uncomplicated chronic alcoholism, *J Comp Asst Tomogr* 13:395-398, 1989.

51. Rosa A, Demiati M, Cartz L, Mizon JP: Marchiafava-Bignami disease, syndrome of interhemispheric disconnection, and right-handed agraphia in a left-hander, *Arch Neurol* 48:986-988, 1991.

52. Chang KH, Cha SH, Han MH et al: Marchiafava-Bignami disease: serial changes in corpus callosum in MRI, *Neuroradiol* 34:480-482, 1992.

53. Galluci M, Bozzao A, Splendiani A et al: Wernicke encephalopathy: MR findings in five patients, *AJNR* 11:887-892, 1990.

54. Galluci M, Bozzao A, Splendiani A et al: Follow-up in Wernicke's encephalopathy, *Neuroradiol* 33(suppl):594-595, 1991.

55. Schroth G, Wichmann W, Valavanis A: Blood-brain-barrier disruption in acute Wernicke encephalopathy: MR findings, *J Comp Asst Tomogr* 15:1059-1061, 1991.

56. Yokote K, Miyagi K, Kuzuhara S et al: Wernicke encephalopathy: follow-up study by CT and MR, *J Comp Asst Tomogr* 15:835-838, 1991.

57. Donnal JF, Heinz ER, Burger PC: MR of reversible thalamic lesions in Wernicke syndrome, *AJNR* 11:893-894, 1990.

58. Truwit CL, Denaro CP, Lake JR, DeMarco T: MR imaging of reversible cyclosporin A-induced neurotoxicity, *AJNR* 12:651-659, 1991.

58a. Vaughn DJ, Jarvik JG, Hackney D et al: High-dose cytarabine neurotoxicity: MR findings during the acute stage, *AJNR* 14:1014-1018, 1993.

59. Paakko E, Vainionpaa L, Lanning M et al: White matter changes in children treated for acute lymphoblastic leukemia, *Cancer* 70:2727-2733, 1992.

60. Ball WS Jr, Prenger EC, Ballard ET: Neurotoxicity of radio/chemotherapy in children: pathologic and MR correlation, *AJNR* 13:761-776, 1992.

61. Ashdown BC, Boyko OB, Uglietta JP et al: Postradiation cerebellar necrosis mimicking tumor: MR appearance, *J Comp Asst Tomogr* 17:124-126, 1993.

62. Schwartz RB, Carvallo PA, Alexander E III et al: Radiation necrosis vs high-grade recurrent glioma: differentiation by using dual-isotope SPECT with ^{201}Tl and ^{99m}Tc-HMPAO, *AJNR* 12:1187-1192, 1992.

63. Kim EE, Chung S-K, Haynie TP et al: Differentiation of residual or recurrent tumors form post-treatment changes with F-18 FDG PET, *RadioGraphics* 12:269-279, 1992.

64. Rorke LB, Zimmerman RA: Prematurity, postmaturity, and destructive lesions in utero, *AJNR* 13:517-536, 1992.

65. Truwit CL, Barkovich AJ, Koch TK, Ferriero DM: Cerebral palsy: MR findings in 40 patients, *AJNR* 13:67-78, 1992.

66. van Bogaert P, Baleriaux D, Christophe C, Szliwowski HB: MRI of patients with cerebral palsy and normal CT scan, *Neuroradiol* 34:52-56, 1992.

67. Birbamer G, Aichner F, Felber S et al: MRI of cerebral hypoxia, *Neuroradiol* 33(suppl):53-55, 1991.

68. Yetkin FZ, Haughton VM, Fischer MR et al: High-signal foci on MR images of the brain: observer variability in their quantification, *AJR* 159:185-188, 1992.

68a. Bots ML, van Swieten JC, Breteler MMB et al: Cerebral white matter lesions and atherosclerosis in the Rotterdam study, *Lancet* 341:1232-1237, 1993.

69. Uhlenbrock D, Sehlen S: The value of T1-weighted images in the differentiation between MS, white matter lesions, and subcortical arteriosclerotic encephalopathy (SAE), *Neuroradiol* 31:203-212, 1989.

70. Yousem DM, Tasman WS, Grossman RI: Proliferative retinopathy: absence of white matter lesions at MR imaging, *Radiol* 179:229-230, 1991.

71. Miller DH, Ormerod IEC, Gibson A et al: MR brain scanning in patients with vasculitis: differentiation from multiple sclerosis, *Neuroradiol* 29:226-231, 1987.

72. Loes DJ, Biller J, Yuh WTC et al: Leukoencephalopathy in cerebral amyloid angiopathy: MR imaging in four cases, *AJNR* 11:485-488, 1990.

73. Coker SB: The diagnosis of childhood neurodegenerative disorders presenting as dementia in adults, *Neurol* 41:794-798, 1991.

74. Kornreich L, Shapira A, Horev G et al: CT and MR evaluation of the brain in patient with anorexia nervosa, *AJNR* 12:1213-1216, 1991.

74a. Tien RD, Felsberg GJ, Ferris NJ, Osumi AK: The dementias: correlation of clinical features, pathophysiology, and neuroradiology, *AJR* 161:245-255, 1993.

75. Brenner DE, Kukull WA, van Belle G et al: Relationship between cigarette smoking and Alzheimer's disease in a population-based case-control study, *Neurol* 43:293-300, 1993.

76. Jack CR Jr, Bentley MD, Twomey CK, Zinsmeister AR: MR imaging-based volume measurements of the hippocampal formation and anterior temporal lobe: validation studies, *Radiol* 176:205-209, 1990.

77. Rusinek H, de Leon MJ, George AE et al: Alzheimer disease: measuring loss of cerebral gray matter with MR imaging, *Radiol* 178:109-114, 1991.

78. Howieson J, Kaye JA, Holm L, Howieson D: Interuncal distance: marker of aging and Alzheimer disease, *AJNR* 14:647-650, 1993.

78a. Early B, Escalona PR, Boyko OB et al: Interuncal distance measurements in healthy volunteers and in patients with Alzheimer disease, *AJNR* 14:907-910, 1993.

78b. de Leon MJ, Golomb J, George AE et al: The radiologic prediction of Alzheimer disease: the atrophic hippocampal formation, *AJNR* 14:897-906, 1993.

79. de Leon MJ, George AE, Reisberg B et al: Alzheimer's disease: longitudinal CT studies of ventricular change, *AJNR* 10:371-376, 1989.

80. Kido DK, Caine ED, Le May M: Temporal lobe atrophy in patients with Alzheimer disease: a CT study, *AJNR* 10:551-555, 1989.

81. George AE, de Leon MJ, Stylopoulos LA et al: CT diagnostic features of Alzheimer disease: importance of the choroidal/hippocampal fissure complex, *AJNR* 11:101-107, 1990.

82. O'Mahoney D, Walsh JB, Coakley D: "Pseudo-Alzheimer's" and primary brain tumor, *Postgrad Med J* 68:673-676, 1992.

83. Förstl H, Burns A, Luthert P et al: The Lewy-body variant of Alzheimer's disease, *Br J Psychiatr* 162:385-392, 1993.

84. Mendez MF, Selwood A, Mastri AR, Frey WH II: Pick's disease versus Alzheimer's disease: a comparison of clinical characteristics, *Neurol* 43:289-292, 1993.

85. Gorelick PB, Chatterjee A, Patel D et al: Cranial computed tomographic observations in multi-infarct dementia, *Stroke* 23:804-811, 1992.

86. Yao H, Sadoshima S, Ibayashi S et al: Leukoariosis and dementia in hypertensive patients, *Stroke* 23:1673-1677, 1992.

87. Cendes F, Leproux F, Melanson D et al: MRI of amygdala and hippocampus in temporal lobe epilepsy, *J Comp Asst Tomogr* 16:206-210, 1993.

88. Jackson GD, Barkovic SF, Duncan JS, Connelly A: Optimizing the diagnosis of hippocampal sclerosis using MR imaging, *AJNR* 14:753-762, 1993.

88a. Holtas S: Neuroradiological approach to the epileptic patient, *Riv Di Neuroradiol* (suppl)2:27-32, 1993.

88b. Jackson GD, Berkovic SF, Duncan JS, Connelly A: Optimizing the diagnosis of hippocampal sclerosis using MR imaging, *AJNR* 14:753-762, 1993.

89. Mark P, Daniels DL, Naidich TP et al: The hippocampus, *AJNR* 14:709-712, 1993.

90. Tien RD, Felsberg GJ, Craine B: Normal anatomy of the hippocampus and adjacent temporal lobe: high-resolution fast-spin-echo MR images in volunteers correlated with cadaveric histologic sections, *AJR* 149:1309-1313, 1992.

91. Rutledge JN, Hilal SK, Silver AJ et al: Study of movement disorders and brain iron by MR, *AJNR* 8:397-411, 1987.

92. Kulisevsky J, Ruscalleda J, Grau JM: MR imaging of acquired hepatocerebral degeneration, *AJNR* 12:527-528, 1991.

93. Inoue E, Hori S, Narumi Y et al: Portal-systemic encephalopathy: presence of basal ganglia lesions with high signal intensity on MR images, *Radiol* 179:551-555, 1991.

94. Kulisevsky J, Pugol J, Balanzo J: Pallidal hyperintensity on magnetic resonance imaging in cirrhotic patients: clinical correlations, *Hepatology* 16:1382-1388, 1992.

95. Pujol JA, Pujol J, Graus F et al: Hyperintense globus pallidus on T1-weighted MRI in cirrhotic patients is associated with severity of liver failure, *Neurol* 43:65-69, 1993.

96. Brunberg JA, Kanal E, Hirsch W, Van Thiel DH: Chronic acquired hepatic failure: MR imaging of the brain at I.5T, *AJNR* 12:909-914, 1991.

97. Mirowitz SA, Westric TJ: Basal ganglial signal intensity alterations: reversal after discontinuation of parenteral manganese administration, *Radiol* 185:535-526, 1992.

98. Silverman CS, Brenner J, Murtagh FR: Hemorrhagic necrosis and vascular injury in carbon monoxide poisoning: MR demonstration, *AJNR* 14:168-170, 1993.

99. Glazer M, Dross P: Necrosis of the putamen caused by methanol intoxication: MR findings, *AJR* 14:168-170, 1990.

100. Chen JC, Hardy PA, Kucharczyk W et al: MR of human post-mortem brain tissue: correlative study between T2 and assays of iron and ferritin in Parkinson and Huntington disease, *AJNR* 14:275-281, 1993.

101. Schenker C, Meier D, Wichmann W et al: Age distribution and iron dependency of the T2 relaxation time in the globus pallidus and putamen, *Neuroradiol* 35:119-124, 1993.

102. Dietrich RB, Bradley WG Jr: Iron accumulation in the basal ganglia following severe ischemic-anoxic insults in children, *Radiol* 168:203-206, 1980.

103. Doraiswamy PM, Na C, Husain MM et al: Morphometric changes of the human midbrain with normal aging: MR and stereologic findings, *AJNR* 13:383-386, 1992.

104. Huber SJ, Chakeres DW, Paulson GW, Khanna R: Magnetic resonance imaging in Parkinson's disease, *Arch Neurol* 47:735-737, 1990.

105. Braffman BH, Gussman RI, Goldberg HI et al: MR imaging of Parkinson disease with spin-echo and gradient-echo sequence, *AJNR* 9:1093-1099, 1988.

106. Savoiardo M, Strada L, Girotti F et al: MR imaging in progressive supranuclear palsy and Shy-Drager syndrome, *J Comp Asst Tomogr* 13:555-560, 1989.

107. Savoiardo M, Strada L, Girotti F et al: Olivopontocerebellar atrophy: MR diagnosis and relationship to multisystem atrophy, *Radiol* 174:693-696, 1990.

107a. Wessel K, Huss G-P, Bruckmann H, Kompf D: Follow-up of neurophysiological tests and CT in late-onset cerebellar ataxia and multiple system atrophy, *J Neurol* 240:168-176, 1993.

108. Raz N, Torres IJ, Spencer WD: Age-related regional differences in cerebellar vermis observed in vivo, *Arch Neurol* 49:412-416, 1992.

109. Murakami JW, Courchesne E, Haas RH et al: Cerebellar and cerebral abnormalities in Rett syndrome: a quantitative MR analysis, *AJNR* 159:177-183, 1992.

110. Riva A, Bradac GB: Atassie cerebellari e spino-cerebellar i primitive progressive, *Riv di Neuroradiol* 5:155-159, 1992.

111. Udaka F, Sawada H, Seriv N et al: MRI and SPECT findings in amyotrophic lateral sclerosis, *Neuroradiol* 34:389-393, 1992.

112. Orita T, Tsurutani T, Izumihara A, Matsunaga T: Coronal MR imaging for visualization of Wallerian degeneration of the pyramidal tract, *J Comp Asst Tomogr* 15:802-804, 1991.

113. Inoue Y, Matsumura Y, Fukuda T et al: MR imaging of the Wallerian degeneration in the brainstem: temporal relationships, *AJNR* 11:897-902, 1990.

PART FIVE

Spine and Spinal Cord

Normal Anatomy and Congenital Anomalies of the Spine and Spinal Cord

S pine and spinal cord examinations comprise a significant and important segment of clinical neuroimaging. Familiarity with normal gross and radiologic anatomy is a prerequisite to understanding the broad spectrum of disorders that affect the spine and spinal cord.

In this chapter the normal gross and imaging anatomy of the spine, spinal cord, and nerve roots, as well as their congenital anomalies, are delineated. Nonneoplastic disorders, including trauma, infection, demyelinating, vascular, and degenerative dis-

eases, are covered in Chapter 20. Tumors, cysts, and tumorlike masses are discussed in the concluding chapter, Chapter 21.

NORMAL ANATOMY
Lumbosacral Spine

The lumbosacral spine has many components. It can be divided into anterior elements (vertebral bodies and intervertebral disks), posterior elements (pedicles, articular pillars, and facet joints), ligaments, soft tissues (e.g., epidural fat and venous plexuses), and neural tissue. Neural tissue in this region includes the conus medullaris and cauda equina, lumbar roots and nerves, and the sacral plexus.

Anterior elements
Vertebral bodies. The lumbosacral spine normally has five lumbar segments and the sacrum, which is composed of five fused segments. Each lumbar segment has a large, somewhat square-shaped vertebral body. The superior and inferior end plates of the vertebral bodies are covered by a fenestrated cartilage to which the intervertebral disks attach (Figs. 19-1 and 19-2).[1]

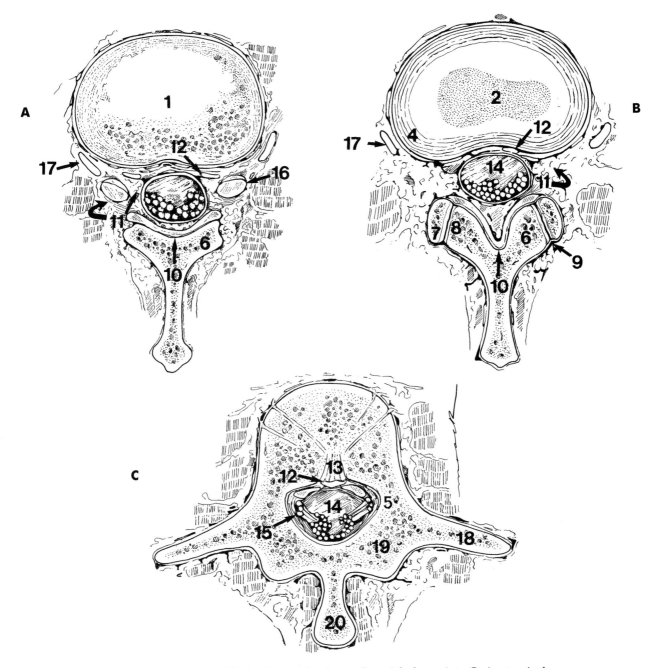

Fig. 19-1. Anatomy of the lumbosacral spine in the axial plane. **A** to **C,** Anatomic drawings through the neural foramen **(A),** intervertebral disk **(B),** and pedicles **(C).**

Each vertebral body has an outer layer of dense, compact cortical bone that surrounds an inner medullary portion composed of bony trabeculae and marrow. The two types of marrow, hematopoietically active (red or cellular) and inactive (yellow or fatty) marrow, are easily distinguished on MR scans. In young children, marrow is typically cellular and appears isointense with paraspinous muscle on T1WI (see Fig. 19-15, B). In patients less than 2 years of age, bone marrow and cartilage may show marked en-

hancement following contrast administration. Mild marrow enhancement persists but gradually diminishes and disappears around age 7 years.[2]

From age 7 to adolescence there is also progressive conversion of red to yellow marrow.[3] This replacement of cellular marrow by fatty marrow results in high signal intensity on T1WI and relatively low signal intensity on standard T2-weighted spin-echo sequences. Inhomogeneous signal is common, and focal fat deposition is seen as localized zones of high

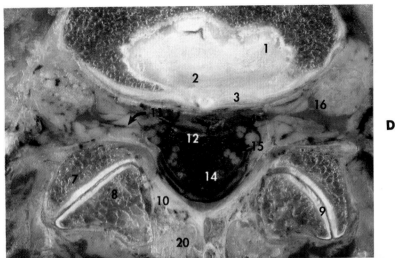

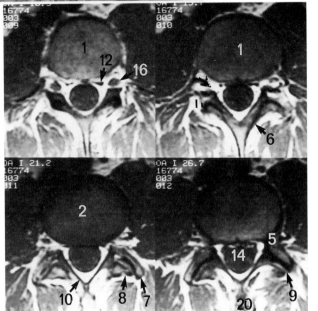

Fig. 19-1, cont'd. D, Axial cryomicrotome section shows gross anatomy at the intervertebral disc level. **E,** Axial T1-weighted MR scans show normal imaging anatomy of the lumbosacral spine. *1,* Vertebral body. *2,* Nucleus pulposus. *3,* Inner anular fibers of disk. *4,* Outer anular fibers of disk. *5,* Pedicles. *6,* Lamina. *7,* Superior articular facet. *8,* Inferior articular facet. *9,* Facet joint. *10,* Ligamentum flavum. *11,* Epidural fat (curved arrow indicates neural foramen). *12,* Epidural venous plexus. *13,* Basivertebral venous plexus. *14,* Thecal sac with roots of cauda equina. *15,* Exiting roots. *16,* Dorsal root ganglia. *17,* Extraforaminal nerve. *18,* Transverse process. *19,* Pars interarticularis. *20,* Spinous process. (**D,** Courtesy V.M. Haughton.)

signal intensity on T1WI (*see* Chapter 20).[4] Marrow in adolescents and adults normally does not enhance following contrast administration.[2]

Intervertebral disks. The intervertebral disks are composed of a central gelatinous core (the nucleus pulposus) surrounded by dense fibrocartilage and fibrous connective tissue (the anulus fibrosus). A normal lumbar intervertebral disk is slightly concave posteriorly, except at L5-S1, where it appears rounded.

The intervertebral disks of infants are typically high signal on T2-weighted scan except for a central low signal area that represents the notochord remnants (*see* Fig. 19-19). Sharpey's fibers are seen at the periphery as low signal intensity regions. Beginning in the second decade of life, a dark band of compact fibrous tissue develops in the disk centrum.[5]

Adult intervertebral disks are slightly hyperdense compared to adjacent muscle on NECT scans. On MR scans, predominately fibrous compact tissue such as Sharpey's fibers and the outer anulus is low signal on both T1- and T2WI, whereas fibrocartilagenous tissue with mucoid matrix such as the nucleus pulposus has high signal intensity on T2WI (Figs. 19-1, *E;* and 19-2, *G*).[5] Age-related changes of disk dessication and degeneration begin in the midteens and continue throughout life (*see* Chapter 20).

Posterior elements. The pedicles and neural arch form the posterior part of the vertebral column. The neural arch is composed of the articular pillars and facet (zygoapophyseal) joints, the laminae, and the spinous processes.

Pedicles. The pedicles are thick, bony pillars that

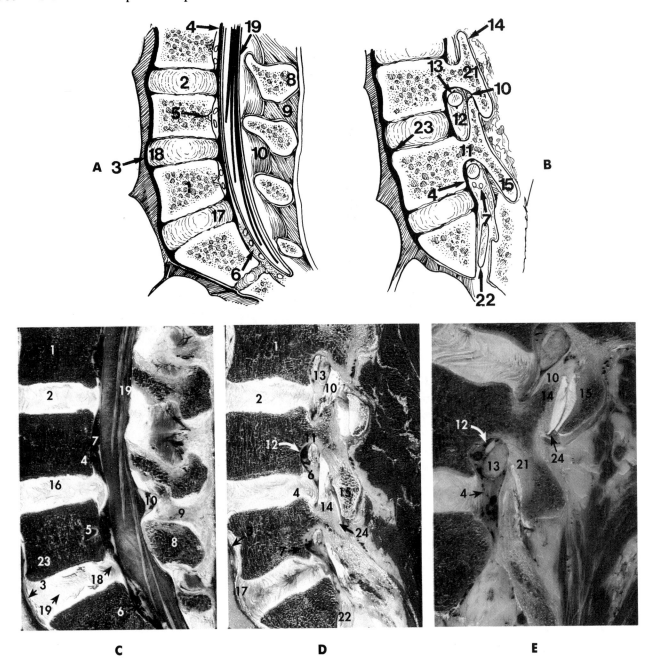

Fig. 19-2. Anatomy of the lumbosacral spine in the sagittal plane is depicted. **A** and **B,** Anatomic drawings show structures in the midline **(A)** and in the neural foramen **(B).** **C** to **E,** Cryomicrotome section shows anatomy in the midline **(C)** and neural foramen **(D).** Close-up view **(E)** of the neural foramen. (C to E, Courtesy V.M. Haughton.)

mostly consist of dense cortical bone. They project posterolaterally from the vertebral bodies, connecting them with the neural arch and forming the spinal canal (Fig. 19-1, *C*).

Articular pillars. The articular pillars consist of the pars interarticularis and the superior and inferior articular facets. The pars interarticularis is a bony plate that extends posteriorly from the pedicle and gives rise to the superior and inferior articular facets.

Facet joints. The facet joints are diarthrodial synovial-lined joints that connect the posterosuperior articular process of a lower vertebra with the posteroinferior articular process of the vertebra above (Figs. 19-1, *B* and *D*; and 19-2, *B* and *D*).[6] A tough, fibrous capsule is present along the posterolateral aspect of each facet joint. There is no fibrous capsule on the ventral aspect of the joint; here, the ligamentum flavum and synovial membrane are the only barriers between the facet joint space and the spinal canal.[7]

The synovial membrane is intimately bound to the

F   **G**   **H**

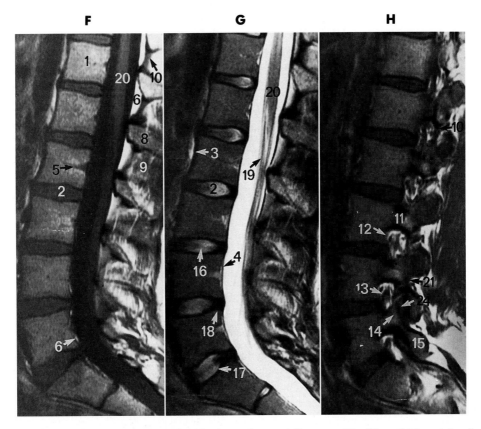

Fig. 19-2, cont'd.   F to **H,** Sagittal high resolution MR scans. T1- **(F)** and T2-weighted **(G)** scans demonstrate normal midline anatomy. **H,** Sagittal T1-weighted scan through the neural foramina shows the relationship of the soft tissues to the surrounding bone and intervertebral disk. *1,* Vertebral body. *2,* Intervertebral disk (nucleus pulposus). *3,* Anterior longitudinal ligament. *4,* Posterior longitudinal ligament. *5,* Basivertebral venous plexus. *6,* Epidural fat. *7,* Epidural veins. *8,* Spinous processes. *9,* Interspinous ligament. *10,* Ligamentum flavum. *11,* Pedicle. *12,* Neural foramen with epidural fat and veins. *13,* Dorsal root ganglion. *14,* Superior articular facet. *15,* Inferior articular facet. *16,* Intranuclear cleft. *17,* Inner anular fibers of disk. *18,* Outer anular fibers of disk. *19,* Cauda equina. *20,* Conus medullaris. *21,* Pars interarticularis. *22,* S1 root. *23,* Sharpey fibers. *24,* Facet joint.

fat in the posteromedial and anterior recesses of the joint space.[6] Synovium and joint space extend a variable distance along the articular processes and under the capsule. The facet joint capsules are richly innervated by sensory fibers that arise from medial branches of the posterior spinal nerve rami.[6]

In the upper lumber spine the articular pillars and facet joints are oriented nearly in the parasagittal plane, whereas they are positioned more obliquely in the lower lumbar region.[1,8] On axial imaging studies the facet joint has a mushroom-shaped appearance; the superior articular facet forms the "cap" and the inferior articular facet and spinal lamina form the "stem" (Fig. 19-1, *E*). On sagittal MR scans the pars interarticularis lies between the more pointed superior articular facet above and the somewhat rounded-appearing inferior articular facet below (Fig. 19-2, *H*).

Laminae and spinous processes. The laminae are comparatively flat bony plates that extend posteriorly from the articular pillars and join together at the midline where they form the root of the spinous process. The spinous processes extend posteriorly and inferiorly from the neural arch (Fig. 19-2, *A*).

Ligaments and soft tissues. In the lumbosacral spine the ligaments, epidural fat, and the epidural venous plexuses form prominent extradural soft tissues that surround the thecal sac and exiting nerve roots.

Ligaments. The anterior (ALL) and posterior (PLL) longitudinal ligaments are thick, dense fibrous bands that extend along the anterior and posterior surface of each vertebral body from the skull base to the sacrum (Fig. 19-2).[9] They connect the vertebral bodies and are attached to the intervertebral disks.

The ALL extends from the basiocciput to S1. It is identified on sagittal T1-weighted MR scans as a very low signal line that is in direct contact with and follows the ventral surface of the vertebral bodies and disks (Fig. 19-2, *A*). The PLL is a thinner band that extends from C1 to the first sacral vertebra.[1] In contrast to the ALL, the PLL does not adhere to the vertebral body.[9] The PLL has a more narrow central segment that widens laterally at the intervertebral disks and attaches firmly to the anulus fibrosus, reinforcing the midline and paramedian zones of the disk.[1]

On midline sagittal MR scans, the PLL is seen as a continuous low signal band that is molded to the posterior disk surface but spans the vertebral body concavities like a bowstring (Fig. 19-2, *G*). Epidural fat and veins are interposed between the PLL and the vertebral body.

The ligamentum flavum (LF) arises from the anterior aspect of the lower margin of one lamina and inserts on the posterior surface of the lamina below.[1] The appearance of the LF on sagittal MR scans varies with its distance from the midline.[10] It is thinnest at the midline where it is seen as an oblique, linear band of low signal that attaches to the superior border of one spinous process and the inferior surface of the next (Fig. 19-2, *F*). On parasagittal scans the LF appears as an inhomogeneous triangle with a narrow base inferiorly and a broader base at its caudal end near the lamina.[10] At the neural foramen it is seen as a curvilinear, low signal structure covering the anterior surface of the facet joint (Fig. 19-2, *H*).

On axial CT and MR studies the LF is seen as a V-shaped structure that covers the facet joint anteriorly and is sometimes filled with fat posteriorly (Fig. 19-1, *E*). On NECT scans the LF is similar in attenuation to muscle; signal on MR is variable because the LF undergoes age-related degenerative change and can calcify or become infiltrated with fat (see subsequent discussion).

Small ligaments, the corporotransverse and transforaminal ligaments, are often found in the neural foramina. These fibrous bands originate from the intervertebral disk and attach to the pedicle, superior articular process, or ligamentum flavum. They reduce the potential space available for nerve roots that traverse the neural foramen.[11]

Epidural fat and veins. Extradural fat surrounds the lumbosacral thecal sac and root sleeves. The epidural fat contains numerous small veins that connect to each other in the midline between the PLL and posterior vertebral body to form the epidural venous plexus.[9] Basivertebral veins traverse the lumbar vertebral bodies and emerge near the midline to drain into this plexus (Figs. 19-1, *C*; and 19-2, *A*).[1]

The lumbar epidural venous plexus is seen as thin, linear, low signal foci on T1- and T2-weighted MR scans (Fig. 19-2, *F*). Enhancement following contrast administration is variable but can sometimes be intense.

Nerves and meninges

Conus medullaris and cauda equina. The distal spinal cord terminates in a slight, diamond-shaped enlargement: the conus medullaris. The conus tip is normally at about the L1-L2 level. The lower spinal nerve roots exit the conus medullaris and pass inferiorly within the thecal sac, forming the cauda equina, or "horse's tail" (Fig. 19-3, *A*).

Using heavily T2-weighted spin-echo sequences (Figs. 19-2, *G*; and 19-3, *G*), MR "myelography" provides detailed definition of the thecal margins, nerve roots, and root sheaths that approaches conventional water-soluble lumbar myelograms and CT-myelography (Fig. 19-3, *E* and *F*).[12] On axial section, the roots of the filum terminale typically lie in a symmetric, crescent-shaped pattern with the lower sacral roots positioned dorsally and the lumbar roots positioned more anterolaterally (Fig. 19-3, *F* and *G*).[13]

Lumbar nerves and neural foramina. Between L1 and L5, the nerve roots exit the spinal canal at about a 45 degree angle. The nerve root axillae are lateral outpouchings of dura and arachnoid that surround the exiting roots (Fig. 19-3, *E*). The motor roots lie ventral to the sensory roots from the thecal sac exit to the dorsal root ganglia.[14] The dorsal root ganglia normally vary considerably in size, and range from 6 mm at L1 to 15 mm at S2.[14]

The pedicles form the superior and inferior borders of the neural foramen; the articular facet and ligamentum flavum form its posterior border (*see* Fig. 19-2, *B*). The anterior border is comprised of the vertebral body superiorly and the intervertebral disk and PLL inferiorly.[15,16]

The normal lumbar neural foramen is widest in its superior aspect and narrows inferiorly. Each lumbar nerve root exits the spinal canal through the superior part of the foramen, above the level of the intervertebral disk. In 90% of cases, the dorsal root ganglion is directly inferior to the pedicle.[14] On sagittal MR scans the fat-filled foramen looks like the head and beak of a bird, with the dorsal root ganglion forming its eye (*see* Fig. 19-2, *H*).

Sacral plexus. The sacral plexus is formed by the ventral rami of the L4-L5 and S1-S4 nerves (Fig. 19-3, *A*). Medial to the psoas muscle, the L4-L5 nerves join to form the lumbosacral trunk. After they exit the spine, the S1-S4 nerves converge in front of the piriformis muscle and join with the lumbosacral trunk to form the sacral plexus. The sciatic nerve (L4-S3) is the continuation of the sacral plexus. The sciatic nerve leaves the pelvis through the greater sciatic foramen to enter the thigh.[17]

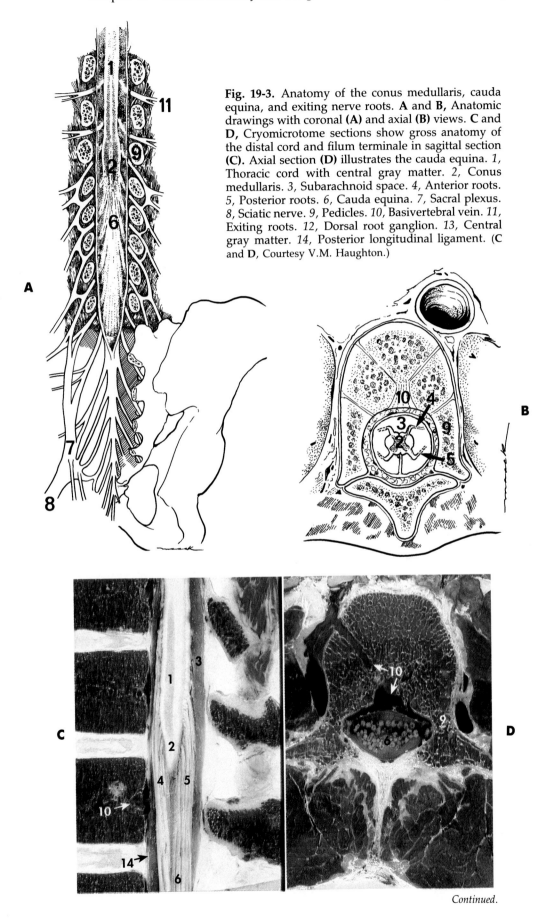

Fig. 19-3. Anatomy of the conus medullaris, cauda equina, and exiting nerve roots. **A** and **B,** Anatomic drawings with coronal **(A)** and axial **(B)** views. **C** and **D,** Cryomicrotome sections show gross anatomy of the distal cord and filum terminale in sagittal section **(C).** Axial section **(D)** illustrates the cauda equina. *1,* Thoracic cord with central gray matter. *2,* Conus medullaris. *3,* Subarachnoid space. *4,* Anterior roots. *5,* Posterior roots. *6,* Cauda equina. *7,* Sacral plexus. *8,* Sciatic nerve. *9,* Pedicles. *10,* Basivertebral vein. *11,* Exiting roots. *12,* Dorsal root ganglion. *13,* Central gray matter. *14,* Posterior longitudinal ligament. (**C** and **D,** Courtesy V.M. Haughton.)

Continued.

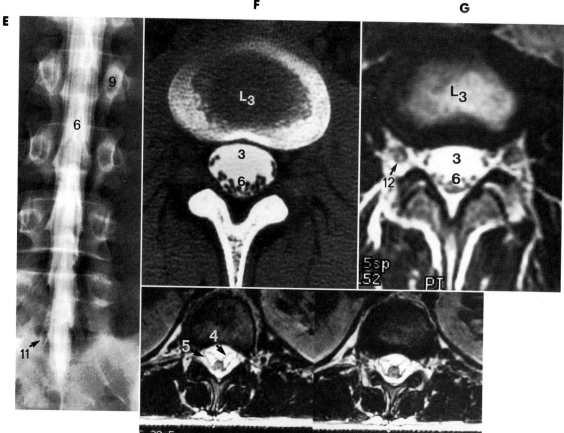

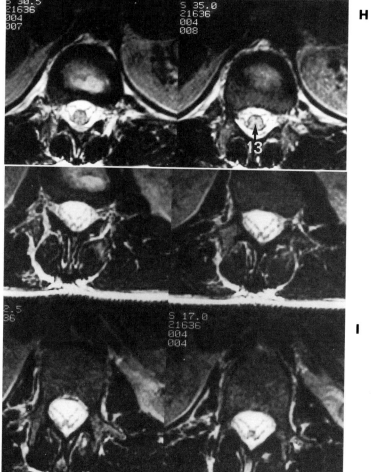

Fig. 19-3, cont'd. E to **I,** Multimodality imaging studies show the conus medullaris and filum terminale. Water-soluble myelogram, AP view **(E).** Axial CT scan **(F)** with intrathecal contrast. Axial T2-weighted MR scan **(G)** through cauda equina. Compare with **F. H** and **I,** Axial T2-weighted MR scans through conus medullaris with "MR myelogram" effect. Compare with **(J),** an axial postmyelogram CT scan of the conus medullaris. *1,* Thoracic cord with central gray matter. *2,* Conus medullaris. *3,* Subarachnoid space. *4,* Anterior roots. *5,* Posterior roots. *6,* Cauda equina. *7,* Sacral plexus. *8,* Sciatic nerve. *9,* Pedicles. *10,* Basivertebral vein. *11,* Exiting roots. *12,* Dorsal root ganglion. *13,* Central gray matter. *14,* Posterior longitudinal ligament.

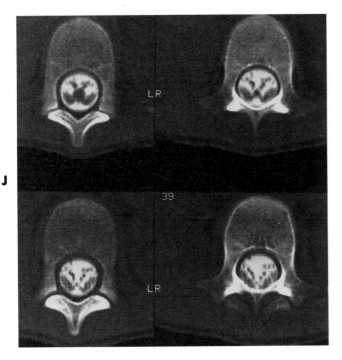

Fig. 19-3, cont'd. J, Axial postmyelogram CT scan of the conus medullaris.

Thoracic Spine

Anterior elements

Vertebral bodies. The dorsally convex thoracic spine consists of twelve vertebrae that gradually increase in size from rostral to caudal (Fig. 19-4, *A*). The weight-bearing vertebral bodies are slightly wedge-shaped from front to back and appear somewhat cone- or triangular-shaped in axial section.[18]

Interverteral disks. The height of the thoracic intervertebral disks is less than either the cervical or lumbar counterparts, but the anulus fibrosus is thicker here.

Posterior elements

Pedicles and laminae. The pedicles project posteriorly from the superior aspects of each vertebral body. The laminae are broad, short, and overlap each other like the tiles on a roof (Fig. 19-4, *B*).[18] The laminae fuse in the midline to form the dorsal canal wall and give origin to the spinous processes. The thoracic spinous processes are long and gracile, extending posteriorly and inferiorly from the spinal canal (Fig. 19-4, *D*).

Articular pillars and joints. Articular processes arise from the superior and inferior aspects of the laminae and form the facet joints. In the thoracic spine, most facet joints lie in the coronal plane. Transverse processes project laterally from the articular pillars between the superior and inferior articu-

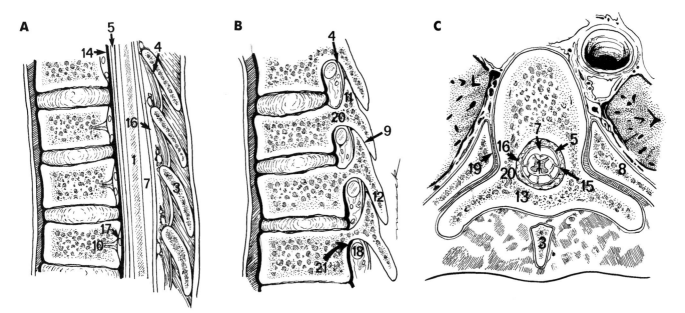

Fig. 19-4. Anatomy of the thoracic spine and spinal cord. **A** to **C,** Anatomic drawings with sagittal midline view **(A),** sagittal view through the neural foramen **(B),** and axial view **(C).** *1,* Spinal cord with central gray matter. *2,* Conus medullaris. *3,* Spinous process. *4,* Ligamentum flavum. *5,* Dura. *6,* Cauda equina. *7,* Subarachnoid space. *8,* Rib. *9,* Facet joints. *10,* Basivertebral venous plexus. *11,* Superior articular facets. *12,* Inferior articular facets. *13,* Lamina. *14,* Posterior longitudinal ligament. *15,* Dentate ligaments. *16,* Epidural fat. *17,* Epidural veins. *18,* Nerve root. *19,* Costovertebral joint. *20,* Pedicle. *21,* Neural foramen.

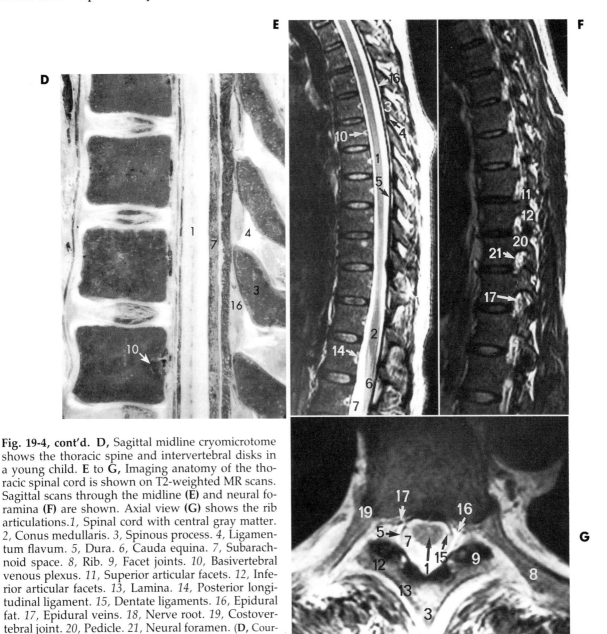

Fig. 19-4, cont'd. D, Sagittal midline cryomicrotome shows the thoracic spine and intervertebral disks in a young child. **E to G,** Imaging anatomy of the thoracic spinal cord is shown on T2-weighted MR scans. Sagittal scans through the midline **(E)** and neural foramina **(F)** are shown. Axial view **(G)** shows the rib articulations. *1,* Spinal cord with central gray matter. *2,* Conus medullaris. *3,* Spinous process. *4,* Ligamentum flavum. *5,* Dura. *6,* Cauda equina. *7,* Subarachnoid space. *8,* Rib. *9,* Facet joints. *10,* Basivertebral venous plexus. *11,* Superior articular facets. *12,* Inferior articular facets. *13,* Lamina. *14,* Posterior longitudinal ligament. *15,* Dentate ligaments. *16,* Epidural fat. *17,* Epidural veins. *18,* Nerve root. *19,* Costovertebral joint. *20,* Pedicle. *21,* Neural foramen. (**D,** Courtesy V.M. Haughton.)

lar facets. The tip of each transverse process from T1 to T10 bears an oval costal facet. Costotransverse joints are formed by the articulation of the rib tubercles and tips of the transverse processes.[19]

Ribs. Ribs articulate with the thoracic vertebrae at two sites. Rib heads articulate with the vertebrae at the disk (Fig. 19-4, *C* and *G*), and the rib tubercle joins with the transverse process at the costotransverse articulation (see previous discussion).[19] At all levels except T1, T11, and T12, demifacets above and below the disk articulate with the rib head to form the costovertebral joint, which is a true synovial joint. The rib heads are therefore helpful landmarks in identifying the intervertebral disk during axial imaging.[19]

Ligaments. The anterior longitudinal ligament is thicker in the thoracic region than in the cervical or lumbar spine.[18] It is also more prominent opposite the vertebral bodies than the disks. The posterior longitudinal ligament is also thicker in the thoracic spine. Other ligaments such as the ligamentum flavum and the interspinous ligaments are not significantly different from their configuration at other spinal segments.[19]

Nerves. A number of rootlets emerge from the thoracic spinal cord and merge to form two roots: a large dorsal sensory root and a smaller ventral motor root (*see* Figs. 19-3, *H* and 19-4, *C*). These descend a

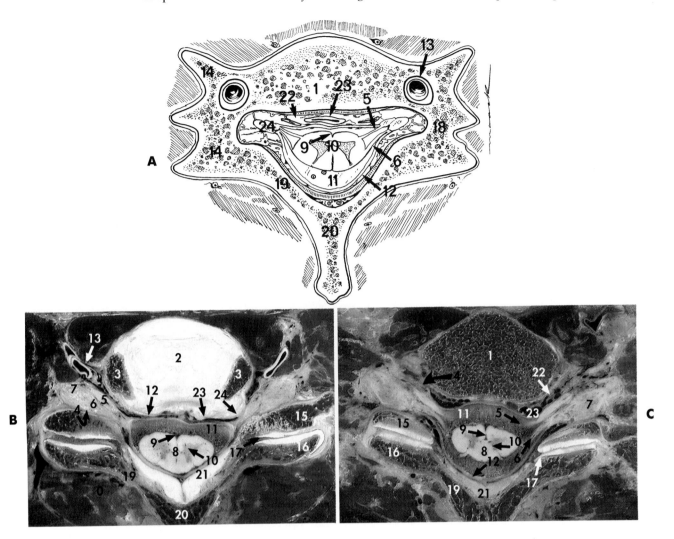

Fig. 19-5. Axial anatomy of the cervical spine and spinal cord. **A,** Anatomic drawing depicting the pedicles and lateral recesses. **B** and **C,** Axial cryomicrotome sections through the C6-C7 interspace and the low vertebral body of C7 are shown. *1,* Vertebral body. *2,* Intervertebral disk. *3,* Uncinate processes. *4,* Neural foramen. *5,* Anterior roots. *6,* Posterior roots. *7,* Ganglion. *8,* Cervical spinal cord. *9,* Ventral median fissure. *10,* Central gray matter. *11,* Subarachnoid space. *12,* Dura. *13,* Vertebral artery in foramen transversarium. *14,* Transverse process. *15,* Superior articular facet. *16,* Inferior articular facet. *17,* Facet joint. *18,* Pedicle. *19,* Lamina. *20,* Spinous process. *21,* Ligamentum flavum. *22,* Epidural fat. *23,* Epidural veins. *24,* Root sleeve. (**B** and **C,** Courtesy V.M. Haughton.)   *Continued.*

variable distance within the subarachnoid space to exit through the neural foramina.[18]

Cervical Spine

The upper two cervical vertebrae differ in size and configuration from the lower five segments.[20] The anatomy and pathology of the craniovertebral junction are discussed in Chapter 12.

C1, the atlas, is a bony ring with ellipsoid, superior articular surfaces that combine with the occipital condyles to form the atlantooccipital joint. The inferior facets are round or oblong and articulate with the superior facets of C2 to form the atlantoaxial joints.

The second cervical vertebra, the axis, is notable because of the dens (odontoid process), a cone-shaped bony prominence that extends superiorly from the C2 body nearly to the clivus.[18] The dens articulates anterosuperiorly with the anterior arch of C1.

C3-C7 are functionally and anatomically quite similar and are therefore discussed together.

Anterior elements

Vertebral bodies and uncovertebral joints (Figs. 19-5 and 19-6). The C3-C7 vertebral bodies are somewhat box-shaped and gradually increase in size from C3 to C7 (Fig. 19-6, *A*). Each has superior pro-

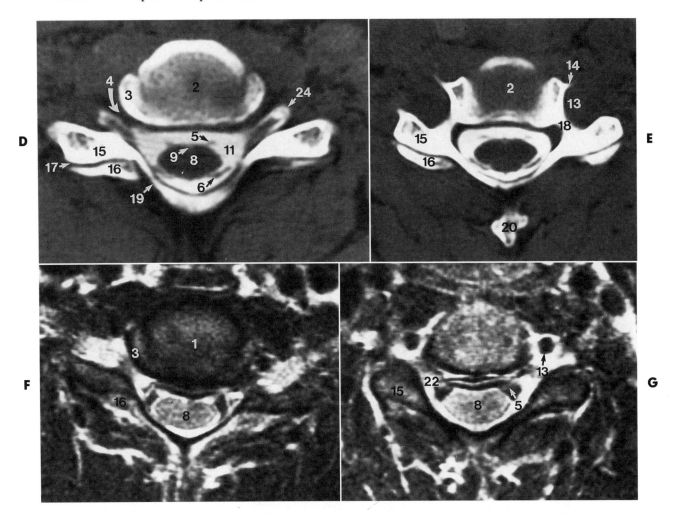

Fig. 19-5, cont'd. D to G, Multimodality imaging studies depict axial anatomy. Axial CT scans (D and E) with intrathecal contrast are shown at the level of the uncovertebral joints and neural foramina (D) and the pedicles (E). F and G, Axial T2-weighted MR scans depict normal cervical spinal cord and soft tissue anatomy. Prominent areas of high velocity signal loss from pulsatile CSF flow are present. 1, Vertebral body. 2, Intervertebral disk. 3, Uncinate processes. 4, Neural foramen. 5, Anterior roots. 6, Posterior roots. 7, Ganglion. 8, Cervical spinal cord. 9, Ventral median fissure. 10, Central gray matter. 11, Subarachnoid space. 12, Dura. 13, Vertebral artery in foramen transversarium. 14, Transverse process. 15, Superior articular facet. 16, Inferior articular facet. 17, Facet joint. 18, Pedicle. 19, Lamina. 20, Spinous process. 21, Ligamentum flavum. 22, Epidural fat. 23, Epidural veins. 24, Root sleeve.

jections, the uncinate processes, that indent the posterolateral margin of the intervertebral disk and vertebral body above, forming the uncovertebral joints (Fig. 19-5, *A*).[21] Some uncovertebral joints are filled with loose connective tissue; others are lined with synovium.[21]

Intervertebral disks. In the cervical spine, the intervertebral disks are kidney bean–shaped structures that are normally somewhat thicker anteriorly than posteriorly (Figs. 19-5, *A* and *F*). These disks have a central amorphous nucleus pulposus and a denser peripheral fibrocartilaginous anulus fibrosus.[20]

Transverse processes and foramina transversaria. The transverse processes project anterolaterally from

the vertebral bodies. The anterior and posterior parts of the transverse processes are connected by a thin bony bar, the costotransverse bar. The canal that is thus created is the transverse foramen. The foramina transversaria contain the vertebral arteries and veins (Fig. 19-5, *B* and *E*).

Posterior elements
Pedicles. The pedicles are short, cylindric structures that project posteriorly and slightly laterally from the vertebral bodies, connecting them to the articular pillars (Fig. 19-6, *B* and *D*).

Articular pillars and facet joints. The cervical articular pillars are rhomboid-shaped bony projections

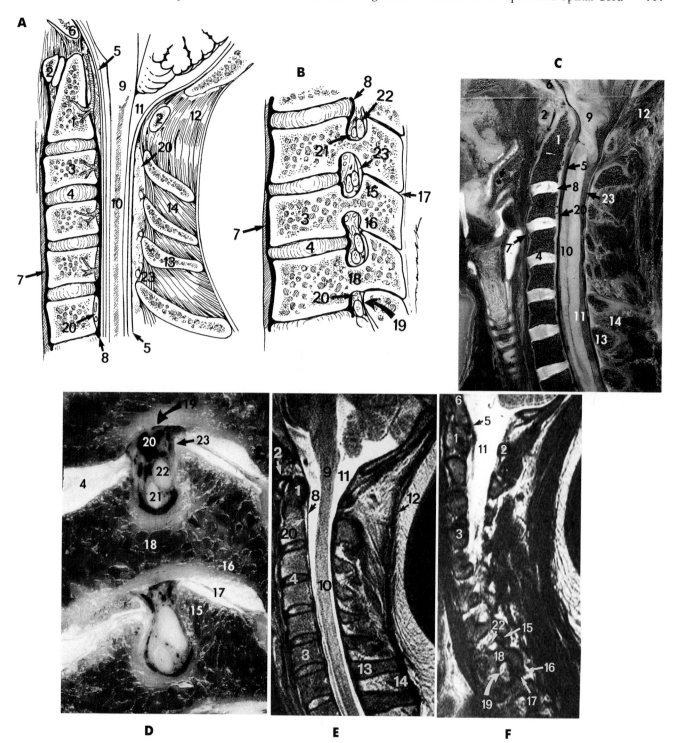

Fig. 19-6. Sagittal anatomy of the cervical spine and spinal cord. **A** and **B,** Anatomic drawings through the midline **(A)** and neural foramina **(B). C** and **D,** Cryomicrotome sections with midline anatomy **(C)** and close-up view of the neural foramen **(D). E,** Midline sagittal T2-weighted MR scan shows the cervical spine and spinal cord. **F,** More lateral scan shows the neural foramina and exiting roots. *1,* Dens with odontoid process. *2,* C1. *3,* Vertebral body. *4,* Intervertebral disk. *5,* Dura. *6,* Clivus. *7,* Anterior longitudinal ligament. *8,* Posterior longitudinal ligament. *9,* Cervicomedullary junction. *10,* Cervical spinal cord with central gray matter. *11,* Subarachnoid space. *12,* Ligamentum nuchae. *13,* Spinous process. *14,* Interspinous ligament. *15,* Superior articular facet. *16,* Inferior articular facet. *17,* Facet joint. *18,* Pedicle. *19,* Neural foramen. *20,* Epidural veins and fat. *21,* Anterior (ventral) roots. *22,* Posterior roots and dorsal root ganglia. *23,* Ligamentum flavum. (**C** and **D,** Courtesy V.M. Haughton.)

that arise at the junction between the pedicle and lamina. The facet joints are formed by the superior and inferior articular facets of adjacent vertebrae (Fig. 19-6, B and D).

In the sagittal plane, the facet joints angle obliquely downward (Fig. 19-6, B and D). On axial section, they are oriented perpendicular to the vertebral body, with the superior articular processes positioned anterior to the inferior ones (Fig. 19-5, B to E). Together the superior and inferior articular facets look like two slightly flattened half-moon-shaped structures with an interposed joint space (Fig. 19-5, E). The facet joints are true synovial joints with a fibrous capsule. The anterior aspect of the ligamentum flavum covers the joints.

Laminae and spinous processes. The cervical laminae are thin bony plates that project dorsally and are fused in the midline, covering the spinal canal (Fig. 19-5, B and C). The spinous processes project posteroinferiorly from the spinolaminar junction (Fig. 19-5, E). The spinous processes are often bifid. C7 has the longest spinous process.

The spinal canal on axial views is roughly shaped like an equilateral triangle (Fig. 19-5). Its anteroposterior diameter varies in size from a normal lower limit of 12 mm in the lower canal to 15 to 16 mm at C1 and C2.[21]

Neural foramina and nerves

Neural foramina. The cervical neural foramina are formed by the vertebral bodies anteriorly, the pedicles above and below, and the articular pillars and ligamentum flavum posteriorly (Fig. 19-6, B and D).

Nerves. The cervical nerve roots extend slightly inferiorly and anterolaterally from the cord at about a 45 degree angle. Cervical nerve roots are located within the root sheath in the inferior half of the neural foramen; the upper half of the cervical neural foramen contains fat and small veins (Fig. 19-6, D).[22] The dorsal roots lie above and behind the ventral nerve roots (Fig. 19-6, B and C). The dorsal root ganglion lies outside the neural foramen between the vertebral artery anteriorly and the superior articular facet posteriorly.[22]

Ligaments and soft tissues

Ligaments. As in the thoracic and lumbar spine, the anterior and posterior longitudinal ligaments connect the cervical vertebrae. Fibers from the PLL diverge from the midline at each disk level, merging with the anulus fibrosus and attaching to the adjacent vertebral end plates.[21] The PLL extends cephalad to merge into the tectorial membrane and dura mater (Fig. 19-6, C). Just behind the dens, the inferior and superior cruciate ligaments merge to form the transverse ligament.[23]

Other cervical ligaments are similar to their thoracic and lumbar counterparts. The interspinous ligament extends between spinous processes (Fig. 19-6, C and E). The ligamentum flavum is continuous along the posterior cervical spinal canal, attaching to the laminae and covering the facet joint capsules (see Fig. 19-5).[21]

Epidural fat and veins. Compared to the lumbosacral region, cervical epidural fat is sparse, whereas the epidural veins are larger. The anterior epidural space contains a prominent venous sinusoidal plexus (Fig. 19-6, A and C). This plexus consists of longitudinal vascular channels that are located in the anterolateral recesses of the epidural space and connected to each other via a network of retrocorporeal veins.[23] The epidural venous plexus communicates anteriorly with the basivertebral venous system. It also forms a venous plexus in each neural foramen that extends through the foramen to surround the vertebral arteries (Fig. 19-6, B and D).[23]

The cervical anterior epidural venous plexus (CAEVP) is visualized on 90% of contrast-enhanced MR scans and is particularly prominent at the C1-C3 level, whereas only 20% of CAEVPs are visualized at C6-C7.[24]

Meninges and Spinal Cord

Meninges

Dura and subdural space. The spinal dura is a dense fibrous tube that encloses the leptomeninges, cerebrospinal fluid, spinal cord, and proximal nerve roots. The dura is continuous cephalad with the inner layer of the cranial pachymeninges (see Chapter 12). The spinal dura extends inferiorly to the second sacral segment, below which it blends into the solid filum terminale externum and attaches to the coccyx.[1] The spinal subdural space is normally very small.

Arachnoid and subarachnoid space. The arachnoid is loosely attached to the inner aspect of the dura. The subarachnoid space lies under the leptomeninges and contains cerebrospinal fluid, spinal cord, conus medullaris, filum terminale internum, and nerve roots. The cervical subarachnoid space is widest at the craniovertebral junction and gradually tapers from the foramen magnum to C2. The subarachnoid space from C3 to C7 ranges from 10 to 15 mm in anteroposterior diameter.[21] The spinal subarachnoid space is continuous cephalad with the intracranial CSF cisterns.

The thoracic subarachnoid space is relatively constant, typically measuring 12 to 13 mm in sagittal diameter. Thin septae extend from the posterior surface of the thoracic cord to the arachnoid. The most prominent and constant of these is the midline septum posticum.[18] Other delicate ligaments, the dentate ligaments, extend laterally from the cord to the arachnoid wall (see Fig. 19-4, G). These fibrous bands func-

Spine MR Imaging *Normal enhancement patterns*
Normally enhance Epidural veins, venous plexus Dorsal root ganglia Meninges (mild) Marrow and disk fibrocartilage (infants, young children only) **Normally do not enhance** Spinal cord Nerve roots Marrow, intervertebral disks (older children, adults)

Congenital Malformations of the Spine and Spinal Cord *Open spinal dysraphism*
Components Incomplete midline closure of mesenchymal, osseous, neural tissue Dorsally dysraphic spine Posterior protrusion of all or part of spinal canal contents Neural tissue exposed **Examples** Myelocele (neural placode flush with surface) Myelomeningocele (protruding placode)

tionally divide the thoracic subarachnoid space into compartments that intercommunicate but may differ in CSF flow rates. This sometimes results in prominent flow-related artifacts that can mimic vascular malformations on MR imaging (*see* Fig. 20-15).

The lumbar subarachnoid space is larger and more variable, ranging from 15 to 20 mm in sagittal diameter.[1]

All of the spinal meninges have a blood supply with a fenestrated capillary endothelium, although their extravascular space is relatively small. This limits the amount of contrast pooling, and thus the spinal meningeal enhancement normally seen on postcontrast T1-weighted MR scans is relatively modest (*see* box, *above*).[25]

Spinal cord

Gross configuration. The cervical spinal cord is somewhat elliptic in cross section, whereas the thoracic cord appears more round. The conus medullaris has a diamond-shaped enlargement before it terminates in the cauda equina. The normal conus in adults ends above L2-L3, typically at the L1-L2 level. This so-called "adult" position is attained during the first few months of life and varies little thereafter.[26]

Cord surface topography is exquisitely delineated on axial T2-weighted MR scans or CT myelograms. A prominent cleft, the ventral median fissure, is seen in the midline anteriorly (*see* Fig. 19-5, *D*); a more shallow dorsal median sulcus is present posteriorly. The dorsolateral sulci lie adjacent to the dorsal nerve roots, and the dorsal intermediate sulci separate the gracile and cuneate fasciculi.[27]

Internal anatomy. Cross sections of the spinal cord delineate the centrally placed gray matter and the surrounding white matter. The central gray matter has a characteristic butterfly or H-shaped configuration that is formed by the dorsal and ventral horns

(*see* Fig. 19-3, *H*).[28] These extend throughout the entire length of the spinal cord. Smaller lateral horns are present from T1 to the conus medullaris. The central gray matter volume appears relatively increased in the cervical and lumbar enlargements.[29]

The spinal cord white matter is divided into three funiculi on each side.[29] The anterior funiculi lie between the ventral median fissure medially and the exit zone for the ventral nerve rootlets. The lateral funiculi lie between the dorsal and ventral spinal nerve roots. The posterior funiculi are the white matter between the dorsal median sulcus and the dorsolateral fasciculus and dorsal horns on each side.[27]

CONGENITAL MALFORMATIONS OF THE SPINE AND SPINAL CORD

An exhaustive description of the numerous congenital malformations that affect the spine and cord is beyond the scope of this text. We discuss the most important entities in two broad categories of congenital malformations, open spinal dysraphism and occult spinal dysraphism. Two other groups of lesions that are also occult dysraphic disorders are the abnormalities of canalization and retrograde differentiation and the split notochord syndromes. We will discuss each of these categories separately, then close our consideration of congenital malformations by summarizing a few miscellaneous but important anomalies.

Open Spinal Dysraphism

The general term "spinal dysraphism" refers to those spinal anomalies that have incomplete midline closure of mesenchymal, osseous, and neural tissue (*see* box, *above*).[30]

In open spina bifida, also called spina bifida aperta or spina bifida cystica, there is a dysraphic spine with posterior protrusion of spinal contents through

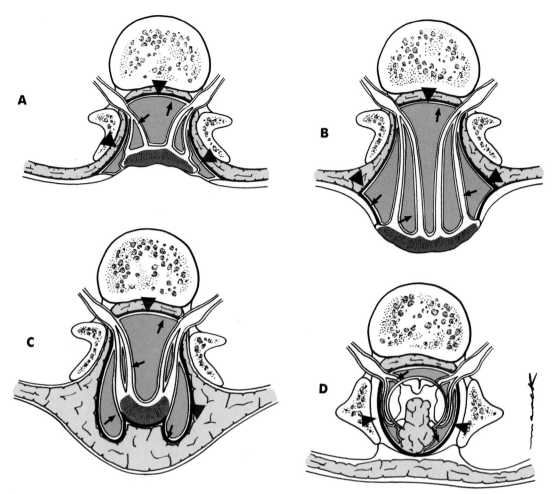

Fig. 19-7. Anatomic drawing depicts myelocele **(A)**, myelomeningocele **(B)**, lipomyelomeningocele **(C)**, and intradural lipoma **(D)**. The neural placode is shown in red **(A to C)**. The lipoma and subcutaneous fat are shown in yellow **(A to D)**. The CSF space is shown in gray, and the dura is indicated by the heavy black line *(arrowheads)*. The pia-arachnoid is shown by the thin black lines *(arrows)*. (Adapted from Barkovich AJ: *Pediatric Neuroimaging,* New York, Raven Press, 1990.)

the dorsal bony defect. In this section we discuss the two forms of open spinal dysraphism, myelocele and myelomeningocele.

Myelocele. Myelocele is a neural tube closure disorder similar in embryogenesis to myelomeningocele (see subsequent discussion). A midline plaque of neural tissue (the neural placode) is flush with the surface laterally. The placode is not covered with skin and is thus open to the air (Fig. 19-7, *A*). The dura is also deficient posteriorly, whereas the pia and arachnoid line the ventral surface of the neural placode and dura. The arachnoid sac thus formed is continuous with the lumbar subarachnoid space.[30]

Myelomeningocele

Etiology and pathology. Myelomeningocele (MM) and myelocele both result from failure of the embryonic neural folds to flex and fuse into a tube (*see*

box).[31] Instead, they persist as a flat plate of unneurulated tissue called the neural placode. The superficial ectoderm does not undergo disjunction from the neural ectoderm and remains in lateral position (*see* Chapter 1).

Bone, cartilage, muscle, and ligament also develop in abnormal position ventrolateral to the neural tissue and remain bifid and everted.[32,33] A midline defect is present, and the everted, elevated neural plate and meninges are continuous laterally with the subcutaneous tissues (Fig. 19-7, *B*). The spinal cord is thus tethered and relatively immobile. The dorsal roots arise from the anterior surface of the neural plate lateral to the ventral roots. Both cross the CSF-filled sac to exit the neural foramina (Fig. 19-8; *see* Fig. 19-7, *B*).[33]

Incidence, age, and gender. Myelomeningocele, anencephaly, and cephalocele are all considered neural tube defects. Together, their incidence in the

Myelomeningocele

Etiology

Neural tube closure defect

Pathology

Dysraphic spine with dorsal protrusion of meninges, CSF, neural tissue; not covered with skin

Location

Nearly always lumbar

Imaging

Intrauterine ultrasound discloses widely open neural arch with flared laminae; meningocele sac; signs of Chiari II malformation ("lemon" and "banana" signs; hydrocephalus and callosal dysgenesis common)

MR, CT nearly always postoperative, show repair; tethered cord often persists

Associated anomalies

Chiari II (virtually 100%)
Syringohydromyelia (30% to 75%)
Hydrocephalus (80%)
Diastematomyelia (30% to 45%)
Callosal dysgenesis

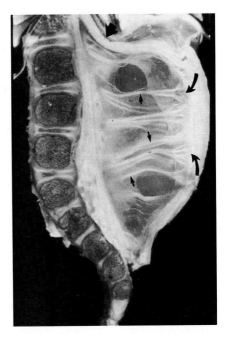

Fig. 19-8. Gross autopsy specimen demonstrates the pathologic findings in myelomeningocele. The spinal cord *(large arrow)* is tethered into a CSF-filled dural sac that protrudes dorsally through a widely dysraphic lumbosacral spine. Note the nerve roots *(small arrows)* that course anteriorly across the sac from the neural placode *(curved arrows).* (Courtesy Royal College of Surgeons of England, *Slide Atlas of Pathology,* Nervous System. Gower Medical Publishing.)

A   **B**

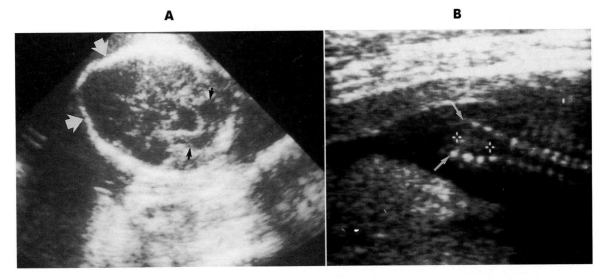

Fig. 19-9. Obstetric ultrasound findings of Chiari II malformation and myelomeningocele are illustrated on these prenatal scans. **A,** Transverse view through the fetal head shows a small posterior fossa with compressed cerebellum around the midbrain forming the "banana sign" *(small arrows).* Note bifrontal concavities, the so-called "lemon sign" *(white arrows).* **B,** Coronal view through the lower fetal spine shows widened lower lumbar and sacral canal with flared posterior elements *(arrows).* (Courtesy C. Sistrom.)

Continued.

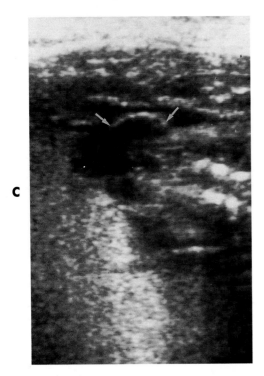

Fig. 19-9, cont'd. C, Coronal view through the lower fetal spine demonstrates the thin-walled sac of a myelomeningocele *(arrows)*. (Courtesy C. Sistrom.)

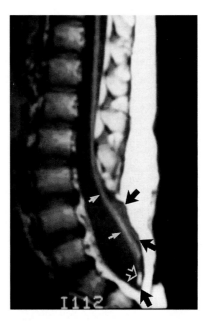

Fig. 19-10. Sagittal T1-weighted MR scan shows a repaired myelomeningocele. The sac *(large arrows)* is now covered with skin; the spinal cord *(small arrows)* remains tethered. A small lipoma is indicated by the outlined arrow.

United States is 1.5 per 1000 live births. Meningomyelocele occurs in 0.6 per 1000 live births. There is a slight female predominance.

Between 90% and 95% of neural tube defects occur in previously unaffected families but previous MM in a sibship increases the risk for all three types of neural tube disorders. Elevated maternal serum alpha-fetoprotein is also associated with an increased incidence of these malformations.[34]

Location. The majority of MMs occur in the lumbosacral region; cervicothoracic MMs are very rare.

Imaging. Untreated myelomeningoceles are almost never imaged except during obstetric ultrasonography. Prenatal sonographic diagnosis of MM is predicated on detecting the spinal dysraphism, seen as an open, widened neural arch with flared laminae (Fig. 19-9, *A*). Other signs are the presence of a spinal myelomeningocele sac and cranial abnormalities associated with Chiari II malformation. (Fig. 19-9, *B* and *C*.[35] Characteristic prenatal sonographic findings include frontal concavities (the so-called lemon sign), hydrocephalus, and a small posterior fossa with compressed cerebellum and no cisterna magna (the "banana sign") (Fig. 19-9, *B*).[35]

Imaging studies of repaired myelomeningoceles typically show a wide dyraphic defect with thinned, flared laminae and a CSF-filled skin-covered sac. The cord and roots are often surgically repositioned

within the spinal canal but usually remain low-lying. Retethering by scarring is common (Fig. 19-10).[32]

Associated anomalies. Chiari II malformation is seen in virtually 100% of MMs (*see* Fig. 2-14). Intracanalicular spinal lipomas are found in nearly three-quarters of patients with MM.[33] Inclusion dermoid or epidermoid cysts are occasionally present.[31]

Hydromyelia, defined as a dilated ependymal-lined central canal, is present in 30% to 75% of patients with MM. Syringomyelia, cord cavitation that is not lined with ependyma, often coexists and is seen in about 20% of these cases.[33] Because these two conditions are difficult to distinguish on imaging studies, they are often grouped together and termed *syringohydromyelia*.

Other CNS abnormalities that are associated with myelomeningocele include hydrocephalus (80%), corpus callosum agenesis, and diastematomyelia (30% to 45%).[33] Non-CNS abnormalities commonly observed in patients with myelomeningocele include congenital scoliosis (20%) or kyphosis (less than 10%), developmental lordosis or kyphoscoliosis (65%), and hip deformities.[32,36]

Occult Spinal Dysraphism

Occult dysraphic defects are skin-covered lesions that have no exposed neural tissue and no visible cystic mass.[37] Although the exact embryologic develop-

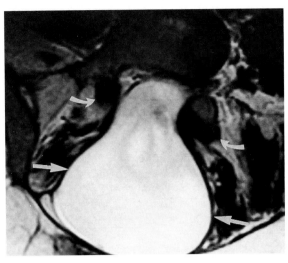

Congenital Malformations of the Spine and Spinal Cord

Occult spinal dysraphism

Components

Dorsally dysraphic spine

Skin covers malformation; neural tissue not exposed

Examples

Meningocele (skin usually intact; sometimes categorized with open spina bifida)

Dorsal dermal sinus

Spinal lipomas

Sometimes also included: tethered cord, split notochord, caudal regression syndromes

---

Fig. 19-11. Axial T2-weighted scan of a congenital simple meningocele shows herniation of CSF-containing meninges (large arrows) through a widely dysraphic spine with everted laminae *(curved arrows)*. The meningocele sac appears featureless and does not contain neural elements. The overlying skin was intact.

---

ment has not been precisely delineated, these defects are thought to result from abnormal fusion or closure of embryonic dorsal midline structures.

Occult spinal dysraphisms are a heterogeneous group of lesions. Meningocele, dorsal dermal sinus, and spinal lipomas are examples (*see* box, *above*).[30] Other anomalies such as tethered conus, tight filum terminale, and the split notochord syndromes are often also associated with occult spinal dysraphism (see subsequent discussion).

Meningocele. Acquired meningocele is a comparatively common laminectomy complication (*see* Fig. 20-60), whereas congenital meningocele is a relatively rare developmental anomaly.

Etiology and pathology. The embryologic origin of congenital meningoceles is unknown. Grossly, a simple meningocele is a protrusion of CSF and meninges through a dorsal spinal defect into the subcutaneous tissue. The overlying skin is typically intact.[31] The meningocele sac is lined by arachnoid and contains only cerebrospinal fluid. No neural tissue is present (*see* box, *right*).

Incidence, age, and gender. Meningoceles are only one-tenth as frequent as myelomeningoceles. Meningoceles occur in 1 per 10,000 live births. There is no gender predilection.[33]

Clinical presentation. A subcutaneous mass that changes size and tension with Valsalva maneuver is typical.[33] Neurologic deficits are uncommon with simple meningoceles.

Location. More than 80% of meningoceles are located in the lumbosacral spine.

Imaging. Imaging studies show spina bifida with a narrow focal defect or a broader lesion with thinned, dorsally everted flared laminae. A sharply demarcated fluid-filled sac that is isodense or isointense with CSF and devoid of neural tissue is present

---

Meningocele, Meningomyelocele, and Lipomyelomeningocele Compared

Meningocele

Dorsal protrusion of meninges, CSF, *no* neural contents

Myelomeningocele

Dorsal protrusion of meninges, CSF *plus* neural contents

Lipomyelomeningocele

Meninges, CSF, neural contents *plus* fat

(Fig. 19-11). The overlying skin is typically intact.[33]

Associated anomalies. Simple meningoceles are rarely associated with other spine or spinal cord anomalies.

Dorsal dermal sinus

Etiology and pathology. Dorsal dermal sinuses are thought to result from faulty neurulation.[38] If disjunction between the superficial and neural ectoderm is faulty, a focal segmental adhesion is created.[32] When the spinal cord later becomes surrounded by mesenchyme and undergoes its ascent relative to the spinal column, this adhesion persists as an elongated epithelial-lined tube connecting the spinal cord with the skin (*see* box, p. 804).[30]

Grossly a dermal sinus tract extends inward from the skin for a variable distance. It may terminate within the subcutaneous tissues or pass through the median raphe or bifid laminae toward the dura.[38] The tract extends into the spinal canal in one-half to two-thirds of all cases.[32]

Incidence, age, and gender. Dorsal dermal sinuses are uncommon lesions. Most are identified in early childhood, although some present as late as age 35. There is no gender predilection.[33]

Clinical presentation. Most congenital dermal sinuses become symptomatic because of infection. Sometimes symptoms arise from the mass effect caused by an associated dermoid or epidermoid tumor.[38] Physical examination discloses a midline dim-

---

Dorsal Dermal Sinus

Epithelial-lined sinus tract from skin; >50% in lumbosacral region; occipital area is second most common site

May terminate in subcutaneous tissue, dura, subarachnoid space, spinal cord, or nerve root; 50% end in dermoid or epidermoid cyst

May terminate several spinal segments from cutaneous ostium

Symptoms usually from infection

Imaging shows tract; underlying spine often dysraphic

---

ple or ostium that is often associated with hyperpigmented patch, hairy nevus, or capillary angioma.[30]

Location. Slightly more than half of all dorsal dermal sinuses occur in the lumbosacral spine. The occipital area is the second most common site, followed by the thoracic spine.[39] A dermal sinus may extend over a considerable distance and terminate several spinal segments away from its cutaneous ostium. The dermatomal level of the cutaneous defect corresponds to the neural ectodermal level of the CNS structure with which it is connected via the tract.[38]

Imaging. NECT scans typically show a relatively hyperdense sinus tract that traverses the subcutaneous fat and passes through a dysraphic or dysplastic lamina into the spinal canal where it penetrates for a variable depth. The tract may merge with the dura, terminate in the subarachnoid space, or traverse the subarachnoid space to terminate in the conus medullaris, filum terminale, a nerve root, or a concomitant dermoid or epidermoid cyst.[31] The subcutaneous portions of dermal sinus tracts and associated intramedullary tumors such as dermoid are easily identified on MR scans (Fig. 19-12); the intraspinal segments may be difficult to delineate unless they are lined by fat.[38]

Associated anomalies. Approximately half of all dermal sinuses terminate in deep dermoid or epidermoid cysts; 20% to 30% of dermoid tumors are associated with dermal sinuses.[31]

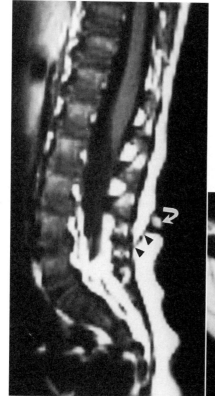

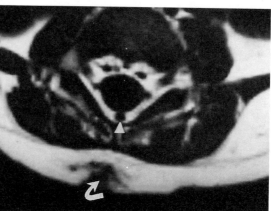

Fig. 19-12. This 18-month-old infant had repeated episodes of meningitis. Sagittal **(A)** and axial **(B)** T1-weighted MR scans show a linear focus of low signal *(arrowheads)* that extends from the skin toward the spine. The sinus tract is surrounded by high signal subcutaneous and epidural fat. A marker capsule delineates the site of a surface dimple *(curved arrow).* Dorsal dermal sinus.

Spinal lipomas. The malformation most frequently associated with all forms of occult spinal dysraphism is lipoma. Spinal lipomas are masses of mature fat and fibrous tissue that are connected with the leptomeninges or spinal cord.[30] Spinal lipomas are divided into the following three principal categories (*see* box, *below*)[31]:

1. Lipomyelomeningocele (84%)
2. Filum terminale fibrolipoma (12%)
3. Intradural lipomas (4%)

Lipomyelomeningocele. Lipomyelomeningocele is a neural tube closure defect. A lipomyelomeningocele is basically analogous to a myelinomeningocele that has superimposed lipomas, fibromuscular capsules, and intact skin (Fig. 19-7, *C*).[33] Lipomyelomeningoceles account for 20% of skin-covered lumbosacral masses and up to half of occult spinal dysraphisms.[31] There is a moderate female predominance.

Most patients with lipomyelomeningocele present before 6 months of age but others may remain undetected into adulthood.[33] Neurogenic bladder, sensory abnormalities, and orthopedic deformities are common presenting symptoms. A large subcutaneous semifluctuant lumbosacral mass is often present on physical examination.

Imaging findings on plain film radiographs include focal spina bifida and widened spinal canal. Segmentation anomalies are common. MR scans disclose a low-lying spinal cord that is continuous dorsally with the neural placode. The nerve roots arise from the placode (not the lipoma) and cross the subarachnoid space to exit the spinal canal.[33] The lipoma itself lies outside the dura and is contiguous with subcutaneous fat (Fig. 19-13).[31,37] Syringohydromyelia is present in 25% of cases.[40]

Lipomyelomeningocele, is *not* associated with Chiari II malformation but has been reported with a Chiari I malformation.[33,40a]

Spinal Lipomas

Three types
Lipomyelomeningocele (84%)
Filum terminale fibrolipoma (12%)
Intradural (subpial) lipoma (4%)

Incidence
Most common lesion with all occult spinal dysraphic disorders; most common cause of tethered cord

Key points
Lipomyelomeningocele is *not* part of the Chiari II malformation; myelomeningocele is
Filum lipomas often incidental, asymptomatic
Intradural lipoma on dorsal cord surface

Filum terminale fibrolipoma. These lipomas may result from faulty retrogressive differentiation.[30] Asymptomatic filum fibrolipomas without tethered spinal cord have been reported in 1% to 6% of random autopsies and are noted incidentally on 0.24% to 5% of lumbosacral MR scans.[41,42] Small lipomas typically occur within the filum itself, whereas larger lipomas are usually found at the lower dorsal dural attachment.[43] Filum fibrolipomas are seen as thin, linear high signal areas on T1-weighted MR scans. The conus medullaris ends at the normal level, i.e., at or above the L1-L2 interspace (Fig. 19-14).

Intradural lipomas. Intradural lipomas are intradural, subpial, juxtamedullary lesions (*see* Fig. 19-7, *D*).[30] The spinal cord is open posteriorly, and the lipoma is situated between the unapposed lips of the placode.[30]

Most lipomas are located in the cervical and thoracic spine. The dorsal cord is the most common site.[30] T1-weighted MR scans show a high signal mass interposed between the central canal of the spinal cord and pia (Fig. 19-15).[30]

Anomalies of Abnormal Canalization and Retrogressive Differentiation

The distal embryonic neural tube normally elongates through the process of canalization and retrogressive differentiation, ultimately forming the conus medullaris, ventriculus terminalis, and the filum terminale.[44] Failure to regress normally results in a spectrum of lesions that includes tethered spinal cord, tight filum terminale syndromes, and caudal spinal anomalies.[30]

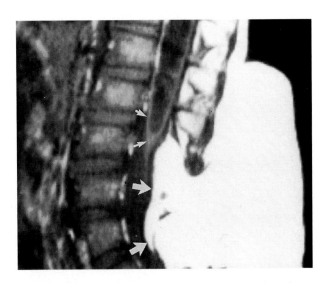

Fig. 19-13. Lipomyelomeningocele (*large arrows*) is shown on this sagittal T1-weighted MR scan. Note spinal cord with hydrosyringomyelia (*small arrows*) tethered into the lipoma (*large arrows*). The lipoma extends posteriorly through a widely dysraphic spine, where it is continuous with the subcutaneous fat. (Courtesy D. Baleriaux; reprinted from *Neuroradiol* 35:375-377, 1993.)

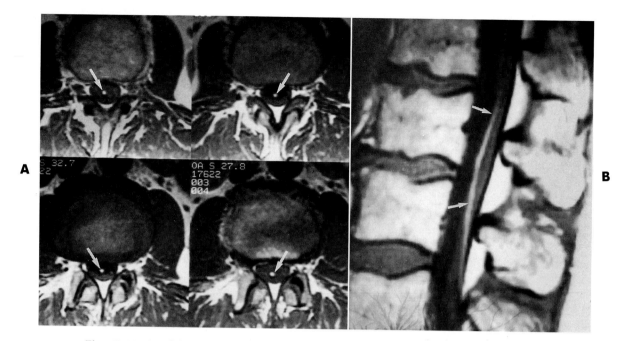

Fig. 19-14. Axial **(A)** and sagittal **(B)** T1-weighted scans in a 52-year-old man with low back pain and no neurologic abnormalities show a "fatty filum" *(arrows)*. The spinal cord is not tethered, and the conus medullaris ended at the normal level. This is probably an incidental finding.

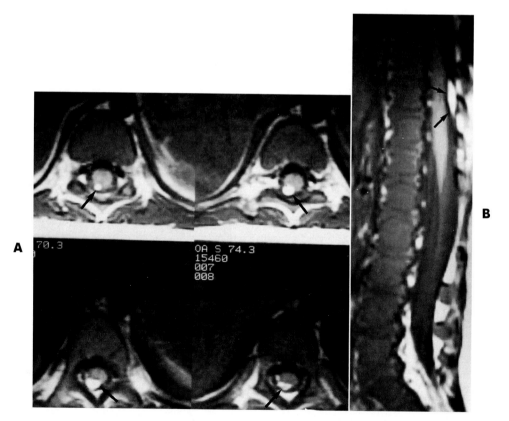

Fig. 19-15. Intradural lipoma in a 2-year-old child with a prominent fatty soft tissue mass at the iliac crest. Axial **(A)** and sagittal **(B)** T1-weighted MR scans show a high signal mass *(arrows)* in the dorsolateral distal thoracic cord. Note conus medullaris terminates at the normal level. Also note low signal in vertebral body marrow, normal at this age because of active hematopoiesis.

Tethered spinal cord and thick filum terminale syndrome

Etiology and pathology. Failure of terminal cord involution or normal nerve fiber lengthening may cause the so-called tight filum terminale syndrome.[33] This syndrome is a complex of neurologic and orthopedic deformities associated with a short, thick filum terminale and low-lying conus medullaris (*see* box, p. 808).[33]

Incidence, age, and gender. Tethered cord is a common feature of many, if not most, spinal malformations, and a thickened filum terminale is usually associated with clinical tethered spinal cord syndrome.[41,45] Reported causes of spinal cord tethering are spinal lipoma (72%), tight filum terminale (12%), diastematomyelia (8%), and myelomeningocele (8%).[44]

Tethered spinal cord and tight filum terminale syndrome can be seen at any age[44]; symptom onset typically begins between 3 and 35 years of age. There is no gender predilection.[33]

Clinical presentation. Symptoms of tethered cord and tight filum terminale vary. Pain, dysesthesias, neurogenic bladder, and spasticity are common.[44] Congenital or developmental kyphoscoliosis is seen in 25%.[31]

Imaging. Imaging findings in tethered cord and tight filum syndromes vary. Plain films may show a dysraphic spine (Fig. 19-16, *A*). Myelography typically shows a low-lying conus without or with a lipoma (Fig. 19-16, *B*). The exiting nerve roots have a

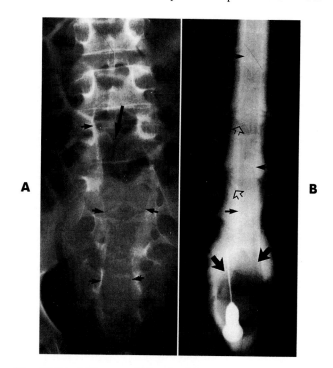

Fig. 19-16. A 12-year-old boy had repeated urinary tract infections and uremia. No cutaneous stigmata were present. AP plain film radiograph **(A)** and myelogram **(B)** show classic findings in tethered cord syndrome. **A,** Plain film shows the entire distal lumbosacral spine is widely dysraphic *(small arrows).* Spina bifida *(large arrow)* is present above the enlarged canal. **B,** Myelogram shows the thinned, elongated spinal cord *(small arrows)* is tethered inferiorly into a prominent mass *(large arrows).* The nerve roots *(open arrows)* are tautly stretched and course superolaterally instead of inferolaterally.

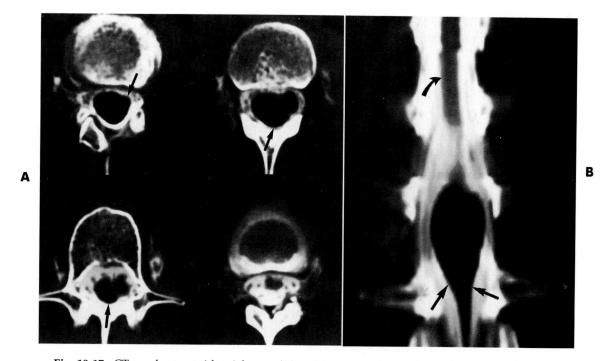

Fig. 19-17. CT-myelogram with axial scans **(A)** and reformatted coronal scan **(B)** shows a stretched spinal cord *(curved arrow)* tethered into a large lipoma *(straight arrows).* (Courtesy R. Jahnke.)

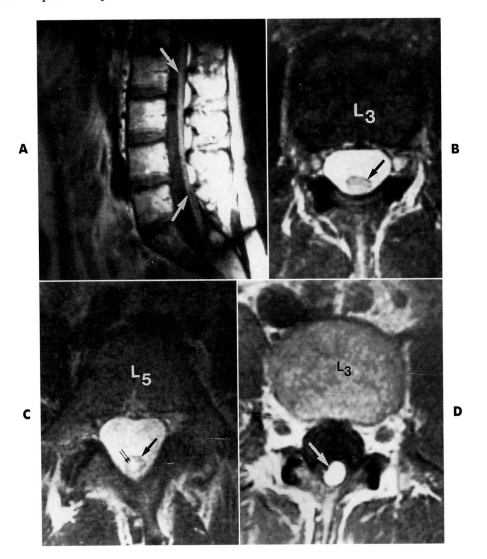

Fig. 19-18. Two cases of tethered spinal cord. Sagittal T1- **(A)** and axial T2-weighted **(B and C)** MR scans show tethered spinal cord *(arrows)*. Note the spinal cord at L2-L3. Normally, only roots of the cauda equina would be present at this level (compare with Fig. 19-3, *F*). The small intramedullary high signal focus at the distal cord **(C,** *double arrows)* represents a small syrinx or possibly a ventriculis terminalis. Axial T1-weighted scan **(D)** in another case shows a tethered spinal cord with lipoma, seen here as a high signal mass *(arrow)*.

Tethered Cord, Thick Filum Syndromes

Terminal embryonic neural tube fails to involute

Back pain, scoliosis common; may have bowel, bladder incontinence

Occult tether may have symptom onset delayed into adulthood

Often associated with other abnormalities (e.g., lipoma, diastematomyelia, myelomeningocele)

Imaging key: axial views because sagittal view can be misleading (lumbar nerve roots usually layer dorsally, can mimic tethered cord)

---

lateral or even "uphill" course in severe cases (Fig. 19-16, *B*). CT-myelography shows a low-lying conus medullaris (below L2), a thickened filum terminale that is greater than 1.5 mm in diameter, and, sometimes, fibrous adhesion bands. The tethered cord may terminate in a lipoma (Fig. 19-17).

On sagittal MR scans, the conus medullaris often appears elongated with no sharp transition between conus and filum. Because roots of the cauda equina are normally layered posteriorly in the thecal sac (*see* Fig. 19-3, *F* and *G*), this can sometimes mimic a tethered cord if only sagittal MR scans are obtained; axial T2-weighted "MR myelograms" are diagnostic (Fig. 19-18).

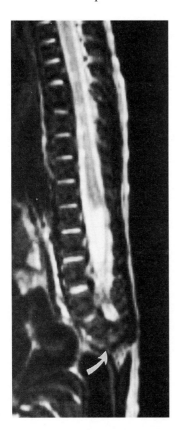

Fig. 19-19. Sagittal T2-weighted MR scan in a newborn with a mild caudal regression syndrome shows the sacrum *(arrow)* ends below S1.

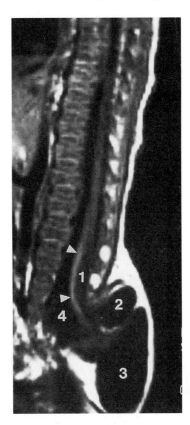

Fig. 19-20. Sagittal T1-weighted MR scan in an infant with a terminal myelocystocele. *1,* Tethered spinal cord *(arrowheads)* with distal hydromyelia. *2,* Meningocele (meninges with subarachnoid space are herniated through a large dorsal defect). *3,* Large terminal cyst, the myelocystocele, bulges below the meningocele and communicates with the dilated central canal of the tethered cord. *4,* Anterior lumbosacral subarachnoid space.

Caudal Spinal Anomalies
Caudal regression syndromes
Terminal myelocystocele
Anterior sacral meningocele
Occult intrasacral meningocele
Sacrococcygeal teratoma

Caudal spinal anomalies. Caudal spinal anomalies are lesions in which malformations of the distal spine, spinal cord, and meninges are associated with hindgut, kidney, urinary bladder, and genitalia anomalies. These include the caudal regression syndromes, terminal myelocystocele, anterior sacral and occult intrasacral meningoceles, and sacrococcygeal teratomas *(see* box).[32,33]

Caudal regression syndromes. The caudal regression syndromes include varying degrees of lumbosacral agenesis combined with other anomalies such as imperforate anus, malformed genitalia, renal dysplasia or aplasia, and sirenomelia (fused lower extremities). They range from absent coccyx usually seen as an isolated incidental finding without neurologic sequelae, to sacral or lumbosacral agenesis (Fig. 19-

19).[33a] In extreme cases, the last intact vertebra is T11 or T12.[32,33]

Terminal myelocystocele. Terminal myelocystocele, also called syringocele, is a localized cystic dilatation of the distal spinal cord. Myelocystocele constitutes between 1% and 5% of skin-covered lumbosacral masses. Terminal myelocystocele consists of posterior spina bifida or partial sacral agenesis and tethered spinal cord with hydromyelia. The cord, meninges, and subarachnoid space protrude into the dorsal subcutaneous plane. The terminal portion of the tethered cord appears ballooned and flared under the subcutaneous fat and enlarged subarachnoid space (Fig. 19-20).[32]

Anterior sacral meningocele. Anterior sacral meningoceles are herniations of meninges through defects in the sacrum, coccyx, or adjacent disc spaces to form a CSF-filled hernia sac within the pelvis.[32] Anterior sacral meningoceles may occur as an isolated defect, as part of the caudal regression syndromes, or as a manifestation of generalized mesen-

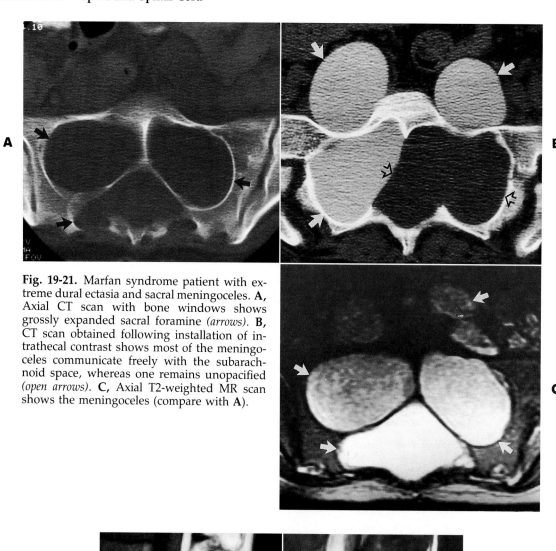

Fig. 19-21. Marfan syndrome patient with extreme dural ectasia and sacral meningoceles. **A,** Axial CT scan with bone windows shows grossly expanded sacral foramine *(arrows).* **B,** CT scan obtained following installation of intrathecal contrast shows most of the meningoceles communicate freely with the subarachnoid space, whereas one remains unopacified *(open arrows).* **C,** Axial T2-weighted MR scan shows the meningoceles (compare with **A**).

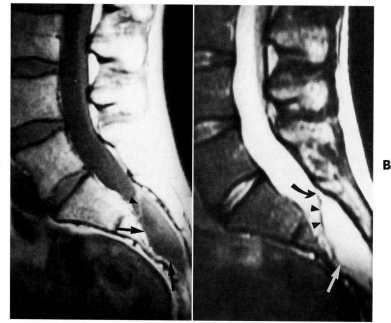

Fig. 19-22. A 24-year-old woman with low back pain had this MR scan. Sagittal T1- **(A)** and T2-weighted **(B)** scans show an intraosseous sacral meningocele *(straight arrows).* Note the dura *(arrowheads)* interposed between the subarachnoid space and the meningocele. A small potential communication site is indicated (**B,** *curved arrow*). Note that the meningocele contents are slightly hyperintense compared to CSF.

Split Notochord Syndromes
Dorsal enteric fistula (most severe)
Dorsal enteric sinus
Dorsal enteric diverticulae
Diastematomyelia
Spinal enterogenous (neurenteric) cyst

Diastematomyelia
Split spinal cord (*not* duplicated cord)
Hemicords in separate (50%) or common (50%) dural tube
Usually between T9-S1 (85%)
Spine nearly always abnormal
Osseous spur in only 50%
Associated with Chiari II malformation, tethered spinal cord, hydromyelia of one or both hemicords

chymal dysplasia such as neurofibromatosis type 1 (NF-1) or Marfan syndrome (Fig. 19-21).[32,46] Widened sacral foramina with smoothly scalloped margins and protruding CSF-filled sacs are present. Occasionally the sacral dura is completely absent.[46a]

Occult intrasacral meningoceles. Occult intrasacral meningoceles are mild dural developmental anomalies in which the arachnoid herniates through a dural defect, expanding and scalloping the bony sacrum.[47,48] These are seen on imaging studies as expansile smoothly marginated, well-delineated cysts that are often slightly higher in signal intensity than CSF within the thecal sac (Fig. 19-22). Symptoms are unrelated to cyst size; cysts that communicate freely with the subarachnoid space are typically asymptomatic whereas noncommunicating cysts are often symptomatic.[48a] Occult intrasacral meningoceles may occur in isolation but are also commonly associated with lipoma, hyperkeratosis, sacral pigmentation, sacrococcygeal dimples, and neurofibromatosis.[47]

Sacrococcygeal teratomas. Sacrococcygeal teratomas are developmental in origin and are the most frequently encountered presacral masses in children.[49] Pathologically, they range from mature teratomas to anaplastic carcinomas.[30] Most are mature teratomas and seen as large, well-encapsulated, heterogeneous pre- or postsacral masses.

Split Notochord Syndromes

This group of anomalies results from splitting of the notochord with a persistent connection between the gut and dorsal ectoderm.[30] The most severe form of split notochord syndrome is the rare dorsal enteric fistula. Other anomalies include diastematomyelia and enterogenous (neurenteric) cysts (*see* box, *above*).

Diastematomyelia
Etiology and pathology. Diastematomyelia is characterized pathologically by sagittal clefting of the spinal cord or filum terminale (*see* box, *above right*). Recent theories postulate that all variants of split spinal cord malformations arise from adhesions between the embryonic ecto- and endoderm. This leads to formation of an accessory neurenteric canal. An endomesenchymal tract condenses around this accessory canal, bisecting the developing notochord and causing two hemineural plates to form.[50] The

result is a split spinal cord, i.e., diastematomyelia (Fig. 19-23, *A*).

The spinal cord is typically split into two halves by a fibrous, bony, or osteocartilagenous septum.[33,37] The cleft typically extends completely through the cord, although partial clefting occasionally occurs. The cord is usually split locally, with a single cord above and below the cleft. The two hemicords are typically somewhat asymmetric. Each hemicord contains a central canal and one set of dorsal and ventral horns and nerve roots.

In 50% of all cases, the two hemicords share a single dural tube; in the remaining half, the hemicords are enclosed in separate dural sacs (Fig. 19-23, *B*).[33] Some authors have proposed a new classification, dividing so-called double spinal cord malformations into Type I and Type II split cord malformations (SCMs). Type I SCMs consist of two hemicords, each contained within its own dural tube and separated by a dura-sheathed rigid osseocartilaginous median septum. A Type II SCM consists of two hemicords contained in a single dural tube with the hemicords separated by a nonrigid fibrous median septum.[50]

Incidence, age, and gender. Diastematomyelia is an uncommon form of occult spinal dysraphism. There is a distinct female predominance.[33] Age at symptom onset varies.

Clinical presentation and natural history. Cutaneous stigmata overlie the spine in 50% to 75% of patients with diastematomyelia. Hair patches, nevi, and lipomas are common, whereas skin dimples and dermal sinuses are less frequently observed.[33] Orthopedic abnormalities such as clubfoot occur in nearly half of all patients, and nonspecific neurologic symptoms are present in 85% to 90% of children with diastematomyelia.[33]

Pain is the predominant symptom in adults with split cord malformations. Symptom onset may be insidious or abrupt, following a fall on the buttocks or low back. Leg weakness and neurogenic bladder are common.[51]

Location. The cleft is located between T9 and S1 in 85% of cases.[52] The lumbar spine is the site of nearly half of these anomalies, a thoracic location is

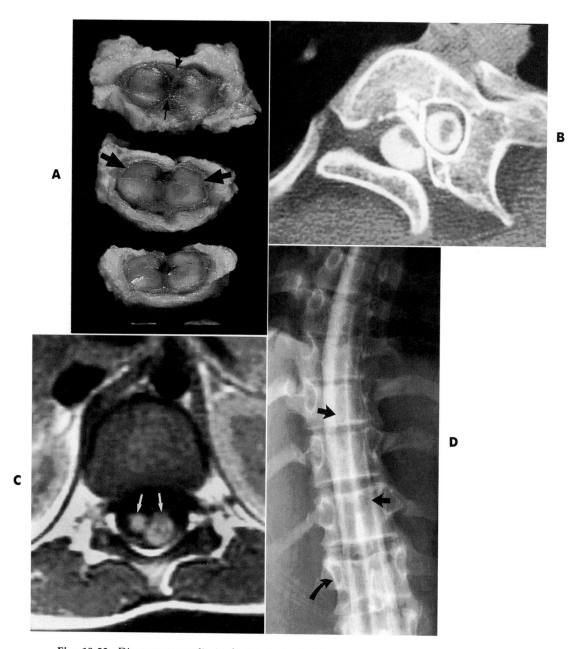

Fig. 19-23. Diastematomyelia is depicted. **A,** Axial gross autopsy specimen shows the two hemicords *(large arrows)* separated by a fibrous septum *(small arrows).* **B,** Axial CT scan with intrathecal contrast shows a grossly abnormal vertebral body with an osseous spur that traverses the entire canal. Two hemicords are clearly seen, each contained within its own dural tube. **C,** Axial T1-weighted MR scan in another case shows two unequal hemicords *(arrows).* **D,** Water-soluble myelogram, AP view, shows two equal hemicords *(straight arrows).* Note scoliosis and butterfly vertebral body *(curved arrow).* (**A,** Courtesy E. Ross.)

seen in 20%, and combined thoracolumbar lesions occur in 15% to 20%.[52] A cervical or basicranial diastematomyelia is very rare.[53] The conus medullaris lies below L2 in three quarters of all cases.

Imaging findings. Plain films and NECT scans show a grossly abnormal osseous spine in nearly all cases of diastematomyelia (Fig. 19-23, *B*) (see subsequent discussion). The hemicords and subarachnoid spaces are well delineated at myelography (Fig. 19-23, *D*), CT-myelography, or on MR scans (Fig. 19-23, *C*).

Associated anomalies. Osseous anomalies are typically striking. At least 85% of patients with diastematomyelia have vertebral body anomalies, including hemivertebrae, block or butterfly vertebrae, and narrow intervertebral disk spaces. Intersegmental laminar fusion with spina bifida is present in 60% of cases.[52] An osseous spur is seen in only half of patients with diastematomyelia. The spur may traverse part or all of the canal and be on or off the midline. The spinal canal itself is abnormally wide with increased interpediculate distance.[33]

Soft tissue anomalies include low-lying or tethered conus with thickened filum terminale (40%) and hydromyelia of one or both hemicords.[31] Between 15% and 20% of patients with Chiari II malformation have diastematomyelia.

Enterogenous cyst
Etiology and pathology. Enterogenous cysts probably result from failure of notochord and foregut separation during formation of the alimentary canal (Figs. 19-24 and 19-25).[54,55]

Grossly, enterogenous cysts are well-delineated, thin-walled, fluid-containing masses (Fig. 19-26, *A*) (*see* box). Their walls are composed of fibrous connective tissue lined by a single layer of columnar or cuboidal epithelial cells. Mucin-secreting goblet cells are often present.[53]

Incidence, age, and gender. Most enterogenous cysts are seen in patients under 40 years of age; peak incidence is during the first or second decade. There is a slight male predominance.[53,54]

Location. The most common location is the tho-

Enterogenous Cyst
Fluid-containing cyst lined by epithelial, goblet cells
Thoracic spine most common site; most cysts anterior to spinal cord
Bony anomalies seen in <50%
Imaging findings: lobulated intradural extramedullary mass; MR variable but usually slightly hyperintense to CSF

Normal development

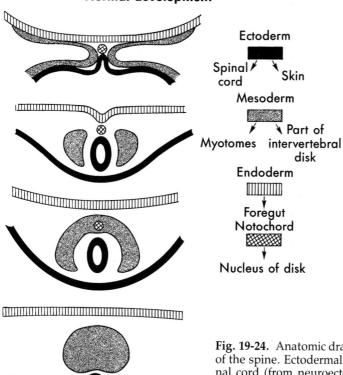

Fig. 19-24. Anatomic drawings depict normal development of the spine. Ectodermal derivatives normally form the spinal cord (from neuroectoderm) and skin (from cutaneous ectoderm). Endodermal derivatives form the foregut and notochord, the precursor of the nucleus pulposus.

Abnormal development

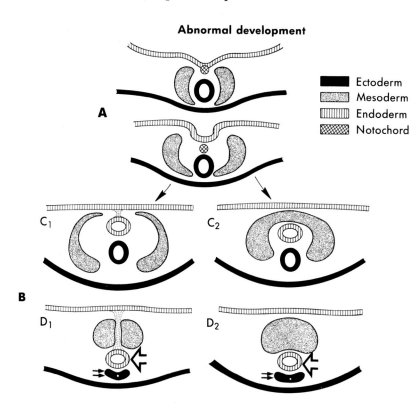

■	Ectoderm
▨	Mesoderm
▥	Endoderm
▩	Notochord

Fig. 19-25. Anatomic drawing depicts possible origin of enterogenous cysts. **A** and **B,** *C1, D1,* Incomplete separation of the notochord and foregut may result in interposition of an endodermal rest, forming a cyst *(open arrow),* which prevents fusion of the vertebral bodies. This results in a split vertebral body with persisting communication between the foregut and the cyst. The spinal cord is compressed *(double arrows).* **A** and **B,** *C2, D2,* An enterogenous cyst *(open arrow)* is shown as an isolated intradural inclusion with subsequent normal vertebral body development.

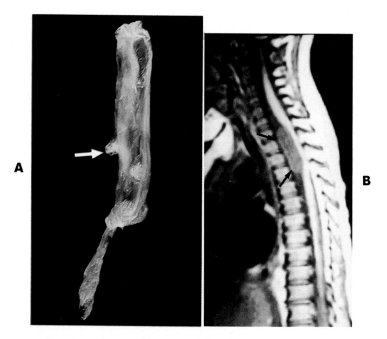

Fig. 19-26. A, Gross pathology of an enterogenous cyst is shown. The thin-walled cyst was filled with clear fluid. The arrow indicates the site of a communication that extended anteriorly through a cleft vertebral body. **B,** Sagittal T1-weighted scan in another case shows a typical enterogenous cyst *(arrows),* seen here as a well-delineated lobulated mass that is interposed between the spinal cord and a normal-appearing spine. The cyst is slightly hyperintense to CSF. (**A,** From archives of the Armed Forces Institute of Pathology.)

racic spine (42%), followed by cervical spine (32%), posterior fossa (13%), and craniovertebral junction (10%). The lumbar spine is a rare site.[53,55] Between 85% and 90% are midline; most are located ventral to the spinal cord or brainstem.[53]

Clinical presentation and natural history. Clinical presentation varies. Pain and myelopathic symptoms are common; septic or chemical meningitis may occur.[33]

Imaging. Myelography typically discloses a sharply marginated intradural extramedullary mass anterior to the spinal cord. CT or CT-myelography shows a well-delineated low density mass. Enterogenous cysts are either iso- or slightly hyperintense compared to CSF on T1-weighted MR scans and slightly hyperintense on proton density and T2-weighted sequences (Fig. 19-26, *B*).[53,54]

Associated anomalies. Vertebral anomalies or associated cleft are seen in 43% of cases.[53]

Differential diagnosis. The differential diagnosis

of enterogenous cyst encompasses a spectrum of intraspinal cystic masses that includes arachnoid cyst (usually dorsal to cord, epidermoid cyst, and inflammatory cyst.

Miscellaneous Malformations

Miscellaneous spine and spinal cord malformations that are briefly reviewed here include the Chiari malformations, hydromyelia and syringomyelia, and spinal manifestations of the phakomatoses (neurocutaneous syndromes).

Chiari malformations. The Chiari malformations are discussed in detail in Chapter 2. Here, we focus on the spinal manifestations of these anomalies.

Chiari I. The Chiari I malformation (ACM I) consists of downward elongation of peglike cerebellar tonsils through the foramen magnum into the posterolateral cervical subarachnoid space behind the upper cervical spinal cord (Figs. 19-27, *A* and *B*).

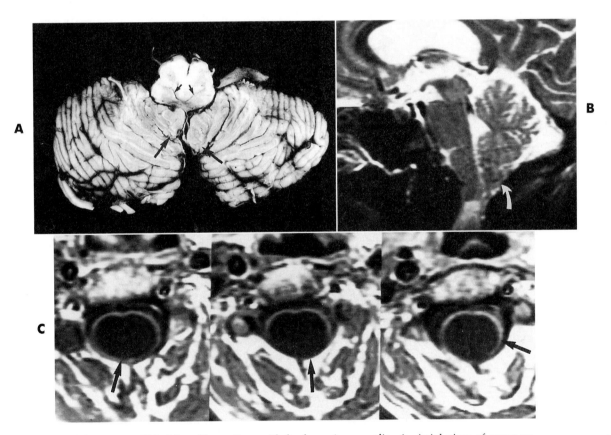

Fig. 19-27. Chiari I malformation with hydrosyringomyelia. **A,** Axial view of gross autopsy specimen shows low-lying tonsils *(large arrows)* and collapsed syrinx *(small arrows)* at the cervicomedullary junction. **B,** Sagittal T1-weighted scan through the craniovertebral junction shows the low-lying, peg-shaped cerebellar tonsil *(arrow).* **C,** Axial T1-weighted scans through the midcervical spine show a large central CSF cavity that grossly expands the cord *(arrows).* Thoracic study (not shown) demonstrated the hydrosyringomyelic cavity extended to the conus medullaris. (**A,** From Okazaki H, Scheithauer B: *Slide Atlas of Neuropathology,* Gower Medical Publishing. **B** and **C,** Courtesy M. Fruin.)

Chiari I malformation is *not* associated with open spina bifida or myelomeningocele. Other than hydrocephalus, ACM I is also *not* associated with brain malformations but it *is* associated with basilar impression (25% to 50%), hydromyelia (25% to 60%) (Fig. 19-27, *B*), and spinal anomalies such as atlantooccipital fusion (10%), partial fusion of C2 and C3 (18%), cervical spina bifida occulta (5%), widened spinal canal (18%, usually from syringohydromyelia), and Klippel-Feil syndrome (5%).[56,57]

The etiology of Chiari I malformations is unclear. Congenital Chiari I malformations may or may not be related to tissue compression caused by disproportion between neural and bony structures at the foramen magnum.[58] So-called acquired Chiari I malformations, seen as isolated tonsillar displacement into the upper cervical canal, have been reported following lumboperitoneal shunting or repeated lumbar punctures.[59,60]

Chiari II. Spinal abnormalities in the Chiari II malformation (ACM II) consist of inferior herniation of the medulla with elongated fourth ventricle and vermis displaced inferiorly into the cervical (occasionally the thoracic) canal behind the cervical spinal cord.[56]

Myelomeningocele is seen in virtually 100% of patients with ACM II (*see* Fig. 2-14). Other commonly observed spinal anomalies include incomplete C1 ring (70%), hydromyelia (50%), syringomyelia (20%), and, occasionally, diastematomyelia.[33,56]

Hydromyelia and syringomyelia

Etiology and pathology. Hydro- and syringomyelia can be congenital or acquired (e.g., posttraumatic syrinx). The pathogenesis of congenital hydromyelia is debatable. The dysraphic theory suggests that a neural tube closure defect is responsible, whereas the hydrodynamic theory maintains that disturbed CSF outflow from the fourth ventricle is responsible. Syringomyelia then supervenes as the dilated ependymal canal ruptures into the spinal cord parenchyma.[61]

Pathologically, hydromyelia is simply ependymal-lined distention of the central canal, whereas syringomyelia is defined as CSF dissection through the ependymal lining to form a paracentral cavity.[62] In practice, these two conditions often coexist and intercommunicate. Because even the histologic distinction between hydro- and syringomyelia is sometimes difficult and because their appearances on imaging studies are usually indistinguishable, these entities are often grouped under the term *hydrosyringomyelia.*[63] This term describes any pathological cavity that occupies the substance of the spinal cord, whether or not it is continuous with the central canal.[63]

Hydrosyringomyelia can be communicating or noncommunicating. Between 15% and 20% of syrinxes are anatomically continuous with the fourth ventricle via the obex. These so-called communicating syrinxes are typically associated with hydrocephalus and occur with subarachnoid hemorrhage, meningitis, and leptomeningeal carcinomatosis.[62]

Nearly 80% of syrinxes are noncommunicating, i.e., they are separated from the fourth ventricle by a syrinx-free segment of spinal cord.[62] Noncommunicating syrinxes occur with both Chiari I and Chiari II malformations, as well as with acquired disorders such as spinal cord trauma, intramedullary tumors, and extramedullary compressive lesions.[62] Most syrinxes that occur with Chiari II malformations are associated with hydrocephalus; those seen with Chiari I malformation typically are not.[62]

Location. Hydrosyringomyelia can occur at any location. The cervical cord is the most common overall site.[63] Syrinxes associated with Chiari I malformation are most often cervical or cervicothoracic; neoplastic syrinxes occur mostly in the cervical spinal cord (*see* Chapter 21). Congenital benign thoracic syrinxes occur but are uncommon. Posttraumatic syrinxes occur at all levels.[63,64]

Clinical presentation and natural history. Classic clinical features include sensory (pain and temperature) disturbances, muscular atrophy or weakness, diminished deep tendon reflexes of the upper extremities, and spastic paraparesis.[64] These findings are encountered relatively infrequently. Approximately 80% of patients complain of stiffness in the legs and weakness in the legs or hands; pain is a presenting complaint in less than 50%.[62] Scoliosis is common, particularly in patients with Chiari malformations.[64] Many, although by no means all, untreated syrinxes gradually enlarge.

Imaging findings. The classic MR imaging finding in syringohydromyelia is an enlarged cord with a central or slightly eccentric fluid-filled cavity that parallels CSF in signal intensity (Fig. 19-27, *C*).[63] A sharp interface between the normal cord and syrinx is typical.[61] Metameric haustrations, or a "beaded" shape, are typical of Chiari-associated hydromyelia.[61] Occasionally, frank septations are present. Increased signal intensity around the syrinx on T2WI probably represents cord gliosis, edema, or myelomalacia.[63] Benign syrinxes do not enhance following contrast administration.[65]

Neurocutaneous syndromes. Both type 1 and type 2 neurofibromatosis (NF-1 and NF-2) have spine and cord manifestations (*see* Chapter 5).

Neurofibromatosis type 1. The diffuse osseous and dural dysplasia that is characteristic of NF-1 results in numerous spine and cord manifestations. Scoliosis, wide spinal canal with patulous dural sac, and meningoceles are characteristic (Fig. 19-28; *see* Fig. 5-13). Neurofibromas of exiting roots are common (*see* Fig. 5-14). Malignant nerve sheath tumors (malignant

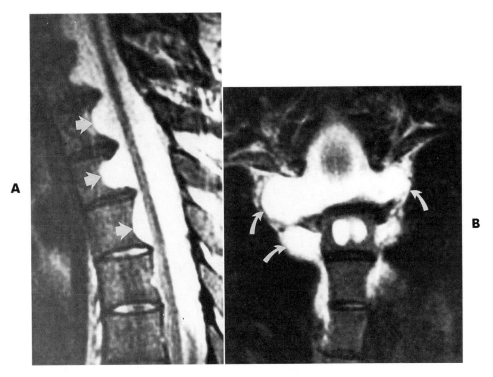

Fig. 19-28. Sagittal **(A)** and coronal **(B)** T2-weighted MR scans in a patient with neurofibromatosis type 1 (NF-1) and gross dural ectasia show multilevel posterior vertebral scalloping *(straight arrows)* and lateral thoracic meningoceles *(curved arrows).*

neurofibroma, neurofibrosarcoma) occur in 2% to 5% of cases.[66] An increased incidence of non-CNS tumors such as leukemia and pheochromocytoma also occurs in patients with neurofibromatosis.[31]

Spinal cord lesions are much less frequent in NF-1 compared to NF-2. Intramedullary hyperintensities on T2WI may represent the same type of glial hamartomatous proliferations that are seen in the brain (*see* Fig. 5-15). Spinal cord neoplasms are rare; when they occur they are typically low-grade astrocytomas.

Neurofibromatosis type 2. NF-2 is characterized by multiple schwannomas and meningiomas. Spinal nerve schwannomas occur in 20% of cases and are approximately equally divided between cervical, thoracic, and lumbar roots (*see* Fig. 5-17, *D*). Approximately 70% are intradural extramedullary lesions, 15% are completely extradural, and 15% are both intra- and extradural (dumbbell schwannomas). Multiple lesions are common (*see* Figs. 5-22 and 5-23). Schwannomas cannot reliably be distinguished from neurofibromas on the basis of imaging findings alone.[66]

Other neoplasms seen in NF-2 patients include spinal, as well as multiple intracranial, meningiomas (*see* Figs. 5-18, *G*; and 5-20, *E*). Spinal cord neoplasms are also common. Ependymoma is the most frequent tumor (*see* Figs. 5-17, *E*; 5-20, *D* and *F*; and 5-22, *B*). It is unclear whether patients with NF-2 develop cord astrocytomas.

Von Hippel-Lindau syndrome. Von Hippel-Lindau syndrome (VHL) is an autosomal dominant, multisystem disorder with renal carcinoma, pheochromocytoma, and cysts of the pancreas, kidney, and epididymis. Hemangioblastomas of the cerebellum, brainstem, and spinal cord, as well as retinal angiomatosis, are typical (*see* Fig. 5-37). Multiple CNS hemangioblastomas are considered diagnostic of VHL.[67] Between 10% and 30% of spinal cord hemangioblastomas occur in patients with VHL.[68]

REFERENCES

1. Dorwart RH, Sauerland EK, Haughton VM et al: Normal lumbosacral spine. In Newton TH, Pitts DG, editors: *Computed Tomography of the Spine and Spinal Cord,* pp. 93-113, San Anselmo, Clavadel Press, 1983.
2. Sze G, Bravo S, Baierl P, Shimkin PM: Developing spinal column: gadolinium-enhanced MR imaging, *Radiol* 180:497-502, 1991.
3. Zawin JK, Jaramillo D: Conversion of bone marrow in the humerus, sternum, and clavicle: changes with age on MR images, *Radiol* 188:159-164, 1993.
4. Hajek PC, Baker LL, Goolar JE et al: Focal fat deposition in axial bone marrow: MR characteristics, *Radiol* 162:245-249, 1987.
5. Yu S, Haughton VM, Lynch KL et al: Fibrous structure in the intervertebral disk: correlation of MR appearance with anatomic sections, *AJNR* 10:1105-1110, 1989.
6. Tournade A, Patay Z, Krupa A et al: A comparative study of the anatomical, radiological, and therapeutic features of the lumbar facet joints, *Neuroradiol* 34:297-261, 1992.
7. Xu GL, Haughton VM, Carrera GF: Lumbar facet joint capsule: appearance at MR imaging and CT, *Radiol* 177:415-420, 1990.

8. Johnson DW, Farnum GN, Latchaw RE, Erba SM: MR imaging of the pars interarticularis, *AJNR* 9:1215-1220, 1988.

9. Grenier N, Greselle J-F, Vital J-M et al: Normal and disrupted lumbar longitudinal ligaments, *Radiol* 171:197-205, 1989.

10. Ho PSP, Yu S, Sether LA et al: Ligamentum flavum: appearance on sagittal and coronal MR images, *Radiol* 168:469-472, 1988.

11. Nowicki BH, Haughton VM: Neural foraminal ligaments of the lumbar spine: appearance at CT and MR imaging, *Radiol* 183:257-264, 1992.

12. Krudy AG: MR myelography using heavily T2-weighted fast spin-echo pulse sequences with fat presaturation, *AJR* 159:1315-1320, 1992.

13. Wall EJ, Cohen MS, Massie JB et al: Cauda equina anatomy I: intrathecal nerve root organization, *Spine* 15:1244-1247, 1990.

14. Cohen MS, Wall EG, Brown RA et al: Cauda equina anatomy II: extrathecal nerve roots and dorsal root ganglia, *Spine* 15:1248-1251, 1990.

15. Kostelic JK, Haughton VM, Sether LA: Lumbar spinal nerves in the neural foramen: MR appearance, *Radiol* 178:837-839, 1991.

16. Kostelic JK, Haughton VM, Sether L: Proximal lumbar spinal nerves in axial MR imaging, CT, and anatomic sections, *Radiol* 183:239-241, 1992.

17. Gierada DS, Erickson SJ, Haughton VM et al: MR imaging of the sacral plexus: normal findings, *AJR* 160:1059-1065, 1993.

18. LaMasters DL, deGroot J, Haughton VM, Williams AL: Normal thoracic spine. In Newton TH, Potts DG, editors: *Computed Tomography of the Spine and Spinal Cord*, pp. 79-91, San Anselmo, Clavadel Press, 1983.

19. El-Khoury GY, Whitten CG: Trauma to the upper thoracic spine: anatomy, biomechanics, and unique imaging features, *AJR* 160:95-102, 1993.

20. LaMasters DL, deGroot J, Williams AL, Haughton VM: Normal craniocervical junction. In Newton TH, Potts, DG, editors: *Computed Tomography of the Spine and Spinal Cord*, pp. 31-52, San Anselmo, Clavadel Press, 1983.

21. LaMasters DL, deGroot J, Williams AL, Haughton VM: Normal cervical spine. In Newton TH, Potts DG, editors, *Computed Tomography of the Spine and Spinal Cord*, pp. 53-78, 1983.

22. Daniels DL, Hyde JS, Kneeland JB et al: The cervical nerve and foramina: local coil MR imaging, *AJNR* 7:129-133, 1986.

23. Flannigan BD, Lufkin RB, McGlade C et al: MR imaging of the cervical spine: neurovascular anatomy, *AJNR* 8:27-32, 1987.

24. Gelber ND, Ragland RL, Knorr JR: Gd-DTPA enhanced MRI of cervical anterior epidural venous plexus, *J Comp Asst Tomogr* 16:760-763, 1992.

25. Haughton VM: Unenhanced and enhanced MRI of the spine, *MRI Decisions*, pp. 2-9, March/April, 1992.

26. DiPietro MA: The conus medullaris: normal US findings throughout childhood, *Radiol* 188:149-153, 1993.

27. Solsberg MD, Lemaire C, Resch L, Potts DG: High-resolution MR imaging of the cadaveric human spinal cord: normal anatomy, *AJNR* 11:3-77, 1990.

28. Beuls E, Gelan J, Vandersteen M et al: Microanatomy of the excised human spinal cord and the corticomedullary junction examined with high-resolution MR imaging at 9.4 Tesla, *AJNR* 14:699-404, 1993.

29. Maillot C: Functional anatomy of the cord, *Riv di Neuroradiol* 5(suppl 2):11-16, 1992.

30. Barkovich AJ, Naidich TP: Congenital anomalies of the spine. In Barkovich AJ: *Pediatric Neuroimaging*, pp. 227-271, New York, Raven Press, 1990.

31. Naidich TP: The pediatric spine and cord: developmental and congenital abnormalities, *Categorical Course on Spine and Cord Imaging*, pp. 1-15, American Society of Neuroradiology, 1988.

32. Naidich TP, Rayband C: Congenital anomalies of the spine and spinal cord, *Rev di Neuroradiol* 5(suppl 2):113-130, 1992.

33. Naidich TP, McLone DG, Harwood-Nash DC: Spinal dysraphisms. In Newton TH, Potts DG, editors: *Computed Tomography of the Spine and Spinal Cord*, pp. 299-353, San Anselmo, Clavadel Press, 1983.

33a. Pang D: Sacral agenesis and caudal spinal cord malformations, *Neurosurg* 32:755-779, 1993.

34. Filly RA, Callen PW, Goldstein RB: α-Fetoprotein screening programs: what every obstetric sonologist should know, *Radiol* 188:1-9, 1993.

35. Robbin M, Filly RA, Fell S et al: Elevated levels of amniotic fluid α-Fetoprotein: sonographic evaluation, *Radiol* 188:165-169, 1993.

36. Westcott MR, Dynes MK, Remer EM et al: Congenital and acquired orthopedic abnormalities in patients with myelomeningocele, *RadioGraphics* 12:1155-1173, 1992.

37. Korsvik HE, Keller MS: Sonography of occult dysraphism in neonates and infants with MR imaging correlation, *RadioGraphics* 12:297-306, 1992.

38. Barkovich AJ, Edwards M SB, Cogen PH: MR evaluation of spinal dermal sinus tracts in children, *AJNR* 12:123-129, 1991.

39. Wright RL: Congenital dermal sinuses, *Prop Neurol Surg* 4:175-191, 1971.

40. Brophy JD, Sutton LN, Zimmerman RA et al: Magnetic resonance imaging of lipomyelomeningocele and tethered cord, *Neurosurg* 25:336-340, 1989.

40a. Grijalvo CA, Bank WO, Balériaux D et al: Lipomyeloschisis associated with thoracic syringomyelia and Chiari I malformation, *Neuroradiol* 35:375-377, 1993.

41. Uchino A, Mori T, Ohno M: Thickened fatty filum terminale: MR imaging, *Neuroradiol* 33:331-333, 1991.

42. Okumra R, Minami S, Asato R, Konishi J: Fatty filum terminale: assessment with MR imaging, *J Comp Asst Tomogr* 14:571-573, 1990.

43. Moufarrij NA, Palmer JM, Hahn JF, Weinstein MA: Correlation between magnetic resonance imaging and surgical findings in the tethered spinal cord, *Neurosurg* 25:341-346, 1989.

44. Raghavan N, Barkovich AJ, Edwards M, Norman D: MR imaging in the tethered spinal cord syndrome, *AJR* 152:843-852, 1989.

45. Tortori-Donati P, Cama A, Rosa ML et al: Occult spinal dysraphism: neuroradiological study, *Neuroradiol* 31:512-522, 1990.

46. Raftopoulos C, Pierard GE, Rétif C et al: Endoscopic cure of a giant sacral meningocele associated with Marfan's syndrome: case report, *Neurosurg* 30:765-768, 1992.

46a. Smith MD: Large sacral dural defect in Marfan syndrome, *J Bone Joint Surg* 75A:1067-1070, 1993.

47. Doty JR, Thomason J, Sinods G et al: Occult intrasacral meningocele: clinical and radiographic diagnosis, *Neurosurg* 24:616-625, 1989.

48. Muras I, Cioffi FA, Punzo A, Bernini FP: The occult intrasacral meningocele, *Neuroradiol* 33(suppl):492-494, 1991.

48a. Davis SW, Levy LM, LeBihan D et al: Sacral meningeal cysts: evaluation with MR imaging, *Radiol* 187:445-448, 1993.

49. Wetzel LH, Levine E: MR imaging of sacral and presacral lesions, *AJR* 154:771-775, 1990.

50. Pang D, Dias MS, Ahab-Barmada M: Split cord malformation: Part I: A unified theory of embryogenesis for double spinal cord malformations, *Neurosurg* 31:451-480, 1992.

51. Pang D: Split cord malformation: Part II: Clinical syndrome, *Neurosurg* 31:481-500, 1992.

52. Hilal SK, Marton D, Pollack E: Diastematomyelia in children: radiographic study of 34 cases, *Radiol* 112:609-621, 1974.

53. Gao P-Y, Osborn AG, Smirniotopoulous JG et al: Intraspinal and posterior fossa enterogenous cysts: imaging and pathologic spectrum, *AJNR*, in press.

54. Brooks BS, Durall ER, El Gammal T et al: Neuroimaging features of neurenteric cysts: analysis of nine cases and review of the literature, *AJNR* 14:735-746, 1993.

55. LeDoux MS, Faye-Peterson OM, Aronin PA et al: Lumbosacral neurenteric cyst in an infant, *J Neurosurg* 78:821-825, 1993.

56. Naidich TP, McLone DG, Harwood-Nash DC: Malformations of the craniocervical junction. In Newton TH, Potts DG, editors: *Computed Tomography of the Spine and Spinal Cord*, pp. 355-366, San Anselmo, Clavadel Press, 1983.

57. Ulmer JH, Elster AD, Ginsberg LE, Williams DW III: Klippel-Feil syndrome: CT and MR of acquired and congenital abnormalities of the cervical spine and cord, *J Comp Asst Tomogr* 17:215-224, 1993.

58. Stovner LJ, Bergan U, Nilsen G, Sjaasted O: Posterior cranial fossa dimensions in the Chiari I malformation: relation to pathogenesis and clinical presentation, *J Neurosurg* 35:113-118, 1993.

59. Chumas PD, Armstrong DC, Drake JM et al: Tonsillar herniation: the rule rather than the exception after lumboperitoneal shunting in the pediatric population, *J Neurosurg* 78:568-573, 1993.

60. Sathi S, Steig PE: "Acquired" Chiari I malformation after multiple lumbar punctures: case report, *Neurosurg* 32:306-309, 1993.

61. Sze G: MR imaging of the spinal cord: current status and future advances, *AJR* 159:149-159, 1992.

62. Milhorat TH, Miller JI, Johnson WD et al: Anatomical basis of syringomyelia occurring with hindbrain lesions, *Neurosurg* 32:748-754, 1993.

63. Sherman JL, Barkovich AJ, Citrin CM: The MR appearance of syringomyelia: new observations, *AJNR* 7:985-995, 1986.

64. Isu T, Iwasaki Y, Akino M, Abe H: Hydromyelia associated with a Chiari I malformation in children and adults, *Neurosurg* 26:591-597, 1990.

65. Slasky BS, Bydder GM, Niendorf HP, Young IR: MR imaging with gadolinium-DTPA in the differentiation of tumor, syrinx, and cyst of the spinal cord, *J Comp Asst Tomogr* 11:845-850, 1987.

66. Varma DGK, Moulopoulos A, Sarat S et al: MR imaging of extracranial nerve sheath tumors, *J Comp Asst Tomogr* 16:448-453, 1992.

67. Murota T, Symon L: Surgical management of hemangioblastoma of the spinal cord: a report of 18 cases, *Neurosurg* 25:699-708, 1989.

68. Avila NA, Shawker TH, Choyke PL, Oldfield EH: Cerebellar and spinal hemangioblastomas: evaluation with intraoperative gray-scale and color doppler flow US, *Radiol* 188:143-147, 1993.

20

Nonneoplastic Disorders of the Spine and Spinal Cord

In this chapter we consider benign acquired disorders of the spine and spinal cord, beginning with infection and demyelinating diseases and concluding with degenerative diseases and trauma.

INFECTION
Spondylitis and Diskitis

Early diagnosis is crucial in the management of spine infections because delayed treatment can lead to increased morbidity and mortality.[1,2] We begin this section by focussing on pyogenic and tuberculous spondylitis and diskitis, then turn our attention to epidural abscess and meningitis. We conclude by discussing spinal cord abscesses (*see* box).

Pyogenic spondylitis. Infective spondylitis involves one or more of the extradural components of the spine. It most often affects the vertebral bodies (osteomyelitis), but the posterior elements, intervertebral disks, epidural spaces, and paraspinous soft tissues can also be affected.[3]

Etiology and pathology. A spectrum of bacterial, fungal, or parasitic organisms can cause infectious spondylitis. *Staphylococcus aureus* is the most common pyogenic organism in adults, accounting for approximately 60% of infections; *Enterobacter*, a frequent genitourinary pathogen, accounts for 30%.[4] Other common organisms include *Escherichia coli*, *Salmonella*, *Pseudomonas aeruginosa*, and *Klebsiella pneumoniae*.[3]

Routes of entry are hematogenous spread, contiguous spread, and direct inoculation of the patho-

---

Spine Infections

Spondylitis > diskitis > epidural abscess >> cord abscess

Most common cause of infectious spondylitis: *S. aureus*

Incidence rising (drug abuse, immunocompromised patients)

Usually hematogenous (arterial, not Batson's plexus)

Initial site

    Children: disk space first, then vertebrae

    Adults: subchondral vertebral body, then disk space

Imaging

    Plain films normal early in disease course

    "Hot" (hyperintense) disk on T2-weighted MR

    Disk, adjacent bone often enhance

    Soft tissue mass common; ±epidural abscess, meningitis

---

gens. Systemic bacteremia, typically from a cutaneous, urinary tract or pulmonary infection, is the most common source. Hematogenous spread typically occurs via arteries; the vertebral veins (Batson's plexus) play a comparatively limited role.[5] Contiguous spread from an adjacent soft-tissue infection (e.g., paraspinous muscle or retropharyngeal abscess) is less common. Direct contamination from open wounds, penetrating foreign bodies, diagnostic procedures, or surgery is rare.

In adults, infection begins in the subchondral portion of the vertebral body, then spreads to the disk space and further along the vertebral body in a subligamentous fashion.[5] In children, the intervertebral disk is richly vascularized and may serve as the initial site, whereas, in adults, disk infection is invariably caused by direct spread from contiguous vertebrae or soft tissues.[3,4]

Incidence, age, and gender. Infectious spondylitis is uncommon, accounting for only 5% of all cases of pyogenic osteomyelitis. Bacterial vertebral osteomyelitis typically affects adults in the 6th and 7th decades. Immunocompromised patients and drug abusers are at increased risk. There has been a major increase in reported incidence of spinal osteomyelitis in the last decade.[3,6] There is a slight male predominance.[3,4]

Location. Although pyogenic spondylitis can occur anywhere, the lumbar spine is the most common site, followed by the thoracic spine. The sacrum and cervical spine are less commonly involved.[4]

Clinical presentation and natural history. Symptoms vary widely. Pain and malaise are common. The patient may be either febrile or afebrile. The erythrocyte sedimentation rate and white blood cell count

are often mildly elevated.[4] Neurologic deficit and signs of cord compression may occur, with infection spread into the epidural space.[4]

Imaging findings. Plain film radiographs are usually normal for the first 8 to 10 days following symptom onset. Abnormalities such as disk-space narrowing and end plate erosions are often subtle and not detected until relatively late in the disease process (Fig. 20-1, *A*). Radionuclide bone scans are sensitive but nonspecific indicators of early disease.[6]

CT scans may also be normal early in the disease course. Disk-space narrowing, cortical bone loss, and paraspinous soft tissue mass can be seen but are usually present only after moderately severe changes have occurred.[6]

MR findings are characteristic. T1-weighted sequences typically show a narrowed disk space and low signal intensity in the adjacent vertebral bodies that reflects increased extracellular fluid within the marrow.[3,6] Subligamentous or epidural soft tissue masses and cortical bone erosion are common (Fig. 20-1, *B*). Postcontrast studies show enhancement of the infected disk space and osteomyelitic bone (Fig. 20-1, *B*). Paraspinous abscess, epidural extension, and associated meningeal inflammation are easily delineated on these studies (Fig. 20-2).[1,2]

T2-weighted sequences show high signal in the affected disk space and vertebral bodies. The "nuclear cleft" that is typically seen as an area of decreased signal intensity in the middle of the disk is effaced.[3]

Differential diagnosis. The differential diagnosis of pyogenic spondylitis includes granulomatous spondylitis (see subsequent discussion), intervertebral osteochondrosis, calcium pyrophosphate crystal deposition disease, and axial neuroarthropathy. In rare circumstances, metastatic disease can cause changes that are virtually identical to those of infection.[7] Occasionally, severe degenerative disk disease is accompanied by secondary spine changes that can also simulate infection.[3]

Granulomatous spondylitis and miscellaneous spondylitides

Etiology and pathology. Granulomatous reaction occurs with a spectrum of bacterial, viral, parasitic, and fungal infections, as well as some tumors, autoimmune diseases, and idiopathic disorders.[3] Granulomatous spondylitis is most commonly caused by *Mycobacterium tuberculosis* (Fig. 20-3). Other organisms that may be implicated include bacilli of the *Brucella* genus, typically *B. melitensis* (Fig. 20-4).[8]

Fungal spondylitis is uncommon but is increasing with the rising numbers of immunocompromised and debilitated patients.[3] Some fungal infections such as blastomycosis and aspergillosis are indistinguishable from tuberculous spondylitis on imaging studies; oth-

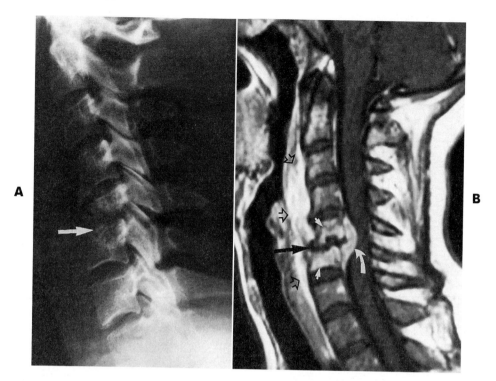

Fig. 20-1. Lateral plain film radiograph **(A)** and sagittal postcontrast T1-weighted MR scan **(B)** in a 44-year-old woman drug abuser show classic findings of vertebral osteomyelitis. The C5-C6 interspace is narrowed, and the end plates of the vertebral bodies appear irregular *(large arrow)*. The marrow enhances **(B,** *small arrows)*, consistent with osteomyelitis. Subligamentous prevertebral soft tissue mass **(B,** *open arrows)* and epidural phlegmon **(B,** *curved arrow)* are also present. Subluxation secondary to ligamentous laxity is seen.

ers such as actinomycosis, cryptococcosis, and coccidiodomycosis cause patchy vertebral body destruction or sclerosis with relative disk sparing.[3]

Parasitic spondylitis is rare. For example, only 1% of echinococcus infections involve bone; when they do, the spine is the common site.[3]

Incidence, age, and gender. Although pulmonary tuberculosis has decreased, the incidence of bone and joint tuberculosis remains unchanged.[9] Tuberculous spondylitis now accounts for 6% of new extrapulmonary tuberculosis cases.[10]

In developing countries, tuberculous spondylitis is a disease of children, whereas in North America and Europe it is most prevalent in middle-aged adults. The mean age at diagnosis is between 40 and 45 years compared with pyogenic osteomyelitis where the peak incidence is in the sixth to seventh decades.[9] Debilitation, immunosuppression, alcoholism, and drug addiction are predisposing conditions.[3] There is no gender predilection.

Location. The lower dorsal and lumbar spine are affected in nearly three quarters of all cases of tuberculous spondylitis; the cervical spine is an uncommon site.[11] Nearly 90% of cases have at least two affected vertebral bodies; 50% have three or more levels affected.[9,11] "Skip" lesions are common.[3] Para-

spinous abscesses are present in 55% to 95% of cases.[9] Occasionally, tuberculous spondylitis affects only one vertebral body, sparing the adjacent disk. Tuberculosis can affect only part of a vertebral body. The transverse processes and posterior elements are sometimes also involved.[3]

Brucellar spondylitis can be focal or diffuse. In focal disease, osteomyelitis is localized to the anterior aspect of an end plate. Lower lumbar involvement is common in brucellar spondylitis, whereas tuberculous spondylitis is most common in the lower thoracic and upper lumbar spine.[8]

Clinical presentation and natural history. Tuberculous spondylitis is typically more indolent than pyogenic osteomyelitis. Onset is often insidious, and symptom duration frequently ranges from months to years.[9] Untreated patients develop progressive vertebral collapse with anterior wedging and gibbus formation.[10]

Imaging findings. Plain film findings in tuberculous spondylitis include bone destruction in nearly all cases and associated soft tissue masses in most. Reactive sclerosis is not a feature on initial presentation in Caucasian patients but early sclerosis is seen in approximately 50% of non-Caucasian patients. Loss of disk height is present in more than three quarters of

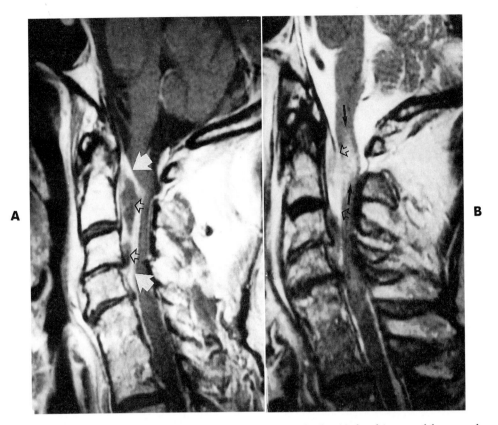

Fig. 20-2. A 65-year-old man with an infected IV site had a 10-day history of fever and chills followed by an increasing sensory deficit that proceeded to paraplegia. **A,** Postcontrast sagittal T1-weighted MR scan shows a frank epidural abscess with enhancing borders *(large arrows)* and central low density nidus *(open arrows).* **B,** Sagittal T2-weighted sequence shows the abscess *(open arrows).* Focal high signal *(solid arrows)* at the cervicomedullary junction is probably secondary myelitis. Loculated pus was removed at surgery.

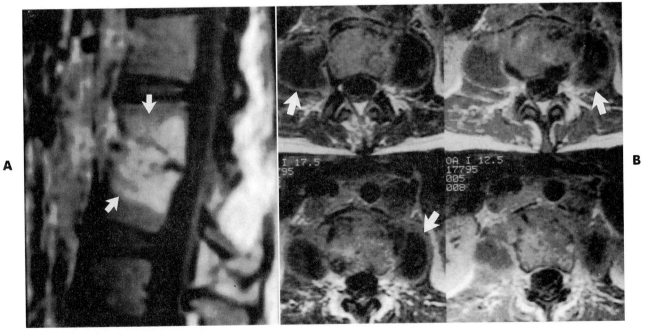

Fig. 20-3. Sagittal **(A)** and axial **(B)** contrast-enhanced T1-weighted MR scans in a 32-year-old man with tuberculous discitis, spondylitis, and psoas abscesses. The affected disk and end plates enhance intensely and homogeneously **(A,** *arrows).* Multiloculated psoas abscesses are present **(B,** *arrows).*

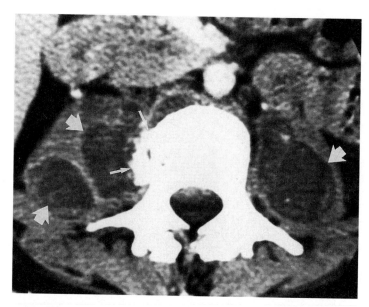

Fig. 20-4. Axial CECT scan in a 52-year-old man shows bilateral psoas abscesses *(large arrows)*. Bone windows (not shown) disclosed osteomyelitis. Note irregular anterior, lateral end plates *(small arrows)*. Brucella abscesses were drained at surgery.

patients; vertebral body fusion eventually occurs in most cases.[10]

CT scans characteristically show extensive bony destruction and large paraspinous abscesses that are relatively disproportionate to the amount of bone destruction. Epidural extension and subligamentous spread are also frequently present.[3,9]

MR scans invariably show loss of cortical definition of the affected vertebrae. However, affected vertebrae are often at least partially maintained in pyogenic spondylitis (Fig. 20-3, *C*). T1WI often shows infection spread beneath the longitudinal ligaments to involve adjacent vertebral bodies.[9] The disks are sometimes relatively spared, particularly in relationship to the degree of bone destruction. The posterior elements are commonly involved.[9]

Differential diagnosis. The major differential diagnosis of tuberculous spondylitis is pyogenic vertebral osteomyelitis or other spondylitides such as brucellosis, actinomycosis, and hydatid disease (Fig. 20-4). Tumor is also a diagnostic consideration when a paraspinal mass is associated with bone destruction.[9]

Epidural and Subdural Infections

Epidural abscess
Etiology and pathology. Spinal epidural abscess (SEA) typically results from direct hematogenous seeding of the epidural space from a cutaneous, pulmonary, or urinary tract source.[5] *Staphylococcus aureus* is by far the most common organism responsible for spine infections of all types.[12]

Two basic stages are observed in SEA. Initially,

there is thickened inflamed tissue with granulomatous material and imbedded microabscesses. This represents a "phlegmonous" stage (*see* Fig. 20-1, *B*).[13] In the second stage a collection of liquid pus forms a frank abscess (Fig. 20-5, *see* Fig. 20-2).[12]

Incidence, age, and gender. Spinal epidural abscesses are uncommon, representing approximately one case per 10,000 hospital admissions in tertiary institutions.[13] However, the incidence of SEA is now increasing significantly.[14] All ages are affected; the mean age is 50 to 55 years.[14,15] There is a moderate male predominance in reported cases of SEA.[12-15]

Location. All areas of the spine are affected. SEAs are often extensive; in one third of cases the infection extends over more than six vertebral segments.[12] Concomitant diskitis or osteomyelitis is seen in 80%.[12]

Clinical presentation and natural history. Fever and localized tenderness are common early symptoms but symptoms are often nonspecific.[13] Predisposing conditions include diabetes mellitus, intravenous drug abuse, multiple medical illnesses, and trauma.[14] If left untreated, severe neurologic deficits and death may occur.[13]

Imaging findings. Plain spine radiographs may disclose osteomyelitis and disk space narrowing (*see* Fig. 20-1, *A*). Myelography or CT-myelography demonstrates an extradural soft tissue mass with blockage of normal CSF flow.[14]

MR scans typically show an extradural, soft tissue mass that is iso- to hypointense compared to spinal

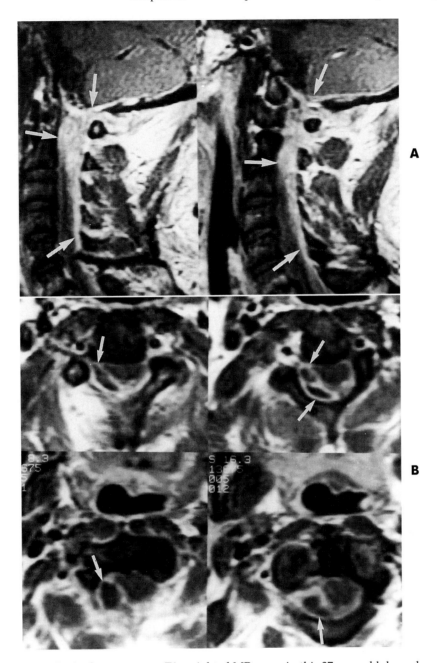

Fig. 20-5. A, Sagittal postcontrast T1-weighted MR scans in this 37-year-old drug abuser show a large, enhancing epidural phlegmon *(arrows).* Cephalad extension into the cisterna magna is present. **B,** Axial scans show thin enhancing rims *(arrows)* surrounding hypointense fluid collections. Phlegmon and frank abscesses were found at surgery.

cord on T1WI and hyperintense on proton density- and T2-weighted sequences *(see* Fig. 20-2, *B).*[13] Coexisting low signal changes in adjacent vertebral bodies are often seen on T1WI with high signal intensity in the intervertebral disks and vertebral bodies on T1-weighted sequences.[14]

Three patterns are observed following contrast administration. Diffuse homogeneous or slightly heterogeneous enhancement is seen in 70% of cases *(see* Fig. 20-1, *B).*[14] This most likely represents the phleg-

monous stage of SEA. The second most frequent finding is a thick or thin enhancing rim that surrounds a liquefied low signal pus collection, seen in 40% of cases *(see* Fig. 20-2, *A).* This represents a frank necrotic abscess.[14] In some cases, a combination of both patterns is observed *(see* Fig. 20-5).[13]

Subdural abscess. Spinal subdural abscesses (SSA) are rare. The relative paucity of reported cases of SSA compared to intracranial subdural abscesses has been ascribed to absence of venous sinuses in the spine, the wide epidural space acting as a "filter," and the centripetal direction of spinal blood flow.[16]

Clinical presentation is nonspecific; symptoms may mimic those of acute transverse myelitis, spinal epidural abscess, epidural hematoma, pyogenic spondylitis, and neoplasm.[16] Imaging studies disclose an intraspinal space-occupying mass, often without features that would localize the lesion to the subdural compartment.[16]

Meningitis, Myelitis, and Cord Abscess

Intradural spinal inflammatory disease includes meningitis and myelitis. The diagnosis of uncomplicated meningitis is typically established by lumbar puncture, whereas imaging studies may be more helpful in diagnosis myelitis.

Meningitis. Spinal meningitis can be caused by bacterial (pyogenic, granulomatous), fungal, parasitic, or viral organisms.[3] Pyogenic leptomeningitis is the most common bacterial infection of the spinal axis. The majority of these cases occur as a manifestation of cerebral meningitis.[3]

Granulomatous, pyogenic, and aseptic meningitides are all seen as contrast-enhancing tissue that surrounds the spinal cord and nerve roots.[17] Three patterns are seen,[17] as follows:

1. Delicate, smooth, linear enhancement outlining the cord, nerve roots, or meninges (Fig. 20-6)
2. Discrete nodular foci on the surface of these structures
3. Diffusely thickened soft tissue that appears as an intradural filling defect

There is no correlation between enhancement pattern and disease severity or specific responsible organism.[17]

Myelitis. The term *myelitis* should be restricted to inflammatory diseases of the spinal cord, whereas "myelopathy" is a more general term that is applied to cord dysfunction from noninflammatory sources (e.g., spondylitic or compressive myelopathy, radiation myelopathy).[18]

Several infectious agents can cause myelitis. Viral infections typically affect the gray matter. Herpes, coxsackie, and polio viruses are the most common agents, although HIV-related myelitis is increasing in frequency.[18] Epidural abscess and chronic meningeal infections such as tuberculosis and fungal meningitis may also cause a secondary myelitis (*see* Fig. 20-2, B).[5,17] Post-infectious and post-vaccinal myelopathies also occur (see subsequent discussion).

Imaging findings are typically nonspecific and resemble other noninfectious inflammatory and demy-

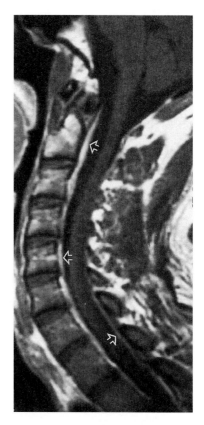

Fig. 20-6. Sagittal postcontrast T1-weighted MR scan in this 26-year-old woman with low-grade fever following lumbar surgery shows diffusely thickened, enhancing meninges *(arrows)*. CSF showed mildly elevated protein, mild pleocytosis, and no organisms. Probable aseptic meningitis.

elinating disorders (see subsequent discussion). Focal or diffuse increased intramedullary signal on T2-weighted MR scans, with or without mass effect, is typical. Enhancement following contrast administration can be seen in some cases.[17]

Intramedullary abscess. In contrast to brain abscess, frank pyogenic spinal cord abscesses are extremely rare. The few reported cases may represent focal venous infarcts that are complicated by bacterial colonization.[3]

DEMYELINATING DISEASES
Multiple Sclerosis

Etiology and pathology. The general etiology and pathology of multiple sclerosis (MS) are detailed in Chapter 17. Spinal cord plaques are an almost universal autopsy finding in patients with MS; in some cases the spinal cord is the earliest affected site.[19] Plaques occur preferentially in the dorsolateral cord and do not respect boundaries between specific tracts or between gray and white matter (Fig. 20-7).[19]

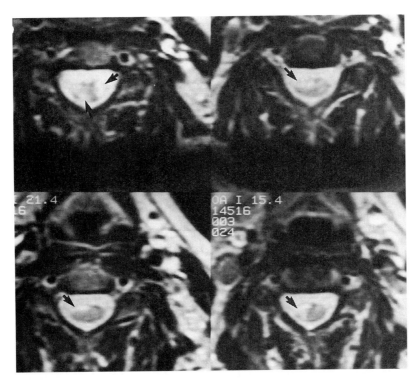

Fig. 20-7. Axial T2-weighted MR scans in a 46-year-old woman with long-standing multiple sclerosis and cervical myelopathy show multifocal white and gray matter high signal intensity foci *(arrows)*.

A   **B**

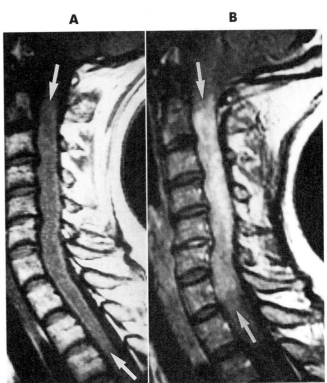

Fig. 20-8. This 43-year-old woman with a 3-month history of optic neuritis and right arm weakness developed sudden onset of rapidly progressive sensory deficit and upper extremity weakness. Pre- **(A)** and postcontrast **(B)** sagittal T1-weighted MR scans show diffuse cervical cord enlargement that extends from C2 to C7 and enhances moderately *(arrows)*. The patient developed severe bilateral optic atrophy and quadriparesis. Follow-up scans 3 years later (not shown) demonstrated diffuse cord atrophy. Neuromyelitis optica (Devic syndrome).

Incidence, age, and gender. MS is a worldwide disease, although the greatest prevalence is in temperate zones such as the United States and Canada, Great Britain, and northern Europe. Disease onset is typically between 15 and 50 years, with a peak in the third and fourth decades. There is a distinct female predominance, particularly in children and adolescents with MS.[20]

Location. Spinal cord plaques can be found at any segment. In later stages, plaques are evenly distributed; in early disease there is a distinct predilection for the cervical spinal cord.[19] An MS variant, *Devic disease* (also called neuromyelitis optica), is a rapidly progressive fulminant demyelination that is restricted to the optic nerves and spinal cord (Fig. 20-8).[20a]

Imaging findings. Spinal MR is not required for confirmation when a definite diagnosis of MS has been made on clinical grounds. However, in patients with isolated myelopathy and a clinical suspicion of demyelinating disease, brain MR is recommended as the first screening imaging study.[21] If such patients have a normal brain scan, MR examination of the spinal cord is appropriate (Fig. 20-8).

The most common finding on T2-weighted MR scans is one or more elongated, poorly marginated, hyperintense intramedullary lesions, particularly if focal or generalized cord atrophy is identified on T1WI.[21] Acute demyelinating lesions may have mass effect and enhance following contrast administration (Figs. 20-8 and 20-9).[20]

Acute Transverse Myelopathy

Acute transverse myelopathy (ATM) is sometimes termed *acute transverse myelitis*. In its most dramatic form, ATM is characterized by an acutely developing, rapidly progressing lesion that affects both halves of the cord. ATM is not actually a true disease but a clinical syndrome with diverse causes (*see* box).[22]

Etiology and pathology. Several neuropathological processes may give rise to ATM. Some cases develop with active infection; others occur as a post-infectious demyelinating disorder (acute disseminated encephalomyelitis, or ADEM) (Fig. 20-10).

Acute Transverse Myelopathy
Etiology

Acute infection
Post-infection
Post-vaccination
Autoimmune (SLE, MS)
Systemic malignancy

ATM sometimes may follow vaccination or be seen with immune disorders such as systemic lupus erythematosus (SLE) and multiple sclerosis (MS). Acute or subacute myelopathy sometimes occurs as a complication of systemic malignancy similar to limbic encephalitis.[18,22] Some cases of ATM with sudden onset may be caused by vascular occlusion and are more accurately characterized as spinal cord infarcts (see subsequent discussion). The precise etiology in most cases remains unknown.[23]

Incidence, age, and gender. The estimated annual incidence of ATM is approximately one case per million.[22] ATM occurs in all age groups. There is no gender predilection.

Location. Any segment can be affected, although there is a slight predilection for the thoracic cord.[23] Multilevel involvement is typical.[22,23]

Clinical presentation and natural history. In the typical case, there is no prior history of neurologic abnormality.[22] Time from symptom onset to maximum deficit ranges from less than 1 hour to 17 days.[23] Sensory levels are typically in the thoracic region.[23] Prognosis in most cases is poor, and severe residual neurologic deficits are common.[22]

Imaging findings. The major role of neuroimaging is to identify treatable conditions that can mimic ATM. These include acute disk herniation, hematoma, epidural abscess, or compression myelopathies.[22]

During the acute phase, MR scans are normal in approximately half of all ATM cases and nonspecific in the remainder.[23] Focal cord enlargement on T1- and poorly delineated hyperintensities on T2-weighted scans are the most commonly identified abnormalities (Fig. 20-10).[22] Enhancement following contrast administration occurs in some cases.

Miscellaneous Myelopathies

Radiation myelopathy. Radiation myelopathy is a rare but serious complication of therapeutic irradiation (*see* box, p. 830). The following three criteria for establishing the diagnosis of radiation myelopathy have been established[24]:

1. The spinal cord must have been included in the radiation field
2. The neurologic deficit must correspond to the cord segment that was irradiated
3. Metastasis or other primary spinal cord lesions must be ruled out

Four distinct clinical syndromes of radiation myelopathy have been described, of which chronic progressive radiation myelopathy (CPRM) is the most common form identified on imaging studies.[24-26]

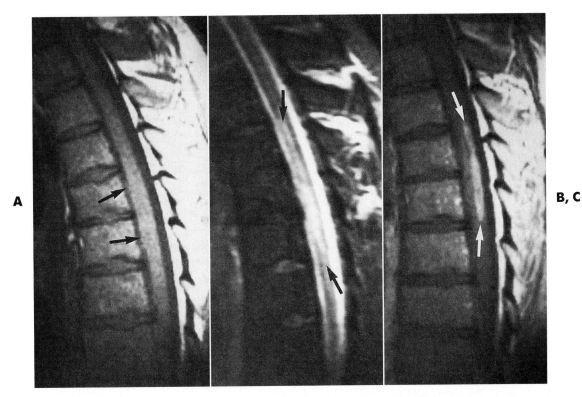

Fig. 20-9. This 42-year-old man with a 3-month history of lower extremity weakness had sudden onset of a rapidly ascending sensory level and paralysis. **A,** Sagittal T1-weighted MR scan shows enlargement of the midthoracic spinal cord *(arrows).* **B,** Sagittal T2-weighted scan shows intramedullary high signal *(arrows).* **C,** T1WI following contrast administration shows patchy enhancement *(arrows).* Biopsy for possible spinal cord neoplasm disclosed multiple sclerosis.

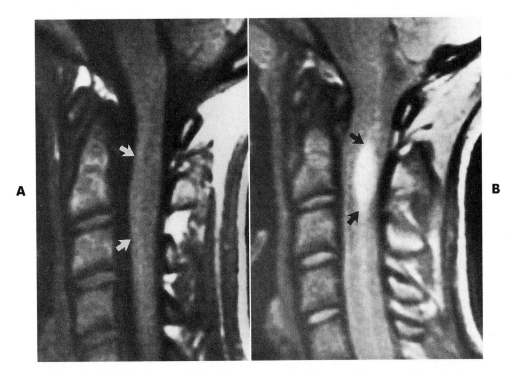

Fig. 20-10. This 16-year-old girl had a two-week history of right arm and leg numbness and tingling following a flulike illness. Sagittal T1- **(A)** and proton density-weighted **(B)** MR scans show enlargement of the upper cervical cord **(A,** *arrows)* with high signal intensity on PDWI **(B,** *arrows).* Acute transverse myelopathy.

Most cases of CPRM are seen following radiotherapy of nasopharyngeal carcinomas. The most commonly affected area is therefore the cervical spinal cord. The latent period between termination of irradiation and symptom onset varies from 3 to 40 months, although most cases occur between 9 and 20 months.[25]

Imaging findings vary. When MR scans are obtained more than 3 years after symptom onset, cord atrophy without abnormal signal intensity is seen.[26] Scans performed within 8 months of symptom onset typically disclose long-segment hyperintensity on T2WI, with or without associated cord swelling and enhancement following contrast administration (Fig. 20-11).[26]

AIDS-related myelopathy. AIDS-related myelopathy is probably related to direct injury of neurons by the HIV virus, although secondary demyelination of the posterior and lateral columns also occurs.[18]

Compressive myelopathy. Some investigators have described intramedullary high signal intensity foci on proton density- or T2-weighted MR scans in cases of moderate to marked spinal stenosis (*see* Fig. 20-31, *D*).[27] This can occur secondary to degenerative disk disease or spondyloarthropathy and is probably related to focal cord ischemia. Some cases resolve following decompressive surgery.[27] Serotonergic mechanisms have been implicated in the deleterious secondary events accompanying spinal cord compression injury.[28]

Miscellaneous causes of compressive myelopathy include mass effect from primary or secondary spine tumors or other epidural lesions such as epidural abscess.[18] The myelopathy frequently associated with vascular malformations and fistulae is probably produced by venous congestion combined with direct compression from dilated spinal veins.[29]

Degenerative and toxic myelopathies. Miscellaneous causes of spinal cord dysfunction include the inherited and acquired degenerative disorders such as Friedreich ataxia and other spinocerebellar degenerations, amyotrophic lateral sclerosis, toxic diseases (e.g., chronic alcoholism), and metabolic disorders (e.g., vitamin B_{12} deficiency).[18]

VASCULAR DISEASES
Normal Vascular Anatomy

A brief description of normal functional anatomy is necessary before delineating the various vascular diseases that involve the spine and spinal cord (*see* box, p. 831).

Spinal arteries. The spinal cord blood supply consists of one anterior and two posterior spinal arteries. At the lower cervical cord and upper two thoracic segments, the anterior spinal artery (ASA) is supplied by two to four anterior radicular arteries that arise from the vertebral, deep cervical, superior intercostal, and ascending cervical arteries. Radicular arteries are less prominent in the midthoracic cord. The thoracolumbar region is supplied by the ASA, also known as the artery of Adamkiewicz (Fig. 20-12). The cauda equina is supplied by lower lumbar, iliolumbar, and lateral sacral arteries.[30]

Via centrifugal branches from deep penetrating arteries the ASA provides approximately 70% of the

---

Miscellaneous Myelopathies
Etiology

Congenital spinocerebellar degeneration syndromes (e.g., Friedrich ataxia)
Radiation
AIDS
Compression (HNP, spinal stenosis, tumor)
Vascular malformations
Toxic/metabolic (alcoholism, vitamin B_{12} deficiency)

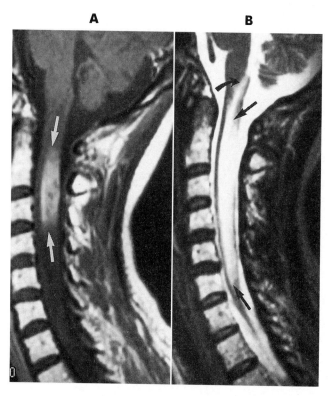

A   **B**

Fig. 20-11. This patient had onset of bilateral upper extremity weakness 3 months following radiation therapy. **A,** Postcontrast sagittal T1-weighted MR scan shows cord enhancement *(arrows).* **B,** Sagittal T2WI shows diffuse cord swelling and intramedullary high signal intensity *(arrows)* that extends cephalad to the medulla *(curved arrow).* Presumed radiation myelopathy. Note high signal in vertebral bodies caused by fatty marrow replacement.

cord blood supply, including the corticospinal tracts and all the gray matter (except for the posterior horns).[31] Within the cord interior there are no anastomoses, and these central penetrating vessels are essentially end arteries.[31]

The posterior aspect of the spinal cord is surrounded by an arterial network that forms a plexus dominated by the two posterior spinal arteries (PSAs). The PSAs supply approximately 30% of the cord, including the posterior horns, posterior columns, and a peripheral rim of white matter.[31] They do this in a centripetal fashion via numerous peripheral perforating arteries that are richly interconnected by anastomotic channels. The spinal cord "watershed zone" is located along the periphery of the gray matter at the border between these centrifugal (ASA) and centripetal (PSA) circulations.[31]

Vascular Disease of the Spinal Cord

Aneurysm, AVM, infarct much less common than in brain

Aneurysm extremely rare except with AVM
Infarct 2° to atherosclerosis, aortic dissection, disk herniation, trauma, hypertension, etc.
Venous infarct (?Foix-Alajouanine syndrome)

Spinal cord vascular supply

One anterior, two posterior spinal arteries
Anterior spinal artery (Adamkiewicz) supplies 70% of cord
Many end arteries, comparative few collaterals
"Watershed zone" at periphery of central gray matter

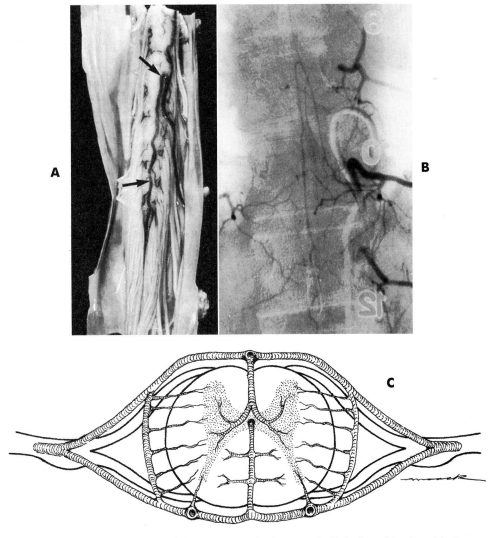

Fig. 20-12. Normal anatomy of the anterior spinal artery. **A,** Spinal cord *in situ* with dura reflected shows the anterior spinal artery and its major branches *(arrows).* **B,** Selective angiogram of the left T10 segmental artery shows the characteristic "hairpin" turn of the anterior spinal artery (of Adamkiewicz). **C,** Anatomic drawing shows spinal cord vascular supply.

The lateral aspect of the spinal cord is supplied by an arterial network located between the anterior and posterior nerve roots. It typically has numerous axial dorsoventral anastomoses.[32]

Extradural venous spaces and spinal veins

Extradural venous spaces. An extensive network of anastomosing, interconnecting, extradural venous channels extends from the skull base to the sacrum. The anterior longitudinal venous plexus is particularly prominent in the upper cervical and lumbar regions (*see* Chapter 19).[32,33] Basivertebral venous plexuses drain the vertebral bodies, and radicular veins accompany nerve roots as they exit the neural foramina.[34]

Spinal veins. Spinal venous drainage occurs via intrinsic and extrinsic venous systems. The intrinsic venous system is composed of numerous sulcal and axial veins that form a network that interconnects with numerous vertical and transmedullary anastomotic channels. The extrinsic system is formed by a pial venous network that collects the intrinsic perforators, longitudinal collector veins that lie anterior and posterior to the cord, and radicular veins.[32]

Aneurysms

Etiology and pathology. Spinal aneurysms (SAs) are localized, saccular dilatations of spine or spinal cord arteries. They are usually, but not invariably, associated with intramedullary spinal cord arteriovenous malformations (AVMs).[35]

Incidence, age, and gender. Compared to their intracranial counterparts, isolated SAs are extremely rare.[36a] SAs have been identified in 20% of patients with intramedullary AVMs. Patients are typically between the ages of 10 and 40 years; the mean age is 18.5 years. There is no gender predilection.[35]

Location. The intramedullary AVMs associated with SAs are equally divided between the cervical and thoracic spinal cord. SAs are almost always located on one of the main high-flow vessels feeding the AVM; nearly 70% are found on the anterior spinal artery.[35] In contrast to intracranial aneurysms, SAs do not usually occur at bifurcation points.[36a]

Clinical presentation. Symptoms are due to SAH in 85% of cases and progressive neurologic deficits in 15%. Recurrent hemorrhage is common in untreated cases.[35]

Imaging. Angiography is the definitive imaging study. Diagnostic criteria for SA include (1) visualization of an arterial vessel outpouching during the initial arterial phase and (2) selective injections with multiple views to rule out dilated vessels or overlapping loops that might mimic aneurysm.[35]

Vascular Malformations

Vascular malformations of the spine and spinal cord are uncommon lesions. Most are arteriovenous malformations (AVMs) or arteriovenous fistulae (AVFs). Cavernous angiomas and capillary telangiectasias are less common; venous angiomas are rarely, if ever, encountered.

Arteriovenous malformations and arteriovenous fistulae

Pathology and classification. AVMs have a true nidus of pathological vessels interposed between enlarged feeding arteries and draining veins.[37] AVFs drain directly into enlarged venous outflow tracts.[38]

Spinal AVMs have been subdivided into four general categories: Type I is a dural arteriovenous fistula. Type I AVMs are primarily found in the dorsal aspect of the lower thoracic cord and conus medullaris. Most type I AVMs consist of a single transdural arterial feeder that drains into an intradural arterialized vein. The draining vein often extends over multiple segments.[39] Type I AVMs typically affect men between their fifth and eighth decades.[38] Nearly 60% are spontaneous, whereas approximately 40% are caused by trauma.[40] Progressive neurologic deterioration, probably caused by chronic venous hypertension, is typical.[39]

Type II AVMs, so-called glomus malformations, are intramedullary AVMs in which a localized compact vascular plexus is supplied by multiple feeders from the anterior or posterior spinal arteries. Type II AVMs drain into a tortuous, arterialized venous plexus that surrounds the spinal cord. These AVMs are usually located dorsally in the cervicomedullary region.[38] Most occur in younger patients with acute onset of neurologic symptoms secondary to intramedullary hemorrhage.[38]

Type III AVMs, the so-called juvenile type, are large, complex vascular masses that involve the cord and often have extramedullary or even extraspinal extension. Multiple arterial feeders from several different vertebral levels are common.

Type IV AVMs are intradural extramedullary arteriovenous fistulas. These lesions are fed by the anterior spinal artery and lie completely outside the spinal cord and pia mater. There is no intervening small vessel network, and the fistula drains directly into an enlarged venous outflow tract of variable size. Most type IV AVMs are anterior to the spinal cord and are fed by the anterior spinal artery. Most occur near the conus medullaris. Type IV AVMs occur in patients between their third and sixth decades. Progressive neurologic deficits are typical.[38]

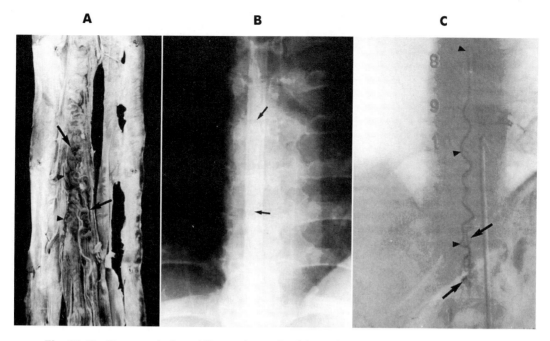

Fig. 20-13. Gross pathology **(A)**, myelography **(B)**, and angiography **(C)** of spinal cord AVM *(arrows)*. Note the enlarged anterior spinal artery *(arrowheads)*. (**A,** Courtesy Royal College of Surgeons of England, *Slide Atlas of Pathology,* Gower Medical Publishing, 1988.)

Incidence, age, and gender. AVMs are the most common spinal vascular anomaly, accounting for between 3% and 11% of spinal space-occupying lesions.[41] Age at symptom onset and gender vary with AVM type (see previous discussion). The most common AVM is type I, i.e., dural arteriovenous fistula. Type III, or juvenile, AVMs are rare.

Location. Location varies with specific AVM type (see previous discussion). The thoracolumbar area is the most common location overall and the site of slightly over half of AVMs (Fig. 20-13, *A*); 40% of AVMs occur in the cervical spinal cord.[37]

Clinical presentation and natural history. Clinical presentation and natural history also vary with AVM type. Paresis, sensory changes, bowel and bladder dysfunction, and impotence are common symptoms. Hemorrhage is seen in approximately 50% of cases.[37] Venous hypertension may be important in the development of cord symptoms.[41a]

Imaging findings. Myelography may show filling defects caused by the enlarged vessels (Fig. 20-13, *B*). Cord atrophy is common.

MR imaging may show foci of high-velocity signal loss within the enlarged vessels (Fig. 20-14). The cord is sometimes atrophic, and high signal intensity is often observed on T2-weighted scans.[42] Hemorrhagic residua may be present. AVM "mimics" are caused by dephasing from turbulent CSF flow or CSF flow-

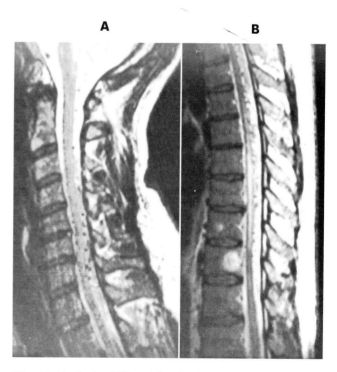

Fig. 20-14. Sagittal T2-weighted MR scans of the cervical **(A)** and thoracic **(B)** regions show multifocal areas of high-velocity signal loss (flow voids) dorsal to the spinal cord caused by an AVM. Note thoracic cord atrophy and myelomalacia, seen as intramedullary hyperintensity in **B**. (Courtesy W.T.C. Yuh.)

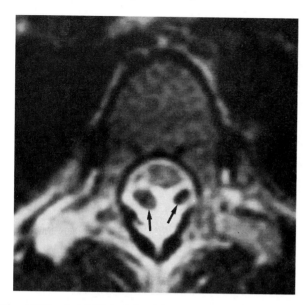

Fig. 20-15. Axial T2-weighted MR scan shows discrete regions of high-velocity signal loss *(arrows),* caused by CSF flow artifacts. The patient was neurologically normal.

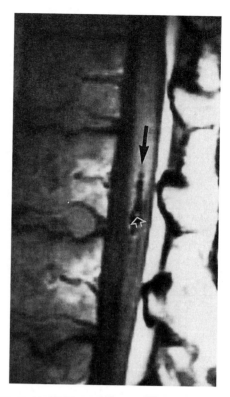

Fig. 20-16. Sagittal T1-weighted MR scan in a patient with lower extremity weakness shows a hypointense conus lesion *(black arrow)* surrounding a tiny high signal focus *(white arrow).* Presumed cavernous angioma.

ing at different rates within functionally separate compartments created by the dentate ligaments and septum posticum around the thoracic spinal cord (Fig. 20-15).

Spinal angiography is the definitive diagnostic procedure for the evaluation of spinal AVMs *(see* Fig. 20-13, *C).* Initial global (intraaortic) injection is followed by selective catheterization of the appropriate vessels to assess site and feeding pedicles, flow pattern, venous drainage, and hemodynamic effects (e.g., vascular steal).[40]

Cavernous angiomas

Pathology. Spinal cord cavernous angiomas are similar to intracranial cavernous angiomas. Grossly, these lesions are typically soft, spongy, well-circumscribed dark red or reddish-brown masses. Microscopically, cavernous angiomas consist of blood-filled endothelial-lined spaces lined by thickened, hyalinized walls that lack elastic fibers and smooth muscle.[43] Localized hemorrhages of different ages may be present. Calcification is rare.[44]

Incidence, age, and gender. Spinal cord cavernous malformations are extremely rare. They typically become symptomatic between the third and sixth decades. There is a 2:1 female predominance.[44]

Location. One large series reports the thoracic cord as the site of slightly more than half of cavernous angiomas, with the cervical cord the next most common location.[43] Multiple lesions occur but are uncommon.[44]

Clinical presentation and natural history. Intra-medullary spinal cord cavernous angiomas usually cause sensorimotor symptoms with progressive painful paraparesis. Clinical course varies from slowly progressive symptoms to acute quadriplegia.[44]

Imaging. Spinal angiography is typically normal. Findings on MR scans include residua of subacute and chronic hemorrhage characterized by mixed high- and low-signal components. The typical appearance is a small high signal focus on both T1- and T2-weighted or gradient-refocussed scans (Fig. 20-16). If a typical spinal cord lesion is identified on MR scans, the brain should be studied using gradient-refocussed sequences to screen for asymptomatic intracranial lesions.[45]

Capillary telangiectasias and venous malformations. Capillary telangiectasias of the pons, medulla, and spinal cord are often found incidentally at autopsy but are rarely identified on imaging studies. Venous malformations are also common brain anomalies but are rarely, if ever, observed in the spinal cord.

Infarction

Arterial infarction

Etiology and pathology. The blood supply to the entire spinal cord depends primarily on three longi-

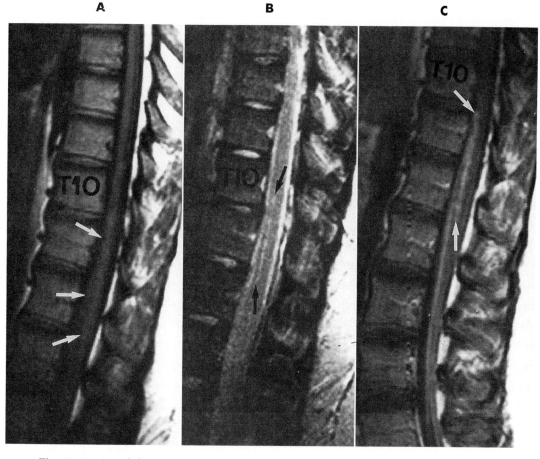

Fig. 20-17. An adolescent had sudden onset of lower extremity paraplegia following vigorous exercise. **A,** Sagittal T1-weighted MR scan shows distal cord enlargement *(arrows)*. **B,** Sagittal T2WI shows high signal intensity *(arrows)*. **C,** Postcontrast T1WI shows patchy enhancement. CSF studies were normal. Presumed cord infarct. (Courtesy D. Mendelsohn.)

tudinal arterial trunks: a single anterior spinal artery and paired posterior spinal arteries (see previous discussion).[46] Collateral flow is comparatively limited, and any pathologic process that interferes with this crucial blood supply may result in ischemia or infarction.[46]

Spontaneous anterior spinal cord infarction primarily affects individuals with severe atherosclerotic disease or aortic dissection. Other reported etiologies include syphilis, vasculitis, fibrocartilagenous emboli from disk herniation, cervical subluxation, hypotension, hematologic disorders, pregnancy, diabetes, thrombophlebitis, trauma, and tuberculosis.[47,48]

Incidence, age, and gender. Spinal cord infarction is extremely rare. Patient age in reported cases ranges from 15 to 75 years.[47]

Location. Most cord infarcts occur at the upper thoracic region or thoracolumbar junction. The extent of involvement ranges from a single segment to multiple levels.[46]

Clinical presentation and natural history. Clinical symptoms vary. The classic ASA infarct presents with sudden onset of flaccid para- or quadriparesis with or without burning and lancinating pain. Dissociated sensory loss with preserved touch, vibration, and position sense is common.[49]

Imaging. T1-weighted MR scans in acute cord infarction may demonstrate an enlarged cord (Fig. 20-17, *A*). Central or anterior intramedullary high signal is typically present on T2WI (Fig. 20-17, *B*). Enhancement following contrast may be initially absent but occurs a few days to a few weeks following symptom onset (Fig. 20-17, *C*).[48-50] Follow-up scans may show focal cord atrophy with myelomalacia and residual high signal intensity on T2WI.[50]

Venous infarction. Little is known about venous ischemia, infarction and their potential relationships to myelopathy.[50a] The disorder called *Foix-Alajouanine syndrome,* also known as subacute necrotic myelitis,

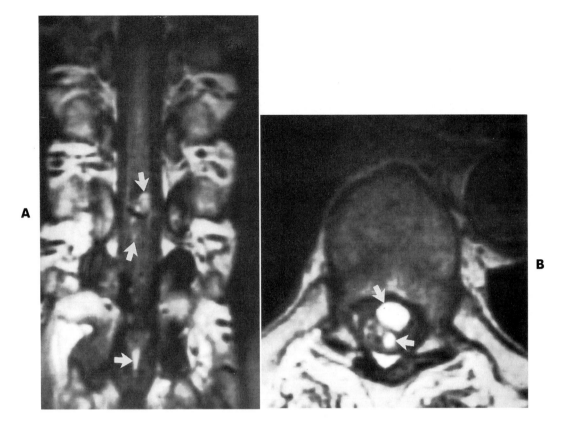

Fig. 20-18. A 78-year-old man had a 2-year history of slowly progressive lower extremity weakness with sudden onset of paraplegia. Coronal **(A)** and axial **(B)** T1-weighted MR scans show intra- and extramedullary high signal foci *(arrows)* mixed with hypointense areas. Surgery disclosed multiple thrombosed thick-walled veins draining a probable AVM. Possible Foix-Alajouanine syndrome.

may be secondary to venous stagnation, thrombosis, and infarction.[32] Pathologic studies in these cases show enlarged, thick-walled tortuous veins that are often thrombosed. Coagulative necrosis that involves both gray and white matter is typical.[51] MR studies suggest a vascular malformation with serpentine filling defects, thrombosed vessels, and cord edema (Fig. 20-18).

DEGENERATIVE DISEASES

The widespread prevalence of patients with back and neck pain makes the spine one of the most frequently requested neuroimaging examinations. Patients with low-back pain have a significant impact on health care costs, particularly in the United States.[52] Some authors estimate that up to 80% of all adults have low-back pain at some time in their lives and that a herniated nucleus pulposus is the cause in only a small percentage of these cases.[53]

In this section we discuss the pathology and imaging of degenerative spine disease. We begin with a discussion of normal age-related changes in the intervertebral disks and vertebral bodies. We then delineate the spectrum of disk herniations, facet arthroses and spinal stenosis, and the spectrum of imaging

findings in the post-operative spine, including the so-called "failed back" syndromes. We conclude our discussion by briefly considering back pain in children.

Normal Aging and Disk Degeneration

Normal aging is a complex physiologic process that encompasses various degrees of gross anatomic and biochemical changes in the entire diskovertebral complex.[54] Whether a distinction can or should be made between normal aging and disk degeneration is controversial.[54-56] What is clear is that age-related changes in the MR appearance of both the intervertebral disks and vertebral bodies normally occur in asymptomatic individuals.[54,55,57-60]

Normal disc microarchitecture and MR signal intensity. Sharpey's fibers and the outer anular rings consist of well-organized collagen fibrils with low signal intensity on both T1- and T2-weighted sequences.[61] The central disk contains two basic tissues: wispy fibrocartilage from the inner anulus and the gelatinous matrix of the nucleus pulposus. These two disk regions are inseparable on routine spin-echo MR scans; both have high signal intensity on T2WI. After childhood, an intranuclear "cleft" composed of

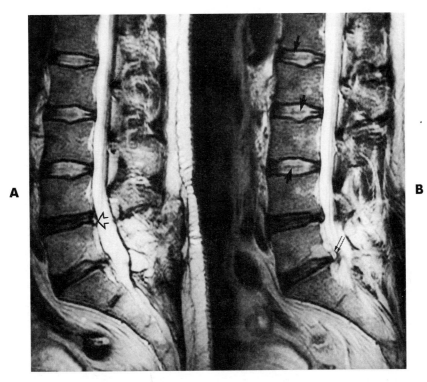

Fig. 20-19. Sagittal T2-weighted MR scans in this 38-year-old man show normal high signal intensity in the upper three intervertebral disks. Note the low signal intranuclear "cleft" (**B,** *single arrows*). The L4-L5 and L5-S1 disks are comparatively hypointense, indicating increasing collagen content and decreasing disk hydration. The L4-L5 disk is bulging and has a small high signal intensity focus in the posterior anulus (**A,** *arrow*), consistent with circumferential anular tear. There is a small central L5-S1 HNP (**B,** *double arrows*).

fibrous transformation of the previously gel-like matrix is seen on T2WI (*see* Chapter 19).[61]

Normal disk aging. Both morphologic and chemical changes occur in the intervertebral disks with normal development and aging. These are in turn reflected by changes on MR scans, particularly T2-weighted sequences.

In children, a transition occurs between the immature nucleus pulposus seen in newborns and the adult configuration. In the newborn, the nucleus pulposus is fibrocartilaginous with little fiber evident on gross anatomic sections. The nucleus appears grossly homogeneous except for a small primitive notochordal remnant.[58,62]

During the first and second decades of life, fibrous tissue initially develops near the dorsal or ventral margin of the nucleus pulposus and spreads toward the center. The notochordal remnants are obliterated, and the distinction between nucleus pulposus and anulus fibrosus is gradually lost. In adults, especially after age 30, there is an indistinct boundary between the nucleus pulposus and inner anulus fibrosus.[58]

Physiologic aging in the nucleus pulposus is related to specific chemical changes in the intervertebral disk. These are a decrease in water-binding ca-

pacity, disintegration of large molecular proteoglycans, and increase in collagen content.[63]

In the first decade of life, the nucleus pulposus contains 85% to 88% water, and the anulus fibrosus contains 75%. In adulthood, the water content of both is about 70%.[55] With aging, the collagen content of the anulus increases from 20% of dry weight to over 25%. The total proteoglycan content of the nucleus decreases with age as the disk becomes more fibrous.[55]

MR imaging of disk aging. Intervertebral disk signal intensity on MR scans is related to the water content of the nucleus pulposus and fibrocartilage of the inner anulus.[55] In the neonate and young child, the nucleus has a very high signal intensity on T2-weighted images and is sharply demarcated from the anulus.[62] With maturation, this demarcation is gradually lost as the nucleus and the inner anulus become more fibrous.[55] Both the nucleus and inner anulus have high signal intensity on T2WI, but the outer anulus is hypointense at all ages.[55] A fibrous plate also develops in the disk equator. This is seen on T2-weighted MR scans as a central transverse band of reduced signal intensity in the nucleus pulposus (Fig. 20-19).[58]

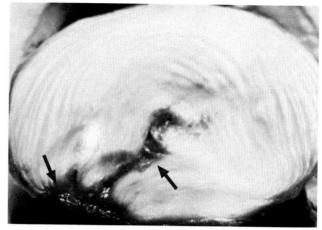

Fig. 20-20. Pathology of radial anular (type II) tear of the anulus fibrosis. Vascularized tear *(arrows)* extends through the outer anulus into the nucleus pulposus. (Courtesy G. Momberger.)

A, B

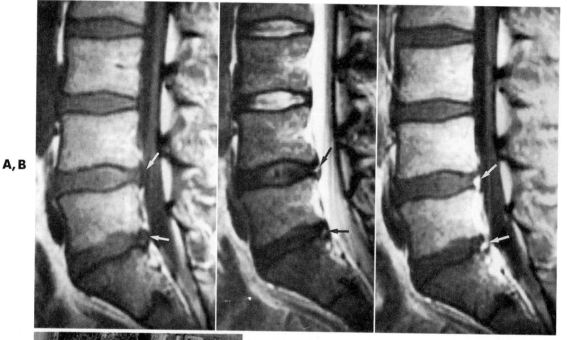

C

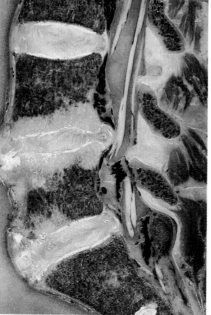

D

Fig. 20-21. Imaging findings of anular tears are shown on the MR scans of this 38-year-old man with low back pain and no previous surgery. **A,** Sagittal T1-weighted scan shows normal disk heights and slight posterior bulging of the L4-L5 and L5-S1 intervertebral disks *(arrows).* **B,** Sagittal T2WI shows these disks are comparatively hypointense. Small high signal foci are seen in the outer anulus of both disks *(arrows).* **C,** Postcontrast T1WI shows these areas enhance *(arrows),* probably due to vascularized granulation tissue in the anular tears. **D,** Sagittal cryomicrotome section demonstrates age-related degenerative changes in the vertebral bodies and intervertebral disks. Note loss of height and posterior bulging of the L4-L5 and L5-S1 disks. There is also fatty marrow replacement adjacent to both degenerated disks, seen here as yellow deposits replacing the red marrow. (**D,** Courtesy V. Haughton.)

Both aging and degeneration affect disk signal intensity.[55] These are clearly not independent variables, and distinguishing between the two is sometimes difficult.[54] Diminishing signal intensity on T2WI reflects increasing collagen content (Fig. 20-19).[58] This occurs both with maturation and degeneration.

Anular tears. Tears of the anulus fibrosis also occur with aging. Three distinct types have been described. Concentric (type I) tears are caused by delamination of longitudinal anular fibers. Radial (type II) tears involve all layers of the anulus from the nucleus to the disk surface (Fig. 20-20). Transverse (type III) tears involve the insertion of Sharpey fibers into the ring apophysis.[62]

Transverse and concentric anular tears are common in adult disks whether or not degenerative changes are present in the nucleus pulposus. These tears are probably incidental findings.[59,62] The significance of radial anular (type II) tears is controversial; some authors have implicated these tears with accelerated disk degeneration.[55,61]

The most common imaging finding with anular tear is high signal intensity on T2-weighted MR scans (Fig. 20-21, *B; see* Fig. 20-19). Enhancing foci on postcontrast T1-weighted sequences are sometimes identified (Fig. 20-21, *C*).

Disk degeneration. Disk degeneration, defined as diminished signal on T2-weighted MR scans combined with loss of disk space height, is common in asymptomatic patients (*see* box, p. 840). Early disk degeneration may also occur without a loss in disk height or signal intensity on T2WI.[61] Another sign of disk degeneration is intradiskal gas (vacuum disk phenomenon). This is seen on CT scans as extremely low density collections within the disk itself.[62] Degeneration or bulging of at least one lumbar disk is seen in 35% of patients between 20 and 39 years of age and in virtually all patients over 60 years of age.[56]

Vertebral body and marrow space changes with aging. With maturation, there is gradual conversion of red (hemopoietically active) marrow to yellow (inactive) marrow (*see* Chapter 19). Further changes in the vertebral body marrow occur with disk degeneration; signal intensity changes in the marrow adjacent to the vertebral end plates is a common observation on MR scans (Fig. 20-21, *D*).

Two types of marrow changes are associated with degenerative disk disease. In the so-called type 1 change, there is decreased signal intensity on T1- and increased signal intensity on T2-weighted scans. Histopathologic examination in these cases shows disruption and fissuring of end plates and vascularized fibrous tissue. In the so-called type 2 change, increased signal intensity is present on T1-weighted

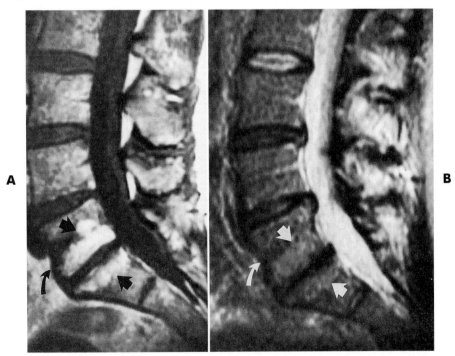

Fig. 20-22. Sagittal T1- **(A)** and T2-weighted **(B)** MR scans in a 56-year-old woman with low back pain show multiple dessicated disks. Note high signal intensity in the subchondral marrow around the L5-S1 interspace (**A,** *large arrows*). The marrow signal is mildly hyperintense on T2WI (**B,** *large arrows*). These so-called type II changes represent fatty replacement of vascular marrow (compare with Fig. 20-21, *D*). There is also a focus of dense bony sclerosis that is low signal on both sequences *(curved arrows).*

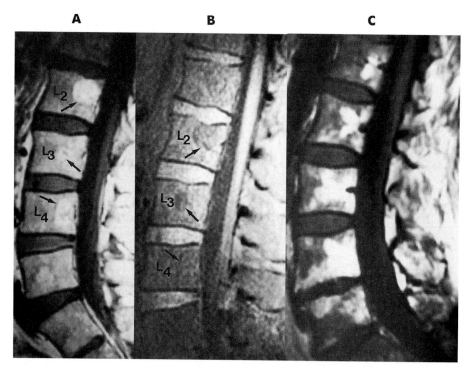

Fig. 20-23. Focal fatty marrow replacement is illustrated on these two scans. **A,** Sagittal T1WI in this 63-year-old man shows multiple round "hot spots" (high signal intensity foci) in the vertebral bodies *(arrows).* **B,** Repeat scan with fat suppression shows the high signal foci are now low signal *(arrows).* **C,** Sagittal T1-weighted scan in a 73-year-old woman with osteoporosis shows very patchy fatty marrow replacement. There was no evidence of systemic disease or malignancy.

scans with isointense or slightly increased signal on T2-weighted sequences. Type 2 changes represent fatty marrow replacement (Figs. 20-22 and 20-23).[60]

Marrow changes are sometimes more focal and can resemble vertebral body hemangiomas on T1WI (Fig. 20-23, *A*); fat suppression sequences are helpful in distinguishing these two entities (Fig. 20-23, *B*). Occasionally, fatty marrow replacement is diffusely patchy, resulting in mottled, inhomogeneous-appearing vertebral bodies (Fig. 20-23, *C*). If dense vertebral sclerosis occurs in response to degeneration of an adjacent intervertebral disk, the affected subchondral marrow is low signal on both T1- and T2-weighted scans.

Spondylosis, Arthrosis, and Spinal Stenosis

Spondylosis
Etiology and pathology. The primary pathologic finding in spondylosis is osteophytosis. Osteophytes are bony excrescences that originate near the margin of vertebral bodies or facet joints.[64]

Vertebral body osteophytes probably result from weakening of anular fibers with disk bulging and traction on Sharpey fibers. Osteophytes typically develop where these fibers attach to the vertebral body, usually several millimeters from the diskovertebral junction.[65]

Disk Degeneration
Dessication, degeneration are part of normal aging Begins in teens, 20's Anular tears, bulges, even herniations often asymptomatic and frequent in older adults

Schmorl's nodes, herniation of disk material through the end plate into the vertebral body, are common manifestations of spondylosis.[64]

Incidence, age, and gender. Spondylosis and osteophytosis increase with advancing age. The prevalence of osteophytes in patients 50 years of age or older is estimated at 60% to 80%. Men are more frequently affected than women; individuals engaged in occupations that require heavy physical labor are more often affected.[65] Schmorl's nodes are seen in up to 75% of the normal population.[64]

Location. Although any spinal segment can be involved, the lumbar and cervical areas are the most common sites, whereas the thoracic spine is often less frequently and less severely involved. In the cervical spine the levels that are most frequently affected by both disk herniation and chronic spondylosis are C6-C7 (60% to 75%) and C5-C6 (20% to 30%).[66] In the

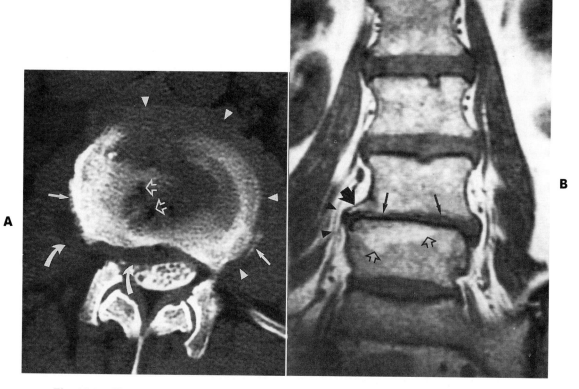

Fig. 20-24. Degenerative spondylosis. **A,** Axial post-myelogram CT scan shows low density in the intervertebral disk (vacuum disk phenomenon) *(open arrows)*, marginal osteophytes *(small arrows)*, and bulging disk *(arrowheads)*. Asymmetric protrusion of disk material to the right, extending into the neural foramen and extraforaminal soft tissues *(curved arrows)*, represents a moderate-size disk herniation. **B,** Coronal T1-weighted MR scan in another case shows thinned L4-L5 disk space *(small black arrows)*, lateral osteophytes *(large arrow)*, and degenerative marrow changes *(open arrows)*. Some lateral subluxation of L4 on L5 is present. Note the right L4 nerve root *(arrowheads)* draped over the osteophyte.

lumbar spine, L4-L5 and L5-S1 are the most commonly and most severely affected sites. Multilevel disease is common in both the cervical and lumbar regions.

Imaging findings. Imaging findings in spondylosis include Schmorl's nodes, osteophytes, and end plate sclerosis (Fig. 20-24). Schmorl's nodes are seen on CT scans as end-plate sclerotic areas surrounding lucencies that represent interbody herniation of disk material.

Vertebral body osteophytes are bony spurs or ledges that originate several millimeters from the diskovertebral junction and extend first in a horizontal and then in a vertical direction (Figs. 20-24, *B,* and 20-25, *A*).[65] Facet osteophytes are seen on axial images as mushroom-like facet overgrowths with subchondral sclerosis. Sagittal scans through the neural foramina show posterosuperior bony narrowing, often combined with ligamentum flavum laxity that further narrows the foramen (Fig. 20-25, *B*).

Differential diagnosis. Osteophytes should be distinguished from syndesmophytes. Syndesmophytes

are slender, vertically oriented ligamentous calcifications and osseous excrescences that extend from the margin of one vertebral body to another.[65] Syndesmophytes are often associated with facet joint ankylosis and are one of the imaging hallmarks of ankylosing spondylitis.[64] Osteophytes should also be distinguished from the sweeping, asymmetric lateral bony excrescences of psoriasis and Reiter syndrome and the flowing ossifications of diffuse idiopathic skeletal hyperostosis (DISH).[65]

Arthrosis, facet joint disease, and synovial cysts
Etiology and pathology. The articular processes of the spine form synovium-lined articulations, the apophyseal joints (*see* Chapter 19). Osteoarthritis is seen pathologically as fibrillation and erosion of articular cartilage, partial or complete denudation of the cartilagenous surface, and new bone formation.[65]

Juxta-articular cysts, also known as "synovial cysts" or "ganglion cysts," sometimes form next to degenerated facet joints (Table 20-1).[67] Cyst contents range from serous or mucinous fluid to semisolid ge-

Fig. 20-25. A, Axial post-myelogram CT scan shows left lateral recess narrowing *(curved arrow)* secondary to vertebral body osteophyte *(small arrows)*. Note partially calcified *(double arrows)*, broad-based disk bulge *(open arrows)*. **B,** Sagittal T1-weighted MR scan in another patient shows normal L3-L4 and L4-L5 neural foramina *(curved arrows)*. Facet arthrosis and lax ligamentum flavum *(small arrows)* narrows the L5-S1 neural foramen and mildly compresses the exiting L5 root *(large arrow)*.

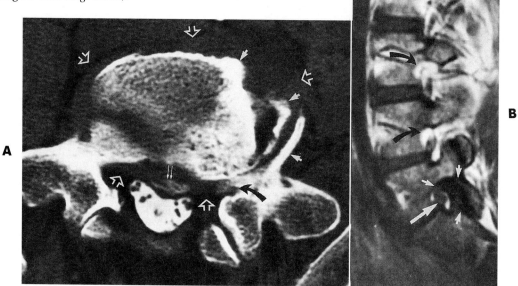

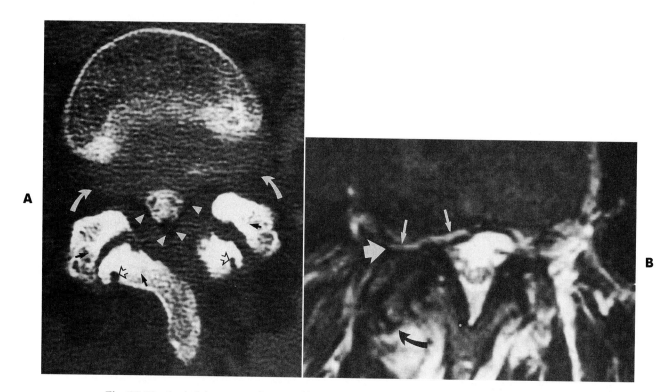

Fig. 20-26. A, Axial post-myelogram CT scan shows eburnation *(small arrows)* and cystic changes *(open arrows)* around both articular facet joints. Ligamentum flavum degeneration and laxity narrows the canal posteriorly *(arrowheads)*, whereas spondylolisthesis with disk bulge *(curved arrows)* narrows the canal anteriorly. **B,** Axial T2-weighted MR scan in another patient shows severe facet arthrosis with "mushroom"-shaped facet spurs *(curved arrow)*. The neural foramen *(large arrow)* is markedly narrowed by the facet arthrosis and a lateral disk herniation *(small arrows)*.

Table 20-1. Spine Cysts

Lesion	Location	Incidence	Pathology	Imaging findings	Comments
Synovial cyst	Adjacent to degenerated facet joint, may be multiple	Common	Synovium-lined cyst	Mass posterolateral to thecal sac; density/signal vary with contents	Contents vary from clear fluid to mucinous to hemorrhagic
Arachnoid cyst Extradural Intradural	Thoracic spine, dorsal to cord; usually single	Rare	Arachnoid-lined	Canal ±expanded, pedicles thinned; ≅CSF density/signal; may be severe cord compression	If cyst communicates with thecal sac, only finding on CT-myelogram is cord compression, anterior displacement
Arachnoid pouch/ diverticulum	Root sleeve dilatation; often multiple	Very common	Dura + arachnoid	Bulbous dilations of root sleeve; can mimic HNP, tumor; fill with intrathecal contrast injection; do not enhance after I.V. contrast	
Meningocele Lateral	All levels; thoracic most common	Common with NF-1, Marfan's	Dura + arachnoid	CSF-filled outpouching; posterior vertebral body scalloping, enlarged neural foramina	Kyphoscoliosis, other signs of NF-1 often present
Intraosseous	Sacrum	Uncommon	Arachnoid	Scalloped sacrum; cyst similar to CSF	
Traumatic pseudomeningocele	Cervical most common	Uncommon	Not lined by meninges	"Empty root sleeve" secondary to root avulsion	Intraspinal cyst can occur, cause mass effect
Perineural cyst ("Tarlov" or "Rexed" cyst)	Root sleeve at dorsal root ganglion	Uncommon	Nerve fibers, ganglion cells in cyst wall	May look like nerve root tumor	

latinous tissue. They may also contain blood, hemosiderin, or even air.[68,69]

Incidence and age. Facet degeneration begins in the first 2 decades of life.[66] Facet arthrosis (apophyseal joint osteoarthritis) is seen in the majority of adults and is virtually universal in patients over 60 years of age.[65,66,70]

Location. The middle and lower cervical spine and the lower lumbar spine are most commonly affected; facet disease is uncommon in the thoracic region.[64] The lower lumbosacral spine is the most common site for synovial cysts; the cervical region is an uncommon location.[67]

Imaging. Imaging findings of facet arthrosis on plain film and NECT scans include joint space narrowing, bone eburnation, and osteophytosis (Fig.

20-26, *A*).[65] Sagittal and thin-section axial MR scans are particularly helpful in delineating the effect of facet hypertrophy on the neural foramina (*see* Fig. 20-26, *B*; Fig. 20-25, *B*).[71,72]

Juxtaarticular cysts display a spectrum of imaging findings. Cyst density on NECT scans varies from hypo- to hyperdense compared to the adjacent ligamentum flavum (Figs. 20-27 and 20-28). Signal on MR scans is also variable. Some cystic contents resemble CSF, whereas others may be high signal or show hemorrhagic residua and fluid-fluid levels (Figs. 20-29, *A* and *B*).[68,69,73] Some synovial cysts also have a solid component; both the solid component and cyst capsule may enhance following contrast administration.[74]

Occasionally, synovial cysts erode bone or present

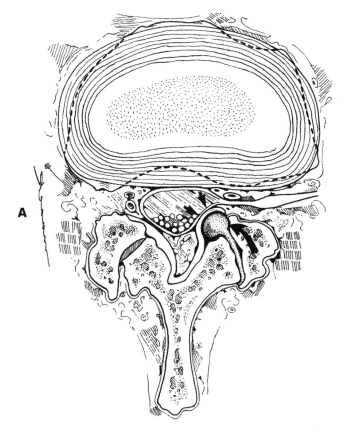

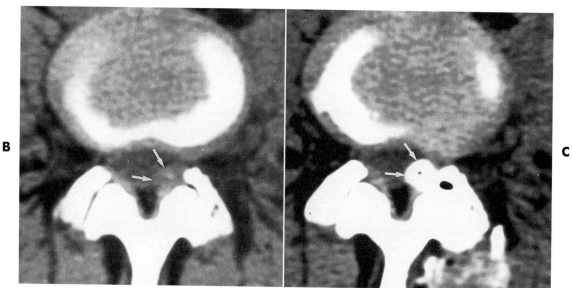

Fig. 20-27. A, Anatomic drawing illustrates a synovial cyst *(curved arrow)*. Note postero-lateral compression of the thecal sac *(small arrows)*. **B,** Axial NECT scan shows a slightly hyperdense mass adjacent to the left facet joint *(arrows)*. **C,** CT scan obtained following contrast injection into the facet joint shows the mass *(arrows)* fills with contrast, indicating the cyst communicates with the joint space. Synovial cyst was removed at laminectomy.

as a neural foraminal lesion and resemble an epidural or nerve root tumor (Fig. 20-28).[75] Therefore the major differential diagnosis of lumbar synovial cyst is a large migrated free disk fragment and cystic nerve root tumor.[76]

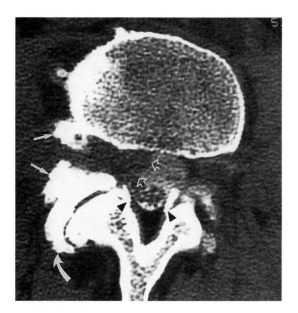

Fig. 20-28. Axial post-myelogram CT scan shows severe degenerative facet disease with "mushroom cap" arthrosis (*curved arrow*). Vertebral body and facet osteophytes (*small arrows*) narrow the neural foramen. Ligamentum flavum ossification is present (*arrowheads*), contributing to the canal and neural foraminal stenosis. A low density soft tissue mass occupies the neural foramen and compresses the thecal sac (*open arrows*). A large juxtaarticular (synovial) cyst was removed at surgery.

Spinal stenosis
Etiology and pathology. Spinal stenosis can be congenital, acquired, or result from a combination of congenital abnormalities with superimposed degenerative changes (*see* box).[64]

Congenital stenosis occurs with short pedicle syndromes. Here, the pedicles typically are thick and reduced in anteroposterior diameter. Minimal disk bulges or spondylotic changes superimposed on a congenitally small canal can produce severe neurologic deficits (Fig. 20-30). Other congenital spinal stenoses occur with achondroplasia and inherited metabolic disorders such as Morquio syndrome.[64]

| **Spinal Stenosis** |
| *Etiology* |
| **Congenital** |
| Morquio syndrome |
| "Short pedicle syndrome" |
| **Acquired/degenerative** |
| Spondylosis |
| Facet disease ± synovial cyst |
| Ligamentous degeneration ± spondylolisthesis |
| Disk bulge/herniation |
| Spondylolysis with spondylolisthesis |
| **Miscellaneous** |
| Ligamentous ossification/calcification (e.g., OPLL) |
| Epidural lipomatosis |

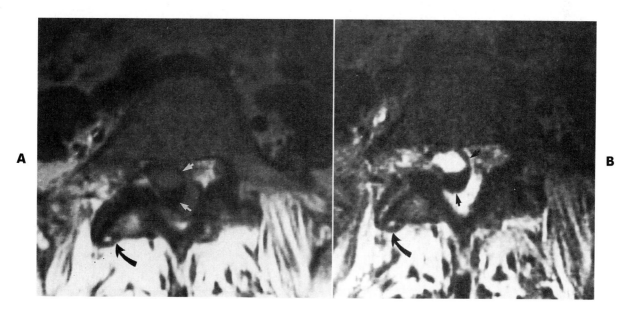

Fig. 20-29. Axial T1- **(A)** and T2-weighted **(B)** scans show severe facet arthrosis (*curved arrows*) and a mixed signal juxtaarticular cyst (*small arrows*). Hemorrhagic synovial cyst was removed at surgery.

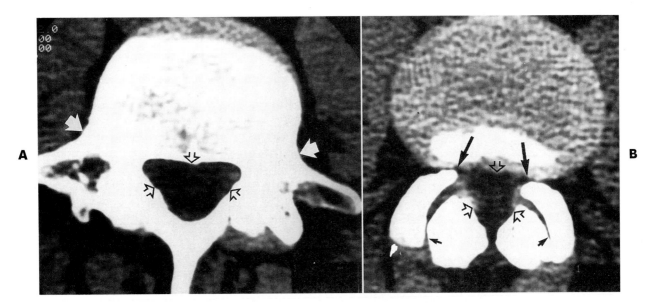

Fig. 20-30. Congenital lumbar spinal stenosis is shown on the axial NECT scans of this 32-year-old man. **A,** The pedicles *(large arrows)* are short, thick, and broad. The spinal canal *(open arrows)* is small. **B,** Mild superimposed disk bulge *(large arrows)* and slight facet subluxation *(small arrows)* cause moderately severe narrowing of the canal *(open arrows).*

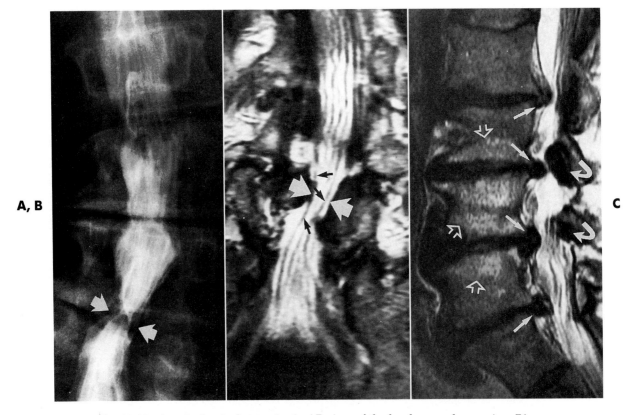

Fig. 20-31. Acquired spinal stenosis. **A,** AP view of the lumbar myelogram in a 76-year-old man shows degenerative subluxation, severe degenerative changes, and moderately severe spinal stenosis *(arrows).* **B,** Coronal T2-weighted MR scan with MR "myelogram" effect shows the severe stenosis *(large arrows)* and crowding of the cauda equina roots *(small arrows).* **C,** Sagittal T2WI shows multilevel HNPs *(small arrows)* and facet arthrosis *(curved arrows)* with anterior and posterior canal narrowing. Note high signal intensity in marrow *(open arrows)* adjacent to the degenerated disks. Type I change.

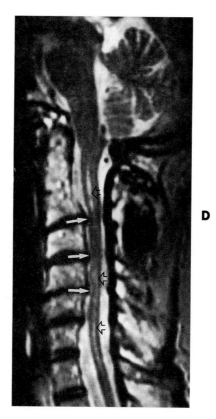

Fig. 20-31, cont'd. D, Sagittal T2-weighted MR scan in a patient with long-standing cervical degenerative disease and myelopathic symptoms. Multilevel spinal stenosis is present *(solid arrows)*. Note high signal in the moderately atrophic cord *(open arrows)*. This probably represents myelomalacic changes secondary to chronic cord compression; syrinx is the other diagnostic consideration (note normal position of the cerebellar tonsils, therefore Chiari I is not present). Postoperative studies following surgical decompression showed no change.

Acquired (degenerative) spinal stenosis is typically caused by spondylosis, disk bulges or herniations, ligamentous degeneration, spondylolysthesis, or a combination of these disorders (Fig. 20-31). Decreased disk and facet joint stability results in abnormal motion and ligamentous laxity, leading to a cascade of progressive degenerative processes that includes accelerated spondyloarthritis and inward buckling of adjacent ligaments, further reducing canal and neural foraminal size.[66]

Incidence and age. The precise incidence of spinal stenosis in the general population is unknown, although numerous studies have shown asymptomatic back disease is common, and its prevalence increases with age. Between 4% to 28% of CT or MR scans in asymptomatic patients show changes of lumbar stenosis.[77]

Location. In its broadest sense, spinal stenosis can affect the canal, lateral recesses, neural foramina, or a combination of these locations. The lumbar and cervical regions are most commonly affected.

Imaging findings. Myelography, CT, CT-myelog-raphy, and MR imaging all show reduced diameter of the thecal sac (Fig. 20-31). Multiple anterior extra-dural defects from osteophytes, bulging or herniated disks, or both, typically narrow the subarachnoid space at the intervertebral disk spaces. In extreme cases, the subarachnoid space is completely effaced; with high-grade lumbar stenosis, the transiting nerve roots may become so edematous and redundant that they mimic vascular malformation (Fig. 20-32). Chronically, severely compressed nerve roots may also enhance following contrast administration.[77a]

In the cervical spine, secondary spinal cord changes can sometimes be seen at the point of maximal compression (see Fig. 20-31, *D*). These are identified as intramedullary high foci on T2WI and probably represent edema, inflammation, vascular ischemia, myelomalacia, or gliosis. Some of these changes may resolve following decompressive surgery.[78]

Ligamentum flavum degeneration and laxity often encroaches on the canal posterolaterally. Facet arthrosis combined with disk space reduction may se-

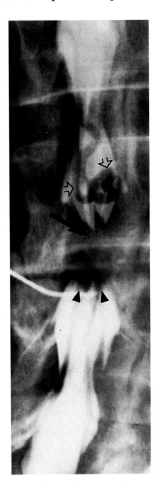

Fig. 20-32. AP view of a lumbar myelogram with very high-grade stenosis *(large arrow)* secondary to a large disk herniation. Note that the edematous, tortuous roots *(open arrows)* above the high-grade stenosis somewhat resemble a vascular malformation. The "feathered" appearance of the contrast column *(arrowheads)* at the stenosis is characteristic of an extradural mass such as HNP or tumor *(see* Fig. 21-1).

verely narrow the intervertebral foramina, compressing the exiting nerve root (Fig. 20-33).[78a]

Spondylolysis and spondylolisthesis

Etiology and pathology. Spondylolysis is a fibrous cleft within the pars interarticularis; spondylolisthesis is the slippage of one vertebral body in relationship to an adjacent vertebral body.[79]

The etiology of spondylolysis is controversial. Some authors regard spondylolysis as a congenital defect; others believe it is acquired secondary to trauma or repetitive high-impact exercise (see subsequent discussion). Spondylolisthesis often accompanies spondylolysis but can also be caused by ligamentous laxity and acute trauma.[79]

Incidence and age. Spondylolysis occurs at all ages and is seen in approximately 5% of the general population. Spondylolysthesis is also common.[79]

Location. Two thirds of spondylolyses occur at L5; 30% are at L4. Most are bilateral. Multilevel spondylolysis is rare.[79] L4-L5 and L5-S1 are the most common locations for spondylolisthesis. Age-related degenerative subluxations due to ligamentous laxity are also common in the cervical spine.

Imaging findings. Plain films findings of spondylolysis are lucent defects in the pars interarticularis with or without forward slippage of the upper vertebral body. NECT scans typically show bilateral pars defects, seen as irregular lucent clefts oriented nearly in the coronal plane (Fig. 20-34, *A*). If significant spondylolisthesis has occurred, the anteroposterior canal diameter is increased; severe cases show a "double canal" appearance (Fig. 20-34, *B*). The interposed disk is nearly always degenerated and bulging but rarely herniates (see Fig. 20-26, *A*). The neural foramina are deformed and variably narrowed.

In some cases of traumatic spondylolysis acquired from repeated high-impact activities, bone scintigraphy with single photon emission computed tomography (SPECT) may identify lesions not seen on planar imaging studies (see subsequent discussion).[80]

Miscellaneous stenoses and degenerative disorders. Calcification and ossification in spinal ligaments may cause spinal stenosis and compressive radiculomyelopathy. The two most common posterior spinal ligaments that ossify are the posterior longitudinal ligament and the ligamentum flavum.

Ossification of the posterior longitudinal ligament (OPLL). OPLL is a dense, ossified strip or plaque of variable thickness along the posterior margins of the vertebral bodies and intervertebral disks.[65] OPLL is an uncommon disorder that was originally described in the Japanese literature. The prevalence of OPLL in Japan is approximately 2%, the highest of any nation. OPLL is therefore often called the "Japanese disease."[81] Sporadic cases have been reported worldwide.[65]

OPLL is most common in the midcervical (C3-C5) and the midthoracic (T4-T7) spine.[65] Individuals with OPLL may be entirely asymptomatic, but others have reported various neurologic symptoms.

On NECT scans, the ossified strip that characterizes OPLL is typically separated from the vertebral body by a thin radiolucent zone.[65] Multilevel involvement is characteristic. Sagittal T1- or proton-density weighted MR scans show increased signal intensity from the fatty marrow of thickly ossified lesions; axial imaging is necessary to demonstrate thinly ossified OPLL.[81] The differential diagnosis of OPLL includes calcified HNP and calcified meningioma, although the shape and multilevel involvement of OPLL are characteristic.[81]

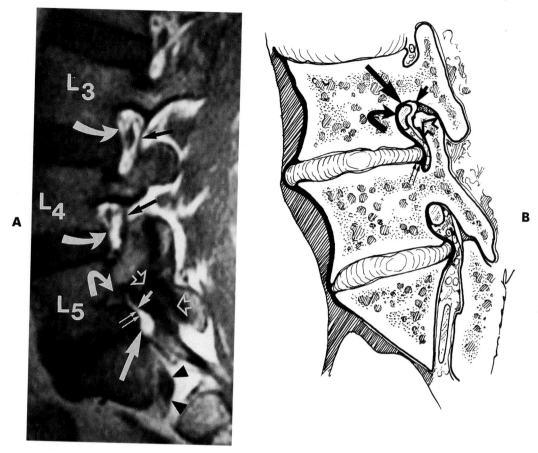

Fig. 20-33. A, Sagittal T1-weighted MR scan through the neural foramina shows normal L3-L4 and L4-L5 foramina *(slightly curved arrows)*. The ligamentum flavum *(black arrows)* at these two levels is normal. The L5-S1 foramen *(large arrow)* is severely narrowed by a combination of facet arthrosis *(open arrows)*, ligamentum flavum laxity *(small single arrow)*, and a lateral disk herniation *(double arrows)*. The S1 root *(arrowheads)* exits normally, whereas the L5 root *(tightly curved arrow)* is severely compressed. The patient had symptoms of right L5 neuropathy. **B,** Sagittal anatomic drawing shows similar degenerative changes at the L4-L5 neural foramen *(straight arrow)*. The foramen is narrowed by a combination of ligamentum flavum laxity *(small arrow)*, facet arthrosis *(open arrow)*, and disk bulge *(double arrows)*. Note severe compression of the exiting L4 nerve root *(curved arrow)*.

Ossification of the ligamentum flavum (OLF). Calcification or bone deposition in the ligamentum flavum and hyperostosis at its osseous attachments has been described. In the Far East, OLF is one of the most common causes of posterior thoracic spinal cord compression.[82]

Ankylosing spondylitis. Ankylosing spondylitis (AS) is a common rheumatologic disorder of adults, with an estimated incidence of 1.4% in the general population. There is disease-specific inflammation at the site of ligamentous insertions into bone.[83] The sacroiliac joints and the lumbar spine are the most commonly affected sites. Fracture/dislocation and spinal stenosis can cause attendant neurologic compromise.[83]

Disk Bulges and Disk Herniation

Disk bulges
Etiology and pathology. As the nucleus pulposus loses its turgor and the elasticity of the anulus diminishes, the disk bulges outward beyond the vertebral body margins.[63]

Incidence, age, and gender. Bulging of at least one lumbar disk is common in patients over 20 and frequently occurs in asymptomatic individuals.[57] Mild bulging of a cervical disk is also a common incidental finding.[66]

Imaging findings. Plain film findings of disk degeneration are indirect and include loss of intervertebral disk height, intradiskal gas (vacuum disk phenomenon), and end-plate osteophytes. On axial

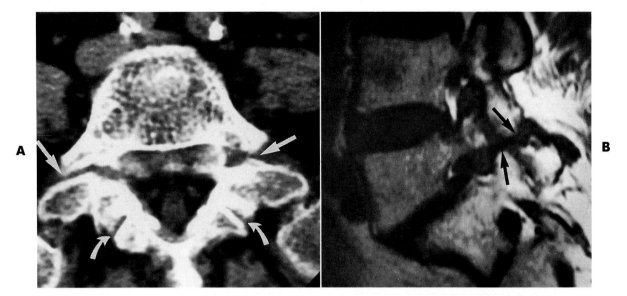

Fig. 20-34. Two cases illustrate imaging findings of spondylolysis with spondylolisthesis. **A,** Axial NECT scan shows bilateral pars interarticularis defects (spondylolysis), seen as the lucent clefts *(large arrows)* oriented nearly in the coronal plane. The facet joints are indicated by the curved arrows. The spinal canal is elongated from anterior to posterior, indicating significant spondylolysthesis. **B,** Sagittal T1-weighted scan in another case shows a pars interarticularis defect *(arrows)*. Spondylolysis with mild spondylolisthesis is present.

NECT and MR scans, a small bulging disk initially appears as loss of the normal posterior disk concavity (*see* Fig. 20-30, *B*). Moderate bulges are seen as diffuse, nonfocal protrusion of disk material beyond the adjacent vertebral end plate (*see* Fig. 20-25, *A*). Disk bulges are typically circumferential, broad-based, and symmetric. Decreased disk height and signal intensity are often seen on T2-weighted MR scans.

Disk bulges with coexisting anular tears are common in asymptomatic adults and are seen as areas of increased signal intensity on T2WI (*see* Fig. 20-19). Enhancement following contrast administration is seen in some anular tears because vascularized granulation tissue is present (Fig. 20-21, *C*).[84]

Disk herniation
Etiology and pathology. Herniation of the nucleus pulposus (HNP) through an anular defect causes focal protrusion of disk material beyond the margins of the adjacent vertebral end plate (*see* Fig. 20-19).

Incidence, age, and gender. Disk herniations are common; by age 60, nearly one third of asymptomatic patients have one or more lumbar HNPs.[57]

Location. Approximately 90% of lumbar disk herniations occur at L4-L5 or L5-S1.[63] Ninety-three percent are inside the spinal canal; 3% are predominately located in the intervertebral foramen, and 4% are extraforaminal (far lateral HNPs).[85]

In the cervical spine, C6-C7 is the site of 60% to 75% of HNPs, whereas C5-C6 accounts for 20% to

30% of cases.[66] The thoracic spine accounts for less than 1% of diskectomies.[86] Approximately 15% of asymptomatic adults have thoracic HNPs on MR imaging studies.[87]

Imaging findings. NECT, CT myelography, and MR have equivalent diagnostic accuracy in the diagnosis of lumbar HNP.[52] Myelographic findings in patients with HNPs include extradural deformity or displacement of the contrast-filled thecal sac, elevation, deviation, or amputation of the root sleeve, and edema of the affected nerve (Fig. 20-35).

NECT scans of HNPs typically show a soft tissue mass with effacement of the epidural fat and displacement of the thecal sac (Fig. 20-36). CT with intrathecal contrast nicely depicts the extradural mass caused by a herniated disk and clearly delineates its relationship to the spinal cord and proximal nerve roots (Fig. 20-37).

MR imaging exquisitely delineates HNPs and the relationship to adjacent soft tissues. Both T1- and T2-weighted sequences are useful (Fig. 20-38); sagittal and axial scans often add complementary information.

MR findings of HNP are focal, asymmetric protrusion of disk material beyond the confines of the anulus (Fig. 20-39). Because disk herniations rarely occur in the absence of a radial (type II) anular tear,[62] high signal in the posterior anulus is often seen on sagittal T2-weighted scans, although HNPs themselves are usually low signal (*see* Figs. 20-19 and 20-

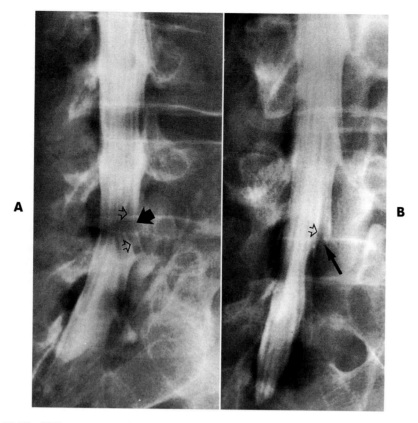

Fig. 20-35. Oblique views of two water-soluble lumbar myelograms show classic signs of disk herniation. **A,** An extradural defect *(large arrow)* is present at the L4-L5 interspace. The L5 nerve root *(open arrows)* is displaced and edematous. **B,** Another case shows root sleeve elevation and amputation *(black arrow)* from herniated disk. Note funnel-shaped enlargement of the elevated, edematous nerve *(open arrow)*.

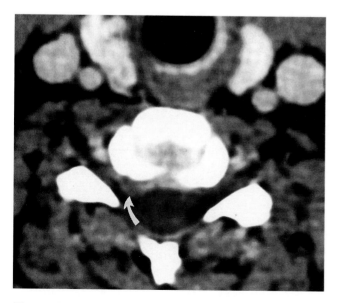

Fig. 20-36. Axial CECT scan shows a typical cervical HNP *(arrow)*.

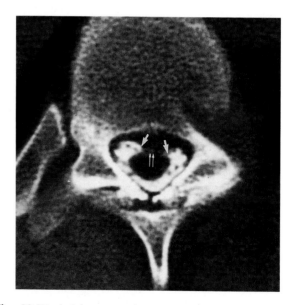

Fig. 20-37. Axial postmyelogram CT shows a herniated thoracic disk *(single arrows)* that displaces the thecal sac and compresses the spinal cord *(double arrows)*.

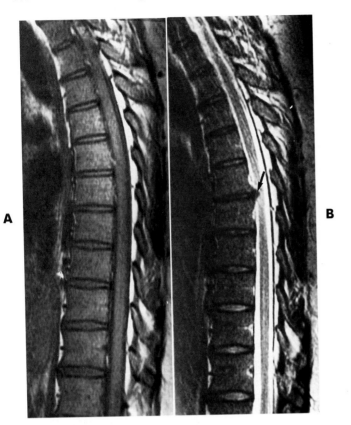

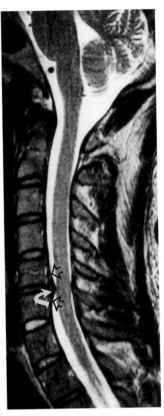

Fig. 20-38. Sagittal T1- **(A)** and T2-weighted **(B)** MR scans show the advantage of using both sequences for spine imaging. The T1WI shows the spine and disks particularly well, but the T2WI (MR "myelogram") depicts the HNP, which is nearly invisible on the T1WI.

Fig. 20-39. Sagittal T2-weighted MR scan shows a classic cervical HNP. The C5-C6 disk height is reduced and a small fragment *(curved arrow)* protrudes beyond the anulus. Note elevation of the posterior longitudinal ligament *(open arrows)*.

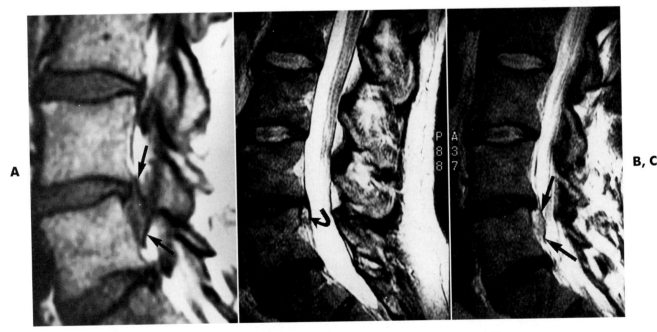

Fig. 20-40. This 42-year-old man experienced sudden onset of back pain following exertion. **A,** Sagittal T1-weighted MR scan shows disk fragments behind the L5 vertebral body *(arrows)*. **B** and **C,** T2WIs show the herniated disk *(curved arrow)* and inferior migratory fragments *(straight arrows)*. Note the high signal on T2WI, probably caused by associated edema. Symptoms resolved with conservative therapy.

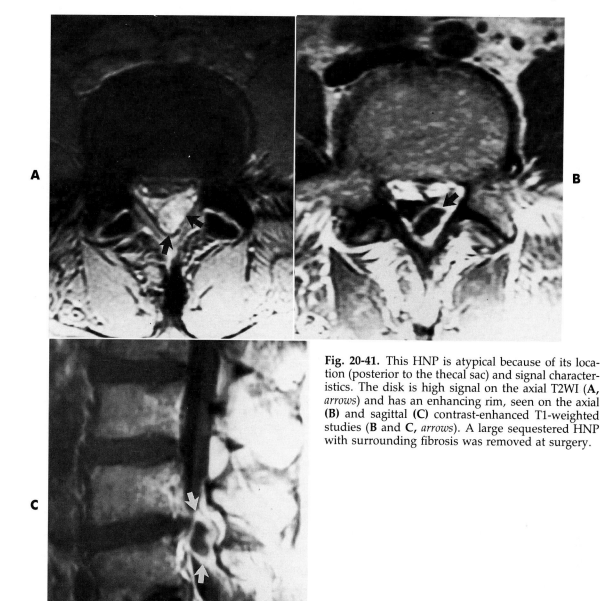

Fig. 20-41. This HNP is atypical because of its location (posterior to the thecal sac) and signal characteristics. The disk is high signal on the axial T2WI (**A,** *arrows*) and has an enhancing rim, seen on the axial (**B**) and sagittal (**C**) contrast-enhanced T1-weighted studies (**B** and **C,** *arrows*). A large sequestered HNP with surrounding fibrosis was removed at surgery.

20, *B*). Sagittal MR scans exquisitely depict the relationship of HNPs and degenerated facets to exiting nerve roots within the neural foramina (*see* Fig. 20-33).

Disk material can detach and migrate away from the parent disk. These so-called free fragments are easily detected on MR scans (Fig. 20-40). Cephalad and caudad extension occur approximately equally.[88]

Uncommon MR findings of HNPs include atypical signal intensity or unusual location. Some HNPs are high signal intensity on T1- or T2WI (Figs. 20-40, *B* and *C*, and 20-41, *A*). Ring enhancement following

contrast administration is sometimes seen with vascularized extruded fragments (Fig. 20-41, *B* and *C*).[89]

Unusual locations include extraforaminal HNP, atypical migratory disk patterns, and contrast enhancement. Sometimes disk herniation occurs completely outside the canal (so-called far lateral herniations) (Fig. 20-42). Occasionally, disk fragments are sequestered posterior to the thecal sac (Fig. 20-41).[90] Sometimes they migrate down a root sleeve (Fig. 20-43). Rarely, they penetrate the posterior longitudinal ligament and extend intradurally (Fig. 20-44). Vascularized disk fragments can occasionally enhance in-

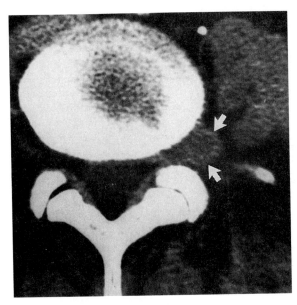

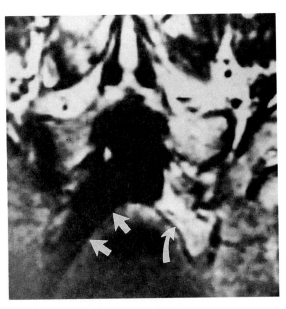

Fig. 20-42. Axial NECT scan in this patient with left anterior thigh pain shows a soft tissue mass *(arrows)* lateral to the left L3-L4 neural foramen. He had two previous CT scans; both were interpreted as normal. Review showed the lesion on both studies. Far lateral HNP was found at surgery.

Fig. 20-43. Coronal T1-weighted MR scan shows normal fat-filled S1 foramen on the left side *(curved arrow)*. The right S1 foramen is filled with low density soft tissue *(straight arrows)* that extends from the thecal sac into the pelvis. Preoperative diagnosis was nerve sheath tumor. Multiple migratory disk fragments were removed at surgery.

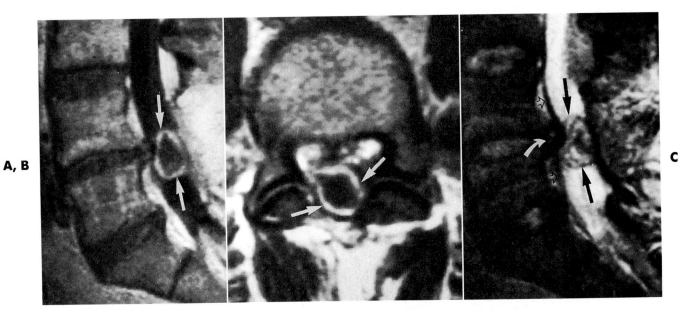

A, B

C

Fig. 20-44. Sagittal **(A)** and axial **(B)** postcontrast T1-weighted MR scans show a ring enhancing mass *(arrows)* in the thecal sac. Sagittal T2WI **(C)** shows the intermediate signal mass *(large arrows)*. The posterior longitudinal ligament *(open arrows)* is elevated by a small L4-L5 HNP *(curved arrow)*. Preoperative diagnosis was schwannoma. Intradural disk herniation was found at surgery. (From R. Wasserstrom et al, *AJNR* 14:401-404, 1993.)

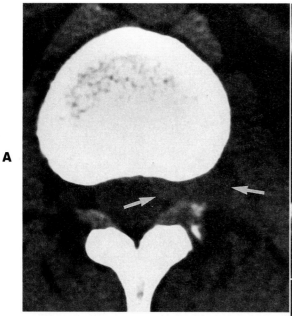

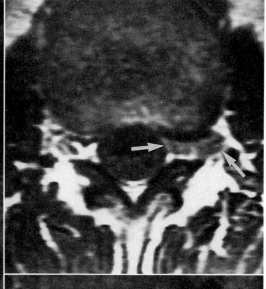

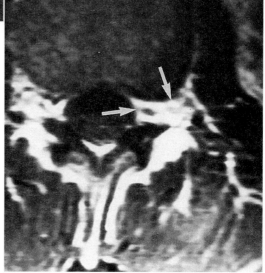

Fig. 20-45. A, Axial NECT scan shows a soft tissue mass *(arrows)* in the left neural foramen and extraforaminal area. **B,** Axial T1-weighted MR scan shows the intermediate signal mass *(arrows)*. **C,** Postcontrast T1WI shows the mass enhances strongly and uniformly *(arrows)*. Preoperative diagnosis was nerve root tumor. Surgery disclosed herniated, vascularized disk material.

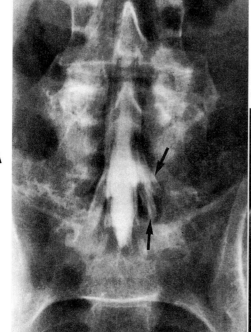

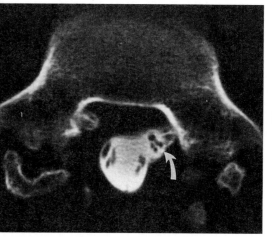

Fig. 20-46. AP view of **(A)** lumbar myelogram and **(B)** postmyelogram axial CT scan in two cases shows a conjoined nerve root *(arrows)*.

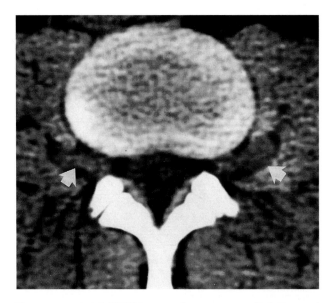

Fig. 20-47. Axial NECT scan shows two well-delineated rounded masses *(arrows)* along both exiting nerve roots. Dilated root sleeves (arachnoid diverticulae).

tensely following contrast administration. In all these cases, an HNP may closely resemble a neoplasm such as ependymoma or nerve root tumor.[89]

Contrast enhancement has limited use in the MR examination of the unoperated spine because unenhanced scans are diagnostic in most cases of lumbosacral disk degeneration or spinal stenosis. Occasionally, findings not identified on routine scans become apparent following contrast administration. Approximately 5% of patients will have abnormally enhancing intrathecal nerve roots (neuritis); 70% of these cases are associated with HNPs or disk bulges.[91,91a] In the cervical spine, contrast administration increases foraminal and epidural tissue conspicuity and may be helpful in difficult diagnostic cases.[84,102]

Differential diagnosis. The differential diagnosis of HNP includes normal variants such as conjoined nerve root, dilated root sleeve, and perineural cysts (Figs. 20-45, 20-46, and 20-47). Nerve root tumors such as schwannoma or neurofibroma may cause a foraminal or extraforaminal mass that can mimic a herniated disk (*see* Chapter 21).

Normal Postoperative Spine

"Normal" postoperative changes occur in both the osseous spine and soft tissues.

Osseous manifestations. Bony alterations vary with the specific surgical procedure. They range from simple laminotomy, in which a small focal defect or discontinuity in the neural arch is present, to wide laminectomy and partial or complete facetectomy. Fusions range from lateral or posterolateral bone grafts between the transverse and articular processes

to interbody fusions that cross the intervertebral disk space.[92]

Osseous abnormalities, including failed fusion, are initially imaged using plain films (with flexion and extension views) and thin-section CT with bone reconstruction algorithms. MR is helpful in delineating associated soft tissue lesions and defining the relationship of bony abnormalities to the thecal sac, spinal cord, and nerve roots.

Soft tissue changes. Alterations that are normally seen in the postoperative spine include epidural scarring or fibrosis, as well as changes in the intervertebral disk, paraspinous soft tissues, and nerve roots. Changes in the adjacent vertebral end plates and marrow are uncommon.[93]

Epidural fibrosis. Some degree of epidural fibrosis occurs after virtually all laminectomies and diskectomies.[94,95] NECT scans typically show effacement of epidural fat by soft tissue that is isodense with paraspinous muscle. The thecal sac is often retracted toward the scar and laminotomy site.

On MR scans epidural scar enhances immediately following contrast enhancement. Enhancement degree varies with postoperative interval. Epidural fibrosis enhances most strongly on imaging studies that are obtained less than 1 year following surgery[94,96]; some enhancement may persist for years after operation.

Disk space changes. Intervertebral disk space undergoes little change in MR signal intensity after uncomplicated diskectomy.[93] Following contrast administration, enhancement of the posterior anulus is seen in over 80% of asymptomatic diskectomy patients, whereas enhancement within the central disk space normally occurs in less than 20% of cases.[93]

Paraspinous soft tissues. Disruption of normal soft tissue planes between fat and muscle is typical. Fat grafts are seen as very low density areas without significant mass effect.[92] Occasionally, there may be focal protrusion of dura and CSF through a laminectomy defect and a postoperative meningocele is formed.

Nerve roots. Pre- and postoperative enhancement of the dorsal root ganglia and distal nerve roots is normal because these structures do not possess a blood-nerve barrier.[97] Enhancement of one or more intrathecal nerve roots following contrast administration is also normal on MR scans obtained within 6 months after surgery.[95]

Vertebral body changes. End plate erosions are not a common feature of uncomplicated diskectomy and disk space curettage typically does not change the MR signal of the adjacent vertebral body marrow. Postcontrast marrow enhancement adjacent to the operative site is common with diskitis but is rarely observed in asymptomatic patients.[93]

"Failed Back" Syndromes

Patients with so-called failed back surgery syndrome (FBSS) constitute a difficult management problem for clinicians and pose special diagnostic challenges for radiologists. In this section we consider the imaging spectrum of abnormalities encountered in FBSS.

Etiology and pathology. There are many causes for FBSS (*see* box). Some are related to the surgery; others are not. Surgically related causes for FBSS include epidural hematoma, recurrent HNP at the operated site, diskitis and osteomyelitis, epidural scar, arachnoiditis, and meningocele or CSF fistula.[98]

Common nonsurgical causes of FBSS are HNP at a nonsurgical site, facet arthrosis, spinal stenosis, spondylolysis with or without spondylolisthesis, and referred pain from other areas such as hip disease. Less common causes of FBSS include conus medullaris or filum terminale tumor, pelvic neoplasms, and nonneoplastic cysts such as intrasacral meningocele, intradural arachnoid cyst, or facet joint (synovial) cyst. Spinal, meningeal, or, especially, nerve root inflammation are also potential causes of FBSS.[99]

Incidence. FBSS reportedly occurs in 10% to 40% of patients following low back surgery.[92,100] Immediate postoperative complications such as epidural hematoma, retained fragment, or acute disk reherniation are relatively uncommon. Delayed complications such as diskitis and osteomyelitis are rare, seen in 1% to 3% of cases.[93]

Of all potential causes for FBSS, spondylosis, arthrosis, and recurrent HNP at the same or a different level are probably the most common etiologies.[92] The role of epidural fibrosis in FBSS is controversial. Epidural fibrosis occurs in most postoperative spines but neither the amount of scar nor the degree of contrast enhancement has been directly correlated with the clinical syndrome.[99,101]

Neuritis, identified as intrathecal enhancement of one or more nerve roots, is seen in approximately 20% of FBSS.[92] Although early postoperative root enhancement is common in asymptomatic patients, persistent enhancement beyond 6 to 8 months has a high correlation with clinical symptoms.[99]

Other causes of FBSS are uncommon. Arachnoiditis is now comparatively rare. Occult filum terminale tumor such as schwannoma or ependymoma is seen in less than 1% of cases, but the conus medullaris should nevertheless be imaged on all routine lumbosacral MR scans, as well as on myelograms and CT-myelograms.

Imaging findings. Persistent or recurrent symptoms in the immediate postoperative period are usually caused by epidural hematoma, retained fragment, or recurrent HNP. All appear as nonspecific extradural mass effects on both CT-myelography and MR scans (Fig. 20-48). Distinction between these entities on MR scans may be especially difficult during the first few days or weeks following surgery (Fig. 20-49).

In the subacute and chronic stage, the most criti-

"Failed Back" Surgery Syndrome*

Very common

Recurrent/persistent HNP at operated site
HNP at other site
Epidural scar/fibrosis (?role)
Facet arthrosis/spinal stenosis

Common

Neuritis
Referred pain from nonspinous site

Uncommon

Diskitis/osteomyelitis/epidural abscess
Arachnoiditis
Conus tumor
Thoracic, high lumbar HNP
Epidural hematoma

*Excluding secondary gain, other nonmedical causes.

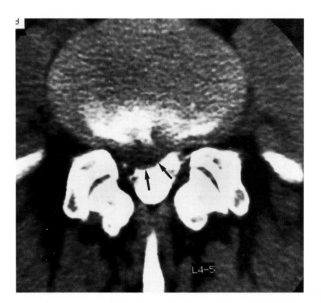

Fig. 20-48. Failed back surgery syndrome (FBSS). This patient complained of severe right leg pain immediately following diskectomy. Postmyelogram CT scan obtained 2 hours after surgery shows a large central-right extradural soft tissue mass (*arrows*) compressing the thecal sac. Preoperative diagnosis was retained disk fragment or epidural hematoma. Epidural hematoma was found at reexploration. No disk material was present.

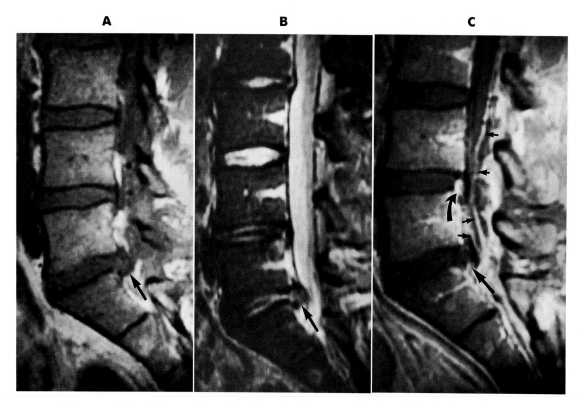

Fig. 20-49. This 32-year-old man had a right L5 radiculopathy that remained unchanged following L4-L5 and L5-S1 diskectomies. MR scan was obtained 6 days after surgery. Sagittal T1- **(A)** and T2-weighted **(B)** scans show a possible L5-S1 recurrent HNP *(arrows).* Sagittal T1-weighted scan **(C)** obtained following contrast administration shows most of the mass enhances *(large straight arrow).* Note enhancement at the posterior anulus of L4-L5 *(curved arrow),* a normal postoperative finding. Nerve root enhancement *(small arrows)* is striking but is also normal up to 6 months following surgery. Reexploration disclosed only hemorrhage and surgical changes.

cal imaging issue is recurrent HNP versus epidural scar because the former may warrant reoperation, whereas the latter does not. NECT is less specific than either CECT or MR.[96] Findings suggestive of disk on NECT scans include mass effect, contiguity with the disk space, density greater than 90 Hounsfield units (HU), gas or calcium collection, and nodularity, whereas scar more often lacks mass effect, is located above or below the disk space, and has a linear configuration.[100]

Disk can be distinguished from epidural fibrosis on 80% of CECT studies.[96] Disks are typically seen as areas of decreased attenuation with a peripheral rim of enhancement, whereas scar demonstrates homogeneous enhancement.[100]

Conventional pre- and postcontrast MR scans are 96% accurate in differentiating disk from scar[102]; special sequences such as fat-suppressed scans are typically not required (Fig. 20-50).[103] Mature, organized epidural scar enhances consistently and intensely on early postinjection T1WI, whereas disk material usually—although not invariably—does not enhance

immediately following contrast administration (Fig. 20-51).[102,103a] Signal intensity is less helpful in distinguishing these two entities.[96]

A spectrum of imaging changes are seen in postoperative arachnoiditis. Myelographic findings of mild arachnoiditis are blunting of the caudal nerve root sleeves, segmental nerve root fusion, and small irregularities of the thecal sac margin.[104] Multisegmental nerve root fusion with root sleeve obliteration, intradural scarring, and loculation is seen with moderate arachnoiditis (Fig. 20-52). Severe adhesive arachnoiditis may cause a myelographic block.[104]

On axial postmyelogram CT scans, nodular or cordlike intradural masses are seen with moderately severe disease (Fig. 20-53, *A*). Sometimes the nerve roots are annealed against the dura and the thecal sac appears empty or featureless (naked sac sign) (Fig. 20-53, *B*). MR findings of arachnoiditis include intradural fibrosis, nerve root clumping, loculation and sacculation, root retraction, and adhesions (Fig. 20-54).

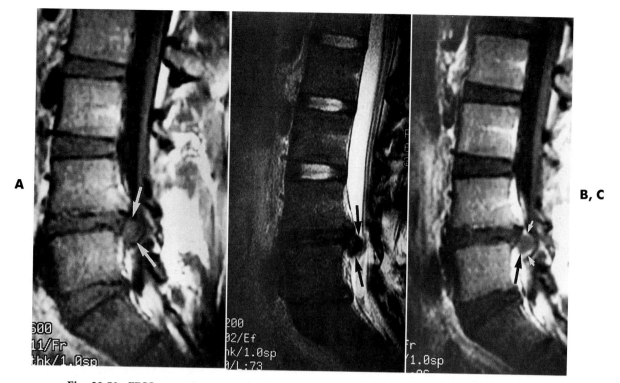

Fig. 20-50. FBSS secondary to recurrent HNP. Sagittal T1- **(A)** and T2-weighted **(B)** MR scans show recurrent L4-L5 HNP. The disk fragment *(arrows)* is isointense with the parent disk on both sequences. Postcontrast sagittal T1WI **(C)** shows peripheral enhancement *(small arrows)*, but the central mass *(large arrows)* remains low signal intensity. Recurrent HNP surrounded by epidural fibrosis was found at surgery.

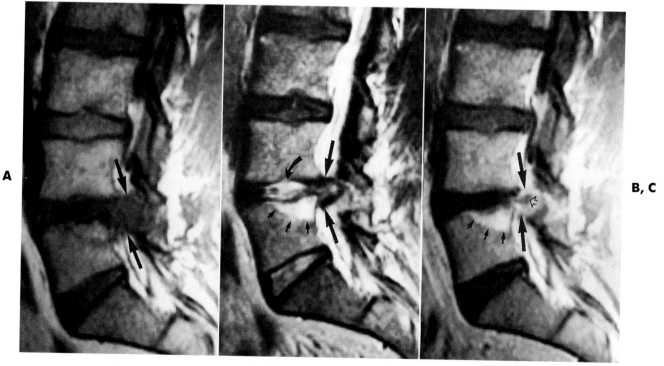

Fig. 20-51. Sagittal pre-contrast T1- **(A)** and T2-weighted **(B)** MR scans in this patient with FBSS show a large soft tissue mass at the L4-L5 interspace *(large arrows)*. Note high signal in the nucleus pulposus **(B,** *curved arrow)* and adjacent marrow **(B,** *small arrows)*. Postcontrast T1WI **(C)** shows all of the mass enhances *(large arrows)* except for a small central portion *(open arrow)*. The disk space does not enhance, but the adjacent marrow *(small arrows)* shows some increased signal intensity. Surgery disclosed a large amount of epidural scar surrounding a small retained disk fragment. There was no evidence for diskitis or osteomyelitis.

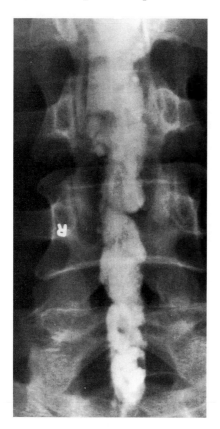

Fig. 20-52. Myelographic findings of moderately severe arachnoiditis on an AP view. Note sacculation, effacement of root sleeves, intradural adhesions, and focal scarring.

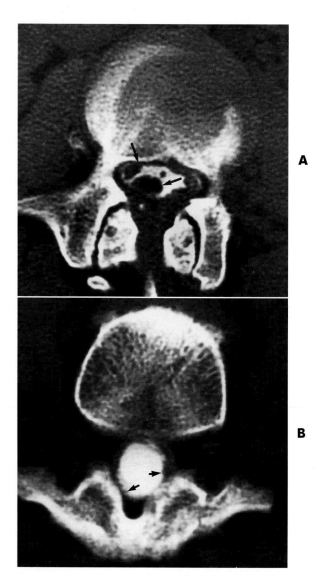

Fig. 20-53. Two cases illustrate CT-myelographic findings of arachnoiditis. **A,** Intradural fibrosis with clumped nerve roots *(arrows).* **B,** Featureless, "naked" thecal sac caused by retraction and adhesion of nerve roots *(arrows)* to the lateral dural wall.

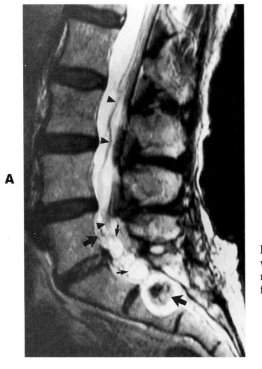

Fig. 20-54. MR findings of arachnoiditis. Sagittal T2-weighted MR scan **(A)** shows thickened, clumped nerve roots *(arrowheads),* sacculation *(small arrows),* and intradural fibrotic masses *(large arrows).*

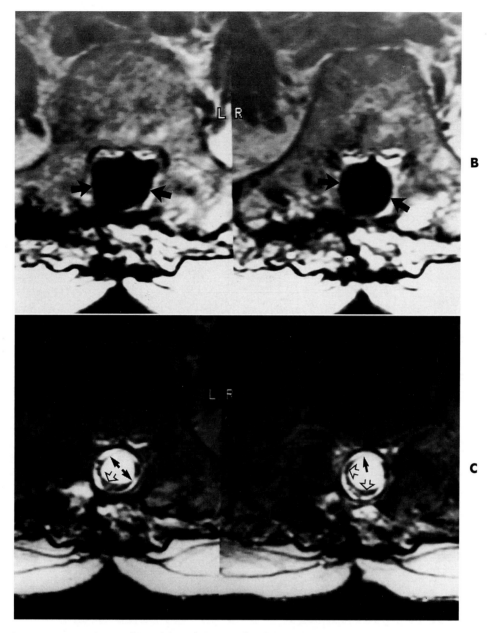

Fig. 20-54, cont'd. Axial T1- (**B**) and T2-weighted (**C**) MR scans in another case show a relatively featureless sac (**B,** *arrows*) with loculated intradural cyst (**C,** *solid arrows*) and retracted, scarred roots (**C,** *open arrows*) (compare with Fig. 20-53, *B*).

Postoperative osteomyelitis can be identified on both CT and MR studies (Figs. 20-55 and 20-56). Contrast-enhanced MR is particularly helpful for delineating diskitis and epidural abscess (Fig. 20-56). Postcontrast T1-weighted scans also show abnormal nerve root enhancement, a relatively common cause of FBSS (Fig. 20-57).

Conus medullaris or filum terminale tumors may be overlooked unless the thoracolumbar junction is routinely imaged on myelograms or MR studies (Fig.

20-58). Other masses that can be overlooked or complicate lumbar surgery and cause postoperative symptoms include synovial cysts and pseudomeningoceles (Figs. 20-59 and 20-60).

Back Pain in Children

In contrast to adults, low back pain in children is uncommonly caused by facet arthroses, spinal stenosis, disk herniation or desire for secondary gain, and often indicates serious disease (*see* box, p. 866).

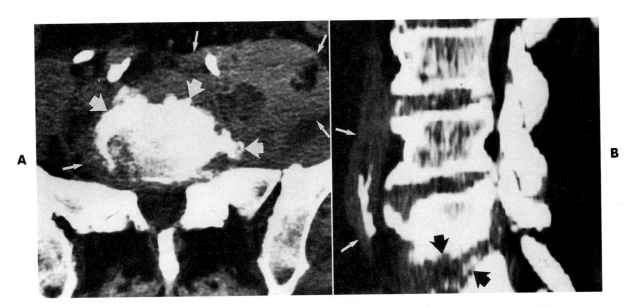

Fig. 20-55. FBSS secondary to postoperative diskitis and osteomyelitis. **A,** Axial NECT scan shows irregular erosion and end plate destruction *(large arrows)* with psoas abscesses *(small arrows).* **B,** Sagittal midline reformatted scan shows the irregular end plates *(large arrows)* and paravertebral soft tissue mass *(small arrows).*

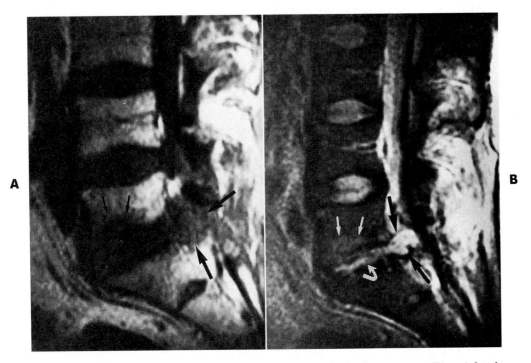

Fig. 20-56. FBSS with diskitis and epidural abscess. **A,** Sagittal precontrast T1-weighted MR scan shows low signal marrow *(small arrows)* and a soft tissue mass *(large arrows)* at the L5-S1 interspace. **B,** Sagittal T2WI shows high signal in the disk space *(curved arrow)*, marrow *(small arrows)*, and soft tissue mass *(large arrows).*

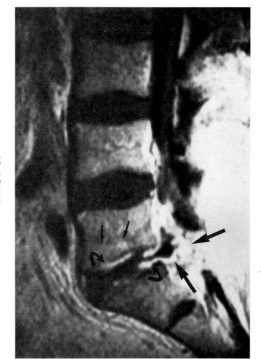

Fig. 20-56, cont'd. C, Sagittal T1WI following contrast administration shows enhancement in the disk space *(curved arrows)* and marrow *(small arrows)*, and around a loculated low signal fluid collection *(large arrows).*

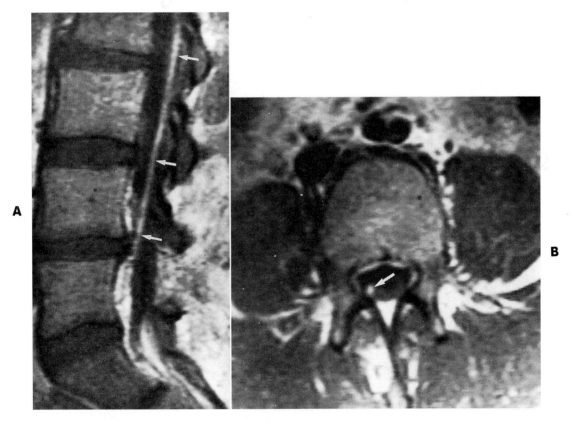

Fig. 20-57. FBSS secondary to neuritis. Postcontrast sagittal **(A)** and axial **(B)** T1-weighted MR scans show enhancing L4 nerve root *(arrows).* (From Jinkins JR, Osborn AG et al, *AJNR* 14:383-394, 1993.)

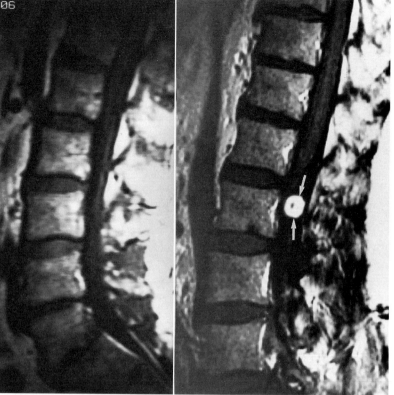

Fig. 20-58. This 46-year-old man had persisting low back pain 1 year after L4-L5 and L5-S1 diskectomies for bulging disks. **A,** First sagittal T1-weighted MR scan was interpreted as normal. Note suboptimal view of conus. **B,** Repeat study with contrast enhancement obtained 3 months later shows a conus medullaris mass *(arrows)*. A schwannoma was found at surgery. The patient's symptoms completely resolved after tumor removal.

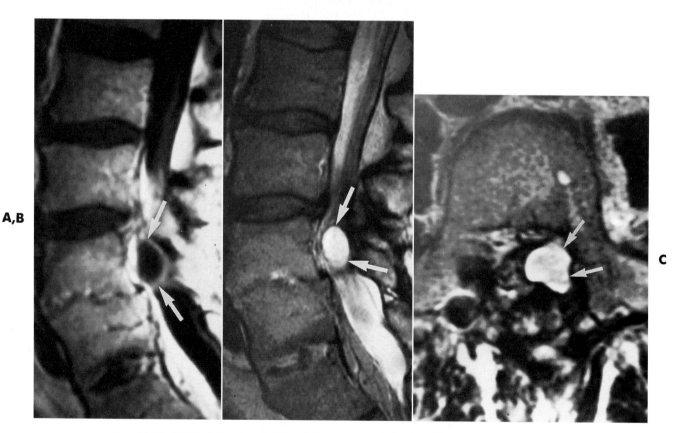

Fig. 20-59. FBSS following L4-L5 diskectomy and fusion. Sagittal postcontrast T1-weighted MR scan **(A)** shows an enhancing cystic mass *(arrows)*. Sagittal **(B)** and axial **(C)** T2WIs show the well-delineated cystic mass *(arrows)* has high signal intensity. Juxtaarticular (synovial) cyst was found.

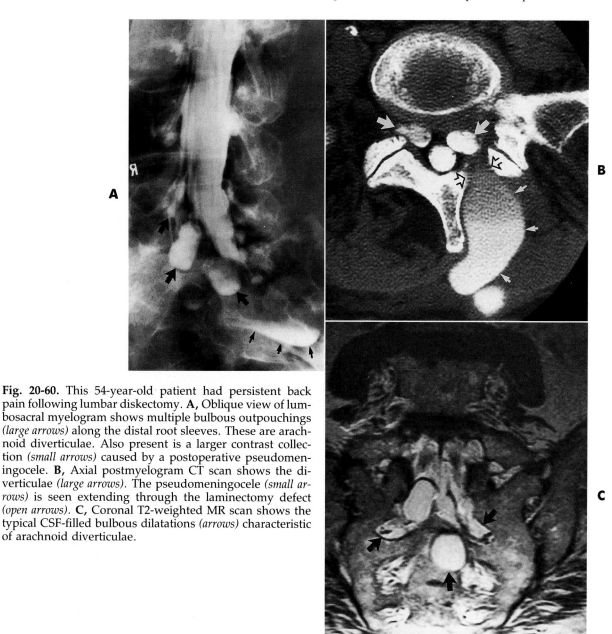

Fig. 20-60. This 54-year-old patient had persistent back pain following lumbar diskectomy. **A,** Oblique view of lumbosacral myelogram shows multiple bulbous outpouchings *(large arrows)* along the distal root sleeves. These are arachnoid diverticulae. Also present is a larger contrast collection *(small arrows)* caused by a postoperative pseudomeningocele. **B,** Axial postmyelogram CT scan shows the diverticulae *(large arrows)*. The pseudomeningocele *(small arrows)* is seen extending through the laminectomy defect *(open arrows)*. **C,** Coronal T2-weighted MR scan shows the typical CSF-filled bulbous dilatations *(arrows)* characteristic of arachnoid diverticulae.

Congenital anomalies. Occult spinal dysraphic disorders can cause painful scoliosis. Low back pain is also often seen with thick filum terminale and tethered conus medullaris *(see* Chapter 19).

Trauma. Spondylolysis and spondylolisthesis are common. Overuse injuries secondary to repetitive, unrepaired microtrauma are frequent, particularly in athletes engaging in high-impact sports (Fig. 20-61).[105] Pars interarticularis stress fractures and "limbus" fractures of the vertebral body ring apophysis are common injuries.[106] An avulsed, displaced arc-

uate end-plate fragment with attached disk material is present (Fig. 20-62).[107]

Infection. Diskitis and osteomyelitis are most commonly found in children younger than 10 years old.[105]

Disk herniation. Disk herniation in prepubescent children is rare, but its prevalence in adolescents is increasing. It nearly always occurs acutely with sudden exertion and is therefore a traumatic injury rather than a degenerative one (see previous discussion).

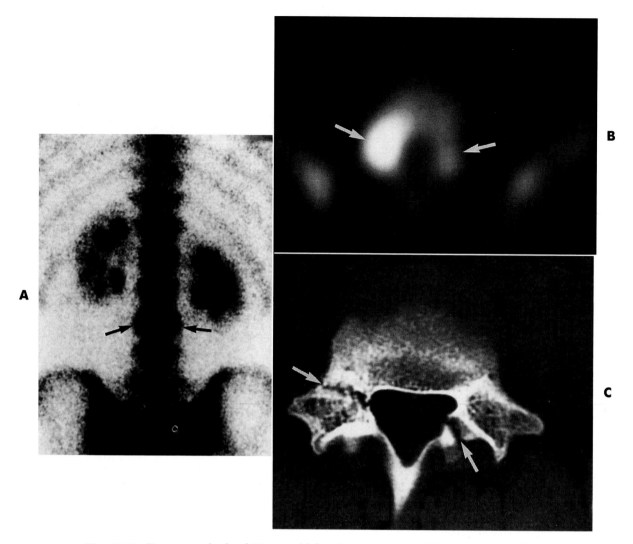

Fig. 20-61. Two cases, both of 13-year-old female gymnasts with low back pain, illustrate imaging findings with stress fractures. **A,** Radionuclide bone scan shows abnormal uptake at the L3 pedicles *(arrows)*. **B,** Tomographic SPECT scan in the second case shows abnormal uptake in the articular pillars *(arrows)*. **C,** NECT scan shows bilateral stress fractures *(arrows)*.

Back Pain in Children*

Congenital malformation (occult dysraphism, tethered cord, diastematomyelia, hydromyelia)
Systemic disease (e.g., sickle cell anemia)
Overuse injury with stress fracture
Avulsion fracture of ring apophysis with detached disk fragment (HNP otherwise uncommon in children)
Spondylolysis, spondylolisthesis
Scheuerman disease
Diskitis, osteomyelitis
Tumor (spinal column, spinal cord)
Referred pain (check kidneys, hips, etc.)

*Not factitious; disease usually real; to be taken seriously.

Scheuerman disease is a common disorder that consists of vertebral body wedging, end-plate irregularities, and narrowed disk spaces with or without disk herniation. Intravertebral disk herniation (Schmorl's nodes) are commonly associated with Scheuerman disease.[105]

Neoplasms. Benign neoplasms and tumorlike lesions in children that may cause back pain include osteoid osteoma, osteoblastoma, and aneurysmal bone cyst; primary osseous malignant tumors include Ewing sarcoma and lymphoma. Pain is also a frequent early presenting symptom in children with intramedullary spinal cord tumors such as astrocytoma or ependymoma *(see Fig. 21-45).*[108]

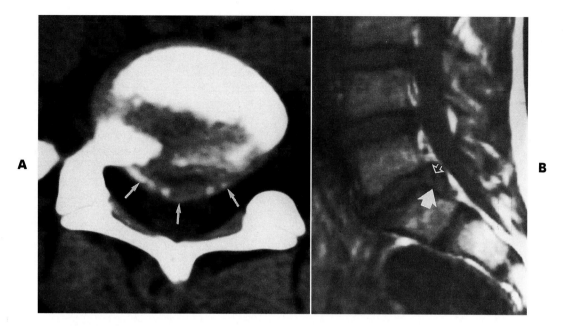

Fig. 20-62. This 12-year-old basketball player had a twisting fall. **A,** Axial NECT scan shows an avulsed ring apophysis with accompanying disk fragment *(arrows).* **B,** Sagittal T1-weighted MR scan shows the disk *(large arrow)* with central, very hypointense area representing avulsed cortex *(open arrow).*

Miscellaneous. Hip disorders, systemic abnormalities such as sickle cell disease, and gastrointestinal or genitourinary problems can cause back pain.

TRAUMA

In this section, we briefly consider the role of CT and MR imaging in evaluating the patient with spine trauma, particularly soft tissue injury.

Mechanisms of Spine Injury

There are four basic types of spine injury: flexion and extension injuries, axial loading (compression) injury, and rotational injury. Each type of injury has manifestations that are relatively site-specific for different regions of the spine.[109]

Flexion injury. Flexion injury is common in the cervical and thoracic spine and at the thoracolumbar junction. Flexion injury typically results in anterior wedging and vertebral body fractures.[109] With sufficient force, disruption of the posterior longitudinal ligament and interspinous ligaments occurs. Facet distraction and anteroposterior subluxation is also common with severe injury.

Extension injury. Extension injury is particularly common in the cervical region. The most common abnormality is posterior element fracture. With sufficient hyperextension, the anterior longitudinal ligament ruptures and subluxation may occur.

Axial loading. These are compressive and vertical force injuries. Typical examples include cervical axial loading from diving injury and thoracolumbar loading from jumping injury. Axial loading commonly results in vertebral body compression (burst) fractures. Lateral element fractures and compression injury (e.g., articular pillar fractures of the cervical spine) are also common.

Rotation injury. Rotation injury is rarely isolated and usually occurs in combination with flexion-extension injury.[109] Lateral mass fractures and facet subluxations are common. Uncovertebral fracture dislocations are frequent manifestations of cervical spine rotation injury.

Osseous Spine Injury Patterns

Cervical spine

C1 (atlas). Atlantooccipital dislocation is often, but not invariably, fatal. A dens to basion distance greater than 12.5 mm on lateral plain film radiographs should suggest this rare injury.[109a] The most common injury to C1 is a bilateral vertical fracture through the neural arch. This so-called *Jefferson fracture* is a burst fracture that involves both the anterior and posterior arches (Fig. 20-63). The patient is neurologically intact unless the transverse ligament is also disrupted.[110] Instability may be present with flexion-extension.[111]

Rotatory *atlantoaxial dislocation* is rare. Here, the at-

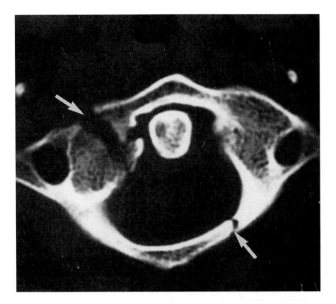

Fig. 20-63. Axial NECT scan shows the anterior and posterior arch fractures of the C1 ring *(arrows)*, also known as a "Jefferson" fracture. The transverse ligament is intact, and the relationship between the axis and dens remains normal.

las is rotated more than 45 degrees and the facets are often locked. Nontraumatic C1-C2 rotational subluxation can occur with various lesions such as rheumatoid arthritis. C1-C2 subluxation can result from tonsillitis and pharyngitis and is a cause of torticollis in children.

C2 (axis). Odontoid (dens) fractures usually occur at the base of the dens. Horizontal dens fractures can be subtle on axial CT scans, and reformatted sagittal and coronal views are particularly useful (Fig. 20-64). The so-called Hangman's fracture is caused by hyperextension resulting in bilateral neural arch fractures (traumatic spondylolysis) (Fig. 20-65). The odontoid and its attachments are intact. Typically there are bilateral C2 pedicle fractures with separation of the neural arch from the C2 body. Anterior subluxation of the C1-C2 complex is common, but spinal cord damage is rare.

C3-C7. Typical flexion injuries include simple wedge fracture of one or more anterior vertebral bodies. Unless the posterior longitudinal ligament (PLL) is disrupted or there is axial loading, retropulsed vertebral body is usually absent.[110] If hyperflexion oc-

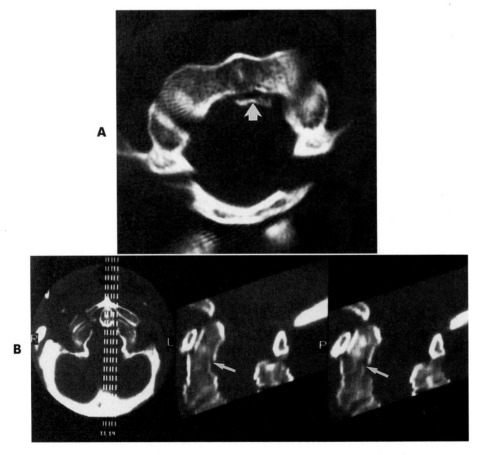

Fig. 20-64. An elderly nursing home resident had a fall. **A,** Axial NECT scan shows some C1-C2 rotation and a bone fragment behind the C2 body *(arrows)*. **B,** Sagittal reformatted scans show the dens is fractured *(arrows)* and displaced posteriorly.

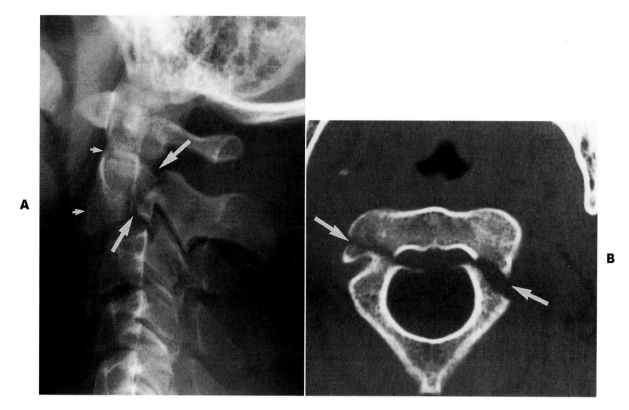

Fig. 20-65. A, Lateral plain film shows traumatic spondylolysis (Hangman's fracture) of C2 *(large arrows)*. Note anterior displacement of the C1-C2 body complex *(small arrows)*. **B,** Axial NECT scan shows the fracture extends through the pedicles and inferior C2 body *(arrows)*. The patient was neurologically intact.

curs, the PLL and interspinous ligaments are disrupted. The posterior aspect of the affected intervertebral disk space is often widened. Facet fracture-subluxation can also occur with flexion injury (Fig. 20-66). Other fractures that occur with flexion injury are the *"clay-shoveler's" fracture* (avulsed spinous process, usually C6 or C7) and the *"teardrop"* or *"burst" fracture*. Posterior vertebral body displacement with spinal cord injury is common with burst injuries.[110] Vertical compression from diving injury can also cause burst fractures of the mid- and lower cervical spine.[109]

Extension injuries often disrupt the anterior longitudinal ligament (ALL), widening the anterior aspect of the affected intervertebral disk space. Prevertebral soft tissue swelling is often present. Avulsion fractures of the anterior vertebral bodies and articular pillar compression fractures are common. Nerve root compression and spinal cord injury without obvious fracture-dislocation can occur with extension injury.[110]

Thoracic spine. Thoracic fractures are less common than cervical and thoracolumbar junction injury. *Thoracic "burst" fractures* can occur with severe axial loading. Because the ribs and sternum act as stabiliz-

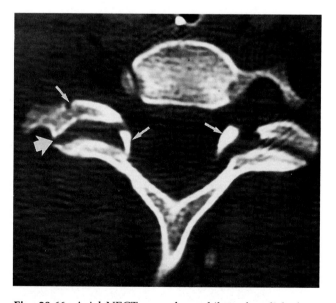

Fig. 20-66. Axial NECT scan shows bilateral pedicle fractures *(small arrows)* with some distraction of the superior and inferior articular facets on the right, seen as joint space widening *(large arrow)*.

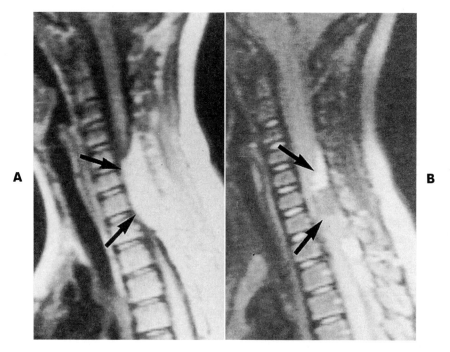

Fig. 20-67. This 3-year-old child with quadriparesis following cervical spine injury had normal plain film examination (not shown). Sagittal T1- **(A)** and proton density-weighted MR scans **(B)** show a large subacute epidural hematoma *(arrows)*. The scan was obtained 5 days after the injury.

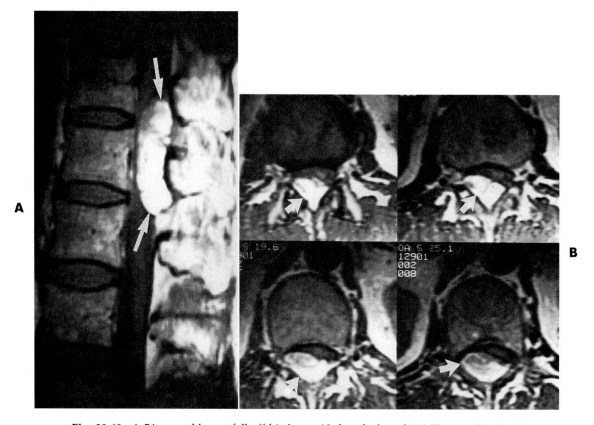

Fig. 20-68. A 54-year-old man fell off his horse 10 days before this MR scan. Study was obtained because of bilateral lower extremity weakness and sphincter incontinence. Sagittal **(A)** and axial **(B)** T1-weighted scans show a large extraaxial high signal mass *(arrows)* with severe cord compression. Epidural hematoma was removed at surgery.

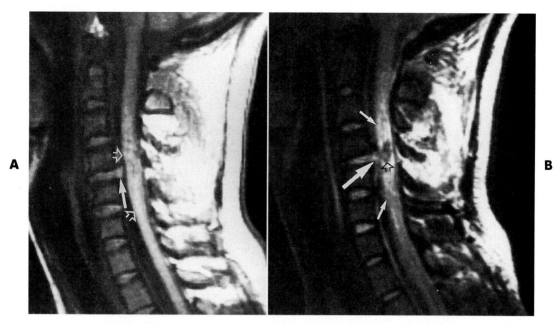

Fig. 20-69. A 32-year-old man was quadriplegic following an automobile accident. Plain films and NECT scan showed no fracture, but mild C4-C5 subluxation with slight widening of the posterior interspace was seen. MR scan was obtained 6 hours after injury. **A,** Sagittal T1-weighted MR scan shows traumatic disk herniation *(large arrow)* with focally enlarged spinal cord *(open arrows)*. **B,** Sagittal proton density-weighted study shows the disk herniation *(large arrow)* and cord contusion, seen here as edema *(small arrows)* surrounding a focal hypointense area *(open arrow)*. The anterior and posterior longitudinal ligaments are disrupted.

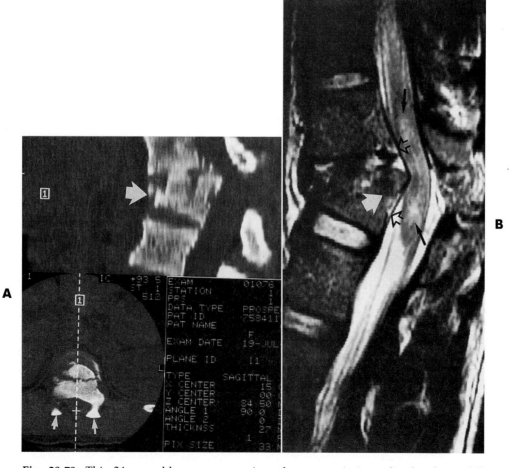

Fig. 20-70. This 24-year-old woman experienced paraparesis immediately after a fall while rock climbing. **A,** Axial NECT scan shows "naked" facets *(small arrows)*, characteristic for severe facet distraction. The sagittal reformatted image shows the thoracolumbar "burst" fracture *(large arrow)* with acute traumatic kyphosis. **B,** Sagittal T2-weighted MR scan shows the deformed spinal canal with retropulsed vertebral body fragment *(large arrow)* impinging on the conus. Note conus edema *(small arrows)*, but no focal intramedullary hematoma is identified. The posterior longitudinal ligament *(open arrows)* is intact.

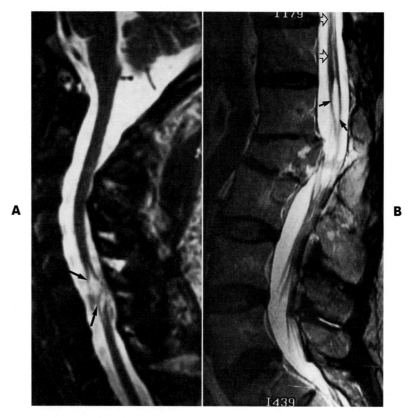

Fig. 20-71. Use of MR imaging to assess long-term sequelae of traumatic spinal cord injury. **A,** Sagittal T2WI in this 33-year-old quadriplegic man shows cord transection *(arrows)* and atrophy. **B,** Sagittal T2-weighted scan in this 28-year-old woman paraplegic with an old thoracolumbar burst fracture shows proximal cord atrophy with myelomalacia *(open arrows).* A small focal syrinx *(small arrows)* is present.

ing forces, thoracic fractures are usually stable, unless multiple rib or sternal fractures are present.[110]

Thoracolumbar junction. The majority of thoracolumbar fractures occur between T12 and L2. Nearly 75% are *compression fractures,* with anterior wedging of one or more vertebral bodies and intact posterior elements. Approximately 20% of thoracolumbar injuries are *fracture-dislocations* in which there is a wedge or burst fracture of the vertebral body combined with facet injury (see subsequent discussion). The facets can be fractured, subluxed, perched, dislocated, or locked.[110]

Soft Tissue Injury

MR is particularly helpful when neurologic deficits are disproportionate to the observed injury. In children, significant spinal cord injury can occur without obvious fracture-dislocation. MR depicts cord contusion and edema, and detects extraaxial lesions such as epidural hematoma (Fig. 20-67). In adults, soft tissue lesions such as epidural hematoma (Fig. 20-68) and traumatic disk herniation with cord compression or contusion (Fig. 20-69) are best delineated with emergent MR imaging.

In many cases of spine trauma the optimal imaging sequence combines thin-section high-resolution axial CT scans using multiplanar reconstruction (Fig. 20-70, *A*) with MR evaluation of the spinal cord and paraspinous soft tissues (Fig. 20-70, *B*). The precise location of bone fragments can be identified on CT, whereas soft tissue injury to the intervertebral disk, ligaments, and spinal cord is exquisitely delineated with MR.

Long-term sequelae of spinal cord trauma such as cord transection, traumatic syrinx, myelomalacia, and meningocele are well delineated using high-resolution MR imaging (Fig. 20-71).

REFERENCES

1. Sklar EML, Post MJD, Lebwohl NH: Imaging of infection of the lumbosacral spine, *Neuroimaging* 3:577-590, 1993.
2. Post MJD, Sze G, Quencer RM et al: Gadolinium-enhanced MR in spinal infection, *J Comp Asst Tomogr* 14:721-729, 1990.
3. Sharif HS: Role of MR imaging in the management of spinal infections, *AJR* 158:1333-1345, 1992.
4. Brant-Zawadzki M: Infections. In Newton TH, Potts DG, editors: *Modern Neuroradiology, vol 1: Computed Tomography of the Spine and Spinal Cord,* pp. 205-229, 1983.
5. Mark AS: MRI of infections and inflammatory diseases of the spine, *MRI Decisions* pp. 12-26, March/April 1991.

6. Thrush A, Enzmann D: MR imaging of infectious spondylitis, *AJNR* 11:1171-1180, 1990.

7. Resnick D: Inflammatory diseases of the vertebral column, *Categorical Course on Spine and Cord Imaging,* pp. 51-49, American Society of Neuroradiology, 1988.

8. Sharif HS, Aideyan OA, Clark DC et al: Brucellar and tuberculosis spondylitis: comparative imaging features, *Radiol* 171:419-425, 1989.

9. Smith AS, Weinstein MA, Mizushima A et al: MR imaging of characteristics of tuberculosis spondylitis vs. vertebral osteomyelitis, *AJNR* 10:619-625, 1989.

10. Boxer DI, Pratt C, Hine AL, McNicol M: Radiological features during and following treatment of spinal tuberculosis, *Br J Radiol* 65:476-479, 1992.

11. Arabi KM, Al Sebai MW, Al Chakaki M: Evaluation of radiological investigations in spinal tuberculosis, *Intl Orthopaedics (SICOT)* 16:165-167, 1992.

12. Numaguchi Y, Rigamonti D, Rothman MI et al: Spinal epidural abscess: evaluation with gadolinium-enhanced MR imaging, *RadioGraphics* 13:545-559, 1993.

13. Sandhu FS, Dillon WP: Spinal epidural abscess: evaluation with contrast-enhanced MR imaging, *AJNR* 12:1087-1093, 1991.

14. Nussbaum ES, Rigamonti D, Standiford H et al: Spinal epidural abscess: a report of 40 cases and review, *Surg Neurol* 38:225-231, 1992.

15. Kricun R, Shoemaker EI, Chovanes GI, Stephens HW: Epidural abscess of the cervical spine: MR findings in five cases, *AJR* 158:1145-1149, 1992.

16. Bartels RH, deJong TR, Grotenhuis JA: Spinal subdural abscess, *J Neurosurg* 76:307-311, 1992.

17. Gero B, Sze G, Sharif H: MR imaging of intradural inflammatory diseases of the spine, *AJNR* 12:1009-1019, 1991.

18. Scotti G, Righi C, Campi A: Myelitis and myelopathies, *Riv di Neuroradiol* 5 (suppl 2): 49-52, 1992.

19. DeLaPaz R: Demyelinating disease of the spinal cord. In Enzmann D, DeLaPaz R, J Rubin, editors: *Magnetic Resonance of the Spine,* pp. 423-436, 1990, St. Louis, Mosby.

20. Osborn AG, Harnsberger HR, Smoker WRK, Boyer R: Multiple sclerosis in adolescents: CT and MR findings, *AJNR* 12:521-424, 1990.

20a. Donati PT, Fondelli MP, Rossi A et al: La neuromielite ottica, *Riv di Neuroradiol* 6:53–59, 1993

21. Larsson E-M, Holtäs S, Nilsson O: Gd-DTPA-enhanced MR of suspected spinal multiple sclerosis, *AJNR* 10:1071-1076, 1989.

22. Holtas S, Basibuyuk N, Frederiksson K: MRI in acute transverse myelopathy, *Neuroradiol* 35:221-226, 1993.

23. Austin SG, Zee C-S, Waters C: The role of magnetic resonance imaging in acute transverse myelitis, *Can J Neurol Sci* 19:508-511, 1992.

24. Zweig G, Russell EJ: Radiation myelopathy of the cervical spinal cord: MR findings, *AJNR* 11:1188-1190, 1990.

25. Michikawa M, Wada Y, Sano M et al: Radiation myelopathy: significance of gadolinium-DTPA enhancement in the diagnosis, *Neuroradiol* 33:286-289, 1991.

26. Wang P-Y, Shen W-C, Jan J-S: MR imaging in radiation myelopathy, *AJNR* 13:1049-1055, 1992.

27. Takahashi M, Yamashita Y, Sakamoto Y, Kojima R: Chronic cervical cord compression: clinical significance of increased signal intensity on MR images, *Radiol* 173:219-224, 1989.

28. Siegal T, Siegal T: Serotonergic manipulations in experimental neoplastic spinal cord compression, *J Neurosurg* 78:929-937, 1993.

29. Narita Y, Watanabe Y, Hoshino T et al: Myelopathy due to large veins draining recurrent spontaneous caroticocavernous fistula, *Neuroradiol* 34:433-435, 1992.

30. Elksnis SM, Hogg JP, Cunningham ME: MR imaging of spontaneous cord infarction, *J Comp Asst Tomogr* 15:228-252, 1991.

31. Friedman DP, Flanders AE: Enhancement of gray matter in anterior spinal infarction, *AJNR* 13:983-985, 1992.

32. Rodesch G, Lasjaunias P, Berenstein A: Functional vascular anatomy of the spine and cord, *Riv di Neuroradiol* (suppl 2):63-66, 1992.

33. Gelber ND, Ragland RL, Knorr JR: Gd-DTPA enhanced MRI of cervical anterior epidural venous plexus, *J Comp Asst Tomogr* 16:760-763, 1992.

34. Czervionke LF, Daniels DL, Ho PSP et al: Cervical neural foramina: correlative anatomic and MR imaging study, *Radiol* 169:753-759, 1988.

35. Biondi A, Merland JJ, Hodes JE et al: Aneurysms of spinal arteries associated with intramedullary arteriovenous malformations. I. Angiographic and clinical aspects, *AJNR* 13:913-922, 1992.

36. Schmidt RH, Grady MS, Cohen WS et al: Acute cauda equina syndrome from a ruptured aneurysm in the sacral canal, *J Neurosurg* 77:945-948, 1992.

36a. Rengachary SS, Duke DA, Tsai FY, Kragel PJ: Spinal artery aneurysm: case report, *Neurosurg* 33:125–130, 1993.

37. Rodesch G, Lasjaunias P, Berenstein A: Embolization of spinal cord arteriovenous malformations, *Riv di Neuroradiol* 5(suppl 2):67-92, 1992.

38. Anson JA, Spetzler RF: Classification of spinal arteriovenous malformations and implications for treatment, *BNI Quarterly* 8:2-8, 1992.

39. Nichols DA, Rufenacht DA, Jack CR Jr, Forbes GA: Embolization of spinal dural arteriovenous fistula with polyvinyl alcohol particles: experience in 14 patients, *AJNR* 13:933-940, 1992.

40. Beaujeux RL, Reizine DC, Casasco A et al: Endovascular treatment of vertebral arteriovenous fistula, *Radiol* 183:361-367, 1992.

41. Naidich TP, McLone DG, Harwood-Nash DC: Vascular malformations. In Newton TH, Potts DG, editors: *Modern Neuroradiology, vol 1: Computed Tomography of the Spine and Spinal Cord,* pp. 397-400, 1983.

41a. Tomlinson FH, Rüfenacht DA, Sundt TM Jr et al: Arteriovenous fristulas of the brain and spinal cord, *J Neurosurg* 79:16–27, 1993.

42. Masaryk TJ, Ross JS, Modic MT et al: Radiculomeningeal vascular malformations of the spine: MR imaging, *Radiol* 164:845-849, 1987.

43. Ogilvy CS, Louis DN, Ojemann RG: Intramedullary cavernous angiomas of the spinal cord: clinical presentation, pathological features, and surgical management, *Neurosurg* 31:219-230, 1992.

44. Anson JA, Spetzler RF: Surgical resection of intramedullary spinal cord cavernous malformations, *J Neurosurg* 78:446-451, 1993.

45. Bourgouin PM, Tampieri D, Johnston W et al: Multiple occult vascular malformations of the brain and spinal cord: MRI diagnosis, *Neuroradiol* 34:110-111, 1992.

46. Yuh WTC, March EE, Wang AK et al: MR imaging of spinal cord and vertebral body infarction, *AJNR* 13:145-154, 1992.

47. Friedman DP, Flanders AE: Enhancement of gray matter in anterior spinal infarction, *AJNR* 13:983-985, 1992.

48. Mikulis DJ, Ogilvy CS, McKee A et al: Spinal cord infarction and fibrocartilagenous emboli, *AJNR* 13:155-160, 1992.

49. Takahashi S, Yamada T, Ishii K et al: MRI of anterior spinal artery syndrome of the cervical spinal cord, *Neuroradiol* 35:25-29, 1992.

50. Hirono H, Yamadori A, Komiyama M et al: MRI of spontaneous spinal cord infarction: serial changes in gadolinium-DTPA enhancement, *Neuroradiol* 34:95-97, 1992.

50a. Henderson FH, Crockard HA, Stevens JM: Spinal cord oedema due to venous stasis, *Neurorardiol* 35:312–315, 1993.

51. Enzmann DR: Vascular diseases. In Enzmann DR, DeLaPaz R, Rubin J, editors, *Magnetic Resonance Imaging of the Spine*, pp. 510-537, 1990, St. Louis, Mosby.

52. Thornbury JR, Fryback DG, Turski PA et al: Disk-caused nerve compression in patients with acute low-back pain: diagnosis with MR, CT myelography, and plain CT, *Radiol* 186:731-738, 1993.

53. Deyo RA, Loeser JD, Bigos SJ: Herniated lumbar intervertebral disk, *Ann Int Med* 112:598-603, 1990.

54. Modic MT, Herfkens RJ: Intervertebral disk: Normal age-related changes in MR signal intensity, *Radiol* 166:332-334, 1990.

55. Sether LA, Yu S, Haughton VM, Fischer ME: Intervertebral disk: normal age-related changes in MR signal intensity, *Radiol* 177:385-388, 1990.

56. Czervionke LF: Lumbar intervertebral disc disease, *Neuroimaging Clin N Amer* 3:465-486, 1993.

57. Boden SD, Davis DO, Dina TS et al: Abnormal magnetic resonance scans of the lumbar spine in asymptomatic patients, *J Bone Joint Surg* 72:403-408, 1990.

58. Yu S, Haughton VM, Ho PSP et al: Progressive and regressive changes in the nucleus purposes, part II. The adult, *Radiol* 169:93-97, 1988.

59. Yu S, Sether LA, Ho PSP et al: Tears of the anulus fibrosus: correlation between MR and pathologic findings in cadavers, *AJNR* 9:367-370, 1988.

60. Modic MT, Steinberg PM, Ross JS et al: Degenerative disk disease: assessment of changes in vertebral body marrow with MR imaging, *Radiol* 166:193-199, 1988.

61. Schiebler ML, Grenier N, Fallon M et al: Normal and degenerated intervertebral disk: in vivo and in vitro MR imaging with histopathologic correlation, *AJR* 157:93-97, 1991.

62. Yu S, Haughton VM, Sether LA et al: Criteria for classifying normal and degenerated intervertebral disks, *Radiol* 170:523-526, 1989.

63. Williams AL, Haughton VM: Disc herniation and degenerative disc disease. In Newton TH, Potts DG, editors: *Modern Neuroradiology, vol 1, Computed Tomography of the Spine and Spinal Cord*, pp. 231-249, 1983.

64. Helms CA, Vogler JB III: Spinal stenosis and degenerative lesions. In Newton TH, Potts DG, editors: *Modern Neuroradiology, vol 1, Computed tomography of the Spine and Spinal Cord*, pp. 251-266, 1983.

65. Resnick D: Degenerative diseases of the vertebral column, *Radiol* 156:3-14, 1985.

66. Russell EG: Cervical disk disease, *Radiol* 177:313-325, 1990.

67. Bergleit R, Gebarski SS, Brunberg JA et al: Lumbar synovial cysts: correlation of myelographic, MR, and pathologic findings, *AJNR* 11:777-779, 1990.

68. Awwad EE, Martin DS, Smith KR Jr, Buchotz RD: MR imaging of lumbar juxtaarticular cysts, *J Comp Asst Tomogr* 14:415-417, 1990.

69. Jackson DE JR, Atlas SW, Mani JR, Normal D: Intraspinal synovial cysts: MR imaging, *Radiol* 170:527-530, 1989.

70. Fletcher G, Haughton VM, Ho K-C, Yu S: Age-related changes in the cervical facet joints: studies with cryomicrotomy, MR, and CT. *AJNR* 11:27-30, 1990.

71. Grenier N, Kressel HY, Schiebler ML et al: Normal and degenerative posterior spinal structures: MR imaging, *Radiol* 165:517-525, 1987.

72. Yousem DM, Atlas SW, Goldberg HI, Grossman RI: Degenerative narrowing of the cervical spine neural foramina: evaluation with high-resolution 3DFT gradient-echo MR imaging, *AJNR* 12:229-236, 1991.

73. Liu SS, Williams KD, Drayer BP et al: Synovial cysts of the lumbosacral spine: diagnosis by MR imaging, *AJNR* 10:1239-1242, 1989.

74. Yuh WTC, Drew JM, Weinstein JN et al: Intraspinal synovial cysts: magnetic resonance evaluation, *Spine* 16:740-745, 1991.

75. Gorey MT, Hyman RA, Black KS et al: Lumbar synovial cysts eroding bone, *AJNR* 13:161-163, 1992.

76. Kiely MJ: Neuroradiology case of the day: lumbar synovial cyst, *AJR* 160:1336-1339, 1993.

77. Kent DL, Haynor DR, Larson EB, Deyo RA: Diagnosis of lumbar spinal stenosis in adults: a metaanalysis of the accuracy of CT, MR, and myelography, *AJR* 158:1135-1144, 1992.

77a. Jinkins JR: Gd-DTPA enhanced MR of the lumbar spinal canal in patients with claudication, *J Comp Asst Tomogr* 17:555-561, 1993.

78. Mehalic TF, Pezzuti RT, Applebaum BI: Magnetic resonance imaging and cervical spondylitic myelopathy, *Neurosurg* 26:216-227, 1990.

78a. Houser OW, Onofrio BM, Miller GM et al: Cervical neural foraminal canal stenosis: computerized tomographic nyelography diagnosis, *J Neurosurg* 79:84-88, 1993.

79. Rothman SLG, Glenn WV: Spondylolysis and spondylolisthesis. In Newton TH, Potts DG, editors: *Modern Neuroradiology, vol 1, Computed Tomography of the Spine and Spinal Cord*, pp. 267-280, 1983.

80. Ryan PJ, Evans PA, Gibson T, Fogelman I: Chronic low back pain: comparison of bone SPECT with radiography and CT, *Radiol* 182:849-854, 1992.

81. Otake S, Matsuo M, Nishizawa S et al: Ossification of the posterior longitudinal ligament: MR evaluation, *AJNR* 13:1059-1067, 1992.

82. Sugimura H, Kakitsubata Y, Suzuki Y et al: MRI of ossification of ligamentum flavum, *J Comp Asst Tomogr* 16:73-76, 1992.

83. Fox MW, Ootrio BM, Kilgore JE: Neurologic complications of ankylosing spondylitis, *J Neurosurg* 78:871-878, 1993.

84. Ross JS, Modic MT, Masaryk TJ: Tears of the anulus fibrosus: assessment with Gd-DTPA-enhanced MR imaging, *AJNR* 10:1251-1254, 1989.

85. Siebner HR, Faulhauer K: Frequency and specific surgical management of far lateral lumbar disc herniations, *Acta Neurochi (Wien)* 105:124-131, 1990.

86. Robertson HJ, Menoni RM, Aprill CN, Smith RD: CT and MRI scans in thoracic intradural disc herniation, *Neuroradiol* 33(suppl):331-332, 1991.

87. Williams MP, Cherryman GR, Husband JE: Significance of thoracic disc herniation demonstrated by MR imaging, *J Comp Asst Tomogr* 13:211-214, 1989.

88. Schellinger D, Mang HJ, Vidic B et al: Disk fragment migration, *Radiol* 175:831-836, 1990.

89. Wasserstrom R, Mamourian AC, Black JF, Lehman RAW: Intradural lumbar disk fragment with ring enhancement on MR, *AJNR* 14:401-404, 1993.

90. Lutz JD, Smith RR, Jones HM: CT myelography of a fragment of a lumbar disk sequestered posterior to the thecal sac, *AJNR* 11:610-611, 1990.

91. Jinkins JR: MR of enhancing nerve roots in the unoperated lumbosacral spine, *AJNR* 14:193-202, 1993.

91a. Toyone T, Takahashi K, Kitahara H et al: Visualization of symptomatic nerve roots, *J Bone Joint Surg* (Br) 75–B: 529-533, 1993.

92. Mall JC, Kaiser JA, Heithoff KB: Postoperative spine. In Newton TH, Potts DG, editors: *Modern Neuroradiology, vol 1, Computed Tomography of the Spine and Spinal Cord*, pp. 187-204, 1983.

93. Boden SD, Davis DO, Dina TS et al: Postoperative diskitis: distinguishing early MR imaging findings from normal postoperative disk space changes, *Radiol* 184:765-771, 1992.

94. Glickstein MF, Sussman SK: Time-dependent scar enhance-

ment in magnetic resonance imaging of the postoperative lumbar spine, *Skeletal Radiol* 20:333-337, 1991.

95. Boden SD, Davis DO, Dina TS et al: Contrast-enhanced MR imaging performed after successful lumbar disk surgery: prospective study, *Radiol* 182:59-64, 1992.

96. Bundschuh CV, Stein L, Slusser JH et al: Distinguishing between scar and recurrent herniated disk in postoperative patients: value of contrast-enhanced CT and MR imaging, *AJNR* 11:949-958, 1990.

97. Bobman SA, Atlas SW, Listerud J, Grossman RI: Postoperative lumbar spine: contrast-enhanced chemical shift MR imaging, *Radiol* 179:557-562, 1991.

98. Ruscalleda J: Postoperative spine, *Riv di Neuroradiol* 5(suppl 2):93-100, 1992.

99. Jinkins JR, Osborn AG, Garrett D Jr et al: Spinal nerve enhancement with Gd-DTPA: MR correlation with the postoperative spine, *AJNR* 14:383-394, 1993.

100. Huftle MG, Modic MT, Ross JS et al: Lumbar spine: postoperative MR imaging with Gd-DTPA, *Radiol* 167:817-824, 1988.

101. Carvellini P, Curri D, Volpin L et al: Computed tomography of epidural fibrosis after discectomy: a comparison between symptomatic and asymptomatic patients, *Neurosurg* 23:710-713, 1988.

102. Ross JS, Masaryk TJ, Schrader M et al: MR imaging of the postoperative lumbar spine: assessment with gadopentetate dimeglumine, *AJNR* 11:771-776, 1990.

103. Mirowitz SA, Shady KL: Gadopentetate dimeglumine-enhanced MR imaging of the postoperative lumbar spine: comparison of fat-suppressed and conventional T1-weighted MR scans, *AJR* 159:385-389, 1992.

103a. Nguyen CM, Haughton VM, Ho K-C, An HS: MR contrast enhancement: an exerimental study in postlaminectomy epidural fibrosis, *AJNR* 14:997–1002, 1993.

104. Johnson CE, Sze G: Benign lumbar archnoiditis: MR imaging with gadopentetate dimeglumine, *AJNR* 11:763-770, 1990.

105. Afshani E, Kuhn JP: Common causes of low back pain in children, *RadioGraphics* 11:269-291, 1991.

106. Wagner A, Albeck MJ, Madsen FF: Diagnostic imaging in fracture of the lumbar vertebral ring apophyses, *Acta Radiol* 33:72-75, 1992.

107. Epstein NE, Epstein JA, Mauri T: Treatment of fractures of the vertebral limbus and spinal stenosis in five adolescents and five adults, *Neurosurg* 24:595-604, 1989.

108. Robertson PL: Atypical presentations of spinal cord tumors in children, *J Child Neurol* 7:360-363, 1992.

109. Brant-Zawadzki M, Post MJD: Trauma. In Newton TH, Potts DG, editors: *Modern Neuroradiology, vol 1, Computed Tomography of the Spine and Spinal Cord,* pp. 149-186, 1985.

109a. Bulas DI, Fitz CR, Johnson DL: Traumatic atlantooccipital dislocation in children, *Radiol* 188:155–158, 1993.

110. Manaster BJ: *Handbook of Skeletal Radiology,* pp. 264-279, Chicago: Yearbook Medical Publishers, 1989.

111. Panjabi MM, Oda T, Crisco JJ III: Experimental study of atlas injuries, *Spine* 16:S460-465, 1991.

21

Tumors, Cysts, and Tumorlike Lesions of the Spine and Spinal Cord

---

Extradural Tumors, Cysts, and Tumorlike Masses
  Benign Tumors
  Cysts and Other Benign Tumorlike Masses
  Malignant Tumors
Intradural Extramedullary Tumors, Cysts, and Tumor-
like Masses
  Benign Tumors
  Cysts and Other Benign Tumorlike Masses
  Malignant Tumors
Intramedullary Tumors, Cysts, and Tumorlike Masses
  Tumors
  Cysts and Tumorlike Masses

Spinal cord tumors and tumorlike masses are traditionally classified by location into three categories,[1,2] (see box, p. 877, top left) as follows:

1. Extradural lesions (lesions of the osseous spine, epidural space, and paraspinous soft tissues)
2. Intradural extramedullary lesions (lesions that are inside the dura but outside the spinal cord)
3. Intramedullary lesions (spinal cord cysts and tumors)

EXTRADURAL TUMORS, CYSTS, AND TUMORLIKE MASSES

Extradural masses occur outside the spinal dura and typically arise from the osseous spine, intervertebral disks, and adjacent soft tissues. General imaging hallmarks of an extradural mass lesion are focal displacement of the thecal sac and its contents away from the mass (Fig. 21-1, *A*). Myelography shows extrinsic compression of the thecal sac. Myelographic "block" (sometimes the redundant term, *complete block,* is used) occurs with large lesions and is seen as a displaced thecal sac with obliterated subarachnoid space and compressed spinal cord. The border between the lesion and the head of the contrast column has a poorly delineated "feathered" appearance (Fig. 21-1, *B* and *C*).[2] MR scans clearly show the dura draped over the mass (Fig. 21-1, *D*). In some cases a crescent of displaced epidural fat can be seen capping the lesion (*see* Fig. 21-16, *B* and *C*).

The most common benign extradural masses are degenerative and traumatic lesions such as disk herniations, osteophytes, and fractures (*see* Chapter 20).

Classification of Spine Lesions by Anatomic Compartment

Extradural masses

Location: outside thecal sac

Tissues: osseous spine, epidural space, paraspinous soft tissues

Examples: herniated disk, spondylitic spurs, fractures, metastases

Classic myelogram appearance: thecal sac extrinsically compressed; if block, interface between lesion and contrast column is poorly defined with "feathered" appearance at level of obstruction

Intradural extramedullary masses

Location: inside thecal sac but outside cord

Tissues: nerve roots, leptomeninges, CSF spaces

Examples: nerve sheath tumors, meningiomas

Classic myelogram appearance: intradural filling defect outlined by sharp meniscus of contrast; spinal cord deviated away from mass; ipsilateral subarachnoid space enlarged up to mass

Intramedullary masses

Location: inside spinal cord

Tissues: cord parenchyma, pia

Examples: astrocytoma, hydrosyringomyelia

Classic myelogram appearance: diffuse, multisegmental smoothly enlarged cord with gradual subarachnoid space effacement

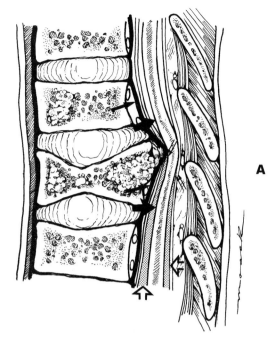

Fig. 21-1. Imaging features of an extradural mass. **A,** Anatomic diagram, lateral view, depicts a pathologic compression fracture with spinal cord compression. The dura *(small arrows)* and spinal cord *(large arrows)* are displaced. The subarachnoid space is filled with intrathecal contrast *(gray area: open arrows)*. Gradual tapering of the contrast column with a "feathered" appearance *(double arrows)* is present. Cephalad flow of contrast is blocked by the compressive lesion, and the CSF distal to the obstruction *(shown in white)* is unopacified.

Continued.

The most common neoplastic extradural mass is metastasis. In this section, we consider neoplasms, cysts, and tumorlike masses of the osseous spine and paraspinal soft tissues.

Benign Tumors

Hemangioma

Pathology. Vertebral hemangiomas (VHs) are slow-growing benign primary neoplasms of capillary, cavernous, or venous origin. The most common histologic type is cavernous hemangioma. These lesions are composed of mature thin-walled vessels and large blood-filled endothelial-lined spaces.[3,4] The dilated vessels are interspersed among longitudinally oriented trabeculae that appear reduced in number but are thicker in diameter.[5] VHs vary from predominantly fatty lesions (Fig. 21-2, *A*) to hemangiomas comprised largely of vascular stroma with little or no adipose tissue *(see box, right).*[4]

Incidence, age, and gender. Hemangiomas are found in 10% to 12% of all autopsies, making VH the most common benign spinal neoplasm.[3] The peak incidence is in the fourth to the sixth decades. Asymptomatic hemangiomas occur equally in men and

Hemangioma

Vascular/fatty stroma with sparse but thick trabeculae

Usual location: part or all of vertebral body

Common incidental finding at MR (round "white spot" on T1WI), CT ("polka dot" vertebral body)

Most are asymptomatic; can expand, cause pathologic fracture, epidural mass with cord compression

Differential diagnosis: fatty marrow replacement

women but there is a female predominance with symptomatic lesions.[6]

Location. Nearly 75% of all osseous hemangiomas occur in the spine.[3] The lower thoracic and lumbar regions are the most common sites.[5] Multiple lesions are seen in 25% to 30% of cases.[6,7]

Most hemangiomas are located in the vertebral body. Lesion extent is variable (Fig. 21-2). Some lesions involve only part of the vertebral body, whereas others affect the entire medullary space. Hemangi-

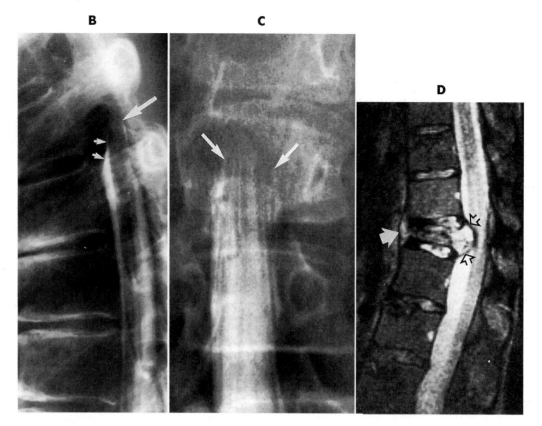

Fig. 21-1, cont'd. B and **C,** Myelographic findings of extradural mass are shown. Lateral view **(B)** shows an extradural mass effect *(small arrows)* with block of contrast flow *(large arrow)*. AP view **(C)** in another case shows the ill-defined "feathered" appearance at the head of the contrast column *(arrows)*, caused by an extradural mass with block. **D,** Sagittal T2-weighted MR scan in a patient with metastatic breast carcinoma and a high signal intensity pathologic compression fracture *(large arrow)* shows the dural displacement *(open arrows)* that is characteristic of an extradural mass effect.

oma isolated to the neural arch is uncommon, but 10% to 15% of vertebral body VHs have concomitant involvement of the posterior elements (Fig. 21-3).[3] Most epidural hemangiomas occur secondarily as extensions of expanding intraosseous lesions.[8] Completely extraosseous hemangioma is rare, accounting for only 1% to 2% of all VHs.

Clinical presentation and natural history. Approximately 60% of VHs are asymptomatic lesions that are discovered incidentally on imaging studies.[6] Pain is the presenting complaint in 20%.[6] In most patients with VHs, back pain is related to other etiologies, not the hemangioma.[4] Approximately 20% of VHs present with progressive neurologic deficits or symptoms of acute spinal cord compression. Progression of an asymptomatic or painful lesion to a neurologically symptomatic one is rare, occurring in less than 5% of cases.[6]

VHs usually become symptomatic when pathologic compression fracture or epidural extension occurs. Symptom onset is often, although not invariably, acute and is probably secondary to hemorrhage with sudden increase in mass effect.[8] Pregnancy may

exacerbate some lesions.[8a] Some authors report fatty VHs are usually clinically inactive, whereas those with imaging findings suggesting a more vascular stroma have the potential to cause spinal cord compression.[4]

Imaging findings. Plain film radiographs show lytic foci with honeycomb trabeculation or thick vertical striations.[5] NECT scans show a lucent lesion with typical "polka dot" densities in the medullary space that represent the coarsened vertical trabeculae characteristic of VHs. VHs range in size from small, localized lesions (Fig. 21-2, *C*) to hemangiomas that involve the entire vertebral body (Fig. 21-2, *B*). Myelography or CT-myelography in cases with extraosseous extension show an extradural mass (Fig. 21-4, *B*). Angiographic findings vary from normal to intense hypervascular stain on selective segmental spinal angiograms.[4]

MR imaging findings vary. Most VHs are seen as round, relatively well-delineated vertebral body lesions that are high signal intensity on both T1- and T2-weighted sequences (Fig. 21-4, *A*). The hyperintense stroma surrounds foci of very low signal inten-

A   **B**   **C**

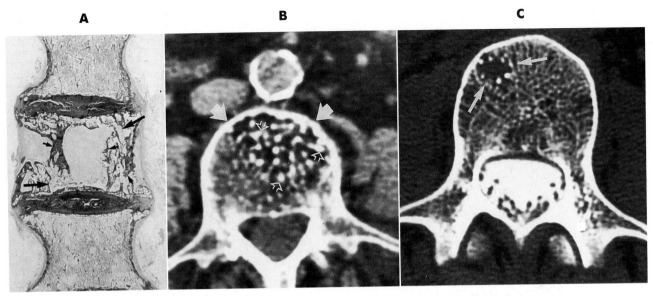

Fig. 21-2. Pathology and imaging findings of typical vertebral body hemangiomas. **A,** Gross pathology specimen shows a classic hemangioma. Note marrow replacement by fatty stroma *(large arrows)* and fewer but strikingly thickened trabeculae *(small arrows).* **B** and **C,** Axial CT scans show typical hemangiomas. This hemangioma **(B)** *(large arrows)* occupies nearly the entire vertebral body. Note "polka-dot" appearance caused by the thickened trabeculae seen in axial section *(open arrows).* Post-myelogram CT scan **(C)** in another patient shows a very small incidental focal hemangioma *(arrows).* (A, From archives of the Armed Forces Institute of Pathology.)

sity, representing the thickened vertical trabeculae (Fig. 21-3, *B*).

Some VHs are predominately low signal on T1WI. These lesions often enhance following contrast administration and may be associated with an extradural soft tissue mass. Histologically, these VHs contain predominately vascular rather than fatty stroma.[4]

Differential diagnosis. The major differential diagnostic consideration on MR scans is focal fatty marrow replacement or hemangioma. VHs typically have high signal intensity on both T1- and T2WI, whereas fatty lesions become hypointense on standard T2-weighted spin echo images. VHs that are mostly fatty can be indistinguishable from fatty marrow replacement; both are clinically indolent lesions that are common causes of vertebral body "white spots" seen incidentally on MR scans. Fat suppression sequences are helpful in distinguishing fatty marrow replacement from VHs that are primarily vascular.

Osteoid osteoma (Table 21-1)

Pathology. Osteoid osteoma is a benign skeletal neoplasm that has a central nidus of interlacing osteoid and woven bone mixed with loose fibrovas-

A

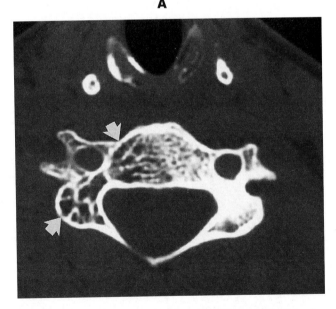

Fig. 21-3. Hemangioma that involves the vertebral body, pedicle, and articular pillar of C5. **A,** Axial NECT scan shows the lesion *(arrows).* (Courtesy M. Fruin.)

Continued.

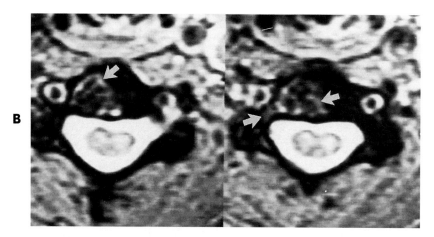

Fig. 21-3, cont'd. B, Axial T2-weighted MR scans show the high signal stroma *(arrows)*. (Courtesy M. Fruin.)

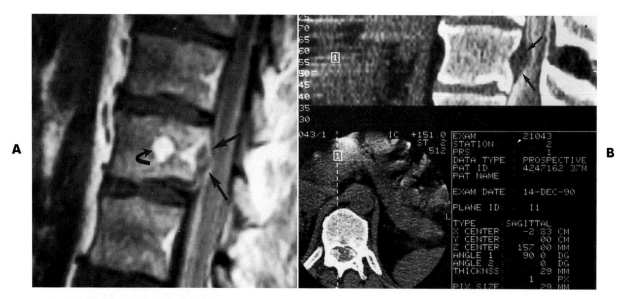

Fig. 21-4. This 42-year-old man had a 48-hour history of back pain and leg weakness followed by sudden onset of paraplegia and incontinence. **A,** Sagittal postcontrast T1-weighted MR scan shows a high signal lesion in the vertebral body *(curved arrow)* and an extradural soft tissue mass with enhancing rim *(straight arrows)* that is compressing the conus medullaris. **B,** Post-myelogram CT scan with reformatted sagittal image shows the extradural mass *(arrows)*. Surgery disclosed extradural hemangioma with acute hemorrhage.

cular stroma.[9,10] Osteoid osteomas are sharply demarcated from surrounding bone and are surrounded by varying degrees of osteosclerosis.[9] Associated paraosseous soft tissue masses occasionally occur with extremity lesions but have not been reported in the spine.[11]

The nidus of an osteoid osteoma rarely exceeds 1.5 to 2.0 cm in diameter[9]; larger lesions are typically categorized as osteoblastoma, although the distinction between these two entities is not always clear.[10]

Incidence, age, and gender. Osteoid osteoma is a relatively common lesion that accounts for approxi-

mately 12% of benign skeletal neoplasms.[9] Osteoid osteomas represent approximately 6% of benign spine tumors.[5]

Patients with osteoid osteoma are usually young. Osteoid osteomas are rarely seen beyond 30 years of age.[5] Approximately half of all cases present between the ages of 10 and 20 years.[9,10] The male:female ratio is 2-4:1.[5,9,10]

Location. Osteoid osteoma may occur in virtually any location; the lower extremity is the site for more than half of all lesions. Approximately 10% of osteoid osteomas are found in the spine. The most commonly

Table 21-1. Benign osseous tumors and tumorlike lesions of the spine

Lesion	Location	Incidence	Age	Imaging
Hemangioma	Vertebral body (T, L>C)	Most common	All	CT: "polka dot" body MR: "hot spot" on T1WI
Osteoid osteoma	Neural arch (L, C>T)	Common (10% in spine)	10 to 20 years	Dense sclerosis, lucent nidus, lesion <2 cm
Osteoblastoma	Neural arch (C>L, T; sacrum)	Uncommon (40% in spine)	<30 years	Expansile lytic mass; ± matrix mineralization
Giant cell tumor	Vertebral body (sacrum >>vertebrae)	Uncommon	20s to 40s	Lytic, expansile, destructive, highly vascular
Osteochondroma	Spinous, transverse processes (10% to 12% multiple)	Common (rare in spine)	5 to 30 years	Pedunculated/sessile lesion; periosteum, cortex, marrow in continuity with host bone; cartilaginous cap ± Ca^{++}
Aneurysmal bone cyst	Posterior elements (C, T most common)	Rare (20% in spine)	80%<20 year	Multiloculated, expansile; eggshell-like rims; blood products with fluid-fluid levels; highly vascular

affected region is the lumbar spine, and the usual site is the neural arch. Vertebral body lesions are unusual.[9]

Clinical presentation and natural history. Pain is the presenting symptom in over 95% of cases[10]; 75% of patients report pain relief following salicylate administration.[9] Symptom duration ranges from 1 month to several years, with an average length of 15 to 16 months.[10] Scoliosis is common in patients with spinal osteoid osteomas.[5]

Imaging findings. Bone scintigraphy reveals focal activity on both immediate and delayed images.[9] Spinal osteoid osteomas may be difficult to identify on plain film radiographs because these are often normal or may demonstrate only subtle osteosclerosis.[9] NECT scans typically show dense sclerosis of the facet, pedicle, or lamina surrounding a lytic lesion that may have a central calcific nidus (Fig. 21-5).[5,9]

MR imaging of osteoid osteoma has been reported in only a few cases. Spinal lesions have variable signal. The nidus is typically low to intermediate in signal intensity on both T1- and T2-weighted MR scans.[9,11] Some osteoid osteomas enhance following contrast administration.[11]

Osteoblastoma (Table 21-1)
Pathology. Osteoblastoma, also known as giant osteoid osteoma, occupies a histologic continuum

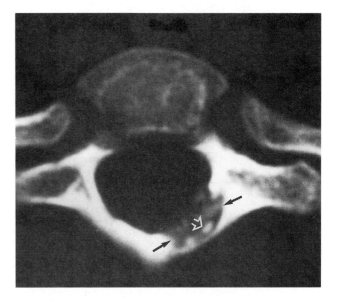

Fig. 21-5. Axial NECT scan in this 15-year-old girl with neck pain shows a typical osteoid osteoma in the T1 lamina. Note thickened, sclerotic bone surrounding a lucent nidus (*black arrows*). Some central calcifications (*open arrow*) are present. Osteoid osteoma.

with osteoid osteoma. Osteoblastomas are typically 2 cm or greater in size; smaller lesions are usually classified as osteoid osteomas.[5]

Incidence, age, and gender. Osteoblastomas are uncommon neoplasms, accounting for approximately 1% of primary bone tumors. The reported age range is from 5 to 50 years, with an average age at presentation of 19.5 years. More than 80% of all patients are symptomatic by age 30.[12] The male:female predominance is approximately 2.5-1.[12]

Location. Whereas only 10% of osteoid osteomas occur in the spine, approximately 40% of all osteoblastomas are located here. Nearly 40% are found in the cervical spine, 23% in the lumbar spine, 21% in the thoracic spine and 17% in the sacrum. Two thirds are confined to the posterior elements; one third extend anteriorly to involve the vertebral body. Osteoblastomas are nearly always solitary lesions.[12]

Clinical presentation and natural history. Pain is the most common presenting symptom, seen in 80% of cases.[12] Neurologic deficit and scoliosis are sometimes observed. Although osteoid osteomas are biologically nonprogressive lesions, osteoblastomas often enlarge.[13] Occasionally, these lesions have atypical histologic features and may behave aggressively. About 10% recur following surgical excision.[14]

Imaging findings. Plain films and NECT scans typ-ically show a well-defined scalloped or lobulated lytic expansile mass arising from the neural arch. Approximately one half of spinal osteoblastomas are predominantly lucent; the remainder display varying degrees of matrix mineralization.[12] A thin bony or sclerotic rim with soft tissue extension is a common appearance (Fig. 21-6, *A*).[5] Intermediate signal intensity on T1WI with mixed high signal foci on T2WI and a wide band of reactive sclerosis have been reported on MR scans (Fig. 21-6, *B*).[14]

Differential diagnosis. The differential diagnosis of spinal osteoblastoma is osteoid osteoma, aneurysmal bone cyst, and giant cell tumor. Aggressive tumors can resemble osteosarcoma.

Giant cell tumor (*see* Table 21-1)

Pathology. Grossly, giant cell tumors are lytic, expansile, locally aggressive primary benign bone tumors that extend to the cortex but rarely transgress the periosteum.[5] Histologically, giant cell tumors contain sinusoidal vessels with hypervascular stroma. Hemorrhage is common; matrix mineralization is rare.[5,15] Monocyte-macrophages and multinucleated giant cells are common.[5]

Incidence, age, and gender. Giant cell tumors comprise approximately 5% of primary bone tumors. Most patients are in the second through the fifth de-

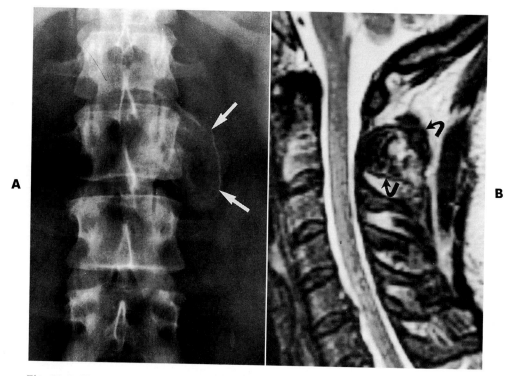

Fig. 21-6. Two cases of osteoblastoma. **A,** AP plain film radiography in this 23-year-old woman shows an expansile lesion of the left L2 pedicle and transverse process. Note thin bony rim *(arrows)*. **B,** Sagittal T2-weighted MR scan in a 29-year-old woman shows a mixed signal mass *(curved arrows)* in the C2 spinous process. Osteoblastoma was found at surgery in both cases. (**A,** Courtesy B.J. Manaster.)

cades; the peak incidence is in the third decade. There is a female predominance in giant cell tumors involving vertebrae other than the sacrum.[5]

Location. Most giant cell tumors occur at the ends of long bones, characteristically around the knee. Giant cell tumors of the spine are uncommon, accounting for only 3% to 7% of these tumors. Most occur in the sacrum; other vertebral segments are rarely involved.[5]

Clinical presentation and natural history. Pain and neurologic deficits are common presenting symptoms.[16] Local recurrence following incomplete resection is common, and some giant cell tumors are biologically aggressive lesions. Malignant transformation occurs in approximately 10% of cases.[17]

Imaging findings. Plain film radiographs and NECT scans typically disclose a lytic, expansile, destructive sacral or vertebral mass (Fig. 21-7). Angiography often demonstrates hypervascularity. MR scans show a mixed-signal, multicompartmented cystic mass that frequently contains blood degradation products.[15]

Differential diagnosis. The differential diagnosis of giant cell tumor in the spine is osteoblastoma and aneurysmal bone cyst.

Osteochondroma (*see* Table 21-1)

Etiology and pathology. Osteochondroma, also known as osteocartilaginous exostosis, arises through lateral displacement of epiphyseal growth cartilage.

This results in formation of a bony excrescence with cartilaginous-covered cortex and a medullary cavity contiguous with that of the parent bone.[18] Osteochondromas grow from their tips as the cartilage undergoes ossification.[18] Histologically, the cartilaginous cap and underlying bone in an osteochondroma are identical to normal bone.

Incidence, age, and gender. Osteochondromas are common lesions, comprising 8% to 9% of all primary bone tumors and slightly more than one third of benign tumors.[18] The mean age of patients with multiple spinal osteochondromas is 21 years, whereas solitary osteochondromas have a mean age at presentation of 30 years.[18] The male:female predominance is 1.5-2.5:1.[18]

Location. Osteochondromas affect mostly long bones; only 1% to 4% of solitary osteochondromas arise in the spine. The spinous or transverse processes are the most common location.[17] Approximately half occur in the cervical spine; C2 is the most commonly affected segment. The thoracic region is the next most common location. Multiple osteochondromas account for 12% of all cases. Approximately 10% of patients with hereditary multiple osteochondromas have spinal lesions.[18]

Clinical presentation and natural history. Osteochondromas rarely cause neurologic symptoms. Malignant transformation occurs in about 1% of solitary and 10% of multiple osteochondromas.[18]

Imaging findings. Plain film radiographs may show a sessile or pedunculated bonelike projection. On NECT scans the cortex of the parent bone flares into the cortex of the osteochondroma, with which it is contiguous. The cartilaginous cap often contains calcific foci (Fig. 21-8).[18] MR scans show mixed signal intensity on both T1- and T2WI.[17]

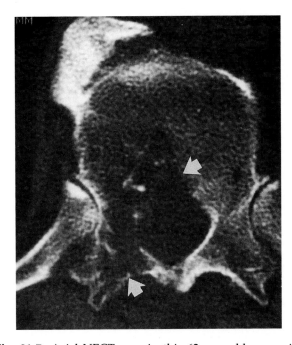

Fig. 21-7. Axial NECT scan in this 62-year-old man with midback pain shows a lytic, destructive lesion that involves the T11 vertebral body, pedicle, and neural arch *(arrows).* No other lesions were present. Giant cell tumor was found at surgery.

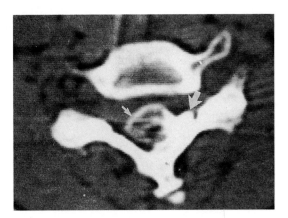

Fig. 21-8. Axial NECT scan shows a cauliflower-like calcified lesion with a mineralized cap *(small arrow)* and a densely ossified base *(large arrow)* that is continuous with the underlying cortical lamina. Osteochondroma (osteocartilagenous exostosis). (Courtesy B.J. Manaster.)

Miscellaneous benign tumors. Other primary bone neoplasms rarely involve the spine. Occasionally, chondromyxoid fibromas, malignant hemangioendotheliomas, and hemangiopericytomas occur in the axial skeleton.[5]

Cysts and Other Benign Tumorlike Masses

Several benign nonneoplastic tumorlike masses can cause an extradural mass. These include the following:

1. Aneurysmal bone cyst
2. Eosinophilic granuloma
3. Epidural lipomatosis
4. Angiolipoma
5. Nonneoplastic cysts such as synovial and arachnoid cysts

Aneurysmal bone cyst (*see* Table 21-1)

Etiology and pathology. Aneurysmal bone cyst (ABC) is a benign, nonneoplastic lesion of unknown etiology.[19] Between 30% and 50% of ABCs are associated with a preexisting osseous lesion such as chondroblastoma, giant cell tumor, osteoblastoma, nonossifying fibroma, or fibrous dysplasia.[20] Some ABCs may represent a vascular anomaly induced by trauma or hemorrhagic infarction of the precursor lesion. Rapid expansion may obliterate the underlying abnormality, leaving behind the blood-filled cavities that are characteristic of ABCs.[20]

Grossly, ABCs are multiloculated, expansile, highly vascular osteolytic lesions that often contain blood degradation products. Histologically, ABCs consist of thin-walled, blood-filled cavities that lack normal endothelium and elastic lamina.[21] Solid portions of the lesion contain benign spindle cells in a collagenous stroma. Multinucleated giant cells are commonly observed.[19]

Incidence, age, and gender. ABCs are uncommon and represent less than 1% of primary bone tumors. Nearly 80% occur in patients less than 20 years of age, whereas 85% of patients with giant cell tumors are 20 years or older.[5] There is a slight female predominance.

Location. ABCs occur in all parts of the skeleton. The metaphyses of long bones are the most common sites.[20] Approximately 20% are found in the spine; the cervical and thoracic regions are the most common locations.[5] ABCs typically occur in the posterior elements but often expand secondarily into the pedicles and vertebral body. Neural canal encroachment is common.[21] Involvement of contiguous vertebrae may occur.[17]

Clinical presentation and natural history. Pain and swelling are the most common overall presenting symptoms.[19] Spinal ABCs may cause cord compression and pathological fractures.[21] Recurrence following surgical resection is common.

Imaging. Plain films and NECT scans show an osteolytic lesion surrounded by expanded, thinned, eggshell-like cortical bone (Fig. 21-9, *A*). A soft tis-

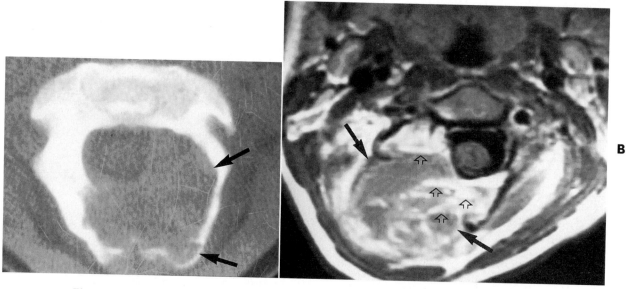

Fig. 21-9. Two cases of aneurysmal bone cyst. **A,** Axial NECT scan in a 6-year-old girl shows a lytic, scalloped, expansile mass in the C2 neural arch (*arrows*). **B,** Axial T1-weighted scan in an 11-year-old girl shows an expansile mass in the articular pillars and neural arch. Note bone expansion (*large arrows*) and multiseptated cysts with fluid-fluid levels (*open arrows*). Aneurysmal bone cysts with hemorrhage were found in both cases. (**B,** Courtesy R.J. Facco.)

sue mass is often present (Fig. 21-10, *B*).[5] Matrix calcification is absent.[21] Myelography shows an extradural mass effect; large lesions can cause a contrast block (Fig. 21-10, *A*). Most ABCs are very hypervascular at angiography (Fig. 21-10, *C*).[19] MR scans typically demonstrate a lobulated, multiseptated lesion with fluid-fluid levels and blood degradation products (Fig. 21-9, *B*).[21]

Differential diagnosis. The major differential diagnosis of a cystic expansile posterior element mass is ABC versus osteoblastoma. The presence of fluid-fluid levels is suggestive of ABC but also occasionally occurs with other lesions such as giant cell tumor, telangiectatic osteosarcoma, chondroblastoma, and nonneoplastic cyst with fracture.[19-21]

Eosinophilic granuloma (*see* Table 21-1). Eosinophilic granuloma (EG) is a benign, nonneoplastic disorder of which Langerhans cell histiocytosis is one manifestation (*see* Chapter 15). EG in the spine is seen as a lytic lesion without surrounding sclerosis. EG is a classic cause of a single collapsed vertebral body,

so-called vertebra plana (Fig. 21-11). Spine EGs most commonly occur between the ages of 5 and 10 years; EG is very rare over age 30 years.[17] EG is typically hyperintense on T2-weighted MR scans, although signal on T1WI is variable. Strong enhancement following contrast administration is seen.[21a]

Epidural lipomatosis
Etiology and pathology. Epidural lipomatosis (EL) is excessive deposition of unencapsulated fat in the epidural space. EL occurs as part of the central or truncal lipomatosis associated with both exogenous and endogenous hypercortisolemia.[22] The majority of symptomatic cases are associated with chronic steroid use; occasionally, ELs occur in morbidly obese patients, and a few cases have no definable etiology.[23,24] Asymptomatic EL is not uncommon in classic pituitary dependent Cushing disease and is even more common in the ectopic adrenocorticotropic hormone (ACTH) syndrome.[22]

Incidence, age, and gender. EL is rare. Most reported cases have occurred in males.[23,24]

Location. Approximately 60% of EL cases occur in the thoracic spine and 40% in the lumbar spine; combined thoracolumbar involvement also occurs and is

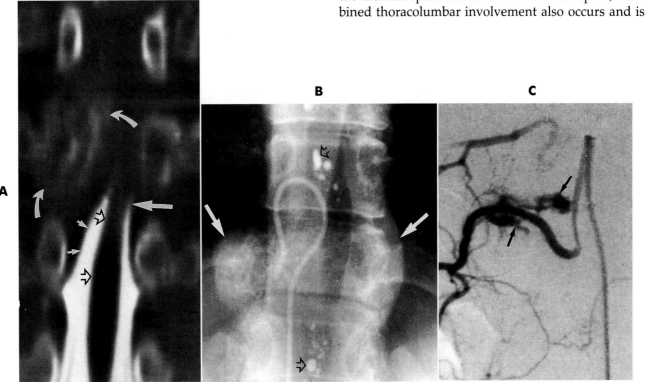

Fig. 21-10. A 17-year-old woman with back pain had these imaging studies. **A,** Coronal reformatted post-myelogram CT scan shows typical findings of an extradural mass. The contrast-filled thecal sac *(small arrows)* and spinal cord *(open arrows)* are displaced. Cephalad flow of contrast is blocked *(large arrow).* Note destructive, expansile mass in the pedicle at this level *(curved arrows).* **B,** Scout view for spinal angiography shows the T11 vertebral body is compressed, the pedicle is destroyed, and an adjacent focal soft tissue mass *(large arrows)* is present. Retained contrast *(open arrows)* from previous Pantopaque myelogram is present. **C,** Selective angiogram of the right T11 segmental artery shows a vascular stain *(arrows).* Aneurysmal bone cyst was found at surgery.

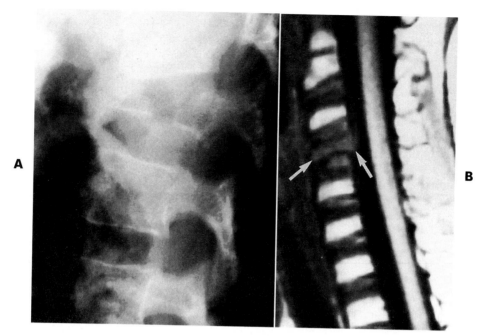

Fig. 21-11. Typical imaging findings in spinal eosinophilic granuloma illustrated in two cases. **A,** Lateral plain film shows "pancaked" L1 vertebral body. **B,** Sagittal T1-weighted MR scan in 10-year-old boy with torticollis shows the C4 vertebral body marrow is replaced by low signal soft tissue *(arrows)* (compare with the high signal seen in the adjacent normal vertebral bodies). Some loss of height of the vertebral body is present, i.e., there is mild vertebra plana.

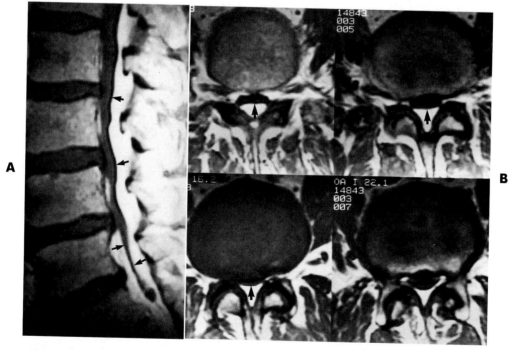

Fig. 21-12. Sagittal **(A)** and axial **(B)** T1-weighted MR scans show severe lumbosacral epidural lipomatosis, seen as widespread high signal surrounding the thecal sac. Note thecal sac compression *(small arrows).*

seen in 16% of cases. Cervical EL has not been reported.[24]

Clinical presentation and natural history. Weakness and back pain are the most frequent presenting complaints, seen in two thirds of all patients with EL. Radicular pain, numbness, and dysesthesias occur in half the cases.[24] EL may resolve after cessation of exogenous corticosteroid administration, suppressive therapy, or bilateral adrenalectomy.[22] Seventy-eight percent of patients undergoing multilevel laminectomy improve after surgery, but reported mortality in operated patients is 22%.[24]

Imaging findings. Myelographic findings range from normal to block.[23,24] CT and MR scans show increased extradural fat and diminished subarachnoid space (Fig. 21-12).[23]

Spinal angiolipoma

Pathology. Spinal angiolipomas (SAs) are benign neoplastic-like lesions composed of mature adipocytes and abnormal blood vessels that vary from capillary to sinusoidal, venular, or arterial in size.[25] SAs are considered a separate entity from the more common lipoma.[26]

Incidence, age, and gender. SAs are very rare, accounting for 0.14% to 1.2% of spinal axis tumors.[25,26] Symptom onset is typically in the fifth decade. There is a slight female predominance.[25]

Location. SAs are almost always epidural, although a few intramedullary lesions have been reported.[25] The thoracic spine is the most common site. Most SAs are dorsal or dorsolateral to the cord.[26]

Clinical presentation. Back pain, lower extremity numbness or paresthesias, and leg weakness are common. Bowel or bladder dysfunction is present in half of all cases. Some patients experience symptom onset during pregnancy.[25]

Imaging findings. Myelograms typically show a thoracic extradural mass or block. CT scans demonstrate a low- or intermediate-density epidural soft tissue mass that enhances following contrast administration.[27] SAs are typically iso- or hyperintense on T1WI and hyperintense on T2WI. Diffuse homogeneous enhancement is typical.[26] A few angiolipomas extensively infiltrate the adjacent vertebral body.[26]

Cysts. Several different types of spinal cysts can cause an extradural mass effect. Synovial (juxta-articular) cysts are rare causes of extradural mass effects. These cysts are nearly always associated with facet degeneration and are discussed in Chapter 20. Congenital and acquired arachnoid cysts are uncommon but important nonneoplastic causes of extra- and intradural mass effects.

Extradural arachnoid cysts. Extradural arachnoid cysts (EACs) are CSF-filled outpouchings of arachnoid that protrude through a dural defect.[28,29] EACs can be congenital or acquired. Two thirds occur in the mid to low thoracic spine; 20% are found in the lumbosacral region and 9% at the thoracolumbar junction. Cervical EACs are uncommon.[29]

EACs cause a spectrum of symptoms. Painless progression of either flaccid or spastic para- or quadriparesis with initial relative sparing of sphincter tone is typical. Kyphosis with localized or radicular pain may develop.[29] Imaging studies typically show a long-segment CSF-equivalent thoracic extradural mass that causes spinal cord compression or myelographic block. Secondary bony changes include widened interpedicular distance, scalloping of vertebral bodies, or pedicle thinning and erosion (Fig. 21-13).[28]

The differential diagnosis of EAC includes traumatic meningocele and lateral thoracic meningocele. Traumatic meningoceles typically have a large extraspinal component that extends through the neural foramina. Lateral thoracic meningoceles are usually associated with neurofibromatosis type 1 (NF-1) and widespread dural ectasia.[29]

Malignant Tumors

By far the most common extradural malignant neoplasm is metastasis. Primary extradural malignant neoplasms are uncommon. Chordoma, Hodgkin and non-Hodgkin lymphoma, and sarcomas such as Ewing sarcoma, chondrosarcoma, and osteogenic sarcoma are examples of primary extradural malignant spine tumors.

Chordoma

Etiology and pathology. Chordomas originate from intraosseous notochordal remnants (*see* box). Grossly, chordomas are locally invasive, lobulated,

---

Chordoma

Arise from intraosseous notochordal remnants
Two types: typical and chondroid chordoma
Any age; peak incidence is 50 to 60 years
Preferential location for both ends of axial skeleton
    50% sacrum/coccyx
    35% skull base
    15% vertebral bodies
NECT scans show lytic, destructive lesion; Ca^{++} in 30% to 70%; soft tissue mass often associated
Inhomogeneous signal on MR; typical chordomas are often very hyperintense on PD/T2WI

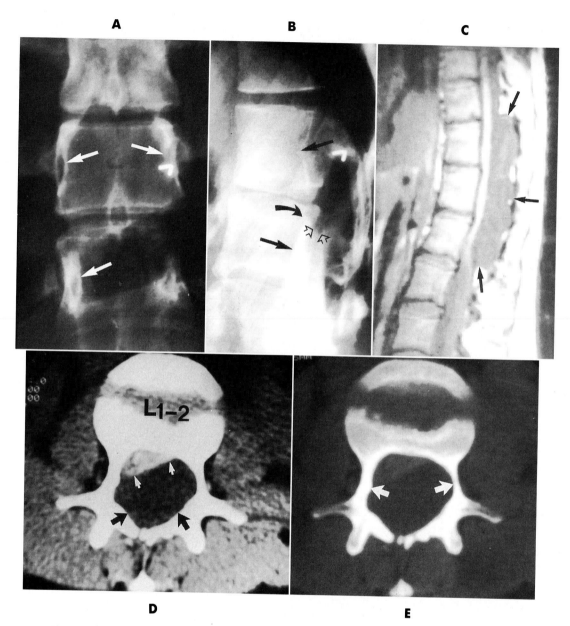

Fig. 21-13. Extradural arachnoid cyst. **A,** AP plain film radiograph shows expansion of the lower thoracic canal, seen as widened interpediculate distance and thinned pedicles *(arrows).* **B,** Lumbar myelogram, lateral view, shows the widened canal with posterior vertebral body scalloping *(large arrows).* The contrast column is displaced anteriorly, and cephalad contrast flow is blocked *(curved arrow).* The "feathered" appearance *(open arrows)* is characteristic of an extradural mass. **C,** Sagittal T1-weighted MR scan shows the lobulated mass *(arrows)* is isointense with CSF. Note anterior displacement and thinning of the thoracic cord. **D,** Post-myelogram CT scan at the L1-L2 level shows the thecal sac is displaced anteriorly and compressed *(small arrows)* by a low density intraspinal mass *(large arrows).* **E,** Bone window shows the enlarged canal and markedly thinned pedicles *(arrows).* (Courtesy W.R.K. Smoker.)

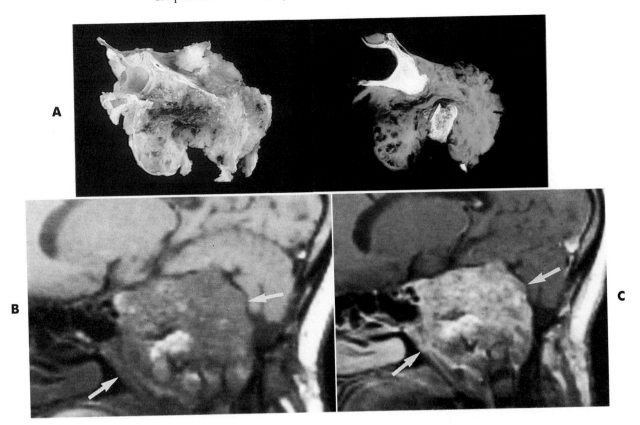

Fig. 21-14. Skull base chordoma. **A,** Sagittal gross pathology *(left)* and specimen radiograph *(right)* show the inhomogeneous-appearing, destructive cartilaginous-like clivus mass. Pre- **(B)** and postcontrast **(C)** sagittal T1-weighted MR scans show a large mixed signal, destructive, strongly enhancing mass *(arrows).* (**A,** From Okazaki H, Scheithauer B: *Slide Atlas of Neuropathology,* Gower Medical Publishing, 1988. **B** and **C,** Courtesy N. Yue.)

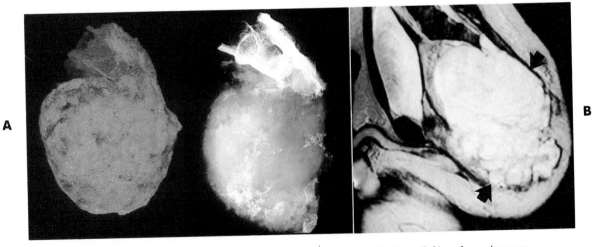

Fig. 21-15. Sacrococcygeal chordoma. **A,** Sagittal gross pathology *(left)* and specimen radiograph *(right)* show the typical bulky, destructive inhomogeneous soft tissue mass that is characteristic of chordoma. **B,** Sagittal T2-weighted MR scan in another case shows the lobulated lesion *(arrows)* is extremely hyperintense. (**A,** From Okazaki H, Scheithauer B: *Slide Atlas of Neuropathology,* Gower Medical Publishing, 1988. **B,** Courtesy B.J. Manaster.)

Continued.

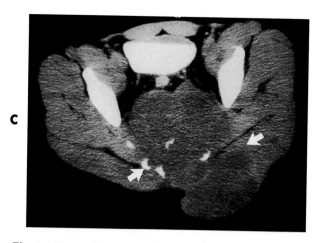

C

Fig. 21-15, cont'd. C, Axial NECT scan shows a low density lytic destructive sacral mass *(large arrows)* with some residual bone or calcification within the lesion. (Courtesy B.J. Manaster.)

gelatinous-appearing masses (Figs. 21-14, *A;* and 21-15, *A*). Chordomas are separated into two pathologic subsets: typical chordomas and chondroid chordomas.[30] In typical chordomas, vacuolated physaliphorous cells with variable amounts of intracytoplasmic mucin are embedded in pools of extracellular mucin. In chondroid chordomas, this watery, gelatinous matrix is replaced by cartilaginous foci.[31] Mitotic activity and cellular pleomorphism are typically absent in both subtypes.[30]

Incidence, age, and gender. Chordomas are rare tumors. They account for only 1% to 2% of primary malignant bone tumors, although chordoma is the most common primary sacral neoplasm.[32] Chordomas can occur at almost any age, but the peak incidence is in the sixth decade.[30] There is a 2:1 male predominance.[17]

Location. Chordomas typically—although not invariably—arise in the midline of the spinal column at any location from the clivus to the coccyx.[33] Over 85% are found in the skull base or sacrum. Approximately half of all chordomas originate in the sacrum or coccyx. Another 35% arise within the skull base, typically in the clivus near the sphenooccipital synchondrosis.[30] Less than 15% of chordomas occur in the vertebral bodies. More than one vertebral segment is often involved. Completely extradural, extraosseous vertebral chordomas have been reported but are very rare.[30]

Clinical presentation and natural history. Chordomas are typically slow-growing neoplasms; symptoms vary with location.

Imaging findings. NECT scans commonly show a lytic, destructive skull base or sacral lesion (Fig. 21-15, *C*). Mixed solid and cystic components are frequent. Calcification occurs in 30% to 70% of cases.[5] An associated anterior or lateral soft tissue mass is often present.

Typical chordomas have inhomogeneous, predominately low signal intensity on T1-weighted MR scans (*see* Fig. 21-16; Fig. 21-14, *B*) and equal or exceed CSF signal intensity on proton density- and T2-weighted sequences (Figs. 21-15, *C;* and 21-16, *C*).[17] Chondroid chordomas typically have shorter T1 and T2 relaxation times than typical chordomas.[30,31] Enhancement following contrast administration varies from little to striking (Fig. 21-14, *C*).

Differential diagnosis. The major differential diagnosis of sacral chordoma is giant cell tumor and metastasis from occult primary neoplasms such as renal cell or thyroid carcinomas. Other tumors that can enlarge and erode sacral segments are ependymoma and schwannoma.[32] Clivus chordomas must be distinguished from other central skull base destructive masses (*see* Chapter 12).

Lymphomas. Lymphoma can involve the spine and epidural soft tissues (Fig. 21-17). Non-Hodgkin lymphoma accounts for over 85% of cases; Hodgkin lymphoma is much less common. Most spinal lymphomas occur between 40 and 60 years of age.[17] Mean age at diagnosis is 58 years; there is a strong male predominance.[34] The biologic behavior of spinal NHL is similar to extranodal lymphomas at other sites.[34] Median survival is 22 months, although nearly half the patients survive more than 3 years with appropriate radiation and chemotherapy.[34,35]

Imaging findings in spinal extradural lymphoma are nonspecific. NHL can cause bone destruction and hyperostosis.[17] Spinal cord compression occurs in up to 6% of patients with NHL during their disease course.[34] Epidural extension is best delineated on MR scans. Spinal lymphoma is typically low signal on T1- and inhomogeneously hyperintense on T2-weighted MR scans.[17]

Sarcomas. Primary spinal sarcomas are rare. Ewing sarcoma, osteogenic sarcoma, chondrosarcoma, and fibrosarcoma occasionally involve the spine.

Ewing sarcoma. Ewing sarcoma (ES) accounts for 7% to 15% of all primary bone malignancies.[5] The peak incidence is in the second decade; there is a definite male predominance. The spine is a rare site for primary ES; most spinal ESs represent metastatic tumor from another site of origin.[5] The vertebral bodies and epidural space are the most common locations.

Imaging findings of ES are nonspecific. An eroded vertebral body associated with a large paraspinal soft

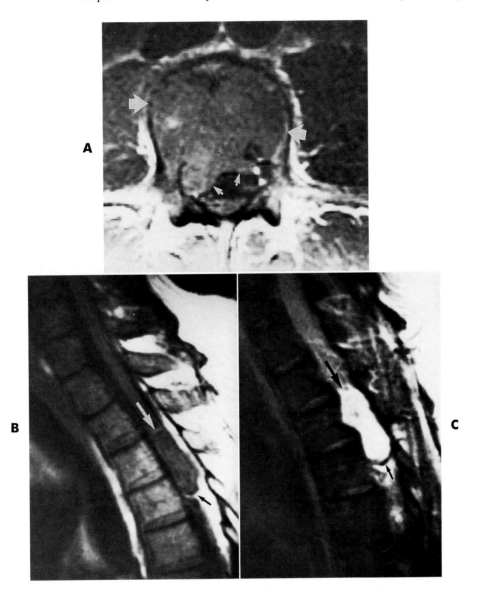

Fig. 21-16. Two cases of vertebral body chordoma illustrate MR findings of this tumor. **A,** Axial T1-weighted MR scan in this 35-year-old man with low back pain and suspected lumbar disk herniation show a destructive vertebral body mass *(large arrows)* with epidural extension *(small arrows)*. **B** and **C,** Sagittal T1- **(B)** and T2-weighted **(C)** MR scans in another case show a lobulated neural foraminal mass *(large arrows)* in the upper thoracic spine. The mass becomes very hyperintense on the long TR/long TE scan. Note the displaced epidural fat *(small arrows)* capping the tumor and indicating its location in the extradural compartment. Chordoma was found in both cases.

tissue mass is typical. ES is usually hypo- to isointense with muscle on T1- and hyperintense on T2-weighted MR scans (Fig. 21-18).[17]

Osteosarcoma. Osteosarcomas account for approximately 20% of all sarcomas but rarely affect the spine.[5] The peak age is 10 to 25 years and there is a slight male predominance.[17] Osteosarcomas occur with increased frequency in previously irradiated bone or in patients with Paget disease. Imaging studies show mixed osteolytic and sclerotic changes with matrix calcification (Fig. 21-19).[5]

Chondrosarcoma. Chondrosarcomas are half as frequent as osteosarcoma. Most patients are middle-aged or older adults and there is a 2:1 male predominance. Chondrosarcomas may arise from malignant degeneration of solitary osteochondromas (1%) or hereditary multiple exostoses (20%).[5] Lytic lesions with sclerotic margins and variable matrix calcification occur in rings and arcs *(see* Chapter 12). Associated soft tissue masses are common and local extension to an adjacent vertebra may occur.[17]

Fibrosarcoma. Fibrosarcomas are rare primary

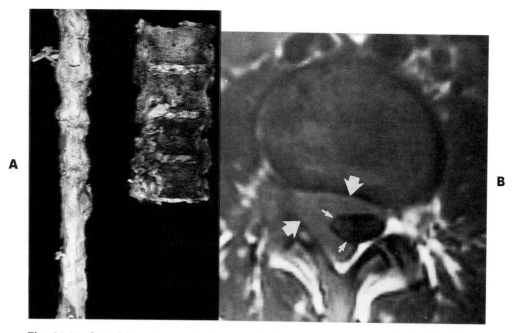

Fig. 21-17. Spinal lymphoma. **A,** Gross pathology specimen shows extensive osseous and epidural tumor. Non-Hodgkin lymphoma. **B,** Axial T1-weighted MR scan in another case shows epidural non-Hodgkin lymphoma *(large arrows)* with thecal sac compression *(small arrows).* (**A,** Courtesy Rubinstein Collection, University of Virginia.)

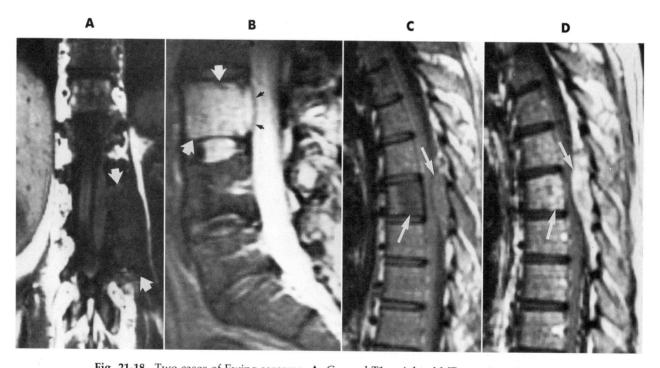

Fig. 21-18. Two cases of Ewing sarcoma. **A,** Coronal T1-weighted MR scan in a 12-year-old girl with Ewing sarcoma shows an extensive paravertebral soft tissue mass (arrows) that extends through the neural foramina into the spinal canal, displacing and compressing the thecal sac. **B,** The mass is hyperintense on the sagittal T2WI *(large arrows).* Note dural displacement *(small arrows)* caused by the epidural mass effect. Sagittal pre- **(C)** and postcontrast **(D)** T1WIs in another case show the vertebral body and epidural lesion *(arrows)* enhances strongly. Note cord compression.

malignant bone tumors. Fibrosarcomas occur in a wide age range; there is no gender predilection.[5] Imaging studies typically show a lytic, destructive, somewhat expansile mass without matrix calcification.[5] Primary spinal fibrosarcomas are extremely rare.

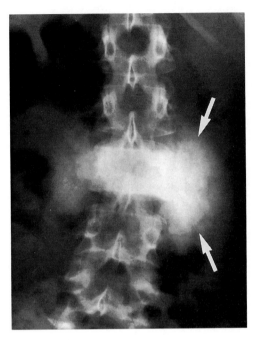

Fig. 21-19. AP plain film radiograph shows osteogenic sarcoma of L3 with large "sunburst" tumor matrix calcification and large soft tissue mass *(arrows)*. (Courtesy B.J. Manaster.)

Plasmacytoma and multiple myeloma (myelomatosis). Plasmacytoma is a solitary lesion, whereas myelomatosis has multiple lesions (Fig. 21-20).

Multiple myeloma (MM) is a monoclonal proliferation of malignant plasma cells that usually affects the bone marrow.[36] The peak incidence is during the sixth decade. The spine is the most common location, and epidural involvement is frequent.[37] The vertebral bodies are the most common site.

Both focal and diffuse lesions occur in MM. Plain film radiographs and NECT scans show focal or diffuse lytic defects. MR signal varies. Most lesions are hypointense to adjacent marrow and iso- or slightly hyperintense compared to muscle on T1WI (Fig. 21-20, *B*).[37,38] MM is typically hyperintense on T2WI. Fat-suppressed and T2-weighted sequences are helpful studies in delineating lesion extent.[37]

Metastatic disease

Pathology. In adults, approximately half of all spine metastases with epidural spinal cord compression arise from breast, lung, or prostate cancer (Fig. 21-21, *A*). Other frequent primary tumors include lymphoma, melanoma, renal cancer, sarcoma, and multiple myeloma.[39] Spine metastases in children are most often caused by Ewing sarcoma and neuroblastoma, followed by osteogenic sarcoma, rhabdomyosarcoma, Hodgkin disease, soft tissue sarcoma, and germ cell tumors.[40]

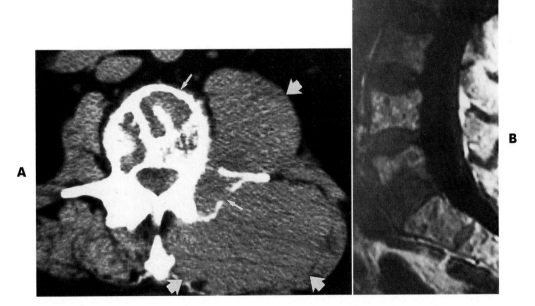

Fig. 21-20. A, Axial NECT scan in this 55-year-old man with back pain shows a large paravertebral soft tissue mass *(large arrows)* with associated bone destruction *(small arrows)*. No other lesions were present. Biopsy disclosed plasmacytoma. **(B),** Sagittal T1-weighted MR scan in a 78-year-old woman with multiple myeloma shows extensive multifocal replacement of fatty marrow by low signal soft tissue. Note multiple compression fractures.

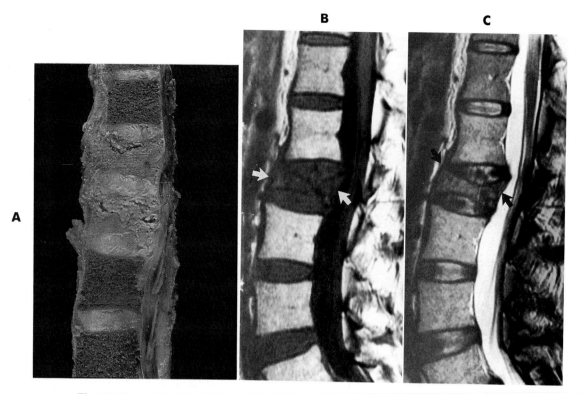

Fig. 21-21. A, Gross pathology specimen shows spine metastases from lung carcinoma. Note marrow replacement and pathologic compression fractures. Sagittal T1- **(B)** and T2-weighted **(C)** MR scans in a 42-year-old woman with treated breast carcinoma show typical findings of sclerotic vertebral body metastases. Note pathologic compression fracture *(arrows)* and complete replacement of fatty marrow by low signal tumor *(arrows)*. Compare to the other vertebral bodies with diffusely fatty marrow (secondary to radiation therapy). **(A,** Courtesy B. Horten.)

Incidence, age, and gender. Metastatic disease is the most common extradural malignant spine tumor in adults. Autopsy studies disclose epidural (vertebral) metastases in 15% to 40% of patients dying of disseminated cancer.[41] Middle-aged and elderly adults are most often affected. Approximately 5% of children with solid malignant tumors develop spinal epidural metastasis with cord compression.[40] There is no overall gender predilection.[17]

Location. Pediatric metastatic tumors typically invade the spinal canal via the neural foramen, causing circumferential cord compression *(see* Fig. 21-18, *A).*[40] In adults, the initial site is in the vertebral body, typically the posterior aspect; epidural space and pedicle lesions are usually secondary to vertebral involvement.[42] The paraspinous soft tissues are also frequently affected.

Spine metastases in adults are distributed according to the location of red bone marrow.[42,43] All vertebral levels can be involved, although the lower thoracic and lumbar spine are the most frequently affected sites.[42,43]

Clinical presentation. Pain and progressive neurologic deficits are common. Cord compression is among the most dreaded complications. If left untreated, metastatic epidural compression inexorably progresses, causing paralysis, sensory loss, and sphincter incontinence.[39]

Imaging findings. Most metastases are osteolytic, although breast and prostate cancer can cause osteoblastic or sclerotic lesions. Pedicle destruction is the most common plain film finding.[42] Other frequent abnormalities include multifocal lytic vertebral body lesions, pathologic compression fracture, and paraspinous soft tissue mass. A subtle but useful plain film clue to epidural metastatic disease is an indistinct posterior vertebral body margin.[44]

Myelography typically discloses extradural mass effect or block *(see* Fig. 21-1, *B* and *C).* Lumbar puncture below the level of a high-grade stenosis or block can cause rapid neurologic deterioration from "coning" of the spinal cord at the level of the block.[41]

Bone scintigraphy is very sensitive in detecting altered local metabolism in areas of skeletal remodeling associated with metastatic deposits. Only a 5% to 10% change in lesion to normal bone area is needed.[43] This compares favorably with the 40% to 50% destruction typically required for lesion detection on plain film radiographs. However, bone scans are nonspecific and can be abnormal in cases of trauma, infection, and degenerative disease.[41] Very aggressive metastatic disease can also have a false-negative scan.[43]

Single photon emission computed tomographic (SPECT) images are sometimes helpful in differentiating between benign and malignant lesions. Lesions with focal or diffuse uptake in the body are usually benign; lesions with both body and pedicle uptake are usually metastatic. Lesions in the apophyseal joints and lesions with an intervening normal pedicle between body and posterior element uptake are typically benign.[45]

NECT scans readily define osteolytic or osteoblastic lesions, although intrathecal contrast is required to delineate the precise extent of epidural disease.[5]

MR imaging is even more sensitive than bone scintigraphy in detecting vertebral metastases.[43] MR also exquisitely and noninvasively delineates epidural and paraspinous soft tissue involvement. Cord compression is easily evaluated.

Four MR patterns of vertebral metastatic disease are seen, as follows:

1. Focal lytic
2. Focal sclerotic
3. Diffuse inhomogeneous
4. Diffuse homogeneous

The most common pattern is multifocal lytic lesions that are characterized by low signal intensity on T1- and high signal intensity on T2-weighted sequences (*see* Fig. 21-1, *D*).[41] Sclerotic lesions are hypointense on both T1- and T2WI (*see* Fig. 21-21, *B* and *C*). Both diffuse inhomogeneous and homogeneous lesions show low signal intensity on T1WI and high signal intensity on T2-weighted sequences.[43]

Contrast-enhanced MR is not routinely required in the evaluation of suspected spinal metastatic dis-

ease.[41] The degree and pattern of enhancement following contrast administration varies. Some lesions may enhance avidly, whereas others may not enhance at all. Lesions in the same patient may also behave differently.[41] Some enhance to isointensity and therefore are difficult to detect unless precontrast studies or fat-suppressed sequences are used.[41]

Distinguishing between benign (i.e., osteoporotic) and pathologic (i.e., metastatic) vertebral body compression fractures is usually possible on MR scans (*see* box). Chronic benign fractures typically have marrow signal intensity that is isointense with normal vertebrae on all sequences. Pathologic fractures show comparatively low signal intensity on T1- and high signal intensity on T2-weighted sequences.[46]

INTRADURAL EXTRAMEDULLARY TUMORS, CYSTS, AND TUMORLIKE MASSES
Benign Tumors

Intradural extramedullary masses arise inside the dura but outside the spinal cord. By convention, nerve root tumors are grouped with the intradural extramedullary masses. Nerve sheath tumors and meningiomas account for 80% to 90% of all intradural extramedullary neoplasms.[47] Other benign tumors are uncommon. The general imaging features of intradural extramedullary masses are illustrated in Fig. 21-22.

Nerve sheath tumors
Pathology. Two main types of nerve sheath tumors are found in the spine: schwannoma (also known as neurinoma or neurilemoma) and neurofibroma. The Schwann cell is the proliferating neoplastic element in both lesions. A third type of neurogenic spinal tumor, ganglioneuroma, is relatively rare (*see* box, p. 897).

Schwannomas are lobulated, grossly encapsulated, well-circumscribed round or oval tumors that often show cystic degeneration, hemorrhage, and xanthomatous changes (*see* Chapter 15). Schwannomas arise eccentrically from their parent nerve (Fig. 21-23). Nerve fibers do not course through the tumor but are confined to the capsule.[48] Microscopically, schwannomas are composed of densely packed, highly ordered spindle cells (the so-called Antoni type A) or more loosely textured myxoid stroma (Antoni type B).[49] Primary malignant peripheral nerve sheath tumors occur but are very rare.

Neurofibromas are unencapsulated, fusiform, less well-delineated lesions. Plexiform-type neurofibromas occur in patients with neurofibromatosis type 1 (NF-1). Necrosis and cystic degeneration are rare in neurofibromas. Neurofibromas usually cannot be dissected from the parent nerve because it typically runs

---

Benign Versus Pathologic Compression Fracture

Benign (osteoporotic) compression fracture

Signal similar to other vertebral bodies (in elderly, marrow is usually high signal on T1WI, low on T2WI)

Signal is relatively uniform

Fat-suppression scans helpful

Pathologic compression fracture

Lesions often multiple

Signal usually different from other vertebral bodies

Often hypointense on T1WI, hyperintense on T2WI

Signal usually heterogeneous

Pedicle involvement common

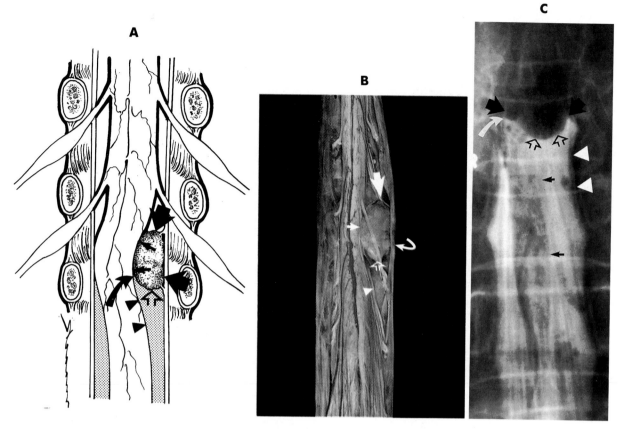

Fig. 21-22. Classic pathologic and imaging findings of an extramedullary intradural mass (in this case, a meningioma). **A,** Anatomic drawing shows the mass *(large arrows)* displaces the spinal cord *(small arrows)* and enlarges the ipsilateral subarachnoid space *(arrowheads)*. A sharp, crescentic interface is formed between the contrast column and undersurface of the mass *(open arrow)*. The subarachnoid space is blocked *(curved arrow)*, and CSF above the block remains unopacified. **B,** Gross pathology of a typical spinal meningioma illustrates these findings. The mass *(large arrow)* is intradural. The spinal cord *(small arrow)* is displaced away from the mass, and the ipsilateral subarachnoid space *(arrowhead)* is enlarged. The interface between CSF and the undersurface of the mass forms a sharply delineated border *(open arrow)*. The curved arrow indicates the theoretical level of a myelographic block. **C,** Lumbosacral myelogram, AP view, in a 59-year-old woman with a 3-year history of spastic paraparesis. Note block *(curved arrow)*, sharp interface *(open arrows)* formed by contrast meniscus abutting the mass *(large arrows)*. The ipsilateral subarachnoid space is enlarged *(arrowheads)*, and the spinal cord *(small arrows)* is displaced away from the mass. Compare with Fig. 21-22, **A.** (**B,** From Okazaki H, Scheithauer B: *Slide Atlas of Neuropathology,* Gower Medical Publishing, 1988.)

through the lesion and nerve fibers are dispersed throughout the tumor.[48,50]

Microscopically, neurofibromas are composed of Schwann cells and fibroblasts. The bulk of the tumor volume consists of intercellular collagen fibrils in a nonorganized mucoid or myxomatous matrix.[49,50]

Ganglioneuromas are uncommon, benign spinal tumors that can occur in either the spinal cord or peripheral nerve roots. Grossly, ganglioneuromas are well-delineated masses that have a distinct whorled appearance. Microscopically, ganglion cells, Schwann cells, and nerve fibers are identified.[51]

Incidence, age, and gender. Nerve sheath tumors

the most common intradural extramedullary spinal neoplasm, accounting for 25% to 30% of all cases.[5,47] Schwannomas are slightly more common than neurofibromas.[49]

Both schwannomas and neurofibromas usually become symptomatic in the middle decades. In general, both sexes are equally affected, although there is a slight female predominance with schwannomas.[5,52] Between 35% and 45% of patients with nerve root tumors have neurofibromatosis.[49]

Location. Most nerve sheath tumors arise from dorsal sensory roots.[17] Depending on their origin along the root, nerve sheath tumors can be intradural

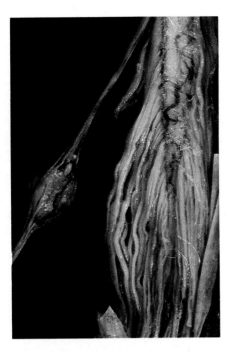

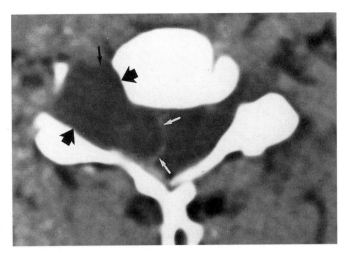

Fig. 21-24. Axial NECT scan shows cervical neural foraminal enlargement *(large arrows)* from a "dumbbell" low density mass *(small arrows)*. Schwannoma.

Fig. 21-23. Gross pathology of spinal nerve root schwannoma. Note the well-delineated, encapsulated mass with nerve fascicles displaced around the tumor. (From Okazaki H, Scheithauer B: *Slide Atlas of Neuropathology,* Gower Medical Publishing, 1988.)

(70% to 75%), extradural (15%), or combined intra- and extradural "dumbbell" masses (15%). Less than 1% of these tumors occur inside the spinal cord.[17]

The distribution of nerve sheath tumors throughout the spine is fairly uniform with a slight lumbar predominance.[5] Multiple lesions are reported in 1% to 55% of cases and are common in neurofibromatosis.[53]

Clinical presentation and natural history. Clinical symptoms are often indistinguishable from those associated with disk herniation.[50,53] Pain and radiculopathy are the most frequent presenting symptom, followed by paresthesias and limb weakness. Some intradural nerve sheath tumors can compress the spinal cord with resulting myelopathic symptoms. Occasionally, cauda equina nerve root tumors cause subarachnoid hemorrhage, although SAH is more commonly caused by ependymoma (see subsequent discussion).[54]

Schwannomas almost never become malignant, whereas sarcomatous transformation occurs in 4% to 11% of patients with neurofibromatosis.[50]

Imaging findings. Osseous changes are common on plain films. The most common findings are pedicle erosion and enlarged neural foramen. Paraspinous soft tissue masses are common with "dumbbell" and extradural lesions. Kyphoscoliosis and so-called "ribbon ribs" are seen with neurofibromatosis. Posterior vertebral body scalloping can occur with in-

Nerve Sheath Tumors
Most common intradural extramedullary mass
Types
Schwannoma, neurofibroma; ganglioneuroma, neurofibrosarcoma are rare
Primarily seen in middle-aged adults
Variable location
Intradural extramedullary (70% to 75%)
"Dumbbell" (15%)
Extradural (15%)
Intramedullary (<1%)
Multiple lesions common with neurofibromatosis
Clinical symptoms can mimic disk herniation
Imaging findings
Enlarged neural foramen common, Ca^{++} rare
75% isointense, 25% hyperintense on T1WI
>95% hyperintense on T2WI ("target" appearance common)
Virtually 100% enhance

tradural lesions but is more commonly due to dural ectasia than neoplasm.[5,55]

Myelography discloses an intradural extramedullary mass that is sharply delineated by a meniscus of contrast abutting the lesion. The spinal cord is displaced away from the mass. Large tumors can obstruct the flow of contrast beyond the lesion (so-called complete block).

NECT scans show bone erosion (Fig. 21-24). Density varies from hypo- to slightly hyperdense. Calcification and hemorrhage are rare.[5,56] MR findings vary. Nearly 75% of nerve root tumors are isointense compared to spinal cord on T1WI (Figs. 21-25, *A;* and

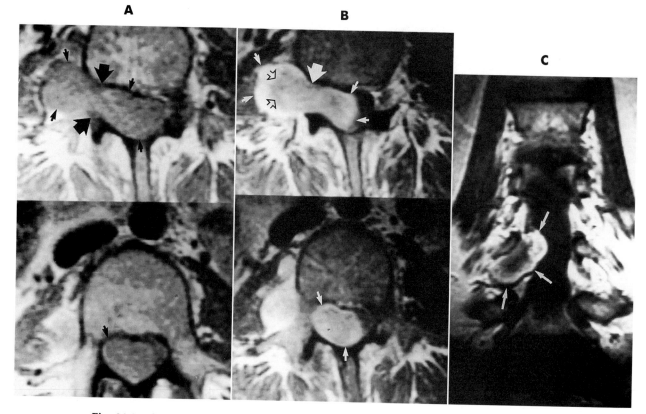

Fig. 21-25. MR findings of solitary spinal schwannoma. Axial pre- **(A)** and postcontrast **(B)** T1-weighted scans show enlarged neural foramen *(large arrows)* and lobulated "dumbbell" combined intra- and extradural soft tissue mass *(small arrows)*. The mass is isointense with adjacent muscle on T1WI and shows strong enhancement following contrast administration. Note that the periphery of the tumor enhances more intensely than the center **(B,** *open arrows)*. Coronal post-contrast T1WI **(C)** in another case shows a typical "dumbbell" schwannoma *(arrows)*. Compare with Fig. 21-23.

21-26, *A*), whereas 25% are hypointense.[57] More than 95% are hyperintense on T2-weighted sequences (Fig. 21-26, *B*).[47,56,57] A "target" appearance with a hyperintense rim and hypointense center is often seen on T2WI and contrast-enhanced T1-weighted scans of neurofibromas. This corresponds histologically to peripheral myxomatous and central fibrocollagenous tissue.[49,51]

In schwannoma, there is no direct correlation between Antoni A and Antoni B tissue types and features recognized on MR scans.[58] Approximately 40% of spinal schwannomas have a cystic component.[56] Cystic, hemorrhagic, or necrotic degeneration is seen as hyperintense and variably inhomogeneous central signal intensity on T2WI (Fig. 21-26, *B*).[49]

Virtually all nerve sheath tumors enhance following contrast administration, regardless of histology.[56] Patterns vary from homogeneously hyperintense (Fig. 21-27) to inhomogeneous, cystic-appearing masses.[59]

Schwannomas and neurofibromas cannot reliably be distinguished on MR scans, and benign tumors can mimic malignant nerve sheath tumors when cystic, hemorrhagic, and necrotic degeneration is present.[49]

Differential diagnosis. The differential diagnosis of spinal nerve root tumor varies with location. The major differential diagnostic consideration with an intradural nerve root tumor is meningioma (see subsequent discussion). Conus and filum terminale ependymomas are sometimes indistinguishable from schwannoma; occasionally, an ependymoma occurs as an isolated spinal nerve root tumor.[60] Other intradural extramedullary neoplasms such as epidermoid or dermoid tumor and metastasis should also be considered.

Intradural disk herniation is rare but it can mimic schwannoma (*see* Fig. 20-44).[61] Diffuse nerve root enlargement can occur in the benign hypertrophic neuropathies and with malignant disorders such as metastatic tumors and non-Hodgkin lymphoma (see subsequent discussion).

Both the so-called dumbbell and completely extradural nerve root tumors have a more limited differ-

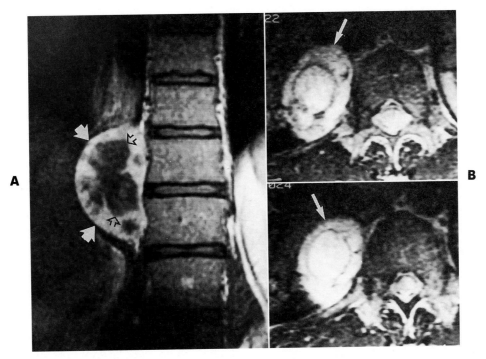

Fig. 21-26. A Coronal postcontrast T1WI shows an extradural paraspinal schwannoma with characteristic enhancing periphery *(large arrows)* and more central low signal foci *(open arrows).* **B,** Axial T2-weighted scans show both segments are hyperintense *(arrows).*

Spinal Meningioma

Most are typical benign meningiomas
Second most common cause of spinal tumor
Classic patient is a middle-aged woman
Most common location: thoracic spine
90% are intradural extramedullary
Imaging findings
  Bone erosion, Ca^{++} rare
  Most are isointense with cord on T1- and T2WI
  Moderate contrast enhancement
  +/− dural "tail"

ential diagnosis. Occasionally, vertebral chordomas or ependymomas, both typically slow-growing tumors, extend through and expand the neural foramina. Approximately 5% of spinal meningiomas are both intra- and extradural.[62] Conjoined nerve roots, root sleeve cysts, ganglion cysts, and foraminal or extraforaminal disk herniations are common benign lesions that can resemble nerve sheath tumors *(see* Figs. 20-45 and 20-47).[63]

Meningioma
Pathology. Most spinal meningiomas are benign.[62] Aggressive tumors and hemangiopericytomas are rare *(see* box).[5]

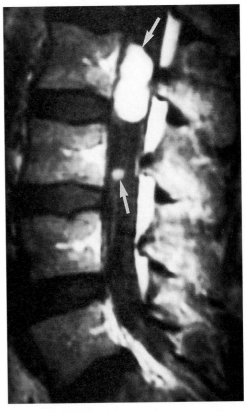

Fig. 21-27. Sagittal postcontrast T1-weighted scan in a 47-year-old man with NF-2 shows multiple enhancing lesions in the cauda equina *(arrows).* Multiple schwannomas were found at surgery.

A **B**

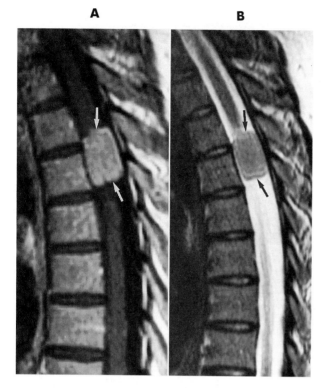

Fig. 21-28. A 24-year-old woman had progressive lower extremity weakness. Postcontrast sagittal T1- **(A)** and T2-weighted **(B)** MR scans show an enhancing, well-demarcated intradural mass *(arrows)* in the midthoracic spine. Typical meningioma.

Incidence, age, and gender. Meningiomas are second only to nerve sheath tumors in frequency, accounting for approximately 25% of all spinal tumors. The ratio of spinal to intracranial meningiomas is about 1:8. The peak incidence is in the fifth and sixth decades. In one large series, the mean age at presentation was 56 years, with ages ranging 13 to 82 years.[62] More than 80% of spinal meningiomas occur in women.[5,62] Multiple spinal meningiomas are rare.

Location. Ninety percent of spinal meningiomas are intradural, whereas 5% each are "dumbbell" or extradural lesions (*see* Fig. 21-22, *B*). Most occur lateral to the spinal cord.[62] The thoracic spine is the most common site (80%), followed by the cervical spine (15%). The lumbar spine is an uncommon location.[62] Multiple spinal meningiomas are rare.[63a]

Clinical presentation and natural history. Motor and sensory deficits are presenting symptoms in 90% and 60% of patients, respectively. Sphincter dysfunction and pain (local, radicular, funicular) occur in about 50% of cases.[62]

Spinal meningiomas are slow-growing neoplasms, and complete tumor removal is achieved in the vast majority of patients. Less than 10% experience tumor recurrence.[62] Aggressive tumors and malignant degeneration are extremely rare.

Imaging appearance. Plain films are usually normal. Bone erosion is uncommon.[5] Calcification is rare and is visible in only 1% to 5% of cases.[62]

Myelography demonstrates a mass localized to the intradural, extramedullary compartment (*see* Fig. 21-22, *C*). The subarachnoid space on the side of the lesion is widened, and the spinal cord and nerve roots are displaced away from the mass. A sharp meniscus is seen where contrast caps the lesion. Large lesions may block cephalad contrast flow.

NECT scans may disclose an extradural or "dumbbell" mass that is iso- or moderately hyperdense compared to muscle. Intradural tumors typically require intrathecal contrast for adequate delineation, although intravenous contrast administration is helpful in some cases.

MR scans demonstrate most intradural meningiomas, clearly delineating their extension and relationship to the spinal cord.[62] Most meningiomas are isointense with the spinal cord on both T1- and T2-weighted sequences (Fig. 21-28, *B*).[62] Moderate, relatively homogeneous enhancement is seen following contrast administration (Fig. 21-28, *A*).[64] Most spinal meningiomas have a broad-based dural attachment[47]; a dural "tail" sign is seen in some cases.[64] Occasionally, densely calcified meningiomas are profoundly hypointense on MR and show only minimal contrast enhancement (Fig. 21-29).

Paraganglioma. Spinal paragangliomas are rare tumors that are found in the cauda equina and filum terminale.[65] Paraganglioma is a tumor of paraganglia, the accessory organs of the peripheral nervous system.[66] Pheochromocytoma of the adrenal medulla is the most common paraganglioma. Extraadrenal paragangliomas occur most often in the carotid body, glomus jugulare, mediastinum, and paraaortic region.[66]

Spinal paragangliomas are seen as an intradural extramedullary cauda equina mass. These are well-encapsulated masses that are isointense with cord on T1- and iso- to hyperintense on T2-weighted scans. Hemorrhage with heterogenous signal intensity is common. Paragangliomas are highly vascular tumors that enhance strongly following contrast administration and therefore appear similar to other cauda equina tumors such as schwannoma or ependymoma (Fig. 21-30). Adjacent blood vessels are seen as serpentine enhancing structures above and below the mass.[65]

Cysts and Other Benign Tumorlike Masses

Epidermoid cyst. Epidermoid cysts are uncommon. They comprise between 0.5% and 1.0% of all spinal tumors but account for up to 10% of intraspinal tumors in children.[67]

Intraspinal epidermoid cysts can be congenital or acquired. Congenital epidermoids most often arise

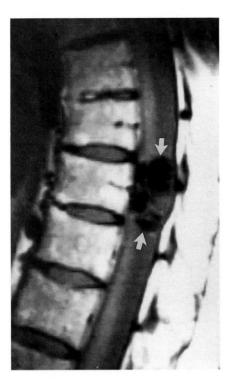

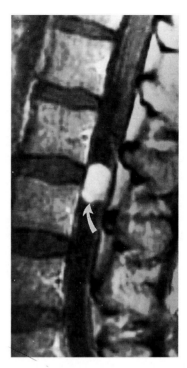

Fig. 21-29. Sagittal T1-weighted MR scan in this 77-year-old woman with persistent low back pain and leg weakness following L4-L5 discectomy shows a very hypointense midthoracic mass *(arrows)*. A densely calcified meningioma was removed at surgery.

Fig. 21-30. Sagittal postcontrast T1WI in a patient with low back pain shows an intensely enhancing cauda equina mass *(curved arrow)*. Paraganglioma was found at surgery. The imaging appearance is similar to schwannoma and ependymoma.

from heterotopic embryonic rests or focal expansion of a dermal sinus *(see* Chapter 19).[68] These cell rests are formed from epithelial tissue that becomes displaced during neural tube closure.[69]

Acquired tumors account for approximately 40% of intraspinal epidermoids and are considered a late complication of lumbar puncture (LP).[69] LPs performed with nonstylet needles or ill-fitting trochars have been implicated.[69] Epidermal elements are implanted into the spinal canal and slowly grow, resulting in an extramedullary intradural mass that usually adheres to the nerve roots and pia-arachnoid.

With acquired epidermoid cysts, the time interval between LP and tumor diagnosis ranges from 1 to more than 20 years.[69] Symptoms include progressive back or radicular pain, hamstring spasm, lordosis, and gait abnormalities.[69]

Imaging findings are variable. Congenital epidermoids often have associated epidermal defects such as spina bifida and hemivertebrae, whereas acquired lesions lack osseous abnormalities.[68] Myelography shows an intradural extramedullary mass. Congenital epidermoids usually occur at the conus or cauda equina[70]; acquired cysts are found in the lower lumbar region.[68] Signal intensity on MR scans varies but is typically iso- or slightly hyperintense compared to CSF on all sequences (Fig. 21-31).

Dermoid cyst. Intradural dermoid tumors are considered one of the congenital midline cystic tumors. Dermoids originate from epithelial inclusions within the neural groove and are therefore developmental in origin, not true neoplasms.[71] Spinal dermoids are uncommon lesions overall but account for nearly 20% of intradural tumors seen during the first year of life. One half are intramedullary and one half are located in the extramedullary intradural compartment. The lumbar spine is the most common site.[70] Dermoids have a variable imaging appearance but usually resemble fat. Spinal dermoids can rupture, resulting in multifocal high signal areas on T1-weighted MR scans.[71]

Neurenteric cyst. Neurenteric (NE) cysts are uncommon congenital nonneoplastic intradural cysts usually located in the thoracic spine anterior to the spinal cord *(see* Chapter 19).[71a]

Arachnoid cyst. Intradural arachnoid cysts are rare. Their etiology is unclear; developmental abnormality, trauma, hemorrhage, and inflammation have been suggested.[72] The thoracic spine is the most common site. Nearly 80% of intradural arachnoid cysts arise near the septum posticum and are located posterior to the spinal cord (80%). Most com-

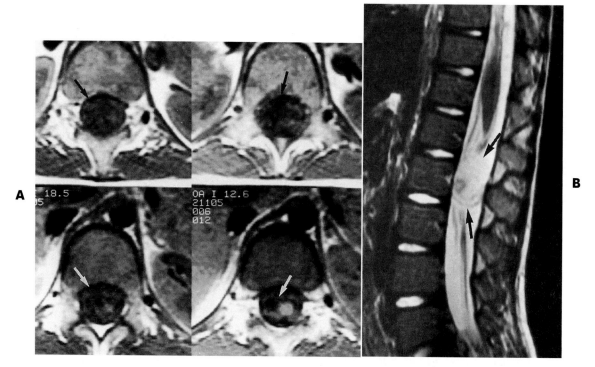

Fig. 21-31. Axial T1- **(A)** and sagittal T2-weighted **(B)** MR scans in an 11-year-old boy with back pain. A conus medullaris and filum terminale mass is present *(arrows)*. The lesion is nearly isointense with CSF and is therefore difficult to identify, particularly on the T1WIs. Epidermoid cyst was found at surgery. The patient had a lumbar puncture at 2 years of age so this is probably an acquired implantation epidermoid tumor.

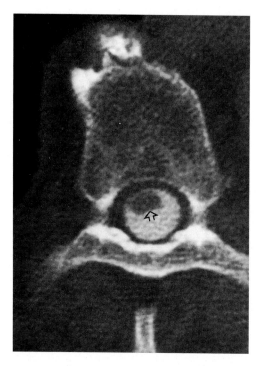

Fig. 21-32. Axial post-myelogram CT shows the spinal cord is compressed and displaced anteriorly *(arrow)*. Surgery disclosed an intradural arachnoid cyst that communicated freely with the thoracic subarachnoid space. The cyst is difficult to identify because it is opacified with contrast but the displaced, dorsally compressed cord is typical for this lesion.

municate with the subarachnoid space and opacify following intrathecal contrast administration.[73] CT-myelography typically shows a compressed thoracic cord that is displaced anteriorly (Fig. 21-32). Signal intensity on MR scans is like CSF. Therefore, MR may fail to demonstrate intradural arachnoid cysts unless the cord appears displaced and flattened.[73]

Hypertrophic neuropathies. Hypertrophic neuropathies such as Dejerine-Sottas disease (familial idiopathic hypertrophic neuropathy) and Charcot-Marie-Tooth disease (also known as peroneal muscular atrophy) can cause intra- and extradural "onion bulb" enlargements that resemble the multiple spinal nerve root tumors of neurofibromatosis.[74]

Other rare nonneoplastic causes of diffuse nerve root enlargement or thickening include toxic neuropathy, inflammatory neuritis, sarcoidosis and histiocytosis (Fig. 21-33) *(see* box).

Malignant Tumors

The most common malignant extramedullary intradural tumors are spinal leptomeningeal metastases and non-Hodgkin lymphoma.

Metastases

Pathology and etiology. Metastatic tumor in the spinal subarachnoid space can arise from CNS and

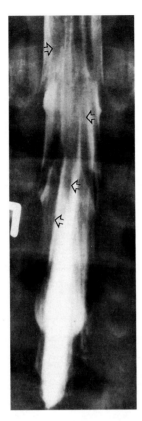

Fig. 21-33. AP lumbar myelogram in a patient with upper and lower extremity weakness. The patient had lymphoma and was treated with radiation therapy and vincristine. There is marked thickening of the cauda equina *(arrows).* CSF studies showed elevated protein but no malignant cells. Probable toxic neuropathy.

| **Diffusely Thickened Nerve Roots** |
| *Differential Diagnosis* |

Common
Carcinomatous meningitis
Lymphoma
Leukemia

Uncommon
Toxic neuropathy
Neuritis
Multiple nerve root tumors (usually nodular)

Rare
Sarcoidosis
Histiocytosis

---

non-CNS sources. Cerebral glioblastoma, anaplastic astrocytoma, ependymoma, and posterior fossa medulloblastoma (PNET-MB) are the most common CNS primary tumors that metastasize to the spinal subarachnoid space.[75] Other CNS sources include pineal tumors (e.g., germinoma and pineoblastoma) and choroid plexus neoplasms. Choroid plexus papilloma and choroid plexus carcinoma can spread via the CSF.

Non-neuraxis neoplasms that are prone to seed the subarachnoid space are carcinomas of the lung or breast, melanoma, and hemopoietic neoplasms, mainly lymphoma and leukemia (Fig. 21-34).[75]

Incidence, age, and gender. Disseminated spinal leptomeningeal metastatic tumor is rare. Intensified therapy of systemic malignancies combined with prolonged patient survival and sensitive imaging techniques such as contrast-enhanced MR are contributing to increased recognition of this entity.[75]

Age of patients at diagnosis varies with tumor type. CNS malignancies with leptomeningeal dissemination occur in younger patients (mean: 37 years), whereas spinal subarachnoid space metastases from small cell lung carcinoma occurs much later (mean:

60 years).[75] Leptomeningeal tumor spread from ependymoma and medulloblastoma is typically seen in children.

Location. The lumbosacral subarachnoid space is the most frequent site. Multiple lesions are common and vary from diffuse sheetlike infiltration of the arachnoid membrane or neoplastic coating of the conus and cauda equina (Fig. 21-34) to nodular deposits scattered throughout the subarachnoid space (Fig. 21-35).[75]

Clinical presentation and natural history. Early symptoms are often nonspecific. Cauda equina syndrome, monoparesis, radicular or low back pain, paresthesia, and gait disturbances occur. CSF cytology is positive in 75% of cases, although false-negative CSF studies sometimes occur, particularly in patients with small cell lung carcinomas.[75]

Prognosis is poor. Death occurs within 4 months in 80% of patients.[75]

Imaging findings. Plain films may show multifocal osseous metastases or pathologic compression fracture. Myelography and CT-myelography show the following four major patterns of leptomeningeal tumor spread[75]:

1. Nodular or plaquelike deposits intimately related to the conus and cauda equina (*see* Figs. 21-34 and 21-35)
2. Focal, discrete lumbosacral mass lesions (Fig. 21-36)
3. Clumping and crowding of diffusely thickened lumbar nerve roots, causing a striated myelographic appearance
4. Root sleeve obliteration, sometimes with expansion of the axilla and ganglion caused by tumor implants

MR without contrast enhancement may be normal. Thickened roots or nodular lesions that are isointense

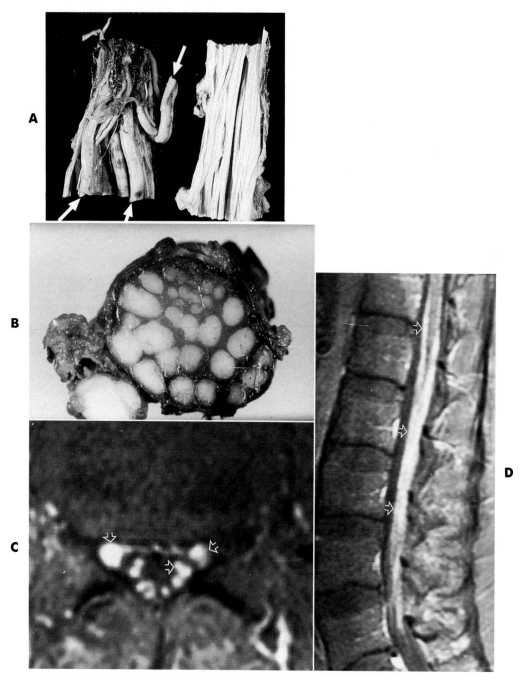

Fig. 21-34. Gross pathology and imaging of diffuse leptomeningeal tumor. **A,** Diffuse rope-like thickening of the cauda equina is present *(arrows)*. Normal case is shown on the right for comparison. **B,** Axial section through the cauda equina shows the thickened nerve roots. Axial **(C)** and sagittal **(D)** post-contrast fat-suppressed MR scans in another patient show diffusely enlarged enhancing nerve roots *(arrows)*. Both cases are non-Hodgkin lymphoma. (**A** and **B,** Courtesy Rubinstein Collection, University of Virginia; **C** and **D,** Courtesy J. Curé.)

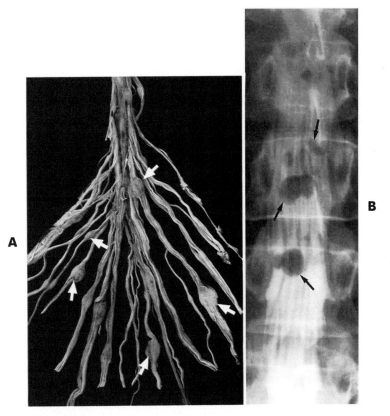

Fig. 21-35. Gross pathology and imaging of nodular metastases. **A,** Gross pathology specimen shows multiple discrete nodular implants on the cauda equina *(arrows).* **B,** Lumbosacral myelogram, AP view, in another case shows multiple sharply circumscribed rounded intradural filling defects *(arrows).* Metastatic melanoma. (**A,** From Okazaki H, Scheithauer B: *Slide Atlas of Neuropathology,* Gower Medical Publishing, 1988.)

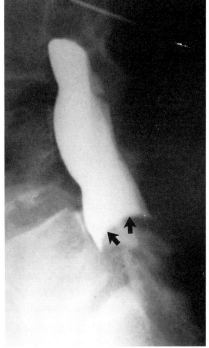

Fig. 21-36. Lumbosacral myelogram, lateral view, shows a discrete focal intradural mass at the mid-L5 level. The mass is capped by a meniscus of contrast *(arrows).* Focal metastatic tumor mass was found at surgery.

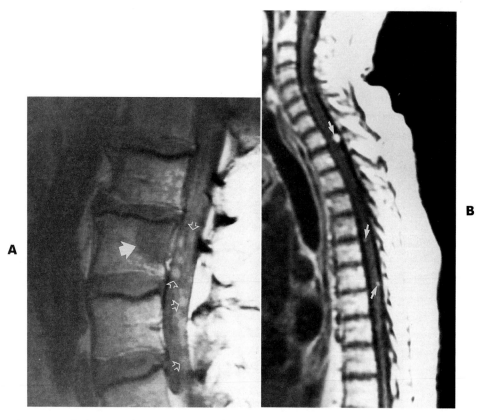

Fig. 21-37. Two cases demonstrate MR findings with intradural metastases. Sagittal **A,** T1-weighted MR scan in a 58-year-old man with known metastatic oat cell carcinoma show numerous small nodular intradural masses *(open arrows).* The lesions are somewhat difficult to identify on these unenhanced scans. Note the vertebral body lesion *(large arrow).* **B,** Postcontrast sagittal T1WI in another patient shows multiple enhancing lesions *(arrows).*

with spinal cord are seen in some cases (Fig. 21-37, *A*). Enhancement of intradural extramedullary metastases following contrast administration is often dramatic. Even small nodular metastases usually enhance strongly and are easily delineated on postcontrast T1-weighted sequences (Fig. 21-37, *B*). Leptomeningeal tumor spread along nerve roots can also be readily demonstrated.[76]

INTRAMEDULLARY TUMORS, CYSTS, AND TUMORLIKE MASSES
Tumors

Intramedullary masses are lesions of the spinal cord. Most are malignant neoplasms, and 90% to 95% of all spinal cord tumors are gliomas. Of the spinal cord gliomas, over 95% are ependymomas and low-grade astrocytomas. Other primary spinal cord tumors such as hemangioblastoma are rare. Paragangliomas occasionally occur in the conus medullaris or filum terminale. Spinal cord (subpial) lipomas are considered congenital malformations (*see* Chapter 19).

Common nonneoplastic cysts and tumorlike spinal

cord masses include hydrosyringomyelia (*see* Chapter 19), hematomyelia (*see* Chapter 20), and noninfectious inflammatory diseases such as multiple sclerosis and transverse myelitis (*see* Chapter 20). The general imaging features of intramedullary masses are illustrated in Fig. 21-38.

Ependymoma
Etiology and pathology. Spinal ependymomas arise from ependymal cells lining the central canal or its remnants and from the cells of the ventriculus terminalis in the filum terminale (*see* box, p. 909).[60] Intramedullary lesions are typically cellular ependymomas. Grossly, these tumors appear as a soft red or grayish-purple mass. They are often sharply circumscribed.[77] Cystic degeneration occurs in most cases and hemorrhage is common, particularly at the tumor margins.[77,78] Symmetric cord expansion is typical.[78a]

Myxopapillary ependymomas occur exclusively in the conus medullaris and filum terminale. These are slow-growing tumors that may attain large size, filling and expanding the lumbosacral canal and neural foramina. Grossly, these tumors are fleshy, sausage-

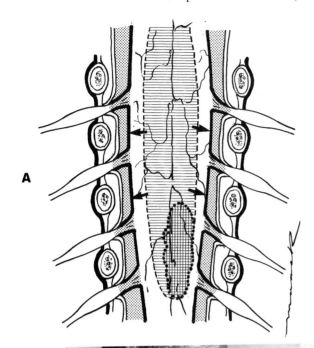

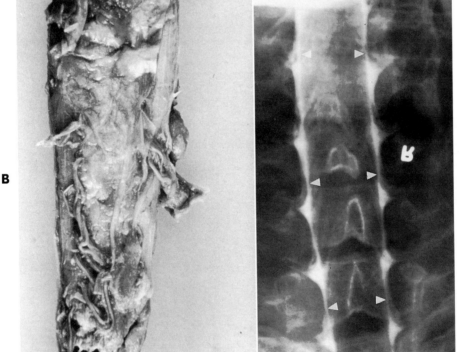

Fig. 21-38. General pathologic and imaging features of an intramedullary mass. **A,** Anatomic drawing illustrates the diffuse multisegmental cord enlargement that is typical of an intramedullary mass (in this case, a cystic astrocytoma). Note reduced subarachnoid space *(arrows)*. **B,** Gross pathology specimen of a cervical astrocytoma shows a diffusely enlarged spinal cord. **C,** Cervical myelogram, AP view, demonstrates classic myelographic findings seen with an intramedullary mass. The spinal cord is diffusely enlarged and has a sausage-like appearance *(arrows)*. (In this particular case, the etiology was benign congenital hydrosyringomyelia, not neoplasm.)

shaped, moderately vascular lesions. Hemorrhage and cystic degeneration are common. Microscopically, typical myxopapillary ependymomas show cellular areas that often display rosettes and pseudorosettes. These are intermixed with papillary regions containing a vascular core embedded in a mucoid matrix.[79]

Incidence, age, and gender. Ependymomas account for 60% of glial spinal cord tumors and comprise 90% of primary tumors in the filum terminale and cauda equina.[80] Ependymomas are the most common in-

tramedullary tumor in adults.[77] The mean age at presentation for intramedullary ependymomas is 43 years.[77] There is a slight female predominance. Mean age at presentation for myxopapillary ependymomas of the cauda equina region is 28 years. There is a slight male predominance with this histologic subtype.[79]

Location. Ependymomas occur most often in the conus medullaris and filum terminale.[17] Myxopapillary ependymoma is most commonly found in this location, whereas the cervical cord is the most common site for intramedullary ependymoma.[77] These are usually cellular or mixed ependymomas.[78] Occasionally, cellular ependymomas also occur at the conus medullaris or cauda equina.

Clinical presentation and natural history. Pain localized to the back or neck is the presenting complaint in 65% of patients with intramedullary ependymomas. Mild, objective neurologic deficits are usually present on physical examination. Because these tumors are usually well-circumscribed, slowly growing neoplasms, antecedent history is often long and recurrence is rare following complete excision.[77,78a]

Myxopapillary ependymomas typically present with low back, leg, or sacral pain. Leg weakness and sphincter dysfunction are seen in only 20% to 25% of patients. Delays in diagnosis are common; average duration of symptoms before the correct diagnosis is established is 2.4 years.[79] Most myxopapillary ependymomas are slow-growing neoplasms, although some sacral and presacral lesions behave aggressively and metastasize to the lymph nodes, lungs, and bone.[79]

Imaging findings. Plain films show widened canal or bone destruction in 20% of cases.[79] Myelography of intramedullary ependymoma discloses nonspecific cord widening. Multisegmental lesions are common.[77]

Small conus medullaris and filum terminale ependymomas are seen as well-delineated intradural masses with a contrast "meniscus" around the tumor (Fig. 21-39).[79] A contrast block may be present. Large myxopapillary ependymomas can fill the entire canal.

CT may show only nonspecific canal widening; scalloped posterior vertebral bodies and neural foraminal enlargement occur with large lesions.

MR imaging shows a widened cord or filum terminale mass (Fig. 21-39). Most ependymomas are isointense compared to cord on T1WI.[81] Mixed signal lesions are seen if cyst formation, tumor necrosis, or hemorrhage has occurred. Ependymomas typically become hyperintense on T2-weighted sequences (Fig. 21-39, *B*). Hypointensity at the tumor margin on T2WI is common in intramedullary tumors and is suggestive of—but not pathognomonic for—ependymoma.[78]

Virtually all ependymomas enhance strongly fol-

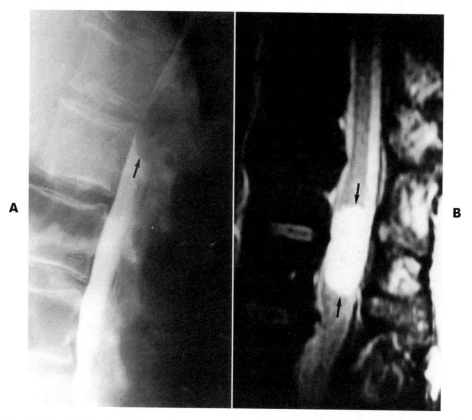

Fig. 21-39. A 56-year-old man with low back pain that radiated into the lower extremities had a lumbosacral myelogram to "rule out disk herniation." **A,** Lateral view of the myelogram shows a sharply circumscribed intradural mass at the distal conus medullaris *(arrow).* **B,** Sagittal T2-weighted MR scan shows the well-delineated mass *(arrows)* is hyperintense compared to the spinal cord. A small myxopapillary ependymoma was found at surgery.

Spinal Ependymoma

Histology and location
   Cellular ependymoma (anywhere, but usually cervical cord)
   Myxopapillary ependymoma (exclusively in conus medullaris and cauda equina)
Most common spinal cord tumor overall; most common intramedullary tumor of adults
Usually in middle-aged patients
Conus ependymomas are slow-growing, may become extremely large and erode bone
Imaging findings
   Vertebral body scalloping common with large conus lesions; may enlarge neural foramina
   Hemorrhage common; cysts also frequent
   Usually isointense with cord on T1-, hyperintense on T2WI
   Enhances strongly, somewhat inhomogeneously

lowing contrast administration (Figs. 21-40 and 21-41).[81] Contrast-enhanced scans clearly delineate tumor extent and are helpful in distinguishing neoplastic cyst from benign syrinx (Fig. 21-42, C to E).[82]

Differential diagnosis. The major differential diagnosis for intramedullary ependymoma is cord astrocytoma. Ependymomas often hemorrhage (Fig. 21-42, A and B) and are typically more sharply delineated than astrocytoma, but there is no specific pattern that permits reliable differentiation between these two common intramedullary tumors.[83]

The differential diagnosis of small conus and filum ependymomas is schwannoma (see Fig. 21-27). Imaging findings of these two entities are often indistinguishable. Other tumors such as ganglioglioma and paraganglioma occur in the filum terminale but are rare (see Fig. 21-30). Large myxopapillary ependymomas that cause sacral destruction can be confused with aneurysmal bone cyst, chordoma, and giant cell tumor.[80]

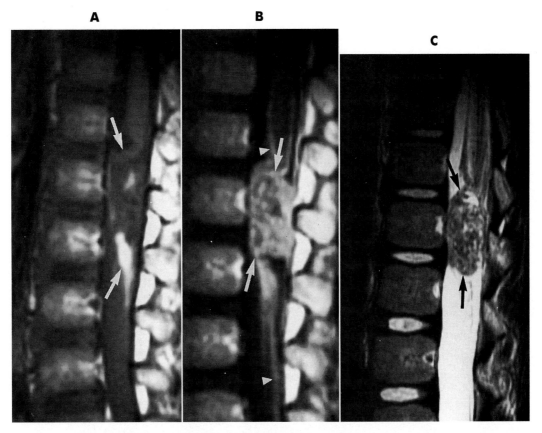

Fig. 21-40. A 7-year-old boy had a 10-day history of severe low back pain. Aspirin failed to relieve the pain, and this MR scan was obtained after lumbar puncture disclosed subarachnoid hemorrhage. **A,** Sagittal precontrast T1WI shows a mixed iso- and hyperintense conus medullaris mass *(arrows).* **B,** Sagittal postcontrast T1WI shows the mass *(large arrows)* enhances strongly but somewhat heterogeneously. Note diffuse leptomeningeal enhancement along the distal thoracic spinal cord and cauda equina *(arrowheads).* **C,** Sagittal T2WI exquisitely delineates the mass, seen here as a heterogeneous rounded lesion *(arrows)* that is mostly isointense with spinal cord. Cellular ependymoma with hemorrhage was found at surgery.

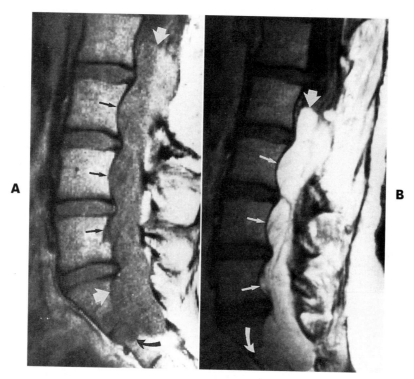

Fig. 21-41. Sagittal pre- **(A)** and postcontrast **(B)** T1WI show an extensive lobulated, strongly enhancing mass *(large arrows)* that fills the lumbosacral canal from L2 to S2. Note posterior vertebral scalloping *(small arrows)* and neural foraminal enlargement *(curved arrow)*. Myxopapillary ependymoma. (From the Armed Forces Institute of Pathology.)

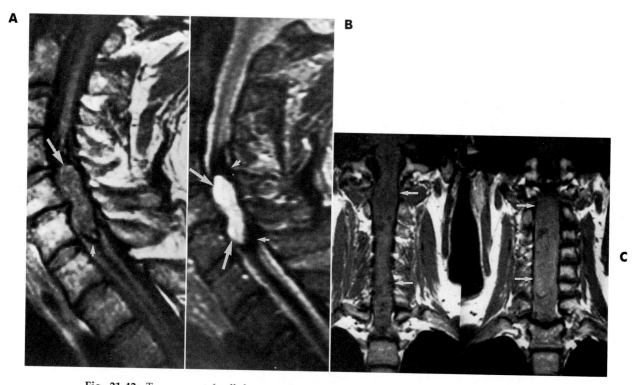

Fig. 21-42. Two cases of cellular ependymoma in the cervical spinal cord. Sagittal T1- **(A)** and T2-weighted **(B)** MR scans show a well-circumscribed intramedullary mass *(large arrows)* that is isointense with cord on T1- and hyperintense on T2WI. The extensive peripheral low signal area *(small arrows)* is hemorrhage, very characteristic of this tumor. Coronal pre-contrast T1WIs **(C)** in another case of ependymoma shows the cervical cord is diffusely enlarged from the cervicomedullary to the cervicothoracic junctions *(arrows)*.

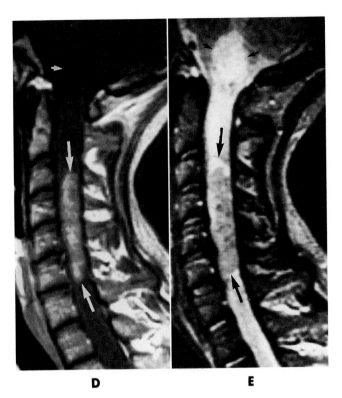

D   **E**

Fig. 21-42, cont'd. Postcontrast sagittal T1WI **(D)** shows part of the tumor enhances *(large arrows).* **E,** Sagittal T2WI shows the lobulated somewhat heterogeneous hyperintense mass *(large arrows).* The cystic cord enlargement above and below the lesion was nonneoplastic. **(C to E,** Courtesy J. Jones.)

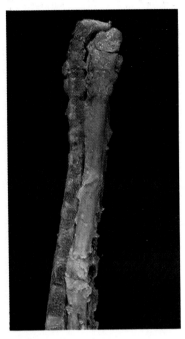

Fig. 21-43. Gross pathology of a typical spinal cord astrocytoma shows the multisegmental enlargement characteristic of this tumor. Note extensive posterior vertebral scalloping caused by this slowly growing mass. (Courtesy B. Horten.)

Astrocytoma

Pathology. In contrast to their intracranial counterparts, most spinal cord astrocytomas are low-grade tumors (Kernohan grades I and II).[5] Anaplastic astrocytomas are uncommon, accounting for only 15% to 25% of all cases. In children, 85% to 90% are low-grade tumors.[84] In adults, almost 75% are low-grade neoplasms.[85] Only 0.2% to 1.5% of spinal cord astrocytomas are glioblastoma multiforme *(see* box).[86,87]

Grossly, intramedullary astrocytomas diffusely expand the spinal cord (Figs. 21-43 and 21-44). Intratumoral cyst formation is common, and associated syrinxes are frequently observed. Tumor cysts are smaller, more irregular, and are often eccentrically positioned within the cord, whereas benign cysts are rostral or caudal to the tumor, have smooth walls, and cause symmetric cord expansion.[88]

Microscopically, most spinal cord astrocytomas are low-grade fibrillary astrocytomas. Nonneoplastic neurons are identified in the pathological specimens of many spinal cord astrocytomas, indicating that at least some microscopic tumor infiltration occurs with these lesions.[85]

Incidence, age, and gender. Astrocytomas account

Spinal Cord Astrocytoma
Usually low-grade fibrillary astrocytoma; anaplastic astrocytoma, GBM rare
Second most common spinal cord tumor overall; most common cord tumor in children
Cause of low back pain, painful scoliosis in children
Imaging findings
Long, multisegment intramedullary mass typical, causes diffuse cord expansion
Interpediculate distance widened, pedicles thinned
Usually iso- to hypointense on T1-, hyperintense on T2WI
Cysts common, often extensive
Virtually 100% enhance

for approximately 30% of spinal cord gliomas, second only to ependymomas.[17] Astrocytoma is the most common intramedullary tumor in children. Median age at presentation is 21 years (range 9 months to 70 years). There is no gender predilection.[84]

Location. The cervical spinal cord is the most common site, closely followed by the thoracic cord. Multisegmental involvement is the rule, and many intramedullary astrocytomas involve both regions.[85]

Clinical presentation and natural history. Pain is a frequent early presenting symptom. The pain is

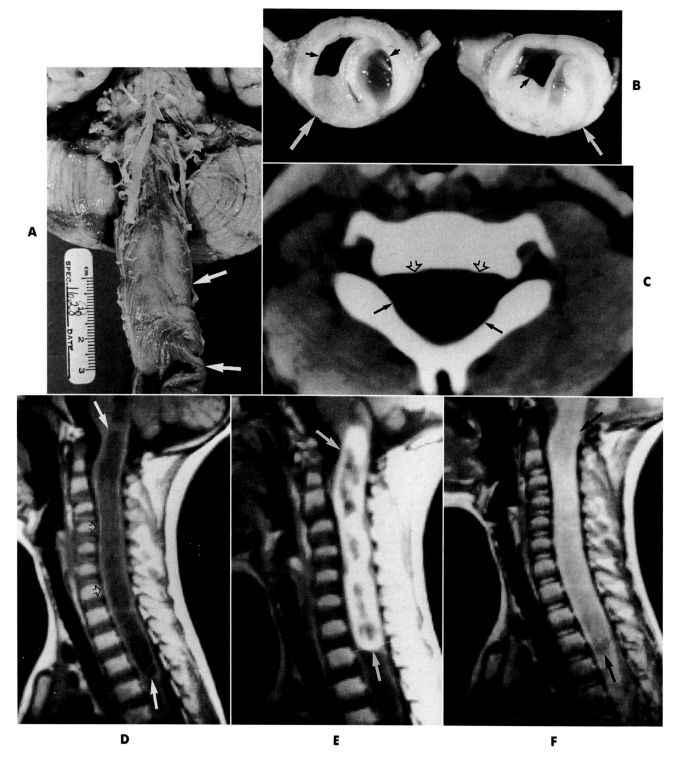

Fig. 21-44. These cord astrocytomas illustrate the gross and imaging characteristics of neoplastic syrinx. **A,** Frontal view of gross specimen shows diffusely expanded cervical spinal cord *(arrows)*. **B,** Axial section shows tumor nodule *(large arrows)* and associated cyst *(small arrows)*. **C,** Axial NECT scan shows expanded cervical canal with posterior vertebral scalloping *(arrows)*. **D** and **E,** Sagittal pre- **(D)** and postcontrast **(E)** T1WIs in this 2-year-old with torticollis show cystic expansion of the cervical cord **(D,** *arrows)* with enhancement following contrast administration **(E,** *arrows)*. **F,** Sagittal proton density-weighted sequence shows the cyst contents are hyperintense compared to CSF. Syrinx with astrocytoma was found at surgery. (**A** and **B,** Courtesy E. Ross; **C** to **E,** From the archives of the Armed Forces Institute of Pathology.)

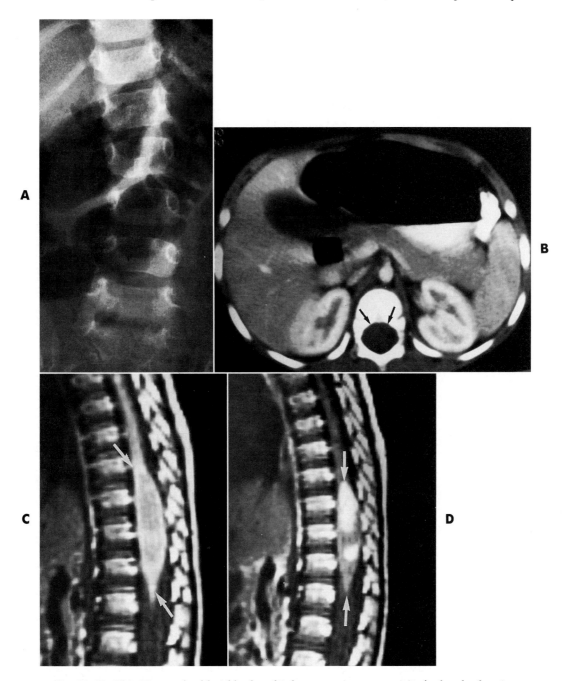

Fig. 21-45. This 22-month-old girl had multiple emergency room visits for low back pain. Upper gastrointestinal series was normal. **A,** Plain film shows scoliosis but is otherwise unremarkable. **B,** Axial CECT scan obtained for possible renal abnormalities disclosed an enlarged, featureless thoracic spinal canal *(arrows)*. **C,** Sagittal precontrast T1-weighted MR scan shows an enlarged distal thoracic spinal cord *(arrows)*. **D,** Postcontrast T1WI shows patchy enhancement *(arrows)*. Low-grade fibrillary astrocytoma was found at surgery.

most commonly and characteristically local, occurring along the spinal axis in the bony segments overlying the tumor. Recurrent abdominal pain can also be the presenting symptom of a spinal cord tumor. As symptoms or signs of neurologic dysfunction are often lacking early in the disease course, diagnostic delays are common (Fig. 21-45).[89]

In general, spinal cord astrocytomas are low-grade slowly growing neoplasms. Long recurrence-free survivals are common, particularly in younger patients.[84]

Imaging findings. Plain films are often normal or show only mild scoliosis (Fig. 21-45, *A*). Widened interpedicular distances are seen in a few cases.[5] My-

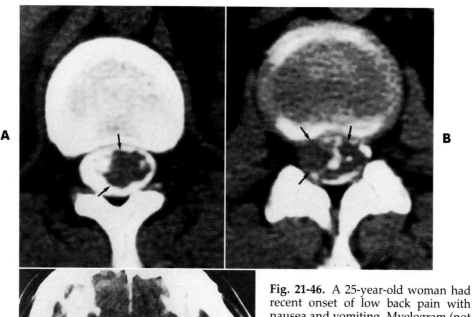

Fig. 21-46. A 25-year-old woman had recent onset of low back pain with nausea and vomiting. Myelogram (not shown) disclosed a conus medullaris mass. **A** and **B,** Axial post-myelogram CT scans showed an enlarged conus medullaris with thickened anterior and posterior roots *(arrows).* **C,** CECT brain scan showed diffuse basilar leptomeningeal enhancement *(arrows)* and moderate hydrocephalus. No parenchymal mass was identified. Laminectomy disclosed spinal cord glioblastoma multiforme. Autopsy showed no evidence for primary brain tumor, but diffuse carcinomatous meningitis was present.

elography typically demonstrates nonspecific multisegmental cord enlargement. NECT scans may show a widened canal.

MR imaging is now the diagnostic procedure of choice in evaluating possible spinal cord tumors. Astrocytomas are iso- to slightly hypointense on T1WI and hyperintense on T2-weighted sequences *(see* Fig. 21-44, *C* to *F).* Despite their low histologic grade, essentially all spinal cord astrocytomas enhance following contrast administration (Fig. 21-45, *C* and *D).* [81,82] Tumor, syrinx, and cysts can be delineated on these studies *(see* Fig. 21-44, *C* to *F).* [90]

The rare spinal cord glioblastoma has a striking propensity to spread throughout the CNS. Nearly 60% of patients have CSF tumor dissemination (Fig. 21-46). [86]

Hemangioblastoma
Pathology. Grossly, the typical spinal cord hemangioblastoma has a highly vascular nodule with an extensive cyst that diffusely enlarges the cord *(see*

box). Prominent leptomeningeal vessels are usually present. Microscopically, spinal hemangioblastomas are characterized by densely vascular tissue that consists of thin-walled, closely packed blood vessels interspersed with large pale stromal cells. [91]

Incidence, age, and gender. Hemangioblastomas are rare, accounting for 1% to 5% of all spinal cord tumors. [92] Symptom onset is typically in the fourth decade; more than 80% of patients are symptomatic before the age of 40 years. [92]

Location. Seventy-five percent of spinal hemangio-blastomas are intramedullary, and another 10% to 15% have combined intramedullary and extramedullary-intradural components. Extramedullary hemangioblastomas are often attached to the dorsal spinal cord pia. Extradural hemangioblastomas are rare. [93]

Half of all hemangioblastomas occur in the thoracic cord; the cervical region is the site for 40%. [5] Eighty percent of cord hemangioblastomas are solitary lesions.

Spinal Cord Hemangioblastoma

Vascular nodule with benign intramedullary cyst is most common
Rare (1% to 5% of cord tumors)
Symptom onset usually between 30 and 40 years
One third have Von Hippel-Lindau syndrome
85% intramedullary or combined intramedullary/extramedullary-intradural
50% thoracic, 40% cervical
Imaging findings
    Angiography shows dense vascular stain, prominent draining veins
    Usually isointense to cord on T1, hyperintense on T2WI
    Foci of high-velocity signal loss common

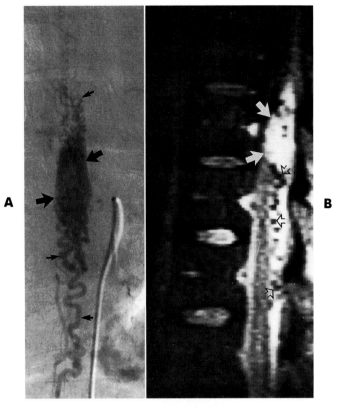

Fig. 21-47. Spinal cord hemangioblastoma is illustrated in two cases. **A,** AP view of a spinal cord angiogram shows an intensely vascular mass *(large arrows)* that had a prolonged vascular stain. Note prominent draining veins *(small arrows)*. **B,** Sagittal T2-weighted MR scan in another case shows a hyperintense midthoracic mass *(large arrows)* on the dorsal surface of the compressed spinal cord. Note numerous foci of high-velocity signal loss *(open arrows)*.

Clinical presentation and natural history. Sensory changes, typically impaired proprioception, is the most common presenting symptom.[92] Approximately one third of patients with spinal cord hemangioblastoma have von Hippel-Lindau syndrome (VHL) *(see* Chapter 5). Retinal or cerebellar involvement typically precedes spinal cord symptoms in these patients.[92] Hemangioblastomas enlarge slowly. If left untreated, progression to para- or quadriplegia may occur.[93]

Imaging findings. Dilated tortuous feeding arteries and draining pial veins can be seen at myelography in approximately 50% of cases.[94] Angiography discloses a highly vascular mass with dense, prolonged tumor stain and prominent draining vessels (Fig. 21-47, *A*). MR often demonstrates diffuse cord expansion with high signal intensity on T2WI and prominent foci of high-velocity signal loss (Fig. 21-47, *B*). Cyst formation or syrinx is seen in 50% to 70% of cases.[92] The tumor nodule in spinal cord hemangioblastoma enhances strongly following contrast administration (Fig. 21-48).

Miscellaneous primary spinal cord neoplasms. Primary spinal cord tumors other than ependymoma, astrocytoma, and hemangioblastoma are rare. Oligodendroglioma is occasionally found in the spinal cord; nonglial neoplasms such as ganglioglioma and intramedullary schwannoma occur here but are also very uncommon.[95]

Metastases. Intramedullary metastases are rare. Most spinal cord metastases are to the pia (Fig. 21-49). Pial metastases are seen on postcontrast T1-weighted MR scans as a thin rim of enhancement along the cord surface.[96] Focal nodular pial and intraparenchymal lesions occur but are less common

than carcinomatous meningitis. Common primary malignancies are breast and lung carcinomas, lymphoma, leukemia, and malignant melanoma.[96]

Cysts and Tumorlike Masses

Sometimes nonneoplastic intramedullary lesions cause focal or diffuse cord expansion. Intramedullary cysts that can mimic spinal cord tumor include congenital and acquired hydrosyringomyelia, inflammatory cysts, and hematomyelia *(see* Chapter 20). Nonneoplastic tumorlike masses that occasionally may be difficult to distinguish from neoplasm are myelitis and demyelinating diseases *(see* Chapter 20).

Myelographic findings in these cases are nonspecific and CT-myelography is often noncontributory. MR imaging without and with contrast enhancement is helpful because benign syrinxes do not enhance, whereas virtually all cord neoplasms do. Contrast-enhanced MR scans permit subcategorization of tumor-associated cysts into intratumoral cysts and nonenhancing extratumoral cysts.[97] MR also localizes a spinal mass to its specific compartment of origin and delineates lesion extent.

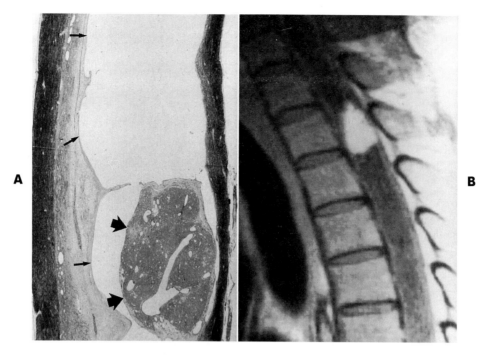

Fig. 21-48. **A,** Gross pathology specimen of a spinal cord hemangioblastoma shows the solid nodule *(large arrows)* and cyst *(small arrows).* **B,** Sagittal postcontrast T1WI in another case shows a large syrinx with intensely enhancing nodule. Cystic hemangioblastoma was found at surgery. (**A,** From Okazaki H, Scheithauer B: *Slide Atlas of Neuropathology,* Gower Medical Publishing, 1988. **B,** From the archives of the Armed Forces Institute of Pathology.)

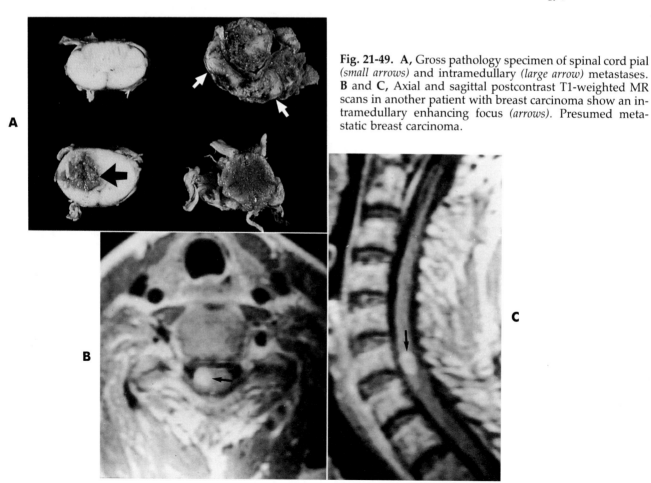

Fig. 21-49. **A,** Gross pathology specimen of spinal cord pial *(small arrows)* and intramedullary *(large arrow)* metastases. **B** and **C,** Axial and sagittal postcontrast T1-weighted MR scans in another patient with breast carcinoma show an intramedullary enhancing focus *(arrows).* Presumed metastatic breast carcinoma.

REFERENCES

1. Bazan C III: Imaging of lumbosacral spine neoplasms, *Neuroimaging Clin N Amer* 3:591-608, 1993.

2. Shapiro R: *Myelography* (ed 4), pp. 345-521, Chicago: Yearbook Medical Publisher, 1984.

3. Yochum TR, Lile RL, Schultz GD et al: Acquired spinal stenosis secondary to an expanding thoracic vertebral hemangioma, *Spine* 18:299-305, 1993.

4. Laredo J-D, Assouline E, Gelbert F et al: Vertebral hemangiomas: fat content as a sign of aggressiveness, *Radiol* 177:467-472, 1990.

5. Dorwart RH, LaMasters DL, Watanabe TJ: Tumors. In Newton TH, Potts DG, editors, *Computed Tomography of the Spine and Spinal Cord,* pp. 115-147, San Anselmo, Clavadel Press, 1983.

6. Fox MW, Onofrio BM: The natural history and management of symptomatic and asymptomatic vertebral hemangiomas, *J Neurosurg* 78:36-45, 1993.

7. Djindjian M, Nguyen J-P, Gaston A et al: Multiple vertebral hemangiomas with neurological signs, *J Neurosurg* 76:1025-1028, 1992.

8. Golwyn DH, Cardenas CA, Murtagh FR et al: MRI of a cervical extradural cavernous hemangioma, *Neuroradiol* 34:68-69, 1992.

8a. Tekkök IH, Açikgöz B, Sǎglams S, Önol B: Vertebral hemangioma symptomatic during pregnancy: report of a case and review of the literature, *Neurosurg* 32:302-306, 1993.

9. Kransdorf MJ, Stull MA, Gilkey FW, Moser RP Jr: Osteoid osteoma, *RadioGraphics* 11:671-696, 1991.

10. Klein MH, Shankman S: Osteoid osteoma: radiologic and pathologic correlation, *Skeletal Radiol* 21:23-31, 1992.

11. Wood ER, Martel W, Mandell SH, Crabbe JP: Reactive soft-tissue mass associated with osteoid osteoma: correlation of MR imaging features with pathologic findings, *Radiol* 186:221-225, 1993.

12. Nemoto O, Moser RP JR, Van Dam BE et al: Osteoblastoma of the spine: a review of 75 cases, *Spine* 15:1272-1280, 1990.

13. Boriani S, Capanna R, Donati D et al: Osteoblastoma of the spine, *Clin Ortho Rel Res* 278:37-45, 1992.

14. Syklawer R, Osborn RE, Kerber CW, Glass RF: Magnetic resonance imaging of vertebral osteoblastoma: a report of two cases, *Surg Neurol* 34:421-426, 1990.

15. Aoki J, Moriya K, Yamashita K et al: Giant cell tumors of bone containing large amounts of hemosiderin: MR-pathologic correlation, *J Comp Asst Tomogr* 15:1024-1027, 1991.

16. Shikata J, Yamamuro T, Shimizu K et al: Surgical treatment of giant-cell tumors of the spine, *Clin Ortho Rel Res* 278:29-36, 1992.

17. Post MJD: Primary spine and cord neoplasms. In *Categorical Course on Spine and Cord Imaging,* pp. 58-70, American Society of Neuroradiology, 1988.

18. Albrecht S, Crutchfield JS, Segall GK: On spinal osteochondromas, *J Neurosurg* 77:247-252, 1992.

19. Cory DA, Fritsch SA, Cohen MD et al: Aneurysmal bone cysts: imaging findings and embolotherapy, *AJR* 153:369-373, 1989.

20. Manaster BJ: *Handbooks in Radiology: Skeletal Radiology,* pp. 1-106. Chicago, Yearbook Medical Publishers, 1989.

21. Munk PL, Helms CA, Holt RG et al: MR imaging of aneurysmal bone cysts, *AJR* 153:99-101, 1989.

21a. De Schepper AMA, Ramon F, Van Marck E: MR imaging of eosinophilic granuloma: report of 11 cases, *Skeletal Radiol* 22:163-166, 1993.

22. Doppman JL: Epidural lipomatosis, *Radiol* 171:581-582, 1989.

23. Quint DJ, Boulos RS, Sanders WP et al: Epidural lipomatosis, *Radiol* 169:485-490, 1988.

24. Fessler RG, Johnson DL, Brown FD et al: Epidural lipomatosis in steroid-treated patients, *Spine* 17:183-188, 1992.

25. Preul MC, Leblanc R, Tampieri D: Spinal angiolipomas: report of three cases, *J Neurosurg* 78:280-286, 1993.

26. Pagni C, Canavero S: Spinal epidural lipoma: rare or unreported? *Neurosurg* 31:758-764, 1992.

27. Mascalchi M, Arnetoli G, Al Pozzo G et al: Spinal epidural angiolipoma: MR findings, *AJNR* 12:744-745, 1991.

28. Goyal RN, Russell NA, Benoit BG, Belanger JMEG: Intraspinal cysts: a classification and literature review, *Spine* 12:209-213, 1987.

29. Rohrer DC, Burchiel KJ, Gruber DP: Intraspinal extradural meningeal cysts demonstrating ball-valve mechanism of formation, *J Neurosurg* 78:122-125, 1993.

30. Sebag G, Dubois J, Beniaminovitz A et al: Extraosseous spinal chordoma: radiographic appearance, *AJNR* 14:205-207, 1993.

31. Sze G, Vichanco LS II, Brant-Sawadzki MN et al: Chordomas: MR imaging, *Radiol* 166:187-191, 1988.

32. Wetzel LH, Levine E: MR imaging of sacral and presacral lesions, *AJR* 154:771-775, 1990.

33. Yuh WTC, Flickinger FW, Barloon TJ, Montagomery WJ: MR imaging of unusual chordomas, *J Comp Asst Tomogr* 12:30-35, 1988.

34. Perry JR, Deodhare SS, Bilbao JM et al: The significance of spinal cord compression as the initial manifestation of lymphoma, *Neurosurg* 32:157-162, 1993.

35. Lyons MK, O'Neill BP, March WR, Kurtin DJ: Primary spinal epidural non-Hodgkin's lymphoma: report of eight patients and review of the literature, *Neurosurg* 30:675-680, 1992.

36. Moulopoulos LA, Varma DGK, Dimopoulos MA et al: Multiple myeloma: spinal MR imaging in patients with untreated newly diagnosed disease, *Radiol* 185:833-840, 1992.

37. Rahmouni A, Divine M, Mathieu D et al: Detection of multiple myeloma involving the spine: efficiency of fat-suppression and contrast-enhanced MR imaging, *AJR* 160:1049-1052, 1993.

38. Libshitz HI, Malthouse SR, Cunningham D et al: Multiple myeloma: appearance at MR imaging, *Radiol* 182:833-837, 1992.

39. Byrne TN: Spinal cord compression from epidural metastases, *NEJM* 327:614-619, 1992.

40. Klein SL, Sanford RA, Muhlbauer MS: Pediatric spinal epidural metastases, *J Neurosurg* 74:70-75, 1991.

41. Kamholtz R, Sze G: Current imaging in spinal metastatic disease, *Sem Oncol* 18:158-169, 1991.

42. Algra PR, Hermans JJ, Valk J et al: Do metastases in vertebrae begin in the body or pedicles? Imaging study in 45 patients, *AJR* 158:1275-1279, 1992.

43. Algra PR, Bloem JL, Tissing H et al: Detection of vertebral metastases: comparison between MR imaging and bone scintigraphy, *RadioGraphics* 11:219-232, 1991.

44. Olcott EW, Dillon WP: Plain film clues to the diagnosis of spinal epidural neoplasm and infection, *Neuroradiol* 35:288-292, 1993.

45. Even-Sapir E, Martin RH, Barnes DL et al: Role of SPECT in differentiating malignant from benign lesions in the lower thoracic and lumbar vertebrae, *Radiol* 187:193-198, 1993.

46. Baker LL, Goodman SB, Perkash I et al: Benign versus pathologic compression fractures of vertebral bodies: assessment with conventional spin-echo chemical-shift and STIR MR imaging, *Radiol* 174:495-502, 1990.

47. Li MH, Holtas, Larsson E-M: MR imaging of intradural extramedullary tumors, *Acta Radiol* 33:207-212, 1992.

48. Kim SH, Choi BI, Han MK, Kim YI: Retroperitoneal neurilemoma: CT and MR findings, *AJR* 159:1023-1026, 1992.

49. Varma DGK, Moulopoulos A, Sara AS et al: MR imaging of extracranial nerve sheath tumors, *J Comp Asst Tomogr* 16:448-453, 1992.

50. Barboriak DP, Rivitz SM, Chew FS: Sacral neurofibroma, *AJR* 159:600, 1992.

51. Sakai F, Sone S, Kiyono K et al: Intrathoracic neurogenic tumors: MR-pathologic correlation, *AJR* 159:279-283, 1992.

52. Friedman DP, Tartaglino LM, Flanders AE: Intradural schwannomas of the spine: MR findings with emphasis on contrast-enhancement characteristics, *AJR* 158:1347-1350, 1992.

53. Hanakita J, Suwa H, Nagayasu S et al: Clinical features of intradural neurinomas in the cauda equina and around the conus medullaris, *Neurochir* 35:145-149, 1992.

54. Bruni P, Esposito S, Oddi G et al: Subarachnoid hemorrhage from multiple neurofibromas of the cauda equina: case report, *Neurosurg* 28:910-913, 1991.

55. Mitchell GE, Louri H, Berne AS: The various causes of scalloped vertebrae with notes on their pathogenesis, *Radiol* 89:67-74, 1967.

56. Ishii N, Matsuzawa H, Houkin K et al: An evaluation of 70 spinal schwannomas using conventional computed tomography and magnetic resonance imaging, *Neuroradiol* 33:542, 1991.

57. Hu HP, Huang QL: Signal intensity correlation of MRI with pathological findings in spinal neurinomas, *Neuroradiol* 34:98-102, 1992.

58. Demachi H, Takashima T, Kadoya M et al: MR imaging of spinal neurinomas with pathological correlation, *J Comp Asst Tomogr* 14:250-254, 1992.

59. Shen WC, Lee SK, Chang CY, Ho WL: Cystic spinal neurilemmoma on magnetic resonance imaging, *Neuroradiol* 34:447-448, 1992.

60. Moser FG, Tovia J, LaSall P, Llana J: Ependymoma of the spinal nerve root: case report, *Neurosurg* 31:962-964, 1992.

61. Wassertrom R, Mamouriam AC, Black JF, Lehman RAW: Intradural lumbar disk fragment with ring enhancement on MR, *AJNR* 14:401-404, 1993.

62. Solero CL, Fornari M, Giombini S et al: Spinal meningiomas: review of 174 operated cases, *Neurosurg* 25:153-160, 1989.

63. Emamian SA, Skriver EB, Henriksen L, Cortsen ME: Lumbar herniated disk mimicking neuroma, *Acta Radiol* 34,fasc. 2:127-129, 1993.

63a. Chaparro MJ, Young RF, Smith M et al: Multiple spinal meningiomas, *Neurosurg* 32:298-302, 1993.

64. Matsumoto S, Hasu K, Uchino A et al: MRI of intradural-extramedullary spinal neurinomas and meningiomas, *Clinical Imaging* 17:46-52, 1993.

65. Levy RA: Paraganglioma of the filum terminale: MR findings, *AJR* 160:851-852, 1993.

66. Araki Y, Ishida T, Ootani M et al: MRI of paraganglioma of the cauda equina, *Neuroradiol* 35:232, 233, 1993.

67. Caro PA, Marks HG, Keret D et al: Intraspinal epidermoid tumors in children: problems in recognition and imaging techniques for diagnosis, *J Ped Orthopaed* 11:288-293, 1991.

68. Pena CA, Lee Y-Y, Van Tassell P et al: MR appearance of acquired epidermoid tumor, *AJNR* 10:597, 1989.

69. Machida T, Abe O, Sasaki Y et al: Acquired epidermoid tumor in the thoracic spinal canal, *Neuroradiol* 35:316-318, 1993.

70. Mathew P, Todd NV: Intradural conus and cauda equina tumors: a retrospective review of presentation, diagnosis, and early outcome, *J Neuro Neurosurg Psychiatr* 56:69-74, 1993.

71. Barsi P, Kenéz J, Várallyay, Gergely L: Unusual origin of the subarachnoid fat drops: a ruptured spinal dermoid tumor, *Neuroradiol* 34:343, 344, 1992.

71a. Brooks BS, Duvall ER, El Gammal T et al: Neuroimaging features of neurenteric cysts: analysis of 9 cases and review of the literature, *AJNR* 14:735-746, 1993.

72. Stern Y, Spiegelmann, Sadeh M: Spinal intradural arachnoid cysts, *Neurochir* 34:127-130, 1991.

73. Dietemann JH, de la Palavesa MMF, Kastler B et al: Thoracic intradural arachnoid cyst: possible pitfalls with myelo-CT and MR, *Neuroradiol* 33:90-91, 1991.

74. Masuda N, Hayashi H, Tanabe H: Nerve root and sciatic trunk enlargement in Déjérine-Sottas disease: MRI appearances, *Neuroradiol* 35:36-37, 1992.

75. Schuknecht B, Huber P, Büller B, Nadjmi M: Spinal leptomeningeal neoplastic disease, *Eur Neurol* 32:11-16, 1992.

76. Sze G: Magnetic resonance imaging in the evaluation of spinal tumors, *Cancer* 67:1229-1241, 1991.

77. McCormick PC, Torres R, Post KD, Stein BM: Intramedullary ependymoma of the spinal cord, *J Neurosurg* 62:523-532, 1990.

78. Nemoto Y, Inoue Y, Tashiro T et al: Intramedullary spinal cord tumors: significance of associated hemorrhage at MR imaging, *Radiol* 182:793-796, 1992.

78a. Epstein FJ, Farmer J-P, Freed D: Adult intramedullary spinal cord ependymomas: the result of surgery in 38 patients, *J Neurosurg* 79:204-209, 1993.

79. Schweitzer JS, Batzdorf U: Ependymoma of the cauda equina region: diagnosis, treatment, and outcome in 15 patients, *Neurosurg* 30:202-207, 1992.

80. Moelleken SMC, Suger LL, Eckardt JJ, Batzdorf U: Myxopapillary ependymoma with extensive sacral destruction: CT and MR findings, *J Comp Asst Tomogr* 16:164-166, 1992.

81. Parizel PM, Balériaux D, Rodesch G et al: Gd-DTPA-enhanced MR imaging of spinal tumors, *AJNR* 10:249-258, 1989.

82. Sze G, Stimac GK, Bartlett C et al: Mutticenter study of gadopentetate dimeglumine as an MR contrast agent: evaluation in patients with spinal cord tumors, *AJNR* 11:967-974, 1990.

83. Freitag H-J, Zanella F, Zeumer H: MR-Klassifikation intramedullär tumoren, *Klin Radiol* 1:224-228, 1991.

84. Sandler HM, Papadopoulos SM, Thornton AF Jr, Ross DA: Spinal cord astrocytomas: results of therapy, *Neurosurg* 30:490-493, 1992.

85. Epstein FJ, Farmer J-P, Freed D: Adult intramedullary astrocytomas of the spinal cord, *J Neurosurg* 77:355-359, 1992.

86. Ciappetta P, Salvati M, Capoccia G et al: Spinal glioblastomas: report of seven cases and review of the literature, *Neurosurg* 28:302-306, 1991.

87. Helseth A, Mork SH: Primary intraspinal neoplasms in Norway, 1955 to 1986, *J Neurosurg* 71:842-845, 1989.

88. Brunberg JA, DiPietro MA, Venes JL et al: Intramedullary lesions of the pediatric spinal cord: correlation of findings from MR imaging, intraoperative sonography, surgery, and histologic study, *Radiol* 181:573-579, 1991.

89. Robertson PL: Atypical presentations of spinal cord tumors in children, *J Child Neurol* 6:360-363, 1992.

90. Slasky BS, Bydder GM, Niendorf HP, Young IR: MR imaging with gadolinium-DTPA in the differentiation of tumor, syrinx, and cyst of the spinal cord, *J Comp Asst Tomogr* 11:845-850, 1987.

91. Silbergeld J, Cohen WA, Maravilla KR et al: Supratentorial and spinal cord hemangioblastomas: gadolinium-enhanced MR appearance with pathologic correlation, *J Comp Asst Tomogr* 13:1048-1051, 1989.

92. Murota T, Symon L: Surgical management of hemangioblastomas of the spinal cord: a report of 18 cases, *Neurosurg* 25:699-708, 1989.

93. Avila NA, Shawker TH, Choyke PL, Oldfield EH: Cerebellar and spinal hemangioblastomas: evaluation with intraoperative gray-scale and color Doppler flow US, *Radiol* 188:43-147, 1993.

94. Kattenberger DA, Shah CP, Murtagh FR et al: MR imaging of spinal cord hemangioblastoma associated with syringomyelia, *J Comp Asst Tomogr* 12:495-498, 1988.

95. Pagni CA, Canavero S, Gaidelti E: Intramedullary "holocord" oligodendroglioma: case report, *Acta Neurochir* (Wien) 113:96-99, 1991.

96. Chamberlain MC, Sandy AD, Press GA: Spinal tumors: gadolinium-DTPA-enhanced MR imaging, *Neuroradiol* 33:469-474, 1991.

97. Lim V, Sobel DF, Zyroff J: Spinal cord pial metastases: MR imaging with gadopentetate dimeglumine, *AJNR* 11:975-9;82, 1990.

Index